Principles and Practice of
Nursing Management and Administration

Principles and Practice of
Nursing Management and Administration

For BSc and MSc Nursing
(As per the Syllabus of Indian Nursing Council)

SECOND EDITION

Jogindra Vati
PhD (Nursing) MSc (N) (Gold Medalist) MA (Public Administration)

Professor-cum-Principal
SGHS College of Nursing
Mohali, Punjab, India

Formerly Faculty at
National Institute of Nursing Education (NINE)
Postgraduate Institute of Medical Education and Research (PGIMER)
Chandigarh, India

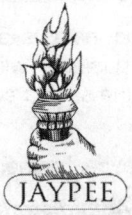

JAYPEE BROTHERS MEDICAL PUBLISHERS
The Health Sciences Publisher
New Delhi | London

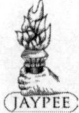
Jaypee Brothers Medical Publishers (P) Ltd

Headquarters

Jaypee Brothers Medical Publishers (P) Ltd
4838/24, Ansari Road, Daryaganj
New Delhi 110 002, India
Phone: +91-11-43574357
Fax: +91-11-43574314
Email: jaypee@jaypeebrothers.com

Overseas Offices

J.P. Medical Ltd
83 Victoria Street, London
SW1H 0HW (UK)
Phone: +44 20 3170 8910
Fax: +44 (0) 20 3008 6180
Email: info@jpmedpub.com

Website: www.jaypeebrothers.com
Website: www.jaypeedigital.com

© 2020, Jaypee Brothers Medical Publishers

The views and opinions expressed in this book are solely those of the original contributor (s)/author (s) and do not necessarily represent those of editor (s) of the book.

All rights reserved. No part of this publication may be reproduced, stored or transmitted in any form or by any means, electronic, mechanical, photocopying, recording or otherwise, without the prior permission in writing of the publishers/editors.

All brand names and product names used in this book are trade names, service marks, trademarks or registered trademarks of their respective owners. The publisher is not associated with any product or vendor mentioned in this book.

Medical knowledge and practice change constantly. This book is designed to provide accurate, authoritative information about the subject matter in question. However, readers are advised to check the most current information available on procedures included and check information from the manufacturer of each product to be administered, to verify the recommended dose, formula, method and duration of administration, adverse effects and contraindications. It is the responsibility of the practitioner to take all appropriate safety precautions. Neither the publisher nor the author (s)/editor (s) assume any liability for any injury and/or damage to persons or property arising from or related to use of material in this book.

This book is sold on the understanding that the publisher is not engaged in providing professional medical services. If such advice or services are required, the services of a competent medical professional should be sought.

Every effort has been made where necessary to contact holders of copyright to obtain permission to reproduce copyright material. If any have been inadvertently overlooked, the publisher will be pleased to make the necessary arrangements at the first opportunity. The **CD/DVD-ROM** (if any) provided in the sealed envelope with this book is complimentary and free of cost. **Not meant for sale.**

Inquiries for bulk sales may be solicited at: jaypee@jaypeebrothers.com

Principles and Practice of Nursing Management and Administration

First Edition: 2013

Second Edition: **2020**

ISBN: 978-93-90020-01-0

Printed at Sanat Printers

*I dedicate this piece of the 2nd edition venture
to the glory of God, "The Almighty"
Without whom I am nothing
&
To my family
For their endless support and encouragement*

Preface to the Second Edition

It gives me great contentment to present the second edition of the book *Principles and Practice of Nursing Management and Administration* on successful completion of seven years of steady progress. The wide acceptance and warmly acknowledgment by a vast family of its readers, including students and the nursing community, encouraged me to bring out a major revision in the second edition.

In the present scenario, the nursing administrators both present and future requires continuous and updated knowledge in developing a science of nursing management and preparing future nurse administrators and managers. Advancement in high technology and globalization poses several challenges for the nursing institutions to prepare nurse managers, who can access, synthesize and evaluate information, communicate effectively with patients and with their team members to make clinical decisions. There is a need for competent nurse managers and administrators, who can plan, organize, manage staff and other resources, communicate as well as guide students and clients by applying various innovative methods and principles of management in any health care setting.

The role of nurse managers is changing with the advancement of communication technology, changes in curriculum designs and syllabi, change in the health system, and an upcoming variety of nursing programs. We need nurse administrators who need to be dynamic and fully convergent with various management modalities and the latest concepts of administration and management to achieve the overall objective of nursing administration and management.

To achieve the professional competence in nursing management, both present–future, and to meet the requirements of the nursing students at degree level and provide a reference book for postgraduate level, the efforts have been made to make the illustrations, diagrams, flowcharts, and content matter more specific and significant for better understanding of users. Moreover, a well-accepted style of the book, with 'Chapter Outline', 'Learning Outcome' in the beginning, and 'Chapter Highlights' and 'Review Questions' at the end of each chapter are provided in the present edition for an easy to understand and quick recall approach. The main goal to revise this book is to present a clear, interesting, systematic, and thoroughly teachable material on nursing administration and management.

The best efforts have been made to bring out comprehensive, simplified, and evidence-based book to nursing students and faculty that would help them to develop their competencies in nursing administration and management practice as nurse managers. I hope that this book will provide an excellent resource to students undergoing graduate and postgraduate nursing courses, and practice nurses who would engage themselves in the rewarding activity of management, who are the future and pillars of our nursing profession, and responsible for its development to fulfill their managerial role.

Some of the key features of the 2nd edition of this book are as follows:

Updated Content

The emphasis has been made on clarity and accuracy of the content in the updated material with recent information is inserted in different chapters. Some of the topics are added to cover the syllabus of graduate and postgraduate nursing courses.

Organization of Book

The present edition of the book has 11 sections covering 62 chapters. Each chapter begins outlining the content to cover in the chapter and learning outcome, which is expected from each learner after going through the whole chapter. To recall the subject matter, at the end of the chapter is provided with chapter highlights, and for self-assessment, review questions covering essay type, short answer, and Multiple Choice Questions (MCQs). Some of the chapters are rearranged in different Sections in the present edition to make the learning linked to relevant topics. The book includes Glossary and Index at the end.

Figures, Tables, Flowcharts

All the illustrations in the present edition are redrawn and made the necessary changes wherever required. Only the important diagrams are in the revised edition to enrich the students with a lot of material in a short space.

User-Friendliness

The book is made user-friendly by using different levels of headings, subheadings, and italicized words to help the users to have in-depth study of subject and quickly revising by adding 'Chapter Highlights' and scope for self-assessment by adding Review Questions of essay type, Short answered, and MCQs at the end of each chapter, that makes the book truly user-friendly.

In short, the revised edition is a comprehensive text of *Principles and Practice of Nursing Administration and Management* meant primarily for students undergoing graduate and postgraduate nursing courses, but also to practice nurses working in hospitals, community, and teaching nursing institutes at all levels. The management students of other disciplines and different courses would also find it useful.

Jogindra Vati

Preface to the First Edition

The nursing administration requires a continuous change particularly after the dawn of high-tech and globalization in India. This has created several challenges for the nursing organizations and also put a demand for professionally trained nurse managers. Efficient utilization of human, physical and technological resources has become an essential requirement for the success of any health organization and so for the nursing organizations. The nurse managers who are energetic, dynamic and fully convergent with the environment of management and the latest concepts and practices of management can achieve this. It can be said that nursing organization is like an orchestra team. It is for the management to make music or a noise out of it. If there is an effective and efficient management, the result is sweet and melodious music; otherwise the result is chaotic and awful noise.

To achieve the professional competence, nurse managers, both present and future are required to be fully equipped with foundation of nursing management and principles of management particularly those which have their applications in Indian scenarios. A comprehensive understanding of bases of management and planning process will increase their competency. Moreover nursing management is an integral part of baccalaureate education, graduate education. A number of nurses are involved in managerial activities in hospital, community, educational institutions and other settings.

This requires the availability of integrated basic reading of materials to them. The present text makes an attempt to give comprehensive approach to the foundation of nursing management and can be treated as the framework of nursing service management. The efforts in this book have been aimed at articulating and systematizing the defined framework or foundation for management of nursing services. The book provides a comprehensive introduction to nursing management for undergraduate, graduate, and practice nurses. At the master's level the text provides not only substantive content related to management but also practical applications based on evidences and author's experiences in teaching nursing management at various educational levels. The chapters have been sequenced to facilitate ease in reading and understanding.

THE ORGANIZATION OF THE TEXTBOOK

This textbook is divided into ten units, with each unit focusing on one of the major domains of nursing management.

Unit 1: Framework of Nursing Management and Administration focusing on introducing the students to the concept of nursing, nursing management and administration and related ethical, legal issues. There is also a detailed description of standards in nursing and quality assurance and quality management in subsequent chapters. Trends and issues related to nursing practice and management provides the broad outlook of nursing management. The role of regulatory body and accreditation and nursing audit gives a strong base for essence of nursing management, has been included in the section of the textbook.

Unit 2: Planning is the one of the important elements of the nursing management. This unit has been divided into eight chapters. Each chapter is discussed elaborately. Mission, philosophy, vision, aims and objectives are the pillars of planning. Strategic planning, plans serve as a framework for decisions and are important to avoid waste, confusion and errors. More detailed information is provided in the process of decision-making and problem-solving. Qualitative method of planning and management by objectives are emphasized in this section.

Unit 3: Health Care Delivery System and Planning Process moves the students into the greater understanding of Indian Administrative System, Health System in India and Fundamentals of Health Planning. The information is provided on National Health Planning, Planning Commission, Five Year Plans, National Health Committees, National Health Programmes and National Health Policies.

Unit 4: Organizing next to the planning provides in-depth presentation of organizing and organization. The basics of organization structure and organization charts are discussed in details. This part covers topics like committees, coordination, organizational climate, organizational effectiveness which is the important aspects of organizing. Conflict management and organizational change management is also newer concept in nursing management and a challenge to nurse managers.

Unit 5: Human Resource Management and Staffing addresses overview of personnel management and administration. This unit has been divided into 14 chapters. Staff which is the most distinct and important component of any health organization is covered under fundamentals of staffing. Staffing norms and staffing patterns are elaborated in Indian context. Nursing Manpower planning is considered as being central in personnel administration; various aspects of manpower planning process are presented at national and organizational level and also highlighted various approaches of forecasting nursing manpower requirements. Job analysis gives the opportunity to design and redesign the job structure to the nurse managers is discussed in detail. It highlighted how to conduct job analysis and develop job descriptions. This part of the book tries to clear the fog surrounding the recruitment, selection, retaining employees, placement, and allocation, promotion, transfers, staff development, and performance appraisal process. Assignment, scheduling and nursing care delivery system form one of the core aspects of this part of the book. How to reduce staff turnover and absenteeism for the improvement of unit staffing aspect is also touched. Since an organizational environment is vital for the staff satisfaction, reduction of turnover and to increase output, the chapters like personnel policies, discipline and grievances, and occupational health and safety are written in a lucid and organized way.

Unit 6: Directing the heart of the nursing management process, helps the nurse managers to supervise and control the activities of nursing staff. This unit comprises of seven chapters and focuses on fundamentals of directing, effective supervision, motivation, communication, public relation, human relation, and collective bargaining.

Unit 7: Leadership major attributes and one of the most effective tools of managerial accomplishments and for successful nursing organization. It includes the chapters on nursing leadership, group dynamics, power and politics, team management, time management and stress management. Leadership chapter familiarizes with the background and classical studies on leadership and exemplified with evidences. Various methods for development of leaders and their leadership behaviors are discussed in detail. Group dynamics the study of groups and group processes is a separate chapter of this unit of the book. It covers various aspects of groups, group dynamics, group norms and group cohesiveness and thus provides well grounded knowledge for the nurse managers. Power and politics inextricably interwoven with the fabric of an organization's life are discussed in detail. It describes various techniques of managing organizational politics. Team management, time management and stress management are the reflections of an effective leadership quality of a nurse manager, provides related theoretical dimensions in subsequent chapters.

Unit 8: Material Management unfolds concepts, principles and procedures of material management. This unit has four chapters and focusing on procurement, inventory control and planning equipment and supplies. The procurement process and the key steps in the process of purchasing are highlighted. There is a detailed description of inventory, inventory management and accounting system, inventory control, types of inventory costs, inventory classification and models. Various aspects and nursing activities in relation to equipment and supplies management is the focus of this section.

Unit 9: Fiscal Management the life blood of the administration, critically examine the usefulness of fiscal management and administration, budget, budgetary process, audit, health economics, economics evaluation techniques, and critical pathways and health care reforms in controlling the utilization of resources. Nursing finance, health care financing and steps of planning budget has the focus in the introductory chapter; Budget and budgeting process, nursing budget, Zero Base Budgeting, Performance budgeting, Programme Planning Budgeting System and Midterm appraisal is also included in subsequent chapters. Knowledge of the cost determination which is necessary to keep a check on the cost of product, services /control on wastages, accounting which aims at keeping records of various transactions and used to study the various aspects of cost, internal and external audit is discussed in detail. Health economics a subject of increasing significance which is based on principle that resources are scarce relative to the demands made on them and economic evaluation techniques has been elaborated.

Unit 10: Nursing Informatics an emerging field of integrating information and computer science with nursing to enable nurses to collect and manage data, process data into information and knowledge, and make knowledge-based decisions about patient care. This part has been divided into five chapters and the readers are provided with the information on concept of nursing informatics, information technology, patients' records, electronic records, information system, and communication system including e-nursing, telemedicine and telenursing.

It is hoped that this book would be able to create an improvement and objective criticism will be appreciated and incorporated in the later editions of this treatise.

Jogindra Vati

Acknowledgments

The work of the revised edition is indeed a great task to complete and would have been impossible without the blessings of God, the Almighty's immense unconditional grace and love showered upon me throughout my life and for giving me strength, and perseverance to pursue and accomplish it.

I appreciate the feedback given by my reviewers, colleagues, and nurse administrators and managers. I owe special thanks to all of them. I will be grateful to my colleagues, friends, teachers who shaped my career in nursing and enriched my teaching experience in nursing management and research. I owe my thanks to my departmental staff and sustained encouragement from my well-wishers and nursing community in particular. I offer special thanks to my students, who continue to be my guides for teaching in nursing. I continue to value inspirations to work given by them and recognize their feelings towards my progress in life.

As always, I remained indebted to particular Ms S Samual, Former Principal, College of Nursing, National Institute of Nursing Education (NINE), Postgraduate Institute of Medical Education and Research (PGIMER), Chandigarh, Dr (Ms) S Baltej, Ex-Faculty, NINE, PGIMER, Chandigarh, Professor in Nursing, and Former Dean, Akal College of Nursing, Eternal University, Baru Sahib, Himachal Pradesh, Dr Saroj Sharma, Ex-Faculty, NINE, PGIMER, Chandigarh, all are my mentors from whom I had an opportunity to learn nursing management.

I am highly thankful to Shri Jitendar P Vij (Group Chairman) of M/s Jaypee Brothers Medical Publishers (P) Limited, who has been highly supportive and encouraging me to complete the project. Many special thanks to Mr Ankit Vij (Managing Director), Mr MS Mani (Group President), Dr Madhu Choudhary (Publishing Head–Education), Ms Pooja Bhandari (Production Head), Ms Samina Khan (Executive Assistant to Publishing Head–Education), Ms Dolly Dominic (Development Editor), Ms Seema Dogra (Cover Visualizer), Mr Binay Kumar (Proofreader), Mr Deepak Saxena (Typesetter), Mr Manoj Pahuja (Graphic Designer) and the whole team of M/s Jaypee Brothers Medical Publishers (P) Limited, who have encouraged, guided and provided time to time support for revising this book and demanding high quality, and time-bound 2nd edition of the book.

Projects like this one take time and certainly require support. My family deserves much of the credit for the gifts of their love, wisdom, and work ethics, which endured and inspired me in my difficult times, keep me motivating and putting up my endless revising this particular book.

Contents

Section 1: Nursing as a Profession: Framework for Management

1. Concept of Nursing   3
- Development of Nursing as a Profession   3
- Definitions of Nursing   5
- Concepts of Nursing   5
- Nursing as a Profession   6
- Characteristics of a Professional Nurse   7

2. Regulatory Bodies   10
- Regulatory Body   11
- Types of Regulatory Bodies in Nursing   12
- Trained Nurses Association of India   14
- Student Nurses Association of India   16

3. Trends and Issues in Nursing   18
- Trends in Nursing   18
- Factors Affecting Trends in Nursing   20
- Issues in Nursing   22
- Future Issues in Nursing   23

4. Ethics and Ethical Issues in Nursing   27
- Ethics and Ethical Theories   27
- Principles and Rights Related to Ethics   29
- Code of Ethics and Professional Conduct   31
- Ethical Committee   34
- Ethical Issues and Ethical Decision-Making   35

5. Consumer Protection Act and Rights of Special Groups   38
- Legal System   38
- Consumers Protection Act   40
- Rights of Special Groups   41

6. Legal Aspects and Legal Issues in Nursing   48
- Legal Aspect in Nursing   48
- Regulation of Nursing Practice   50
- Legal Safeguard for Nurses in Practice   50
- Legal Responsibilities in Nursing   51
- Dealing in Specific Conditions   53
- Dealing With Medicolegal Cases   54

Section 2: Introduction to Nursing Management and Health Care Delivery System

7. Introduction to Nursing Management and Administration   59
- Concept of Management   59
- Nursing Management   61
- Administration   62
- Administration Versus Management   63
- Nature/Characteristics of Management   64
- Importance of Management   64
- Levels of Management in Hospital Nursing Services   65
- Functions of Nursing Management and Administration   66
- Principles of Nursing Management   67
- Role of Nurse as a Manager   68

8. Management Theories and Models   73
- Evolution of Management Thought   73
- Classical Theories of Management   73
- Neoclassical Theories of Management   75
- Modern Management Theories   79

9. Indian Administrative System and Health Care Delivery System   84
- Influences of the British Government   84
- Indian Constitution   85
- The Preamble   85
- Administrative System of India   86
- Health-care Delivery System in India   90
- Development of Modern Health System   90
- Organization of the Health-care Delivery System   91

10. Fundamentals of Health Planning   96
- Health Planning   96
- Regulatory Bodies   97
- National Health Plan   98
- National Health Committees   101

11. National Health Policies   107
- National Health Policies   107

Section 3: Planning Process

12. Fundamentals of Planning   123
- Planning   123
- Planning Process   127
- Types of Planning   128
- Advantages of Planning   129
- Limitations of Planning   129

13. Mission, Philosophy and Objectives   132
- Mission and Purpose   132
- Philosophy   133
- Objectives   134

14. Strategic Planning, Operating Plans and Planning New Venture   140
- Strategic Planning   140
- Operating Plan   142
- Planning New Venture   146

15. **Innovation in Nursing and Planning for Change** — 149
    - Innovation in Nursing 149
    - Planning for Change 153

16. **Program Evaluation Review Technique, Activity Plan, Management by Objectives, and Benchmarking** — 159
    - Program Evaluation and Review Technique 160
    - Activity Plan (Gantt Chart) 161
    - Management by Objectives 162
    - Benchmarking 164

Section 4: Fundamentals of Organization, Planning and Organizing Hospital Nursing and Ancillary Services

17. **Organization and Organization Structure** — 171
    - Basics of Organization 171
    - The Formal and Informal Organization 174
    - Organization Theories 175
    - Minimum Requirements for an Organization 176
    - Organization Structure 177
    - Types of Organization 178

18. **Organizational Climate and Organizational Effectiveness** — 184
    - Organizational Climate 184
    - Organizational Effectiveness 188

19. **Planning of Hospitals and Patient Care Units** — 192
    - Planning of Hospital 196
    - Planning of Patient Care Unit (PCU) 200

20. **Ward Management and Methods of Patient Assignment** — 208
    - Ward Management 208
    - Methods of Patient Assignment 215

21. **Planning and Organizing Ancillary Services** — 221
    - Planning and Organizing Central Sterile Supply Department Services 221
    - Planning and Organizing Laundry Services 223
    - Planning and Organizing Dietary Services/Kitchen 224
    - Planning and Organizing Laboratory Services 226

22. **Planning for Emergency and Disaster Management** — 230
    - Emergency and Disaster Management 230
    - Planning for Emergency and Disaster Management 235

Section 5: Human Resource Management and Staffing

23. **Human Resource Management** — 245
    - Human Resource Management 245
    - Recruitment 246
    - Selection 250
    - Deployment 253
    - Retention 255
    - Promotion 257
    - Demotion 258
    - Transfer 259
    - Superannuation 260

24. **Human Resource Management in Nursing Services** — 264
    - Human Resource Management in Hospital Nursing Services 264
    - Human Resource Management in Community Health Nursing Services 272

25. **Fundamentals of Staffing: Staffing, Philosophy, Staffing Study, and Norms** — 281
    - Staffing 281
    - Philosophy of Staffing 285
    - Staffing Study/Estimation of Nursing Staff Requirement 285
    - Staffing Norms and Normative Approaches 287

26. **Nursing Activities, Patient Classification System, and Scheduling** — 293
    - Nursing Activities and Activity-based Approaches 293
    - Patient Classification System and Patient Dependency-Related Approaches 296
    - Scheduling 299

27. **Categories and Job Description** — 306
    - Categories of Nursing Personnel 306
    - Job Description 308

28. **Personnel Policies** — 322
    - Personal Policies 322
    - Organization of Personnel Policies 324
    - Formulation of Personnel Policies 324

29. **Staff Development and In-service Education** — 326
    - Staff Development 326
    - Staff Development Models 327
    - Staff Development Methods 329
    - Staff Development Programs 329
    - In-service Education 330

30. **Career Planning, Development and Opportunities** — 336
    - Career Planning 336
    - Career Planning and Development 337
    - High Power Committee Recommendations on Career Development-Related Issues 338
    - Nursing as a Career, Career Positions, and Opportunities in Nursing 339
    - Nursing Career Development Opportunities and Practices 340

31. **Performance Appraisal** — 343
    - Performance Appraisal 343
    - Approaches to Performance Appraisal 345

- Performance Appraisal Process 345
- Methods of Performance Appraisal 346
- Guidelines for Effective Performance Appraisal 348

32. Discipline and Grievance Procedure 349
- Discipline 349
- Indiscipline 350
- Employee Grievance 352

33. Stress Management 356
- Work Stress 356
- Sources of Stress 357
- Consequences of Workplace Stress 359
- Approaches to Stress Management 359
- Nurse Managers' Role in Stress Management 361
- Tips for Reducing Stress at Workplace 361

34. Occupational Health and Safety 363
- Occupational Health and Safety 363
- Occupational Hazards 364
- Prevention of Occupational Hazards 366
- Nurses' Role in the Prevention of Occupational Hazards/Diseases 368

Section 6: Directing and Leading

35. Directing and Motivation 373
- Directing 373
- Motivation 376
- Motivation and Performance 377
- Models of Motivation 378
- Motivational Theories 379
- How to Create a Motivating Climate? 380
- Role of Nurse Managers to Motivate Staff 381

36. Communication 383
- Communication 383
- Communication Process 384
- Types of Communication 385
- Channels of Communication 387
- Effective Communication 388
- Communication Pattern in Nursing 389

37. Effective Supervision 392
- Supervision 392
- Supervision Styles 394
- Forms of Supervision 394
- Responsibilities of a Nurse Supervisor 395
- Role of a Nurse Supervisor 395
- Essential Qualities of a Nurse Supervisor 396
- Steps of Supervision 397
- Techniques and Tools Used for Supervision 397
- Tips for Effective Supervision 399

38. Nursing Leadership 402
- Significance of Leadership 402
- Leadership 403
- Leadership and Management 403
- Theoretical Approaches to Leadership 404
- Effective Leadership 406
- Leader and Leadership Development 408

39. Conflict Management 412
- Organizational Conflict 412
- Conflict Management 415

40. Collective Bargaining, Unions, and Professional Associations 419
- Collective Bargaining 419
- Health-care Laws 421
- Employee Unions 422
- Professional Associations 423

Section 7: Organizational Behavior and Human Relations

41. Fundamentals of Organizational Behavior, Human Relations, Public Relations, Publicity, and Public Education 429
- Organizational Behavior 430
- Human Relations 432
- Public Relations 433
- Publicity and Public Education 435

42. Group, Group Formation, and Group Dynamics 438
- Group and Group Formation 438
- Group Dynamics 442

43. Power, Organizational Politics, Lobbying, and Advocacy 446
- Power 446
- Organizational Politics 448
- Lobbying and Advocacy 450

44. Team Management and Time Management 454
- Team Management 455
- Time Management 458
- Effective Time Management 461

Section 8: Material Management

45. Material Management: Concept, Principles, and Procedures 469
- Material Management 469
- Procedure of Material Management System 472

46. Equipment Management, Planning Equipment and Supplies, and Condemnation 476
- Equipment and Supplies 476
- Planning of Equipment and Supplies 480
- Condemnation of Equipment 483

47. Procurement and Purchasing 485
- Procurement 485
- Purchasing 488

48. Inventory Control and Inventory Accounting System 490
- Inventory Control 490
- Inventory Control System 496

Section 9: Controlling

49. Fundamentals of Controlling — 501
- Controlling 501
- Principles of Effective Control 503
- Steps in the Controlling Process 504
- Limitation of Control 504

50. Quality Assurance and Quality Management — 506
- Historical Perspectives of Quality Assurance 506
- Quality Assurance and Quality Management 507
- Total Quality Management 511
- Quality Circle 512
- Models of Quality Assurance and Quality Management 512
- Quality Evaluation Systems in Health Care 514
- Six Sigma in Healthcare 515

51. Nursing Service Standards — 520
- Nursing Standards 521
- Taxonomy of Standards 521
- Setting and Measuring Quality Standards 523
- Role of Nurse Administrators in Developing Standards 525
- Barriers and Constraints in Developing Nursing Standards 526
- Developed Nursing Practice Standards 526
- Role of Regulatory Bodies in Regulating Nursing Standards 527
- ANA Standards of Nursing Service 531
- ANA Standards of Care/Practice 531
- Professional Responsibility and Accountability 535
- Nursing Practice 535
- Communication and Interpersonal Relationships 535
- Valuing Human Beings 535
- Management 536
- Professional Development 536

52. Nursing Audit — 537
- Nursing Audit 537
- Nursing Audit Process 540
- Role of Nurse Managers in Nursing Audit 541

53. Accreditation — 543
- Accreditation 543
- Types of Accreditation Agencies in India 545
- National Assessment and Accreditation Council 545
- INC as an Accreditation Body 546
- Accreditation of Hospitals 549

Section 10: Fiscal Management

54. Financial Management, Financial Planning, and Financial Audit — 557
- Financial Management 557
- Financial Planning 560
- Financial Audit 561

55. Budget and Budgetary Process — 565
- Budget 565
- Budgeting 568
- Budgetary Process 575
- Nursing Budget 576
- Midterm Appraisal 577
- Program Planning Budgeting System 577

56. Cost Accounting and Health Economics — 581
- Concept of Cost 581
- Accounting 585
- Cost Accounting 586
- Health Economics 587

57. Economic Evaluation Techniques — 594
- Cost Analysis 594
- Cost-benefit Analysis 598
- Cost-effectiveness Analysis 601
- Cost-utility Analysis 603
- Cost Consequences Analysis 604

58. Critical Pathways and Health Care Reforms — 607
- Critical Pathways 607
- Healthcare Reforms 609

Section 11: Nursing Informatics

59. Nursing Informatics, Information Technology, Use of Computers and Telecommunications — 617
- Nursing Informatics 617
- Information Technology 622
- Use of Computers 624
- Telecommunications 626

60. Documentation System: Nursing Records and Recording, Reports and Reporting, and Correspondence — 629
- Documentation System 630
- Records and Recording 634
- Reports and Reporting 636
- Correspondence 638

61. Information Systems: Management Information and Evaluation System, Health Information and Management System, and Nursing Information System — 641
- Information System 641
- Management Information and Evaluation System 642
- Health Management Information System 643
- Nursing Information System 645
- Computer-based NIS 646

62. Use of Communication Technology: e-Learning, Telemedicine, Telenursing — 648
- The e-Learning 648
- Telemedicine 652
- Telenursing 655

Glossary — 661
Index — 665

Nursing as a Profession: Framework for Management

1. Concept of Nursing
2. Regulatory Bodies
3. Trends and Issues in Nursing
4. Ethics and Ethical Issues in Nursing
5. Consumer Protection Act and Rights of Special Groups
6. Legal Aspects and Legal Issues in Nursing

CHAPTER 1

Concept of Nursing

CHAPTER OUTLINE

- Development of Nursing as a Profession
- Definitions of Nursing
- Concept of Nursing
  - Concepts of Modern Nursing
  - Nursing as an Academic Discipline
  - Nursing as a Practice Science
- Nursing as a Human Science
- Nursing as a Profession
  - Meaning and Definitions of Profession
  - Characteristic of Profession
  - Is Nursing a Profession?
- Characteristics of a Professional Nurse

LEARNING OUTCOMES

After completion of this chapter, the learner will be able to:

- Understand the development and changing the concept of nursing
- Identify essential components of modern nursing
- Discuss nursing as an academic discipline, a science, and a profession
- Describe the essential characteristics of a profession
- Identify criteria of a profession
- Differentiate between profession and vocation
- Enumerate characteristics of a professional nurse

KEY TERMS

Nursing, modern nursing, profession, vocation, the ayurvedic system of medicine, discipline, regulation, autonomy, status, prestige, power, professional nurse

INTRODUCTION

Nursing is compassion personified and has a long and rich heritage. Nurses with their unique, divergent opinions, and talents have made many valuable individuals and collective contribution to society. Nursing originated independently and existed many centuries without contact with modern medicine.

DEVELOPMENT OF NURSING AS A PROFESSION

Historical Development

Nursing has developed over the last 100 years. There have been many variations in the rate of development even though there are similarities in the basic pattern. The events are divided into four phases: the early period, the years up to World War II in which a basic pattern was more or less standardized, the war years that gave an impetus to nursing education, and the year after independence marked by the development of public health nursing and start of degree programs in nursing.

Phase I

It is the early period of evolution of nursing: the period in which the foundation of nursing took place. The history of nursing begins with the history of humankind, ancient eastern and western cultures, and religion. There is hardly any available literature on the ancient history of nursing, and caring sick in primitive times. However, through myths, songs, and archeologists, it has been found that the primitive man had the skill of massaging, fermentation bone setting, amputation, hot and cold bath, and heat to control hemorrhages. Temples and houses of worship were to take care of sick people.

Under the Ayurvedic system of medicine (3000 BC), there was a mention of "Upacharika" means "Nurse" in a book written by Sushruta (1400 BC) on surgery and years later by "Charaka" on internal medicine describing qualities of Upacharika. According to Charaka, Upacharika should be pure or clean in physical appearance and mental hygiene (Shuchi), should have the competency and willing to care (Daksha), and should be co-coordinator with the patient and doctor (Anuraktha), and should be intelligent (Buddhiman).

In "Siddha" system of medicine (700–600 BC), the nurse was like the one who attends the patient, is cool headed and pleasant in her demeanors, does not speak ill of anybody, is strong and attentive enough fulfill the requirements of the sick, and follows the instructions of the doctor. During King Ashoka period (264 BC), there were a large number of hospitals for the sick and also provide for the education and training of women for that purpose. After the Mogul period, the nursing in India was looked upon as servants work due to various reasons such as the low state of women, the system of "pardha" among Muslims, caste system among Hindus, illiteracy, poverty, political unrest, and language difference.

Phase II

Phase after early period up to World War II in which a basic pattern was more or less standardized. During this period, nursing development in India took place in three dimensions: civilian nursing, missionary nursing, and military nursing.

Civilian nursing: Civilian nursing in India dates back to 1664 with upcoming of Government General Hospital at Madras during British Raj. Midwives training school granted certificates of "diploma in midwifery" for passed students and "sick nursing" for failed students in 1854. The training of civilian nurses for the hospital started in 1871. The first batch of six nurses came out as "diploma in midwifery nursing."

Missionary nursing: Missionary nursing training brought fully qualified Indian nurses. Due to cultural barriers, deep-seated caste system and degrading and unworthy attitude of people toward nursing Hindu and Muslims girls were not allowed to do work, and they were holding back, so Christian girls were encouraged to do nursing. Christianity introduced a new aspect of nursing and thus transforming nursing to a higher level and raising it to professional standing. The dawn of modern nursing dates from the late 1700s through 1853.

Mission hospitals came up in different parts of India at about the same time. Religion prevented Hindu and Muslim girls from joining, so only Christian girls could be trained first. The Dufferin fund: Queen Victoria noticed this trend and asked Lady Dufferin (whose husband was in government service) to take an interest in the care of children and women. She had raised a fund named Dufferin Fund in 1885 and started the "National Association" for supplying aid by women to Women of India.

Military nursing: Shortly after the criminal war, in which Florence Nightingale played a notable role, she sent a questionnaire to all British Military establishments in India to obtain morbidity and mortality rate among soldiers in the hospitals attached to Indian Cantonments. Recommendations made by Florence Nightingale led to the beginning of organized nursing in India. Military nursing developed in India during the first world war, when British officers informed need of nurses to take care of British officials and soldiers. After that, many events took place in nursing.

Indian Army Nursing Services started in 1888. Ten fully certified nurses from Florence Nightingale's arrived in Bombay to lead nursing in India on 21st February 1888. There is a record of staring at the school of nursing in India in 1891. However, the low status of women, caste system, illiteracy, poverty, and language differences were the barriers or the difficulties that hinder in the progress of nursing.

Phase III

Phase III starts from the war period to the preindependence period that gave an impetus to nursing education. In 1927, Indian Military Nursing services formed with 12 matrons, 18 sisters, and 25 staff nurses, and during the Second World War, nursing services were expanded in India and overseas under the direction of the chief principal matron. A 3-year training program was carried out in preliminary training schools in selected military hospitals. They were awarded a certificate as "registered nurse" after successful completion of training. **Figure 1.1** depicts the nursing developed as a profession from historical period to the preindependence period.

Phase IV

Phase IV is the period after independence. During the first 10 years of independence, there has been considerable development in all fields of social welfare; nursing has been one of them. There were many opportunities for nurses especially for improving their knowledge and conducting research studies and widen their horizons and career in India and abroad.

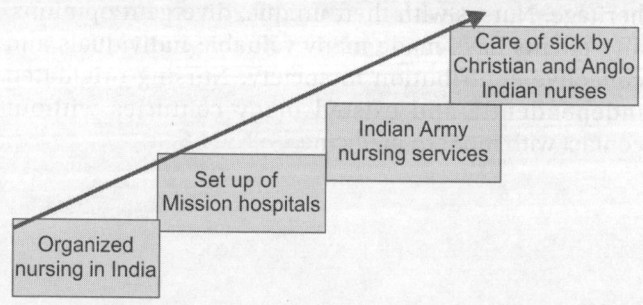

Fig. 1.1: Milestone in nursing before independence period.

DEFINITIONS OF NURSING

- According to Virginia Henderson (1966), ICN (1973), the function of a nurse is to help a sick or a healthy individual to perform those activities that contribute to his or her health, its recovery, and peaceful death. These activities he or she may perform without assistance or help to become self-independent as rapidly as possible.
- International Council of Nurses (2010) define nursing as collaborative care required for all persons of all ages, either sick or well. Its focus is on preventive, promotive, and caring of sick, disabled, and dying. The main nursing roles are in promoting a safe environment, advocacy, education, management, and research and participation in formulating health policy.
- American Nurses Association viewed the functions of nursing to protect, promote, and optimize health and abilities; to prevent illness and injury, early diagnosis, and treatment of diseases; and to communicate and advocate healthcare to the community at large, individually, and to the family.

CONCEPTS OF NURSING

A review of literature from the late 1970s until the present poses a query whether nursing is concerned with the care, core, coordination, an intellectual activity, a science, or an academic discipline, and a profession. Let us discuss one by one.

Concept of Modern Nursing

The dawn of modern nursing dates from the late 1700s to 1853. During pre-Christianity period, there was a great emphasis on caring and the way of caring for sick and suffering people. The concept of care, however, continued during the middle-age period, and during that time, nuns and monks were rendering care with devotion. During this period, the transformation of nursing to a higher level took place and raised the standard of nursing professional.

The concept of modern nursing is based on the spiritual philosophy and has focused on "health maintenance" and "restoration" (Nightingale, 1860). According to this philosophy, nursing is a search for truth to find out answers to health-care questions and discovering and using Gods' law of healing in nursing practice. The main focus was on health maintenance through proper nutrition, hygiene, and shelter. There are three components of modern nursing are as follows (Fig. 1.2):
1. **Care:** Caring is dealing with human beings under stress, frequently over long periods. The caring component is to provide comfort and support.
2. **Cure:** The cure is concerned with the promotion of health and healing. It focuses on the diagnosis treatment of the client.
3. **Coordination:** Nursing needs to share the responsibility for the health and welfare of all the people in the community and participates in the program designed

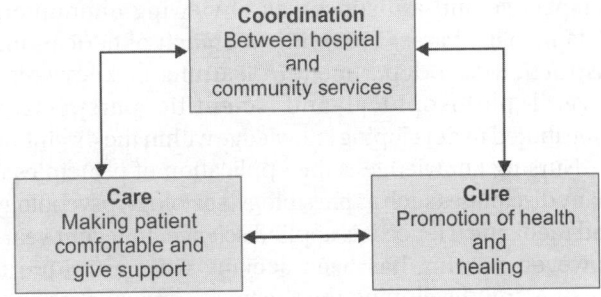

Fig. 1.2: Components of modern nursing.

to prevent illness and maintain health. In the hospital, it coordinates with medical and other professional and technical services. Professional nurse supervises, teaches, and directs all those involved in nursing care.

In modern nursing, the role of professional nurse ranges from rendering patient care to planning and implementation of health services for direction and supervision of others who give care to the patients. Thus administrative skills have become indispensable in providing creative and need-based patient care.

Nursing as an Intellectual Activity

Clark viewed nursing as an intellectual activity. According to her, there are two ways of looking at nursing: (1) nursing as a collection of tasks, and (2) nursing as a particular kind of interpersonal interaction.

Nursing as a Collection of Tasks

The first view is that the nursing as a collection of tasks or procedures, which requires some skills per the direction of doctors whose functions they exist to assist.

Nursing as a Particular Kind of Interpersonal Interaction

The second view describes nursing as a particular kind of interpersonal interaction, which has specific goals and involves particular kinds of activities. Its focus is on physical and emotional responses of people toward illness, treatment, and disability, and its goals are as follows:
 i. To enable people to maximize their potentials for health
 ii. To enhance their ability to cope with the illness and disability
 iii. To promote physical and mental comfort, healing, and recovery.

This perspective of nursing gives it intellectual touch that needs the use of clinical judgment and skill by applying the steps of the nursing process.

Nursing as an Academic Discipline

A discipline is "a branch of knowledge ordered through the theories and methods evolving from more than one worldview of the phenomenon of concern" (Parse, 1997, p. 74). It is a field of inquiry characterized by a unique perspective and a distinct way of viewing phenomena (Adam, 1985; Parse, 1999). It is a branch of educational instruction or a department of learning or knowledge. Several philosophical and scientific perspectives contributed to developing knowledge within the discipline.

Nursing knowledge is the application of principles of many disciplines such as physiology, sociology, psychology, and medicine. Hence it is applied science. In recent years, however, nursing has been seeking what a unique to nursing and developing those aspects into an academic discipline. Following are the areas that can identify nursing as a distinct discipline:
- An identifiable philosophy
- Conceptual framework
- Acceptable methodological approaches for the development of knowledge (Oldnall, 1995)
- The body of knowledge is developed within designated boundaries and guides the pursuit, development, and dissemination of that knowledge.

Nursing as a Practice Science

Whether nursing was a basic science or applied science was the debate in the early years. The goal of basic sciences is the attainment of knowledge. In contrast, applied science is one that uses the knowledge of basic sciences for some practical end. In practice sciences, research is largely clinical and action oriented. Thus, as an applied or practice science, nursing requires research that is applied and clinical (Fawcett, 1999).

Nursing as a Human Science

Nursing is also considered as a human science as it examines various issues related to behavior and culture as well as of biology and physiology. Evidence revealed that there is an association among related factors that affect human health and illness (Gortner, 1993).

NURSING AS A PROFESSION

Meaning and Definition of a Profession

The word "profession" is a derivative of "profess," which means "to proclaim something publicly." Profession professes or proclaims to know something better than the people they serve and who thus need their service. A profession has been viewed differently by different schools of thought.

The Australian Council of Professions (2004) viewed a profession as a group of individuals who follow ethical standards, have social acceptance, and special knowledge and skills. They have undergone specialized training to apply their knowledge and skills in rendering care.

According to Boone (2001), professions should have scientific and philosophical facts acquired through inquiry and research. The professional differs from other vocations—the professionals directed toward unique public service based on the scientific or philosophical knowledge and specialized skills that require from professional training.

Characteristics of a Profession

The characteristic of a profession has a long list, and various authors have their views.

According to Southern Illinois University (2004), a profession has:
- A body of special knowledge
- Specialized training in applying special knowledge
- The standards of practice
- The sense of responsibility toward the public, clients, and other team members.

General Characteristics of Profession

1. **Autonomy:** Professions need to be autonomous. It means that the professions have a high degree of control of their affair, have the freedom to exercise professional judgment, and can make independent judgments about their work. To have professional autonomy, other members of the profession must evaluate the activities and decisions of members of the profession. The concept of autonomy includes judgment and also the self-interest and continuous evaluation of ethics and procedures from within the profession itself.
2. **Regulation:** Professions have their regulatory bodies, whose function are to define, promote, oversees, support, and regulate the affairs of its members. There may be several such bodies as professional associations or councils. These are self-regulating and independent from government.
3. **Legitimacy:** All professions have power and clear legal authority over some activities.
4. **Status:** Professions have high social status in the society due to their social service to society and client. All professions require having technical, specialized and highly skilled workers, and needing professional expertise. Professional qualification, degree, and licensure are required to enter the profession.
5. **Theoretical knowledge-based skill:** Professionals should have extensive theoretical knowledge at least 3 years at university. The clinical skills must practice by theoretical knowledge.
6. **Licensed practitioners:** Professionals are required to enroll or register with the licensing body to practice or to get a job in that profession.
7. **Code of ethics and professional conduct:** A code of ethics is important to govern the activities of each profession. These codes require behavior and practice. It refers to personal moral obligations of an individual. The code of ethics defines high standards of behavior about the services provided by them. These codes are mandatory by profession and are acknowledged and accepted by the community.

Is Nursing a Profession?

There have been many debates about whether nursing a profession rather than an occupation. However, for nursing to be recognized as a profession by the society it should serve, and it must demonstrate an ongoing basis that meets the criteria of a profession:

- Nursing requires knowledge; judgment; and skills based on biological, sociological, psychological, and other allied sciences including medical and nursing sciences.
- Nurses are providing unique services to the public through hospitals, community, and in other settings. They are licensed to practice in nursing through State Nursing Councils.
- Nursing has a knowledge base. Nursing theorists and nurse researchers are contributing to the knowledge bases and thus providing the evidenced-based nursing.
- The registered nurses are accountable for their negligence in the care and thus accountable for the public through legal regulations and licensures.
- Nursing education is both theory and practical based. It is mandatory to apply scientific rationale in rendering care. Hence the basis of professional nursing is on scientific knowledge, skills, and abilities.
- Nursing in India with limited autonomy, have administrative positions at State and Center Level are comparable with other medical administrators.
- Professional organizations share common values.
- Today both men and other background groups are entering in nursing. Recruitment and placement of registered nurses are on a regular basis like other government employees.
- Trained Nurses Association of India and the Indian Nursing Council had published a code of ethics for nurses. Many of the values are identified within the codes, thus establishing legal requirements.
- Nursing thus accomplished much in the way of establishing its body of knowledge, the scope of practice, research base, and code of ethics. However, it needs to continue to struggle with maintaining autonomy over its nursing practice.

Hence, Nursing is a profession that focuses on helping individuals, families, and communities to attain and maintain optimal health and functioning and recover from diseases. Each nurse irrespective of his or her qualification or position has a definite part to play as the member of the nursing profession. Thus nursing is a profession, an academic discipline, and a science. **Table 1.1** depicts characteristics of a profession, discipline, and science applicable to nursing.

Professional nurses create a physical, social, and spiritual environment to prevent illness, to promote health through teaching—the nursing personnel coordinate with other health professions in caring for the clients. The primary function of the nurses is to serve humanity for the existence of the nursing profession. Need for the nursing service is universal. Professional nursing has the dedication to serve irrespective of nationality, race, creed, color, politics, or social status.

CHARACTERISTICS OF A PROFESSIONAL NURSE

The word "nurse" is derived from the Latin word "nutritious," meaning nourishing. According to Virginia Henderson, a complete nurse is one who has thoroughly mastered nursing technical skills but who uses his or her emotional and technical responses in a unique design that suits the peculiar needs of the person whom he or she serves.

1. **Personal characteristics:** Good nurses should be caring, have compassion, respect for self and others, and respect the person, his or her feelings, rules, culture, creed, and religion. He or she is impartial and maintains the confidentiality of the patients. They should have patience with patients, health team members, family members, confidence in herself and her knowledge. He or she should also be physically, mentally, spiritually, and emotionally healthy.
2. **Commitment:** The professional nurse should commit those he or she serves. He or she should follow a code of ethics and maintain standards of care, have ethical and moral values, the role of being a good nurse, and doing the right things and in the progression of the profession of nursing.
3. **Knowledgeable:** The professional nurse should have the knowledge base and have a thorough knowledge of nursing, basic sciences, and principles of nursing. He or she should be competent in performing all types

TABLE 1.1: Characteristics of profession, discipline, and science.

Profession	Discipline	Science
➢ Vocation/occupation	➢ Education, research, service	➢ Research experimental investigation
➢ Specialized knowledge and skills	➢ Defined knowledge boundaries	➢ A unified body of knowledge
➢ Methods based on scientific principles	➢ Evidence-based theory	➢ Experimental investigation
➢ The institution of higher learning	➢ Pursuit, development, dissemination of knowledge	➢ Observation, identification, and description of phenomena
➢ Higher ethical standards	➢ Academic freedom for faculty and students	➢ Assurance of human rights
➢ Expanding body of knowledge	➢ The distinct theoretical body of knowledge	➢ A unified body of knowledge
➢ Autonomous functioning	➢ The classroom and the laboratory	➢ The laboratory
➢ Continuous study	➢ Pursuit of knowledge	➢ The pursuit of solutions and answers
➢ Service to society	➢ For the betterment of society	➢ Health needs of society

of nursing procedures and willing to enhance the skills and knowledge.
4. **Technical skills:** Nurses need to be competent in delivering nursing care and traditional care to advanced nursing care. There should not be any negligence or errors in his or her part.
5. **Patient centeredness:** The professional nurse should be patient oriented and provide care according to priority.
6. **Communication skills:** Nurses should have excellent communication skills especially listening. She should communicate with the clients and family. She should follow the principles and channel of communication effectively while working with health personnel in a team. She should have the ability to express, both verbally and nonverbally, in ways that are appropriate to cultures and situations.
7. **Advocacy:** The professional nurse strongly advocates for the patients, empowering others. She makes clear what is ethically and legally right.
8. **Emotionally strong:** The nurses should be emotionally mature to deal with all types of patients. Since nursing is stressful, he or she should have the ability to accept suffering and death without letting it get personal.
9. **Empathetic:** Nurses should be empathetic to the pain and suffering of the patients and sympathetic toward their experience as a patient. It is one of the important qualities to be a nurse.
10. **Critical thinking:** A professional nurse makes appropriate and right decisions for the care and plan and evaluates the outcome. The nurse should continually ask questions, clarify information, and consider a variety of options before taking any decision.
11. **Interpersonal skills:** Nurses are central to the care and link health personnel in caring for patients. She coordinates all the activities and hence should have a good interpersonal relationship with the health team as well as with the patient and their families.
12. **Problem-solving skills:** The nurses need to identify the problems encountered while caring for or managing the patients and should have the skill to solve those problems systematically and also involve the patient in deciding his or her care. Make him or her understand the alternatives and in selecting the best one.

CHAPTER HIGHLIGHTS

- The history of nursing begins with the history of humankind. It took various developmental stages to be a profession.
- The root of nursing is in mythology, ancient eastern and western cultures, and religion.
- Nurse (Upacharika) was one of the wings of treatment, traced back in the sacred books of Sushruta and Charaka, and the one who attends patients, mentioned in all the Indian systems of medicine.
- Christianity introduced a new aspect on nursing to transform it to a higher level and raising it to a professional standing.
- Nursing is committed to promote health of sick and healthy individuals, families, and communities to meet national health goals.
- Nursing is a professional service for enabling a person to maintain and sustain health and well-being.
- Regulation, autonomy, status, and legitimacy are the general characteristics of a profession; nursing skills based on theoretical knowledge, licensed practitioners, and code of ethics are other important features of a profession.
- Apart from personal characteristics, a nurse should be committed to service, patient centered, knowledgeable, empathetic, and emotionally mature; she or he should possess various skills such as technical, communication, advocacy, interpersonal, and professional solving skills and should have therapeutic and professional interpersonal relationship and critical thinking to take professional decisions.

REVIEW QUESTIONS

I. Essay Type Questions
1. Define nursing. Discuss the historical development of nursing.
2. Is nursing a profession? Discuss.
3. Describe the concept of modern nursing.
4. Enumerate characteristics of a professional nurse.

II. Short Notes
1. Phases in nursing development
2. Criteria to be a profession
3. Nursing as an academic discipline
4. Nursing as human science
5. A professional nurse

III. Multiple Choice Questions
1. The Ayurvedic system of medicine dates back in:
   a. 1000 BC b. 1400 BC
   c. 2000 BC d. 3000 BC
2. The Siddha system of medicine dates back in:
   a. 1000 BC b. 700–600 BC
   c. 264 BC   d. 200 BC
3. The dimension(s) in nursing development in India is/are:
   a. Missionary nursing
   b. Civilian nursing and missionary nursing
   c. Civilian, missionary, and military nursing
   d. Civilian nursing
4. The nursing training in Madras started during the year:
   a. 1871 b. 1888
   c. 1664 d. 1606
5. The modern nursing in India dates from:
   a. Late 1700s through 1853
   b. 1600s through 1700

Chapter 1: Concept of Nursing

    c. 1500s through 1600
    d. 1400s through 1500

6. When did Indian Military Nursing Services form?
    a. 1871
    b. 1891
    c. 1905
    d. 1927

7. In which year 10 fully certified nurses from Florence arrived in Bombay to lead nursing in India?
    a. 1885
    b. 1888
    c. 1890
    d. 1894

8. Who was the superintendent of first modern training school for nurses?
    a. Atkinson
    b. Dufferin
    c. Victoria
    d. Kelly

9. "Nursing as a collection of tasks or procedures" is one of the concepts of nursing as:
    a. An academic discipline
    b. An intellectual activity
    c. A practice science
    d. A human science

10. One of the characteristics to be a profession that "to have a high degree of control of their affair, have the freedom to exercise professional judgment and can make independent judgments about their work" is:
    a. Status and prestige
    b. Power
    c. Self-regulation
    d. Autonomy

Answer Keys

1. d   2. b   3. c   4. c   5. a   6. d   7. b
8. a   9. b   10. d

SUGGESTED READING

1. Adam E. Towards more clarity in terminology: framework, theories, and models. J Nurs Educ. 1985;24:151-5.
2. Asa K. Professional ethics and collective professional autonomy—a conceptual analysis. Ethical Pers. 2005;12(1):67-97.
3. Australian Council of Professions. About Professions Australia: Definition of a Profession 2004. Available from http://www.professions.com.au/defineprofession.html.
4. Available from http://www.eu.wikipedia.org/wiki/Profession.
5. Available from http://www.icn.cn/abouticn.htm. International Council of Nurses.
6. Available from http://www.victorianweb.org/history/crimea/florrie.html.
7. Available from https://www.dovepress.com/the-senior-living-lab-an-example-of-nursing-leadership.
8. Available from https://www.icn.ch/nursing-policy/nursing-definitions.
9. Boone T. Constructing a profession, professionalization of exercise physiology online. Int Electron J Exercise Physiol. 2001;4(5):May, ISSN 1099-5862. Available from http://www.css.edu/users/tboone2/asep/ConstructingAprofession.html.
10. Buckley JW, Buckley MH. The Accounting Profession. Melville, Los Angeles, 1974. Quoted by Perks, p. 4.
11. Bullock A, Butt M. The New Fontana Dictionary of Modern Thought. London: Harper-Collins; 1999. p. 689.
12. Burbules N, Densmore K. The limits of making teaching a profession. Education Pol. 1991;5(1):44-63.
13. Connelly, L. Use of theoretical frameworks in research. Medsurg Nurs. 2014;23(3):187.
14. Donaldson SK, Crowley DM. The discipline of nursing. Nurs Outlook. 1978;26(2):113-20.
15. Gerald L. Occupational Monopoly and Modern Medicine. London: Tavistock; 1983.
16. Gortner SR. Nursing syntax revisited: A critique of philosophies said to influence nursing theories. Available from https://www.readbyqxmd.com/read/8288417/nursing-s-syntax-revisited-a-critique-of.
17. Hood LJ, Leddy SK. Leddy & Pepper's Conceptual Bases of Professional Nursing, 5th edition. Philadelphia: Lippincott, William & Wilkins; 2003.
18. Joel LA. Kelly's Dimensions of Professional Nursing, 9th edition. New York: McGraw-Hill/Appleton & Lange; 2003.
19. Latham SR. Medical professionalism: A parsanian view. Mt Sinai J Med. 2002;69:393-9.
20. Leddy SK. Leddy's & Pepper's Conceptual Bases of Professional Nursing, 5th edition. Philadelphia: Lippincott, Williams & Wilkins; 2003.
21. Logan J, Franzen D, Pauling C, Butcher HK. Achieving professional hood through participation in professional organizations. In Haynes L, Boese T, Butcher H (Eds). Nursing in contemporary society: Issues, trends, and transition to practice. Upper Saddle River, NJ: Prentice Hall; 2004.
22. Nightingale Florence. Notes on Nursing. 1860. Full text online. Accessed 14 August 2007.
23. Nurse. The Oxford English Dictionary, 2nd edition 10. Oxford University Press; 1989. pp. 603-4.
24. Oldnall AS. Nursing as an emerging academic discipline. J Adv Nurs. 1995;21:605-12.
25. Parse RR. Nursing: The discipline and the profession. Nurs Sci Quart. 1999;12(4):275-6.
26. Parse RR. The language of nursing knowledge: Saying what we mean. In: King IM, Fawcett J (Eds). The Language of Nursing Theory and Metatheory. Indianapolis, Center Nursing Press; 1997.
27. Southern Illinois University. Engineering as a Profession. [Online] Available from http://civil.engr.siu.edu/intro/profession.htm.
28. Wilkinson A. A brief history of nursing in India and Pakistan. Am J Nurs. 1958;58(11):1514.

CHAPTER 2

Regulatory Bodies

CHAPTER OUTLINE

- Defining Regulation, Regulatory System, and Professional Body
- Regulatory Body
  - Meaning and Definition
  - Aims of Regulatory Bodies of Nursing
  - Objectives of Regulatory Bodies of Nursing
  - Role of Professional and Regulatory Bodies
- Types of Regulatory Bodies of Nursing
  - Indian Nursing Council
  - State Nursing Councils
  - Examinations Boards and Universities
- Trained Nurses Association of India
- Student Nurses Association of India

LEARNING OUTCOMES

After completion of this chapter, the learner will be able to:
- Understand the concept of regulatory system and professional body
- Define the terms regulation, regulatory body, and professional body
- Discuss the aims, objectives, and the role of regulatory and professional bodies
- Describe various types of regulatory bodies of nursing
- Familiarize with Trained Nurses Association of India (TNAI) and Student Nurses Associations (SNAs)

KEY TERMS

Regulatory system, professional body, regulatory body, Indian Nursing Council, State Nursing Council, Trained Nurses Association of India

INTRODUCTION

Nurses are considered to be the heart and soul of health-care settings, the front-line caregiver to clients. Supporting nurses through their critical entry into the profession is not only good for the development of the nurse and the employer, but it is most important to the good of the patient. Regulation implies the intervention of the government to accomplish an end beneficial to its citizens. Each state has regulatory bodies, which provide a vital role to ensure the public right to quality health-care service, and to support and assist professional members.

Health professionals such as nurses, doctors, pharmacists, and many others are regulated and licensed by regulatory bodies as required by legislation. Nursing regulatory bodies receive their authority from legislation. It is mandatory for nurses to register with state nursing regulatory body as a registered nurse and registered midwife and takes licensure to practice.

Regulation

The word "regulation" means rules and restrictions. Each organization frames its rules and regulation to the employees. These are the boundaries that need to be followed by each of the employees. The regulations are also to have control over the conduct. Professional regulation is the means to maintain order, consistency, and control in the profession and its practice. It is concerned with the promotion of the profession as well for the welfare of society.

Regulation is about the improving standards of education for nursing, standards of practice and care of patients. It concerns with the position and status of the nursing profession in the society and the power of the profession to govern its affairs. The regulation of nursing, in other words, is at the very heart of the future of the profession itself.

Regulatory System

The regulatory system is a system that provides for the enrichment of care through improved standards of education for the development of practice and the creation of codes of conduct and ethics. It is like a cardiovascular system of the body. As a human cardiovascular system is vital to life, a nursing regulatory system is also concerned with the lifeblood of the profession and its destiny. In India, the nursing profession has established its regulatory system through regulatory bodies.

Professional Body

A professional body is a group of professionals who are responsible for maintaining the legitimate practice of the profession. Professional bodies maintain standards of professional education. According to the Australian Council of Professions, a professional body must represent a profession, comprises practitioners of the related field. The Wikipedia (2004) refers to it as an organization, usually nonprofit, that protects the interest of both the public and of professionals. It protects the public by maintaining and enforcing standards of training and ethics, certifies professional qualification, and also maintains academic discipline.

REGULATORY BODY

Meaning and Definition

A regulatory body is an external organization that has been empowered by legislation to supervise and control the educational process and outputs. Its primary purpose is to protect the interest of the public. These are the authorized bodies to make rules and regulations. Statutory bodies give this authority.

Health professionals such as nurses, doctors, pharmacists, and many others are regulated and licensed by regulatory bodies as required by legislation. All nurses are required to register and get licensure to practice with State Nursing Regulatory Body.

Aims of Regulatory Bodies of Nursing

The following list shows the aims of regulatory bodies:
- The setting, monitoring, and enforcing essential standards
- Improving and sustaining education, training, and practice
- Providing a framework for nursing practice
- Providing legitimacy, protection, and support to nurses
- Promoting regulation of the profession
- Encouraging nurses to participate in and influence public debate on health policy
- Ensuring that each of its practitioners is accountable to the public for nursing practice
- Providing comparable labor regulations to guarantee and safeguard the working and systems of remuneration for practitioners.

Objectives of Regulatory Bodies of Nursing

The list below shows the objectives of regulatory bodies:
- To protect the public by ensuring qualified and competent practitioners in nursing through certification, registration, and licensure
- To define scope and standards of education, training, and practice
- To reflect and be responsive to the country's healthcare needs
- To develop codes of ethics, professional conduct, and job classification and its validation measures such as tests, certification, recommendation, and disciplinary proceedings
- To provide equitable, fair, and responsible regulation through standards for practicing and developing criteria for assessing them, regulatory processes and the right to appeal from the decision of the regulatory body
- To maintain and update knowledge, skill, and attitude of professionals
- To prepare strict regulation and place an effective monitoring mechanism such as antiragging measures.

Role of Professional and Regulatory Bodies

Each national/state regulatory body receives their authority from legislation, thus providing a vital role:
- To ensure the public's right to quality health-care service by:
  - Setting and enforcing standards of nursing practice
  - Monitoring and enforcing standards for nursing education
  - Monitoring and enforcing standards of nursing practice
  - Setting requirements for registration of nursing professionals.
- To support and assist professional members by:
  - Safeguarding the interest of the public
  - Safeguarding the interest of the professional practitioners through association
  - Safeguarding its self-interest through having act to maintain its own privileged and powerful position as a controlling body.

Functions of Nursing Regulatory Bodies

Regulatory bodies exercise a high degree of control and influence over professional affairs. It has the legal power to regulate the profession. It has varied functions (**Fig. 2.1**):
1. Accreditation of nursing institutes
2. Registration of nurses within their respective state
3. Setting standards for education and practice
4. Developing a Code of Conduct and Ethics
5. Setting registration norms and procedures
6. Setting criteria for expanding the scope of the profession
7. Ensuring competent and ethical practices by nurses
8. Safeguard the public by communicating the professional development and ensuring the services through qualified and certified nurses
9. Taking appropriate action against incompetent and unethical members and also against members impaired by alcohol, drugs, or a mental condition
10. Regular reporting to the government in particular cases such as the ground of termination of a nurse from employment.

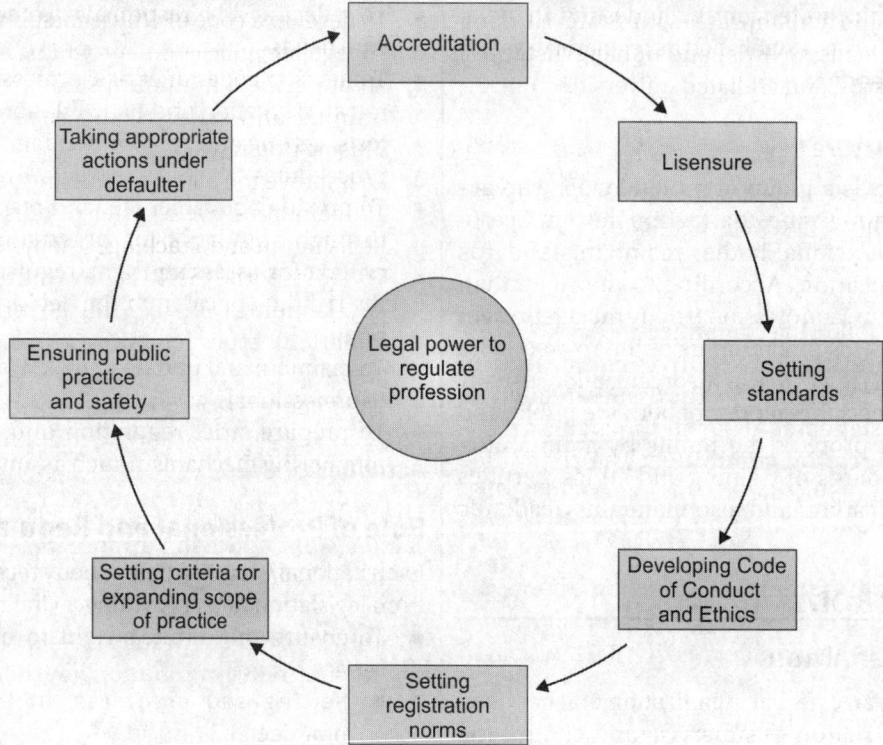

Fig. 2.1: Function of nursing regulatory body.

TYPES OF REGULATORY BODIES IN NURSING

Like industrial dispute laws, nurses govern by Code of Ethics, adopted by International Council of Nurses (ICN), Indian Nursing Council (INC), and Trained Nurses Association of India (TNAI), and also by rules of a particular hospital/institution. Thus the individual nurse governs for her professional activities by central, state, hospital/institution, and association laws and regulations as well as judicial rulings.

Indian Nursing Council (INC)

Introduction

The existing legislative regulations of nursing and nurses' associations comprised mainly INC Act of 1947 as amended by Act no. LXXV 1950 and by Act no. LXV, 1957. The INC is an independent statutory body under Ministry of Health and Family Welfare under the INC Act, 1947 (XLVIII of 1947) of parliament. The main aim to establish INC is to establish a uniform standard for nurses, midwives, and health visitors. The ordinance of the INC act passed on December 31st, 1947. The council constituted in 1949.

INC Regulations

The council has its regulation called the INC Regulations. It consists of 12 parts that describe the terms and conditions for regulation:
1. Part I describes time and place of business for meetings of the council.
2. Part II is about the conduct of the business meeting of the council.
3. Part III describes minutes of the council.
4. Part IV is regarding election of members of the council.
5. Part V is on resignation and filling of casual vacancies.
6. Part VI describes the tenure of office and powers and duties of officials.
7. Part VII describes the executive committee.
8. Part VIII has a description of committees.
9. Part IX describes tenure of office and powers and duties of secretary and staff.
10. Part X has a description regarding inspection of examinations and training institutions.
11. Part XI is about finance and accounts.
12. Part XII is about sales of publications.

Aims and Objectives of INC

Following are the aims and objectives of INC:
- To regulate training policies and programs in nursing
- To bring about standards of nursing training courses
- To set and monitor minimum standards of nursing education and practices
- To recognize nursing qualification of foreign universities/institutions
- To promote research in nursing
- To maintain the Indian nursing register for registration of nursing personnel and training programs.

Purposes of INC

The purposes of INC are as follows:
- To set standards and regulate all types of nursing education
- To prescribe a minimum requirement for different nursing programs

- To coordinate and collaborate with State Nursing Registration Councils (SNRCs) and nursing institutes, examination boards, and affiliated universities.

Organization Structure

It has 1 President, Vice President, Secretary, Assistant Secretary, and 15 other office staff **(Fig. 2.2)**.

Committees

INC constituted the following committees:
- **Executive committee:** Executive committee of the council to deliberate on the issues related to maintenance of standards of nursing programs.
- **The nursing education committee:** The committee is constituted to deliberate on the issues concerned mainly with nursing education and policy matters concerning nursing education.
- **Equivalence committee:** It is to deliberate on the issues of recognition of foreign qualifications, which is essential for registration under Section 11(2)(a) or (b) of the INC Act, 1947, as amended.
- **Finance committee:** Finance committee is another important subcommittee of the council, which decides upon the matters about finance of the council regarding budget, expenditure, implementation of central government orders concerning service conditions, etc.

Functions of INC

The council is responsible for the regulation and maintenance of a uniform standard of training for nurses, midwives, auxiliary nurse midwives (ANMs), and health visitors. Various functions are as follows:
- To set and monitor the standard of nursing education for all categories of nurses
- To recognize the qualifications for registration and employment in India and abroad
- To recognize foreign degree/diploma/certificate in nursing on a reciprocal basis
- To approve the registration of Indian and Foreign Nurses possessing the foreign qualification
- To withdraw the recognition of the institution, if it fails to maintain its standards.

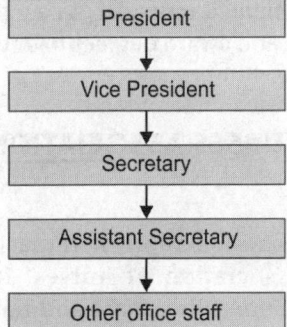

Fig. 2.2: Organization structure of Indian Nursing Council.

- To develop a code of ethics and professional conduct
- To regulate policies and programs about nursing
- To prescribe a minimum standard of education and training and syllabus and regulations for various nursing programs
- To improve the quality of nursing education
- To maintain a live register of nurses through Nurses Registration and Tracking system
- To advise the SNRCs, examining boards, state governments, and central government in various important issues regarding nursing education in the country
- To promote research in nursing.

Activities of INC

The prime responsibility of INC is to set the norms and standards for education, training, research, and practice within the relevant legislative framework. Various activities of INC are as follows:
- **Activities related to state nursing councils, school of nursing, and examination board**
    - Prescribing of syllabi
    - Implementation of syllabi
    - Recognition of qualifications
    - Maintenance of register nurses in India
    - Collection of data from schools of nursing
    - Advises on the matters proposed as when by the State Nursing Councils and nursing institutions.
- **Activities related to Government of India**
    - Sanctioning of budget and grant in aid
    - Sanctioning of the scales of pay and allowances of the offices and staff of the council
    - Collection of information from State Nursing Services and school of nursing having special projects
    - Declaration under Sections 10, 14, and 15 of INC act.
- **Activities in support with World Health Organization and other organizations**
    - Development of (1) teaching material for quality assurance model, (2) nursing practice standards, (3) curriculum for HIV/AIDS and ART, (4) strategic framework for advance standard and investment plan for advancing standards of nursing education and practice, (5) module for training of nurses in providing outreach services during disaster and for facilitators, and (6) module in nursing care in emergency.
    - Organizes a training program for trainers for teaching faculty in Integrated Management of Neonatal and Childhood Illnesses (IMNCI).
    - Constitution of National Consortium for PhD in Nursing with six study centers.
- **Miscellaneous activities**
    - Operational management and regulation of services in the interest of society

- Keeps up to date with tracking international development
- Understanding research in various relevant fields
- Responsible for the corporate governance of nurses and the nursing profession by the issue of discipline
- Promotion of health and health-care proposing and commenting on planned legislation, as well as proactively advising, altering, and offering suggestions to the government on matters affecting the nursing profession
- E-learning-HIV
- Publications
- Organizing conferences and workshops.

State Nursing Councils

Introduction

The State Nursing Registration Council (SNRC) is autonomous except that they do not have the power to prescribe the syllabi for courses to recognize examining bodies and to regulate reciprocity are now vested in the INC.

Indian Nursing Council delegated laws and regulation to State legislation-State Nursing Registration Acts to create uniformity in the standards established by states for the practice of nursing and to control activities and conducts of all government employees by government service conduct rules. There are 28 state nursing councils/examination boards or bodies in India as of January 2018 **(Table 2.1)**.

Functions of SNRC

The list below shows the functions of SNRC:
- Inspect and accredit schools/training institutes of nursing in their states
- Conduct the examinations
- Prescribe rules of conduct
- Maintain registers of nurses, midwives, ANMs, and health visitors in the state
- Issue license (registration certificate) and to ensure the maintenance of standards as laid down by INC.

Coordination with INC

The following list shows the coordination with INC:
- To be affiliated to INC, SNC must register a person.
- SNRC must implement syllabus prescribed by INC.
- Meeting of state registrars with INC to discuss various problems.
- SNRC checks the unethical practices with INC such as dishonest use of certificates, getting registration by false or by an unrecognized person, representation of registration as a medical practitioner, defect in character, bad conduct along. Decides and takes disciplinary action against defaulters.

Examination Boards and Universities

The respective SNRC conducts examination and award degree and certificates to General Nursing and Midwifery candidates and Auxillary Nursing Midwives, respectively, through approved examination boards/itself/university. The approved affiliated university in each state conducts the examination and award degrees to undergraduate and graduate nursing.

TABLE 2.1: List of State Nursing Councils.

S. No.	State Nursing Councils
1.	Andhra Pradesh Nurses, Midwives Council, Vijayawada (Andhra Pradesh)
2.	Arunachal Pradesh Nursing Council, Papum Pare (Arunachal Pradesh)
3.	Assam Nurses Midwives and Health Visitor Council, Guwahati (Assam)
4.	Chhattisgarh Nursing Council, Raipur (Chhattisgarh)
5.	Delhi Nursing Council, LNJP Hospital, New Delhi
6.	Goa Nursing Council, Bambolim (Goa)
7.	Gujarat Nursing Council, Ahmedabad (Gujarat)
8.	Haryana Nursing Council, Panchkula (Haryana)
9.	Bihar Nurses Registration Council, Patna (Bihar)
10.	Himachal Pradesh Nurses Registration Council, Shimla (Himachal Pradesh)
11.	Jammu and Kashmir State Paramedical and Nursing Council, Jammu
12.	Jharkhand Nurses Registration Council, Ranchi (Jharkhand)
13.	Karnataka State Nursing Council, Bengaluru (Karnataka)
14.	Kerala Nurses and Midwives Council, Thiruvananthapuram (Kerala)
15.	Madhya Pradesh Nurses Registration Council, Bhopal (Madhya Pradesh)
16.	Maharashtra Nursing Council, Mumbai (Maharashtra)
17.	Manipur Nursing Council, Imphal West (Manipur)
18.	Meghalaya Nursing Council, Shillong (Meghalaya)
19.	Mizoram Nursing Council, Dwarpui, Aizwal (Mizoram)
20.	Orissa Nurses and Midwives Council, Bhubaneswar (Orissa)
21.	Punjab Nurses Registration Council, Mohali (Punjab)
22.	Rajasthan Nursing Council, Jaipur (Rajasthan)
23.	Tamil Nadu Nurses and Midwives Council, Chennai (Tamil Nadu)
24.	Telangana State Nurses, Midwives, Auxiliary Nurse Midwives and Health Visitors Council, Hyderabad (Telangana)
25.	Tripura Nursing Council, Agartala (Tripura)
26.	Uttar Pradesh Nurses and Midwives Council, Lucknow (Uttar Pradesh)
27.	Uttarakhand Nurses Midwives Council, Dehradun (Uttarakhand)
28.	West Bengal Nursing Council, Kolkata (West Bengal)

Source: http://www.indiannursingcouncil.org/pdf/SNRC_%20web.pdf as on 09.01.2018.

TRAINED NURSES ASSOCIATION OF INDIA

Introduction

Trained Nurses Association of India is the national professional association of nurses. It began as an Association of Superintendents and has its beginning as "Trained Nurses Association" in 1908 in a decision taken at the annual conference of Association of Nursing Superintendents at Bombay founded in 1905, at Lucknow. Later on, association inaugurated in 1909. Florence Mac Haughton joined as the first president of TNAI. On June 16th, 1917, the association registered under the Registration Act no. XXI of 1860. The Association of Nursing Superintendents and Trained Nurses' Association clubbed together in 1922 as the Trained Nurses Association of India. The association has established within its jurisdiction the following organizations: Health Visitors' League (1922), Midwives and Auxiliary Nurse-Midwives Association (1925), and SNA (1929–1930). TNAI's first issue of Nursing Journal of India has got published in 1910.

The first state branch inaugurated in Delhi in 1949. After that, state branches inaugurated in Madras, Bombay, Uttar Pradesh, and West Bengal (1950). Later on Bihar (1953), Punjab (1953), Andhra Pradesh (1954), Assam, and Madhya Pradesh (1957) branches established. In 1969, separate state branches were formed in Haryana, Himachal Pradesh, and Punjab after these states attained separate statehood. In 1971, North Zone and North-East Zone Branches were formed. At present all northeastern states, namely Assam, Meghalaya, Mizoram, Manipur, Nagaland, and Arunachal Pradesh, have separate state branches. Lakshadweep and Sikkim are the states in which TNAI branch is yet to establish.

Affiliation of TNAI

TNAI has the affiliation with other associations/organizations:
- **International Council of Nurses (ICN) affiliation:** TNAI remained affiliated with International Nursing Council as an 8th Association in the world from 1912 to May 1995. However, due to the paucity of funds, it became difficult to pay the heavy subscription it stands disaffiliated from the ICN.
- **Affiliation with Commonwealth Nurses Federation:** TNAI had a membership with Commonwealth Nurses Federation.
- **Affiliation with Government Committees and Councils:** The views submitted by TNAI considered as the most authentic for the nursing profession in processing the findings of official committees such as the Bhore Committee and Mudaliar Committee. TNAI played an important role in the High Power Committee on Nursing and Nursing Profession (Report: 1987). The Central Council of Health (CCH) also consults TNAI for its recommendations on various aspects of the profession. The TNAI has many activities and its links with the INC for the promotion of nursing education and other aspects of the profession.
- **Affiliation with other organizations:** It has an affiliation with other associations such as Indian Red Cross Society, Indian Public Health Association, Association for Social Health, Indian Hospital Association, Federation of Delhi Hospital Welfare Societies, Tuberculosis Association of India, Indian Leprosy Association, and National Institute of Public Cooperation and Child Development.

Philosophy of TNAI

TNAI believes that good health is a fundamental right of every person, and it is the responsibility of health professionals including nurses to provide optimum health of each section of society.

Aims

- To upgrade and standardization of nursing education
- To improve living and working conditions for nurses
- To register the qualified nurses as members.

Organization Structure

TNAI has its officers, executive, and council members.
- **TNAI officers:** President, 4 Regional Vice Presidents, Secretary General, 3 Assistant General Secretaries, and 1 Honorary Treasurer.
- **The executive council:** It comprises all TNAI officers, Former President TNAI Principal, Presidents of State Branches (10), Secretaries of State Branches (10), Hony Secretary of Health Visitor League (HVL), and Hony Secretary of Midwives and Auxillary Nurse Midwife Association.
- **The council members:** It comprises all TNAI officers, Presidents of State Branches and UTs (30), Secretaries of State Branches and UTs (30), 3 co-opted members, 2 ex officio members, Hony Secretary of HVL, and Hony Secretary of Midwives, and Auxillary Nurse Midwife Association.

Membership

TNAI has its registered life members that include registered nurses and retired nurses having certificates of training, religious sisters, health visitors, ANMs, and multipurpose health workers.

Activities of TNAI

The list below shows the activities of TNAI:
- Organizing workshops and conferences
- Granting scholarships and welfare funds
- Granting railway concessions to TNAI members
- Publishes nursing journal, textbooks, and bulletins to SNA unit
- Support disaster-affected area nurses at individually, state, national, or international level
- Addressing and advocating issues of nurses welfare to government
- Social welfare activities through Social-Economic Welfare Committee
- Association with funding agencies to generate funds
- The inception of the central institute of nursing and research, daycare center, and elderly care home
- **Recruitment agency:** Government accredited recruitment agency to the nurses seeking employment within the country and abroad
- Jointly working on baby-friendly hospital initiative, disaster preparedness, the role of nurses in policy

making regarding the care of the elderly, human rights, nursing ethics, and rights of children.

Associate Organizations

Health Visitor League

Health Visitor League is an associate organization of TNAI.

Objectives of HVL
- To uphold the dignity and honor of lady health visitors
- To bring spirit de corps among the LHVs
- To discuss professional-related issues and problems
- To improve the standard of education and practice.

Midwives and Auxillary Nurse Midwives Association

Objectives
- To uphold the dignity and honor of midwives and ANM
- To bring spirit de corps among the midwives and ANM
- To discuss professional-related issues and problems
- To improve the standard of education and practice.

Christian Nurses League of the Christian Medical Association of India

Christian Nurses League is an affiliated association of TNAI.

Objectives
- To promote cooperation and encouragement to Christian Nurses
- To help to secure high efficiency in nursing education and service
- To cooperate and work with CMAI.

STUDENT NURSES ASSOCIATION OF INDIA

Introduction

The Student Nurses Association (SNA) is the organization of Student Nurses in India. It established in 1929 at the time of the Annual Conference of the TNAI. The Nursing Superintendent of the Government General Hospital, Madras, Miss LN Jeans, was the first Honorary Organising Secretary of this Association. Its first unit established at the General Hospital, Madras, followed by Christian Rainy Hospital, Madras and the Presidency General Hospital, Calcutta.

Its units increase an almost three-fold increase and seven times increase in membership by August 2001 and till 31.08.2009; its membership strength raised to 102,207, state branches to 33, and SNA units to 1,002. It has full-time SNA secretary/advisor and also deputy general secretary.

Objectives of SNA

- To help the students to uphold the dignity and ideals of the nursing profession for which they are qualifying
- To promote a cooperative spirit among students
- To furnish nurses in training with the advice in their course leading to the qualification
- To aid in the overall development of nursing students
- To encourage optimal achievement in the professional role of the nurse
- To help in participating in educational and other co-curricular activities
- To provide Foundations of National Student Nurses Association (FNSNA) scholarship, awards, and conferences.

Membership

All student nurses including BSc Nursing, General Nursing, and Midwifery, Auxillary Nurse Midwives/Multipurpose Health Worker (female) are eligible to register in the Association through Director/Principal, Principal tutor nursing of college/school of nursing with onetime payment.

Activities of SNA

- Organizes SNA exhibition
- Fundraising
- Awarding special prizes to deserving candidates
- Organizes annual meets for the student nurses.

CHAPTER HIGHLIGHTS

- The regulatory system is concerning with improving standards of education and practice and creating codes of conduct.
- A professional body constitutes a group of professionals responsible for maintaining the legitimate practice.
- A regulatory body is an authorized body that makes rules and regulation, supervises, and controls the educational process and outputs.
- Indian Nursing Councils, State Nursing councils, Examination Bodies, Universities, and Trained Nurses Association of India are the important regulatory bodies in nursing.

REVIEW QUESTIONS

I. Essay Type Questions
1. Define regulatory system and regulatory body. Enlist its objectives.
2. Describe the role of professional and regulatory bodies.
3. Explain the important functions of regulatory bodies.
4. Discuss the role of the Indian Nursing Council in regulating nursing.
5. Discuss the main activities of the Trained Nurses Association of India.

II. Short Notes
1. Indian Nursing Council
2. State Nursing Registration Council
3. Trained Nurses Association of India
4. Student Nurses Association of India

Chapter 2: Regulatory Bodies

III. Multiple Choice Questions

1. A body that is empowered by legislation to supervise and control the education process and output is:
   a. Professional body
   b. Regulatory body
   c. Nursing association
   d. Corporate body

2. In which year, the ordinance of Indian Nursing Council Act passed?
   a. 1947 b. 1949
   c. 1950 d. 1957

3. Which part of INC regulation describes finance and accounts?
   a. Part II b. Part VII
   c. Part IX d. Part XI

4. The main purpose of Nurses Registration and Tracking system is to:
   a. Develop a code of ethics
   b. Approve registration of nurses
   c. Maintain a live register of nurses
   d. Set standards of nursing

5. Which committee of INC deals with matters related to recognition of foreign qualification for registration?
   a. Executive b. Nursing education
   c. Equivalence d. Finance

6. Which nursing regulatory body prescribes minimum qualification and other requirement for nursing programs?
   a. Indian Nursing Council
   b. State Nursing Council
   c. Trained Nurses Association of India
   d. University/Examination body

7. Of which nursing program(s), the State Nursing Council conducts examination and award degree/diploma?
   a. ANM and GNM b. Post-Basic BSc
   c. BSc (N) d. MSc (N)

8. In which year, TNAI has its beginning?
   a. 1905 b. 1908
   c. 1909 d. 1917

9. When did TNAI publish its first issue of Nursing Journal of India?
   a. 1925 b. 1922
   c. 1917 d. 1910

10. Who was the first honorary Organizing Secretary of Student Nurses Association?
    a. Mac Haughton b. LN Jeans
    c. Margaret Johan d. RA Kaur

Answer Keys

1. b   2. a   3. d   4. c   5. c   6. a   7. a
8. b   9. d   10. b

SUGGESTED READINGS

1. Available from http://medical-dictionary.thefreedictionary.com/National+Student+Nurses+Association.
2. Available from http://rajyasabha.nic.in/bills-ls-rs/2006/LXXIX_2006.pdf.
3. Available from http://updates.highereducationinindia.com/2009/single-regulatory-body-to-oversee-1163.php Union Health Ministry suggest setting up a single regulatory body, by the name 'National Council for Human Resources in Health (NCHRH)' to oversee the medical education system in India.
4. Available from http://www.authorstream.com/Presentation/spk123spk123-237563-role-regulatory-bodies-nursing-education-ppt-powerpoint/.
5. Available from http://www.cna.nurses.ca.
6. Available from http://www.dauniv.ac.in/notices/Indian_Nursing_Council_Act_-_1947.pdf.
7. Available from http://www.educationmaster.org/news/new-regulatory-body-train-doctors-paramedics.html Staff Writer New regulatory body to train doctors, paramedics. [Accessed July 2009].
8. Available from http://www.google.com.
9. Available from http://www.indiaedunews.net/Today/Regulatory_bodies_to_implement_strict_anti_ragging_measures_7796/Regulatory bodies to implement strict anti-ragging measures. [Accessed March 2009].
10. Available from http://www.indiannursingcouncil.org/bsc_007.pdf.
11. Available from http://www.indiannursingcouncil.org/gnm_007.pdf.
12. Available from http://www.indiannursingcouncil.org/msc_007.pdf.
13. Available from http://www.indiannursingcouncil.org/pbbsc_007.pdf.
14. Available from http://www.indiannursingcouncil.org/snrc.pdf.
15. Available from http://www.nihfw.org/ndc-nihfw/html/Legislations/TheIndianNursingCouncil.htm.
16. Available from http://www.nursingworld.org/affi.
17. Available from http://www.tnaionline.org.
18. Available from http://www.tnaionline.org/snaintro.htm.
19. Cherian A. A Handbook of Trained Nurses Association of India. New Delhi: TNAI; 1980. pp. 125-30.
20. Harvey L. Analytic Quality Glossary. Quality Research International. Available from http://www.qualityresearchinternational.com/glossary/.
21. The role of professional bodies in higher education quality monitoring. https://www.qualityresearchinternational.com › Harvey papers. [Accessed on 14.12.2019].
22. Indian Nursing Council Act 1947 Act No. of Year: ACT NO. 48. https://www.indiannursingcouncil.org › pdf › inc-act-1947. [Accessed on 15.12.2019].
23. Ralph C. Regulation and empowerment of Nursing. Int Nurs Rev. 2002;40(2):58-60.
24. The Trained Nurses Association of India. Handbook of the Trained Nurses Association of India. New Delhi, 2000.
25. Wikipedia, 2004, Professional Body. Available from http://en.wikipedia.org/wiki/Professional_body, updated 11 November 2004.

3

Trends and Issues in Nursing

CHAPTER OUTLINE

- Trends in Nursing
  - Trends in Nursing Services
  - Trends in Nursing Education
- Factors Affecting Trends in Nursing
- Issues in Nursing
  - Issues Related to Nursing Services
- Issues Related to Nursing Education
- Future Issues in Nursing
  - Future Nursing Practice Issues
  - Future Issues in Nursing Administration
  - Future Issues in Nursing Education
  - Ways to Meet Challenges

LEARNING OUTCOMES

After completion of this chapter, the learner will be able to:
- Understand the concept of trends in nursing
- Describe trends in nursing
- Discuss major trends in nursing education
- Enlist factors affecting trends in nursing
- Identify issues in nursing service and education
- Identify future issues in nursing and ways to meet challenges

KEY TERMS

Trends in nursing, current issues, future issues, differentiated nursing practice, competencies, competency models, nursing practice model, nursing nomenclature

INTRODUCTION

Nursing has traditionally been the profession that carries out medical regimes, provides nursing care, and assesses and treats the patients in the context of his or her environment. Nursing has a long and rich heritage; nurses with their unique, divergent opinions, and talents have made many valuable individuals and collective contributions to the society within the total health-care environment. Due to modernization, globalization, and liberalization, there is a rapid change in general and nursing education from the past.

TRENDS IN NURSING

A trend in nursing is a change that is taking place in present days in any field of nursing, which affects the profession as a whole. A trend means a change or movement in a particular direction. It also denotes general directions and tendencies especially of events of opinions or movements in a particular direction.

It is the general direction toward which the different nursing events have moved and are moving as well as the opinions in and around nursing and tendencies that we find in and about our profession. It also means a change currently taking place in any area of nursing and influencing the profession. Many changes took place in nursing services, administration, and nursing education.

Trends in Nursing Services

Trends in nursing services are multidimensional directly or indirectly related to nurses, their roles, nursing education, and nursing services **(Table 3.1)**.

1. **Nature of care:** In the past, the focus was on a traditional type of care. Now more emphasis is on evidence-based practice. The trends in caring may continue by evidence in the future.
2. **Type of nursing care:** At present, the emphasis is on specialized nursing care, e.g. caring for patients suffering from cardiovascular, respiratory as compared to past that was an emphasis on general nursing. In future, the focus of nursing care as well the nurses would be trained for super specialty care.
3. **Use of information technology:** There is an advancement in technology in the present era, which was lacking in the past, and due to this, there are many

TABLE 3.1: Trends in nursing services: past, present, and future.

Trends in nursing services	Past	Present	Future
Type of nursing	Military nursing	Civilian Govt. hospital-based nursing	Private hospital-based nursing
Nursing agency	By western nurses Christian and Anglo Indian nurses	By Indian nurses irrespective of caste, creed, and religion	By Indian nurses irrespective of caste, creed, and religion
Focus on nursing care	Basic patient care	Quality assurance	Quality assurance, standards
Nature of care	Traditional care	Evidence-based care	Research-oriented evidence-based care
Type of nursing care	General nursing	Specialized-nursing	Super specialized nursing
Use of information technology	Lacking	Computerization	Advanced
Marital status of nurses	Unmarried nurses	Majority of married nurses	Majority of married nurses
Uniform attire	Western type	Indian culture	Indian culture
Shift duty pattern	Split shift duties 8-hour duties	Straight shift duties	Straight shift duties
Assignment of nurses	Functional assignment	Functional assignment Patients assignment	Patients assignment
Role	Basic role	Multiple roles	Multiple roles
Nurse practitioner	Dependent role	Independent practitioner	Independent practitioner
Attendance of in-service education	Lacking	Mandatory and organized	Self-motivated and organized
Awareness among nurses	Ignorant about their rights	Well aware of their rights Participation in association	Well aware of their rights Participation in association
Leadership styles	Autocratic	Democratic	Participative, transformational transactional
Turnover	Less	Increasing	Debatable
Nursing institutions	Recognized and unrecognized schools of nursing (certificate nurses)	Recognized schools/colleges of nursing (Diploma nurses) Degree and postgraduate nurses	Recognized schools/colleges of nursing (Diploma nurses) Degree and postgraduate nurses
No. of schools/colleges of nursing	Few	Mushrooming of schools/colleges of nursing	Stabilization of schools/colleges of nursing

changes in the curriculum as well in the practice area. These days, the hospital uses computer-based information technology such as Hospital Information System and Computerized Record System.

4. **Marital status of nurses:** In the past, nurses used to be unmarried, gradually; the majority of nurses are married; and in the future, the same trend will continue.
5. **Uniform attire:** Earlier the image of nurses was due to uniform attire that was of a western type, and in a white shade with cap, now the trend has been changed, and the uniform is per the Indian culture and different shades. There is no uniform shade of uniforms for nurses throughout India.
6. **Shift duty pattern:** In the past, nurses used to work in split shift duties or 8-hour duties; now mostly all the hospitals follow straight shift duty pattern, which is convenient for nurses, and this trend may continue shortly.
7. **Assignment of nurses:** In most of the hospitals, nurses carry out the functional assignment. In the present scenario, nurses have both functional and patient's assignment. In the future, nurses may be assigned patients to give holistic or individualized care.
8. **Role of nurses:** Nurses' role in the past was hospital oriented. However, now they have multiple, expanded, and specialized roles in a different setting.
9. **Nurse practitioners:** In the past, nurses had dependent jobs, now trends to prepare nurses as independent practitioners, and this trend will continue in future as well.
10. **Participation in staff development:** Presently nurses take the initiative and active part in national and international conferences seminars and workshops as compare to the past.
11. **Awareness among nurses:** In the past, the majority of nurses were not even aware of their rights, but now nurses are aware of their rights and negotiate through their associations and societies to redress their grievances.
12. **Leadership styles:** Nurse leaders exercise autocratic type leadership style in the past. But at present, they believe in democratic and participatory leadership. It may continue in future as well.
13. **Turnover:** The trend of turnover is also changing. In the past, there was not much turnover in nursing. The evidence shows that at present, there is a turn over in nursing and the future, it is questionable or debatable.
14. **Nursing institutions:** Both unrecognized and recognized institutions were prevailing in the past, but at present, it is mandatory to take approval from nursing councils and university before starting new courses in nursing, and this trend will continue.

15. **Number of schools and colleges:** There were very few schools/colleges of nursing imparting training program in the past, but at present, there is mushrooming of schools/colleges of nursing, and in future, there will be a nursing institution per demand.

Trends in Nursing Education

Since the philosophy of nation, education, organization, and nursing influences nursing education, the trends also go on changing per the requirement. The changes take place regarding curriculum, teaching-learning methods, education quality, and standardization, educational technology, student status, and nurse teachers. Some of the salient trends in nursing education are as follows:

1. **Changing focus from cure to care:** Due to shifting on promotive and preventive aspect of care, there is a need for more workforce. Therefore the nursing curriculum of various courses is revised per the need of national health policy and national education policy.
2. **Change in admission criteria:** Per the need of society and nation, the recruitment criteria regarding minimum qualification and conditions, a method of recruitment and selection in nursing courses, are different compared with the previous one. Presently nurses get employment through merit and apply online.
3. **Improved teaching-learning methods:** The nursing teachers these days rely on group methods, simulation, problem-based learning, reflective learning, demonstration, and other interacting methods to teach theory and practical compared to traditional classroom methods.
4. **Advanced educational technology:** Now the education technology approaches used both types: hardware approach and software approach as well as system approach to provide a scientific base to nursing education and to make education more productive, instructions more powerful, and useful to make equal and immediate access to education.
5. **Comprehensive evaluation:** Presently the focus of evaluation is a continuous and comprehensive evaluation. Formative and summative evaluations are well appreciated. Efforts are made to make clinical evaluation more objective by using objective structured clinical examination and on various aspects in the clinical areas.
6. **Emphasis on interpersonal and human relation:** Nurses are paying attention to critical thinking, interpersonal relationship, communication, understanding self, and clients while making correct nursing diagnoses and making the decision for nursing intervention.
7. **The emergence of specialization and research:** Due to advancement in medical and allied professions, specialties and subspecialties are emerging. The nursing institutions have already taken the lead to prepare specialized nurses to render care in super specialty areas. Due to an emphasis on evidence-based nursing practice and different research methodologies, action research is gaining importance. Many research projects are being taken up by the nurse faculty by getting funds from different agencies.
8. **Gaining national importance:** The nursing education has gained importance nationally like other educational and professional programs. Private nursing institutions are coming up in all the states of India.
9. **Opportunities for higher studies:** Comparatively, currently many nursing both government and approved private nursing institutions are offering nursing programs.
10. **Improved student status:** In the past, the student was given the student status, being working like employed nurses; now they are viewed as student nurses rather than nursing students.
11. **Uniform attire:** There is a change in color and type of uniform attire of students in different programs. There is no uniformity.
12. **Accreditation of nursing institutions:** Differing from the past, the nursing institutions are regularly accredited by the licensing authority, state nursing council, university, and state government and follow procedures per guidelines to start a program.
13. **Standardization and quality of education:** Standardization and quality of education are debatable issues in nursing. Eminent nurse administrations discuss in forums, conferences, and seminars to find the way to tackle these issues.

FACTORS AFFECTING TRENDS IN NURSING

1. **Changing the health scenario of government:** The government made efforts to deliver the healthcare to both the rural and urban community especially slums, vulnerable under National Health Mission and National Health Programmes. National Health Policy, 2017, has focused toward the attainment of the highest possible level of well-being and affordable quality secondary and tertiary health-care services to everyone and to achieve universal health coverage by ensuring availability of free and comprehensive primary health services to people of all ages. The creation of "National Institute for Transforming India (NITI)" Aayog in place of Planning Commission aims at sustainable developmental goals with a bottom-up approach.
2. **Changing demographics:** The alarming increase in elderly population will impact on the health-care services and nursing. The increased lifespan of people with chronic illnesses will pose further challenges. There is a need that increased nursing workforce with geriatric nursing preparation to deal with them.
3. **Change in health-care delivery system:** Transition is taking place in the health-care system and in the hospitals that affect the role of nurses at the top, supervisory, and operational level in hospitals **(Box 3.1)**.

Chapter 3: Trends and Issues in Nursing

Box 3.1: Transition in health-care system.

Curative	Preventive approach
Specialized care	Primary healthcare
Medical diagnosis	Patients' emphasis
Discipline stovepipes	Program stovepipe
Professional identity	Team identity
Trial and error →	Evidence-based practice
Self-regulation	Questioning on profession
Focus on quality	Focus on costs
Public	Private
High tech	Humanistic-Telecommunication
Competition	Cooperation
Need to supervise	Coaching, mentoring
Hierarchies	Decentralized approach

4. **Impact of globalization:** With globalization, there is the narrowing of distance; the risk of disease transmission has increased; and its care has become imminent, and hence there is a need for knowledge transfer to deal with these problems. Nursing education must, therefore, become more internationally focused on disseminating information and benefiting from this change. Hence the need for curriculum revision focused on international health and clinical modalities.

5. **Advancement in technology:** With the advancement of technology, old techniques, methods of treatments, procedures, and activities have completely become obsolete. New technology facilitates diagnosis, decision-making, and research although these technologies pose constant learning challenges for all. However, advancement in technology always saves time and improves quality care.

   In the hospital, more documentation will be done directly on a computer, often at the patient's bedside. Wireless handheld computers will enable doctors and nurses to be close at hand, even far away. Personal digital assistants (PDAs) and other electronic organizers will help nurses' access information and manage time. Computerized records, informally called CPRs (computerized patient records), and CMRs (computerized medical records), or OLPRs (online patient records) will be common. Nurses must have thorough knowledge to manage advanced information and technology. Therefore, there is a need for curriculum revision keeping in mind various clinical modalities, information system, and patient monitoring devices, which is must for the safety of patients.

6. **Impact on medical tourism:** The concept of medical tourism is coming up. More and more stakeholders are working on it, if it is so the nursing education and nursing practice will require focusing on specialization, quality education, and practical oriented.

7. **Advances in medical, paramedical, and allied professions:** Growing specialization and super specialization in medical and allied professions have brought the development of new tests, diagnostic procedures, medicines, and machines. There is also focus on quality-oriented services. So the nurses also need to be trained accordingly to keep pace with the medical and allied professionals' current knowledge in the nursing field that has to be improved.

8. **Informatics and efforts to standardize and unify nursing language:** Informatics, the study of how to use computers to capture the data, is proved to be better for clinical and research purposes, and it is growing and on demand. Various programs are required to take decisions for nursing care.

9. **Case management, disease management, and telehealth-care expansion:** More nurses will become involved in disease management and case management through telenursing to keep costs down by helping people with chronic illnesses and improve their health status through close monitoring, early intervention, and use of resources.

10. **Diverse responsibilities:** Nurses at all the levels in hospitals, homes, and communities are accountable for the diagnosis, prevention, and management of various health problems. Primary healthcare, patient education, health promotion, rehabilitation, self-care, and alternative methods of healing are the added responsibilities. To carry out such responsibilities, the nurses need to have diverse skills, and they need to prepare to gain and enhance their competencies in related roles. It also affects nursing education preparation.

11. **Educated consumers:** Education and technology advancement brings about a growing awareness of health needs among people. They are becoming aware of their rights, so nursing needs are to be directed according to their health needs.

12. **Changing women' role:** The status of nurses as women is improving in society. They are now independent and can take independent decisions for themselves and their clients.

13. **International influence:** The international organizations and their influence encouraged nurses to participate in international conferences and workshops. Most of the nurses are on deputation for undergoing training programs in abroad sponsored by WHO, INC, etc. International Council of nurses promotes sharing ideas, whereas WHO, USAID, etc. assist in research, education, and publications.

14. **Changing the focus of nursing:**
    - *Regulatory requirements:* It is mandatory for nurses to prove their values to both customers and their employers, showing how they impact on patient outcomes.
    - *Changing role:* The nursing role is changing with the advancement of technology. Therefore nurses at managerial and supervisory level need to have managerial skills, organizational skills, leadership, critical thinking, delegation, and supervision, and communication skills are required for the nurses working at different levels.

- *Shared governance:* Nurses must take part in decision-making to make rules and develop procedures, manuals, and standard operative procedures for nursing care.
- *Specialization:* It is an era of specialization and nurse demand for clinical nurse experts, so nursing educational preparation has to be a focus on this direction.
- *Nursing shortage threatens patient care:* More demand with fewer nurses threatens patient care. Ways need to find out to attract and retain nurses.
- *Nursing education goes online:* Various courses of nursing education will go online in the future.
- *Standards and practice guidelines:* This is a high time to have the standards in nursing and practice models, protocols, and guidelines that should aim to reduce useless or harmful practices.
- *Evidence-based care:* Evidence-based care on research and clinical studies can be analyzed to come to the consensus about what are the best approaches to specific conditions from outcome and cost perspectives. These best approaches often are referred to as benchmarks or best practices. The nurses need to acquaint with various types of research methodology, evidence-based nursing practice, action research, etc. and thus call for appropriate planning nursing education curriculum.
- *New ethical concerns:* Now the focus is on end-of-life care, technological advancements in the treatment of infertility, genetic testing that challenges the traditional ethical and societal values regarding conception, birth, death, and dying. Law is now more consumer friendly, and nurses must know ethical and legal issues.
- *Complementary and alternative therapies:* There is a great focus on promoting health through complementary and alternative therapies such as yoga, ayurveda, meditation, and other.
- *Healthy working environment:* New regulations, laws, and organizations are making an effort to make the working environment healthy so that nurses can work better and stress free.

ISSUES IN NURSING

Issues Related to Nursing Services

1. **Administrative Issues**
   - The insufficient contribution of nurses to health-care development due to few positions for nurses at the state and national levels
   - Inadequate nursing leadership and strategic management
   - Inappropriate nurse to population/patient ratio
   - Inadequate preparedness of the nursing workforce
   - Inadequate recognition of nurse's status in the health-care system
   - Limited active involvement of professional organizations
   - Limited career progression at all levels
   - Limited role and authority of INC in nursing development due to limited roles prescribed in the Indian Nursing Council Act, 1947: inconsistency in state nursing councils and Indian Nursing Council and insufficient information system in nursing: a shortage of staff at the INC and state nursing councils.

   Figure 3.1 depicts some of the major administrative issues.

2. **Practice Issues**
   - Poor quality of care due to a shortage of nursing workforce and other reasons
   - Limited competency of nurses due to too many categories of nurses with overlapping roles
   - Unclear roles and responsibilities of nurses
   - Inadequate continuing education system and staff development methods
   - Ineffective clinical preparation and supervision during training and limited utilization of evidence and research
   - Insufficient clinical nurse specialist and independent nurse practitioners
   - Inadequate infrastructure and facilities
   - Inadequate standards and guidelines for nursing practice
   - Ineffective regulation of nursing workforce
   - Lack of motivation to provide effective care.

Issues Related to Nursing Education

1. **Uniformity and standardization of nursing education:** The nursing workforce available is less per demand to meet the future health-care needs and challenges. Numbers of nursing institutions are coming up to prepare nurses of different levels. There is limited involvement of nurses at the policy level.
2. **The gap between theory and practice:** There is a gap between theory and practice. The students that they learn in the class are not the same as available in the

---

- Nursing service standards and quality care
- Accreditation of hospitals and institutions
- Shortage and brain drain of nurses
- Phasing out schools of nursing
- Lack of leadership
- Professional autonomy
- Independent nurse practitioners
- Preparation of nurses for using information technology
- Nursing care evaluation
- Nursing records and documentation
- Staff development/programes
- Ethical and legal issues
- Nursing audit system
- Renewal of registration
- Job descriptions
- Working conditions

Fig. 3.1: Major issues related to nursing service.

practice settings. Thus they became theory oriented rather than skill oriented.

3. **Changing teaching modalities:** Since the nurse teachers are expected to teach through interactive methods and simulations. But how far the teachers are expert in using these teaching modalities? It is a big question in front of nursing planners. Therefore, to put into practice these types of modalities, there is a need to have expert teachers and well oriented with these modalities to bring out expected teaching outcome.
4. **Educational preparation:** There is a need to prepare competent students with adequate knowledge, attitude, and skill. The infrastructure, e.g. adequate library facility, clinical facilities, articles, etc., is lacking in most of the nursing institutions, which even if available, it is not utilized properly.
5. **Lack of competent teachers:** Having qualified and competent nurse teachers is a major issue at present. They should have rich experience of clinical with update knowledge of system and technology used for patient care.
6. **Lack of promotional avenues and team spirit among teachers:** In most of the nursing institutions, the carrier ladder of nursing faculty is poor, and there is a lack of team spirit among them. They have less opportunity to have higher positions that may create frustrations among them.
7. **Inadequate infrastructure:** Inadequate library facilities, transport facilities, poor nursing lab facilities, and inadequate hostel facilities need attention.
8. **Lack of work culture:** There is a need to develop a work culture among teachers and students who are lacking.
9. **Quality of nursing education:** The quality of nursing education is in jeopardy due to an inadequate national nursing educational plan, development, and evaluation system. The criteria for evaluating quality will be through student competencies shortly.

FUTURE ISSUES IN NURSING

Future Nursing Practice Issues

The identified future nursing practice issues are differentiated nursing practice, competencies, practice models, and a nursing classification to keep pace with international nursing standards **(Fig. 3.2)**.

1. **Differentiated nursing practice:** Differentiated nursing practice is the nursing role by education, experience, and competence (Boston, 1990). Efforts to place the right nurse with the right competencies with the right patient at the right cost become the goal of health-care professionals.
2. **Defining and implementing differentiated nursing practice:** Defining and implementing differentiated nursing practice is a very challenging task, as there is a shortage of staff and a growing demand for accountability.

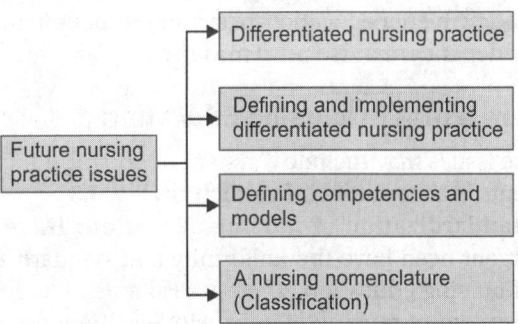

Fig. 3.2: Future nursing practice issues.

3. **Defining competencies and models:** Competency refers to what an individual is capable of performing. It includes cognitive skills such as decision-making and interpersonal skills and psychomotor or technical skills associated with nursing procedures. There is a need to explore which type of competency model and what competencies for the nurses will work out in the Indian setting. There is a need to have an innovative practice model focused on differentiated nursing practice.
4. **A nursing nomenclature (classification):** Naming or describing phenomena in nursing is nursing nomenclature. It is the language of nursing that addresses nursing diagnosis, nursing interventions, nursing outcomes, and classification is the systematic arrangement or a structured framework of these phenomena. The most common classification system adopted by the American Nurses Association is:
    - *North American Nursing Diagnosis Association (NANDA):* It contains 71 concepts and 143 items.
    - *Nursing Intervention Classification (NIC):* It is having 486 interventions organized into 30 classes and 7 domains.
    - *Nursing Outcome Classification (NOC):* It includes 247 individual-level outcomes, 7 family outcomes, and 6 community outcomes.
    - *Omaha System:* It includes an assessment component—problem classification scheme, intervention component—intervention scheme, and an outcome component—problem rating scale for outcome.

Future Issues in Nursing Administration

The important issues in nursing administration are related to cost of healthcare affecting nursing, the challenge of managed care, the impact of health-care policy and regulation, nursing shortage, opportunities for lifelong learning, and significant advances in nursing science and research.

The issues recognized by Indian Nursing Council are renewal of nursing registration, diploma versus degree in nursing for registration to practice in nursing, specialization in clinical areas, nursing care standards, staffing pattern/nurse–patient ratio, conduct of nursing research, nursing audits, and higher education for senior positions in nursing and independent nurse practitioners.

Future Issues in Nursing Education

Future issues may include a system of nursing education, students, teachers, and infrastructure (**Fig. 3.3**).

1. **Standardization of nursing education:** There is an urgent need have the uniformity and standardization of nursing education. There is also a need to develop a system of ranking of university-level preparation of nurses regarding the competency of the graduates, world-class research facilities, well-stocked library, and so on (Samuel, 2012).
2. **Practice-oriented education system:** The nursing education system should be practice oriented. As we know, the nursing profession has a social obligation to the public to meet their general, and specialized care needs as well as the public expects that a nurse has the expert knowledge and skills to ensure safe care.
3. **Well planned, mix, and match teaching methods:** Pedagogies have been changed and replaced by newer methods such as problem-based learning, competency-oriented education, and use of skill laboratories will improve the teaching-learning process but cannot replace teachers and clinical experiences. There is a need to work on a well-planned, wise, mix, and match methods.
4. **Competent students' preparation:** There is a need to prepare competent students with adequate knowledge, attitude, and skill. The infrastructure, e.g. adequate library facility, clinical facilities, articles, etc., which is lacking in most of the nursing institutions, if available, not utilized properly.
5. **Preparation of competent teachers:** The nurse teachers should have rich experience of clinical with update knowledge of system and technology used for patient care. The nurse teacher must undergo in-service training on the use of modern education technology, human relation, communication methods, reflective teaching-learning methods, and team building.
6. **Promotional avenues for teachers:** There is a need for a better career ladder for nursing faculty with appropriate positions and salary structures.
7. **Adequate infrastructure:** There should be proper library facilities, transport facilities, poor nursing lab facilities, and hostel facilities both students and faculties.
8. **Work culture:** Emphasis should be made to develop work culture among teachers and students who are lacking.
9. **Quality of nursing education:** There is a need for reviewing educational system-imparting knowledge, developing skill, and inculcating a positive attitude to care, which is must for quality nursing education. The selection of students needs objective criteria and transparency.

Ways to Meet Challenges

INC has recommended various solutions to improve the overall scenario of nursing services including practice, administration, and education in India:
- Strengthen the involvement of nurses in health and nursing policy formulation and planning
- Empower nursing leaders
- Development and implementation of quality assurance models and system in nursing
- Ensure nursing workforce management as an integral part of human resource planning and health system development
- Enhance nursing autonomy in practice
- Enforce implementation of recommended norms on nurse-patient ratio
- Produce advanced practice nurses
- Ensure appropriate facilities and adequate equipment and supplies
- Promote evidence-based practice and nursing research
- Establish a continuing nursing education system
- Improve pay scales, incentives systems, and working conditions
- Ensure the quality of nursing education by strengthening nursing programs, increasing qualified nurse educators, and allocate appropriate resources to maximize efficiency and effectiveness.

CHAPTER HIGHLIGHTS

- A trend means a change or movement in a particular direction. A trend in nursing is a change that is taking place in present days in any field of nursing, which affects the profession as a whole.
- Trends in nursing include areas such as nursing care, nurses, research, administration, use of information technology, nursing education, infrastructure, etc.
- The trends in nursing education are related to curriculum, teaching-learning methods, education

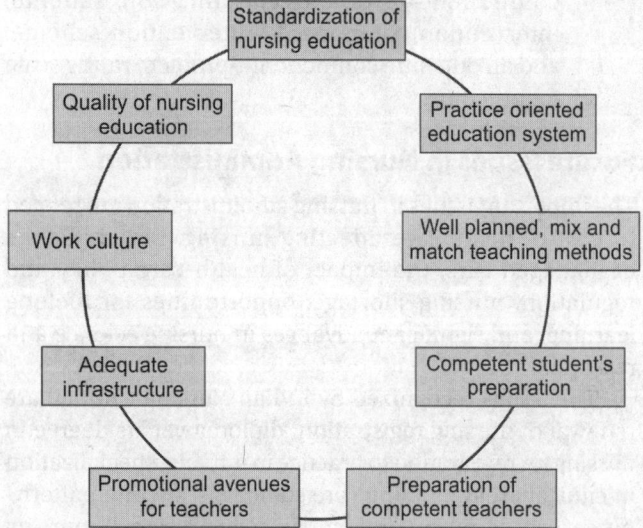

Fig. 3.3: Future issues in nursing education.

quality, and standardization, educational technology, student status, nurse teachers, etc.
- The important influencing factors for the trend is technology advancement, health-care delivery system, advancement of nursing, the diverse responsibilities of nurses, educated consumers, shortage of nurses, etc.
- The major issues in nursing education are uniformity and standardization of education, the quality nursing education gap between theory and practice, change in the traditional teaching-learning methods, educational preparation, lack of competent teachers, inadequate infrastructure, etc.
- Future issues in nursing practice would be related to planning and implementing differentiated practice, defining competencies, development of nursing practice models, and defining nursing nomenclature.
- Future issues in nursing education would be related to quality nursing education, practice-oriented nursing education, well-planned mix and match teaching methods, competent students' and teachers' preparation, etc.
- Poor quality of care and nursing education are the major issues at present, and INC recommended various solutions to improve the overall scenario of nursing services in India.

REVIEW QUESTIONS

I. Essay Type Questions
1. Define trends in nursing and describe trends in nursing service.
2. Discuss trends in nursing education.
3. Describe factors affecting trends in nursing.
4. Enumerate issues in nursing service.
5. Explain future major issues in nursing education.

II. Short Notes
1. Trends in nursing.
2. Enumerate future issues in nursing service.
3. Issues in nursing education.
4. Ways to meet challenges in nursing.

III. Multiple Choice Questions
1. The term used for general direction and tendency of movement in a particular direction is:
   a. Development b. Trend
   c. An issue d. Challenge
2. The pattern of shift duty of nurses at present followed by most hospitals is:
   a. Straight shift duty
   b. 8-hour shift duty
   c. 12-hour shift duty
   d. Split shift duty
3. The method of using computers to gather the data is better for clinical and research purposes are:
   a. Case management
   b. Telehealth
   c. Informatics
   d. Computers and technology
4. The differentiated nursing practice is:
   a. The structuring nursing roles by education, experience, and competence
   b. Nursing practice using cognitive, interpersonal, and technical skills
   c. Redesigning nursing practice
   d. Structure framework of nursing diagnosis, nursing interventions, and nursing outcomes
5. How many interventions are there in Nursing Intervention Classification System?
   a. 71 b. 143
   c. 247 d. 321
6. Which classification system has problem rating scale for measuring outcome of care given?
   a. NANDA b. NOC
   c. NIC d. OMHA
7. Which term addresses individual's capability in performing a task?
   a. Nomenclature b. Competency
   c. Intervention d. Standard
8. Which category of population poses challenges to nursing services due to change in demographics?
   a. Children b. Adolescent
   c. Adult d. Elderly

Answer Keys
1. b   2. a   3. c   4. a   5. c   6. d   7. b
8. d

SUGGESTED READING

1. Anderson RD, Sweeney SD, William AT. An-introduction-to-management-science-quantitative … (n.d.); 2000. [Online] Available from https://www.coursehero.com/file/14221925/An-Introduction-to-Management-Science-Q. [Accessed on 16.11.2019].
2. Bateman ST, Snell AS. Management: Building Competitive Advantage. New York: Irwin McGraw-Hill; 1999.
3. Bellock JP, O'Neil, Ethics: Nursing around the World: Cultural Values and … (n.d.). [Online] Available from http://ojin.nursingworld.org/MainMenuCategories/ANAMarketplace/ANAPeriodicals/OJ. [Accessed on 09.02.2019].
4. Bose R. Nursing administration and services-suggestion for improvement in management effectiveness. Nurs J India. 1994;LXXXV(11):201-2.
5. Bulechek G, Butcher H, Dochterman J, Wagner C (Eds). Nursing Interventions Classification (NIC), 6th edition. St. Louis, MO: Elsevier; 2013. [Online] Available from http://www.nursing.uiwa.edu/centers/cncce/.
6. Ethics: Nursing Around The World: Cultural Values And … (n.d.). [Online] Available from http://ojin.nursingworld.org/MainMenuCategories/ANAMarketplace/ANAPeriodicals/OJ. [Accessed on 09.02.2019].
7. Halstead JA, Rains JW, Boland DL, May FE. Reconceptualizing baccalaureate nursing education: Outcomes and competencies for practice in the 21st century. J Nurs Educat. 1996;35(9):413-6.
8. Henry B, Lorensen M, Hirschfield MJ. Management and leadership by nurses. World Health Forum. 1994;15(2):153-7.
9. Indian Nursing Council. Indian Nursing Council Act, 1947. New Delhi (Amended in 1950 and 1957).

10. ICN. An analysis of nursing priorities worldwide. Int Nurs Rev. 1994;41(4):115-7. [Online] Available from http://www.ncbi.nlm.nih.gov/pubmed/7928139.
11. Indian Nursing Council. Golden Jubilee Celebration: Nursing in the New Millennium. New Delhi: Daryaganj, Jaina Offset Printers; 2000.
12. Indian Nursing Council. Syllabus and regulations: Diploma in general nursing and midwifery. INC: New Delhi, 2001.
13. Joglekar KS. Hospital Wards Management: Professional Adjustments and Trends in Nursing. Bombay: Vohra Medical Publications; 2000.
14. Kingma M. Professional and socioeconomic issues: Separate but interdependent. Int Nurs Rev. 1993;40(3):85-8, 94. [Online] Available from http://www.ncbi.nlm.nih.gov/pubmed/8330955.
15. Korniewicz DM, Palmer MH. The preferable future for nursing. Nurs Outlook. 1997;45(3):108-13.
16. McCloskey J, Bulchek G (Eds). Nursing Intervention Classification (NIC): Iowa International Project, 3rd edition. St. Louis, MO: Mosby; 2002.
17. Trends and issues in nursing - SlideShare. https://www.slideshare.net › rsmehta › 12-trends-and-issues-in-nursing. [Accessed on 10.02.2019].
18. O'Neale M, Kurtz S. Certification: Perspectives on competency assurance. Semin Perioperative Nurs. 2001;10(2):88-92.
19. Porter-O'Grady T. Profound change: 21st-century nursing. Nurs Outlook. 2001;49(4):182-6.
20. Samuel SA. Nursing education: Opportunities and challenges. TNAI Bull. 2012;1(10). [Online] Available from http://www.tnaionline.org/Nov_12/6.htm.
21. Scoble KB, Russell G. Vision 2020, Part 1: Profile of future nurse leader. JONA. 2003;33(6), 324-30.
22. Subbaraman R, Thomas B, Sellappan S, Chandra S, Jayabal L, Raja A, … Swaminathan S. Tuberculosis patients in an Indian mega-city: Where do they live and where are they diagnosed? PLoS One. 2017;12(8):e0183240.
23. The government of India. Report of Health Survey and Development Committee Recommendations. New Delhi: Govt. of India; 1964.
24. Vati J, Das K, Walia I. Leadership behaviour of nurses. Nurs Midwifery Res J. 2004;1(1):24-31.
25. Vati J, Walia I. Staff and professional development methods used by hospital nurses of north India. Nurs J India. 2001;LXXXXII(2):38-40.
26. Vati J. Organization and administration of nursing services in district hospitals of north India. Unpublished Ph.D. in Nursing Theses; 1992.
27. Zerwekh J, Claborn JK. Role transitions. In Nursing Today: Transition and Trends, 4th edition. Philadelphia: Saunders; 2002.

4
Ethics and Ethical Issues in Nursing

CHAPTER OUTLINE

- Ethics and Ethical Theories
  - Concept of Ethics
  - Nursing Ethics
  - Types of Ethics
  - Ethical Theories
- Principles and Rights Related to Ethics
  - Principles of Ethics
  - Principles-based Ethics
  - Rights of Patients Supported by Ethics
  - Nurses' Rights
- Code of Ethics and Professional Conduct
  - Purposes of Code
  - Purposes of Code of Ethics
  - Codes of Ethics and Professional Conduct
- Ethical Committee
- Ethical Issues and Ethical Decision-making
  - Ethical Issues
  - Ethical Decision-making
  - Role of Nurse Managers in Dealing Ethical Issues

LEARNING OUTCOMES

After completion of this chapter, the learner will be able to:
- Understand the concept of ethics and nursing ethics
- Describe types of ethics
- Describe ethical theories
- Enlist principles of ethics
- Appreciate principles-based ethics
- Enumerate rights of patients supported by ethics
- Describe the nursing code of ethics and professional conduct
- Elaborate on the role of the ethical committee (EC)
- Discuss ethical dilemmas and ethical decision-making
- Describe the role of nurse managers in ethical issues

KEY TERMS

Ethics, nursing ethics, ethical theories, principles of ethics, rights of patients, code of ethics, professional conduct, ethical dilemma, ethical decision-making, ethical issues

INTRODUCTION

Advancement in the globalization, modernization, and technology has an impact in nursing. Increased complexity in the professional role and awareness among the clients for their rights required nurses to pay attention to understand and follow strictly ethical responsibilities about their jobs and clients.

ETHICS AND ETHICAL THEORIES

Concept of Ethics

The word *ethics* is the derivative of the Greek word "ethos," which refers to "character." According to Webster's New Collegiate Dictionary ethics is "the science of moral duty or the science of ideal human character." Beauchamp (2001) viewed it as "a generic term for various ways of understanding and examining the moral life." Ethics is what is good or valuable for all people. Values form conduct, or the behavior of a person and values reflect the ethics that a person follows in his personal, societal, and professional life (**Fig. 4.1**).

Nursing Ethics

Nursing ethics is applied ethics focussed on both patient and nurse problems related to the nursing profession: the practice of nurses, exemplified in the codes of ethics and standards of nursing practice. These ethics provide

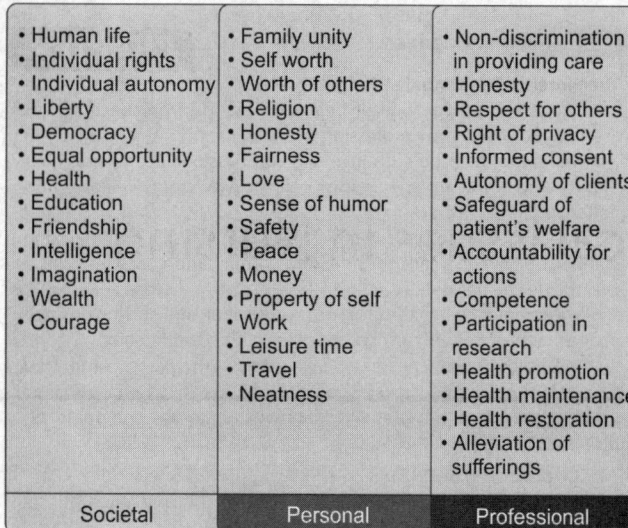

Fig. 4.1: Types of values.

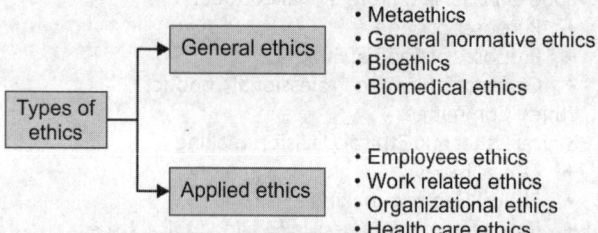

Fig. 4.2: Types of ethics.

field of human endeavor, such as warfare, medicine, nursing, journalism, and so on, in an attempt to resolve these ethical issues and to show, in particular situations and circumstances, what would be the right course of action to take. These are also known as bioethics or biomedical ethics.

a. *Employees ethics:* These ethics are concerning moral laws that bind the working community together. Code of ethics, well-defined policies and procedures, and procedures to resolve ethical dilemmas are examples of this type of ethics. Through these ethics, professional groups set standards of practice in the organization.

b. *Work-related ethics:* These types of ethics are concerning duty consciousness. The staff is obliged to perform the assigned duties.

c. *Organizational-related ethics:* Organizational ethics in health-care setting comprises of professional and moral conduct such as commitment, conflict resolution through negotiation, and acceptance for organizational change. Mission, vision, governance, and leadership are examples of organizational ethics.

d. *Health-care ethics:* These ethics are related to problems and issues in healthcare.

Ethical Theories

Ethical principles derive from normative ethical theories. These theories are of six types—deontology, utilitarianism, rights ethical theory, casuist ethical theory, virtue ethical theory, and ethics of care theory.

1. **Deontology theory:** The word "deontology" derives from the Greek words for duty (*deon*) and science (or study) of (*logos*) "the study of duty or obligation" and refers to duty and obedience at center of all ethical decisions. This theory guides and assesses our choices of what we ought to do. It provides a basis for special duties and obligations to a particular individual emphasizing universal standards and impartiality.

2. **Utilitarianism:** This theory is on the moral values of action, and action is directed by the utility or outcome. The utility is a pleasure or happiness versus pain or suffering, as the satisfaction of preferences. This theory predicts the consequences of action and emphasizes universal standards and impartiality.

   a. *Act utilitarianism:* In act utilitarianism, a person performs the acts that benefit the most people, regardless of personal feelings or societal constraints such as laws.

   b. *Rule utilitarianism:* It is concerned with the rule of fairness, and it is by laws to get the maximum benefit.

3. **Rights ethical theory:** According to this theory, society sets forth the rights, which are considered ethically right, since a large number of people consensus it.

4. **Casuist ethical theory:** The casuist ethical theory compares an ethical dilemma with other ethical

a framework for assessing situations and interactions between and among care providers and their patients or clients.

Types of Ethics

Ethics are of two types—general ethics and applied ethics (Fig. 4.2).

1. **General ethics:** General ethics consider the morality of human acts in general, irrespective of any particular field of application, occupation, or profession. These are of two types—metaethics and general normative ethics.

   a. *Metaethics:* Metaethics is the study of the meaning of moral terms and how they use in moral discourse. These ethics attempt to establish what we as human beings should or should not do, should or should not be, and should or should not nurture or sustain.

   b. *General normative ethics:* The general normative ethics determine the moral quality of human acts and the way in which they give reasons to deal with moral matters. The word "normative" refers to guidelines or norms, and these ethics are derived from normative ethical theories like Kantian ethics, Virtue ethics, and Utilitarian ethics and so on.

2. **Applied ethics:** Applied ethics are general principles of normative ethics applied systematically to ethical issues. These ethics arise within a given specialized

dilemmas of a similar nature. It allows one to determine the severity of the situation and to create the best possible solution according to others' experiences.
5. **Virtue ethical theory:** This theory judges a person by his or her character rather than by action. The character behaviors include moral values, reputation, and motivation of a person. Autonomy, beneficence, and confidentiality are examples of normal behavior.
6. **Ethics of care theory:** Care theory explains what makes actions right or wrong. It is one of a cluster of normative ethical theories developed by feminist in the second half of the 20th century. This theory emphasizes the importance of communication and relationships build up in a community or within a family.

PRINCIPLES AND RIGHTS RELATED TO ETHICS

Principles of Ethics

A principle is a basic foundational belief that guides actions. Ethical principles are statements of human obligations or duties that are generally accepted. These are an expression of normative ethical systems. These are of three types:
1. **Principles of global ethics:** Global ethics are the most controversial the least understood. The principles of global ethics include global justice as reflected in international laws, society before self/social responsibility, environmental stewardship, interdependence, and responsibility for the "whole," and reverence for place.
2. **Principles of personal ethics:** The principles of personal or morality ethics reflect general expectations of any person in any society, acting in any capacity. These principles instill during childhood. The examples of these principles are concern for well-being of others, respect for the autonomy of others, trustworthiness and honesty, and preventing harm to others are the principles of personal ethics.
3. **Principles of professional ethics:** The principles of professional ethics provide rules of conduct and standards of behavior of professionals, developed by professional associations as codes of ethics. These include impartiality, objectivity, openness, full disclosure, confidentiality, the duty of care, fidelity to professional responsibilities, and avoiding a potential or apparent conflict of interest.

All the nurses before entering to their practice take the Florence Nightingale Pledge, a modified Hippocratic Oath, arranged by Mrs. Lystra E. Gretter and her committee for the Farrand Training School for Nurses, Detroit as a token of esteem for the Founder of Modern Nursing. The Trained Nurses Association of India (TNAI) has also proposed a pledge for the Indian nurses that depict the ethics required for the nursing profession **(Box 4.1)**.

> **Box 4.1:** Nurses pledge.
>
> **The Florence Nightingale Pledge**
> "I solemnly pledge myself before God and in presence of this assembly to practice my profession with dedication.
> I will serve mankind with love and compassion, recognizing their dignity and rights irrespective of color, caste, creed, religion and nationality.
> I will endeavor to update my knowledge and skill and maintain standard of nursing care to individual, family and community as a member of the health team.
> I will uphold the standard of nursing education and nursing practice in all aspects of holistic care as a member of the health team.
> I will hold in confidence personal matters of my clients committed to my care and also fulfill my responsibilities as a citizen.
> I will refrain from any activity that will harm my personal and professional dignity as a Nurse."
>
> **Pledge proposed by TNAI**
> "I solemnly pledge myself before God and in presence of this assembly to practice my profession with dedication.
> I will serve mankind with love and compassion, recognizing their dignity and rights irrespective of color, caste, creed, religion and nationality.
> I will endeavor to update my knowledge and skill and maintain standard of nursing care to individual, family and community in all settings and in all aspects of holistic care as a member of the health team.
> I will hold in confidence personal matters of my clients committed to my care and help them to develop confidence in care rendered by me.
> I will refrain from any activity that will harm my personal and professional dignity as a Nurse.
> I will actively support my profession and strive towards its advancement.
> I will fulfill my responsibilities as a citizen and encourage change towards better health."

Principles-based Ethics

Principles-based ethics is a systematic method of resolving ethical problems that involve reflection on general principles of ethics. These principles are also applicable in healthcare and have its implications in nursing **(Fig. 4.3)**.
1. **Autonomy:** Autonomy means control of people over their lives by their lifestyle. It refers to a person's independence, self-determination, and self-reliance. Autonomy provides a scope in nursing to display respect for all persons and support the patient's right to informed consent.
2. **Informed consent:** Informed consent is the derivative of the concept of autonomy. A patient must get an adequate amount of information about his or her health condition, and he or she is free to decide about his or her treatment. Typically, informed consent involves informing the patient (or relative) about the recommended procedure, its risks, benefits, and alternatives.
3. **Justice:** The justice principle states that ethical theories should prescribe actions that are fair to those involved. Justice means fairness or equity in dealing. It can be ensured by providing nursing care to all the patients and as per priority based on clients at greater risk.

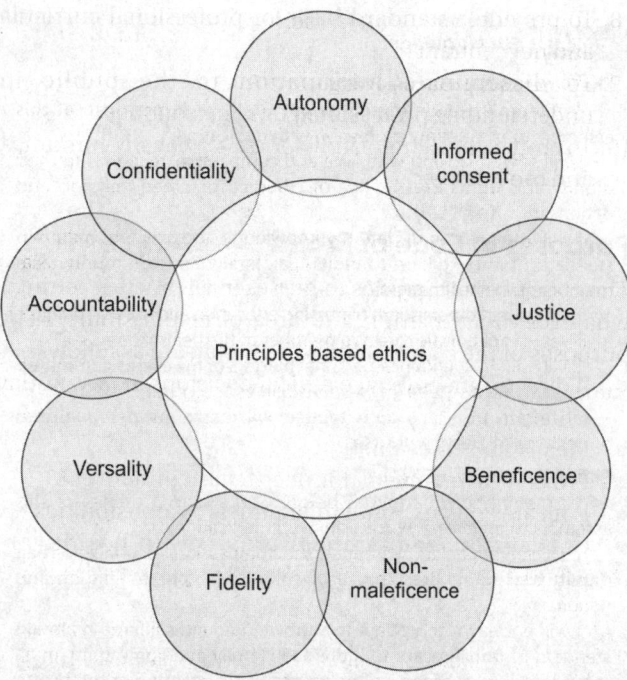

Fig. 4.3: Principles-based ethics.

Professionally trained nurses are educated to consider the individual, the family, and the social context of patients in providing nursing care. They need to recognize the importance of understanding the values, beliefs, and health practices of patients with different backgrounds to provide care to the patients and should be very fair to give equal weight age as for as the care part is concerned.

4. **Beneficence:** The principle of beneficence ethics directs what to do and what is good and avoids harm. It also states that we should attempt to generate the largest ratio of good over evil possible in the world.
5. **Nonmaleficence/Do no harm:** It deals with situations in which none of the choices is beneficial. In this situation, a person should choose to do the least harm possible and to do harm to the fewest people. The dichotomy between the beneficence and nonmaleficence principles is the foundation for "risk/benefit" analysis.
6. **Fidelity:** Fidelity means faithfulness, i.e. striving to keep promises. According to this principle, a person should fulfill his or her duties and obligations honestly. Fidelity stands for the proposition that nurses keep their patients' interests in mind, maintain trust and confidence, and they give care to patients with faithful attention.
7. **Veracity:** It means to tell the truth. Be honest with the patients, families, and peers. Nurses need to be honest while giving dealing with the patients and their family members.
8. **Accountability:** It is the process in which individuals are answerable for their action and have the obligation (duty) to act. The nurses are also bound by professional codes to be accountable to them, clients and their families, the nursing profession, employers, and to the general public.
9. **Confidentiality:** Confidentiality means privacy of the information of a person. It is the right of an individual patient either disclose or not his or her personal, identifiable medical information. Without the consent of the patient, his or her information cannot disclose to anyone physician' record and insurance personnel as necessary. The patient has the right to sue on disclosing his or her confidentiality.

Rights of Patients Supported by Ethics

Patient or client in the health-care system has his or her ethical or legal rights. There are four types of patient's ethical rights—rights of personal dignity, right to individualized care, right to assistance toward independence, and right to complaint and obtain changes in care (**Fig. 4.4**).

1. **Rights of personal dignity:** These rights describe the personal dignity of the patients while caring for them. Maintain the personal dignity of the patient by considering him as a human being. Calling by name that he or she chooses to have, maintaining privacy, modesty by knocking on closed doors, pulling curtains, providing appropriate garments, and helping him to have the best possible appearance through careful attention to personal hygiene and personal care are examples of maintaining patient's dignity. Have good attitudes toward the patients by listening to the thoughts and concerns of the patient, explaining expectations and new situations, and accepting his feelings as real without judging them right or wrong.
2. **Right to individualized care:** Every patient has right according to his or her needs and lifestyle, e.g. a nurse can consider patient's preferences and way of getting nursing procedure; alter if possible, visiting hours to help to maintain an important family bond, or plan diet modifications to fit the patient's cultural background.
3. **Right to assistance toward independence:** It is the ethical right of a patient that he or she should be helped

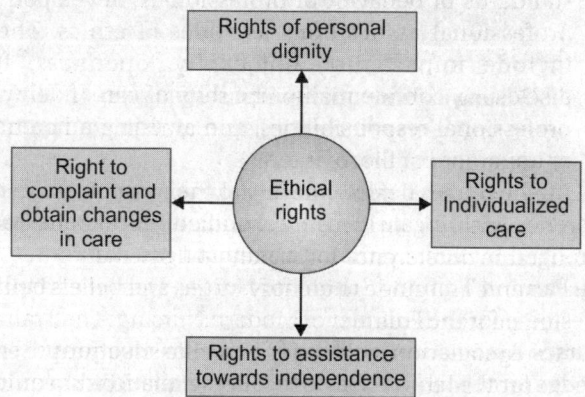

Fig. 4.4: Patients' rights supported by ethics.

to be independent in carrying out activities of daily living of building their self-esteem and encouraging them. Few examples allow the patient to perform self-care wherever possible, take care of the interest of the patient, and take extra time to give instructions or directions carefully to the patient.

4. **Right to the complaint and obtain changes in care:** The patient has the right to complain when care has not been of high quality and to obtain changes that are important to improve the quality of care.

Nurses' Rights

Since the nurses have duties toward patient care, ward management and education of patients, they should also have the rights. Fagin has listed the nurses' rights concerning significant matter, which are as follows:

- The right to find dignity in self-expression and self-enhancement through the use of our special abilities and educational background
- The right to recognize for contribution through the provision of an environment for its practice and proper professional economic rewards
- The right of the work environment, which will minimize physical and emotional stress and health risks
- The right to control what is professional practice within the limits of the law
- The right to set standards for excellence in nursing
- The right to social and political action on behalf of nursing and healthcare.

CODE OF ETHICS AND PROFESSIONAL CONDUCT

The code is a collection of laws or a system of rules and regulations. A code adopted by profession is to regulate the profession and to promote high standards of competence among its members, whereas *Code of ethics* is often a formal statement of an organization's values on certain ethical and social issues derived from the dignity and rights of the patient as a person. These are the indicators of acceptance of the trust and have the responsibility the patient places in the profession.

Purposes of Code

The following list shows the purposes of code:
1. To provide a means to establish, maintain, and improve the standard of practice
2. To form formal guidelines to take actions
3. To compare between ethical and unethical behaviors
4. A frame of reference for making judgments
5. To serve as a guide to identify values and beliefs behind ethical standards
6. To regulate conduct in more specific situations
7. To provide the basis for regulating relationship among nurse, patient, coworkers, society, and profession
8. To provide a standard base for professional curricula and new entrant
9. To disseminate information to the public in understanding professional nursing conduct
10. To protect the rights of individuals, families, community, and the nurse.

Purposes of Code of Ethics

The code of ethics applies to nurses in all practice settings, whatever their position and area of responsibility. The purposes of the code of ethics in nursing are as follows:
- It directs nurses to take ethical decisions in day-to-day situations
- Means for self-evaluation
- Provides a framework for peer-review initiatives
- Educates nurses about their ethical responsibilities
- Conveys the commitment of nurses to health-care professionals and public toward service.

Codes of Ethics and Professional Conduct

Codes of ethics adopted by different countries such as International Council of Nurses, the American Nurses Association, the Canadian Nurses Association, and by nurses in Australia. Code of Ethics for Nurses in India adopted was complementary to the International Council of Nurses (ICN) Codes for Nurses (1993).

Trained Nurses Association of India's Nurses Ethical Behavior and Professional Conduct

The Trained Nurses Association of India addresses the ethical behavior of nurses and professional conduct as follows:
1. Only those procedures, which are taught and learned through prescribed educational programs and on the job training, should be carried out on patients/clients.
2. Irrespective of caste, creed, religion, and sex, every person would be helped and cared to attain/maintain the optimum levels of health.
3. Each patient/client should respect as a person at all levels of health and illness or otherwise.
4. Take informed consent from the patient (or a relative) before performing or subjecting him or her to any treatment investigation per policy of the institute.
5. Information about the patient/client should not be divulged and should be shared selectively with his or her permission with those involved in the care.
6. In an emergency, apply every possible life-saving measures, prompt, and appropriate medical help.
7. Record all practice attempts in the patient chart or any other record book.
8. A nurse must question/clarify and refuses to carry out a participating in a treatment/procedure about which in any way he or she is in doubt and is, according to the nurse, likely to harm or exploit the patient or client and herself or himself.

9. Advocate the health policies/programs that would help to safeguard the patient's/client's interest and ensure the nurse's self-protection.
10. Ensure the protection of an individual customer's rights to healthcare.
11. Whenever there is a change in the health-care policy, the health issues are likely to re-emerge, and nurses are required to face new challenges with a moral vigilance that would prove ethical conduct in a given situation.
12. Nurses collectively create or influence the policies in the making to remain as an authentic health-care voice within the social contract that is in keeping with the moral conscience of the nursing profession.

Code of Conduct Related to Doctor Nurse Professional Relationship

Indian Medical Association and Trained Nurses Association of India developed a code of conduct regarding doctor–nurse professional relationship. The main aim of doctor–nurse professional relationship is to create a congenial working environment where nurse and doctors can make decisions in an assertive manner related to patient care. It is mandatory for doctors and nurses to follow a code of ethics in rendering patient care. It mentions that:

1. "Doctors to follow MCI Ethics regulations in general including
   a. Physicians must recognize and promote the practice of nursing as a profession and should seek their cooperation wherever required.
   b. In case of running of a nursing home by a physician and employing nurses, the ultimate responsibility rests on the physician, (3) to employ nurses in all health sectors.
2. Nurses to adhere to International code of ethics and professional conduct developed by the International Council for Nurses (1973) and Indian Nursing Council (2006). It also states that:
   a. Doctor and nurse relationships must be on ethical and professional concerns for better patient care.
   b. The goal of this partnership is on shared responsibility and accountability for increasing quality of care and patient safety.
   c. Although nurses carry out the prescription given by doctors as a part of their job, at the same time, they are bound to contradict with the same in the case of interfering with the standard of patient care and professional nursing standards. An ethical doctor should neither expect nor insist that nurses blindly follow his or her orders contrary to set standards of good ethical, medical, and nursing practice.
   d. In emergencies, when prompt action is a necessary and concerned doctor is not available, a nurse may be justified in acting of his or her own for the safety of the patient per standing order and institution protocol. This protection and insulation are everyone's right under Section 92 of Panel Code Act.

Code of Ethics and Professional Conduct (2006)

According to INC, following are the codes for nurses:

I. Code of ethics and professional conduct
- To inform both the nurse and society of the minimum standard for professional conduct
- To provide regulatory bodies a basis for decisions regarding standards of professional conduct
- To help to protect the rights of individuals, families, and community and also the rights of the nurse.

II. Code of Ethics for Nurses
- The nurse respects the uniqueness of each patient
- Gives care to each patient irrespective of caste, creed, gender, religion, culture, and economic status
- Renders care to individual patient keeping in mind his beliefs, values, and culture
- Appreciates the place of the individual in the family and community and facilitates the participation of significant others in the care
- Develops and promotes a trustful relationship with each patient as an individual
- Identifies the ability of each patient or individual to plan nursing interventions.

1. To respect the rights of individuals or patients as a part of care and help to make decisions for the care.
   - Gives appropriate and accurate information to decide on various choices for the care
   - Respects the decisions made by an individual(s) regarding their care
   - Provides accurate information regarding the availability of health services
   - Protects vulnerable population by informing about the provision of health service especially to them.
2. The nurse respects an individual's right to privacy, maintains confidentiality, and shares information judiciously.
   - Respects the individual' right to privacy of their personal information
   - Maintains confidentiality of privileged information except in life-threatening situations and uses discretion in sharing information
   - Takes informed consent and maintains anonymity for quality assurance/academic/legal reasons
   - Limits the access to all personal records to authorized persons only.
3. Nurse maintains competence to render quality nursing care.
   - Only registered nurses must provide nursing care
   - Nurse strives to maintain the standard of nursing care
   - Takes initiative to participate in continuing education and avails opportunities for self-development
   - Participates in research concerning ethical issues for the development of nursing.

4. Nurse obliges to practice keeping in mind the nursing ethics and code of ethics.
   - Follows the ethics and professional conduct codes
   - Familiarizes with relevant laws and practices by the law of the state.
5. The nurse is obliged to work harmoniously with members of the health team.
   - Appreciates the team efforts in rendering care
   - Works as a health team member and coordinates with other health professionals to accomplish the objective of patient care.
6. Nurse maintain trust in the society in rendering care.
   - Demonstrates personal etiquettes and professional attributes in all dealings.

Code of Professional Conduct for Nurses

1. Professional responsibility and accountability Nurse
   - Recognizes the value of self and has a self-understanding
   - Practices standard of personal conduct
   - Carries out responsibilities within the framework of professional boundaries
   - Is accountable for maintaining practice standards
   - Is accountable for own decisions and actions
   - Is being compassionate
   - Is responsible for continuous improvement of current practices.
2. Nursing practice
   - Provides quality care to the clients
   - Maintains equality and dignity in rendering care
   - Respects healthy traditional and cultural practices and discourages the harmful ones
   - Provides accurate health-related information to individuals and families to take their decisions in healthcare
   - Encourages individuals and their family to participate in the care
   - Ensures safe practices
   - Consults, coordinates, collaborates, and follows up appropriately when individuals' care needs exceed the nurse's competence.
3. Communication and interpersonal relationships
   - Maintains an effective therapeutic interpersonal relationship with clients
   - Maintains an effective interpersonal working relationship with team members and respect them
   - Inculcates teal spirit and appreciates the professional role
   - Coordinates and cooperates with team members to accomplish the goal of rendering care.
4. Be a human being and value it
   - Protects individuals from harmful and unethical practice
   - Considers relevant facts while taking conscious decisions in the best interest of individuals
   - Encourages and supports individuals in their right to speak for themselves on issues affecting their health and welfare
   - Respects and supports choices made by individuals.
5. Related to management
   - Ensures proper allocation and maximum utilization of available resources
   - Supervises and guiding student nurses and caretakers
   - Uses judgment about individual competence while accepting and delegating responsibility
   - Facilitates conducive work culture to achieve institutional objectives
   - Communicates effectively following appropriate channels of communication
   - Participates in performance evaluation
   - Conducts nursing audits
   - Participates in policy making by the principle of equity and accessibility of services
   - Believes in participatory management to find out the needs of individuals to make a recommendation to policy makers and funding agencies.
6. Professional advancement
   - Protects human rights while pursuing the advancement of knowledge
   - Contributes to the development of nursing practice
   - Searches and implements evidence-based practices
   - Updates and improves own knowledge and skills in nursing
   - Contributes to advancing professional knowledge by conducting research studies.

Code of Ethics for Supervisors of Nursing Service Personnel

The nursing supervisors are committed to:
1. Recognize that all personnel, above, beside, or below have an inherent desire to do good work and to be useful and respected citizens.
2. Recognize merit in the suggestions and thinking of others.
3. Be firm in dealing with all other associates in the nursing profession. Recognizing that she is in an important position, she will assume responsibility for her own mistakes and will refrain from shifting blame to others.
4. Have understanding and application of business principles, personally, and to the guidance of her personnel in the understanding and application of business principles.
5. The development of personal progress in medicine and the resultant changes in the equipment and nursing procedures and to the recommendation and institution of methods and equipment that give promise of increasing quality of nursing service, lowering costs, and improved working conditions.

6. A realization and constant awareness of supervision's function to improve nursing service by helping personnel to a maximum of satisfaction from life and work.
7. Cognizance of the fact that personnel are desirous of a supervisor who is worthy of respect and possessed of a good moral character, good citizenship, and integrity; a supervisor who supports and promotes an uplifting influence in her personal and upon the community.

ETHICAL COMMITTEE

An EC is a group of persons comprising health-care professionals and nonmembers who are officially responsible for promoting ethical practices and code of ethics, protects the dignity, rights, safety, and well-being of trial subjects and particular care to protect vulnerable participants. It is advisory and takes decisions regarding ethics and resolves ethical issues and dilemmas in practice, administration, education, and research.

ECs in India

Mostly in Indian hospitals and institutions, ECs are to review biomedical research proposals, to improve the quality of research, and to safeguard the rights and safety of human study subjects.

Indian Council for Medical Research (ICMR) initiated formulation of the EC in India and prepared its first official guidelines to form an ethics committee in February 1980 for conducting research that provided membership criteria and standards for an ethical standard for review. ICMR issued guidelines for bioethics for research in medical, epidemiology, and public health in 2002 and revises in 2006.

It is mandatory to get approval for any biomedical research on human participants by the Institutional Ethical Committee (IEC)/institutional review board (IRB) before its initiation. Therefore each institution should have its ethics committee under Amendment 2005 of the Drugs and Cosmetics Act, 1940,

ICMR developed guidelines for preparing standard operating procedures (SOPs) for Institutional Ethics Committee (IEC) for Human Research in collaboration with the Forum for Ethics Review Committees of Asia Pacific (FERCAP). The Forum for Ethics Committee Review in India (FERC) has been set up under FERCAP.

It is compulsory to register IEC with the Central Drugs Standard Control Organization (CDSCO) per rule passed by the government of India per General Statutory Rule, 72 E dated February 8, 2013 and required re-registration per notification 2016. Ethics committees are concerned with serious adverse events reporting and compensation in cases of deaths occurs during clinical trial, and care of participants injured during research.

Functions and Activities of Ethics Committee

1. **Research:**
   - Validates research proposal from the technical, scientific, statistical, and ethical point of view
   - Examines adherence of principles of research ethics, i.e. autonomy, beneficence, nonmaleficence, and justice in planning, conducting, and reporting in the proposal
   - Reviews informed consent process (audiovisual [AV] recording of consent as per office order dated Nov. 19, 2013; and AV consent in cases of vulnerable population and research on new chemical entities per General Statutory Rule, 611E dated July 31, 2015)
   - Examines (1) risk–benefit ratio, (2) distribution of burden and benefits, and (3) provision of appropriate compensation
   - Examines compliance with all regulating requirements, applicable guidelines, and laws
   - Decides to solve actual or anticipated ethical dilemmas in research.
2. **Quality of care:** Evaluates the quality of care by keeping in mind the ethical principles and rights of patients in various areas. The some of areas of care include the art of bedside care, relief of suffering, cure of disease, incidence, trend over time of iatrogenic disease, cost to patient in terms of tests, drugs, other costs, prompt attention to the needs of the patient, and care of the seriously ill, dying, and dead patients.
3. **Education:** Plans and conducts in-service training programs, seminars/workshops/mini-conferences on various topics related to biomedical ethics, ethical principles, rights of patients, code of ethics, and quality research.
4. **Other roles of the ethics committee:**
   - Policy development
   - Providing consultation in cases of ethical dilemma and resolving ethical conflicts
   - Preparing guidelines, manual on bioethics, principles of ethics, code of ethics, a method of dealing with ethical dilemmas, etc. for staff
   - Preparing guidelines to patients, families regarding their rights, responsibilities, means of seeking redress for any harm
   - Disclosure of diagnosis
   - Diagnosis of brain death
   - Requesting permission to harvest organs for transplantation
   - Informed consent process
   - Guiding and supporting patients, families, and health-care providers
   - Conducting surveys regarding any malpractices/deficiency in care practices
   - Setting a supportive framework/forum to guide and monitor the proper functioning of a forum for redress of complaints from patients, families, employees

- Resolving conflicts about what is right things to do to patients at the end of life
- Getting feedback regarding the functioning of the EC.

Composition

The members of the EC should have commitment and knowledge to bioethics, research, and subjects. The committee should be multidisciplinary. The hospital EC must ensure representatives from the administrators, clinicians (from medical, surgical, nursing, and another discipline), social worker, priest/philosopher, lawyer, rehabilitation personnel, a layperson from the community, and statistician. Each department should also constitute a departmental EC to deal with its respective ethical issues. The size of EC may vary according to the size of the institution and function of ECs.

According to guidelines for preparing SOPs for IEC for Human Research by ICMR, the committee should have seven to nine members and maximum 12–15. The minimum five members are required to compose a quorum. The IEC for research should comprise the following members:
- The chairperson who should preferably be from outside the institution
- A deputy chairman if needed
- One to two basic medical scientists
- One to two clinicians from various institutes
- One legal expert or retired judge
- One social scientist/representative of the nongovernmental voluntary agency
- One philosopher/ethicist/theologian
- One layperson from the community
- Member-Secretary who generally belongs to the same institution
- If required subject expert from a related discipline.

According to ICMR Ethical Guidelines (2006), there is a need for periodical training national and international ethical guidelines and regulations for EC members.

Duration

The committee is constituted by the Head of Institution initially for 2–3 years.

Meeting Procedure

Committee meetings held on scheduled intervals as prescribed and also as and when required. The chairperson chairs the session, and member secretary is the convener who organizes meetings, maintains records, writes and prepares minutes of the meetings, and gets it approved by the Chairman and communicates to all concerned.

ETHICAL ISSUES AND ETHICAL DECISION-MAKING

Ethical Issues

The ethical issue or dilemma is a conflicting situation in selecting one alternative from two courses of action having similar significant consequences. There is no set procedure to resolve an ethical dilemma. It requires critical thinking and knowledge of ethical principles and ethical theories to resolve ethical dilemmas.

Ethical Decision-making

It is a process of taking appropriate decision to resolve an ethical dilemma. There are many decision-making models. Rational decision-making model proposed by Herbert Simon and summarized by Ham and Hill. This model involves the selection of the alternative, which will maximize. The following are the steps taken for the decision-making:
- Define the problem, need, or opportunity
- Gather information and find out the relevancy of an ethical dilemma
- Search and evaluate various possible means of solving the problem
- Select the most promising of the options evaluated
- Implement the selected option
- Evaluate action about the problem defined in stage 1.

Role of Nurse Managers in Dealing Ethical Issues

- Have introspected regarding her own moral values and basic belief about rights, duties, and goals of human beings
- Create awareness among nurses about bioethics through discussions and formal education sessions
- Conduct unit-wise ethical rounds
- Follow guidelines of bioethics
- Participate in IEC meetings
- Monitor organizational and departmental policies related to ethics
- Develop an effective therapeutic and working relationship
- Develop and implement a team approach
- Identify any ethical issue and solve by using the appropriate method.

CHAPTER HIGHLIGHTS

- Ethics means a moral duty or ideal human character based on values and principles of life.
- Nursing ethics is applied ethics focus on both patients and nurses problems related to the nursing profession. There are two types of ethics—general and applied.
- Deontology, utilitarianism, rights ethical theory, casuist ethical theory, virtue ethical theory, and ethics of care theory form the theoretical base for developing ethical principles.
- Ethical principles are statements of human obligations or duties that are generally accepted. There are principles of personal, professional, and global ethics.
- Autonomy, informed consent, justice, beneficence, nonmaleficence/do not harm, fidelity, veracity, accountability; confidentiality is principle-based ethics.

- Rights of personal dignity, the individualized care, assistance toward independence, right to the complaint, and obtain changes in care are important ethical rights of a patient.
- Code of ethics is an organization's values on certain ethical and social issues derived from the dignity and rights of the patient as a person. These are adopted internationally and nationally by nursing councils and nursing associations.
- The EC is advisory and takes decisions regarding ethics and resolves ethical issues and dilemmas in practice, administration, education, and research.
- Ethical decision-making is a process of taking appropriate decision to resolve an ethical dilemma. Nurse managers can play an important role in managing ethical issues by taking appropriate actions through critical thinking and applying ethical principles and ethical theories.

REVIEW QUESTIONS

I. Essay Type Questions
1. Define nursing ethics and describe different types of ethics.
2. Briefly describe ethical theories.
3. Write principles-based ethics.
4. Define the ethical dilemma and discuss the ethical decision-making process.

II. Short Notes
1. Principles of ethics
2. Rights of patients supported by ethics
3. Ethical committee
4. Role of a nurse manager in ethical issues

III. Multiple Choice Questions
1. A study of moral duty or an ideal human character refers to:
   a. General ethics   b. Applied ethics
   c. Meta-ethics   d. Ethics
2. The theory of utilitarianism is useful in:
   a. Predicting the consequences of an action and emphasize universal standards and impartiality
   b. Guiding and assessing our choices of what we ought to do
   c. Protecting rights set forth by a society
   d. Judging a person by his character deviated from his normal behavior
3. The principle of ethics that means "tells the truth"; be honest with the patients, families, and peers is:
   a. Fidelity   b. Nonmaleficence
   c. Veracity   d. Beneficence
4. The ethical theory that compares a current ethical dilemma with examples of similar ethical dilemmas and their outcomes is:
   a. Casuist ethical theory
   b. Virtue ethical theory
   c. Rights ethical theory
   d. Ethics of care theory
5. In a situation where a client is helped to become independent in carrying out activities of daily living of building self-esteem and encouraging him is an example of:
   a. Rights of personal dignity
   b. Right to individualized care
   c. Right to assistance toward independence
   d. Right to the complaint and obtain changes in care

Answer Keys
1. d   2. a   3. c   4. a   5. c

SUGGESTED READING

1. American Medical Association. Patient Confidentiality. [Online] Available from http://www.ama-assn.org/ama/pub/category/4610.html. [Accessed on 18.2.2018].
2. American School Counselor Association. The Ethical Decision-Making Model 1996. [Online] Available from http://www.schoolcounselor.org/Ethics/ethics_d.html. [Accessed on 18.2.2018].
3. Barbara JD. Moving forward: A new code of ethics. Nurs Outlook. 2002;50:97-9.
4. Beauchamp TL, Childress JF. Principles of Biomedical Ethics, 4th edition. New York: Oxford University Press; 1994.
5. Cooper RW, Frank GL, Hansen MM, et al. Key ethical issues encountered in healthcare organizations—the perceptions of staff nurses and nurse leaders. JONA. 2004;34:149-56.
6. Code of Conduct: Doctor Nurse Professional Relationship. [Online] Available from http://www.tnaionline.org/news/Announcement/code-of-conduct-doctor-nurse-professional-relationship/112.html [Accessed January 2018].
7. Ethical Principles. [Online] Available from http://peds.ufl.edu/ethics_course/Ethics,%20Ethical%20Principles.htm. [Accessed on 18.6.2018].
8. Available from https://cwru.pure.elsevier.com/en/publications/ethics-and-palliative-care-. [Accessed on 13.12.2018].
9. Holmes DR, Firth B, James A. Conflict of interest. Am Heart J. 2004;147:228-37.
10. Financial Literacy (unit 1) Flashcards | Quizlet. (n.d.). [Online] Available from https://quizlet.com/147871551/financial-literacy-unit-1-flash-cards/. [Accessed on 14.12.2018].
11. Hunt G (Ed). Ethical Issues in Nursing. London: Routledge; 1994.
12. Indian Nursing Council. Code of Ethics and Professional Conduct. New Delhi: INC; 2006.
13. International Council of Nurses. ICN Code for Nurses: Ethical Concepts Applied to Nursing. Geneva: Imprimerie Populaires; 1983.
14. Kadam R, Karandikar S. Ethics committee in India: Facing the challenges! Perspect Clin Res. 2012;3(2):50-6.
15. Kuyare M, Taur SR, Thatte UM. Establishing institutional ethics committees: Challenges and solutions–a review of the literature. Indian J Med Ethics. 2014;11(3):181-85.
16. Pandya SK. Hospital Ethics Committee. Indian J Med Res. 1996;4(2):51-6.
17. Raanan G, Ann L. Principles of Health Care Ethics. Chichester: John Wiley & Sons; 1994.

18. Rajput VJ, Bekes CE. Ethical issues in hospital medicine. Med Clin N Am. 2002;86:869-86.
19. Ridley A. Beginning Bioethics. New York: St. Martin's Press; 1998.
20. Rosemarie T. New Perspectives in Healthcare Ethics: An Interdisciplinary and Cross-cultural. Prentice Hall: Approach Publisher; 2007.
21. Rumbold G. Ethics in Nursing Practice. Balliere Tindall; 1999.
22. Simpson J, Weiner E (Eds). The Oxford English Dictionary, 2nd edition. Clarendon Press; 1989.
23. Singh S. Procedures & operations of Institutional Ethics Committees in public sector hospitals in Delhi, India. Indian J Med Res. 2009;130:568-9.
24. Spencer EM. A new role for institutional ethics committees: Organizational ethics. J Clin Ethics. 1997;8:372-6.
25. Pandya SK. Principles of health care ethics. Indian Journal of Medical Ethics. 1995;3(2):5.
26. Thatte UM, Marathe PA. Ethics committees in India: Past, present, and future. Perspect Clin Res. 2017;8(1):22-30.
27. Turner MH. A toolbox for healthcare ethics program development. J Nurs Staff Dev. 2003;19:9-15.
28. University of Washington School of Medicine. Ethics Committees, programs, and Consultation. [Online] Available from Ethics%20Committees%20and%20Ethics%20Consultation_%20Ethical%20Topic%20in%20Medicine.html. [Accessed on 13.12.2018].

CHAPTER 5

Consumer Protection Act and Rights of Special Groups

CHAPTER OUTLINE

- Legal System
  - Definitions and Purposes of Law
  - Sources of Public Laws
  - Types of Laws
  - The Judicial Process
- Consumers Protection Act
- Rights of Special Groups
  - Rights of Children, Women, Aging People
  - Rights of People Living with HIV/AIDS in India
  - Rights of Persons with Disability

LEARNING OUTCOMES

After completion of this chapter, the learner will be able to:
- Understand concept and purposes of law
- Describe different types and sources of law
- Describe the Consumers Protection Act
- Discuss the rights of special groups

KEY TERMS

Legal system, judicial system, Consumers Protection Act, Special groups, rights, HIV patients, disability, aging

INTRODUCTION

Nurses are expected to deliver appropriate and high-quality nursing care. Advanced knowledge, skills, and critical thinking are required to render the care as per the individual needs of each patient. The nurse's job is complex in the present advanced medical technology and therapies, not explicitly defined increase legal challenges and issues. Nurses need to have thorough knowledge about the law, Consumer Protection Act, and rights of special groups to prevent any legal suits, and to protect clients.

LEGAL SYSTEM

The word "Law" is a derivative of an Anglo-Saxon term means "*lay down*" or "*fixed*". The law means a rule; it constitutes rules of human conduct that binds society and guides for their actions.

It is a legal document setting forth rules governing a particular kind of activity.

Definitions

- The law means the rule of conduct, which is established and enforced by an authority. These laws, which prevent extremes behavior so that one can live without fear for oneself or one's property.
  —*Sullivan and Decker, 2001*
- Law exists if it is externally guaranteed by the probability of coercion (physical or psychological) to bring about conformity or avenge violation, and is applied by a staff of people holding themselves especially ready for that purpose.
  —*Max Weber*
- Law is "a system of rules, a union of primary and secondary rules"
  —*Hart*
- Law is rules and regulations to govern society. As such people create law and law regulates all persons.
  —*Guido, 2001*
- Laws are those rules made by humans who regulated social conduct in a formally prescribed and legally binding manner, based upon concern for fairness and justice.
  —*Abbas, AD*

Purposes of Law

- **To establish standards:** Laws establish the standards as a guidepost for minimally acceptable behavior in the society; but not unacceptable behaviors that injure a person or damage their property, e.g. crime.

- **To maintain orders:** Laws help in maintaining order by establishing standards. These are important in civil society.
- **To resolve disputes:** Society, a group of people living with different needs, wants, values and views have some or other forms of disputes. Laws resolve those disputes formally.
- **To protect liberties and rights:** Laws protect the liberties and rights of persons from violation from persons, organization.
- **To safeguard and protect the interest of people:** Laws safeguard and protect the interest of people through its judicial machinery and Acts.

Sources of Laws

- **Constitutional law:** The Constitution defines various fundamental rights, directive principles, and duties of citizens. There are six fundamental rights in our constitution. These are right to equality, freedom, right against exploitation, religion, cultural and educational rights, and the right to constitutional remedies. Violations result in punishments as prescribed in Indian Penal Code, subject to the discretion of the judiciary.
- **Statutory laws:** The elected legislative bodies of State or statutory (administrative) bodies formulated these laws such as Indian Nursing Council and passed by the legislation of the state.
- **Administrative laws:** These laws consist of rules and regulation established by administrative agencies and the executive branch of a government execute it.
- **Common laws:** It is a body of legal principles, created by judicial decisions made in the courts.

Types of Laws

There are various ways of classifying laws. The most common laws are civil and criminal laws.

Civil Laws

Civil laws are the laws of private rights and duties, dealing with disputes between individuals and organizations. These disputes are:

Breach of contract: A contract means an agreement between parties. The legal agreement is enforced by the law and those who sign the agreement enter into a legal contract. Law decides the breach of contract and penalty for the breach according to its severity.

Tort: Tort means a legal wrong committed intentionally or unintentionally against a person or rights, or property. Torts further categorizes into unintentional, intentional and quasi-intentional torts **(Fig. 5.1)**.
- **Unintentional torts:** These are accidental actions that cause injury to another person or property due to negligence and malpractice. *Negligence* is a tort which depends on the existence of a breach of the duty of care owed by one person to another. *Malpractice* is a type of negligence, a legal act performed improperly (misfeasance), or a failure to act results in harm to another party (nonfeasance).
- **Intentional torts:** These torts are a deliberate action to cause injury to a person or property. These torts can fall under criminal law depending on the violation of the standards of care. Assault, battery, false imprisonments are the intentional torts.
  - *Assault* is a form of a crime of violence against another person.
  - *The battery* is intentional touching or doing unjustified harm. The battery also differs from assault in that it does not require the victim to be in apprehension of harm. It may be criminal or civil.
  - *False imprisonment* is intentionally restraining another person without any legal right to do so.
- **Quasi-intentional torts:** It usually involves situations of communication; often violates a person's reputation, personal privacy or civil rights. Defamation, slander, libel, and fraud are some of the quasi-intentional torts.
- *Defamation* means issuing a false statement about another person to harm intentionally or unintentionally.
- *Slander* involves making of defamatory statements usually an oral (spoken) representation that harms a third person's reputation. *Libel* involves making of defamatory statements in a printed medium such as magazine or newspaper. *Fraud* is a crime or offense of deliberately deceiving another to damage another- to obtain property or services.

Criminal Laws

Criminal laws are the laws of public rights and duties; creates and controls the wrongs committed by a person(s). Crime is the act of a violation of duty or breach of the law, punishable by the state by fine or imprisonment. Criminal law involves the imposing state sanctions for crimes committed by individuals so that society can achieve justice and peaceable social order.

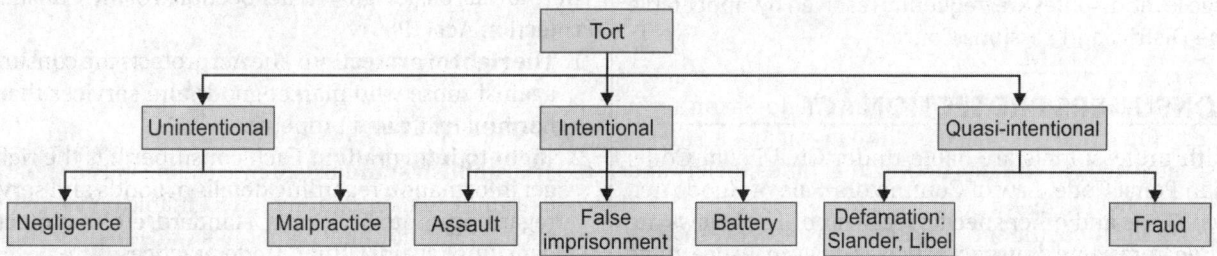

Fig. 5.1: Types of tort laws.

The Judicial Process

Both civil and criminal laws are set up under the Indian Penal Code, Criminal Procedure Code, etc. Hearing of all civil and criminal cases is at three levels: at national level by the Supreme Court of India, at state level by the High Courts, at district level by the district courts and the session courts.

The Supreme Court of India

The Supreme Court of India is the National Judiciary. It has its original, appellate and advisory jurisdiction. Article 32 of the Indian Constitution gives extensive original jurisdiction to the Supreme Court regarding enforcing fundamental rights. The head of the Supreme Court is Chief Justice, who works with 30 judges and more.

It issues directions, orders or writs, including writs like habeas corpus, mandamus, prohibition, quo warrantor. The Supreme Court has the power to direct transfer of any civil or criminal case from state court to another or from a court subordinate to another State High Court.

Public Interest Litigation (PIL): The Supreme Court also deals with matters of interest public at large. In that case, an individual or a group of people can file a Writ Petition at the filing counter or can address the letter to the Chief Justice.

The High Court

The High Court is the State Judiciary. There are 24 High Courts in all states and union territory of India, and out of that four high courts are shared or common. Each High Court comprises of 94 judges including 23 additional judges. Each High Court has powers of jurisprudence on all lower courts within its jurisdiction. It deals with civil and criminal cases if lower courts are not able to satisfy the clients.

District and Session Courts

The District and Session Courts comprise the highest level of courts in a District for Civil and Criminal cases respectively and may be trial courts of original jurisdiction, applying both federal and state laws.

Each district of the State has a District and Session Judge. A District court deals with civil cases and Sessions Courts with criminal cases. Sub-district or munsif courts deal with civil cases. The courts of Magistrates functioning under the Sessions Judge deals with lesser criminal cases. Panchayat or Lok Adalat deals with the disputes of the village level; disputes are frequently resolved by, appealable to the District and Sessions Court.

CONSUMERS PROTECTION ACT

Health professionals are liable under Civil Penal Code, Indian Penal Code, Law of Contractors, Sale of Goods Act, Law of Torts and other specific legislation. These laws are not free from some drawbacks such as delay in justice, huge legal fees, and limited access to courts, difficulties involved in proving both negligence and cause.

The Consumers Protection Act (COPRA) 1986 of India is a legal instrument aimed at better social justice. Indian Parliament passed this Act to safeguard and protect the interest of consumers. CPA aims at simplification of procedures for seeking redressal of grievances of patients or their relatives without any court fee in all over India except in the State of Jammu and Kashmir. Main objectives of CPA are: (i) to protect the rights of consumers, (ii) to redress their complaints, and (iii) to resolve their disputes. It is preventive and compensatory.

Who are Consumers?

"Consumer" refers to "goods" and "services" and has different definitions.

About "Goods", the consumers are the persons who either buy/agree to buy any goods/already paid the amount/partly paid/promised to pay or any user other than persons who buy goods/use goods with the approval of purchaser.

About "Service", the consumers are the persons who hire or utilize any services either paid/promise to pay/partly paid/partially promised/under any system of deferred payment or any beneficiary other than hired/availed services with the approval of such person. The patients are service consumers in healthcare settings. These consumers fall into three categories:

Patients of Government Hospitals

Patients availing free medical care in general wards are not consumers, but patients availing medical care in private wards of these hospitals are consumers as they are hiring services for a consideration.

Patients of Charitable Hospitals

The patient of charitable hospitals is a consumer when he pays for the medical treatment either partially or in full, but he is not a consumer when he does not pay at all.

Patients of Nursing Homes and Private Practitioners

Patients of nursing homes and private practitioners are covered under the act because they satisfy the definition of consumer and service as given under section 2 (1) (d) (ii) and 2(1)(0).

Basic Rights of Consumers

There are six basic rights under Section 6 of the Consumers Protection Act (1986):
1. **The right of protection:** The Act protects the consumers against those who market goods and services that are harmful to life and property.
2. **Right to information:** Each consumer has the right to get information regarding details of goods and services regarding its quality, purity, standard, etc. to protect the consumer against unfair trade practices.

3. **The right of assurance:** The consumers have the right to get assurance regarding goods and services for its access at competitive prices.
4. **The right of interest:** The consumers have the right to hear/assure to consider their interest at the appropriate forum.
5. **Right to seek grievance redressal:** The consumers have the right to file a complaint against any unfair practices and their exploitation.
6. **Right to consumer education:** The consumers have the right to get information regarding their rights.

Grievance Redressal Mechanism

Grievance mechanism under CPA operates at three different levels, district, State, and Central levels:

District Consumer Court/Forum

It is set up in each district of State by State Government. The district judge heads it. The consumer can approach district consumer court if the complaint involves the payment of compensation up to ₹ 20 lakh.

State Consumer Commission

It is set up by each State. Consumers can file complain if compensation for complaint is above ₹ 20 lakh but less than one crore.

National Consumer Commission

It is set up by the Central Government. Consumers can file complain if compensation is above one crore.

A consumer can file complaint against to whom goods or services sold/delivered, agree to sell/deliver, or such services provide/ agreed to provide or the person who is working in a Voluntary Consumer Organization/in Central Government, State/UT Administration/consumers of same interest, and the legal heir of representatives upon the death of the consumer.

The complaint must file within 2 years from the date on which cause of action has arisen. However, a complaint can be entertained after the period if the complainant had sufficient cause for not filing the complaint within such period by recording its reason for condoning such delay.

RIGHTS OF SPECIAL GROUPS

Rights of Children

In India, children population (472 million ages 0–18 years) represents more than 39% of the total population of the country according to the 2011 census. They belong to a vulnerable group and need special protection and care; to protect from exploitation, prevent from diseases, to fulfil their basic survival needs, and education needs; freedom from any discrimination and so on. The description of these rights is in The Indian Constitution and The Indian Penal Code, and other Acts/scheme framed time to time which specifies the rights of children such as the Juvenile Justice Act (2000), Prohibition of Child Marriage Act (2006), and the Integrated Child Protection Scheme.

The constitution, children, have the following rights:
- Compulsory free elementary education up to 6 years of age
- Education opportunity by parents up to age 14 years
- Equal treatment to children for their development without any discrimination
- The protection of children against exploitation, risky health employment, social injustice, and any violence
- Basic needs and human rights protection for all juvenile children of 16 years of age under the Juvenile Justice Act
- Protection of boys (up to 21 years of age) and girls (up to 18 years of age) against child marriage under the Prohibition of Child Marriage Act (2006)
- Provision of child safety under Integrated Child Protection Scheme (2009–10)

Indian Penal Code (1860) covers the protection of children:
- Protection against any criminal action by the normal children below seven years and mentally disabled children up to 12 years
- Protection of boys (of 16 years) and girls (of 18 years) against offenses like kidnapping, abduction, etc.
- Protection of an unmarried girl child below 16 years against giving consent for sex.

Rights of Women

Constitutional Rights

These are the rights provided under the provision of the constitution of India to safeguard and protect the dignity of women and to uplift their status.

Under Fundamental Rights

a. **Rights for equality:** Article 14 mentions equality before the law for women
b. **Prohibition of discrimination:** There is no discrimination of women concerning caste creed, religion, place of birth or any other as per Article 15
c. **The right of positive discrimination in favor of women:** There is special provision for women and children by the State
d. **Rights for equality in public employment:** There is a provision of equal opportunities without any discrimination as per Article 16 (1,2)
e. **The right of personal or life freedom:** All have right of personal or life liberty as per procedure under Article 21
f. Right to the prohibition of traffic in human beings and forced labor under Article 23.

Under the Directive Principles of State Policy

a. Rights of equality in livelihood, equal pay for equal work, and not to abuse the health and strength of workers under Article 39
b. The Right of justice and conditions of work and maternity relief under Article 42.
c. The right of uniformity in civil code for all under Article 44.

Under Fundamental Duties of Citizens
a. The right of the dignity of women under Article 51-A (e)
b. Reservation of one-third seat for women belong to SC/ST category in the direct election in every Panchayat, and Municipality, 1/3rd of offices of chairpersons for women in Panchayat and Municipality under Article 243 (D and T).

Legal Rights to Women

These are the legislative measures enacted by the State to ensure equal rights to women against any social discrimination or any violence especially to working women under Indian Penal Code and special laws for crimes against women.

Crimes Covered Under Indian Penal Code (IPC)
a. **Rape:** A rapist under Section 376 IPC shall be punished by imprisonment either for a term of not less than seven years or may be extended to life imprisonment, and shall also be liable to fine
b. **Kidnapping and abduction for different purposes:** Under Section 363-373, any person who is abducting a minor/women for begging/prostitution, will award punishment imprisonment and monetary
c. **Women homicide for dowry, dowry deaths or attempts:** If a homicide occurs by women within seven years of marriage; the guilty will award punishment with imprisonment under Section 302/304-B IPC
d. **Mental and physical torture:** There is a provision that a person either a husband or relative for mentally or physically torturing women will get an award of punishment either imprisonment or monetary fine under Section 498-A IPC
e. **Molestation:** If a person intentionally tough or likely to outrage is liable to get punishment either imprisonment or monetary fine under Section 354 IPC
f. **Sexual harassment:** If a person intends to insult the modesty of a woman verbally or any other communication or interfere with her privacy, is liable to get punishment either imprisonment or monetary fine under Section 509 IPC

Special Laws for Crimes Against Women
a. **The Dowry Prohibition Act (1961):** This act has the provision to prohibit any request, payment or acceptance of dowry at, before or any time after marriage from women is liable to get punishment either imprisonment or a monetary fine
b. **The Suppression Immoral Traffic Act (SITA) (1956):** This Act is premier legislation to prevent trafficking for commercial sexual exploitation and deals with the status of sex workers. According to this Act, prostitutes can practice their trade privately but cannot legally solicit customers in public, but organized prostitution (brothels, prostitution rings, pimping, etc.) means of living is illegal
c. **Domestic Violence Act (2005):** This Act protects women from all forms of domestic violence including physical, verbal, emotional, sexual, or economic actual or threatening
d. **The Act of the Sexual Harassment of Women at Workplace (Prevention, Prohibition and Redressal) (2013):** This Act protects women at their workplace either public or private, school or college students, patients in hospitals from sexual harassment
e. **The Hindu Marriage Act (1955):** This act was enacted to amend and codify the law relating to marriage among Hindus. This act had the provision of monogamy and allowed divorce on certain specified grounds and also provided equal rights to both man and woman for marriage and divorce
f. **The Marriage Laws (Amendment) Bill (2013):** This Act is the amendment in Hindu Marriage Act, 1955, in Chapter II, section 13B, subsection (2); and Special Marriage Act, 1954, in chapter III, section 28, in subsection (2) to provide a better safety to wife and adequate maintenance of children of diverse
g. **The Maternity Benefit Act, 1961 (Amended in 2016):** This Act protects the employment of women serving an organization having 10 or more employees during the maternity period and provides maternity and other benefits. Amendments in this Act have been made several times to make it more beneficial to women workers. According to the Maternity Benefit (Amendment) Bill, 2016, the maternity leaves are extended up to 26 weeks for two surviving children and 12 weeks for more than two surviving children. The adopting or commissioning mothers also have the provision of availing 12 weeks maternity leave. There is also a compulsory provision of Creche in an organization having 50 and more than 50 employees
h. **MTP Act (1971) and MTP Amendment Act (2002):** The MTP, 1971 Act has a provision of preventing illegal abortion; to provide for the termination of certain pregnancies by registered medical practitioners. This Act was amended in 18th December 2002 and called The Medical Termination of Pregnancy Amendment Act (2002) with the substitution of a mentally ill person; a specified place for termination of pregnancies, and award of the punishment
i. **The Equal Remuneration Act (1976):** This Act has the provision for equal remuneration to men and women workers for the same or similar work and prevention of discrimination, on the ground of sex, against women in employment and service conditions
j. **National Commission for Women Act (1990):** This Act was enacted on 30th August 1990 to investigate and examine, matters relating to safeguards provided for women under the Constitution and other laws; to review, monitor, evaluate these laws time to time and recommend amendments and to suggest remedial legislative measures against affected women
k. **PCPNDT Act (2003):** The Pre-Conception and Pre-Natal Diagnostic Techniques (Prohibition of Sex Selection) Act is to prohibit sex selection after conception also to

regulate prenatal diagnostic techniques to detect genetic abnormalities, metabolic disorders, chromosomal abnormalities, certain congenital malformation, sex-linked disorders. To prevent misuse of using sex selection for female feticide, the Act has penalty provision under various sections

l. **Empowerment of Women (2016):** The national policy on the empowerment of women is ensuring equal rights and opportunities for women the family, community, and workplace. The priority areas include health, education, economy, agriculture, industry, labor, employment, service sector, science and technology, governance and decision making; violence against women, enabling environment, etc.

Rights of Aging People/Senior Citizen

Aging is a natural phenomenon characterized by many physical, physiological, psychological and social changes. According to Law in India, a person who is above 60 years of age is an elderly or a senior citizen. The population of elderly or old people in India is about 104 million (about 9% of total population) as per population census 2011 and expected to increase to 173 million by 2026 as per projection by UN Population Fund and HelpAge India. The elderly population above the age of 80 years is also growing fast and will increase Due to improving living conditions and lifestyle, advancement of health care, science, and technology, the estimated life expectancy at birth has increased to approximate 68 years and will increase in future. The age dependency is also increasing and is 14.2% in 2011 as compared to 10.9% in 2001.

Most of the older people have a locomotor and visual disability and at least is suffering from heart disease, hypertension, asthma, diabetes, and depression. Due to a change in social structure, most of the older people are living separately from their children, and are independent socially and financially. They face numerous difficulties in health and care, employment, financial, housing, social network, protection and so on. Other issues such as the social security system, health care, empowerment, and protection of fundamental rights need urgent attention. Hence, it is important to have sound policies and Laws and Acts to protect the elderly or senior citizens against diseases, isolation, elderly abuse, mistreatment, and crime. They need to engage for their active participation in society to lead a quality life.

The Ministry of Social Justice and Empowerment prepares policies and programs for the welfare and maintenance of senior citizens with the collaboration of State, NGOs, and societies and associations. There are the following rights of elderly or aging people:

Constitutional Rights

a. **Right to work, education, and public assistance:** According to Article 41, there is a provision to protect the right to work, education and providing assistance to particular cases including during old age by the State within its capacity.

b. **Right to a standard of living and nutrition:** Article 47 has a provision to raise the standard of living and level of nutrition to improve the health by the State as its primary duty.

Legal Rights

a. **Personal Laws:** Under these laws, the moral duty of children to maintain their parents. These laws are different for different community, e.g.
   - *Hindu Law:* According to the Hindu Adoption and Maintenance Act (1956), it is an obligatory duty of both son and daughter to maintain their aged parents and ask for maintenance if, financial not able to maintain
   - *Muslim Law:* According to Mullah, it is obligatory of both son and daughter to provide maintenance to their father, mother, grandfather, and grandmother
   - *Christian and Parsi Law:* The parents through the Criminal Procedure Code can apply for obligatory maintenance from their son, daughter, including a married daughter

b. **Criminal Procedure Code (1973):** As per this Code, the children, both son and daughter including married daughter have their duty to maintain their parents. It applies to all irrespective of religions and communities.

Government Protection

a. **National Policy for Older Persons (1999):** There is the provision of:
   - *Welfare services for the elderly:*
     - The pension fund for security purpose of people of unorganized sector
     - Old age homes
     - Resource centers and reemployment bureaus
     - Railway/airfare travel concession
     - Legislation for compulsory elderly care
   - *National Council for Older Persons:* This council to set up the Agewell Foundation to make provision of welfare measures to elderly at the national level by The Ministry of Justice and Empowerment.
   - *Helpline for elderly:* Government takes the initiative to provide round the clock helpline for the elderly.
   - Settlement of pension, provident funds, and other benefits at the earliest on superannuation
   - High priority to the health needs of the elderly
   - Discount in income under Income Tax Act
   - Providing Insurance schemes by LIC especially for elderly
   - Annapurna Yojana to provide food of 10 kg for the neglected aged persons
   - Provision of house construction under government scheme (10%) for both urban and rural poor on easy loan

b. **The Maintenance and Welfare of the Parents and Senior Citizen Act (2007):** This Act is applicable

for children (son, daughter, grandson, and grand daughter), heirs, and children living abroad to provide:
- The maintenance of parents and senior citizen of family members who are not able to maintain themselves. The maintenance includes the provision of basic amenities such as food, clothing, residence and medical and treatment
- State level, provision of old age homes of 150 bedded for neglected elderly

c. **The National Policy on Senior Citizens, 2011:** The policy focus on:
- *Income security*
  - Minimum ₹ 1000/- per month for elderly from BPL group under Indira Gandhi National Old Age Pension Scheme. There is a provision of additional pension in case of disability or loss of an adult child
  - A public distribution system for BPL senior citizen
  - Special provision in income tax
  - Provision of loans on reasonable interest rates
- *Health care protection*
  - High priority in health care needs
  - Focus on primary health care
  - Provision of special screening by ASHA for 80+ aged
  - Strengthening the family system to be sensitive towards the care of elderly
  - Health insurances
  - Healthcare fund to meet the expenses after retirement/during old age
  - Special emphasis on mental health problems such as dementia, Alzheimer's disease
  - Care of eyesight problems under National Programme for Control of Blindness
  - Establishment of national and regional institutes for geriatric care by the professionals
  - Expansion of National Programme for Health Care of the Elderly
  - Health insurance coverage especially for 80+ years old
- *Safety and security protection:* Appropriate provision for any elderly abuse and crime against elderly especially widows, disabled, and residing alone, helpline, and police vigilance
- *Shelter protection:* Special provision in a housing scheme, and other facilities
- Post-retirement/re-employment opportunities
- Welfare services such as welfare fund, services by Voluntary organizations, eligibility for government schemes, etc.
- Establishment of National Council

Rights of People Living with HIV/AIDS in India

Constitutional Rights

Under Fundamental Rights

People living with HIV/AIDS have the same rights as all Indian citizens are entitled to fundamental human rights guaranteed by law, without discrimination. These rights are right to education, employment, health, travel, marriage, procreation, privacy, social security, scientific benefits, asylum, etc.

a. **The right of equality of treatment:** Article 14 guarantees the right to equality of treatment to a person suffering from any ailment; nobody can refuse to give treatment to a patient by HIV/AIDS otherwise it is considered a case of discrimination
b. **Right to confidentiality and right to disclosure:** A patient with HIV/AIDS has a right to keep his/her HIV/AIDS status confidential or right to disclose.
c. **Right to protect against discrimination:** Article 15 and 16 protect a person with HIV/AIDS against discrimination.
d. **Employment right and right against discrimination:** HIV/AIDS clients have equal right for job opportunities and employment and cannot be discriminated on the basis of his HIV/AIDS status.
e. **Right to liberty:** Article 21 of the constitution protects the right to life and liberty and ensures their rights to privacy.

Under the Directive Principles of State Policy

a. **Rights of equality in livelihood:** All Indian citizens including HIV/AIDS clients have the right to adequate means of livelihood under Article 39.
b. **Right for justice and humane conditions of work:** HIV/AIDS clients have the right for justice and sympathetic working conditions under Article 42.
c. **Right to improve public health:** Article 47 directs the State to improve public health.

Legal Provision

1. **Drugs and Cosmetic Act (1940 and 2005) and Drug and Cosmetic Rules, 1993:** According to this Act, it is compulsory to test blood and blood products for transfusion for HIV.
2. **Immoral Trafficking Prevention Act (1986):** There is a compulsory medical examination for detection of HIV/AIDS and provisions for compulsory testing of sex workers under this Act.
3. **HIV and AIDs Bill (2016):** It is the amendment of previous HIV/AIDs bill (2014). The Bill is concerning preventing and controlling the spread of HIV and AIDS such as:
   a. *Prohibition of discrimination against HIV positive persons and those living with them:* Positive HIV/AIDs persons and those living with them have protection against any discrimination regarding employment, health care services, residing and renting property, and insurance.
   b. *Right to live in a shared household:* HIV/AIDs positive persons of less than 18 years old have the right to reside in the shared household.
   c. *Prohibition of publishing information or advocating feelings:* No individual can publish or advocate any hatred feeling against HIV positive and those living with them.

d. *Disclosure of HIV status:* No person can disclose HIV status of HIV positive person without his informed consent or if required by a court order. The organization shall keep the records confidently by using data protection measures.

Rights of Persons with Disabilities

According to the Rights of Persons with Disabilities Act, 2016 (No. 49 of 2016), the persons with disability have the following rights:

1. **The right to equality and nondiscrimination:** All persons with disability have the right of equality regarding maintaining dignity and respect for their integrity; freedom to express views by disabled children on the matter affecting, providing an appropriate environment, and personal liberty.
2. **Right to live and social security:** All persons with disabilities have the right for an adequate standard of living and the right to live and have access to all support services. No child with a disability shall separate from his or her parents on the ground of disability except on order of the competent court. The court will decide in case the parents are unable to take care of the disabled child.
3. **Protection from cruelty and inhuman treatment:** All persons with disability have the right to protection against torture, cruelty, inhuman or degrading treatment by taking various measures.
4. **Protection from abuse, violence, and exploitation:** All persons with disability have the right for protection from any abuse, violence, and exploitation by taking various measures; provide legal remedies and take appropriate measures to rescue, protect and rehabilitate victims of such incidents. He/she has the right to apply for protection, the right to free legal aid, and the right to file a complaint.
5. **Right for protection and safety in difficult situations:** Persons with disabilities have equal protection and safety in situations of risk, armed conflict, humanitarian emergencies and natural disasters (under the Disaster Management Act, 2005 for the safety and protection of persons with disabilities).
6. **Rights of education regarding reproductive and family planning:** Persons with disabilities have the right to seek information regarding reproductive and family planning. Any medical procedure that leads to infertility cannot perform without his or her free and informed consent.
7. **The right of getting accessibility in voting:** It shall ensure that all polling stations are accessible to persons with disabilities and all materials regarding the electoral process are easily understandable and accessible to them.
8. **Access to justice:** Persons with disabilities have the right to file complain and access any court, tribunal, authority, commission or any other body having judicial without discrimination by disability. Under the Legal Services Authorities Act, 1987, they have access to any scheme, program, facility or service offered by them equally with others.
9. **The right of legal capacity and equal recognition:** Persons with disabilities have the right, equally with others, regarding property, financial affairs, and have the right to equal recognition everywhere.
10. **Provision for guardianship:** There is a provision of limited guardianship which means a joint decision between the guardian and the person with a disability for a limited period.
11. **Right to education:** All educational institutions shall provide inclusive education to children with disabilities and shall take specific measures to promote and facilitate inclusive education, adult education, and continuing education programs equally with others.
12. **Free education for children with benchmark disabilities:** There is a provision of free education for children with benchmark disabilities between the age of six to eighteen years under Rights of Children to Free and Compulsory Education Act, 2009.
13. **Nondiscrimination in employment:** All persons with a disability shall not discriminate against any matter relating to employment, and there is the provision of loans at concessional rates to facilitate and support employment for them.
14. **Provision of additional benefits:** There is a provision of additional benefits for persons with benchmark disabilities and those with high support needs such as reservation in higher education; an upper age relaxation of five years for admission, in government jobs, in the allocation of land, poverty alleviation schemes, etc.

CHAPTER HIGHLIGHTS

- Law is a body of rules to regulate external human conduct, and the sources of laws are a constitution, statutory bodies, administrative agencies, and court decisions.
- Commonly, there are two types of laws—civil and criminal. The civil laws deal with disputes between individuals, and organizations arise due to a breach of contracts and torts.
- Tort means a legal wrong committed intentionally or unintentionally against a person or rights, or property.
- Assault, Battery, and false imprisonment are examples of intentional torts. And Defamation and Slander fall under the category of quasi-intentional torts.
- The judiciary system to deal with all civil and criminal cases are by the Supreme Court, High Courts, District Courts and Session Courts at national, state, and district level respectively.
- Consumers Protection Act (1986) is a legal instrument to safeguard and protect the interest of consumers.
- There are laws under the constitution of India, The Indian Penal Code, and Acts to protect the rights of people of India and special groups like children, women, people who have HIV/AIDs, disabled and aging people.

REVIEW QUESTIONS

I. Essay Type Questions
1. Define law. Write the importance of laws in nursing.
2. Describe different types of laws.
3. Discuss in detail the Consumers Protection Act.
4. Explain the judicial process of India.
5. Describe the important rights of women.

II. Short Notes
1. Sources of laws
2. Basic rights of consumers
3. Grievance redressal mechanism
4. Rights of children

III. Multiple Choice Questions
1. A legal document that has rules governing a particular kind of activity is:
   a. Morality
   b. Value
   c. Law
   d. Tort
2. The law deals with a legal wrong committed intentionally against a person, his rights, or property is:
   a. Civil law
   b. Constitution law
   c. Criminal law
   d. Contract law
3. An offensive touching of another person is a type of intentional tort:
   a. Assault
   b. Battery
   c. Malpractice
   d. Invasion of privacy
4. Making defamatory statements to harm a third person's reputation is:
   a. Fraud
   b. Libel
   c. Slander
   d. False imprisonment
5. Which of the following law describes fundamental rights, directives principles, and duties of citizens?
   a. Administrative
   b. Common
   c. Statutory
   d. Constitution
6. Which one of the following statements relates to quasi-intentional torts?
   a. Deliberate action to cause injury to a person
   b. The situation that violets the reputation of a person
   c. Accidental action that harms a person or his property
   d. A Legal Act performed improperly
7. Which court at district level deals with criminal cases?
   a. Session Court
   b. District Court
   c. High Court
   d. Lok Adalat
8. Who are *NOT* the service consumers under the Consumer Protection Act?
   a. The patient availing services in nursing homes
   b. The patients availing services in charitable hospitals
   c. The patients availing services in private wards of government hospitals
   d. The patients availing free services in general wards of government hospitals
9. Which one of the following statements means "Right to Information" to a service consumer?
   a. Getting details of services regarding quality, quantity, purity, and standard
   b. Getting information regarding their rights
   c. Getting protection against the services harmful to their life and property
   d. Getting consideration of their interest at the appropriate forum
10. Up to what age the protection of a girl child is against marriage under the Prohibition of Child Marriage Act (2006)?
    a. 16 years
    b. 18 years
    c. 21 years
    d. 23 years

Answer Keys
1. c   2. a   3. b   4. c   5. d   6. b   7. a
8. d   9. a   10. b

SUGGESTED READING

1. Aggarwal A, Chaudhari AP. Medical Profession and Consumer Protection Act. New Delhi: Aapee Publications; 1998.
2. Alexander CH. International Law in India. International & Comparative Law Quarterly. 1952;1(3):289-300.
3. Atkinson LD, Murray ME. Fundamentals of nursing: A nursing process approach. Macmillan Pub. Co.; 1994.
4. Atkinson JM. Private and public protection: Civil mental health legislation. Dunedin Academic Press Ltd; 2006.
5. Banerjee AK. Digest on the Law of Injunctions. New Delhi: Ashok Law House; 1992.
6. Garner BA(Ed). A Dictionary of Basic Legal Terms. West Group; 1999. pp. 120.
7. Burns H. Patient safety: Developing policies for engagement in the prevention of harm to patients. J Am Assoc Coll Nurs. 2004;20(1):4-75.
8. Chaudhuri PK. Medical Profession and Consumer Protection Act. J Indian Med Assoc. 1993;91(7):168-9.
9. Carmi A, Schneider S. Nursing Law and Ethics. Springer. 1985.
10. Edwards RB. Privacy and the Right to Information Act, 2005. [online] Available from http://ijme.in/articles/privacy-and-the-right-to-information-act-2005/?galley=ht [Last accessed November, 2019].
11. Croke EM. Nurses, negligence, and malpractice: An analysis based on more than 250 cases against nurses. Am J Nurs. 2003;103(9):54-63.
12. Furlong S, Glover D. Legal accountability in changing practice. Nursing Times. 1998;94(39):61-2.
13. Enzman Hagedorn MI, Gardner SL. Legal issues in neonatal nursing: considerations for staff nurses and advanced practice nurses. J Obstet Gynecol Neonatal Nurs. 1999;28(3):320-30.
14. Goyal RC. Is a patient a consumer? J Acad Hosp Adm. 1992;4(2):17-25.
15. Heinemann A, Tsokos M, Püschel K. Medico-legal aspects of pressure sores. Leg Med (Tokyo). 2003;5(Suppl 1):S263-6.
16. Jesani A. Laws and health care providers. Centre for enquiry into health and allied themes, Mumbai. 1996.

17. Kozier B, Erb GL, Blais K, et al. Fundamentals of Nursing: Concept, Process, and Practice, 5th edition. Menlo Park: Addition Wesley; 1995.
18. KK Murthy. Medical Negligence and the Law. Indian J Med Ethics. 2007;4(3):116-118.
19. Ramanathan U. Tort Law in India. http://ielrc.org/Content/a0206.pdf. [Accessed on 15.12.2019].
20. Regu M. The nurse, the patient and the law. Nursing J India. 1996;87:273-6.
21. Singh G. Law of Consumer Protection. Jaipur: Bharat Law Publications.
22. Stanford University. The definition of morality. Stanford Encyclopedia of Philosophy. [online] Available from http://plato.stanford.edu/entries/morality-definition/ [Last accessed October, 2019]. Indian Penal Code. [online] Available from http://www.indianlawcds.com/Criminalbareacts/IPC.htm [Last accessed October, 2019].

6 Legal Aspects and Legal Issues in Nursing

CHAPTER OUTLINE

- Legal Aspects of Nursing
  - Importance of Law in Nursing
  - Legal Liabilities in Nursing
  - Legal Issues in Nursing
- Regulation of Nursing Practice
- Legal Safeguard for Nurses in Practice
- Legal Responsibilities in Nursing
- Dealing in Specific Conditions
- Dealing with Medicolegal Cases

LEARNING OUTCOMES

After completion of this chapter, the learner will be able to:
- Understand concept and purposes of law
- Describe different types and sources of law
- Appreciate the importance of law in nursing
- Describe legal liabilities and issues in nursing
- Enumerate laws and issues in specific conditions
- Discuss the regulation of nursing practice
- Explain important legal safeguard for nurses in practice
- Discuss legal responsibilities in nursing
- Describe the ways of dealing with medicolegal cases

KEY TERMS

Law, legal liability, legal safeguard, legal issues, regulation, specific conditions, medicolegal cases

INTRODUCTION

The nurses in the modern era have multifunction in their work setting. In spite of having in the job description, these job activities are not explicitly defined. There is job ambiguity, so in that situation, they need to know about the law and legal issues that can have a positive impact on them in day to day functioning and on their clients who are the recipient of their car. Moreover, in the competitive world and use of advanced technology, nurses have multiple and expanded roles to render high-quality nursing care. To avoid legal suits and to protect clients, nurses should have a good understanding of legal issues, ethical and professional roles, and nursing regulatory mechanisms.

LEGAL ASPECT IN NURSING

Importance of Law in Nursing

Laws are important in nursing as the law protects patients/clients against deliberate and inadvertent injury by a nurse, and also protects nurses against suits if she renders right care.

1. To provide a framework to establish nursing actions in the care of clients those are legal
2. To differentiate the nurses' responsibilities from other health professionals
3. To demarcate the boundaries of independent nursing actions
4. To assist in maintaining standards of nursing practice by making nurses accountable under the law
5. To safeguard and protect the right of self and clients.

Legal Liabilities in Nursing

Liability is a form of a hindrance that causes individuals at a disadvantage. It is a state of accountability or responsibility for doing something. Legal liability is concerned with legal accountability or responsibility for something or any action. Nurses are legally liable or responsible/accountable to render care to the assigned patient. The person is made legally responsible for his or actions. Legal liability involves four elements to establish proof of harming patient: the duty of care, breach of duty, causation, and damages.

1. **The duty of care:** Duty of care is a legal obligation to follow the standard in caring patients.

2. **Breach of duty:** Breach of duty means the failing on the part of nurses to act/care as per standard.
3. **Causation:** Causation is an element of liability to prove that the failure to meet the standard of care which caused the harm to the patient (proof).
4. **Damages:** Damage is a term used for the actual harm to a patient resulting from a definite cause.

Legal Issues in Nursing

The legal issue is a dispute or a legal question that need to deal in the court for deciding as per civil or criminal law. The civil laws resolve most of the legal issues of unintentional, intentional, or quasi-intentional torts, and breach of duty. The major legal issues in nursing practice are as follows (Fig. 6.1):

Nursing Negligence

Nursing negligence is the failure by the nurse to take the appropriate action to protect the patient from harm. A nurse who fails to put side-rails on the sides of the bed of a confused patient or fails to initiate standard safety precautions to prevent patient harm is by the charge of negligence under civil law. If the negligence is gross, complete disregard of client's life dealt under both civil and criminal law. The common examples of negligence are:
- Burns resulting by use of hot water bottle, applying heating pads, administering steam inhalation, and sitz bath
- The incidence of fall among elderly, sedated, preoperatively, postoperatively, confused, dizzy, blind, and semiconscious when nursed without fixing bed side-railing
- Patients had fallen due to a slippery or waxed floor
- Administration of wrong medications, wrong dose of medication, to wrong patients
- Unskilled nurses not able to assess symptoms of shock, respiratory distress
- Injury to patients by using defective apparatus or appliances
- Loss of the unconscious patient's belongings.

Malpractice

Malpractice is negligence by nurses causing an injury or harm to the patients due to professional misconduct or lack of skill in performing standards of care. Nurses need to comply six International "Patient Safety Goals": identifying patients correctly, improving communication, safety of high alert medications, eliminating wrong-site, wrong patient, wrong procedure surgery, reducing the risk of hospital-acquired infections and reducing the risk of patient harm resulting from falls in the clinical practice; failing which can be resulted negligence or malpractice. The common malpractices in nursing practice can be:
- Failure to select an appropriate site by the nurse to administer an intramuscular injection that causes permanent damage to the patient's extremity.
- Failing to obtain a proper informed consent
- Failing to provide patient's safety: physical, social, spiritual, financial, political, emotional, occupational, psychological, educational or other types of failure.

Assault and Battery

Assault is an intentional, unlawful threat or attempts to make bodily contact with another person without that patient's consent. The unconsented touching of the body is the example of an Assult. The battery is an unjustified harmful or offensive touching with the intention of a crime or doing wrong with a person.

The common examples of assault in nursing practice can be threatening patient while not cooperating to do desirable care. Forcibly removing the patient's clothing, administering enema after the patient has refused it, or pushing a patient on to a chair is an example of the battery.

Restraints

Restraints are physical, chemical or environmental measures used to control the physical or behavioral activity of a person or a portion of his/her body. Physical restraints limit a client's least restraint practices and the right to refuse proposed interventions. For example use of the bed, rails are routine in many hospitals and other care facilities. Law requires to use that most involuntary medical restraint when ordered by a physician.

Defamation of Character

Defamation is an intentional tort or the issuance of a false statement about another person, causing harm to a person. Slander is oral defamation of character and libel is a defamation of character in writing. Defamation of character can be grounded both in criminal or civil law based on the amount of harm done to the plaintiff. Nurses who make false statements about the patient or their coworkers have the risk of being sued for slander or libel.

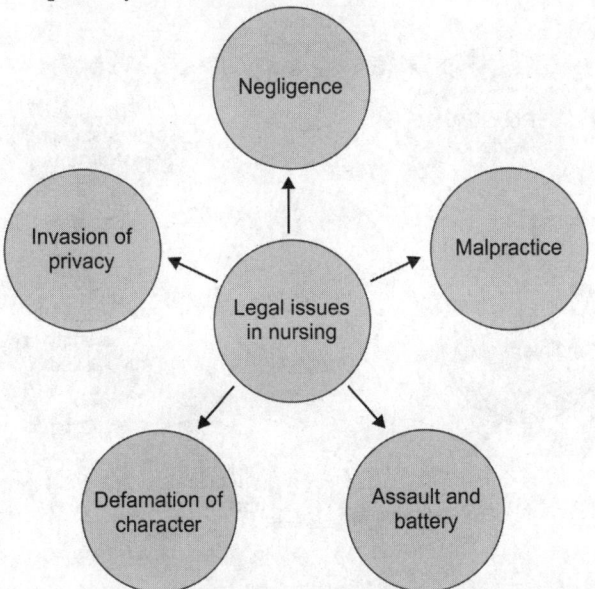

Fig. 6.1: Major legal issues in nursing practice.

Invasion of Privacy

All the information of the patient in any form is considered private, confidential, and legal. Privacy is a human right to maintain autonomy. Certain actions of nurse can constitute an invasion of privacy, e.g. unnecessary exposing patient while assisting for examination, discussing patient information with other people insisting patient to provide information not required, research without the consent of the patient. Any health information of the patient should not disclose unless required by law or given permission by the patient.

Fraud

A person who either practices without registration or fraudulently misrepresenting him or her to obtain a registration to practice nursing is fraud under the law. The misinterpretation of a procedure or treatment may also consider as a fraud.

REGULATION OF NURSING PRACTICE

Nurses are abiding by constitutional laws, professional laws, institutional policies, rules and regulations, standing orders, and precedents to practice nursing. These are:

Licensure to Practice

The INC is a statutory body, which regulates standards of education and practices through licensure. In 1948, the Nursing Council Act came into being as an autonomous body. It was constituted by the Central Government, with the purpose of safeguarding nursing education in the country.

Every State has its own State Nursing Council that pertains to the registration of nurses upon completion of training. On completing training, a nurse must register name and details with the State Nursing Council to indicate status as a registered nurse. Nurses employed for the nursing service required possessing a valid registration certificate issued by respective State Nursing Council with aims at protecting patients by providing qualified nurses. The nurse is responsible for obtaining registration in the respective State Nursing Registration Council. In most of the States, selection of staff nurses is through merit.

Professional Code of Conduct

Nurses abide by the INC Professional Code of Conduct and Code of Ethics, and Code of Ethics by Trained Nurses Association of India in sustaining ethical behavior of nurses (refer Chapter 4). On entering profession formally, they have to take the "Nightingale Pledge" which is a way of stating that they will adhere to professional conduct. They also have to abide by laws relating to Penalty for Misconducts defined by State Councils or Statutory Authorities. The State Council can withdraw the nurse's registration on a temporary or permanent basis and can charge by awarding formal warning, suspension, termination or court charge based on the severity of professional misconduct.

Standards of Care

Each institution/hospital needs to have the policies and procedures defining the standards of care for the nurses of different levels. The department must have policies and standard operative procedures to follow.

The standards of care are inbuilt in the INC code of ethics and professional conduct for nurses, followed by State Nursing Councils. Trained Nurses Association of India also believes that good health is a fundamental right of every person and it is the responsibility of health professionals including nurses to provide optimum health of each and promote high standards of health care to nursing practice.

Standing Orders/Instructions

Hospital policies having standing orders for nurses can regulate nursing practice. Nurses are required to execute prescribed orders. In case of emergency, if the doctor/medical personnel is not available, each nursing service area should have standing instruction or orders for the nurses to carry out.

LEGAL SAFEGUARD FOR NURSES IN PRACTICE

Nurses can legally protect themselves by adopting the following basic guidelines (Fig. 6.2):

Informed Consent

It is an agreement by a patient to accept a course of treatment or procedure after informing risks, benefits, and consequences. The requisites to obtain the informed consent are:
- A patient may give his/her consent if he/she of 18 years age or is a minor of 16 years. Consent if given under fear

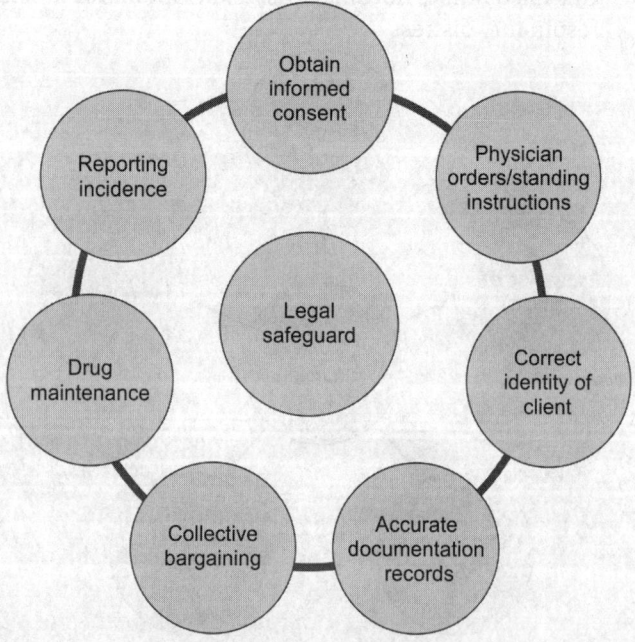

Fig. 6.2: Important legal safeguards for nurses.

of injury, under the misconception of fact is excluded under Section 90 of Indian Penal Code (IPC).
- The Act also excludes consent of a person of unsound mind, intoxicated, and a child below 14 years of age.
- The consent must be voluntary; no forceful measures may be used to obtain it.
- No one should be asked to sign an operation consent form before he has a full understanding of the procedure involved.

If the patient refuses the treatment, document it, sign and witness. In an emergency, if the patient is not in a situation to sign, and no one is with him, the medical officer can take responsibility for authorizing treatment. The nurse is to ensure that consent form is in the file of a patient before any diagnostic or treatment procedure.

Physician Orders/Standing Instructions

Nurses are legally responsible for following the orders of the physician. In that case, the nurse needs to seek clarification from a physician regarding the orders. A nurse who carries out inappropriate orders is liable for the harm experienced by the client.

Correct Identity

Nurses are accountable for the correct identity especially babies born in the hospital are correctly labeled at birth and to ensure that at no time they are placed in the wrong cot or handed to the wrong mothers. Ensure correct identification of patient before giving premedition and performing other procedures.

Accurate Documentation

Accurate and comprehensive records are essential. Records provide legal proof about the treatment of the patient. The records should be accurate, concise and up to date. Verbal orders if carried out should be documented or written as "told over the phone or verbal orders carried out," etc.

Negotiation

Negotiation in collective bargaining is a legal process in which the representative of organization or association of nurses negotiates with employers about matters such as wages, and conditions, etc. Through collective demands for adequate staffing, Indian nurses asserted their legal rights through negotiation with the government.

Drug Maintenance

Checking unlawful use of narcotic drugs is liable to drug dependence. Keep these drugs under lock and key.

Reporting Crimes, Torts, and Unsafe Practices

The nurse may report to a supervisor or other health team members about the practices that endanger the health and safety of patient, employee, or visitor. These are the means of identifying the risks. If the nurse is made responsible for a potential or harmful incidence, she should follow institution policy for reporting.

LEGAL RESPONSIBILITIES IN NURSING

Nurses working at different levels are required to discharge their responsibilities to avoid legal suits:

Administrative and Supervisory Level

The nurses working at the administrative and supervisory levels exhibit various legal responsibilities (**Fig. 6.3**):

a. **Appointment, assignment, and transfer of staff:** Nurse managers must be aware of legal restrictions affecting personnel appointment, placement, and assignment. Nurse supervisor must ensure the availability of staff and transferring nursing based on specialty and experience.

b. **Quality control management:** The nurse managers are required to review the nursing practice periodically and devise the methods for ensuring the quality care and supervisors need to implement. Prepare nursing manual, standard operative procedures, and ward policies, nursing audits and review time to time. These measures/methods must put into action.

c. **Material management:** The quality and quantity of equipment required for basic patient care is the prime responsibility of nurse managers. The supervisor must ensure the adequate supply and maintenance of equipment and supply.

d. **Maintaining proper documentation:** The nurse managers must exercise good record and reporting system. Staff should be instructed to maintain proper records and reports of patients. The staff meetings and rounds should be the regular feature of supervision.

e. **Maintaining public relation:** The nurse manager requires educating the staff to have a positive attitude

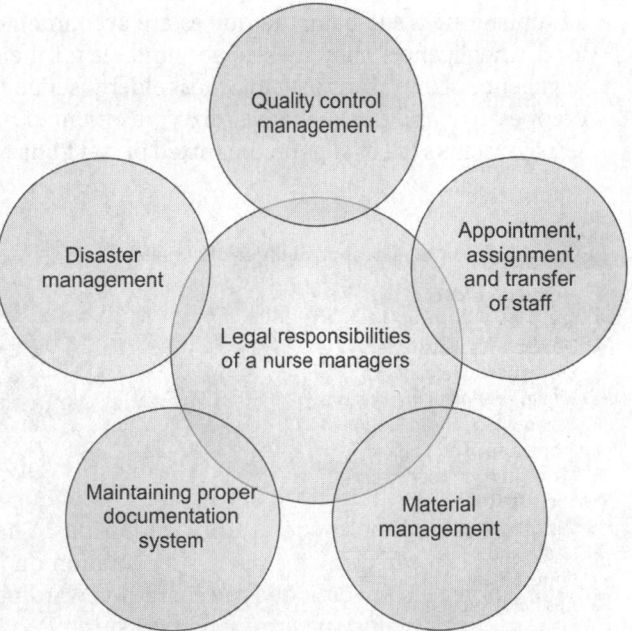

Fig. 6.3: Legal responsibilities of nurse managers.

and good communication with patients, their relatives, and team members.

f. **Disaster management**: Keep a disaster management team ready, in case of any disaster. Prepare and adhere to policies related to disaster management.

g. **Staff management**: Display written instructions in all the nursing units for necessary guidance and protection of staff regarding legal issues. Nurse managers must organize training programs and special lectures to update knowledge and skills of nurses and supervisors on legal aspects in nursing.

At Operational Level

Nurses at the operational level must take great cautions while working. She has legal responsibilities on the following areas **(Box 6.1)**.

a. **Carrying out physician's orders:** Nurses on duty must follow physicians' order or instruction immediately. She must ensure or clarify if any doubts arise.

b. **Transcription of verbal orders:** The nurse must follow the written orders, and should not accept the verbal orders. It is mandatory for the physician to write all the medical orders. At the time of an emergency, the nurses can start treatment on verbal order of physicians, but needs transcription by a physician as soon as possible, usually within 24 hours.

c. **Do not resuscitate (DNR) orders:** In terminally ill patients, the physician must write orders if no effort to resuscitate ("No code" or DNR) or half-hearted effort is to be made to resuscitate (slow code) the patients. Have a written order in this regard.

d. **Prevention of negligence:** The nurses are made liable in case the patient has any negligence against any care. For example, if the patient had burned on applying heating pads to a part of the body or providing a hot water bottle, administering steam inhalation, administering a sitz bath, the nurses are accountable for the negligence. They are also accountable for their negligence of duty if any patient, who is elderly, sedated preoperative and postoperative, dizzy, disoriented or semiconscious fell or slips on the waxed or wet floor.

e. **Maintaining a safe environment:** A safe environment for the patient while in the hospital is required. The environment should be free from pathogenic microorganisms, rodents, and should be clean, well ventilated, noise-free so that patients feel safe and comfortable.

f. **Proper use of equipment:** The nurses should ensure proper availability of equipment, equipment available in working order. Defective and chipped equipment is the cause of harm the patients. The nurse should know the safety features, capabilities, and limitation and hazards of any equipment and monitors while using.

g. **Maintaining proper records:** The nurses are accountable for their performance. Therefore, nurses must document the care with signature. They need to keep medicolegal records under the safe custody of the nurse in each ward and not accessible to the patient's visitors, lawyers, and police without permission. All nurses are legally and ethically obliged to keep in confidence all the information provided in the records.

h. **Intimation of short staff:** If the nurses are assigned to care for more patients than reasonable, they should bring to the notice of nurse supervisor/nurse manager. Otherwise, they will be responsible for any harm resulted to the patient due to a shortage of staff.

i. **Maintaining and using controlled substances:** Nurses must administer controlled drugs on the prescription of a physician. They must store these medicines in a specially locked cupboard and should mark as controlled drugs or poisonous drugs. The nurse on duty must keep the keys of the lock with her/him. Maintain a drug book to make entry of used drugs mentioning the name, registration number of the patient and date and time of administering the drug with signature. Keep 6 R's in mind while administering drugs and two persons must check the drugs, one must be a nursing staff.

j. **Dealing with death and dying patients:** Nurses must be aware of the legal definition of death because they have to document all events that occur when the patient is in their care. Nurses should treat a person (deceased) with dignity and obtain consent for an autopsy for decedent or close family members as per policy. An adult can legally give consent to denote specific organs and nurse may serve as a witness to this decision.

k. **Correct identity of clients:** The nurse has a greater responsibility to have correct identification of a patient. For example, all babies born and unconscious patients must have correct identification. A nurse also must make sure the correct identification of the patient, indication of the site of operation in the records of the patients.

l. **Information regarding absconding patient:** When a patient absconds or run away from the ward without informing the staff, inform immediately to the senior nursing staff, attending the doctor, hospital superintendent, to the local police station, and to relative (if psychiatric patient absconds).

> **Box 6.1: Areas of legal responsibilities of nurses.**
>
> - Physician's orders
> - Verbal orders
> - Do not resuscitate orders
> - Prevention of negligence
> - Administration of medications
> - Maintaining safe environment
> - Proper use of equipment
> - Maintaining proper records
> - Short staff
> - Use of controlled substances
> - Death and dying patients
> - Correct identity of clients
> - Absconding patient

Practice Checklist

Operational level nurses must use a checklist for their actions to prevent any negligence in their duties. A checklist must include the following activities:
1. Protect the rights and safety of patients
2. Communicate with clients by keeping them informed and listening to what they say
3. Maintain a positive interpersonal relationship with the patient
4. Do not make a statement that a patient may interpret as guilt or fault
5. Witness, but not obtained, informed consent for medical procedures
6. Acknowledge unfortunate incidences, report any mishap
7. Document observations immediately while facts are still fresh in mind
8. Be competent in practice; if any doubt, seek advice/help from professional colleagues
9. Practice within the boundaries of professional licensure
10. Use appropriate standards of care/practice standards/protocol/safety standards
11. Follow 6 R's, i.e. right patient, right drug, right time, right dose, right route, and the right technique
12. Document and communicate information regarding patient care and responses
13. Refuse to carry out orders that nurse knows/believes harmful to the patient
14. Have a positive interpersonal relationship with team members, and other health care professionals
15. Be responsible for your acts; know your strengths and weaknesses.

DEALING IN SPECIFIC CONDITIONS

Legal issues can arise in nursing in specific conditions such as dealing with controlled substances, acquired immune deficiency syndrome, deaths and dying patients, in autopsy and organ donations, living wills and healthcare surrogates, and patients' property. The nurse must deal with cautions keeping in mind related laws and policies while nursing the patients.

Use of Dangerous Drugs

The two Acts that control the use of poisons in medicine are Misuse of Drug Act, 1971 and Dangerous Drug Act, 1965 and 1967. Cocaine, heroin, methadone, morphine, opium, pethidine, and hallucinogens are dangerous drugs.

Caring HIV Positive and Acquired Immune Deficiency Syndrome (AIDS) Clients

The care of AIDS and HIV+ (human immunodeficiency virus) client may pose legal implications for nurses. People living with HIV have the same fundamental rights as another citizen of the country. There are certain laws related to HIV/AIDS, if not followed, can create legal issues for nurses:

- Indian Penal Code, Section 280, a Malignant Act likely to spread infection of disease dangerous to life.
- Compulsory blood and blood products testing for transfusion under Drugs and Cosmetic Rules, 1993.
- Appropriate HIV testing before insemination under Insemination Human Act, 1995.
- The Medical Council of India regulation, 2002 states the physician shall not disclose confidential information of patients without his/her consent except required by the court, in case of notifiable diseases, or case of identified serious risk to specific person or community. Hence, confidential information must be protected from HIV+ patients.
- Respect individual's right to privacy under Right of Privacy of a person-Article 21 of the constitution of India.
- An HIV-infected person cannot discriminate against based on contagiousness. Identification of HIV status should not mark on the person's medical record.
- Cannot refuse to care for an AIDS patient.
- Counseling and informed consent before HIV testing.
- Adherence to proper biomedical waste management regulation.

Deaths and Dying

There are many legal issues regarding the definition of death. The law identifies that death occurs when there is a greatly diminished brain function, despite the function of another body organ.

For Undergoing Autopsy and Organ Donation

The nurse must be aware of the policies and procedures of institutions and laws in the state where they are asked to serve as a witness for a person who wishes to give consent for a donation.

Living Wills and Healthcare Surrogates

Living wills are documents instructing the physician to hold or withdraw life-sustaining procedures whose death is imminent. For living-will, there is a need to have two witnesses. The client executes these documents to appoint someone to make healthcare decisions if and when they are no longer able to decide on their behalf, e.g. in terminally ill state and persistently vegetative state. The nurse should be aware of institutional policies with the Patient's Self-determination Act.

Patient's Property

Follow hospital policy for safekeeping of belongings of a patient who is unconscious or in serious condition without their relatives. List all the belongings after confirming by two nurses and put in safekeeping. While a patient is in hospital, the nurse has no right to go through his locker or personal property without his consent unless the patient intends to injure him or others and has the means to do so. In case, the patient dies in the hospital, keep a record of cash and belongings in the property book maintained in the emergency unit. Pack all belongings of patient separately mentioning the color, size, etc. Inform administrative officers.

DEALING WITH MEDICOLEGAL CASES

Medicolegal Case

The medicolegal case (MLC) is a case requiring investigations by law enforcing agencies apart from the medical treatment to fix the responsibility to cause of injury/illness and to assess its health status or the condition. The medicolegal cases have both medical and legal implications. Usually attending doctor in the emergency department has the authority to decide the case as MLC in a situation where the police brought the case, a referred case as MLC from another hospital, or by examining the patients by attending doctor in an emergency. Following type of cases require registering as MLC at the earliest when a doctor suspects it as MLC case or feels the necessity of informing the police or any time during admission:

- The persons who met a roadside accident, factory accidents, unnatural mishaps or any other disaster
- All burn cases of any cause
- Suspected or evident homicides, suicides
- All types of poisoning cases, sexual offenses, and criminal abortions
- Injury cases where there is a likelihood of death shortly
- Any suspected foul play, unnatural deaths, brought as "dead on arrival," found dead, an unconscious patient without any proper history
- A patient who dies immediately after admission
- Death of a patient within 24 hours in the hospital
- Death in OT during MTP, delivery
- Alcohol or drug-related deaths
- Patient absconded from the ward
- An admitted patient who had fall or trauma during stay and treatment in the hospital
- Cases referred by the court or otherwise requiring age certificate.

Guidelines for Dealing Medicolegal Cases and Issues

1. Availability of well-defined guidelines in each department
2. Well equipped with functional monitors, life-saving drugs and resuscitation equipment in the emergency outpatient department (OPD)
3. Send the information to the civil police in writing immediately, on admission and discharge, the death of MLC
4. Make sure that the doctor prepares a medicolegal report of the patient in duplicate with the marking of "Medicolegal Case" and hand over to the security officer on duty. The security officer informs police station and returns the duly filled form with details of police personnel. File the copy in the patient' record
5. Take consent for any medical examination from the patient or legal guardian
6. All clothing worn by injured/deceased, bloodstains, gastric lavage, bullets, vomits material, should be preserved, sealed properly and handed over to police on request after obtaining a proper receipt
7. Take care of all X-rays of MLCs which are of vital importance. Mark "Medicolegal Case" marks at the top of all investigations slips and X-rays requisitions
8. Keep all the information and records of MLC confidential
9. Keep all medicolegal reports and registers in proper safe custody as per institutional policy
10. Collect the required samples/specimen, label, preserve and seal and send for investigation if required
11. Keep an up-to-date chart of the treatment and antidotes of all types of poisoning cases
12. Make the availability of essential investigation facilities
13. Give due care with all the precautions while administering IV fluids and transfusing blood.

CHAPTER HIGHLIGHTS

- Negligence and malpractice, assault, battery, restraints, defamation, fraud, and invasion of privacy are the major legal issues in nursing.
- Indian Nursing Council, State Nursing Council through licensure, code of ethics and professional code of conduct, institutional policies regulate the nursing practice.
- The main safeguard in nursing practice is obtaining informed consent; executing physician orders, the correct identity of patients; documenting all actions regarding patient care; collective bargaining; protect the patient's rights, reporting any incidence.
- Nurses working in different levels have legal responsibilities towards patients including medicolegal cases and in specific conditions.

REVIEW QUESTIONS

I. Essay Type Questions
1. Define the term law. Why are laws important in nursing?
2. Describe different types of laws.
3. What do mean by "liability"? Describe in detail issues arising from liabilities in nursing practice.
4. Write main legal safeguards in nursing practice.
5. Enumerate responsibilities of nurses to avoid legal/issues.

II. Short Notes
1. Guidelines to deal with medicolegal cases
2. Ways to reduce legal liabilities
3. Sources of laws
4. Regulation of nursing practice

III. Multiple Choice Questions

1. A term used for hindering that causes individual at risk is:
   a. Legal issue
   b. Legal liability
   c. Tort
   d. Breach of duty
2. Which type of legal issue occurs if a nurse fails to take appropriate action for the treatment of a patient?
   a. Negligence
   b. Malpractice
   c. Assault
   d. Battery
3. Threatening a patient while not cooperating for the care is an example of:
   a. Malpractice
   b. Invasion of privacy
   c. Battery
   d. Assault
4. Which of the following act of a nurse is considering a fraud?
   a. Unnecessary exposing patient while assisting in the examination
   b. Making a false statement against another person
   c. The misinterpretation of a procedure/treatment
   d. Failing to obtain a proper informed consent
5. A legal process in which representative of organization/association negotiates with the employer for their concerns is:
   a. Professional code of conduct
   b. Collective bargaining
   c. Legal liability
   d. Transcription

Answer Keys

1. b   2. a   3. d   4. c   5. b

SUGGESTED READING

1. Bailey-Allen AM. Changing liability of the nurse over the past decade. Orthop Nurs. 1990;9(2):13-5.
2. Barnabas S. Study to assess the knowledge of legal responsibilities in patient care among nursing graduates. Nurs J India. 2004;95(4):90-1.
3. Garner BA (Ed). A dictionary of basic legal terms. West Group; 1999. pp. 120.
4. Burns H. Patient safety: Developing policies for engagement in the prevention of harm to patients. J Prof Nurs. 2004;20(1):4.
5. Charles SC, Wilbert JT, Franke KJ. Sued and nonsued physicians' self-reported reactions to malpractice litigation. Am J Psychiatry. 1985;142(4):437-40.
6. Carmi A, Schneider S. Nursing law and ethics. New York: Springer-Verlag; 1985.
7. Croke EM. . Nurses, negligence and malpractice. Am J Nurs. 2003;103(9):54-63.
8. Fisher WA. Restraint and seclusion: a review of the literature. Am J Psychiatry. 1994;151(11):1584-91.
9. Furlong S, Glover D. Legal accountability in changing practice. Nurs Times. 1998;94(39):61-2.
10. Gardner SL, Hagedorn ME. Holding nurses accountable. J Obstet Gynecol Neonatal Nurs. 1999;28(3):320-30.
11. Heinemann A, Puschel K. Medico-legal aspects of pressure sore. Legal Medicine. 2003;5 (Suppl 1):263-66.
12. Medico-legal cases-BARC. [online] Available from http://www.barc.gov.in/publications/tb/mg2009.pdf. [Last accessed November, 2019].
13. Khanikor MS. Ethical and legal issues in nursing. Nurs J India. 1996;87(2):33-5.
14. Kozier B, Erb GL, Blais K, et al. Fundamentals of Nursing: Concept, process, and practice, 5th edition. Menlo Park: Addition Wesley; 1995.
15. Lee NG. Legal issues. Am J Nurs. 2000;100(9):57-8.
16. Mock KD. Keep lawsuits at bay with compassionate care. RN. 2001;64(5):83-6.
17. Murthy KK. Medical negligence and the law. Indian J Med Ethics. 2007;4(3):116-8.
18. Ministry of Law and Justice, Government of India. The Right to Information Act-2005, [As modified up to 1st February, 2011] (Act No. 22 of 2005). http://righttoinformation.gov.in/rti-act.pdf. [Accessed on 05.01.2020].
19. Regu M. The nurse, the patient, and the law. Nurs J India. 1996;87(12):273-6.
20. Samuels A. The basis of legal liability of the hospitals. Med Sci Law. 1982;22(2):140-2.
21. Solomon RC. Ethical issues in medical malpractice. Emerg Med Clin North Am. 2006;24(3):733-47.
22. Tingle J. Clinical negligence and the need to keep professionally updated. Br J Nurs. 2002;11(20):1304-6.
23. White G. Informed consent. Am J Nurs. 2000;100(9):83.

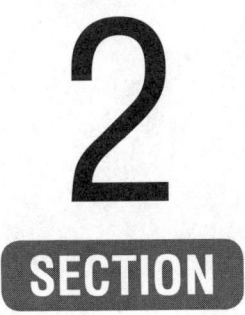

SECTION 2

Introduction to Nursing Management and Health Care Delivery System

- 7. Introduction to Nursing Management and Administration
- 8. Management Theories and Models
- 9. Indian Administrative System and Health Care Delivery System
- 10. Fundamentals of Health Planning
- 11. National Health Policies

CHAPTER 7

Introduction to Nursing Management and Administration

CHAPTER OUTLINE

- Concept of Management
  - Meaning of Management
  - Changing Concept of Management
  - Definitions of Management
- Nursing Management
  - Meaning of Nursing Management
  - Changing Concept of Nursing Management
- Administration
  - Defining Administration
  - Nature of Administration
  - Scope of Administration
  - Importance of Administration
- Type of Administration
- Nursing Service Administration
- Administration vs Management
  - Difference Between Administration and Management
  - Viewpoints Over Administration and Management
- Nature/Characteristic of Management
- Importance of Management
- Levels of Management in Hospital Nursing Services
- Functions of Nursing Management and Administration
- Principles of Nursing Management
- Role of Nurse as a Manager

LEARNING OUTCOMES

After completion of this chapter, the learner will be able to:
- Understand management and administration
- Define nursing management and administration
- Compare nursing management with the nursing process
- Discuss nursing management as a system
- Describe functions of nursing management and administration
- Enlist principles of nursing management
- Discuss the role of the nurse as a manager

KEY TERMS

Management, discipline, process, administration, system, managerial functions, principles

INTRODUCTION

Man is a social animal. He lives in a social group, in communities, and society. All human beings live in organized groups of many kinds such as family, playgroup, workgroup, school, college, office, etc. Each group forms an organization where they work together with some common goal. It may be informal or formal where various group activities are carried out to achieve those common goals.

Management is an essential part of any group activity. It is a primary force within the group or organization which tends to lead it toward the group goal. It is required to plan, organize, coordinate and control all activities of the organization to achieve its objectives.

CONCEPT OF MANAGEMENT

Meaning of Management

The term management has different views. Sometimes it refers to manage the group of managerial personnel in an organization and sometimes viewed as a process to carry out all activities of management. It is a body of knowledge, practice, and discipline. It is also used to lead and to make decisions, whereas for others it is a system of authority or a factor of producing an outcome.

According to Haimann, management is a noun, to accomplish the work from others and a process, to carry out all activities of management, and a discipline which required knowledge, rationales, and skills to manage. Though different authors used it in different ways in a true sense, it is a process.

Management as a Group of People

The management refers to a group of all these persons, who are involved in managerial functions in an organization. Another group of people in the organization is nonmanagerial operational personnel, who are not involved in manual or technical work.

Management as a Discipline

Management is a discipline, as it deals with concepts and principles as characteristics of discipline and these principles have application in managing the organizations. Management is multidisciplinary discipline and derived from other disciplines like sociology, psychology, etc. It is both art and science. Managers make use of the knowledge, skills, techniques, concepts, and principles of management in managing the activities of the organization. It is a science as it has developed principles and techniques that have universal application and also as art as skills are required by the manager to manage.

Management as an Organized Group Activity

Management is an organized group activity as it aims to achieve a particular goal. Group of people puts their maximum effort by utilizing resources effectively to get the maximum output.

Management as a Process

A process includes managerial activities such as planning, organizing, staffing, directing, coordinating, and controlling that are carried out systematically to achieve organizational goals (**Fig. 7.1**).

These activities seem to be independent, but all are interrelated, interactive carried out sequentially to achieve certain objectives. Management is a social process since its major task is to motivate, guide, and lead the people for effective utilization of resources to achieve its goals and objectives.

Changing Concept of Management

Traditional authors viewed management to get the work done, and modern authors viewed management as a process to achieve certain objectives through utilization of human and other resources. Moreover, the concepts mentioned above provide the scope of personnel, efficiency, decisions, and function orientation to the management. The management has various concepts such as traditional, functional, human-relation, and integrating concepts (**Fig. 7.2**).

Definitions of Management

Since different authors used it in a variety of ways and defined it differently, therefore, the term management is not so easy to define. Important definitions of management are:

- Management consists of getting things done through others.
  —*S George*
- Management is a process to plan, organize, direct, and control performance to determine and accomplish the stated objectives by the use of human beings and other resources.
  —*George, R Terry*
- Management is concerned with the internal environment in an enterprise where individuals, working in groups and perform efficiently to attain group goals.
  —*Koontz Harold and Cyril O'Donnell*
- Management is the process of forecast and plan, to organize, to command, to coordinate, and to control.
  —*Henry Fayol*

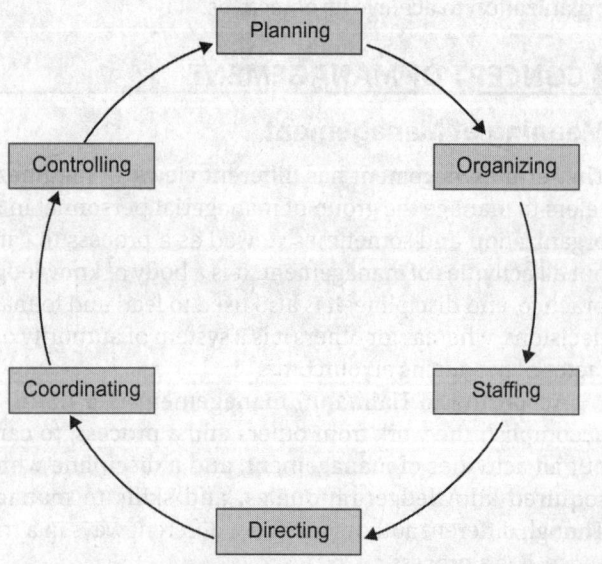

Fig. 7.1: Management process.

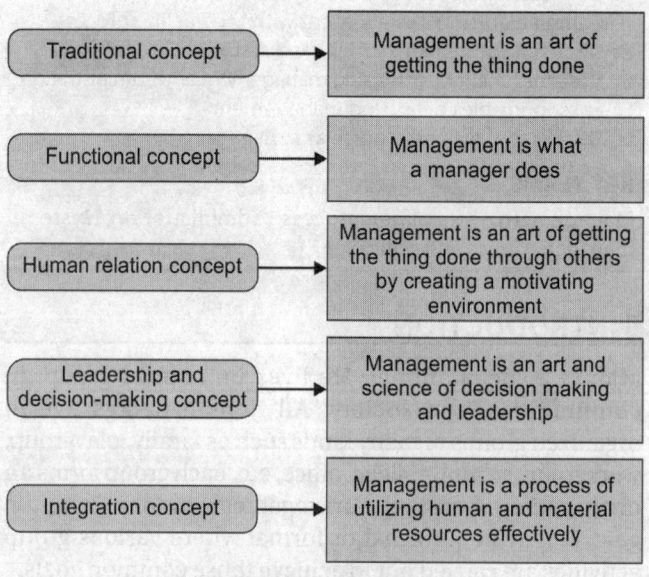

Fig. 7.2: Concepts of management.

NURSING MANAGEMENT

Meaning of Nursing Management

Nursing Management as a Process

Gillies described nursing management as a process and compared with the nursing process. Nursing management, like the nursing process, includes all the steps of data gathering, diagnosing, planning, implementation, and evaluation as shown in **Figure 7.3**.

Nursing Management as a System

Nursing management is a system based on general system theory. A system has a series of interrelated activities carried out schematically.

Nursing management has a series of interrelated events that include inputs of energy, material, and information; the systematic transformation of such input into a preplanned product, patient care; and monitoring of system input and throughput or transformation process to correct system malfunction (**Fig. 7.4**).

Changing Concept of Nursing Management

The concept of nursing management derived from various definitions given by the thinkers of management discipline. These concepts are performance, decision-making, personnel, functions or activity based.

Efficiency or Performance-oriented View

This view emphasizes the relationship between efforts and results to achieve predetermined objectives, i.e. to ensure the best possible nursing care. Nursing management is the art of getting the desired nursing outcome by putting a minimum effort by nurse managers and nurses.

Decision-oriented View

The decision theorists like Peter Drucker, Moore opine that decision making by the managers has a great role in management. Therefore, management is a decision-making process. Nursing management is also a process of making various administrative decisions and controlling nurses working in different positions in the hierarchy for the expressed purpose of attaining the predetermined goal of ensuring the quality of patient care.

Personnel Oriented View

Management is like a process of coordinative efforts of the personnel working in the organizations and management is concerned with personnel management. Nursing management is also aiming to accomplish the work through and with nursing personnel.

Functions Oriented View

Nursing management is a process of forecasting, planning, organizing, coordinating and controlling the work of nursing personnel by nurse managers to achieve organizational goals. It is a process of working through nursing staff members to provide care, cure, and comfort to patients (Gillies DA). The nurse managers are concerned with planning, organizing, utilizing, and controlling all resources effectively so that the best possible nursing care is delivered. They also carry out other decision making and leadership activities.

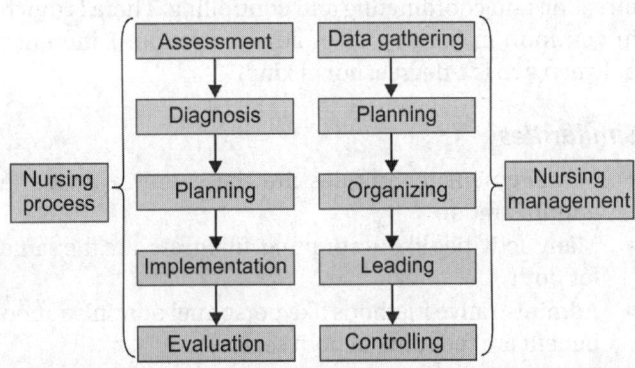

Fig. 7.3: Nursing process vs nursing management.

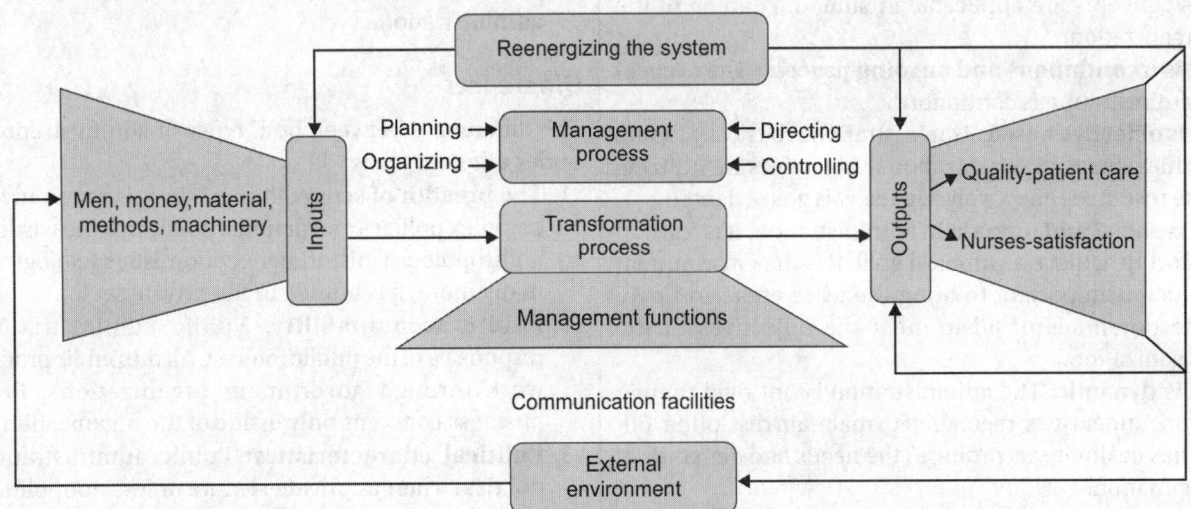

Fig. 7.4: A system approach to nursing management.

ADMINISTRATION

Defining Administration

The word "administration" is a derivative of the Latin word 'Ad + minister, means to manage affairs, or to look after or to care for people. The meaning itself reflects that the administrator regards himself as a servant, to look after, perform all functions.

- Luther Gulick defined administration as getting the things done to accomplish defined objectives.
- Goddard viewed the administration as an enabling process of planning and implementing policy, plans, and rules in a government, the public or private agency through leadership.
- According to Pfiffner, the administration is organizing and directing human and material resources to fulfill its objectives.
- Tiny M Calendar refers administration to perform executive duties of any organization or business.
- Herman Finer also viewed administration to perform actions by one person or a group of persons to accomplish a common purpose set by them or by someone else.
- The administration is a process of administering the managerial activities by exercising its powers and duties in a government or a large institution. In the government sector, the executive branch and in a large institution, a group of managers carry out administrative functions.

Nature of Administration

The administrative process is intellectual, social, dynamic and creative and continuous. It is multidimensional.

1. **It is universal:** The principles of administration are applicable in all types of set up, in every organization for their effective achievement of goals.
2. **It is holistic:** The whole process of administration embraces the organization and its functions.
3. **It is intangible:** The administration is in abstract, but its concepts are applicable in smooth running of the organization.
4. **It is a continuous and ongoing process:** The cycle of administration is continuous.
5. **It is objective based:** Administration is basically for the achievement of organizational objectives by utilizing the resources effectively. Hence, it is goal oriented.
6. **It is social and human:** In administration, it is a group effort to achieve a common goal. It is the environment which is important to bring the team effort and pool the potentials of all to meet the objectives of the organization.
7. **It is dynamic:** The administration is not rigid though work under rules, regulation to maintain discipline. But it has flexibility according to the needs and demands of a situation.
8. **It is creative or innovative:** Administration provides a great scope to invite the creative idea to bring about the changes in the organization.

Scope of Administration

The scope of administration is very wide. It is not only restricted to public administration that deals with three functionaries, i.e. legislative, executive, and judiciary. It covers all the areas like school, hospital, business, etc. It covers all the managerial activities and functional areas of management and administration like personnel, financial, material and production. It is considered as a process to accomplish the goals.

Importance of Administration

- It is lifeblood, brain, and shoulder of an organization
- Its main function is to achieve the objectives
- There is no substitute for good administration
- Good administration brings out organizational growth
- Good administration brings the team together to work
- It provides new innovative ideas to compete globally.

Types of Administration

Usually, the administration is of two types: **Public and Private**. Henri Fayol, Mary P Follett, and Urwick, the management thinkers believe that administration is one and possessing the same fundamental principles and all undertakings require planning, organization, staffing, directing and coordinating and controlling. There is much in common in both types of administration. Difference between two is a degree, not of kind.

Similarities

- Management techniques are the same in both the administration
- Many activities like accounting, filing, etc. are the same for both
- Administrative methods like personnel administration benefit are the same in both sectors
- Both are creative in its effort to make the changes. Achievement of the goal is the same in both types of administration.

Differences

The differences between both types of administration are under different areas:

1. **The breadth of scope:** Public administration involves complex policies and actions. It requires the wisdom of anthropologist, historians, economists, sociologist, and many more. It is limited in the private sector.
2. **Public accountability:** Public administration is responsive to the public interest. All the public processes work through government organizations. Private business concerns only inside of the organization.
3. **Political characteristics:** Public administration is political whereas private is more or less nonpolitical.
4. **Legal entities:** Public administration functions strictly by legal safeguards and also sustains the confidence and trust of the general public and operates within the

framework of general and specific laws limiting freedom of individual action. In the private sector, it has its own rules and regulation but under legal jurisdiction.
5. **Profit motive:** Public administration is characterized by service motive to promote social welfare activities. The profit motive is the main aim in private business.
6. **Tasks and operations:** Public sector has essential services for the welfare of people at large, e.g., police, fire, protection recreation. The private sector has its related tasks and operations.
7. **The principle of consistency of treatment:** Public administration observes the principle of equality, in the private sector, it also observes equality but more often observes discrimination in selling its service.
8. **Anonymity:** In public administration, the officials bore the anonymity and protected from harm, in private it lacks to that extent.
9. **Financial control:** There is external financial control in public administration. This kind of separation is not in private administration.
10. **Social prestige:** Public administration carries a greater social prestige because of the greater opportunity of serving the people that is comparatively less in the private sector.

Nevertheless, public and private administration are not two distinct entities, rather they are two species of the same genus, i.e., administration. Private administration is obliged to function within the framework of general laws, special laws controlling it. However, these days profit motto is no longer the sole driving force.

Nursing Service Administration

It is the process by which nurse manager work through others to achieve nursing organizational goals. It is also a system of activities directed toward the nursing care of patients and includes the establishment of overall goals and policies within the aims of health agency and provision for the organization, personnel, and facilities to accomplish these goals in the most effective and economical manner through coordinating the service with other departments of the institution.

Nursing service administration at any level is the application of the principles of administration for the ultimate purpose of providing nursing service to the individuals. The nurse manager is an effective leader in the nursing service has to manage the nursing workforce and other resources by keeping in mind the training needs of the staff.

ADMINISTRATION VERSUS MANAGEMENT

Difference Between Administration and Management

The term "administration" and "management" used interchangeably. There was no distinction between these two terms till the 1920s. Later on, thinkers viewed administration and management as different entities. The decision-making is the function of administration and execution is the function of management (Oliver). The administration differs from management regarding its nature of functions, scope, authority, level, and directing activities **(Table 7.1)**.

TABLE 7.1: Administration versus management.

Bases	Administration	Management
Nature of function	Formulation of policies, objectives, plans, programs requiring thinking function	It is concerned with implementing plans and policies
Scope	Takes major decisions	Execution of decisions and decides within its framework
Level of authority	Decision-making to carry out strategic and policy decisions	Operational authority to implement administrative decisions
Functional level	Top level	Lower level
Nature of organization	Public sector	Private sectors, business firms having profit-motive
Directive activities	Not directly involved	Directing human efforts at the operational level
Influence on decisions	Through external factors	Through internal factors

Viewpoints Over Administration and Management

There are mainly three viewpoints on administration and management.

The Administration is at a Higher Level than Management

Administration determines goals, objectives, policies, procedures, programs, action plans; management with executive functions, i.e. the direction of human effort to get the work done.

Nursing administration is a process to establish the nursing objectives or purposes, which an undertaking or staffs are to achieve.

Nursing administration deals with planning and developing principles to direct nursing action. Nursing management is the process to execute planned and supervised nursing policy (Milward GE).

According to this concept, the administration is anatomy and management is physiology, as administration determines the basic framework within which the managerial functions are carried out, the administration is the function of top-level managers, management is of middle and lower levels managers. The main focus in nursing administration is to formulate the nursing policies and to determine the nursing objectives, whereas, in management, the nursing policies are executed to achieve the nursing objectives and mostly it is technical.

Management is a Broad Term

According to this concept, the administration is a part of management. Management sets goals and makes policy, whereas, the administration implements those policies.

As compared to nursing management, the nursing administration is less comprehensive and not concerned with routine activities. Nursing administration is concerned with implementing preplanned programs and procedures.

Both Management and Administration Terms can use Interchangeably

There is no difference between administration and management; one can use both the terms interchangeably. The management can categorize as administrative management and operative management.

The top-level administrative management spends more time in formulating policies, programs; middle-level administrative management in executing policies and lower level management in implementing those policies (**Fig. 7.5**).

The administrative management is primarily deal with the policy-making and operative management deals with the execution of policies. The managers of top-level are more concerned for administrative functions than the middle or lower level. Everyone in the nursing organization performs a managerial function. But the managerial functions vary at different levels.

NATURE/CHARACTERISTICS OF MANAGEMENT

1. **Management is a group activity:** Management is a group activity that directs the group to put their efforts to achieve predetermined group goals. Management is also known as a cooperative group.
2. **Management is goal oriented:** Management determines how to achieve organizational goals and objectives.
3. **Management is means:** Management is a factor of outcome that coordinates with other factors of outcome to accomplish predetermined goals. Thus, it is a means to achieve a goal rather an end.
4. **Management is universal:** Management is applicable in all types of organizations either public or private.
5. **Management functions at all levels:** Management operates from top to bottom levels. However, levels differ in its nature of job, activities, techniques, procedures, and scope of authority.
6. **Management is a social process:** The main objective of management is to get the work done through others. They are guided, supervised and controlled by the management to achieve desired goals.
7. **Management is a system of power:** Without authority, management is not possible. Hence, management authority and responsibility at all levels of the organization.
8. **Management is a continuous process:** Management is a continuous process to achieve maximum output with minimum efforts and utilization of resources. There are continuous monitoring and feedback of the processes.
9. **Management is art as well as science:** Management is an art as it uses personal skills and practical knowledge in solving problems. It is a result-oriented. Management requires creativity to get the work done from others; and tries to attain higher and higher goals to reach a higher level of perfection.

Management is also a science because it uses various data gathering methods scientifically and systematically for observation; establishes a relationship between cause and effect, and knowledge gathered can be verified. Practitioners and theorists developed and verified principles of management through continuous efforts.

IMPORTANCE OF MANAGEMENT

Good management is to the organization what health is to the body for the smooth functioning of the organization. Each organization helps increase efficiency, to crystallize its nature, improve research and to attain social goals and in many other ways. Management is the thinking organ that provides vision to the organization. Peter F. Drucker refers to management as the lifeline of every enterprise.

1. **The accomplishment of the organizational goal:** Management determines and accomplishes the goals of the organization and other departments. It is the management to direct all the activities toward the organizational objectives.
2. **Provides innovative vision and mission:** Management keeps itself in touch with changing needs of the

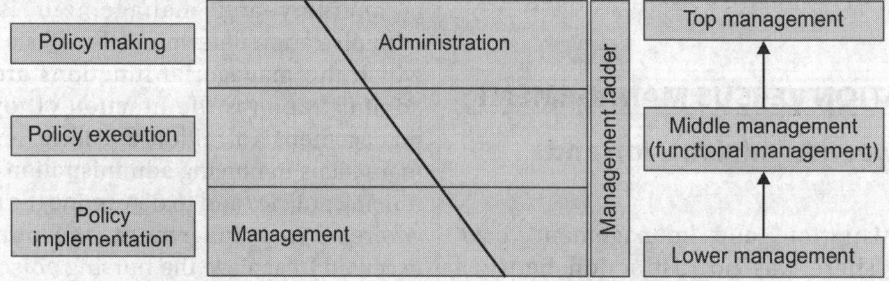

Fig. 7.5: Administration versus management at different levels of management.

society at large and accordingly has the vision for the organization and identify the mission and objectives of the organization and direct all the activities and strategies in that light.

3. **Increases efficiency:** The managers can become more effective by using established guidelines to help, solve problems. Even no manager can control without basing them on plans, that manager should have the organizational authority necessary to accomplish the result expected of them.
4. **Minimizes time and cost:** Effective management economizes time and costs to provide quality services by applying principles of management.
5. **Crystallize nature of management:** Lack of understanding of concepts, principles, and techniques of management makes it difficult to analyze the management job and to train managers. Management, when viewed as human, will help the managers to understand the human dynamics and thus dealing in that way can bring the change in them and can get the maximum output from them.
6. **Effective utilization of resources:** Management ensures the proper and effective utilization of human and other resources by using principles of management and using management techniques to get the maximum performance.
7. **Brings harmony in groups:** It is the management which directs and coordinates the activities of all the individuals working in any organization in the use of materials, methods, and machines. It brings harmony among the group so that they work together with the feeling of belongingness to achieve the organizational objectives.
8. **To improve research:** Since management deals with people and since groups of people are unpredictable and complex, effective research poses a question mark. It also deals with planning activities, the devising control, and grouping of activities, the research in all areas is slow and costly. Hence, managerial techniques can improve upon research or studies to be conducted and how to be conducted. It will help to bring about the evidence to apply in managerial activities to accomplish the organizational goals and objectives.
9. **To attain social goals:** Management coordinates the efforts of people to translate individual goals to social attainment. The organizations are to fulfill the needs of the community at large. So, it is the management that has the vision and strategies toward that direction.

LEVELS OF MANAGEMENT IN HOSPITAL NURSING SERVICES

By hierarchy, their position and relative responsibilities, there are three levels in nursing management. These are top, middle, and lower level (**Fig. 7.6**).

Top Management

In nursing services, Assistant Directors are at the top management at State Directorate level and Chief Nursing Officers or Nursing Superintendent or Matrons in the hospitals. They formulate policies, goals, objectives, and procedures for the nursing services. They are mainly engaged in planning and coordinating functions. They issue the instructions for the lower levels. In the hospital setting, deputy nursing superintendent, assistant nursing superintendents or assistant matrons assist them.

Middle Management

Middle management in nursing is usually the heads of nursing units in the hospitals, and they are at the supervisory level. They are designated as ward sisters or sister grade I, and they report to their seniors.

Nurses at middle management make duty plans of the nursing personnel of lower or operational level, divide the work to them. They follow and implement the policies and guidelines issued to them by the top nursing management. They evaluate operative level nurses and coordinate with other departments and team to ensure that

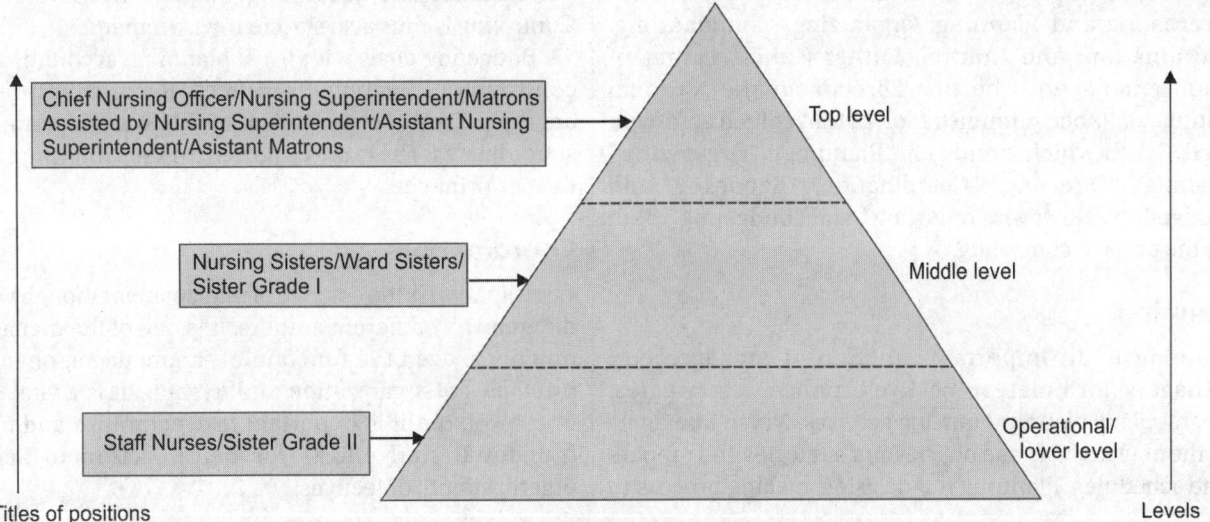

Fig. 7.6: Levels of management in hospital nursing services.

TABLE 7.2: Job responsibilities of different levels in nursing management.

Job responsibilities	Top	Middle	Lower
Formulation of policy	Maximum	Moderate	Minimum
Skill required	Innovative	Persuasive	Technical
Scope	Broad	Large-function	Small/Limited (sub functional)
Area of activity	Setting objectives/goals	Implementation	Operationalize
Nature	Complex	Moderate	Simple
Span of people	Small	Moderate	Large
Evaluation	Difficult	Less difficult	Easy

the best possible patient care. They arrange for necessary materials, equipment for the operative level nurses and provide them with the necessary working and therapeutic environment. They supervise and guide them and also solve their problems. They maintain good human relation in the unit and communicate their problems to the higher level management.

Lower or Operating Management

Operative level management comprises nurses at the operational level designated as staff nurses or sister grade II. They are responsible for patient care. They plan nursing care for the individual patient. They carry out nursing orders given by the next senior and the doctors. They are also known as the first line management. **Table 7.2** depicts the nature of job responsibilities of these levels of management.

FUNCTIONS OF NURSING MANAGEMENT AND ADMINISTRATION

Like management, nursing management/has its own managerial and administrative functions. In the words of Henri Fayol, the process of management has five functions: Forecasting and Planning; Organizing; Commanding; Coordination; and Control. Luther Gulick, Father of Management, and the first Director of the National Institute of Public Administration of USA coined acronym: POSDCORB which stands for "Planning," "Organizing," "Staffing," "Directing," "Coordination," "Reporting," and "Budgeting". However "reporting" and "budgeting" both are the parts of controlling.

Planning

Planning is an important function of management. Managers formulate objectives, policies, strategies, programs for planning nursing services. Nurse Managers set the objectives, frame policies and strategies and prepare time schedules. Planning is a decision-making process to define tasks and to plan resources. It is the responsibility of nursing managers of all level in the organization; the intensity and nature of planning differ.

Organizing

The term organizing means to develop a system for maximum utilization of available resources. Activities are carried out to identify work activities, preparing job descriptions and job responsibilities; assigning and identifying job roles, and developing rationales to organize those activities. It involves totality of activities and authority relationship that constitute organizing functions. According to Allen "organization involves identification and grouping of the activities and distribution of those activities among the staff to accomplish organizational objectives" (Allen et al.).

Staffing

Staffing involves recruiting and developing nurses as per norms. This process includes searching for the talents, recruitment, selection, and deploying them in proper positions and organizing orientation and other skill training program, and appraising them.

Directing and Leading

Directing and leading is a very important managerial function to implement the system effectively. It is concerned with inspiring and encouraging staff, creating understanding among them. Regular supervision, effective communication, and leadership among managers are important ingredients for achieving the organizational objectives. Direction directly deals with guiding, supervising, motivating, and communicating with subordinates.

Controling

Controling is measuring and correcting the performance of staff as per expected performance. It is the process of comparing the actual performance of staff with standard performance and accordingly taking corrective actions. Controling is thus also system measurement.

Budgeting deals with fiscal planning, accounting, and controlling of financial resources. Records and reports are the means of communication between superiors and subordinates. These are important to keep informed about the performance.

Coordination

Coordination is the essence of management though viewed differently by different authors. It is one of the managerial functions, even the function of the manager, one of the principles of organization and to some, it is a vital phase of control. But it is important to synchronize and unifies individual staff efforts for better action to achieve organizational objectives.

PRINCIPLES OF NURSING MANAGEMENT

Principles of nursing management refer to the concept of reality related to the nursing field. These principles provide guidelines for nurse managers to work in their day to day work set up. These principles also serve as ready reckoner for the decisions and actions of nurse managers working at any level in different settings. The principles of nursing management can be derived and applied from the principles given by Henri Fayol, the father of management has given more emphasis on functions of managers and showed regard to human elements with wider perspectives.

Division of Work

This principle means that every employee is given only one type of work to bring about specialization in every activity. The specialization helps in developing staff and thus helps in improving their work efficiency. This principle of management is also called the principle of specialization.

Authority and Responsibility

Authority is one's right for giving orders by position by senior managers to the juniors in the hierarchy, and responsibility is just concerned with performance and not a right. Both authority and responsibility go side by side if authority goes side by side with responsibility. In the same way, if a person is responsible for a particular job, should also give authority.

Discipline

Discipline refers to sincerity, respect, and observance of rules and regulation of an organization. According to this principle, subordinates must respect their superiors and obey their instructions. It must flow and enforced within the hierarchy.

Unity of Command

Every subordinate must receive orders and instructions only from one superior—the unity of command aids in improving the performance of the employee. If an employee is getting orders from many heads; there will be overlapping of orders and instructions and create confusion and conflict. The dual command generates tension, confusion, and conflict, and results in diluted responsibility and blurred communication.

Unity of Direction

According to this principle, one head should give the direction or subordinates must receive orders only from one head-all group activities directed toward the same goal.

Subordination of Individual Interest to General Interest

Of all must be considered in all the circumstances in the organization. The individuals must sacrifice their interest for the common interest. The subordinates can show the general interest through collective bargaining. To achieve this attitude by employees; they should be honest and sincere. There should be regular supervision of employees and agreement over differences in opinions among management and employees.

Fair Remuneration

The remuneration to be paid for the employees should be reasonable, satisfactory and rewarding of the effort. It will reduce the differences between administration and staff and create a pleasing atmosphere in the organization.

Effective Centralization and Decentralization

Centralization means that concentration of authority rests at one place or one level in the organization. Centralization is a situation in which the administration retains most of the decision making power. Decentralization is the downward sharing of authority in the organization.

Scalar Chain

Fayol defines Scalar Chain is the chain of superiors ranging from the ultimate authority to the lowest. The principle suggests that every order, instructions, messages, and the request has to pass through this scalar chain. However, there is a shortcut path known as gangPlank to facilitate quick and easy communication.

Order

It is concerned with the proper and a systematic arrangement of things and people. The place must be allocated to every article and equipment to use effectively. Select suitable persons for a suitable job, and there should be a specific place for everyone according to need.

Equity

Equity means fair and impartial treatment. It is fairness, kindness, and justice. The administration must give and similar treatment to employees of a similar position. There should not be any discrimination with them in respect to age, caste, sex, religion, relation, etc. Creating a positive attitude among managers and subordinates is important. They must constantly apply the correct balance between equity and discipline.

Stability of Tenure

Stability of tenure means that employees should not frequently move from one position to another rather fix the tenure of an employee to a particular position. It will help in creating team spirit and sense of belongingness which ultimately improves the quality of work.

Initiative

Give opportunity to subordinates in initiating the plans. The administration must provide an opportunity for them to give new ideas, experiences, and new methods of work.

Esprit de Corps (Union is a Strength)

It refers to a sense of unity, team spirit, devotion, and cooperation which unites the members of the group. It refers to mutual understanding among employees. It inspires them to work hard. Encouraging subordinates help in developing an informal relationship.

According to Mooney and Reiley, Lyndall Urwick, Davis, and others, additions principles of management are:

1. **Principles of objectives:** According to this principle of management, there must be organizational objectives for the achievement of which everybody in the organization should work. All energy of human resources must be channelized to attain those objectives.
2. **Principle of coordination:** The principle of coordination states that the efforts of the group should be unified and integrated to achieve a common goal.
3. **Span of supervision:** According to this principle, a supervisor must supervise only that number of subordinates that he can properly supervise. The employees' supervision is by nature and type of work.
4. **Principle of planning:** Planning is prerequisite for effective management. According to this principle, planning is must to determine goals and policies and ways of executing.
5. **Principle of motivation:** The principle of motivation implies that the performance of a person depends upon his ability and motivation. Motivation is an urge among subordinates to perform in a better way. Therefore, the motivational system must be flexible, productive, and comprehensive and should be according to the felt needs of the staff.
6. **Principle of exception:** According to this principle, managers have rationalized workload and free from overload.
7. **Principle of participation:** The principle of participation states that there should be the bottom-up approach in management. Employees of operation level should also be involved or consulted while taking important policy decisions. The process of participation will ensure the smooth and effective implementation of various decisions.

ROLE OF NURSE AS A MANAGER

The role of the nurse as a manager is multiple, interrelated, and overlapping. The nurses at all levels play managerial roles to some extent. In general, they are responsible for managing all resources such as personnel, material, standard operative procedures/methods, machinery or equipment and also involved in fiscal management.

Role in Planning Nursing Service

It is the foremost function of management. It allows nurse managers to organize, staff, direct, and control all activities to fulfill all the objectives of the nursing department. Nurse Managers at the top level are concerned with the overall planning of nursing services. They:

- Frame philosophy, mission, long and short-term goals and objectives of nursing services
- Develop various policies, and administrative manuals such as protocols, procedures, rules
- Set nursing standards of care and nursing practice, and also budget for nursing services
- Constitute different committees
- Prepare a master rotation plan, job descriptions, and job specifications of various nursing categories
- Develop a system of maintaining personnel records, and of conducting various administrative meetings, within and with other departments
- Plan various types of in-service education programs and staff development programs, etc.

Role of Nurses in Organizing Nursing Services

- To develop an organizational structure and allocating resources
- To determine, and categorize the activities to be performed by the nurses.
- To create a structure of various positions in the hierarchy for the top to the operational level
- To utilize effectively various resources.

Role in Personnel/Human Resource Management

- Determine number and type of nursing staff required
- Develop job specification, and job descriptions
- Participate in recruitment, selection, placement, allocation, and transferring staff
- Plan and implement induction and orientation programs
- Plan training and staff development programs
- Plan and implement various stress management programs
- Motivate and counsel
- Promote occupational health, safety, and welfare of staff
- Develop health surveillance procedures, periodic health assessment plan and performance appraisal of staff annually and write a confidential report
- Implement universal standard precautions, advocates for proper body postures during any nursing intervention
- Maintain discipline, high morale, and professionalism among staff

- Prepare assignment and work schedules (roster plan/time planning)
- Collective bargaining, negotiation and effective grievance handling procedures.

Directing Role

Directing is the core function of management process to achieve organizational goal. Nurse as a manager supervise and control activities of nursing staff to maintain the healthy working environment. The nurse managers direct, communicate, guide, motivate, and supervise their subordinates time to time to get maximum output from them. They carry out the following role and responsibilities:

- **As a leader:** Leadership is the art of getting others to do something. A nurse manager is responsible for the activities of nurses working under her/him. She/he has to act as a leader of the group and set an example of hard work and dedication empowering subordinates so that they can follow her/his direction with respect. Nurse as a manager can use a bottom-up approach; can synthesis and solve all the issues holistically.
- **As a managerial supervisor:** Nurses are managing and supervising their subordinates. As managerial supervisors, their focus is on balancing weekly workload, administrative procedures, conducting meetings, planning and developing strategies. They are also involved in data collection and audit activities, recruitment and retention issues, and communication by using various methods.
- **As a mentor:** Nurse Managers not only act as a supervisor but also act as a mentor to guide their subordinates in their personal and professional activities. There is a challenge for nurse managers to keep staff motivated in the workplace. Motivation is a means to energize, activate and direct staff toward goal. They need to know the behavior of each staff working under her; encourage them to take the initiative and self-reliance. Provide opportunities, motivating work culture and climate to prove their worth. Give recognition to good work. Delegate, develop, train, brief, and provide a just reward.

Role in Interpersonal Relationship

- **As a figurehead:** A nurse manager has to perform many symbolic functions as a figurehead of the organization or head of the nursing unit. She/he has to sign various papers, attends social functions of the subordinates speak at functions, etc.
- **Liaison officer:** A nurse manager has to maintain contact with higher management and subordinates. She/he has to keep in touch with the external environment, government policies by attending meetings, conferences, functions, etc.
- **Human relationship role:** A nurse manager has an important role in developing human relation in the nursing department. She/he has to recognize the importance of their subordinates as individuals and mutual understanding of their position and fair and impartial in all the matters while dealing with them. Nurse manager should inculcate mutual discussion, exchange of views and good communication among nurses for the accomplishment of organizational goals. They develop their subordinates for promotion and know the details of all the principles, policies and laws.
- **As communicator and coordinator:** The nurse as a manager is central to all the activities and among health team members. Effective communication is important to perform all functions of management. Nurse managers share responsibility for the health and welfare of all people in the community and participate in the programs designed to prevent illnesses and maintain health. They coordinate and synchronize medical and other professionals and technical services that affect patient care. To ensure quality care to patients, the nurse manager has to make a cordial relationship and coordinate with them and imparts information to health team members, public, clients, and relatives.
- **Public relation role:** Nurse as manager tries to deliver and ensure high-quality patient care, develop various information tools, education material and strategies to orient clients and relatives regarding rules and regulation, them about care and other health matters. Nurse managers also ensure that the client is getting all hospital services in a proper way, e.g. dietary services, etc., and hospital environment is clean and infection free. Attend complaints and get feedback and suggestions from them for further improvement in services.

Role in Decision Making

Decision making is the prime function of a nurse manager. Nurse managers have to take many decisions programed or nonprogramed, organizational or personal, routine or strategic, policy and operative, individual or group decision at all levels. They perform the roles as a decision-maker.

- **As an entrepreneur:** A nurse manager performs the role of an entrepreneur to decide about expansion and diversification of department. They have to take many strategic decisions related to sources of resources, funds, other inputs through meetings, and asking suggestions.
- **As a conflict handler:** A nurse manager has to act as an arbitrator in resolving disputes of staff. They can resolve those disputes by establishing a procedural system to allow parties to share their grievances, and use a third party negotiator, exchange, rotate or terminate individuals.
- **As a change manager:** A nurse manager acts as a change manager to bring about innovative changes in the work set up. Managers encourage subordinates to participate in change management. They motivate them by conducting regular meetings, using a participatory

approach and by inviting suggestions from them. They act as a catalyst to mobilize the support of their staff and respect the ideas and suggestions given by them. They delegate appropriate responsibility to capable staff and flexible and strong to take the risk, solve problems and reward the team members for bringing the successful changes.

Role in Material Management

The material in the hospital includes equipment, apparatus, instruments, linen and drugs and medicines, etc. The role of nurse managers in equipment and supplies is to ensure an adequate supply of and to maximize proper utilization and maintenance of equipment and supplies in all nursing units as discussed below:
- Take an active part in estimating demand for equipment and supplies as per hospital policy.
- Develop ward policy and communicate higher authority about the gap in demand and supply.
- Conduct meetings and prepare guidelines for handing and taking over.
- Ensure adequate supply maintain a current inventory of equipment and supplies in functional order
- Condemn nonfunctional and outdated articles
- Have inventory control and maintain a buffer stock
- Send requisition monthly, weekly, as per policy
- Keep enough stock for evening and nights
- Communicate all staff about "out of stock" material
- Maintain proper records and reports of supplies and materials.

Role in Fiscal Management

Nurse manager can play a role related to fiscal management. They prepare a financial plan for each nursing unit by keeping in mind number and type of staff, nurse-patient ratio, and an option for new programs. It should also include variable cost including office supplies repair and maintenance of equipment, etc. Nurse managers also involved in planning budgeting-allocation of resources of the department and evaluation of financial status.

Role in Informatics and Documentation

The role of the nurse as managers in informatics and documentation has emerged as:
- A leader ineffective designing and using health electronic record (HER) system
- Integrator of patient's data
- Partner in decision making
- Advocates for engaging clients and their families.

As an Evaluator and Auditor

Nurse manager performs the role as a nursing auditor and evaluator to control and regulate how nursing services are used and focused on controlling the cost of services provided. Nurse managers use it as a method of measuring performance in all areas through observation, questioning, and records. Nurse managers:
- Conduct regular meetings with audit committee members
- Develop standardized tools to gather data
- Prepare and train auditors for auditing
- Prepare an action plan
- Gather information and analyze
- Prepare report
- Modify action plan if required.

As an Advocate

As an advocate of clients, nurses at the operational level as Nurse Managers play an important role and have a responsibility to protect the human and legal rights. They provide care to all the clients of all age group irrespective of caste, creed, and religion. She informs about the policy of the organization that may conflict their well being with their rights and makes informed decisions by telling pro and cons of a particular treatment and protects the client against receiving inadequate care, etc.

According to Indian Nursing Council (INC) professional Code of Conduct (2006), the nurse as a manager plays important roles as to:
- Ensures appropriate earmark and utilize available resources
- Participates in supervising and teaching nursing students
- Uses judgment for individual competence while accepting and delegating responsibility
- Facilitates conducive and motivating work culture to achieve institutional objectives
- Communicates effectively following appropriate channels of communication
- Participates in performance evaluation; participates in the evaluation of nursing services
- Participates in policy decisions by following the principle of equity and accessibility of services works with individuals to identify their needs.

The heads of nursing units in the hospitals are at the supervisory level and are middle managers. They report to seniors in their departments who are designated as ward sisters or sister grade I. Their main role of ward management are as follows:
- Follow and implement the policies and guidelines issued to them by the top nursing management
- Make duty plans of the nursing personnel of lower level, divide the work to them
- Management of materials, equipment for the operative level nurses
- Coordinate with other departments and team to ensure that the best possible patient care
- Maintain necessary working and therapeutic environment
- Supervise and guide them and also solve their problems
- Maintain good human relation in the unit.

Chapter 7: Introduction to Nursing Management and Administration

Nurses at the operational level designated as staff nurses or sister grade II. In the hospital, the first line management responsible for the patient care. As a manager, they do perform the following roles:
- Plan and make decisions for rendering nursing care
- Carry out instructions given by their superiors and team members about patient care
- Maintain supplies (drugs, medicines, linen, etc.) and equipment
- Coordinate the activities of other departments and health team members, e.g., with dieticians, or physiotherapists in the care of patients and also in the community she coordinates, implement and supervise the activities of national health programmes
- Communicate their problems to the higher level management.

CHAPTER HIGHLIGHTS

- Management is a process of planning, organizing, actuating (directing), and controlling performed to determine and accomplish stated objectives by using human and other resources.
- Management is a continuous dynamic social process that includes goal-oriented group activities and required at all levels of the organization. It is universal and considered both art and science.
- There are three viewpoints on administration and management that administration is a higher level function as compared to management, management is a broad term and includes administration, and both management and administration are same.
- There are three levels in the nursing organization: top, middle and lower level. They all carry out managerial functions.
- Effective management is the key to: i) identify vision and mission, ii) achieve a goal, iii) increase efficiency, iv) minimize time and cost, v) ensure proper utilization of resources, and vi) bring harmony in the group.
- Functions of management are planning, organization, and staffing, directing, coordination, reporting and budgeting.
- Nurse as a Manager has multiple managerial role and responsibilities toward nursing services to accomplish its goal and objectives.

REVIEW QUESTIONS

I. Essay Type Questions
1. Define management and nursing management. Discuss its main characteristics.
2. Describe functions of management and administration in nursing.
3. Describe principles of management applicable in nursing.
4. "Management is the art of getting things done through other people" discuss.
5. Discuss managerial role of a nurse.

II. Short Notes
1. Concept of management
2. Differentiate between administration and management
3. Different levels of nursing management
4. Importance of management
5. Management as an art and science

III. Multiple Choice Questions
1. The management is a process because:
    a. All persons are involved in managerial functions in an organization
    b. It deals with concepts and principles in managing the organization
    c. Some activities are carried out systematically to achieve organizational goals
    d. Efforts are made to get maximum output
2. The concept that views management as a process of utilizing human and material resources is:
    a. Traditional
    b. Functional
    c. Human-relation
    d. Integration
3. The concept that views nursing management like a process of coordinating efforts of nursing personnel working in the organization is:
    a. Decision-oriented
    b. Personnel-oriented
    c. Performance-oriented
    d. Function-oriented
4. Management is universal because:
    a. It determines how to achieve goals and objectives
    b. It directs the efforts of the groups
    c. It operates from top to bottom levels
    d. It is applicable in all organizations
5. The administration is at a higher level than management because:
    a. Administration develops a basic framework and concerns with executive functions
    b. The administration is a part of management
    c. Management deals with the execution of functions
    d. Management sets goals and objectives
6. Which type of skill is required by the top nursing management?
    a. Technical   b. Innovative
    c. Persuasive   d. Human-relation
7. A system for maximum utilization of available resources is known as:
    a. Planning   b. Directing
    c. Organizing   d. Coordinating
8. The basic principle of nursing management which advocates that every employee is given only one type of work to bring specialization in every activity is known as:
    a. Division of work   b. Unity of command
    c. Equity   d. Authority

9. The role of a nurse manager in planning nursing services is revealed by:
   a. Utilizing resources efficiently
   b. Developing job specification and job descriptions
   c. Advocating clients and their families
   d. Framing philosophy, goals, and objectives for the nursing services
10. The principle that refers to mutual understanding, team spirit and cooperation among employees is:
    a. Initiative   b. Equity
    c. Esprit de Corps   d. Discipline

Answer Keys

1. c   2. d   3. b   4. d   5. a   6. b   7. c
8. a   9. d   10. c

SUGGESTED READING

1. Alexander E, Gordon P. Nursing Service Administration. St Louis Mosby Co.; 1962. pp. 91-125.
2. Bose R. Nursing administration and services-suggestions for improvement in management effectiveness. Nurs J India. 1994;85(11):253-5.
3. Breech EFL. Principles and Practice of Management. London: Pitman; 1972. p. 29.
4. Ellis JR, Hartley CL. Nursing in Today's World: Trends, Issues, and Management, 8th edition Philadelphia: Lippincott, William & Wilkins, 2004.
5. Fayol H. General and Industrial Management. London: Sir Issac Pitman; 1949. p. 1.
6. Gillies DA. Nursing Management-A System Approach. Philadelphia, WB: Saunders; 1982. pp. 1-7.
7. Goddard HA. Principles of Administration applied to Nursing Service. Geneva: WHO; 1958. pp. 19-41.
8. Hellriegel D, Jackson SE, Slocum JW. Management: A Competency-Based Approach. 10th edition. Mason, OH: Thomson South-Western; 2005.
9. MacFarland DE. Management Principles and Practices. New York: Macmillan; 1974. p. 6.
10. Marquis BC, Huston CJ. Leadership Roles and Management Functions in Nursing, 3rd edition. Philadelphia: Lippincott William & Wilkins; 2000.
11. Marriner-Tomey M. Guide to Nursing Management, 3rd edition. St Louis: Mosby; 1988.
12. Oliver S. The Philosophy of Management. London: Sir Issac Pitman; 1923.
13. Potter PA, Perry AG. Fundamentals of Nursing. St Louis Mosby Co.; 2001. p. 376.
14. Principles of Management Fayol. [online] Available from http://www.12manage.com/methods_fayol_14_principles_of_management.html. [Last Accessed November, 2019].
15. Rinehart EL. Management of Nursing Care. New York: The Macmillan Co.; 1969. pp. 5-37.
16. Robbins SP, Delenzo DA. Fundamentals of Management, 3rd edition. Upper Saddle River NJ: Prentice Hall; 2001.
17. Shanks MD, Kennedy DA. The Theory & Practice of Nursing Service Administration. New York: McGraw Hill Co.; 1965.
18. Terry GR. Principles of Management. Illinois: Richard; 1960.
19. Weihrich H, Koontz H. Management—A Global Perspective. New York: McGraw Hill 1993. pp. 20-5.
20. Young LC. Nursing Administration from Concepts to Practice. Philadelphia: WB Saunders. 1988. pp. 166-71.
21. Zovko V. Strategic management process in hospitals. World Hosp Health Serv 2001;37(1):2-5.

CHAPTER 8

Management Theories and Models

CHAPTER OUTLINE

- Evolution of Management Thought
- Classical Theories of Management
  - Theory of Bureaucracy
  - Scientific Management Theory
  - Process Management Theories
- Neoclassical Theories of Management
  - Human Relations Management Theories
- Behavioral Sciences Theories
- Modern Management Theories
  - Quantitative Approach
  - Systems Approach
  - Contingency Approach

LEARNING OUTCOMES

- Understand the concept of theories and models
- Discuss various theories related to management
- Apply concepts of management theories in nursing management

KEY TERMS

Theory, model, classical, neoclassical, modern management, bureaucracy, scientific, process, human relation, behavioral, quantitative, systems, contingency approach

INTRODUCTION

Management practice has always existed in some form as early as human civilization, but a systematic study has been started from the 19th century onwards. Before the 19th century, the concept of administration existed in Egypt in 1300 BC, Kautilya in 320 BC, and Roman Catholic, a group of German and Australian public administrators, intellectuals during 16th to 18th century and later on the concept of scientific management emerged. Taylor made the beginning in the early 20th century.

EVOLUTION OF MANAGEMENT THOUGHT

I. Classical Theories of Management
1. *Bureaucratic model:* Max Weber introduced it around 1900.
2. *Scientific management:* Taylor introduced the concept of scientific management around 1910.
3. *Process management:* Henry Fayol and others around 1910 introduce the concept of functional management.

II. Neoclassical Theory of Management
1. *Human relations:* Introduced by Elton Mayo, and others around the 1930s.
2. *Behavioral sciences:* Maslow, McGregor, and others were the contributors for this concept and introduced around the 1940s.

III. Modern Management Theories
1. *Quantitative approach:* This approach is also known as Operational Research Analysis and developed by Taylor around 1950.
2. *Systems approach:* Boulding, Johnson, and others develop this approach after 1950.
3. *Contingency approach:* Lorsch, Lawrence, and others introduced contingency or situational approach to management in the 1970s.

Table 8.1 depicts the management approaches and its contributors.

CLASSICAL THEORIES OF MANAGEMENT

The classical school of thought began in the early nineties. It focuses on efficiency and includes bureaucratic, scientific and process or administrative management theories.

TABLE 8.1: Management approaches and its contributors.

Period	Management approaches	Contributors
1900–1930	Scientific management	Frederick Winslow Taylor
1916–1940	Process management	Henry Fayol, Follett, Mooney, Urwick, Luther Gullick
1920–1938	Operational approach	PW Bridgman
1930–1950	Bureaucratic approach	Max Weber
1930–1940	Human relations approach	Elton Mayo
1940–1950	Social system approach	Chester Barnard
1945–1965	Decision-making approach	Herbert Simon, March, Cyert
1950–1960	Management approach	Peter Drucker
1950–1970	Human behavior approach	Maslow, Herzberg, McGregor, Likert, Blake, and others
1950 onwards	Quantitative approach	Taylor
1960's	System approach	Ludwig von Bertalanffy, Boulding, Hagel Zalia
1970's	Contingency approach	Joan Woodward Lorsch, PR Lawrence, Fredrick Fielder,

Weber's Bureaucratic Management Theory

Bureaucratic management believes rational guidelines such as rules and procedures, hierarchy, and a clear division of labor. The main thinker of bureaucracy is Max Weber. Max Weber (1864–1920), a German Sociologist, is known as the Father of Modern Sociology and the father of bureaucratic management. He developed a working system in the office. He analyzed bureaucracy as the most logical and rational structure for large organizations.

Characteristics of Bureaucracy

Weber described bureaucracy as an "administrative body of appointed officials". Weber focused on dividing organizations into hierarchies and establishing strong lines of authority and control. He looked organization from a closed system perspective. He suggested that organizations should develop comprehensive and detailed standard operating procedures for all routine tasks. The organization must consider specialization while dividing the work and official rules in the administrative process. The bureaucratic model has characteristics of legal-rational bureaucracy which include:

- Distribution of officially designated tasks among the staff with a division of labor and specialization of function
- Organization of roles into hierarchal structures with superiors and subordinates must be clearly defined and should be by legal authority and power
- Formalization of policies and procedures to govern staff behavior and ensures uniformity within the organization
- Encouragement of impersonal attitudes between staff members to maintain a psychological distance between superiors and subordinates (Kelly Joe).

Elements/Principles of the Bureaucratic Model

- A formal hierarchical structure
- Management by rules
- Impersonal order
- Functional specialty
- Selection through merit
- Personal and public ends
- Written documents
- Technically qualified people

Criticism

Behavioral scientists considered it as inhuman and incompatible with the development of a mature personality. This model lacks empirical validity.

Scientific Management Theories

Scientific management approach focuses on the "one best way" to do a job. Frederick Taylor, Frank Gilbreth, and Henry Gantt are the pioneers of this approach.

Taylor and Scientific Management

Frederick W Taylor (1856–1915), an American Engineer, developed scientific management theory. He is a pioneer in management science and known as the Father of Scientific Management. He was born in 1856, in Philadelphia, USA. He conducted a series of experiment and in 1911, published Principles of Scientific Management. The principles developed by Taylor are the guide to practice management. Taylor's approach was from bottom to top level and focused on work simplification, standardization, and thus increasing efficiency and productivity. Taylor's principles of scientific management are given here.

Principles of scientific management

1. Every job should be broken into elements and scientific methods to perform each element rather than the rule of thumb methods
2. Scientific procedure for selection, training, and development of employees
3. There should be cooperation between management and employees by scientific principles
4. Scientifically division of responsibility between management and employees. Management should design, set up, and supervise the work of workers, and workers should be free to do work
5. Both management and employees should try to achieve maximum output in place of restricted output.

Elements of scientific management

- Work measurement studies
- Standardization of tools and equipment
- Scientific selection, placement, and training
- Division of labor
- Cost accounting
- Mental attitude

Time and Motion Studies by Frank and Gilbreth

Frank Gilbreth (1068-1924) and Lillian Gilbreth (1878-1972) are a pioneer of Time and Motion Studies. Frank conducted time and motion studies, and Lillian tried to find the role of human factors at work by understanding the personality and needs of the workers.

They identified elements about time in work which were instrumental in forming operational methods. They believed that prior estimation of time is must to design work methods rather relying upon observation-based time studies. It enabled the manager to break down a job into its parts and streamline the process. They are known for contributions in production and operation management. Gilbreth developed the "laws of motion economy" and related principles of management to deal with employees and designing tools and equipment.

The Gantt Chart by Henry Gantt

Henry L Gantt (1861-1919) believed in the scientific selection of workers and "harmonious cooperation" between labor and management. He developed planning and control techniques by using simple graphics like a bar chart labeled as the Gantt chart to depict relationships between planned and completed work on one axis and elapsed time on the other. He believed in the use of motivational strategies rather than punishment.

Gantt developed a pay incentive system with a guaranteed minimum wage and bonus systems for people on fixed wages. Gantt also focused on the importance of the qualities of leadership and management skills in building effective industrial organizations and emphasized the need for training.

Process Management Theories

Process theories deal with the functions of administrative management. It focuses on managing the organization as a whole instead of managing the individuals. It emphasized the flow of information in the operation of the organization, the manager, and the functions of management and dealt with total management organization. Main thinkers of this school are Henri Fayol and Mary Parker Follett.

Henri Fayol and Process Management

Henri Fayol (1841-1925), was a French Manager and Industrialist born in 1841, in France. He developed a systematic theory of management and a framework for studying management. He is known as "Universalist" and the "Father of Principles of General Management or Functional Management". He was one of the earliest administrative theorists to profound universal principles of the administration who translated his personal experiences into universal truths. He was the father of modern operational management theory. His theory is also known as *Classical Organizational Theory*. The process management has a variety of activities such as technical, commercial, financial, accounting, and managerial.

According to this theory, the functions of process management are to plan, organize, command, coordinate and control various managerial activities. It specifies 14 principles of management.

Fayol used top downward approach He recommended regular meetings of departmental heads and liaison officers to improve coordination of organizational operations. These principles are flexible and can apply for taking decisions in any situation.

Luther Gulick and Administrative Management

Both Gulick and Urwick had rich experience in working of civil services, military organizations, and industrial undertakings. They developed a classical theory of organization which is also known as Administrative Management.

Luther Halsey Gulick (1892-1993), born in Osaka, Japan in 1892, expanded the works of Henri Fayol to build a foundation for management theory. He viewed management functions as universal. He coined a seven-activity acronym, POSDCORB; each letter represents one important function of the manager. It stands for planning, organization, staffing, directing, coordinating, reporting and budgeting. His major contribution was the theory of departmentalization. He identified 4P's: purpose (function), process, persons (clientele), and place as the bases for dividing the work to create departments.

Lyndall Urwick and Administrative Management

Lyndall Urwick (1891-1983) born in Britain in 1891. Urwick defined the organization as determining activities that are necessary for a purpose. His main contribution is in the field of managerial functions and developing general managerial guidelines and principles of management.

NEOCLASSICAL THEORIES OF MANAGEMENT

The neoclassical theory is the extended work to the shortcomings of the classical approaches to management and the beginning of applied research in the area of organizational behavior. It includes management thoughts of human relations school and human resources school.

Human Relations Management Theories

Behavioral or human relations management emerged in the 1920s. Its main concern was on human behavior in the workplace.

George Elton Mayo (1880-1949)

Elton Mayo was an Australian psychologist, sociologist and organization theorist. He is the founder of the Human Relations Movement and is known as the Father of the

Hawthorne Studies. He identified the *Hawthorne Effect* or the bias that occurs when people know that they are being studied or observed. He along with his employees Roethlisberger and Dickinson conducted this study to determine the effect of better physical facilities on workers' output. Some studies were conducted to find out the impact of different situations on the efficiency of workers. The Hawthorne Studies demonstrated the important influence of human factors such as high morale among individuals and group, people-oriented approach to consider people as human beings, and understanding of group attitude and psychology on worker productivity.

Mary Parker Follett and Management Theory

Mary Parker Follett (1868–1933) was born in Quincy, Massachusetts. She was an American social worker and pioneer in the fields of organizational theory and organizational behavior. She emphasized participative decision-making rather than using coercive power. She established a clear-cut channel of communication and was in favor of using depersonalized authority and order in an organization. Three major concepts of Follett's theory were:

- **Universal goal:** The universal goal of organizations is an integration of individual effort into a synergistic whole. Integration is a method of settling conflicts instead of compromise or domination.
- **Universal principle:** It is a circular or reciprocal response emphasizing feedback to the sender considering two-way communications.
- **Law of the situation:** According to the law of the situation, there is no one best way to do anything, but it all depends on the situation. Facts of situation determine the basis of authority and responsibility.

Behavioral Sciences Management Theories

The School of Human Resources represented a substantial progression from human relations in the early 1950s. The contributors of behavioral sciences are Abraham Maslow, Chester Bernard, Douglas McGregor, and Rensis Likert.

Maslow's Theory of Motivation

Abraham Maslow (1908–1970) born in New York, developed the Hierarchy of Needs model in 1940–50s. Maslow was an American psychologist whose theories have been influential in 20th century thought. Maslow's motivation theory known as Need Hierarchy Theory is one of the best known and most influential theories on workplace motivation. This theory is useful for understanding human motivation, management training, and personal development.

According to this theory, human beings have a variety of needs to motivate them to work. These needs are in a *hierarchy, and the man starts satisfying needs step by step. It postulates that satisfied need never motivates human behavior.* Maslow enumerated a wide range of human needs and classified these needs into five categories. Maslow represented these five needs in a hierarchical triangle in a model. He viewed that when the first need is satisfied, then a person moves to next and so on to strive for self-actualization **(Fig. 8.1)**.

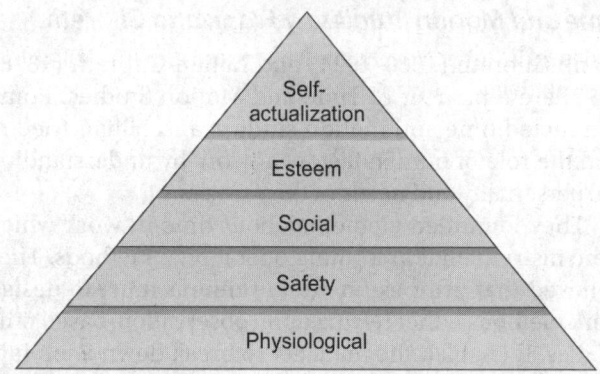

Fig. 8.1: Maslow's "hierarchy of needs" model.

1. **Physiological needs:** These are basic needs required for survival and maintenance of life such as food, clothing, shelter, etc.
2. **Safety needs:** These needs include physical safety against murder, fire, accident, security against unemployment, etc.
3. **Social needs:** These are related to love, affection, belonging to the workgroup, family, etc.
4. **Esteem needs:** These needs ego needs, derived from achievement, mastery, independence, status, dominance, prestige, managerial responsibility, etc.
5. **Self-actualization needs:** These needs are to fulfill the real mission of one's life. These include realizing personal potential, self-fulfillment, seeking personal growth and peak experiences.

The basic core of Maslow's theory is motivation and can apply to motivate employees. The employer in the organization should keep in mind that all human beings have basic needs and a right to strive for self-actualization. The concept of self-actualization provides real meaning, the purpose for employees and the basis for staff development.

Table 8.2 depicts the seventh and eighth need adaptation later on. First four levels are what Maslow called

TABLE 8.2: Hierarchy of need.		
Maslow's Hierarchy of needs	*Adapted in the 1970s*	*Adapted in the 1990s*
➢ Physiological needs ➢ Safety needs ➢ Social needs ➢ Esteem needs ➢ Self-actualization needs	➢ Physiological needs ➢ Safety needs ➢ Social needs ➢ Esteem needs ➢ Cognitive needs (knowledge related) ➢ Esthetic needs (Appreciation and search for beauty, etc.) ➢ Self-actualization needs	➢ Physiological needs ➢ Safety needs ➢ Social needs ➢ Esteem needs ➢ Cognitive needs ➢ Esthetic needs ➢ Self-actualization needs ➢ Transcendence needs (helping others to achieve self-actualization

"deficiency needs" or "D-needs" or deficiency motivators and level 5, and by implication 6 to 8, are growth motivators and relatively rarely found.

Chester Irving Barnard (1886–1961)

Chester Barnard was a telecommunications executive and author of Functions of the Executive, an influential 20th century management book, in which he presented a theory of organization and the functions of executives in organizations. Two of his theories: i) the theory of authority, and ii) the theory of incentives has seven essential rules of communication system. These rules are as follows:

Rules of the communication system
- Definite channels of communication
- Each employee should know and have access to these channels of communication
- Keep communication short and direct
- Adequate skill among person dealing with communication
- No interruption of communication during working hours
- Be honest in communication.

According to Barnard, the organization is a system of discerning coordinating individual activities. He emphasized efficiency and effectiveness as criteria for organizational survival. He divided organization into formal and informal. The informal organization is a part of a formal one. He emphasized on developing a major plan which he labeled as strategic planning.

The key areas of managers to plan are an effective communication system, recruitment, selection, and retaining policies, and employees' motivation. Another major contribution of Barnard is on acceptance of authority. Acceptance theory of authority states that managers only have as much authority as employees allow them to have. Authority flows downward but depends on acceptance by the subordinate. The employees must understand the expectation of the manager and should comply with the directive.

Herzberg's Motivation–Hygiene Theory

Frederick Herzberg (1923–2000), a clinical psychologist and pioneer of "job enrichment". He developed two-factor theory. It identifies five strong motivational factors of job satisfaction (satisfiers) and five job dissatisfaction factors (hygiene factors/dissatisfiers) **(Fig. 8.2)**.

Satisfiers have an association with the growth of employees and task content of the job such as achievement, recognition, works itself, responsibility, advancement, and growth. Hygienic factors or dissatisfiers define the job context such as status, interpersonal relations with supervisor, peers, and subordinates, supervision, company policy and administration, job security, working conditions, salary and personal life, that have little or no relationship to the motivation of job-related behavior.

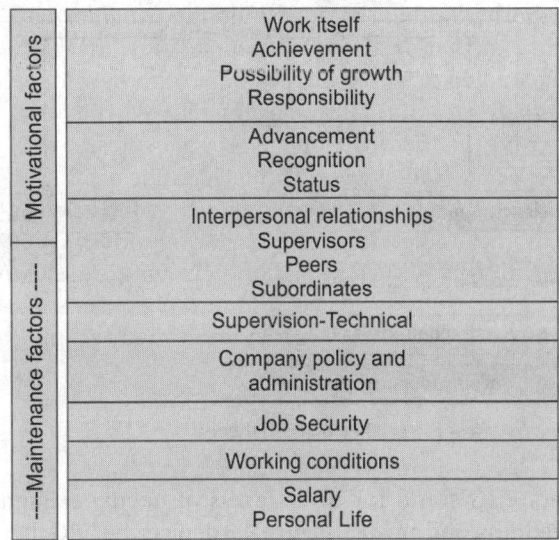

Fig. 8.2: Herzberg's Motivation-Maintenance model.

McGregor Theory X and Theory Y

Douglas McGregor (1906–1964) was an American social psychologist best known for the theory of motivation, i.e. theory X and theory Y. These are two opposing assumptions about human behavior behind every management decision.

i. **Theory X (authoritative management style):** Theory X represents a traditional or narrow view of human nature. The managers think that employees are lazy and dislike work. They avoid taking responsibility and prefers that somebody lead them. That they have no concern with organizational objectives, need constant direction to achieve goals. They need the threat of job loss and financial incentives to work hard. Managers who believe on theory X, generally get poor results. Their management style is authoritarian with repressive style; have tight control without any development. They produce limited, depressed culture.

ii. **Theory Y (participative management style):** Theory Y believes in human relations approach and is adopted most of the modern management thinkers. Y theory assumed that:
   - The persons put efforts as natural as work and play
   - They have self-control and self-direction to achieve organizational objectives
   - Bound to a commitment
   - People are responsible and work with honesty
   - They are innovative and have the problem-solving ability.

Managers who use theory Y, get better results and allow people to grow and develop. Their management style is liberating and developmental, have control for better achievement and continuous improvement through enabling, empowering and giving responsibility.

Alderfer's ERG Theory

ERG theory, proposed by Clayton Alderfer is the extension of Maslow's theory, describes needs as a hierarchy. The

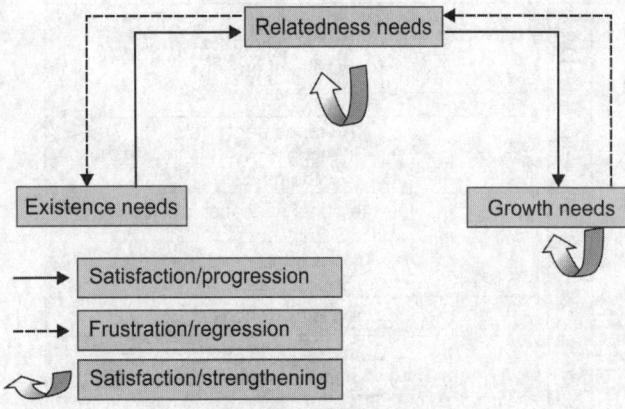

Fig. 8.3: ERG theory.

letters ERG stand for three levels of needs: existence, relatedness, and growth. **Figure 8.3** depicts the ERG theory. It specifies three types of needs as discussed below:

Existence needs: Existence needs is the combination of Maslow's physiological and safety needs.

Relatedness needs: It is the combination of social and esteems needs. These needs are related to a feeling of a sense of identity and position within society.

Growth needs: Growth needs include self-actualization and transcendence needs. These needs are the highest level of needs and concern with growth and attainment of one's potential.

Managers must identify frustration due to the particular need among employees and try to satisfy by using certain motivational techniques to maximize the output.

McClelland's Three Needs Theory

David Clarence McClelland (1917–98), the American Psychologist, is chiefly known for his work on achievement motivation. He was a pioneer for workplace motivational thinking. He developed achievement-based motivational theories and models and advocated competency-based assessment tests to evaluate the performance of employees. His ideas relate closely to Herzberg two-factor theory. Achievement-motivational theory is "three needs theory" developed by McClelland and his associates. According to this theory, people have three types of needs and behave accordingly to fulfill those needs. These needs are:

1. **Need for achievement (nAch):** People who want to achieve something try to attain challenging goals and set new records. They do something different from others. They try to become the best leaders. They believe in hard work and put the effort to succeed.
2. **Need for power (nPow):** Persons who have this type of need are "authority motivated" and they want to have personal status and prestige. They have a strong desire to lead, direct people and want that their ideas should prevail.
3. **Need for affiliation (nAff):** People who have "need for affiliation" are friendly and have good interpersonal relationships with the group. They participate and enjoy social activities. They cooperate and support each other. They feel motivated by being "liked" and "accepted" by others. They prefer to work with people who maintained group harmony and cohesion. Persons having moderate "need for affiliations" are effective managers.

Locke's Goal Setting Theory

Edwin A Locke was a pioneer on "goal setting and motivation theory" based on an idea born out of Aristotle's theory of "final causality," in the late 1960s understands how goals can influence an individual's performance.

In 1990, Locke along with Latham published a theory of "Goal Setting and Task Performance". This theory has five basic principles:

1. **Clear goals:** According to this theory, employees motivated to work if they have clear goals and get appropriate feedback. Goals provide a major source of motivation for the employees to work and to improve performance to achieve the goals. The goals must be productive, clear, measurable, unambiguous, and behavioral and time-bound.
2. **Challenge:** Goals should be explicit and should pose sufficient challenge to the employees.
3. **Commitment:** According to this theory, if the employees are involved in goal setting, they feel more committed rather than if not involved. Employees get motivated and will work hard if they find the goals and tasks are difficult rather than easy.
4. **Performance monitoring and feedback:** Performance monitoring and feedback process are very important to goal setting. Teamwork must be assessed at intervals of time to check its progress and to make modification if required.
5. **Self-efficacy:** Self-efficiency of employees is an important factor to achieve goals. To make employees self-sufficient, arrange a training session.

Expectancy (Three Factors) Theory

Expectancy theory developed by Victor Vroom is a process motivation theory. It deals with motivation and management. According to this theory, motivation is determined by the outcomes that people expect as a result of their actions on the job. It is the combination of effort, which arises from motivation, performance, and outcomes. Vroom hypothesizes that to make a person to be motivated, "effort," "performance" and 'motivation/satisfaction" must be linked. He proposes three variables for positive motivation in his theoretical model **(Fig. 8.4)**:

1. **Valence:** Valence is the value that is attached to the outcome, i.e. the importance given to the expected outcome
2. **Expectancy:** Expectancy is the belief that efforts will influence performance, i.e. increased effort will lead to increased performance and
3. **Instrumentality** is a performance that leads to a specific outcome.

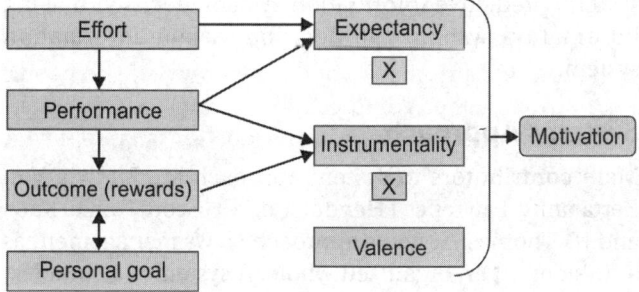

Fig. 8.4: Vroom's expectancy theory model.

Motivation (M) = Expectancy (E) × Instrumentality (I) × Valence (V)

This model holds that job satisfaction follows effective job performance rather than the other way round. Hence, it is important to clarify expectancies about effort and levels of performance and to link rewards with performance outcome to attain the desired level of performance. Managers should be sensitive to employee's expectation and their desires to get rewards. This theory works at times of setting a goal, during a performance appraisal, for taking decisions on salary, and promotion of employees.

Equity Theory (Adams)

John Stacey Adams advocated Equity Theory in 1963 based on job motivation. The basic concept of the theory is on workers' perceptions of the way getting treatment in comparison with others. It also involved feeling and perception as a comparative process. It also states that equality has a direct impact on positive outcomes and motivation among employees.

Equity is a motivational situation where a person compares reward/investment/efforts ratio with ratio enjoyed or suffered by others in the same situation. Specifically, he strives to maintain ratios of his rewards to contributions which are equal to others' ratios. Equity is dependent on comparing own ratio of input/output with a ratio of "referent" others. The concepts of Adams' Equity theory are depicted in **Box 8.1**.

Likert's System 4 Management

Rensis Likert (1903–1981) was an American educator and organizational psychologist. He did extensive research on organizations and management styles. He also developed Likert scale and linking pin model. According to Likert, job oriented supervision was the cause of low productivity and low morale and suggested participative management for decision making. Based on the type of working relationship between superior and subordinates and the degree of involvement of subordinates in the decision-making process, he classified management styles into the four categories:

1. **Exploitive autocratic:** There is no participation of workers with management in decision making due to low confidence in them. They ignore them and use threats and other fear-based methods to achieve the goal.

> **Box 8.1:** Concepts of Adam's equity theory.
>
> $$\text{Equity} = \frac{\text{Outcomes (self)}}{\text{Input (self)}} = \frac{\text{Outcomes (others)}}{\text{Input (others)}}$$
>
> $$\text{Underpayment inequity} = \frac{\text{Outcomes (self)}}{\text{Input (self)}} < \frac{\text{Outcomes (others)}}{\text{Input (others)}}$$
>
> $$\text{Overpayment inequity} = \frac{\text{Outcomes (self)}}{\text{Input (self)}} > \frac{\text{Outcomes (others)}}{\text{Input (others)}}$$
>
> ❖ **Equity:** It is measure fairness by comparing one's balance of input (effort) and outcome (reward), with others input (effort) and outcome (reward).
> ❖ **Underpayment inequality:** The Ratio of input (efforts) and outcome rewards (outcome) of a person is less than others
> ❖ **Overpayment inequality:** When the ratio of one's input (efforts) and outcome rewards (outcome) are more than others.
> ❖ **Inputs:** Inputs are personal characteristics of a person such an effort, loyalty, hard work, commitment, etc.
> ❖ **Outputs:** It refers to all financial rewards

2. **Benevolent authoritative:** There are master and servant type of relationship among superior and subordinates. The subordinates are encouraged for appropriate performance by giving few rewards by top management.
3. **Consultative:** The management has partial confidence in employees and makes maximum use of participative methods, allow them in decision-making for specific decisions. Employees in the organization are closer together and work well together at all levels. The communication is downwards; the upwards communication is cautious.
4. **Participative:** Management has full confidence in employees and encourages group participation and involves them in setting high-performance goals with some economic reward. Employees throughout the organization feel responsible for achieving the organization's objectives.

MODERN MANAGEMENT THEORIES

The origination of the school of modern management thoughts has since 1960. It includes three approaches: quantitative, systems, and contingency approach.

Quantitative Approach

Quantitative approaches include management science approach, operations management, and Management information System approach.

Features

- Problem-solving and decision-making is the prime concern of this approach
- Mathematical models have quantifying variables
- Use of various mathematical symbols to depict managerial problems
- Use of various mathematical tools to solve problems.

Management Science or Mathematical Approach

Management science approach dates back to scientific management of Taylor and his associates. Contributors to this approach are Gilbreth, Gantt, Newman, and Hicks. According to approach, management is a system of the logical process based on scientific research studies.

Various mathematical symbols, equations, and models are used to describe managerial problems and its solutions. Scientific techniques such as mathematical and statistical models are used to provide a quantitative base on this approach.

Mathematical models such as linear programming, Critical Path Methods, Program Evaluation Review Techniques, used to take various managerial decisions like scheduling, budgeting, and staff development. Nowadays, these scientific management techniques are computer-based and more sophisticated. This approach is lacking in the human element and only limited to the decision-making function of management. **Figure 8.5** depicts the problem-solving process approach in quantitative management.

Operations Management

Operation management approach is an application of management science. George B Dontzig was the pioneer of Operation Research approach. This approach can apply them in the managerial situation and less sophisticated than management science. This approach is used to solve the problems concerning service such as human resource management, finance, production, planning, designing, purchasing, etc. The operation management uses tools like linear programming, queuing theory, simulation, and breakdown analysis.

Management Information System

Charles Babbage introduced management information system (MIS) approach. MIS is a computer-based program designed to collect, transmit, process, and store information regarding resources, programs and accomplishment of an organization. The system makes it possible to convert this information into management information for use to make appropriate decisions to solve problems within the organization. It is useful in planning and controlling functions of management by processing data into information—for example, databank information system, predictive information system, decision making information system, and decision making information system.

Systems Approach

Main contributors to system approach are Ludwig Von Bertalanffy, Lawrence J Henderson, W G Scott, Denial Katz, and JD Thomas. Systems approach views management as a "System" of an organized whole. A system is a complex, interrelated and interdependent set of elements which perform common functions to achieve a common goal. It views the organization as a whole, unified and purposeful entity. It looks its effectiveness as a whole, not in parts.

It is an open system that interacts with its internal environment and operates in a larger external environment. Hence, an organization is also a single system of subsystems. Each subsystem has boundaries and includes various inputs, throughput, outputs and feedback to accomplish an overall goal for the subsystem. **Figure 8.6** depicts the elements of each subsystem or a system.

1. **Inputs:** Input is the resources such as raw materials, money, technologies, and people.
2. **Throughput:** Throughput is a process where all resources are aligned moved along and carefully coordinated to achieve the desired goals of the system.
3. **Outputs:** Outputs are the results produced by processes in the system or goals achieved.
4. **Feedback:** Feedback is an ongoing process to ensure that either all resources remain aligned as per plan. The employer takes feedback from various sources such as from employees who carry out processes in the organization, customers/clients using the products and services, and from the external environment (government, society, etc.) that may affect the functioning of the organization.

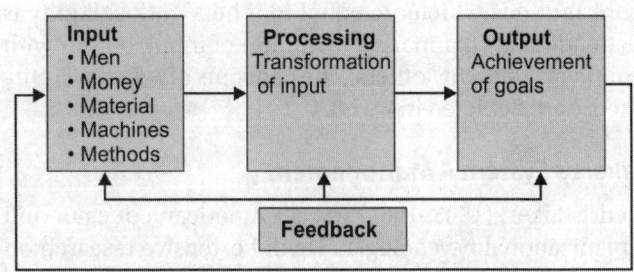

Fig. 8.6: Elements of each subsystem/system.

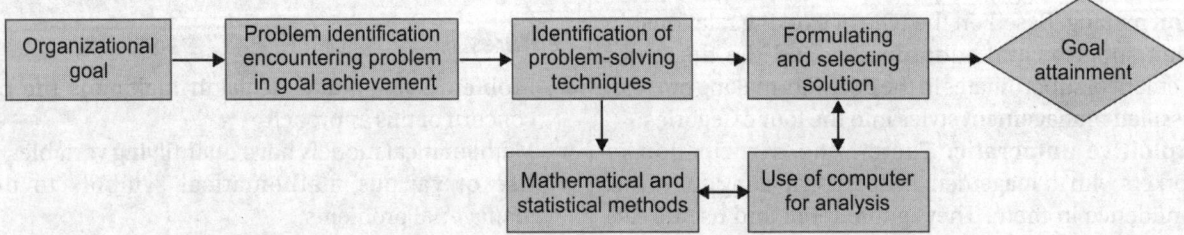

Fig. 8.5: Problem-solving process in quantitative management approach.

Features

- An organization is a system consisting of many subsystems
- All subsystems are mutually interrelated to each other
- Organization as a system depends upon the effective functioning of subsystems
- Measurement of performance of the system in totality rather of its each subsystem
- The system consists of five elements: input, processor, output, controls, and feedback
- The system has an identifiable boundary that distinguishes it from the macro/external environment
- The boundary defines the domain of the system that can be open or closed.
- Social system has open boundaries whereas physical and mechanical systems have closed boundaries.
- Feedback about environmental responses to keep the system in place about its goals and functioning of its subunits
- The organization seeks equilibrium or a stable state both internally and externally.

Contingency or Situational Approach

The concept of contingency or situation in management was emerged quite long back in 1918 by Follett, but related theories were developed in the late 1960s and continue through early 1980s. JW Lorsch and PR Lawrence was the pioneer to contingency approach. According to this theory, management problems are different in different situation need to handle according to a particular situation. It is important for the managers to find out a suitable technique, in a particular situation under particular circumstances that should contribute to attaining the desired managerial goal.

This theory is the extended work of system theory, which views the organization as an open system interacts with the internal and external environment. Various factors of the internal and external environment affect the functioning of the organization. The contingency approach takes into account various factors in the internal and external environment that influence its functioning in a particular situation. Managers develop various methods, design action plans, and tools as per the specific situation. The type of technology, management style, communication system, type of motivation, type of leadership style to be used depends upon the circumstances or situations prevailing at different times.

Features

- Management is situational, and managerial actions entirely dependent upon a particular situation
- No single solution exists in tacking all managerial problems
- Policies, procedures, techniques are affected by internal and external variables. Hence, techniques and control system should be designed to fit in a particular situation
- The type of technology, management style, communication system, type of motivation, and the type of leadership style should be decided according to a particular situation to tackle a problem.
- All principles and methods of management are situational and should not be treated as universal by managers.
- Managers should be situation oriented rather than stereotype.

Fiedler Contingency Theory of Leadership

According to this theory, situational characteristics are the prime contingency factors to determine the effectiveness of leader behavior. Situational characteristics have by three principal factors, i.e. leader-member relationship, task structure, and position power

1. **Leader-member relationship:** Leader-member relationship refers to the personal relationships of the leader with the subordinates.
2. **Task structure:** Task structure includes nature and type of work. It refers to the extent of clarity regarding tasks requirements, standards, documentation and control.
3. **Position power:** It refers to the position in the organization held by the leader and the extent, the leader has the authority to give reward and punishment.

Fiedler identified the effectiveness of a leader's style in the different situation by developing the Least Preferred Coworker (LPC) scale. This scale was to evaluate a manager/leader on a range of scale between positive factors and negative factors about a relationship with coworkers, task structure and position power, and the most effective leadership style to be fitted according to the situation **(Table 8.3)**. A leader must follow "task-oriented" approach in very favorable or very unfavorable situations, and "relation oriented" approach in moderately favorable situations.

Path-goal Theory by Robert House

This theory is also known as the path-goal theory of leader effectiveness, developed by the American psychologist Robert House in 1971 and revised in 1996. This theory is the combination of situational leadership and Vroom's expectancy theory of motivation, based on research.

TABLE 8.3: Leadership style in different contingency/situation factors.

Leader-follower relationship	Task structure	Leader's position power	Most effective leader
Good	Structured	Strong	Low LPC (task-oriented)
Good	Structured	Weak	Low LPC (task-oriented)
Good	Unstructured	Strong	Low LPC (task-oriented)
Good	Unstructured	Weak	High LPC (relation-oriented)
Poor	Structured	Strong	High LPC (relation-oriented)
Poor	Structured	Weak	High LPC (relation-oriented)
Poor	Unstructured	Strong	High LPC (relation-oriented)
Poor	Unstructured	Weak	Low LPC (task-oriented)

(Low LPC: least preferred coworker score is negative; High LPC: least preferred coworker score is positive)

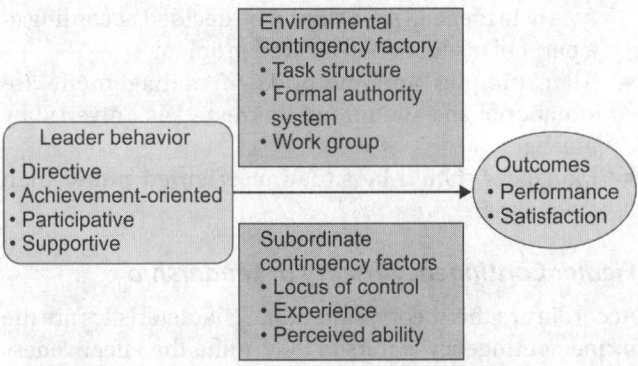

Fig. 8.7: Concepts of path-goal theory.

According to this theory, the leadership style of leaders can determine by contingency factors like characteristics of subordinates (age, ability, acceptance of authority) and environmental factors including nature of the task, structure of the organization. The leader must behave differently in different situations. This theory is an attempt to predict leadership behavior in different situations. There are four leadership styles have emerged from these situation factors, i.e. directive, supportive, participative, and achievement-oriented leadership. **Figure 8.7** illustrates the main concepts of path-goal theory.

Situational Leadership Theory

Heresy and Blanchard propose the situational leadership theory. According to this theory, leaders choose the best course of action based on situational variables.

CHAPTER HIGHLIGHTS

- The management has three stages: classical, neoclassical, and modern approaches.
- The classical approach dealt with bureaucratic, scientific and administrative management thoughts and focused on structure and ways of managing organizations effectively.
- The neoclassical approach deals with human relationships and behavioral sciences based on applied research. Modern management theories emerge from quantitative, system, and contingency streams.
- Taylor developed principles of practice management and Henri Fayol 14 principles and five functions of management. He believed in the top to bottom approach in management.
- Luther Gulick coined a seven-activity acronym, POSDCORB (planning, organization, staffing, directing, coordinating, reporting, and budgeting) and identified 4P's: purpose (function), process, persons (clientele), and place, as the bases for dividing the work.
- Maslow enumerated a wide range of human needs and classified these needs into five categories: physiological, safety, social, esteem, and self-actualization and represented in the hierarchical triangle.
- Herzberg' two-factor theory identifies motivational factors (satisfiers) and maintenance factors (job dissatisfiers), which are separate and distinct from each other.
- Douglas McGregor was best known for the theory of motivation: Theory X (authoritative management style) and Theory Y (Participative management style) depicting two opposing assumptions about human behavior behind every management decision.
- Alderfer's ERG theory describes three types of needs (existence, relatedness, and growth needs) as a hierarchy. Edwin A. Locke was a pioneer in "goal setting and motivation theory" based on five basic principles.
- Equity theory by Adam states that equity is a motivational situation where a person compares reward/investment/efforts ratio with ratio enjoyed or suffered by others in the same situation.
- Likert 4 system theory classified four types of management styles of managers based on the type of working relationship between superior and subordinates and the degree of involvement of subordinates in the decision-making process.
- Modern management theories comprise quantitative, systems, and contingency approaches. Various mathematical symbols, equations, and models are used to describe managerial problems and its solutions in a quantitative approach.
- Systems approach views management as a "System" of an organized whole, having a complex, interrelated and interdependent set of elements known as subsystems which perform common functions to achieve a common goal.
- In the contingency approach, management problems are viewed differently in a different situation and handled according to a particular situation.

REVIEW QUESTIONS

I. Essay Type Questions
1. Enlist various stages of management thought and describe scientific management theory.
2. Discuss the contribution of Henri Fayol in process management.
3. Enumerate important behavioral sciences management theories. Discuss any one theory.
4. Describe the contribution of Elton Mayo and Follett to the development of management thought.
5. Which is the best theory of management in your opinion that you have application in nursing and why?

II. Short Notes
1. Maslow's theory of motivation
2. Systems approach
3. Elements of scientific management
4. The contribution of Chester Barnard
5. The principles of "goal setting and motivation theory".

III. Multiple Choice Questions

1. Fayol has how many principles of management:
   a. 10   b. 12
   c. 14   d. 15
2. FW Tylor is known as Father of:
   a. Modern sociology
   b. Scientific management
   c. Principles of management
   d. Time and motion study
3. Which of the following theory has a rational legal approach?
   a. Bureaucratic
   b. Scientific management
   c. Modern management
   d. Human relation
4. POSDCORB, a seven-activity acronym coined by one of the following thinkers:
   a. Lyndall Urwick   b. McGregor
   c. Locke Edwin A   d. Luther Gulick
5. Purpose, Process, Person, and Place (4P's) are identified as the basis for:
   a. Dividing the work
   b. Span of control
   c. Unity of command
   d. Unity of direction
6. The bias that occurs due to the nonparticipatory observation is known as:
   a. Esprit de corps   b. Hawthorne effect
   c. Confusion   d. Bad management
7. Which theory explains "motivational and maintenance" factors for long-term success of the organization?
   a. Maslow's theory of motivation
   b. Herzberg's motivation-hygiene theory
   c. McGregor theory X and theory Y
   d. Alderfer's ERG theory
8. The style in which management does not allow subordinates to participate in decision making due to low confidence in them is known as:
   a. Exploitive
   b. Benevolent authoritative
   c. Consultative
   d. Participative
9. In which year John Stacey Adams developed equity theory on job motivation?
   a. 1918   b. 1956
   c. 1963   d. 1971
10. Who was the pioneer of human relation movement?
    a. Max Weber   b. Chester Barnard
    c. McGregor   d. Elton Mayo

Answer Keys

1. c   2. b   3. a   4. d   5. a   6. b   7. b
8. a   9. c   10. d

SUGGESTED READING

1. Green GB, Uhl-Bien M. The relationship-based approach to leadership: development of LMX theory of leadership over 25 years: applying a multi-level, multi-domain perspective. Leadership Quarterly. 1995;6(2):219-47.
2. Leader-member Exchange Theory. https://en.wikipedia.org/wiki/Leader%E2%80%93member_exchange_theory. [Accessed on 05.01.2020].
3. Schenkel M, Brazeal D. https://www.questia.com/library/journal/1P3-4159661361/the-effect-of-pro-entrepreneurial-architectures-and. [Accessed on 05.01.2020].

CHAPTER 9

Indian Administrative System and Health Care Delivery System

CHAPTER OUTLINE

- Introduction
- Influences of the British Government
- Indian Constitution
- The Preamble
- Administrative System of India
  - Central Government/Government of India
  - State Government
- District Administration
- Administration of UTS
- Local Self-Government
- Health-care Delivery System of India
  - Introduction
  - Development of Modern Health System
  - Organization of Health-care Delivery System

LEARNING OUTCOMES

After completion of this chapter, the learner will be able to:
- Understand Indian Administrative System
- Discuss Indian Constitution and the preamble
- Describe the administrative system of India
- Depict administrative structure of government at different levels
- Appreciate the evolution of modern health system
- Discuss the organization of the health-care delivery system of different levels

KEY TERMS

Administrative system, Indian constitution, Preamble, health-care delivery system

INTRODUCTION

The administration is of two types—public and private administration. Public administration deals with the activities of the government and private administration refer to the management of private business enterprises. Indian Administration System has passed through various stages to have the present administrative system. During the British period, East India Company did not pay much attention in public administrative till 1773. After that, 'Diwani' set up a system to have a check on servants of the company and developed a code of conduct at supreme and provincial level of governments.

Britishers government had a parliamentary system of administration and appointed civil servants who were trained by them to run the administration. The secretary of state was responsible to British parliament with the power of superintendence and control. Governor General was responsible for smooth running of administration. Indians were for the first time included in administration under Act 1892. Diarchy introduced in the provinces, and the central legislature was bicameral. India became federation of provinces and princely states in 1935. After Quit India Movement, the country had division and became independent in 1947. New Constitution was laid down on 26th January 1950.

INFLUENCES OF THE BRITISH GOVERNMENT

Before 1947, the Britishers government played a negative role. There was no concern for the masses and removing social problems. They followed dividing and rule policy; there was no place for democracy. However, the Britishers' administrative system had a great influence on the present Indian administrative system.

1. **Federal system:** Considering that it would be impossible to run a big country like India administratively from one center, Britishers adopted a federal pattern of the administrative system. India after independence continued the same system.

2. **Parliamentary system:** India continued parliamentary system of government for better administration as British opted.
3. **Independent recruiting body:** Indian administration sets up a separate Union Public Service Commission and State Public Service Commissions for recruiting civil servants. This concept borrowed from Britishers.
4. **Neutrality of civil servant:** During Britishers' Raj, the civil servants were politically neutral. After independence, India also followed the same concept.
5. **The district as a unit of administration:** During British government, collector was head of district administration and was exercising executive, legislative, and judicial powers. After independence, India also followed the same type of administrative setup.
6. **Hierarchical system:** The Britisher's government followed a hierarchical system, a superior-subordinate relationship in the offices, is continued after independence in India.
7. **Local self-government institutions:** British government sets up local self-government institutions for local administration. India after independence also followed the pattern of local self institutions.
8. **Red tapism:** Red tapism is the gift of Britisher's government to Indian administrative setup.
9. **Democratic system:** It is a system "of the people, for the people and by the people" government. India after independence decided to be a democratic country in which the people will be sovereign. This concept is different from the British period.

INDIAN CONSTITUTION

India is a union of 29 states and 7 union territories (UTs) administered directly by the central government and a National Capital Territory (NCT-Delhi). India has a parliamentary system of government. The governance of the republic is regarding the Constitution of India. It is the supreme law of the country and passed in Constituent Assembly of India on November 26, 1949 and enforced on January 26, 1950. The committee under the chairmanship of Dr Babasaheb Ambedkar prepared the Indian constitution.

The Constitution of India is one of the longest written constitutions in the world, containing 395 articles in 22 parts and 8 schedules at the time of its constitution. Article 370 deals with the temporary provisions with respect of the State of Jammu and Kashmir. Total of 93 amendments done in the constitution of India till 2006 and by September 2012, 101 amendments. The last amendment of the constitution was on 8th September 2016.

The Constitution of India is the yardstick for the administration of parliamentary government. The President of India is the constitutional head of the union. According to the Article 79, the Council of the Parliament of the Union consists of the President and two houses, the Council of States (Rajya Sabha), and the House of the People (Lok Sabha). The Rajya Sabha and Lok Sabha are upper and lower houses of the parliament. The Prime Minister is the executive head who has all the executive powers of the government. Lok Sabha is also the House of the People, and the Council of Ministers is responsible.

Every state has a legislative assembly. The certain states have an upper house called State Legislative Council. Governor is the head of a state. Governor heads each state to issue orders. Chief Minister and Council of Ministers advise the Governor for its executive functions. The Council of the Ministers of a state is responsible to the State Legislative Assembly.

There are 7 UTs directly administered by the center. The NCT-Delhi is an exception and is a para-state. It has a legislative assembly with the same system of governance as in case of other states of the country. Pondicherry is such a UT with a legislative assembly.

THE PREAMBLE

The preamble of the Indian Constitution has aspiration, expectation, and aims of the people. It is a written law passed by the Constituent Assembly. It is an act of consolidated regulations that specifies aims, objectives, and philosophy including legislature framework of Indian Republic. Its opening lines are as follows:

We, the people of India, having solemnly resolved to constitute India into a sovereign socialist secular democratic republic and to secure to all its citizens: Justice, social, economic and political; liberty of thought, expression, belief, faith and worship; equality of status and of opportunity; and to promote among them all fraternity assuring the dignity of the individual and the unity and integrity of the nation; in our constituent assembly this twenty-sixth day of November, 1949, do hereby adopt, enact and give to ourselves this constitution.

It indicates the source of constitution, the nature of states, objective, and date of adoption.
1. **Source of constitution:** The source of the constitution is "We, the people of India." It means that the people of India made the constitution without any external power or influence.
2. **Nature of Indian states:** It specifies the nature of the Indian states that are sovereign, socialist, secular, democratic, and republic.
    a. **Sovereign:** It means that India is independent internally and externally. It has its government elected by people and makes a law to govern them.
    b. **Socialist:** It means socialism. According to economic philosophy, socialism that state will own its economy regarding production and distribution, but in India has a mixed economy. It includes private production as well. According to social philosophy, socialism stands for social equality.
    c. **Secular:** Secular means that state has no religion of its own; the people have the right to freedom of conscience, free to express, and propagate the religion of their own.

d. **Democratic:** It is a form of government, which means that people elect the officials of the government to govern them.
e. **Republic:** Republic refers to the head of the state who is either elected directly or indirectly by the people for a fixed tenure.
3. **Objectives of the Indian states:** The objectives of states are to secure justice, equality, liberty, and fraternity to its citizens. The state assures that:
   - People of India will have social, economic, and political justice.
   - They are equal regarding status and getting opportunities.
   - They are free to think, express, belief, faith, and worship of any kind.
   - They assure for individual's dignity, unity, and integrity of the nation.
4. **Date of adoption of constitution:** The constitution drafted by Pandit Jawaharlal Nehru approved and adopted in the Constituent Assembly on 26th November 1949.

ADMINISTRATIVE SYSTEM OF INDIA

According to the constitution, our country has three levels of governments: the central/union government, state, and UTs. Besides these three levels of government, it has local government bodies in rural and urban areas. Ministries and department are run the work of government at three levels, namely Center, State, and District.

At Center/National Level

Central Government/Government of India

The Government of India or the *Union Government* (*Central Government*) is the governing authority of a federal union. It has 29 states, 7 UTs, and a NCT-Delhi. The government is Quasi-Federal Government since it is partly federal and partly unitary.

There are three lists: union list, state list, and concurrent list to exercise powers by both Center and State. The parliament has legislative powers on 97 subjects of the union list and 47 subjects of the concurrent list. But on an emergency, the parliament can make laws on 66 subjects of the state list. The Prime Minister is the head that has a majority in the Lok Sabha of the parliament. The Government of India/Central Government has three sections: the legislature or parliament, the executive, and the judiciary under the headship of the President of India. According to Article 53, all executive powers of the union are exercised by him or through his subordinates.

The Legislature or Parliament

The legislature or parliament is the supreme authority in our country. Indian Administration is carried out by the legislature or parliament. The legislature is responsible for making laws. The President of India heads it. The parliament is bicameral having two houses: Lok Sabha and Rajya Sabha. The President of India elects the members of Lok Sabha and Rajya Sabha, Legislative Assembly of States, and two UTs (Delhi and Puducherry).

1. **The Lok Sabha:** The Lok Sabha is also called the "House of the People" and referred to as the lower house. The Lok Sabha has 552 members as conceived in Article 81 of the Constitution of India. The term of Lok Sabha is 5 years, after which it dissolves automatically and held fresh elections. The citizens of India directly elect the members of the Lok Sabha. There are up to 530 elected members from the states, 20 from the UT, and President of India nominates not more than two members.
At present in Lok Sabha 543 members (530 members from the states and 13 members from the UTs) are elected by voting the President of India elects population of India and two Anglo Indians. The "Speaker" is the presiding officer in the Lok Sabha, who is elected by its members.
2. **The Rajya Sabha:** The upper house or the Rajya Sabha is the "Council of States." The term "Rajya Sabha" is 6 years, and 1/3 members retire every 2 years and replaced by newly elected members. There is a total of 250 members; the state elects 238 members and rests 12 members based on their contribution in the field of art, science, literature, or social services the President of India nominates. Vice President is the ex officio chairman (speaker) of this house and elected by the members of both houses. These houses are concerning making and passing laws. Each prepared bill passes through both the houses and becomes law after the approval by the President.

The Executive

The real executive head is the Prime Minister of India who heads the Council of Ministers and an advisor to the President of India. The President of India has all the constitutional powers but exercises only on the advice of the Prime Minister. The executive section of Government of India consists of President, Vice President, and Cabinet Ministers. The main responsibility of the executive is to pass the laws made by the legislature.

The Judiciary

The third branch of the government of India is the judiciary. Judiciary system of India has on "common law," a single integrated judiciary system with the unified structure of three-tier division. It has judges and courts. Supreme Court of India is apex body in the judiciary. High Courts (HCs) of different states or group of states or a UT and under HCs are hierarchy of subordinate courts such as district and session courts, subordinate judges courts and court of session (criminal), nyaya panchayat, subordinate magistrate, executive magistrate, panchayat adalats, metropolitan magistrate court in metropolitan cities, city civil and session courts, presidency small courts, etc. Apart from courts and judges, it has quasi-judicial bodies such as tribunals (e.g. Central Administrative Tribunal and Armed Forces Tribunal) and regulators.

1. **Supreme Court:** Supreme court of India is the highest court of law in India. It has the final authority to interpret the constitution. It consists of Chief Justice of India and not more than 25 other judges. The President appoints Chief Justice of India who is a citizen of India and having minimum 5 years of experience as a HC judge or an advocate of a HC for a minimum of 10 years.
2. **High Court:** Each state has HC, or by law, parliament may establish a common HC for two or more states and a UT. Each HC has Chief Justice who is appointed by President in consultation of Chief Justice of India, Governor of State, and President also appoints other judges in consultation with Chief Justice of HC and with all mentioned above. The upper age of these officials is 62 years. HC has the power to enforce the fundamental rights, settlement of disputes related to the election of UTs and states legislature, revenue matters and other civil and criminal matters.
3. **Subordinate Court:** Subordinate courts are under HC. These courts have different nomenclature but usually have a uniform organization structure. It includes district and lower courts under the administrative control of HCs.
    i. *District Court:* At the district level, district courts are the judiciary that is directly the HC of respective state. District and session courts are the highest courts in districts, presided over by district and sessions judge. It is a principal court of civil jurisdictions and also a court of sessions that has the power of awarding any sentence including capital punishment. There may be more courts for additional district and sessions judge.
    ii. *Lower Court:* District court has its subordinate courts such as on court of Civil Judge (senior and junior division), court of Chief Judicial Magistrate (senior division for handling criminal cases), and court of Judicial Magistrate (junior division), and many additional courts of Additional Civil Judge (senior division), and additional Chief Judicial Magistrate (senior division). Each court has its judicial independence.
4. **Panchayat Court/Nyaya Panchayat:** Panchayat court also named as nyaya panchayat, gram panchayat, panchayat adalat, or *Kachehri* is the judiciary to deal with the administration of justice at grass root/local/rural level. Panchayat is a judicial component of Panchayat System and has its constitutional status under the 73rd Amendment Act of 1992. It deals with settling disputes of civil cases and also several minor offenses and criminal cases.
5. **Lok Adalat:** It is also known as "People's Court", is a statutory body, established under the Legal Services Authorities Act, 1987 in Article 39-A of the Constitution of India. It provides free, speedy, and competent legal services through negotiations, conciliations, and compromise approach to settling disputes usually of money claims, damages, matrimonial, etc. or cases pending in regular courts under its jurisdiction especially to weaker section. A sitting or retired judicial officer (chairman) along with two other members (usually a lawyer and a social worker) presides over in Lok Adalat. The decision is final if both parties agree. First Lok Adalat was held in 1982 at Junagarh in Gujarat, and now, these are almost functional in every district and taluk/tehsil and are very successful. With the amendment of Legal Services Authorities Act, 1987, there is a provision of a pre-litigation mechanism for conciliation and settlement of disputes related to "public utility services" such as transport services, postal services, services in hospitals, insurances, etc. Permanent Lok Adalat under Section 22B of legal services (Amendment) Act, 2002 decides such matters in most of states and UTs.

Administrative Setup

Central Secretariat

Central secretariat or cabinet secretariat is the administrative machinery at the center level. It constitutes all ministries and departments of the central government. Ministry consists of one or more departments; each department has two or more wings; each wing has two or more divisions; each division has offices comprising some secretariats. The Prime Minister is the political executive head of central secretariat, who is assisted by secretariat staff. Cabinet secretary is the administrative head, who is working under the leadership of Prime Minister. There are other administrative staffs, namely Undersecretary, Deputy secretary, Additional or Joint secretary, who are under Cabinet secretary.

Prime Minister's Office

Prime Minister is the head of an executive branch of government as mentioned above is assisted by Prime Minister's Office (PMO). Before June 1977, the Prime Minister secretariat was PMO. Politically Prime Minister heads PMO, and its administrative head is Principal Secretary. Principal secretary deals with all administrative government files, important documents of PM, and many more functions. There are additional secretaries and joint secretaries under the principal secretary. More than 350 people are working under PMO.

At State Level

State Government

The state government is below the level of central government. There are 29 states in the country, and its state government governs each state. The Governor and Chief Minister head each state. The Chief Minister is also the head of Council Ministers. Governor is the nominal head of state and appointed directly by the President of India for 5 years. The same person can be the head of two or more states. Like the president of India, he or she has certain executive, legislative, and judiciary powers and also certain emergency powers of the state. Each state has different departments for its functioning such as internal security, education, public health, sanitation, agriculture, etc. The units of each state are districts.

Structure of State Government

State government like central government has three sections: the executive, the legislature, and the judiciary.

1. **State executive:** The state executive consists of Governor, the Chief Minister, and Council Ministers. The Chief Minister is the executive head of the state. The executive powers are vested with Governor, and he takes all executive actions in the name of Governor, but the actual executive powers for the functioning of state are with Chief Minister of state and his Council Ministers.
2. **State legislature:** Each state has its state legislature known as a legislative assembly. It comprises of Governor and either one house (unicameral), i.e. legislative assembly or two houses (bicameral), i.e. legislative assembly and legislative council. Seven states have two houses (legislative assembly and legislative council), and rest states have only one house (legislative assembly). The Chief Minister heads legislative assembly/legislative council. Legislative assembly is known as Vidhan Sabha, and the legislative council is known as Vidhan Parishad.
   i. *Vidhan sabha or legislative assembly:* A total number of Members of Legislative Assembly (MLAs) vary from 60 to 500. Each state has a fixed number of MLAs. All states have MLAs. These are elected members by the people of state. Cabinet Minister's nomination is from MLAs.
   ii. *Vidhan parishad or legislative council:* The size of vidhan parishad is not more than one-third of the seats reserved for MLAs. These are the elected by the Governor and are known as Members of Legislative Council (MLCs). MLCs cannot be the member of cabinet ministers.
3. **State judiciary:** High Courts are the supreme authority of judiciary system at the state level. It is an appellate authority for a state or a group of states. High Courts deal with the appeals from the lower courts and also writ petition filed under article 226. High Courts vary in their territorial jurisdictions.

Administrative Setup at State Level

There are three components of government at state level, namely Minister, Secretary, and Executive Head. Minister and the Secretary are the political and administrative head, respectively, of state secretariat, and the directorate is the office of the executive head.

1. **State secretariat:** At the state level, state secretariat comprises ministries and departments. It is headed politically by Chief Minister, and the administrative head of entire state secretariat is *Chief Secretary* who controls the administration of the state. He is an advisor to Chief Minister in all matters. Chief Secretary is assisted by Secretary who is head of one or two departments. The secretariat departments vary in number from 15 to 35. The common departments in states are General Administration, Finance, Home, Jail, Police, Forest, Social welfare, etc. Departments have officers as of central secretariat for a fixed period. State secretariat is concerned with policy making.
2. **Directorates:** The directorate is the office of the executive head. Directorates are the executive branch of state government and are under state secretariat. It is concerned with execution or implementation of policies framed by state secretariat. It provides technical advice to ministers, organizes various in-service education programmes, prepares a budget of the department, etc., and also tries to improve the efficiency of its department by implementing various programs.

District Administration

The districts are territorial divisions of the state. It is a basic unit of administration. It has about 2 million populations. District administration is concerned with various managerial activities of the district. Main functions of district administration are to maintain law and order, administration of criminal and civil justice, revenue administration, and implementation of various developmental and welfare programmes, special programs for weaker sections, development schemes, assisting people at the time of natural disasters and calamities, etc.

1. **Structure:** The structure of the district is of three or four tiers. The law, order, and revenue components are by the district, one or two intermediate levels, and ground level (district, subdivision, tehsil, village level). Community development and Panchayati Raj component is mainly District–Block–Panchayat.

   At the district level, multiple functionaries are working to carry out various functions of the government. District collector or deputy commissioner, district magistrate, and district officers are the officer-in-charge of each district that represents the state governments. Other functionaries under district administration are Superintendent of Police, Assistant Registrar of Cooperative Societies, and District Medical Officers, etc. There are six types of administrative areas at the district level: subdivisions, tehsil, community development blocks, municipality and corporations, villages, and panchayat.
2. **Administrative areas**
   a. **Law, order, and revenue components**
      i. *Subdivisions:* Subdivisions are the units of a district named as Prants. These are the head of each subdivision is an officer-in-charge of IAS rank designated as Subdivisional Officer (SDO), Subdivisional Magistrate, Revenue Divisional Officer, Subcollector, Deputy Collector or Prant-officer in the different states of India. Subdivisions are responsible for general administration, law, and order and

in many states mainly responsible for *land revenue administration*. Subdivisional officer coordinates with District Collector and Tehsildar for revenue matters, whereas for matters relating to law and order, he coordinates with District Magistrate and Station Officer (police).

ii. *Tehsils:* Tehsils or talukas are the administrative areas of each subdivision. Tehsils look after the general administration, treasury, land revenue, land records, and other functions. It has around 200–600 villages. The size of villages range from 500 to 5,000 persons and vary from state to state. More than 65% population of these villages belong to rural areas. *Tehsildar* is the office in charge or chief executive of each tehsil/taluka who acts as an actual revenue collector. There are four types of tehsildar: nonexistence, weak (SDO is resident), stronger (SDO not a resident), and strongest (no SDO). *Naib tehsildars* called *Kanungos* (surveyors) assist tehsildar; *Patwaris* and *Lekhpals* look after revenue, and land records related to work and also maintenance of law and orders in some places. Other officers-in-charge in each tehsil are police inspector, assistants, surgeons, overseers, veterinary officers, agriculture inspectors, and other departmental officers. In some states, in place of *tehsildar*, the position of subdeputy collectors exists.

iii. *Pargana:* Next to *tehsil* is a Circle/Pargana/Firka. The head of Pargana is *Kanungo/Circle Inspector/Revenue Inspector*, who supervises and compiles land records maintained by *Patwaris*. He is the first line supervisor in land administration in the state.

iv. *Villages:* Village is the lowest administrative and fiscal unit of the state. *Patwaris/Karamchari/Patel/Munsif/Lekhpal* is the in charge of one or more villages, whose main role is the maintenance of land records, land measurement, and statistical data at the village level.

b. **Community development and Panchayati Raj component:** The head of community development and Panchayati Raj component at the district level is *District Collector*; at state level, *Development Commissioner*; and at the national level, department of rural development under Ministry of Agriculture and Irrigation.

i. *Blocks:* To run rural community development programmes and schemes, rural area of each district is divided into community development blocks. Each block has a population of one lakh covering 100 villages. *Block development officer (BDO)* is the in-charge of each block who directly works under district collector/SDO. He is responsible for community development programmes concerning irrigation and road construction and management of Panchayat Samiti.

ii. *Circles/villages:* Each block has 10 circles/villages. A village level worker designated as *Gram Sevak* is in charge of each circle.

Administration of UTs

There are 7 UTs in India, namely Andaman and Nicobar Islands, Chandigarh, Dadra and Nagar Haveli, Daman and Diu, Lakshadweep, NCT of Delhi, and Puducherry.

Structure of UTs

Union territories are directly under the control and administration of central or union government except for Delhi and Puducherry. These two UTs are vested with partial statehood and having its legislative assemblies, executive councils of ministers, and the Chief Minister. Rest five UTs has an administrator (either an IAS or an MP) appointed by the President of India designated as either Lieutenant Governor or Chief Commissioner or Administrator. The President of India can appoint Governor of adjoining state as an administrator for the administration of UTs.

Local Government Bodies

1. **Village (rural) administration:** Panchayati Raj is a basic unit of administration. Rural administration works at three levels: at village (gram), tehsil/taluka (block), and district (zila) level.

   a. **At village level/gram level**
   Village/gram panchayat: A village/gram panchayat is an elective and statuary local government body for one or several villages. The size and number of villages per panchayat vary from state to state. It comprises 1 elected *Sarpanch* and 15–20 members. It is concerned with planning and implementation of economic development and social justice programmes, and levy and collection of taxes, etc.

   b. **At tehsil/taluka/block level**
   Block panchayat/panchayat samiti: At block/tehsil level, there is a block panchayat or panchayat samiti. It comprises all Sarpanches of panchayat samiti, MPs, MLAs of the area, SDO of subdivision, and other members from weaker sections. A development block has rural 100 villages of tehsil or taluka and a population of 80,000–120,000.

   c. **At district/zila level**
   Zila panchayat/parishad: The zila panchayat/parishad is the agency of rural local self-government at the district level. It includes all the areas of the district except the smaller urban areas/areas under the authority of municipal corporation (MC)/town panchayat/industrial township. An IAS officer is the chief executive officer (CEO) for administration the zila panchayat appointed by state government. It also includes chief accounts officer, chief planning officer, and one deputy secretary and other elected members of gram panchayat and panchayat samiti.

Main functions of zila parishad/panchayat are overall supervision, coordination, planning, and integration of all developmental, welfare programmes, and schemes at the district level. It works through various standing committees such as general standing committee, Finance, Audit, Planning Committee, Social Justice Committee, Education and Health Committee, Agriculture, and Industries Committee. Each committee has a chairman and other elected members.

2. **City (urban) administration:** There are several types of urban local bodies in India such as MC, municipality, notified area committees (NACs), town area committee (TAC), cantonment board, township, port trust, and special purpose agencies.

   a. **MC/Mahanagar Nigam:** Municipal corporations are the urban local bodies for the administration in metro or large cities and towns such as Delhi, Mumbai, Chennai, and Kolkata. These are established indiscretion of state government by passing act, and in UTs, these are established by parliament acts.

   The state government appoints *Municipal Commissioner* who is the executive head of MC and is the rank of an IAS officer. MC consists of the *standing committee* and *a council*. The council is the deliberative and legislative wing of MC. It has elected members known as *counselors*. The head of council is *a Mayor*, who is assisted by Deputy Mayor. The standing committees are constituted to coordinate and facilitate work of MC.

   b. **Municipality/nagar palika:** Municipalities are the urban local bodies for the administration of smaller cities and towns, set up by respective state government by passing Acts and in UTs these are established by parliament acts. These are municipal committee, municipal board, and municipal council, etc. The head of municipality is the CEO, appointed by state government. The municipality has a deliberative and legislative wing known as council. It has elected members named as *Counselors* and a head called *President* or *Chairman*; who is assisted by Vice-President/Vice-Chairman. There are standing committees to facilitate the work of the municipality.

   c. **NAC/nagar panchayat/nagar parishad:** As the name indicates, these are the local urban bodies, established by notification in state government gazette under the provision of State Municipal Act. NACs are responsible for the administration of areas either underdeveloped or fast-developing town converted into municipality. It is for the population of 11,000–25,000. It is a nominated body.

   d. **Town area committee:** Town area committees are established under separate act by state government for the administration in small towns. It is either wholly elected or wholly nominated by the government or partially nominated and partially elected body. It has limited functions.

   e. **Cantonment board:** Cantonment boards look after the administration of civilian population in cantonment areas. These are directly under the control of union/central government (under Cantonment Act, 2006) through Union Defense Ministry. It has partially elected and partially nominated members; an Ex-officio President, a military officer of the commanding the station; and Vice-President elected from the members. It also has an executive officer, appointed by President of India.

   f. **Township:** These are responsible for the administration of large public sector enterprises for its staff and workers residing near to plant. It has a town administrator, engineers, and other staffs but no elected members.

   g. **Port trust:** These are established by an Act of Parliament, for the protection, safety of ports, and for civic amenities in port areas such as in Kolkata, Mumbai, and Chennai. It has an official chairman and members both elected and nominated.

   h. **Special purpose agencies:** These are the agencies that are established by the government under any of the above-mentioned urban local bodies to look after special or single purpose such as housing boards, city transport trust, urban developmental authorities, and pollution control boards, etc.

HEALTH-CARE DELIVERY SYSTEM IN INDIA

Introduction

According to WHO, the health-care delivery system in every country comprises all organizations, institutions, and resources that put effort to promote, restore, maintain, or improve health. Each health-care delivery system is responsible for improving the health and also to protect the people against financial risk for medical care and for providing care to them with dignity. It is the responsibility of health systems to fulfill the needs of the community, especially the poor. Health is one of the rights of people as well as contribution in economic development and poverty reduction. India has a mixed health-care system. The health-care services are through the public and private sectors. Apart from an allopathic system of medicine, it also has other systems of medicine such as AYUSH.

DEVELOPMENT OF MODERN HEALTH SYSTEM

Health systems have existed since the time of organized form of group living. Initially, the individual practicing medicine and surgery was providing healthcare as a family trade. During ancient time, charitable and public hospitals were the institutions providing health-care services to people. There is also a record of practicing different systems of medicine over the last 4,000 years. The modern health system originated from Europe is the allopathic systems of medicine traced back for the last 300–400 years. Indian health system can be categorized under three phases:

Phase I (1947–1983): The first report on Health Survey and Development Committee (Bhore Committee) formed the landmark in developing health policy and health system in India. It also recommended the three-tiered healthcare system to provide preventive and curative health-care services. According to the Health Policy, the state has the responsibility to provide health services to the people, and they cannot deny such services for want of ability to pay. The public hospitals, individual private practitioners, and family doctors were providing services through Indian systems of medicine.

Phase II (1983–2000): The National Health Policy (NHP; 1983) emphasizes to encourage private initiative in health-care service delivery. So the focus of the state policy shifted to primary healthcare, especially to the rural population.

Phase III (2000–2012): During this phase, there was a shift in the provision of health-care services. There was a plan to utilize the private health sector resources and to liberalize the insurance sector for financing health expenditure. The role of state is now both as a provider and as a financier of health services.

Due to noncompliance of achieving the goals of the first NHP (1983), many health policies emerged. The government followed the decentralization approach in implementing health programs and established two-tier urban health-care system to achieve health goals of the National Policy (2002). The government made efforts to increase public expenditure and health investment to utilize the resources of the private sector to achieve an acceptable standard of good health by 2015.

The government launched the National Rural Health Mission (NRHM) on 12th April 2005 to strengthen rural health with the objective to introduce the Accredited Social Health Activist (ASHA) females to provide the services at the village level. To improve infrastructure and human resources at the subcentre level, integrate vertical health programs at national level, and providing technical support, building capacity, and ensuring availability of doctors in rural areas per Indian Public Health Standards (IPHS) for community health centres (CHCs).

Phase IV (2012–2017): During this phase, the government introduced a 12th Five-Year Plan strategy to achieve its goal for *universal access* to equitable, affordable, and quality health-care services and to revitalize both rural and urban health sectors. The NRHM emerged into National Health Mission (NHM) (2012–2017).

It aims at universal coverage of all villages and towns in the country to strengthen health system both urban and rural and focus on reproductive-maternal-neonatal-child-adolescent health (RMNCH+A), communicable, and noncommunicable diseases. Two major submissions, i.e. NRHM and National Urban Health Mission (NUHM) approved on 1st May 2013 under NHM.

National Urban Health Mission as submission of NHM was launched on 20th January 2014 to improve the health status of urban poor both listed and unlisted living in slums, vulnerable population by addressing their particular health issues. It operates at national government, state government, and city/community level.

Phase V (2017 and onward): During this phase, the government introduced the NHP 2017 and replaced the planning commission with National Institute of Transforming India (NITI) Aayog. The government prepared a three-year agenda to strengthen the existing health system with the objectives to attain universal health coverage of the highest possible level, free and comprehensive and affordable primary healthcare, improved access to secondary and tertiary quality health-care services, and reduction of a poor household's out-of-pocket expenditure on healthcare. The NHP (2017) focuses on:

- Health finance sector
- Health infrastructure and building capacity per IPHS standard norms
- Establishing primary and secondary health-care facilities
- Health management information system
- Strengthening health surveillance system
- Establishing registries for public health diseases
- Integrated health information architecture.

The principle of Team India is the base of NITI Aayog. It has a strategic vision, long-term policies and program framework, implementation, monitoring, and evaluation strategies to achieve the specific goals of Three-Year Health agenda by 2020. It focuses on public and preventive health, quality healthcare, better health outcome, strengthening human resources for health, access to medicines, health research, and reforms in professional regulatory bodies.

The role of private hospitals in urban India through the participation of private hospitals for diagnosis and treatment and by sharing its services such as ambulance services, blood bank, physiotherapy, highlighted to strengthen district hospitals. It also specifies free-of-cost treatment to people with government health insurance and people of below poverty line (BPL).

ORGANIZATION OF THE HEALTH-CARE DELIVERY SYSTEM

A good health system delivers quality services to all people, when, and where they need them. It needs to respond in a balanced way to the needs and expectations of the community at large to improve their health status, to defend them against health threats, and to provide equitable access to people-centered care. Since health is the fundamental right of each, the country has the responsibility for their health. In India, the states are largely independent in matters relating to the delivery of healthcare to the people. The control of the health system is through three main links: Center, state, and local or peripheral.

Organization of Health System at the National Level

The organization of the health system in India at the national level is under the Ministry of Health and Family Welfare (MOHFW). The center makes the policy, plans, guidelines, and assists and coordinates the activities of state health ministries.

Ministry of Health and Family Welfare

The Ministry of Health and Welfare is the official organ of the health system in India. It is responsible for framing the health policy and for all the national health programmes in India. The Union Health Minister, a member of Council of Ministers, is head of MOHFW and holds cabinet rank and assisted by two ministers of state [Health and Family Welfare (H and FW)]. Two departments are under its control: Department of H&FW and Directorate General of Health Services (DGHS).

1. **Department of H&FW:** Department of H&FW deals with health and family welfare-related policies and matters. Health statutory bodies, societies, and autonomous health institutions are under the administrative control of this department. It has about 37 health divisions under its control. The secretary is the head of this department who is assisted by additional and joint secretaries.
2. **The Directorate General of Health Services:** Directorate General of Health Services is a technical wing attached to the office of the Department of H&FW. It provides technical advice regarding public health, medical education, and health-related matters and implementing health schemes. The head of the Directorate is Director General of Health Services, who coordinates with directorates of all states and UTs through its regional offices. It controls the functioning of all central hospitals and deals with health-related matters through its subordinate offices and health institutes. DGHS performs both general and specific functions. The general functions of DGHS are to conduct the survey, planning, coordination, programming, and appraisal of all health matters in the country.

   There are 14 division/departments such as administration, vigilance, tuberculosis, leprosy, public health, etc. under its control. All divisions have staff and specific work allocation. It has nine subordinate offices located at different places all over the country. These offices implement government health policies and provide advice on technical matters.
   1. **Regional office of H&FW:** These offices are at different places throughout the country. These offices coordinate with state for all centrally sponsored Health & Welfare Programmes. There are five units under its control. These are related to Malaria Operation Field Research, Entomology, Malaria, Health Information Field, and regional evaluation team. Each unit has subunits. The organization of each unit is different from other.
   2. **Central drug lab:** The drug and cosmetic control is part of DGHS and drug controller is its head. It lays and enforces the standards and controls the manufacture and distribution of drugs through both central and state government officers under the Indian Drug & Cosmetic Act, 1940.
   3. **Central drug testing lab:** There are seven labs located at different places of India. The statutory lab is at Mumbai. The director is the head of each lab.
   4. **Medical store organization:** DGHS has control over medical store depots for the quality, cost, and supply run by the union government. There are seven medical store depots located in different places. Of seven, three are with Chennai testing lab. Deputy Assistant Director-General is the head of medical store organizations (MSOs). Each MSO has three divisions: office division, store, and accounts division.
   5. **National Centre for Disease Control:** The director is the head of this subordinate office and responsible for all its administrative and technical matters. It is mainly for surveillance to control and prevent communicable diseases. It has 12 divisions of various sections and labs. An office-in-charge is the head of each division, and medical and nonmedical scientists, research officers, and other supporting staff work under the officer-in-charge. The National Centre for Disease Control (NCDC) office has eight branches located at different places covering all states and UTs for surveillance, monitoring, and response. It also has training programs in Public Health, Lab Sciences, etc.
   6. **Central Health Education Bureau:** Preparation of education material for creating health awareness among people is one of the outstanding activities of this bureau. It has five divisions: media, health promotion, school health education, training, and administrative division.
   7. **National Vector Borne Disease Control Programme Directorate:** The directorate of National Vector Borne Disease Control Programme (NVBDCP) is one of the subordinate office or technical division of DGHS. It is an agency to control and prevent six vector-borne diseases. It frames its national guidelines, policies, and strategies to combat vector diseases and provide directions to states for its implementation.
   8. **Rural Health Training Centre:** Rural Health Training Centre (RHTC), which is at Najafgarh, New Delhi, is under DGHS. It is a training center for training to medical interns on rural health under Reorientation of Medical Education (ROME) scheme. It undertakes many training-related activities, providing primary health services, emergency services, and healthcare under NHRM; conducts field research studies; and organizes village health days and so on.

9. **International Health Division:** International airports and all major ports are directly under the control of DGHS. It also coordinates all the activities related to obtaining assistance from international agencies.

Organization of Health System at State Level

The state is independent to decide its health matters. Each state, therefore, has developed its system of health-care machinery, independent of the central government.

State Ministry of Health

The state health minister is the head of the Health Ministry. There is secretariat under the charge of secretary/commissioner (Health and Family Welfare) belonging to the cadre of Indian Administrative Service (IAS). Deputy secretary, undersecretary, and a large number of administrative staff work under Health Secretary.

Department of H&FW

Department of Health and Family Welfare is under the State Ministry of Health. This department deals with the execution of health and family welfare-related policies and matters and implementation of health and family welfare services and national health programmes. It also assists in implementing various national- and state-level health schemes and health programs under NHM. State health statutory bodies, societies, and health institutions are under the administrative control of this department. The state H&FW department performs preventive, promotive, and curative health services to its people. Its organization differs from state to state. It has various departments and subordinate offices under its control such as Directorate of H&FW, NHM, Directorate of AYUSH, Directorate of Homeopathy, Food and Drug Administration, and so on.

The State Health Directorate

Each state has its health-care system. The organization structure of state is a similar pattern to Central Government. The State Directorate of Health Services is a technical wing. Director General of Health Services is the in-charge of State Health Directorate, who report to State Health Secretary/commissioner. Both Directorate of Health Services and Directorate of Medical Education and Research integrated but are separate. Deputy Director, Joint Director, and Assistant Director are under the Director. Few states have the post of Ayurvedic Director and Homeopathy Director in their Health Directorates. The State Health Directorate performs the following functions:

- To study the health problems to identify the health needs of people
- To provide curative and preventive services
- To make provision for control of milk and food sanitation
- To take all the remedial action at the time of the outbreak of communicable diseases
- To establish and maintain central laboratories for the preparation of vaccines
- To promote health awareness among people
- To collect, tabulate, and publish vital statistics
- To promote all the health programs
- To recruit health personnel for rural health services
- Supervision of primary health center (PHC) and staff
- Planning and carrying out surveys on health-related matters
- Establishing training courses, etc.
- To coordinate all health services with other states.

Organization of Health Services at Regional Level

Few states have regional or divisional health services under State Health Directorate. Each zone comprises three to five districts. Usually additional or deputy director is the head of these regional health departments.

Organization of Health System at District Level

The administration of district in India is under the control of a collector or deputy commissioner. He controls six types of administrative areas: subdivisions, tehsil, villages, municipalities, corporate, community developmental blocks, and panchayat.

District health organization has no uniformity in its organizational structure. Each state develops its pattern to suit its policy and convenience. The people at large receive the health-care services through the public sector, private sector, indigenous system of medicines, voluntary health agencies, and vertical health program. However, present organization of health services by public or government sector consists of rural hospitals, subdivisional or tehsil, taluq hospitals, district hospitals, specialist hospitals, and teaching institutions.

a. **District hospitals:** District hospitals provide mostly curative services, has no catchments area, and the team consists of curative staff. The chief medical and health officer/civil surgeon is the head of a district hospital/civil hospital. They are responsible for implementing all the national health programmes per the direction of States and Centre. Deputy medical officers are under Chief Medical Officer (CMO).

b. **Subdivisional/taluk:** At the taluk level, Assistant District Health and Family Welfare Officer (ADHO) is responsible for health-care services of Talukas/subdivisional hospitals. These hospitals converted into CHCs.

c. **Community health center:** For an effective referral, one CHC is to cater the needs of every 80,000–1,20,000 rural populations. It is a functional 30-bedded rural hospital to provide the basic specialty services in general medicine, pediatrics, surgery, obstetrics, and gynecology round the clock. According to norms, it should have 10 staff nurses and 1 public health nurse under block medical officer/senior medical officer/medical superintendent.

It is upgradation of the subdistrict/taluka hospitals or some of the block level PHC.

Each urban-CHC covers a population of 2.5 lakh population (5 lakh for metros). It has 30- to 50-bedded inpatient facilities (100-bedded facilities in metros). It provides curative, and maternal and child health (MCH) services including institutional deliveries, specialties services, and diagnostic facilities.

d. **Primary health centers:** Each PHC has the facility of four to six in patients' beds. It is a center to provide the preventive, promotive, MCH, curative, and other services to a rural population of 20,000–30,000 to cover 25 villages or six subcenters. It is a referral unit of six subcenters and refers cases to the CHC. It varies from state to state. It provides Out Patient Department (OPD), emergency, referral, and in-patient services. According to Indian Public Health Standard, there is a requirement of one HW (female)/auxillary nurse midwife (ANM) for subcenter of the area, one health assistant (male), one health assistant (female)/LHV, and three–four staff nurses and under NRHM two additional staff nurses on contract basis under medical officer-in-charge. The urban PHC caters the needs of 50,000–60,000 urban population including slum population of 20,000–30,000. It provides services through OPDs that run for 8 hours in two shifts from 8 to 12 pm and 4 to 8 pm with flexible timings according to need. Medical officer-in-charge is the head of urban PHC. The workforce includes three staff nurses, one LHV, three to five FHWs/ANMs, and other staff.

e. **Subcenter:** Each subcenter is to give MCH services (including delivery facility with four to five rooms in type B subcenter), family planning, immunization, and other services under different programs to a population of 3,000–5,000 and to cover at least four villages. According to Indian Public Health Standard (2012), there is a requirement of one health worker (HW; male)/Multi Purpose Health Workers (MPWs), and one ANM/HW (female) and an additional ANM/HW (F) on a contract basis to provide outreach services. There is no subcenter the urban community level. Health services catered to the urban community through ASHA, Mahila Arogya Samiti, and ANM female/HW female. They report to Medical Officer (MO) I/C of urban PHC.

CHAPTER HIGHLIGHTS

- Indian administrative system has a great influence of British government in many ways.
- India has a parliamentary system of government. The Constitution of India is the yardstick for the administration of parliamentary government.
- The preamble of the Indian Constitution is a written law passed by the Constituent Assembly.
- India has three levels of governments: national, state, and UTs, and local government bodies.
- The centre and each state government have three branches: legislature (parliament), executive, and judiciary.
- Cabinet secretariat is the administrative machinery at center level. Chief Minister is the political head of each state, and chief secretary is an administrative head of secretariat.
- The modern health system originated from Europe is the allopathic systems of medicine traced back for the last 300–400 hundred years.
- The control of the health system is through three main links: Center, State, and local or peripheral.
- The MOHFW at the national level has two departments: Department of Health and Famly Welfare and DGHS. Thee are many departments and subordinate offices under DGHS.
- Health-care delivery system of state is almost in the center pattern. Director General of Health Services is the head of State Health Directorate.
- Collector or deputy commissioner is the administrative head of a district. He controls various administrative areas. The CMO is the head of a district hospital. It has a link with subdivisions, CHCs, PHCs, and subcenters.

REVIEW QUESTIONS

I. Essay Type Questions
1. Describe Indian administrative system at national level.
2. Discuss in detail the state administration.
3. Explain various stages of development of the modern health system.
4. Describe the health-care delivery system at the national level.
5. Describe the district health-care delivery system.

II. Short Notes
1. Indian Constitution
2. Preamble
3. District administration
4. Local government bodies
5. Health-care delivery system at state level

III. Multiple Choice Questions
1. When did the Indian Constitution lay down?
   a. 1950 b. 1949
   c. 1947 d. 1935
2. India is the union of how many states?
   a. 21 b. 25
   c. 27 d. 29
3. When did the last amendment of the Indian Constitution after 2012?
   a. 2014 b. 2015
   c. 2016 d. 2018
4. What does "sovereign" means?
   a. That people have the right to express feelings and of freedom of consciousness
   b. That India is independent of internal and external forces

    c. That India has social equality
    d. That state has no religion of its own
5. Which is the supreme authority in our country?
    a. Supreme Court   b. The legislature
    c. Executive   d. Judiciary
6. Which of the subordinate court deals with civil cases?
    a. District court   b. Session court
    c. Lower court   d. High court
7. The Legislative Council at State legislature is known as:
    a. Vidhan Sabha   b. Rajya Sabha
    c. Lok Sabha   d. Vidhan Parishad
8. Which subordinate office lay and enforce a standard of drugs?
    a. Regional office
    b. Central drug lab
    c. Central drug testing lab
    d. Medical store organization
9. What is the main function of National Centre of Disease Control?
    a. Health promotion and control of communicable and noncommunicable diseases
    b. Control of vector-borne diseases
    c. Surveillance, monitoring, and response to control and prevent communicable diseases
    d. Coordination with state to all centrally sponsored health programs
10. What is the population coverage of Urban Community Health Centre of Metro cities?
    a. 80,000   b. 1,20,000
    c. 2,50,000   d. 5,00,000

Answer Keys

| 1. a | 2. d | 3. c | 4. b | 5. b | 6. a | 7. d |
| 8. b | 9. c | 10. d | | | | |

SUGGESTED READING

1. Administration of Union Territories in India. https://www.gktoday.in/gk/administration-of-union-territories-in-india/. [Accessed on 05.01.2020].
2. The Constitution of India. http://legislative.gov.in/sites/default/files/coi-4March2016.pdf. [Accessed on 05.01.2020].
3. Preamble of the Constitution of India. https://en.wikipedia.org/wiki/Preamble_to_the_Constitution_of_India. [Accessed on 05.01.2020].
4. [PDF] chapter–3 structure of district administration-Shodhganga. https://shodhganga.inflibnet.ac.in/bitstream/10603/104159/7/07_chapter%203.pdf. [Accessed on 06.01.2020].
5. Constitution of India | National Portal of India. https://www.india.gov.in/my-government/constitution-india. [Accessed on 06.01.2020].
6. District Courts of India - Indian Courts. http://indiancourts.nic.in/districtcourt.html. [Accessed on 06.01.2020].
7. Judiciary. [Online] Available from https://archive.india.gov.in/citizen/lawnorder.php?id=8.
8. List of Socialist States – Wikipedia. (n.d.). [Online] Available from https://en.wikipedia.org/wiki/List_of_socialist_states.
9. Awasthi A, and Maheshwari SR. Public Administration. Agra: Lakshmi Narayan Agarwal Publications, 2006.
10. Park K. Park's Textbook of Preventive and Social Medicine. India: Bhanot Publishers, 2017.
11. Indian Judicial System - Silf. http://www.silf.org.in/indian-judicial-system.php. [Accessed on 06.01.2020].
12. State Government: Structure, Role, and Responsibilities: My India, Mar 12, 2016. [Online] Available from https://www.mapsofindia.com/my-india/government/what-is-state-government-structure-roles-and-responsibilities. [Accessed on 05.01.2020].
13. Government of India, Structure of Government of India. https://www.elections.in/government/. [Accessed on 05.01.2020].
14. Types of urban bodies in India: IAS Point GK Today. [Online] Available from https://academy.gktoday.in/article/types-of-urban-bodies-in-india/. [Accessed on 06.01.2020].

10 Fundamentals of Health Planning

CHAPTER OUTLINE

- Health Planning
  - Defining Health Planning
  - Elements of Health Planning
  - Purposes of Health Planning
  - Health Planning Process
- Regulatory bodies
  - Planning Commission
  - NITI Aayog
- National Health Plans
- National Health Committees

LEARNING OUTCOMES

After completion of this chapter, the learner will be able to:
- Understand the concept of health planning
- Describe features of National Health Planning
- Explain NITI Aayog
- Describe national health plans and Five-Year Plans
- Discuss various committee reports on health

KEY TERMS
Health planning, Five-Years Plans, NITI Aayog, committees

INTRODUCTION

Health planning is part of national development planning. It comprises activities that share the goal of improving health outcomes or improving the efficiency of health services provision or both. Health and socioeconomic developments are so close to each other that it is impossible to achieve one without the other. The health sector is complex with multiple goals, multiple products, and different beneficiaries.

HEALTH PLANNING

Defining Health Planning

Health planning is a process to plan and execute health-related issues by creating an actionable link between health needs and resources. Its nature and scope depend upon time allowable; some evidence-based answerable questions need to address within the process and resources available to support the process within a political and social environment.

A health planning is the predetermined course of action that depends on the nature and extent of health problems and of its goals. Various factors such as the environment of political direction, changing public expectation, new information and evidence about outcomes, and on occasion, media headlines need to consider at the time of health planning.

National Health Planning is "the orderly process of defining national health problems, identifying unmet needs and surveying the resources to meet them, establishing the priority goals that are realistic and feasible to accomplish the purpose of accomplished programme" (WHO, 1971). It is a process of setting national targets and preparing programs and policies that will help achieve those targets—the policies and programs developed in the light of national resources, economy, and priority goals of the country.

Elements of Health Planning

The following list shows the elements of health planning:
- Identifying the health vision and development goals
- Development of policies and programs and strategic plans
- Implementing the strategic health plans
- Monitoring and evaluation.

Purposes of Health Planning

The list below provides the purposes of health planning:
- To improve health services
- To match limited resources with many problems

- To eliminate wasteful expenditure and to avoid the duplication of expenditure
- To develop the best course of action to achieve defined objectives.

Health Planning Process

An effective health planning must start before the actual planning. Clear-cut policies, legislation, and interest of the government must have an effective health plan. The health planning process involves the following steps:

1. **Analysis of the health situation:** It involves the collection, assessment, and interpretation of extensive health information to assess the health or illness status of the population. To identify current health situation, the following information need to collect:
   - Demographic data of population
   - Social and health problems
   - The requirement of human service resources for a population
   - Cost of resources required and the linkages
   - Utilization of resources by population and expected changes in social and health status among users.
2. **Setting goals and objectives:** After analyzing the health situation, it is important to set health goals and objectives. The targets within the time frame are set to compare the performance of current health/illness profile, organizational, and system performance. Both short-term and long-terms goals framed in the light of desirable future outcome within available resources.
3. **Assessing the availability of resources:** It involves identifying and quantifying the requirement of resources per norms to tackle existing health problems and challenges and to implement various health programs and schemes. It also includes finding out the gap between requirement and available resources. These resources are the workforce, money, materials, and methods of delivering and monitoring healthcare.
4. **Determining alternative solutions and setting priorities:** Identify alternative solutions to tackle health problem or challenges. Assess each alternative for its feasibility, cost, effectiveness, and output for comparative purpose. Develop alternate plans to achieve set goals and objectives. Identifying and assessing alternatives needs creativity and thinking process.
5. **Selecting the best alternative solution(s):** Make a comparative statement of all alternatives. Select the best that can address the problems or challenges considering fiscal, political, and other limitations.
6. **Developing and implementing the proposed plan:** Prepare a detailed operational and strategic health plan of the selected alternative. Define clearly performance indicators, the requirement of resource, methods of implementation, monitoring, and evaluation. Implement the proposed plan that needs full cooperation from members of all the levels.
7. **Monitoring:** Plan and develop appropriate managerial and monitoring methods well in advance to assess the intended and unintended consequences of implementation actions. It will help to check that everything is going on per plan and schedule, and finding out any problems or hindrances come across can rectify immediately.
8. **Evaluation and finding gap:** Evaluation is the final step of the planning process after implementing the plan. It involves comparing output/results with the predetermined performance indicators to determine whether the implemented solutions are effective in achieving its health goals and targets. Determine the gap between expected and actual results.
9. **Replanning:** Based on the deficiencies/gap, redefine and replan the goals, objectives, and strategies to achieve the targets.

REGULATORY BODIES

Planning Commission

The Planning Commission in India was set up in March 1950 to formulate, execute and monitor national health plans independently without any interference of cabinet/parliament. The Prime Minister was the Chairman of Planning Commission. The first Five Year Plan (1951-56) drafted under the chairmanship of Planning Commission in 1951. Twelfth Five Year Plan was the last plan of Government of India developed under Planning Commission before its dissolution on October 2011. Various committees appointed time to time during five-year plans. The main focus was to control and eradication of major communicable diseases, strengthening of basic health services, population control, and development of health workforce resources, medical care institutions, medical education, training and research, and promoting Indigenous system of medicine.

NITI Aayog

National Institute of Transforming India (NITI) Aayog is an institute came into existence on 15th January 2015 to replace Planning Commission. The responsibility of formulating, executing, and monitoring of plans of Planning Commission transferred to NITI Aayog with effect from 1st January 2015.

The main objective of NITI Aayog is to achieve sustainable development. It is based on the principle of Team India to formulate a strategic vision and long-term policies and programs through horizontal and vertical cooperation. The focus was on decentralized planning by utilizing expertise based on best practices and model laws. It works on the top-down model. It has specialized, consultancy, and research wing. The specialized wing is Team India or hub of knowledge and innovation. Health and nutrition, women, and child development are one of the social sectors among knowledge and innovative hub.

Structure of NITI Aayog

The Prime Minister of India is an Ex-officio chairman of NITI Aayog. It has:
- Governing Council consisting Chief Ministers of all states (including Delhi and Pudichery) and Lt Governors of Union Territories (UTs) as the members
- Regional Council composed of Chief Ministers of all states and Lt Governors of UTs
- A full-time organization composed of Vice-chairperson nominated by Prime Minister; five full-time members; two part-time members selected from leading universities, research organizations, and leading institutions; four ex-officio members of Union Council of Ministers; a Chief Executive Officer with a rank of Secretary of India; and experts and specialists.
- The committee comprises Prime Minister as a chairperson, Vice-chairperson nominated by Prime Minister, four ex-officio members, three special invitees, four full-time members, Chief Executive Officer, and all Governing Council members.

Functions of NITI Aayog

Following are its functions:
- To foster cooperative and competitive federalism
- To formulate and implement policy and program framework
- To act as a resource center and knowledge and innovative hub
- To evaluate the implemented policies and programs.

NATIONAL HEALTH PLAN

First Five-Year Plan (1951–1956)

The first Five-Year plan based on the Harrod–Domar Model implemented in 1951. The plan was agriculture, community development, communications, and land rehabilitation oriented. Community Development Programme launched in 1952. The focus was on children's health to reduce infant mortality and to control population growth. Various health programs such as BCG vaccination, Community Development Programme, National Malaria Control Programme, National Family Programme, National Leprosy Control Programme, and National Filaria Control Programme launched during this plan. There was seven-point public health programme on provision of water supply and sanitation, control of malaria, preventive healthcare of rural population through health units and a mobile unit, health services for mother and children, health education, self-sufficiency in drugs and equipment, and family planning and population control.

Second Five-Year Plan (1956–1961)

The second Five-Year Plan is Mahalanobis Plan (named after its chief architect). The focus was on rapid industrialization and abolition of the Zamindari system and the creation of cooperatives among the rural poor. Under this plan, various health programs initiated in health sector such as the National Malaria Control Programme converted into National Malaria Eradication Programme (NMEP), Trachoma Control Pilot Project, Root Cause Analysis (RCA) Projects, and Pilot Projects for Eradication of Smallpox.

Third Five-Year Plan (1961–1966)

During the third Five-Year Plan, various sectors such as defense, price stabilization, construction of dams, cement and fertilizers plants, education, etc. were the priority areas. The health programs such as the National Smallpox Eradication Programme, School Health Programme, National Goiter Control Programme, District Tuberculosis Programme, Applied Nutrition Programme, Reinforced Extended Family Planning and Indian Council of Medical Research (ICMR) Director recommended Lippes Loop as safe and effective for a mass program, "Direct" BCG vaccination, and International Postpartum Family Planning Programme are the landmarks during this plan.

Three Annual Plans (1966–1969)

Three annual plans drafted between 1966 and 1968, and emphasis was on agriculture and exports. This period is "Plan Holidays" because of Indo-Pakistan war and failure of the third Five-Year Plan. Due to the crisis in agriculture sector and serious food shortage, a new agricultural strategy.

Fourth Five-Year Plan (1969–1974)

During the fourth Five-Year Plan, the main emphasis was on agriculture growth and hence put slogan "Garibi-Hatao" during 1971. All India Hospitals' Postpartum and Family Planning programme, started in 1970 in addition to other health programs.

Fifth Five-Year Plan (1974–1979)

The fifth plan launched to achieve two main objectives, namely "removal of poverty" (Garibi-Hatao) and "attainment of self-reliance," through the promotion of high rate of growth and better distribution of income. This plan terminated in 1978 (instead of 1979). During the fifth Five-Year Plan, various health programs and initiatives took place. These are National Programme of Minimum Needs, a scheme for setting up 30-bedded rural hospitals, one such hospital for every four primary health centers (PHCs), Integrated Child Development from October 2, 1975, National Programme for Prevention of Blindness, Rural Health Scheme in 1977, Revised Modified Plan for Malaria Eradication and ROME (Re-Orientation of Medical Education) Scheme in 1977, Declaration of Alma Ata underlined the primary health-care approach in 1978.

Sixth Five-Year Plan (1980–1985)

There were two annual rolling plans in 1978 and 1979. The main objectives of the sixth Five-Year Plan were to increase national income and modern technology and ensure a continuous decrease in poverty and unemployment and population control, etc. During this Five-Year Plan, the government launched various programs such as the National Leprosy Eradication Programme and National Guinea-worm Eradication Programme and expanded Family Planning Programme. It also announced National Health Policy (NHP) and a new 20-point program in 1982. World Health Organization released the Global Strategy for Health for All.

Seventh Five-Year Plan (1985–1990)

The objectives of the seventh Five-Year Plan were improving productivity by upgrading technology. This plan emphasized policies and programs, which aimed at the growth and employment opportunities. It laid a greater emphasis on energy and social development. Private sector got priority during this Five-Year Plan.

The Government initiated various health programs such as Universal Immunization Programme, Central Rural Sanitation Programme, National Diabetes Control Programme, AIDS Control Programme, and Blood Safety Programme during this Five-Year Plan. World bank launched a world-wide "Safe Motherhood" campaign in 1987, and our country initiated "Control of Respiratory Infection (ARI) Programme" in 1990 across 14 districts.

Annual Plans (1990–1991 and 1991–1992)

Due to political instability in India, the government did not formulate any Five-Year Plan in 1989–1991. There were only Annual Plans during the year 1990–1991 and 1991–1992. In 1991, due to a crisis in Foreign Exchange reserves, there was a beginning of privatization and liberalization in India.

Eighth Five-Year Plan (1992–1997)

The government of India launched the eighth Five-Year Plan in 1992. The focus was on economic liberalization and modernization of industries. There was a private investment in major public sector undertakings and a greater rural and agricultural development.

The Government initiated various health programs such as the Child Survival and Safe Motherhood Programme and Reproductive and Child Health Programme. ICDS renamed as Integrated Mother and Child Development Services (IMCD) in 1995. The government observed a single-day event for Pulse Polio Immunization in the first and second phases. Family Planning Programme made target free from 1st April 1996 and Revised National Tuberculosis Programme with DOTS introduced as Pilot Project in 1993.

Ninth Five-Year Plan (1997–2002)

The main objectives of the ninth Five-Year Plan were agriculture and rural development, empowerment of women, and providing basic requirements such as health, drinking water, sanitation, etc. The main focus was on quality of life, generation of productive employment, regional balance, and self-reliance.

The Government launched various programs such as National AIDS Control Programme and the National Programme for Control and Treatment of Occupational Diseases in 1998–1999. It also conducted National Family Health Survey-2 in 1998–1999 and adopted National Policy for Older Persons and Health Care for the Elderly (NPHCE) Programme. The country declared Guinea-worm free country in 2000, but there was the emergence of treating severe acute respiratory syndrome (SARS) in 2002.

Tenth Five-Year Plan (2002–2007)

India's 10th Five-Year Plan has been devised to complement and meet the United Nations Millennium Development Goals (MDG) targets. The MDG were issued in 2000 to achieve eight targets to eradicate hunger and poverty and raise the standards of living worldwide by the year 2015 through global cooperation.

This plan highlighted the need to combat poverty ratio, improve literacy rates, and economic growth, etc. during the tenth plan period. The health initiatives were to control population growth and reduce infant and maternal mortality rate. The target was to the universal availability of drinking water, clearing of all major polluted rivers and increase in the forest.

The Government approved National Vector Borne Disease Control Programme approved as Umbrella Programme for prevention of vector-borne diseases. It also launched Vandematarum scheme, Mid-Day Meal Scheme, and oral dehydration with existing formula, Reproductive & Child Health II, Janani Suraksha Yojana, and National Rural Health Mission (2005). World Health Organisation released New Pediatric Growth Chart based on breastfed children in 2006.

There was a plan to set up six institutions in the line of AIIMS under Pradhan Mantri Swasthya Suraksha Yojana (PMSSY) and upgradation of 13 existing Government Medical College Institutions. The Government banned Child Labour as a domestic servant in 2006 and implemented National Programme for Prevention and Control of Deafness (the pilot phase) in 10 states and one UT.

Eleventh Five-Year Plan (2007–2012)

The major objectives of the 11th Five-Year Plan are to increase GDP growth and income generation and to combat poverty and elementary school education in general. The main focus on the health sector was to reduce infant and maternity mortality, total fertility rate (TFR), malnutrition among children of age group 0–3 to half, and anemia among women and girls.

The Government launched various health programs such as National Tobacco Control Programme (NTCP) in 42 districts of 21 States/Union Territories, The Rajiv Aarogyasri Health Scheme especially the poor and underprivileged, National Programme for Prevention and Control of Deafness, and National Rural Drinking Water Supply Programme (NRDWP). It also activated emergency transport services on 108 number and health information—a caller-free telephone service on 104 number.

The Government provided free entitlement to pregnant women in government health institutions under Janani Shishu Suraksha Karyakaram (JSSK) and implemented Total Sanitation Campaign (TSC), Mid-Day Meal Scheme (MDM), and Integrated Child Development Services (ICDS).

Twelfth Five-Year Plan (2012–2017)

Twelfth Five-Year Plan is the last plan of Government of India developed by Planning Commission before its dissolution on October 2011. The vision of the plan was "Faster, Sustainable, and More Inclusive Growth." This plan is more health oriented and set measurable health targets and strategies to achieve by the end of the plan. The main focus is on comprehensive healthcare. The health goals are as follows:

- To reduce infant mortality rate (IMR) to 25/1000 live birth
- To reduce maternity mortality rate (MMR) to 100/100,000 live birth
- To reduce under-five mortality rate to 38/1000 live birth
- To reduce the TFR to 2.1
- To prevent and reduce under-nutrition in children under 3 years to half of National Family Health Survey (NFHS)-3 (2005–2006) levels to 27%
- To reduce anemia among women of age group 15–49 years to 28%
- To raise child sex ratio in the 0- to 6-year age group from 914 to 950
- To reduce annual incidence and mortality of tuberculosis by half
- To reduce prevalence to <1 per 10000 population and incidence to zero in all districts
- To reduce the incidence of malaria (annual parasite incidence) to <1/1,000
- To reduce the prevalence of filariasis to <1% microfilaria in all districts
- To sustain case fatality rate of dengue <1%
- To eliminate kala-azar in all districts by 2015, and <1 case per 10,000 population in all blocks
- To reduce new infection of HIV/AIDS to zero
- To reduce Japanese encephalitis mortality by 30%
- To reduce premature mortality from noncommunicable diseases by 1/4th of Family Health survey-4 levels
  To reduce poor household's out-of-pocket spending as a proportion of private spending on health.

During 12th Five-Year Plan, the Government launched National Urban Health Mission (NUHM)-submission of National Health Mission (NHM) on 20th January 2014 in all cities/towns with a population of more than 50,000 with the aim to improve the health of urban people especially slum dwellers. It also launched Mission Indhradhanush on 25th December 2014 to achieve the target of full coverage of immunization by 2020 to children either unvaccinated or partially vaccinated against 12 life-threatening vaccine-preventable diseases. It implemented National AYUSH Mission (NAM). AYUSH stands for Ayurveda, Yoga and Naturopathy, Unani, Siddha, and Homeopathy.

The Government launched various health programs such as Prevention and Control of Viral Hepatitis Programme and Rashtriya Kishor Swasthya Karyakram (National Adolescent Health Programme) in 2014. It also planned services for early identification and early intervention for children from birth to 18 years to cover any abnormality including disability under Rashtriya Bal Swasthya Karyakram (RBSK).

The government initiated the efforts to reduce the expenditure incurred by patients suffering from cancer and heart diseases through recognized outlets under Affordable Medicines and Reliable Implants for Treatment (AMRIT) program. It rolled out Pradhan Mantri National Dialysis Programme in 2016 under NHM to provide free dialysis services to the poor.

There were many areas under consideration during the 12th Five-Year Plan. These are as follows:

- Transformation of NRHM to NHM
- Building capacity through expansion of teaching and training of health professionals
- A system of Universal Health Coverage (UHC)
- Review of the regulatory system and drug regulation
- Development and strengthening of public health-care system and infrastructures
- Reforming Rashtriya Swasthya Bima Yojana (RSBY) to cover the entire BPL population for health care
- Continue to have mix health system both by the public and private health-care providers
- Computerizing and interlinking all health facilities at all levels and use of mobile technology
- Restructuring of ICDS program
- Proper regulation of public–private partnership to finance health-care services.

Three-Year Action Agenda

Five-Year Plans end in March 2017. The role of NITI Aayog prepared a Fifteen-Year Vision, Seven-Year Strategy, and Three-Year Action Agenda documents. Fifteen-Year Vision and Seven-Year Strategy are under preparation, and Three-Year Action Agenda document (2017–2018 to 2019–2020) is ready. This document has 7 parts and 21 chapters and Health agenda.

Specific Health Goals

The specific health goals are as follows:
- To reduce IMR to 30/1,000 live births
- To reduce MMR to 120/100,000 live births
- To reduce under-five mortality rate to 38/1,000 live births
- To reduce the TFR to 2.1
- To reduce the incidence rate of tuberculosis to 130/100,000

- To reduce the incidence of malaria (annual parasite incidence) to less than 1/1,000 in 90% districts
- To eliminate kala-azar and lymphatic filariasis
- To reduce mortality from noncommunicable diseases
- To reduce out-of-pocket spending to 50% of total health expenditure.

The focus areas of Three-Year Action Agenda are as follows:
- Public and preventive health.
- Quality healthcare by both public and private health institutions.
- Fiscal transfer to better health outcome.
- Strengthening human resources for health regarding quantity and quality.
- Access to medicines, health research, key social determinants of health such as nutrition, drinking water, and sanitation.
- Reforms need to update for medical (Indian system of medicine), nursing, dental councils within 3 years, in a similar line as of the National Medical Council Commission Bill, 2016.
- Opportunity to ASHAs and Anganwadi workers (AWWs) to seek admission in auxiliary nurse midwife (ANM) schools on performance based for career progression.

NATIONAL HEALTH COMMITTEES

Before the NHP framed in 1983, various committees of experts appointed from time to time. The Constitution, Planning Commission, Central Council of Health and Family Welfare, and Consultative Committees attached to the Ministry of Health and Family Welfare render advice on initiating health programs, the requirement of health workforce and other resources in government, voluntary and private sectors based on health needs and demands of the people through health surveys. The reports of these committees form a base to take appropriate actions and help in planning health policies.

Bhore Committee, 1946

The Government appointed a Health Survey and Development Committee in 1943 under the Chairmanship of Sir Joseph Bhore. The main emphasis of the working committee was on the integration of curative and preventive medicine at all levels. It recommended remodeling of health services in India. The important recommendations of this committee are as follows:
1. To integrate preventive and curative services at all administrative levels
2. Development of PHCs in two phases: short-term and long-term plan.
   a. *The short-term plan* included the provision of one PHC for a population of 40,000, supported by secondary health center to coordinate and supervise their functioning. The workforce requirement of each PHC has 2 doctors, 1 nurse, 4 public health nurses, 4 midwives, 4-trained dais, 2 sanitary inspectors, 2 health assistants, 1 pharmacist, and 15 other class IV employees.
   b. **Long-term program (the 3 million plans)**
      It includes the following:
      - Primary health units with 75-bedded hospitals for each 10,000 to 20,000 population
      - Secondary units with 650-bedded hospital, again regionalized around district hospitals with 2,500 beds
      - The inclusion of 3-month training in preventive and social medicine to prepare social physicians
      - Fixing up doctor nurse ratio
      - To start 100 training centers for nurses to train about 7,40,000 nurses by 1977
      - To have a college of nursing to run degree courses in nursing started in 1946
      - Two grades of nurses: senior and junior; for senior grade, the qualification should be matriculation; and for the junior grade, the qualification should be middle school standard
      - Training of public health nursing; male nurses, midwives, and dais as an interim measure till the adequate number of midwives are made available
      - Advance courses in hospital nursing administration, the teaching of nurses, and training of public health supervisors
      - One nurse for 500 populations.

Shetty Committee, 1954

In 1954, the Government constituted Shetty committee under the chairmanship of Attavar Balakrishna Shetty, State Health Minister of Madras, to review the condition of nursing service, emoluments, etc. of the nursing profession to standardize and development of nursing in India. The committee recommendations were as follows:
- Establishment of new schools of nursing with adequate teaching and supervisory staff to trained nurses
- Provision of adequate training for nursing teachers
- Deputation to two to four nurses to undergo higher study and to take up courses in teaching, administration, and public health nursing
- Adequate facility for clinical experience and clinical supervision
- Admission criteria per Indian Nursing Council norms
- Adequate accommodation for nurse students and proper care of their health
- Improvement in nursing education standard
- Two grades of nurses: A fully trained nurse and midwives who have undergone 3.5–4 years training in nursing and midwifery and another auxiliary nurse and midwife of 2 years
- Appointment of Superintendents of Nursing in the offices of Directorates in each state
- A national minimum pay scales for nurses, midwives, and ANMs

- Improvement in working conditions of nurses
- Provision of in-service education programs
- Part-time working facilities for nurses
- Need for the training of male nurses.

Mudaliar Committee, 1962

The Government of India in 1959 appointed another committee to provide guidelines for the Five-Year Plans. This committee is known as the "Health Survey and Planning Committee." Dr AL Mudaliar, Vice Chancellor of Madras University, headed it. This committee appointed to assess the performance in the health sector based on Bhore recommendations. This committee found the conditions in PHCs to be unsatisfactory and suggested the following recommendations:

- Strengthening of existing PHC before the opening of new ones.
- PHC for 40,000 population.
- PHC should provide the curative, preventive, and promotive services.
- Strengthening of subdivisional and district hospitals.
- Each district hospital should have one bed against 1,000 population; Taluk hospital should have 600–800 beds, and each PHC should have 10 beds.
- Lady health visitor (LHV) and midwife should be engaged in providing health education, personal hygiene, and nutrition.
- There should be one ANM for 5,000 population.
- There should be three grade of nurses: Basic nurses with 4 years of training, ANM with 2 years training, and degree nurses.
- The minimum qualification for General Nursing and Midwifery (GNM) should be matriculation or equivalent, and for degree nurses, the minimum qualification should be higher secondary or preuniversity.
- The medium of instruction in GNM course should be preferably in English, whereas in the degree course, it should be in English only.
- Public health nursing should be a part of the nursing curriculum.
- The district hospitals with bed strength with 75–100 can consider for clinical practice for nurse students; there should be provision for free accommodation, free uniform, laundry, free books, and free medical services, and stipend to student nurses.
- Each school of nursing should have an advisory committee and should have its budget.
- Train male nurses for certain jobs.
- There should be short-term special training courses such as pediatric nursing, public health nursing, theatre nursing, psychiatric nursing, nursing administration, etc.
- *Dai* training program.
- Other postbasic training courses such as sister tutor course, operation theater technique, public health nursing, mental disease nursing, and nursing service administration.

Chadha Committee

This committee appointed in 1963 under the chairmanship of Dr MS Chadha who was the Director General of Health Services. The main aim of this committee was to give inputs regarding the maintenance phase of the NMEP. The committee made the following suggestions:

- Basic health workers for NMEP activity.
- Basic health workers as multipurpose workers would perform malaria work and the duties of family planning and vital statistics data collection.
- They would work under the supervision of family planning health assistants.
- Integration of different nursing services.

Mukherjee Committee, 1965

This committee formulated in 1965 under the chairmanship of Shri Mukherjee who was then Secretary of Health to Government of India to review the performance basic health workers per recommendations of the Chadha Committee and develop a strategy in the area of family planning. The following were the committee recommendations:

- A separate staff for the family planning program
- Family planning assistants for family planning-related duties
- Training of nurses and ANMs in family planning
- Basic health workers for other services only.

Separate the malaria activities from family planning.

Mukherjee Committee, 1966

The Government appointed a committee of Health Secretaries in 1966 under the chairmanship of Shri Mukherjee. He was then Union Health Secretary to work out specific health service at the block level and strengthening higher levels of administration. The committee recommendations were as follows:

- One family planning female worker for every two subcenters
- One LHV for 40,000 populations
- One part-time worker for motivation population for acceptance of Intra Uterine Devices (IUD)
- Appointment of education leaders at block and district
- Part-time availability of Government doctors on an incentive basis.

Jungalwalla Committee, 1967

The Government constituted the "Committee on Integration of Health Services" in 1964 under the chairmanship of Dr N Jungalwalla. He was the Director of National Institute of Health Administration and Education. The objective of the committee was to examine various problems related to the integration of health services, the abolition of private practice by doctors in government services, and the service conditions of doctors.

1. The committee recommended that an "integrated health services" is a unified approach for all problems.

It also suggested the integration at all levels of health organization in the country regarding unified cadre, common seniority, recognition of extra qualifications, equal pay for equal work, special pay for special work, the abolition of private practice by government doctors, and improvement in their service conditions.
2. Medical Care and Public Health Programmes under the charge of a single administrator at all levels of hierarchy.

Kartar Singh Committee, 1973

The government of India constituted "Committee on multipurpose workers" under Health and Family Planning in 1972 under the Chairmanship of Kartar Singh and then the Additional Secretary, Ministry of Health and Family Planning, Government of India. The committee constituted to develop a framework for the integration of health and medical services at the peripheral and supervisory levels. The main recommendations of the committee were as follows:

- Amalgamation of various categories of peripheral workers into a single cadre of multipurpose workers (male and female).
- Converting auxiliary nurse midwives into Multipurpose Health Workers-Females (MPW-F) and basic health workers, malaria surveillance workers, etc. to Multipurpose Health Workers-Male (MPW-M).
- Supervision of three to four male MPWs by one male health supervisor and of three to four female MPWs by female health supervisor.
- Converting existing LHVs as female health supervisor.
- The population coverage of one PHC of 50,000 with 16 subcenters (one for 3,000 to 3,500 population).
- Each PHC must have a male and a female multipurpose health worker.

Shrivastav Committee, 1975

The Government of India, Ministry of Health and Family Planning, constituted a committee "Medical Education and Support Manpower" in 1974 to reorient medical education by national needs and priorities to develop a curriculum for health assistants. Based on recommendation, it helped in launching the Rural Health Service Plan in 1977. The following were the recommendations:

- Creation of bands of paraprofessional and semiprofessional health workers from within the community itself
- Three cadres of health workers—multipurpose health workers and health at PHC
- Development of a "Referral Services Complex"
- Establishment of a Medical and Health Education Commission
- Design a curriculum for health assistants.

Mehta Committee, 1983

A Medical Education Review Committee was set up by the Ministry of Health and Family Welfare, under the chairmanship of Dr Shantilal J Mehta, Former Director Jaslok Hospital, on 8th September 1981. It recommended admission eligibility criteria and duration to the undergraduates and postgraduates, residency scheme, measures for improvement, and incentives to the doctors working in rural areas. The committee also recommended establishing universities of Medical Sciences and Medical and Health Education Commission.

Working Group on Medical Education, Training and Manpower Planning, 1984

This working group appointed by Planning Commission to work on the restructuring of organizational setup, workforce planning, and development with special reference to community health management in 1984. It also worked on medical location and ROME Scheme, institutional network with universities of Medical Sciences and Medical and Health Education Commission. The recommendations of the working group were as follows:

- Training and development of auxiliary personnel and paraprofessional personnel
- Basic and preservice training and continuing education in public health and health management
- Undergraduate and postgraduate medical education
- Health-related vocational courses for ANMs, MPHW-Females, MPHW-Males, etc.

Bajaj Committee, 1987

An "Expert Committee for Health Manpower Planning, Production and Management" constituted in 1985 under the Chairmanship of Dr JS Bajaj, the then professor at AIIMS, New Delhi. Following are the major recommendations of this committee:

- Formulation of National Medical and Health Education Policy
- Formulation of National Health Manpower Policy
- Educational Commission for Health Sciences (ECHS) on the lines of UGC
- Establishing Health Science Universities in various states and union territories
- Vocationalization of education at 10+2 levels as regards health-related fields with appropriate incentives
- Carrying out a realistic Health Manpower Survey.

High Power Committee, 1988

The Government of India constituted a High Power Committee on Nursing and Nursing profession on 25th August 1987 and organized convention in 1988. The committee constituted to review and discuss the working conditions of nurses, the status of nurses, and allied matters about the nursing profession in rural and urban areas. The thrust areas were staffing norms, training of all categories, levels of nursing personnel, role nurses, and organization of nursing services at different levels. Key recommendations were as follows:

- Defined policies for nursing services

- Improving the service conditions of nurses
- Standardize job descriptions at the central level
- Reduce working hours to 40 hours in a week; norms for workload, uniformity in pay scales, career development opportunities
- Transport and accommodation facilities to nurses near the working place
- Allowances and welfare facilities; provision of special incentives to recognize meritorious work
- Nurses should be a member of purchase and condemnation committees
- Introduction of specialty courses, continuing and staff development courses
- Renewal of nursing registration after every 5 years
- Independent nursing practice
- Involvement of nurses in policy and decision-making
- Appointment of LHV and ANM after undergoing administrative training
- Upgrading nursing schools and strengthening of Master's programs and Doctorate programs
- Selection of students on merit and aptitude test, adequate teaching and library facilities, accommodation facilities for students
- Regulation of nursing education standards
- Regulation of private nursing home norms
- Constitution of nursing advisory committee or board to advise the government on issues of nursing.

National Commission on Macroeconomics and Health, 2005

National Commission on Macroeconomics and Health constituted under the chairmanship of Shri P Chidambaram, the then Finance Minister of India in April 2004, to review the present health system both in public and private sector and make a recommendation for improvement. Recommendations about human resources for health were as follows:

- Establishment of an additional 225 nursing colleges and upgrade and strengthening the existing ones in another 5–10 years.
- Improvement in the standards of training in medical colleges, nursing schools, and colleges and in those institutions that impart training to paramedical personnel.
- Establishment of a Commission for Human Resource Development and Medical and Health Education.
- Fellowship for teachers working in medical and nursing training institutions.
- At least 1,000 fellowships for research and higher education in various fields of public health, nursing, medical management, etc. for faculty positions in various schools and autonomous bodies. 25% of these should be earmarked for PhD and postgraduate studies and be open to all—government employees, universities, research institutions, etc. alike.
- A live register and database needs to be maintained for all categories of medical and paramedical personnel and regularly updated by the respective professional councils.
- Introduction of a system of re-registration of doctors and nurses once every 5 years and linking re-registration with a minimum number of hours of continuing medical education (CME).
- Every state should focus on nursing for better management and development of human resource for health.
- To start multidisciplinary leadership and management development programs for nurses and midwives.
- Measures should be taken to retain the best and most qualified nurses to serve the health needs of the country.
- Constitution of a high-level task force to examine various aspects of the deteriorating environment in medical colleges and nursing schools. To address issues related to service conditions, payment systems, particularly for specialists, and incentives for stimulating the better quality of training and research.

Arvind Panagariya Committee, 2016

Committees constituted to examine various reforms in Medical Council of India, Homeopathy Central Council and Indian Medicine Central Council of India under the chairmanship of Vice President NITI Aayog in March 2016. A draft of "National Medical Commission Bill" was prepared to replace "Mild Cognitive Impairment (MCI)" with "National Medical Commission." Another committee is constituted under the chairmanship of Vice President NITI Aayog to examine the options for reforms in Homeopathy Central Council and Indian Medicine Central Council are still working on it.

CHAPTER HIGHLIGHTS

- Health planning is a process of undertaking various activities of health-related issues to achieve health goals of improving health outcomes and improving health services provision.
- National Health Planning is a process of setting national targets and preparing programs and policies that will help achieve those targets.
- NITI Aayog is a National Institute of Transforming India based on Team India came into existence on 15th January 2015 to replace Planning Commission.
- The main focus of Five-Year Plans was to control and eradication of major communicable diseases, strengthening of basic health services, population control, and development of health workforce resources, medical care institutions, medical education, training and research, and promoting indigenous system of medicine.
- Five-Year Plans ends in March 2017. The role of NITI Aayog prepared a Fifteen-Year Vision, Seven-Year Strategy, and Three-Year Action Agenda documents.
- Three-Year Action Agenda document (2017–2018 to 2019–2020) has 7 parts and 21 chapters. Under health agenda, Three-Year Agenda specifies specific health goals and focus areas.

Chapter 10: Fundamentals of Health Planning

- Various National Health Committees of experts appointed from time to time. The Bhore Committee was the first committee to take health initiatives. The main emphasis of the working committee was on the integration of curative and preventive medicine at all levels.

REVIEW QUESTIONS

I. Essay Type Questions
1. Define the term "Health Planning." Explain health planning process.
2. Describe 12th Five-Year Plan in detail.
3. Discuss specific health goals and focus areas under Three-Year Action Agenda.
4. Enumerate important recommendations of Bhore's Committee, 1946.
5. Describe the major areas discussed in the High Power Committee.

II. Short Notes
1. Purposes and elements of health planning
2. Mudaliar Committee recommendations
3. National Commission on Microeconomics and Health
4. Structure of NITI Aayog

III. Multiple Choice Questions
1. Which committee is headed by Dr JS Bajaj?
   a. Health Manpower Planning, Production, and Management
   b. Health Survey and Planning Committee
   c. Health Survey and Development Committee
   d. Committee on multipurpose workers
2. When did NITI Aayog come into existence?
   a. 2012 b. 2013
   c. 2014 d. 2015
3. Under whose chairmanship, Planning Commission formulated Five-Year Plans in India?
   a. The President b. Vice President
   c. Prime Minister d. Health Minister
4. During which Five-Year Plan, the National Malaria Control Programme was initiated for the first time?
   a. First Five-Year Plan
   b. Second Five-Year Plan
   c. Third Five-Year Plan
   d. Fourth Five-Year Plan
5. The aim of to launch Affordable Medicines and Reliable Implants for Treatment (AMRIT) programme is:
   a. To reduce the expenditure incurred by patients suffering from cancer and heart diseases
   b. To provide free dialysis services to the poor
   c. To identify and provide early intervention for children
   d. To prevent and control hepatitis
6. When did control of Acute Respiratory Infection Programme start?
   a. 1985 b. 1987
   c. 1990 d. 1993
7. When did revised National Tuberculosis Programme with DOTS introduce as pilot project in our country?
   a. 1992 b. 1993
   c. 1994 d. 1995
8. Which of the following health committee recommended one primary health center for 40,000 populations?
   a. Shetty committee
   b. Chadha Committee
   c. Bajaj Committee
   d. Bhore Committee

Answer Keys
1. a 2. d 3. c 4. b 5. a 6. c 7. b
8. d

SUGGESTED READING

1. Available from Charakasamhita%20ACDP%20%20english_0.pdf. [Accessed February 2018].
2. Health Planning in India - Business Maps of India. https://business.mapsofindia.com/india-planning/health.html. [Accessed on 05.01.2020].
3. Available from [PDF]Action Plan Final PART 1 text - NITI Aayog http://niti.gov.in/writereaddata/files/coop/IndiaActionPlan.pdf. [Accessed on 06.01.2020].
4. Available from http://nposonline.net/fiveyearplans.shtml.
5. Available from http://planningcommission.nic.in/plans/planrel/11thf.htm.
6. Available from http://shodhganga.inflibnet.ac.in/bitstream/10603/48400/7/07_chapter%202.pdf.
7. How to Do to Planning - Free Management Library. https://managementhelp.org/planning/index.htm. [Accessed on 06.01.2020].
8. Available from National Institute of Health & Family Welfare. http://www.nihfw.org/. [Accessed on 05.01.2020].
9. Available from Committee & Commission - Nihfw. http://www.nihfw.org/ReportsOfNCC.aspx. [Accessed on 05.01.2020].
10. Twelfth Five Year Plan - Planning Commission. planningcommission.gov.in › plans › planrel › 12thplan › pdf › 12fyp_vol3. [Accessed on 05.01.2020].
11. Commision on Macroeconomic and Health Primary Health Care in India Review of Policy Plan and Committee Reports. https://www.scribd.com/document/2382877/Commision-on-Macroeconomic-and-Health-Primary-Health-Care-in-India-Review-of-Policy-Plan-and-Committee-Reports. [Accessed on 06.01.2020].
12. [PDF]National Population Policy, 2000 - MoHFW. https://mohfw.gov.in/sites/default/files/26953755641410949469%20%281%29.pdf. [Accessed on 04.01.2020].
13. Health Care Facilities for Pregnant Women and Children – IAS .... https://www.iasabhiyan.com/health-care-facilities-pregnant-women-children/. [Accessed on 06.01.2020].
14. India's Economic Plans: History, Characteristics and Objectives. http://www.economicsdiscussion.net/economic-planning/indias-economic-plans-history-characteristics-and-objectives/6467. [Accessed on 05.01.2020].
15. Five Year Plan for Development of Economy in India. http://www.yourarticlelibrary.com/economy/five-year-plan-for-development-of-economy-in-india/43895. [Accessed on 05.01.2020].

16. National Ayush Mission (NAM)—Vikaspedia. http://vikaspedia.in/health/nrhm/national-health-programmes-1/national-ayush-mission-nam. [Accessed on 06.01.2020].
17. National AYUSH Mission | Ministry of AYUSH | GOI. http://ayush.gov.in/schemes/financial-sanctions/national-ayush-mission. [Accessed on 05.01.2020].
18. [PDF]report of the health survey and development committee-Nihfw. http://www.nihfw.org/Doc/Reports/Bhore%20Committee%20Report%20-%20Vol%20II.pdf. [Accessed on 06.01.2020].
19. The government of India. Report of Health Survey and Planning Committee, (Chairman: Mudaliar). New Delhi: Ministry of Health; 1961.
20. Twelfth Five Year Plan_vol 3.indb - of Planning Commission. [Online] Available from http://planningcommission.gov.in/plans/planrel/12thplan/pdf/12fyp_vol3.pdf. [Accessed January 2016].
21. [PDF]HEALTH21: the health for all policy framework - WHO/Europe. http://www.euro.who.int/__data/assets/pdf_file/0010/98398/wa540ga199heeng.pdf. [Accessed on 06.01.2020].
22. [PDF]WHO_TRS_472.pdf - World Health Organization. https://apps.who.int/iris/bitstream/handle/10665/40905/WHO_TRS_472.pdf;jsessionid=C679552C994DDBECAECDB901D17E2F02?sequence=1. [Accessed on 06.01.2020].

11
National Health Policies

CHAPTER OUTLINE
- National Health Policies
  - National Health Policy 2017
  - National Policy on AYUSH 2002
  - National Population Policy 2002
- National AYUSH Mission
- National Health Mission 2012-2017

LEARNING OUTCOMES
After completion of this chapter, the learner will be able to:
- Describe national health policies
- Discuss National Health Mission (NHM)
- Describe various programs under NHM
- Describe National Ayurveda, Yoga, and Naturopathy, Unani, Siddha, and Homeopathy (AYUSH) Mission

KEY TERMS
Health policies, health mission, national programs, AYUSH Mission

INTRODUCTION

Policy is a system that provides the logical framework and rationality of decision-making for achieving the intended objectives. It consists of statements that guide and provide discretion within the limited boundaries. It sets priorities and guides resource allocations. A national policy is the policy at any level of government that may be formal or precedence over others. Heads of government set it; legislatures and regulatory agencies are empowered by others.

NATIONAL HEALTH POLICIES

Health policy is concerned with the health of the people. It aims at the improving the conditions in which people live. Major health policies are listed in the subsequent pages.

National Health Policy 2017

The Union Cabinet approved the National Health Policy (NHP) 2017 on March 15, 2017, after recognizing the shift in health priorities, growing emergence of sustainability in the health-care industry, increased cost of healthcare, improved economic growth, and the progress made since 2002. This policy emphasizes the provision of comprehensive preventive, promotive, and affordable quality health-care services that should reach everyone. It is concerned with health security and Make in India for drugs and devices. The main goal of NHP 2017 is to attain the highest possible level of well-being and provide affordable quality health-care services to everyone.

1. **Professionalism, integrity, and ethics:** Maintaining the highest professional standards, integrity, and ethics within the regulatory environment.
2. **Equity:** Provision of healthcare to all, irrespective of the gender, social status, caste, disability, or other forms of social exclusion and geographical barriers.
3. **Affordability:** Healthcare must be affordable to people of all sections of our society.
4. **Universality:** Provision of health-care services to the entire population including special groups.
5. **Patient centered and quality of care:** Health-care services should be gender sensitive, effective, safe, and convenient and provided with dignity and confidentiality. It is necessary to implement developed standards and guidelines in all health-care institutions to ensure the quality of healthcare.
6. **Accountability:** There should be financial and performance accountability and transparency in decision-making, both in public and private settings.
7. **Multistakeholder approach:** Health-care sector must have a multistakeholder approach with partnership

and participation from all nonhealth ministries and communities.
8. **Pluralism:** Patients who wish to have can access alternative care, i.e. AYUSH care.
9. **Decentralization:** An appropriate level of decentralization of decision-making should be allowed, keeping in mind the practical considerations and institutional capacity. Community participation in health planning processes should be allowed.
10. **Dynamism and adaptability:** Organization of healthcare should be evidence based.

Objectives

The objectives of NHP 2017 are given below:
1. To achieve universal health coverage by ensuring the availability of free and comprehensive primary health services to people of all ages. It also aims to improve access and affordability to quality secondary and tertiary health-care services.
2. To make health services comprehensive, predictable, efficient, effective, safe, rational, patient centric, and affordable.
3. To enable the public health sector to achieve public health goals.

Specific Goals

The 12 goals of NHP 2017 are listed below:
1. To increase the life expectancy at birth to 70 years by 2025.
2. To estimate the burden of disease and its trend through an index called Disability Adjusted Life Year Index by 2022.
3. To reduce the total fertility rate (TFR) to 2.1 children per woman and the mortality rate of the mother, neonatal, infant, and children under 5 years of age.
4. To achieve the target of HIV/AIDS as 20:20:20 by 2020.
5. To eliminate leprosy, kala-azar, and lymphatic filariasis by 2018.
6. To improve the cure rate of sputum-positive TB cases and reduce the incidence of new cases by 2025.
7. To reduce the prevalence of blindness and the mortality rate of noncommunicable diseases to 25% by 2025.
8. To improve the utilization of health services and immunization coverage by 90% among infants up to 1 year of age by 2025.
9. To provide basic services such as safe and clean drinking water and sanitation to all.
10. To increase the funds allocated to the public health sector and ensure excellent health infrastructure including workforce per Indian Public Health Standards.
11. To establish a health institution for primary and secondary health services.
12. To improve the health surveillance system, health management information system, and information network.

Areas of Policy

The policy is applicable in the following areas:
1. Ensuring adequate investment in public health.
2. Coordinated action on preventive and promotive health through "Health in All" approach as a complement to "Health for All" on priority areas such as the following:
   - The Swachh Bharat Abhiyan
   - Balanced healthy diets and regular exercises
   - Addressing tobacco, alcohol, and substance abuse
   - Preventing accidental traffic mortality
   - Action against gender violence
   - Safety at the workplace
   - Reducing indoor and outdoor air pollution.
3. Changes in health-care services in the following areas:
   - Primary, secondary, and tertiary care
   - Public hospitals
   - Infrastructure
   - Human resource development
   - Urban health
   - National Health
   - Ayurveda, Yoga and Naturopathy, Unani, Siddha, and Homeopathy services.
4. Strengthening national health programmes to achieve specific goals and objectives of the policies:
   - Reproductive-Maternal-Neonatal-Child-Adolescent Health (RMNCH+A) services
   - Child and adolescent health programme
   - Planned strategies to address malnutrition and micronutrient deficiencies
   - Universal immunization program
   - Communicable diseases: control of tuberculosis, control of HIV/AIDS, leprosy elimination, and vector-borne disease control
   - Noncommunicable diseases
   - Mental health
   - Population stabilization.
5. Women's health and gender mainstreaming.
6. Gender-based violence (GBV).
7. Innovative measures (e.g. digital tools) with supportive supervision.
8. In urban areas comprising a population of 30 lakhs, only one trauma management center is available. However, in rural areas, it is one trauma center for a population of 10 lakhs to manage emergency and disaster.
9. Mainstreaming the potential of AYUSH: Linking AYUSH systems with accredited social health activists (ASHAs) and Village Health Sanitation and Nutrition Committees (VHSNCs).
10. Establishing new medical colleges, nursing institutions, and All India Institute of Medical Sciences (AIIMS) by the government.
11. Development of evidence-based standard guidelines of care.
12. Strengthening medical education by:
    - Improving the infrastructure of medical colleges and converting district hospitals into medical colleges

- Establishing new AIIMS
- A common medical entrance test and common exams for licensure for both medical and nursing students
- Periodic licensure, and objectives tests in postgraduate entrance exams, revision of curriculum, and quality education
- Attracting and retaining doctors in remote areas
- Specialist attraction and retention
- Midlevel service providers: Creation of a cadre of midlevel care providers through bridge courses, short courses, etc.

13. Nursing education:
    - Regulation and quality management of nursing education
    - Creation of cadres such as nurse practitioners and public health
    - Specialized courses such as critical care, cardiothoracic, vascular care, neurological care, trauma care, palliative care, and care of terminally ill
    - Establishment of nursing schools and centers of excellence for nursing at the state level
    - Exploring and appointing General Nurse Midwives (GNMs)/graduate nurses in subcenters.
14. Accredited social health activists (ASHAs) play a role in the following:
    - Seeking admission in Auxillary Nurse Midwives (ANM), nursing, and paramedical courses
    - Involving nongovernmental organizations (NGOs) to serve as support and as training institutions for ASHAs
    - Revising and improving the cadre of Mutipurpose health worker (MPHW)—Male.
15. Enhancing paramedical skills by conducting courses and curriculum for superspecialty paramedical care.
16. Public health management cadre.
17. Allocating funds for healthcare from National Health Accounts System.
18. Collaboration with nongovernment sector/engagement with private sectors for capacity building, skill development programs, corporate social responsibility (CSR), mental health-care programs, disaster management, strategic purchasing as stewardship, in immunization programs and disease surveillance, tissue and organ transplantations, Make in India, health information system, etc.
19. Strengthening regulatory framework for medical, clinical, food, drug, medical devices, clinical trials, and pricing for equipment, drugs, and devices.
20. Vaccine safety: Effective regulation, research, and development for manufacturing new vaccines by National Vaccine Policy 2011.
21. Medical technologies.
22. Public procurement involves ensuring access to free drugs and diagnostics through public facilities.
23. Availability of drugs and medical devices: Domestic production of active pharmaceutical ingredient and medical devices under Make in India goal.
24. Antimicrobial resistance.
25. Health technology assessment.
26. Digital health technology ecosystem: A National Digital Health Authority (NDHA) will be set up to regulate, develop, and deploy digital health.
27. Health surveys.
28. Health research.
29. Governance and legal framework.

National Policy on AYUSH 2002

Department of Indian Systems of Medicine and Homoeopathy (ISM & H) was given an independent identity in March 1995 in the Ministry of Health and Family Welfare (MoHFW) by creating a separate department, which was renamed as the Department of Ayurveda, Yoga and Naturopathy, Unani, Siddha and Homeopathy (AYUSH) in November 2003. Sowa Rigpa, a Tibetan system of medicine similar to Ayurveda, was also introduced under AYUSH.

A separate Ministry of AYUSH was formed on November 9, 2014, to develop and propagate the ISM. The objective of setting a separate ministry is to upgrade education standards of ISM; to strengthen research institutions; to develop various schemes for promotion, cultivation, and regeneration of medicinal plants; and to develop drugs standards. The first International Yoga day was celebrated on June 21, 2015, and the Union Ministry of AYUSH launched Mission Madhumeha on the occasion of the first National Ayurveda Day on October 28, 2016.

The November 2003 policy on AYUSH is in place since 2002. Keeping in mind many developments, its importance, and amendment in Acts, the Ministry of AYUSH is drafting a new policy on AYUSH.

Main Objectives of AYUSH Policy 2002

The main objectives of AYUSH 2002 are listed below:
- To promote good health by expanding the outreach of AYUSH healthcare through preventive, promotive, mitigating, and curative interventions
- To improve the teaching and clinical standards of teachers and clinicians
- To ensure affordable and efficacious AYUSH services and drugs
- To integrate AYUSH in health-care delivery system and national health programmes
- To improve the quality of drugs for domestic consumption and export
- To sensitize people at national and international levels, other stakeholders, and providers of health regarding AYUSH
- To develop and utilize these systems.

Strategies/Thrust Areas of Policy

The detailed list provides the various strategies of the policy:
1. **Education and research**
   - Developing regulation to establish new colleges and to start new courses

- Establishment of model colleges and center of excellence or national institutes
- Curriculum revision
- Setting up separate regulatory council for Yoga and naturopathy
- Compulsory reorientation programs for physicians and teachers
- Development of vocational training programs for homemakers, dais, nurses, dietitians, etc.
- Separate entrance examination for undergraduate courses at the state level and unified admission test for postgraduate (PG) courses in Ayurveda and Unani medicine
- Setting up an accreditation system at the central level
- Strengthening studies based on clinical trials and other priority areas.

2. **Medicinal plants**
   - Statutory status for Medicinal Plants Board to regulate the registration of farmers and cooperative societies, transportation, marketing, procurement, and supply to the pharmaceutical industry
   - Establishment of an export authority
   - Focus on research studies of particular areas such as reproductive system of plants, distribution, and storage
   - Research and development on rare and endangered plants.

3. **Intellectual property rights and patents**
   - Creation of a digital library for each system to protect traditional medical knowledge
   - Addressing relevant international fora regarding the need for sharing benefits to the custodian of knowledge and compensation to originators
   - Setting up of a *sui generis* system to provide an incentive to grassroots' innovators to disclose knowledge.

4. **Integration of ISM & H and national health programmes**
   - Integration and the mainstream of ISM & H in health-care delivery system and vertical national health programmes
   - Modification of laws about the practice of modern medicine by ISM practitioners
   - Upgradation of referral ISM hospitals
   - Setting up of specialty centers at primary health center (PHC) and district hospitals, and also Panchkarma and Ksharsutra facilities for treating various disorders in allopathic specialty hospitals with the assistance of the central government
   - Consolidation of infrastructure and raising salary and status of ISM practitioners at the state levels.

5. **Drug standardization and quality control**
   - Time target of 2005 to complete all pharmacopeia work related to all systems of medicine through an activation mechanism
   - Introduction of quality certification scheme for batch-by-batch testing by industry, and financial support for obtaining ISO 9000 certification by ISM
   - Creating new legislation for neutraceuticals and food supplements not covered under drug and food licensing, respectively
   - Setting up quality control centers or recognition on regional basis
   - Amendment of Drugs and Cosmetics Act.

6. **ISM industry**
   - Priority industry status to ISM industry as a green industry
   - Framing guidelines for patents, proprietary medicines, etc.

7. **Revitalization to local/folk health traditions and home remedy kits**
   - Identification, reinforcement, validation, and propagation of folk health traditions related to birth attendants, herbal healers, etc.
   - Implementation of a scheme to identify medicines to be included in the home remedy kits.

8. **Veterinary medicine**
   - The inclusion of homeopathic medicines for treatment of animals under Drugs and Cosmetics Act.

9. **Operational use of ISM in Reproductive and Child Health (RCH) services**
   - Use of Unani and homeopathic drugs in addition to Ayurveda drugs.

10. **Finance, administration, and development of ISM sector**
    - Raising the ISM share in the overall health plan
    - Establishing separate directorates of ISM and autonomy to ISM sector
    - Developing utilization of medicinal plants, the setting of dispensaries, need-based teaching institution in North East and other states, which are rich in medicinal flora and fauna.

11. **Medical tourism**
    - Promotion of Panchkarma and Yoga in hotels and through road shows
    - Development of ISM parks and scheme for accreditation of Panchkarma and Yoga facilities.

12. **Intersectoral cooperation**
    - Linking with other departments such as cultural tourism and railways for promotion and propagation
    - Schemes for the production and sale of medicinal plant products
    - Exploring the introduction of ISM in the school curriculum, and encouraging naturopathy diets and yogic exercises in schools, colleges, and offices.

13. **Exposing both foreign and Indian modern graduates to ISM**
    - Development of modules and courses on Ayurveda and Yoga in medical colleges and institutions
    - Provision of scholarships for PG and doctorate scholars for researching ISM.

14. **Building awareness**
    - Launching of electronic and print media programs on the utility and effectiveness of ISM & H

- Special incentive schemes for colleges and students, especially of management and science courses to work and for innovative ideas to provide awareness
- Utilizing services from NGOs
- Allocation of budget for Information Education and Communication (IEC) on healthy lifestyles and preventive health.

National Population Policy (NPP) 2002

Background

The inception of National Population Policy (NPP) started in 1940 by a "population committee" constituted by the National Planning Committee under the chairmanship of RK Mukherjee. The committee recommended various measures such as increasing the age of marriage and creating awareness among people about safe methods of birth control, which is achieved through communication methods and setting clinics. In 1946, the Bhore committee also made a recommendation to focus on self-control to arrest population growth.

In 1951, the government started a "family planning programme," which was a state-sponsored program in 1951. Later, in 1952, another committee was set up to frame a population policy. A separate committee on "family planning research and programme committee" was recommended, which also focused on self-control as a measure to arrest population growth. However, steps taken to stabilize population became a failure. In 1956, the government set up a central family planning board to deal with these issues, whose main focus was on sterilization.

In the Five-Year Plans, the government recommended various measures. In the first Five-Year Plan, advising people on family planning became an integrated part of health services. Many studies were conducted to gather information regarding factors affecting population growth to find the appropriate method of controlling population growth. Many family planning clinics were started in urban areas during the second Five-Year Plan. In the third and fourth Five-Year Plans, the main focus was on family planning and birth control. However, in the fifth Five-Year Plan (1974–1979), maternal and child health and nutrition services were added under the Population Control Programme.

National Population Policy (NPP) 1976–1977

The government launched the first NPP in 1976–1977, and the family planning programme came up as the family welfare programme and recommended the following measures:
- Legally enforce the minimum age for marriage as 18 years for girls and 21 years for boys
- Freezing the population count of 1971 till 2001
- Financial incentives to those opting for birth control
- Improvement in the educational level of girls
- Performance-based assistance from the center to the state
- Integrating family planning courses in education curriculum
- Use of communication media to motivate rural community
- Associating with voluntary associations to impart family planning programmes
- Group awards for associations/organizations initiating family planning programs
- Involving all government institutions/ministries in family planning programs
- Focus on research studies to generate evidence-based data.

National Health Policy 1983 focused on small family to attain the expected level of population stability. The National Development Council constituted a committee in 1991 to work out population control issues. The committee under the chairmanship of Karunakaran submitted its report in 1993 and recommended to prepare the NPP and suggest guidelines for programs, goals, and monitoring strategies. An expert committee under the chairmanship of MS Swaminathan drafted the NPP, which came up as the NPP 2000.

Objectives of NPP 2000

The government adopted its second National Population Policy on February 15, 2000. It aims at RCH services with an integrated approach consisting of the following objectives:
- The immediate objective was to provide services related to maternal and child and women empowerment after considering the needs for contraception, health-care facilities, and workforce requirement.
- The midterm objective is to reduce the TFR up to 2.1 children per woman by 2010.
- The long-term objective is to stabilize the expected population growth by 2045.

On May 11, 2000, the National Population Commission was formed under the chairmanship of the prime minister to monitor and evaluate the implementation of NPP 2000.

Goals

The NPP possesses sociodemographic-based goals that are required to be achieved by 2010.
- To find the needs for RCH services, facilities, and workforce requirement
- To make school education free and compulsory up to age 14
- To reduce dropouts of both girls and boys at primary and secondary school levels
- To reduce infant mortality rate (IMR) by less than 30/1,000 live births
- To reduce maternal mortality ratio to below 100/1 lakh live births
- To encourage delayed marriage for girls
- To achieve universal immunization of children

- To achieve a target of 80% deliveries in the health institutions and 100% by skilled health professionals
- To provide universal access for counseling, fertility regulation, and contraception services on choice basis
- To achieve 100% registration of births, deaths, marriages, and pregnancies
- To control the spread of AIDS, integrate reproductive tract infection (RTI) and sexually transmitted infection (STI) services with the National AIDS Control Organization
- To prevent and control communicable diseases
- To integrate AYUSH medicine in RCH services
- To promote the norms of small family
- To make family welfare programmes as central to all national health programmes.

Strategic Themes and Action Plans

The subsequent list is about the themes and action plans of NPP 2000:

1. Delegation of planning and program implementation to Panchayati Raj institutions at village level and further delegating administrative, financial, and resource mobilization power to them. The panchayat representative committees are formed to promote the gender-sensitive and multisectoral agenda for population stabilization.
2. Integrating essential services, family planning, and Maternal and Child Health (MCH) services at the village level can be achieved through self-help group, mobile clinics, and counseling services. It also needs to collaborate with voluntary and nongovernment sectors to provide services.
3. Empowering women for improved health and nutrition by creating an enabling environment, opening childcare centers, providing access to drinking water through reward schemes, improving health management, adequate transport, etc.
4. Child health and survival can be achieved through various programs and by setting a national technical committee, baby-friendly hospitals, perinatal audits, breastfeeding, complementary feeding, immunization, control of childhood diseases, etc.
5. Meeting the needs of family welfare services and improving facilities at every level by making the public accountable at all levels, i.e. improving infrastructure and facilities for referral transport and providing special loan schemes, site allocation, etc.
6. Focusing on providing basic healthcare to vulnerable especially the urban slum population, tribes, migrants, and people living in hilly areas. Coordinating with municipal bodies for the provision of water supply, sanitation, and waste disposal, disseminating information through IEC campaigns, and involving men in parenthood.
7. Collaborating with governmental and other organization for advertisement and campaigns, promoting transport, providing preventive RCH services for its employees, and creating a national network to provide free services to clients.
8. Sensitizing people for ISM. It requires training and orientation to ISM & H medical practitioners with regard to RCH services, utilizing their services, and providing advocacy and counseling.
9. Focusing on contraceptive techniques and research on RCH. The government needs to encourage, train, and provide funds to conduct studies on RCH and restructure population research centres.
10. Building geriatric health concerns, which include training urban and rural health centers to provide geriatric care.

Legislation

The government extended the freezing of 1971 census from 2001 to 2026 as motivational measures for states to work fearlessly to attain population stabilization through various population policy initiatives.

Institutional Setup

The new institutional structure is proposed to bring comprehensive and multisectoral coordination of family welfare services and other schemes and programs to stabilize population, which are as follows:

1. **At national level:** A national commission on population at the national level headed by the prime minister oversees and reviews the implementation of policy. It comprised chief ministers of all states and union territories (UTs), central ministers of the Department of Health and Family Welfare (H&FW), and other ministries.
2. **At state and UT level:** A state/UT commission at the state/UT level headed by the chief minister to oversees and reviews the implementation of policy.
3. **Coordination cell:** The planning commission consisted of a coordination cell at that time. Now it is under the National Rural Health Mission (NRHM).
4. **Technology mission:** A technology mission in the Department of H&FW provides technical support to design and monitor the project.

National AYUSH Mission

National AYUSH Mission (NAM) was launched in the 12th plan to implement the participation of states and UTs, with the aim to improve planning, supervision, and monitoring of various schemes under it.

Objectives

- Promote the AYUSH system by upgrading its hospitals and dispensaries and improving facilities at various levels of health-care delivery systems
- Strengthen AYUSH educational system by upgrading and setting these institutions including drug testing labs at state levels

- Facilitate quality control of Allopathic, Siddha, Unani, and Homeopathic (ASU&H) drugs by its enforcement mechanisms
- Maintain the availability of raw materials for preparing ASU&H drugs by adopting better agricultural practices and setting up clusters through various methods
- Develop infrastructure for entrepreneurs.

Components/Activities

1. **Mandatory component:** Mandatory component includes activities related to AYUSH services, its institutions, the medicinal plants of ASU&H, and quality control of the related drugs.
2. **Flexible component:** The flexible component includes various activities such as wellness centers, telemedicine, sports medicine, IEC, research and development, innovations such as public–private partnership, interest subsidy for private institutions, reimbursement, voluntary certification, and market promotion.

Structure/Mechanism

1. **At national level:** At the national level, NAM has a governing body and an appraisal committee. A *National Mission Directorate* is a governing body that is headed by the secretary of AYUSH, a chairperson with eight members including the member secretary of different departments, and may include experts as co-opted members with the approval of the chairperson. Its main role is to approve the State Annual Action Plan (SAAP) recommended by the appraisal committee. The *appraisal committee* constitutes the joint secretary in charge of NAM as a chairperson with eight other members including the secretary member and may also include experts as co-opted members. The main role of this committee is to appraise and submit SAAP to the governing body for approval.
2. **At state level:** At the state level, NAM possesses a governing body and an executive body. The *State AYUSH Mission Society* is the governing body that is headed by the chief secretary, a chairperson with nine members including member secretary, and also experts as co-opted members with the approval of the chairperson. Its main role is to overview the system, review its policies and program implementation, work on requirements, and approve SAAP. The *executive body* headed by the principal secretary/secretary in charge of AYUSH/H&FW as a chairperson and also comprise the vice-chairperson and eight members including the member secretary of different departments and may include experts as co-opted members with the approval of the chairperson. Its main role is to prepare and execute SAAP and administration of society, follow the decision made by the governing body, implement, review, monitor, account, etc.

Program Management Units

Program Management Units (PMUs) are setup at both national and state levels. It comprises management and technical staff. The function of PMUs is to give technical assistance to NAM for its implementation.

Monitoring and Evaluating Cells

Health Management Information System (HMIS) is setup at the center/state for concurrent monitoring and evaluation. It is proposed to have three HMIS managers at the national level and one HMIS at the state level.

National Health Mission (NHM) 2012–2017

National Health Mission is a flagship health sector program to revitalize both rural and urban health sectors to achieve universal access to equitable, affordable, and quality health-care services according to the health needs of people. The framework of the NHM implementation has two major sub-missions, i.e. the NRHM, which was started in 2005 and approved for continuation up to 2017 by the ministry, and the National Urban Health Mission (NUHM), which was approved by the cabinet on May 1, 2013.

Objectives

- To reduce IMR to 25/1,000 live births
- To reduce maternal mortality rate to 1/1,000 live births
- To achieve TFR to 2.1
- To prevent and reduce anemia among women of age-group 15–49 years
- To reduce both morbidity and mortality rates caused by communicable and noncommunicable diseases, injuries, and emerging diseases
  - To reduce the annual incidence and mortality due to TB by half
  - To prevent leprosy to less than 1/10,000 population and its incidence to zero in all districts
  - To reduce the annual incidence of malaria to be less than 1/1,000
  - To reduce the prevalence of microfilaria to less than 1% in all districts
  - To eliminate kala-azar by 2015, i.e. to less than 1 case/10,000 population in all blocks.
- To reduce household's out-of-pocket expenditure on total health-care expenditure.

Components of NHM

The four components of NHM consist of financial management group, strengthening health system, RMNCH+A, and national disease control programmes.

1. **Financial management group:** It deals with financial matters and managing funds to resources. It is under the finance division of the NHM. It manages the funds for state health societies and helps it to setup the financial management group. This division helps districts to build their financial capacity.

2. **Strengthening health system:** The government under the health mission planned to strengthen the health services in both rural and urban sectors in the following areas:
   - Mobile medical units to provide outreach healthcare services
   - Patient Transport Services, to implement National Ambulance services that can be availed on dialing 108/102
   - Infrastructure at all levels of the health system
   - Human resources including doctors, nurses, and specialists under NRHM
   - Provision of free essential drugs and logistics under NHM.

   The government took various initiatives to strengthen these areas by:
   - Adopting Indian public health standards for planning and evaluating health infrastructure and human resources
   - Improving quality standards by defining and implementing clinical protocols and guidelines on RCH
   - Preparing treatment protocols and packages such as Skilled Birth Attendant (SBA) and ANM training protocols, Integrated management of neonatal and childhood illness (IMNCI) package
   - Creating hospital management societies to improve the quality of care
   - Building quality management systems including audits and certification of hospitals and institution.

3. **Reproductive-Maternal-Neonatal-Child-Adolescent Health:** Reproductive-Maternal-Neonatal-Child-Adolescent Health is an important component under NHM concerning maternal and child health. The government launched this program under MoHFW in January 2013 to achieve the goals of the 12th Five-Year Plan and NRHM, so that the millennium developmental goals 4 and 5 are met for healthy mother and child, thus reducing IMR and maternal mortality rate. It is a strategic approach to safeguard the health of women, children, and adolescents. It is based on the "continuum of care" focusing on various stages of life and emphasizes maternal health, child health and immunization, and adolescent health [Rashtriya Kishor Swasthya Karyakram (RKSK)], family planning, the involvement of AYUSH doctors in carrying out the related activities, and aspirational district program.

4. **Communicable and noncommunicable diseases:**
   - National Iodine Deficiency Disorders Control Programme
   - National Vector Borne Disease Control Programme (NVBDCP) to control malaria, dengue, lymphatic filariasis, kala-azar, Japanese encephalitis, and chikungunya in India.
   - Revised National TB Control Programme
   - National Programme for Control of Blindness
   - National Leprosy Eradication Programme
   - Integrated Diseases Surveillance Programme
   - National Mental Health Programme
   - Noncommunicable Disease Programmes
   - Prevention and Management of Burn Injuries Programme.

Framework for Implementation

1. **At national level:** The Mission Steering Group under the chairmanship of the Union Health Minister, Empowered Programme Committee under union secretary (H&FW), and the mission headed by the mission director is responsible for planning, implementing, and monitoring the NHM activities, and a "National Programme Management Unit" is setup, and the National Health Systems Resource Centre is to serve as an apex body for technical assistance to the center and the states.

2. **At state level:** At the state level, the State Health Mission (SHM) would be under the state chief minister, with minister of H&FW as the co-chairperson, principal secretary/secretary as the convener, and other members. The State Health Society will be headed by the chief secretary or development commissioner, with the convener officer designated as the mission director of the SHM. State Program Management Unit (SPMU) will act as the main secretariat for the SHM. The State Health Systems Resource Centre would serve as an apex body for providing technical assistance to the state. The State Institute of Health and Family Welfare is the apex body to train professionals.

3. **At district level:** At the district level, the head of the local self-government would head the District Health Mission (DHM)/City Health Mission (CHM), and the District Health Society (DHS) by the district collector. It recommends the District Program Management Unit (DPMU) would link with a District Health Knowledge Centre (DHKC) for technical assistance and a District Training Center (DTC) for training.

National Rural Health Mission

National Rural Health Mission is a strategy of the government to provide an integrated, comprehensive primary healthcare to the rural people, especially the poor and vulnerable population. The Honorable Prime Minister launched NRHM on April 12, 2005, for 7 years. However, it continued till 2017 as a sub-mission under NHM. It is a framework to implement and attain the goals of NHP 2002. The key national programs are RCH-2, National Disease Control Programmes, and the Integrated Disease Surveillance Project under NRHM. It integrates all vertical health programs run by the Department of H&FW.

Objectives of NRHM

To restructure the delivery mechanism for health toward providing universal access to equitable, affordable, and quality healthcare to attain the targets laid down in NHP 2002.

- Reducing infant mortality rate (IMR) from the current 41 per thousand to 30 per thousand by 2010
- Reducing maternal mortality rate (MMR) from the current 300 per lakh to 100 per lakh by 2010
- Reducing TFR from the current 2.6 to 2.1 by 2010
- Increasing awareness of RTI/STI and HIV/AIDS from the current 36% to 100% by 2010
- Completing immunization
- Improving access to maternal and child health-care services, nutrition, and sanitation
- Doing prevention and control of communicable and noncommunicable diseases
- Strengthening comprehensive primary health-care services
- Achieving population stabilization and balance in the sex ratio
- Mainstreaming of AYUSH
- HIV/AIDS prevention and control efforts.

Aim and Purpose

NRHM aims to correct and enable the health system to effectively handle allocation and to promote policies to strengthen public health management and service delivery in the country. The main objectives are as follows:

- To make public health system accountable, affordable, and accessible by improved management and community action
- To develop pro-people partnerships with the private sector, so that quality health-care services are provided to the poor
- To make health professionals and paramedics deliver quality health services in rural areas.

Strategies of NRHM

The formulating strategies are based on the principles of "Health for All," i.e. equitable distribution, community participation, intersectoral coordination, and appropriate technology at the village, district, state, and national levels. The main focus areas are Family Welfare, AYUSH, nutrition, and sanitation to achieve the NRHM goal.

Action Plan

1. **At community level: ASHA:** The government recommended over 400,000 female ASHAs; one for 1,000 population (flexible for tribal hilly and deserted areas) in 18 high-focus areas with poor health indicators/weak health infrastructure to increase the accessibility to health services.
2. **Strengthening subcenters:** The government recommended an additional ANM at each subcenter and establishing about 21,983 new subcenters per the 2001 population norms. The estimated total requirement for the country is 200,000 ANMs.
3. **Strengthening primary health centers:** The government proposed the availability of three staff nurses against one staff nurse, appointing/posting AYUSH doctors over and above the medical officers posted in PHCs, an additional 24,000 MBBS/AYUSH doctors, and 46,000 staff nurses to provide 24×7 hours of service. It is also proposed to have an additional 4,436 PHCs per the 2001 population norms
4. **Strengthening community health centers:** The government proposed a functional 30-bedded rural hospital at the Community Health Center (CHC) level to provide round-the-clock hospital services with specialist facilities, seven specialists, and nine staff nurses. The plan is to have a separate AYUSH setup and an additional 3,332 CHCs and its upgradation in a phase manner. All CHCs are to be first made the referral units to provide emergency obstetric and newborn care, ensuring the availability of doctors in rural areas.
5. **Strengthening district health plan:** The focus areas of this plan are water supply, sanitation, and hygiene and nutrition under DHM. It integrates all vertical and centrally sponsored schemes. There is one project management unit for all districts of a state.
6. **Strengthening sanitation and hygiene:** It covers the total sanitation campaign, information education, and communication activities, school, household, and public sanitation programs.
7. **Strengthening disease control programmes:** All communicable and noncommunicable disease control and disease surveillance programs are part of DHM. At every level, it is also responsible for supplying generic drugs for common ailments and has the provision of mobile medical unit.
8. **Strengthening public-private partnership:** The government recommended involving the private sector in providing health services and their representation in regulatory bodies and district institutional mechanisms. At every level, the need is to develop clear-cut guidelines and plans for Public-Private Partnership (PPP).
9. **Strengthening health financing mechanism:** The government planned to strengthen the financial mechanisms through an accounting system, standardizing hospital care and services periodically. The need is to have community-based health insurance schemes with the help of Insurance Regulatory and Development Authority (IRDA).
10. **Strengthening reorienting health/medical education:** Strengthening health/medical education is one of the important action plans of the government under NRHM. It emphasizes to have a referral care chain and guidelines and to setup a commission for excellence in healthcare.
11. **Capacity building:** It includes training of ANMs as skilled birth attendants, training, and monitoring of ASHAs, the involvement of medical colleges, improved

career progression for medical/paramedical staff, strengthening of nursing colleges/ANM training schools, and partnership with NGOs and professional bodies.
12. **Ensuring quality and accountability:** Quality and accountability of service delivery are ensured by setting standards by the constituting committees at health centers/hospital levels.

National Urban Health Mission

National Urban Health Mission was approved by the cabinet on May 1, 2013 and was launched on January 20, 2014 by the union health minister as a sub-mission under NHM to improve the health status of urban poor both listed and unlisted living in slums, vulnerable population such as homeless, ragpickers, limekiln workers, and sex workers by addressing their particular health issues.

Urban local self-governments such as municipal corporation, municipality, notified area committee, and town panchayat are the unit of planning. All these urban local governments except municipal corporations are the part of the District Health Action Plan, which has a separate plan of action per the norms for urban areas.

Objectives

- To reduce IMR by 40% (in urban areas); national IMR to 20 per 1,000 live births by 2017
- Forty percent reduction in Under 5 mortality rate (U5MR) and IMR
- To achieve universal immunization in all urban areas
- To reduce the maternal mortality rate and 100% Antenatal care (ANC) coverage (in urban areas) and TFR
- To provide universal access to reproductive health including 100% institutional deliveries
- To achieve all targets of disease control programmes such as National Iodine Deficiency Disorders Control Programme and Revised National Tuberculosis Control Programme.

Strategies

- Strengthening the existing public-sector primary health structure and referral system
- Establishing community-based groups such as Mahila Arogya Samiti (MAS) at the household level
- Having coverage with other schemes and programs such as the Jawaharlal Nehru National Urban Renewal Mission (JNNURM), Rajiv Awas Yojana, Swarn Jayanti Shahri Rozgar Yojana (SJSRY), North Eastern Region Urban Development Programme, School Health Programmes, and Adolescent Reproductive and Sexual Health (ARSH)
- Utilizing other areas of synergy such as Member of Parliament Local Area Development Scheme (MPLADS) and CSR for mobilization of funds to provide health facilities
- Coordinating and integrating various programs implemented by the Ministry of Women Development, e.g. Integrated Child Development Scheme (ICDS), by Human Resource Development for School Health Programmes and Adolescent Reproductive, and Social Health, and by the Ministry of Minority Affairs for multisectoral developmental programs
- Public–private partnership to carry out innovative promotive and preventive actions at the community level, such as water and environmental sanitation, nutrition, and other aspects of health
- Creating revolving fund to provide increased access to healthcare
- Effective tracking, monitoring, and timely intervention system through information technology-enabled services and e-governance at the state level
- Capacity building of health-care providers
- Identifying and prioritizing the most vulnerable urban poor
- Ensuring quality health-care services through quality management and assurance mechanism.

Framework for Implementation

The National Urban Health Mission planned to operationalize at national/center, state, district-city, and community levels.

1. **At national level:** The Mission Steering Group under the chairmanship of Union Health Minister, Empowered Programme Committee under secretary (H&FW), and National Programme Coordinator Committee under mission director is responsible for planning, coordinating, monitoring, and financing programs. A National Program Management Unit is setup to provide technical assistance for implementing and monitoring NUHM.
2. **At state level:** There is an SPMU, the extension of NRHM SPMU, with a separate urban health cell under the state mission director NRHM. There is SHM under the chief minister of state, the State Health Society under the chief secretary, Health Mission Directorate serviced by urban health division will be responsible for planning, monitoring, and financing at the state level.
3. **At city/community level:** The states may either have a separate City Urban Health Mission/City Urban Health Societies or use the existing structure of District Health Society (DHS) (headed by municipal commissioner/District Magistrate (DM)/District Health Mission (DHM) (headed by mayor/chairman) under NRHM, with additional staff. A City Programme Management Unit (CPMU) may also be set up.

Urban Health-Care Delivery System

The services included under Urban Health-Care Delivery System are given below:

1. **At the community level for outreach services:** At the community level, the frontline workers designated as ASHAs, MAS members, and ANMs.
   a. **Accredited Social Health Activist:** The activist is similar to NRHM ASHA and covers 1,000–2,500 beneficiaries between 200 and 250 households located at Anganwadi center, providing doorstep

services at the slum level. She should be a resident of slum and in the age-group of 25–45 years and acts as a link between Urban Primary Health Centre (UPHC) and urban slum population. She is expected to promote desired health-seeking behavior among the urban poor of the assigned area and to extend help to ANM for providing outreach services. They are responsible to MAS.
   b. **Mahila Arogya Samiti:** It is a community group comprising 10–12 women with an elected chairperson and a treasurer supported by ASHA under SJSRY. One MAS is for every 50–100 slums and urban poor households. It forms linkages between UPHC and urban slum population, and its main function is to facilitate health awareness on essential services and monitoring.
   c. **ANM:** One ANM is expected to cover 10,000–12,000 population and four to five ANMs per UPHC. At the community level, she is responsible for providing preventive and promotive health-care services through regular visits and by organizing outreach sessions in coordination with ASHA and MAS members (one routine session monthly and special outreach session weekly along with other health professionals).
2. **At the first level of service delivery**
   a. **Urban Primary Health Centre:** One UPHC is to cover approximately 50,000–60,000 population located near the slum area to cater to the health needs of approximately 25,000–30,000 slum population. Each UPHC should be manned by two doctors, i.e. one regular and another part-time, three staff nurses, one pharmacist, one lab technician, one Lady health visitor (LHV), and four to five ANMs (depending upon the population size) with co-opted AYUSH centre.
3. **At the referral level**
   a. **Urban Community Health Centre:** For referral services, one UCHC-satellite hospital (30–50 beds) for every four to five UPHCs to provide inpatient services including medical care, minor surgical facilities, and facilities for institutional deliveries to a population size of 250,000, and 100 beds for a population size of more than 5 lakhs for metro cities.
4. **Referral linkages:** Existing hospitals, apart from the private hospitals, are also considered the referral linkages for availing different types of health services.
5. **School health services:** School health services for the urban poor population under UPHC are integrated with the existing School Health Program and Scheme.

Programs Under NHM

Programs Under Maternal Health

The five main programs under maternal health are as follows:
1. **Janani Suraksha Yojana:** Janani Suraksha Yojana (JSY) under the overall umbrella of NRHM was launched in April 2005 and proposed by modifying the existing National Maternity Benefit Scheme (NMBS). Although NMBS provides a better diet for pregnant women from below poverty line (BPL) families, JSY integrates cash assistance with antenatal care during the pregnancy period, institutional care during delivery, and immediate postpartum period in a health center by establishing a system of coordinated care by field-level health worker. The JSY is a 100% centrally sponsored scheme. The objectives of this yojana are to reduce the overall maternal mortality ratio and neonatal mortality rate/IMR and to promote institutional deliveries and provide incentives to BPL SC/ST pregnant women delivering in government institutions/accredited private institutions.
2. **Janani Shishu Suraksha Karyakram:** Janani Shishu Suraksha Karyakram (JSSK) scheme was launched on June 1, 2011, with the objective of providing free and no expense delivery to all pregnant women delivering, including cesarean section, in government hospitals. They will provide free medicine, diagnostics, blood, diet, and transport facility from home to back home in case of referral after delivery.
3. **The Pradhan Mantri Surakshit Matritva Abhiyan:** The Pradhan Mantri Surakshit Matritva Abhiyan (PMSA) was launched on June 9, 2016, by the MoHFW, Government of India, to boost health-care facilities to those poor pregnant women (3–6 months' pregnant) who approach the public health institutions. They will provide free health checkup and the required treatment on ninth of every month. Its objective is to reduce maternal mortality rate and IMR, ensuring safe delivery and healthy child, and to make pregnant women aware of their health issues.
4. **Labour Room Quality Improvement Initiative Programme:** The government launched Labour Room Quality Improvement Initiative (LaQshya) Programme to improve the quality of services provided in labor rooms and its operational theaters, so that quality care is provided to both mother and newborn.
5. **Other programs:** The government has initiated other programs such as:
   - Comprehensive abortion care services
   - Provision of RTI and STI services
   - Establishing blood storage centers
   - Village and Nutrition Day
   - Screening for gestational diabetes and hypothyroidism and deworming, etc.

Child and Adolescent Health-Related Schemes/Programs

The five programs of child and adolescent health-related schemes are the following:
1. **Rashtriya Bal Swasthya Karyakram:** Rashtriya Bal Swasthya Karyakram (RBSK) scheme under NHM was launched in 2013 by the MoHFW, Government of India. The aim of this initiative was early detection and treatment of congenital disabilities, diseases,

deficiencies, and development delays including disability for children from birth to 18 years of age, all provided free of cost. Early detection is planned at the delivery point by the attending staff, after 48 hours by ASHA at home, outreach screening by mobile health team (comprises two doctors, ANM/staff nurse, and pharmacy/paramedical) both from 6 weeks to 6 years at Anganwadi center and from 6 years to 18 years at school.

2. **India Newborn Action Plan:** Under Global Strategy for Women's and Children's health, the Government of India launched "Newborn Action Plan" in June 2014, with an aim to eliminate newborn deaths and stillbirths.
3. **Intensified Diarrhea Control Fortnight:** Intensified Diarrhea Control Fortnight (IDCF) is a special campaign/drive started national wide since 2014 for a period of 2 weeks from July to August to prevent and control the risk of childhood diarrhea and will be observed every year during this period to achieve "zero child deaths due to childhood diarrhea," so that IMR and child mortality rate are reduced. It includes a various set of activities related to advocacy, awareness generation, management service, establishing oral rehydration solution (ORS)-zinc corners, distributing ORS by ASHA, screening of undernourished children and treating them, infant and young child feeding activities, handwashing, etc. through capacity building, multisectoral involvement.
4. **Rashtriya Kishor Swasthya Karyakram:** Rashtriya Kishor Swasthya Karyakram, a national health programme for adolescent of age-group of 10–14 years, was launched by the MOHFW on January 7, 2014, to improve nutrition, to improve sexual and reproductive health including menstrual hygiene practices, to prevent injuries and violence, and to improve mental health. It is a community-based interventional program through peer educators and was started in collaboration with other ministries and state governments. It involves the provision of providing guidance and counseling through adolescent-friendly health clinics, supervisory weekly iron and folic acid (IFA) supplements, and twice a year antihelminthic medication to control helminthic.
5. **Mothers' Absolute Affection Programme:** Mothers' Absolute Affection (MAA) Programme, a flagship national program, was launched by the Union Minister of Health and Family Welfare on August 5, 2016, to promote breastfeeding and provide counseling services through the health system.

The Swachh Bharat Mission

The government launched Swachh Bharat Mission (SBM) on October 2, 2014, to eliminate/reduce open defecation and improve sanitation by 2019. It has two sub-missions: the Swachh Bharat Mission–Gramin (SBM-G) for rural areas and the SBM for urban areas. Various Swachh Bharat campaigns/programmes motivate people regarding sustainable sanitation practices, the use of appropriate technologies for sanitation and management of solid and liquid wastes planned at national, state, district, block, and gram panchayat/village, and water sanitation committee. SBM-G replaced Nirmal Bharat Abhiyan 2012.

M-Health Initiation

Union Health Minister of India launched m-Health Initiative Programme, as a part of the Digital India Programme on January 17, 2016, to strengthen public health infrastructure. It consists of four mobile services, namely kilkari, mobile academy, m-cessation, and TB missed call initiative.

1. **Kilkari:** The Hindi word kilkari means "baby's gurgle." It is a program developed by BBC Media Action to deliver free, weekly, and time-appropriate 72 audio messages via mobile and the messages are related to pregnancy, childbirth, and childcare delivery by health-care workers (ASHA) to pregnant mothers in their second trimester till the child becomes 1 year. In the first phase, this program was launched in six states.
2. **Mobile academy:** The mobile academy is another audio-training program developed by BBC Media Action to train ASHA frontline health workers in maternal and child healthcare to use interactive voice response messages on a mobile phone and improve their communication skills.
3. **M-cessation:** It is a campaign to reach out and support those who are willing to quit tobacco use, which is achieved through text messages sent through mobile phones.
4. **TB missed call initiative:** The TB missed call initiative is a helpline/support services to give information, counseling, and treatment to a caller who gives a missed call and the support service return the call to the caller. The service is available in the states of Punjab, Chandigarh, Haryana, and Delhi.

Programs Under National Institute for Transforming India (NITI) Aayog

The various schemes of NITI Aayog are listed below:
1. **Sustainable action for transforming human capital programme:** Under the agenda of cooperative federalism, the NITI Aayog, a "Sustainable Action for Transforming Human Capital (SATH)" program, was launched on July 2, 2016, to identify and build three future role models of health system in collaboration with the respective state governments and implemented with selected McKinsey & Co. & IPE Global Consortium in order to transform the health sector.
2. **Performance index:** NITI Aayog launched performance on health index with MOHFW on December 23, 2016, with the aim to improve health outcome and data collection systems at the state level to get its annual incremental index of health improvements.
3. **Aspirational district programme:** The government launched this program in January 2018 to raise people's

Chapter 11: National Health Policies

standard of living and to improve the India's ranking in human development index by 2022. At present, under NITI Aayog, 117 were identified as aspirational districts by health and nutrition (30% weight), education (30%), agriculture and water (20%), financial consideration (10%), and skill development and basic infrastructure (10%). Overall it has 49 indicators and 13 core indicators related to the health sector. Apart from this index, the government developed health atlas, a diagnostic tool launched on April 14, 2018, guidelines and checklist on health and nutrition, and e-Mitra, a mobile integrated tool kit for providing statistical information regarding RMNCH+A launched on October 22, 2018.

CHAPTER HIGHLIGHTS

- Policy is a system or a statement that guides and provides discretion within the limited boundaries.
- The main goal of NHP 2017 is to attain the highest possible level of well-being and provide affordable quality health-care services to everyone, and the objective is to achieve universal health coverage having many priority areas.
- The main objectives of AYUSH Policy 2002 are to promote good health, improve teaching and clinical standards and drug standards, and provide affordable services. It also aims at integrating its services in the health-care delivery system and sensitizing people to adopt AYUSH services.
- National AYUSH Mission aims to improve planning, supervision, monitoring of various schemes under it.
- The NPP 2000 is a framework aiming at RCH services, with an integrated approach to stabilize the expected population growth by 2045.
- NHM is a program to achieve universal access to equitable, affordable, and quality health-care services per the health needs of both rural and urban people.

REVIEW QUESTIONS

I. Essay Type Questions
1. What do you mean by "policy"? Describe National Health Policy 2017 in detail.
2. Discuss National Policy on AYUSH.
3. Explain the major strategies and action plan of NPP 2000.
4. Describe the framework for implementation of the National Health Mission.
5. Enlist the various maternal and child health-related programs. Describe any one in detail.

II. Short Notes
1. National AYUSH Mission
2. RMNCH+A Program
3. NRHM Action Plan
4. Urban Health-Care Delivery System
5. Janani Suraksha Yojana

III. Multiple Choice Questions
1. The Disability Adjusted Life Year Index is a measure to:
   a. Assess life expectancy
   b. Estimate the burden of disease and its trends
   c. Calculate the total fertility rate
   d. Estimate the cure rate
2. In which year, did the Indian Systems of Medicine and Homeopathy (ISM & H) get an independent identity in the Ministry of Health and Family Welfare?
   a. 1990　　　　b. 1993
   c. 1995　　　　d. 2000
3. What system of medicine is Sowa Rigpa?
   a. Ayurveda　　b. Yoga
   c. Siddha　　　d. Tibetan
4. Who is the head of the executive body of the state AYUSH Mission Society?
   a. Principal Secretary
   b. Chief Secretary
   c. Chief Minister
   d. Health Minister
5. When was the first National Ayurveda Day celebrated?
   a. March 12, 2013
   b. November 9, 2014
   c. June 21, 2015
   d. October 28, 2016
6. Who drafted the National Population Policy 2000?
   a. Karunakaran　　b. MS Swaminathan
   c. RK Mukherjee　 d. Dr JS Bajaj
7. Up to which year the freezing population count of 1971 was extended by both Houses?
   a. 2020　　　　b. 2022
   c. 2024　　　　d. 2026
8. Which one of the following National Health Programmes has the provision of providing free and no expense delivery to all pregnant women?
   a. Janani Suraksha Yojana (JSY)
   b. The Pradhan Mantri Surakshit Matritva Abhiyan
   c. Janani Shishu Suraksha Karyakram (JSSK)
   d. LaQshya Programme

Answer Keys
1. b　　2. c　　3. d　　4. a　　5. d　　6. b　　7. d
8. c

SUGGESTED READING

1. Available from http://dm.nuhru.in/files/NHP-%202002%20-%20Excerpts.pdf. [Accessed on 23.12.2018].
2. Available from http://ijme.in/wp-content/uploads/2016/11/650-5.pdf. [Accessed on 23.12.2018].
3. Available from http://india.gov.in/knowindia/india_at_a_glance.php. [Accessed on 24.12.2018].

4. Available from http://india.gov.in/outerwin.htm?id=http://mohfw.nic.in/NRHM/NRHM(National%20Rural%20Health%20Mission).htm. [Accessed on 24.12.2018].
5. Available from http://ispub.com/IJH/7/1/7116>.
6. Available from http://mohfw.nic.in/np2002.htm National Health Policy. [Accessed on 25.12.2018].
7. Available from http://nhm.gov.in/images/pdf/NUHM/Implementation_Framework_NUHM.pdf. [Accessed on 24.12.2018].
8. Available from http://populationcommission.nic.in/npp.htm. [Accessed on 22.12.2018].
9. Available from http://www.ayush.gov.in/sites/default/files/Draft%20National%20Policy%20on%20AYUSH_1.pdf. [Accessed on 26.12.2018].
10. Available from http://www.gujhealth.gov.in/National_policy.pdf. [Accessed on 24.12.2018].
11. Available from http://www.planningcommission.nic.in/plans/planrel/fiveyr/12th/pdf/12fyp_vol3.pdf. [Accessed on 20.12.2018].
12. Available from https://vdocuments.mx/documents/planning-commission-of-india-sreport-on-universa. [Accessed on 24.12.2018].
13. Govt. of India. National Population Policy 2000. New Delhi: Department of Family Welfare, Ministry of Health & Family Welfare, GOI.
14. Health and Population Policy Initiatives in India. Available from http://www.ghwatch.org/english/casestudies/healthpop_india.pdf. [Accessed on 28.12.2018].
15. Subbaraman R, Thomas B, Sellappan S, et al. Tuberculosis patients in an Indian mega-city: where do they live and where are they diagnosed? PLoS One. 2017;12(8):e0183240.
16. The Government of India. National Population Policy 2000. New Delhi.
17. The Government of India. National Rural Health Mission 2005–2012. Reference Material. Ministry of Health & Family Welfare.
18. The Government of India. National Rural Health Mission: Mission Document. New Delhi: MOHFW; 2005.

SECTION 3

Planning Process

12. Fundamentals of Planning
13. Mission, Philosophy, and Objectives
14. Strategic Planning, Operating Plans and Planning New Venture
15. Innovation in Nursing and Planning for Change
16. Program Evaluation Review Technique, Activity Plan, Management by Objectives, and Benchmarking

CHAPTER 12

Fundamentals of Planning

CHAPTER OUTLINE

- Planning
  - Introduction
  - Concept and Meaning of Planning
  - Definitions of Planning
  - Nature/Characteristics of Planning
  - Elements of Planning
  - Objectives of Planning
  - Principles of Planning
  - Importance of Planning
- Planning Process
- Types of Planning
- Advantages of Planning
- Limitations of Planning

LEARNING OUTCOMES

After completion of this chapter, the learner will be able to:
- Understand the concept and meaning of planning
- Define the term planning
- Discuss the nature, objectives, and principles of planning
- Discuss the importance of planning in management
- Explain the key steps of the planning process
- Describe different types of planning
- Enumerate advantages of planning
- Justify the limitations of planning

KEY TERMS

Planning, managerial functions, intellectual process, rational approach, promise, priorities, primacy, operational planning, long-term and short-term planning, proactive and reactive planning

PLANNING

Introduction

Planning is the major function of management and forms a platform for nursing management for proper preparation (Fig. 12.1). Based on planning, decisions are taken for any action to achieve objectives. Plans guide managers to follow the line of actions to accomplish preplanned goals and objectives.

Concept and Meaning of Planning

Planning determines the line of action, i.e. what action, why and how to take action, when to take action, and who will take action. Thus, the planning is a process that is concerned with the answers of why, what, how, when, and by whom. However, the basic process of planning is the same for all the managers but vary from managers to managers.

Planning guides for the future reduce the overall impact of changes and allow nurse managers to organize and control nursing services and the activities necessary to accomplish the nursing organizational objectives. However, without setting the objectives, there is nothing to organize, direct, or control. Planning is related to this aspect.

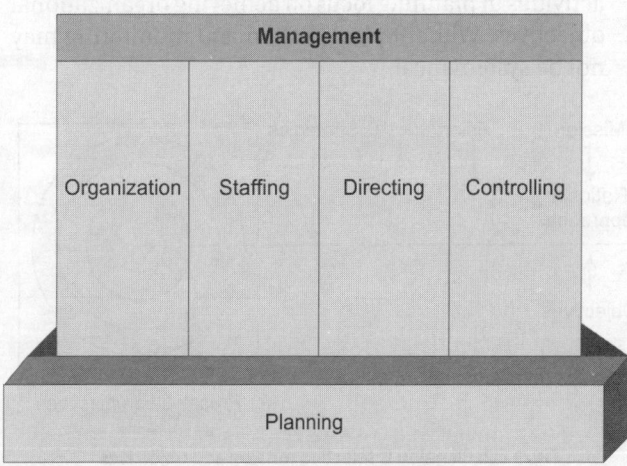

Fig. 12.1: Planning as the foundation of nursing management.

Definitions of Planning

Planning is deciding in advance and looking ahead. According to the Oxford dictionary, planning is the act or process of making plans for something.

- Planning is done by a manager, which involves the selection from among alternatives for the organization in common and each department within it.

  —*Koontz and O'Donnell*

- Planning means the determination of what to do, how and where to do, who and how results to evaluate.

  —*James Lundy*

- It is an organized attempt to anticipate and to make rational arrangement for dealing with the future problem by projecting trends

  —*Dimock and Dimock*

- Planning is an intellectual thinking process. It makes possible the actions to be done to accomplish objectives and requires a nurse administrator to think critically about the implications of taking a particular decision.

Planning is a looking forward and decision-making process to take future action to achieve certain objectives. Planning is a decision-making process to select the best line of action out of alternatives. It is a continuous process of thinking in advance for the future of what is to be done by analyzing and evaluating the various alternative courses of action to select the best possible course of action to achieve the organizational goals. It fills the gap from present to future planned objectives, policies, strategies, procedures, programs, and budgets. Mission, vision, objectives, and strategies achieve goals **(Fig. 12.2)**.

Nature/Characteristics of Planning

The following list details the nature/characteristics of planning:

1. **Planning is goal oriented:** Planning, being goal oriented, focuses on setting organizational goals and objectives and suggests the ways to achieve them. It provides a blueprint for the entire organization to operate. The planning process includes subactivities and determines the future course of actions—all activities in planning focus on achieving organizational objectives. Without plans, action and monitoring may not be systematical.

2. **Planning is a continuous process basic to all managerial functions:** Planning is the foremost function of management and includes various activities. A manager has to plan before doing any activity. It is an ongoing process of making modifications and re-examining and readjustment to changing situations, which is important in directing and controlling as well.

   Planning logically precedes the performance of all other managerial activities. It is the first function of a planner and follows all other managerial functions as depicted in **Figure 12.3**.

   Formulating objectives, policies, procedures, programs, and rules are basic to planning. The output of all managerial activities is when matched with a plan in the controlling process, acts as a basis for replanning or future planning to achieve the desired objectives. It assists in workforce planning and designing training programs for the nursing staff. It lays down the standards or benchmarks of performance for the staff to control their activities.

3. **Planning is futuristic or forward looking:** Planning requires forecasting of future situation in which an organization has to function. It also includes decision-making for the future. Planners develop strategies and action plans by keeping in mind all probable threats and opportunities and try to control it.

4. **Planning aims at efficiency:** Planning is a conscious process to decide in advance about the future course of action to achieve predetermined goals and objectives. Efficiency is measured by looking at the output or the best result produced with lesser input regarding resources such as human resources, money, material, methods, and machinery used for a particular activity.

5. **Planning is a thinking process:** Planning is an intellectual process of creative thinking. It involves vision and foresightedness to decide actions to be done in the future and involves mental faculties by the managers. A manager uses facts, reasonable premises, and constraints, and from these, he or she visualizes and formulates what necessary activities, such as generating key **issue** formulation of proposals, making choices, preparing a budget, implementing, and monitoring, are

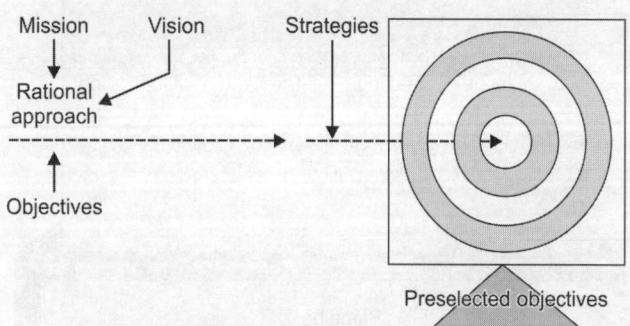

Fig. 12.2: Planning is selecting mission and objectives.

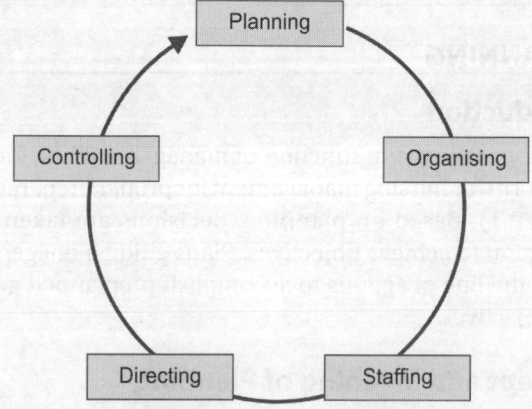

Fig. 12.3: Primacy of planning.

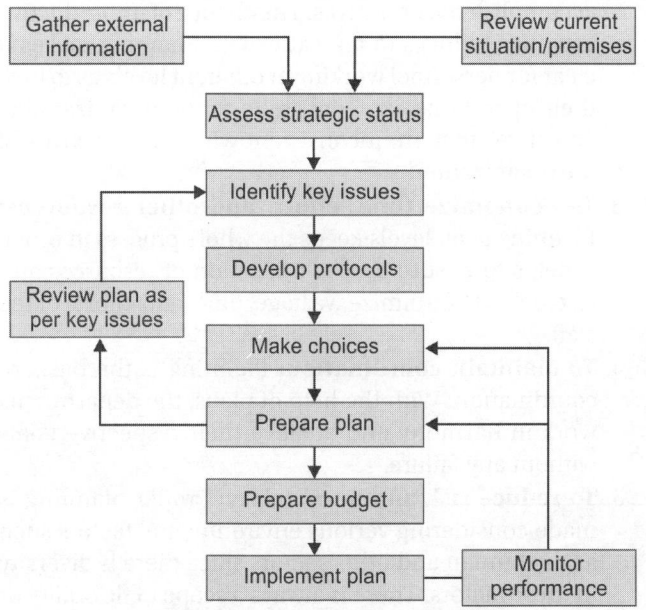

Fig. 12.4: Planning as a critical thinking process.

required to achieve the desired results **(Fig. 12.4)**. One requires thinking process to carry out all these steps. Hence planning is an intellectual process.

6. **Planning is a pervasive function:** Planning being pervasive extends throughout the organization. All levels of managers are involved in planning. Nurse manager at every level has a planning function to perform. The higher level of management is responsible for formulating the overall objectives and actions of the nursing organization. They need to formulate organizational objectives, develop policies and action plans, and draw procedures and programs for the nursing service. Similarly, the block-level nurse managers need to formulate objectives of their block within organizational objectives and also methods of achieving those objectives; ward/nursing unit supervisors formulate objectives of respective units and ways to attain those objectives. At the operational level, nurses frame objectives and develop nursing care plans based on the need of the individual patient–client under their charge. Thus each level of nurse manager contributes toward organizational goals, i.e. to ensure the best possible patient care **(Fig. 12.5)**.

7. **Planning is a dynamic function:** Planning has a scope of flexibility by the needs of customers and changing situations in the internal environment of the organization. Hence it is called a dynamic function. Successful organizations are always ready to cope up with the current situations and plan for the future. The planning process must allow flexibility to meet new challenges. The targets need to revise and require introducing new steps to achieve the said targets.

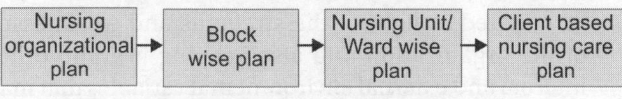

Fig. 12.5: Planning at various levels.

8. **Planning is a social process:** Planning requires consultation and participation. All the employees of the organization should be informed about the planning and coordinated with all concerned involved in planning **(Fig. 12.6)**.

9. **Planning has a rational approach:** The concept of rationality denotes the choice of appropriate means for achieving stated objectives. It is a rational process to select the best course of action from various alternative courses of action. It tries to identify and bridge the gap between the actual status and the desired performance status of various courses of action. There is a need for utilizing various sources to carry out actions. The most appropriate use of these resources is the focus of the rational approach to planning.

10. **Planning is a form of a bridge:** Planning is a form of a bridge that fills the gap between the present and the future. It indicates an open-system approach to planning. Open-system approach of planning indicates that identification of the gap between the current status and the desired status in the future—actions required to bridge the gap influenced by external environmental factors such as political, legal, technical, and social. Managers have to take into account all the external and internal environmental factors.

11. **Planning is a realistic approach to problems:** Planning starts with the formulation of objectives, and action plans are developed to achieve those objectives. The objectives are defined in meaningful and technical terms so that managerial actions could be possible. Various alternatives of action plans are drafted keeping in mind strengths, weaknesses, encountered threats, and opportunities. It selects the most realistic and possible alternative action plan so that the organization can pursue and achieve its objectives successfully.

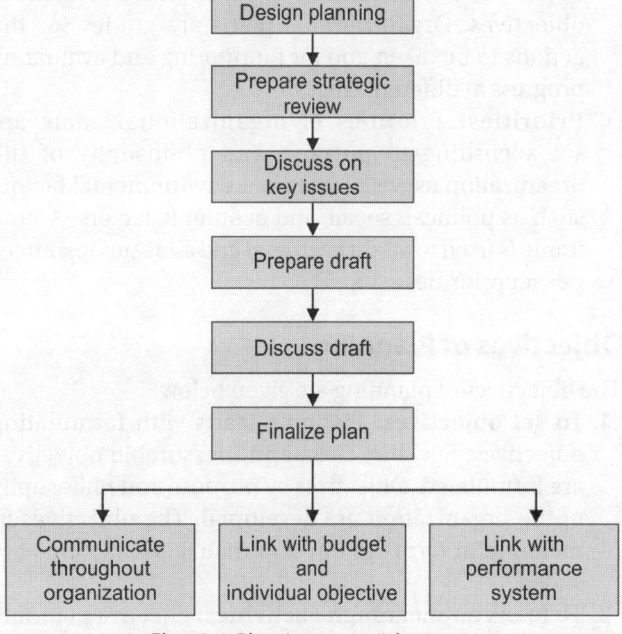

Fig. 12.6: Planning as a social process.

12. **Planning aims at ensuring coordination:** Planning is pervasive and required at all levels of management. Organizational objectives, policies, procedures, and programs are drawn to bind all departments to work in pursuit of attaining the main goals. They all perform their roles and move in the same direction. Planning coordinates what, who, how, why, and where action plans done. If planning is appropriate, the coordination of all activities will be better. Hence planning aims at ensuring coordination.

Elements of Planning

There are six P's required for planning. The elements of planning are as follows:
1. **Purpose:** While planning, purpose or the aim of the organization must be stated clearly and should be specific.
2. **Philosophy:** It provides a statement of belief and values that are basic to all operations of the organization and to achieve the organization's purpose. It should be inconsistent with organizational purpose or mission.
3. **Promise:** It is a process of assessing the strengths and weaknesses of an organization based on knowledge and assumptions of internal and external environmental factors. The management can deal with changing environment by knowing the capability of the organization in comparison to opportunities and threats that are likely to prevail in the organization through strength, weaknesses, opportunities, and threats (SWOT) analysis,
4. **Policies:** They are designated plans or courses of actions in a specific situation. These provide guidelines and constraints for decision-making and preparing action plans. Policies are the frame at the top management usually by the Board of Directors.
5. **Plans:** Action plans are written document reflecting objectives and detailed course of action to achieve objectives. Organizational plans are guides for the actions to be taken and for monitoring and evaluating progress at different stages.
6. **Priorities:** Priorities of organizational goals are set according to purpose and philosophy of the organization as well as external environmental factors such as political, social, and economic factors. A time frame is fixed to attain each goal and allocates resources per set priorities.

Objectives of Planning

The objectives of planning are given below:
1. **To set objectives:** Planning starts with formulating objectives. Specific, clear, and measurable objectives are formulated. Objectives by purpose and philosophy of the organization are developed. The objectives in meaningful terms to develop managerial actions are stated.
2. **To focus on meaningful activities:** Effective planning lays down various courses of action, which are useful to accomplish the objectives. The chance of unproductive activities reduces to a great extent. Planning makes it clear for personnel working at different levels as to how their operations can contribute to the organizational objectives that are inconsistent with the objectives of the organization.
3. **To economize time, effort, and other resources:** Planning at all levels keeps the whole process in order. It helps to ensure proper utilization of resources and also helps to minimize wastage, time, and efforts of the staff.
4. **To maintain coordination:** Planning is the basis of coordination. With the help of plans, the departments work in harmony and achieve their respective goals without any failure.
5. **To reduce risk and uncertainty:** Proper planning is made considering various environmental factors such as the human and other factors since there is diversity in these factors. There is always a scope of flexibility or alternatives in good planning that reduces the risk and uncertainty arising out of them.
6. **To aid in taking decisions:** A planner thinks various plans of action and selects the best among alternative future courses of action according to the priority of the organization.
7. **To ensure proper control:** Planning ensures proper control by laying down performance evaluation methods and measuring the performance of people. The performance and standards are compared, which provide a gap between the actual and the expected performance. It will help to take appropriate measure.
8. **To achieve organizational effectiveness:** During the implementation of plans, it is easy to monitor the effective utilization of resources per plan or not. Proper monitoring improves organizational performance and has scope to explore and to take appropriate corrective measures to improve the effectiveness of the organization.
9. **To promote creativity:** Planning is basically concerned with critical thinking of exploring, selecting, and applying the best alternative to achieve the goal. Thus planning promotes creativity and innovation.
10. **To improve efficiency:** Planning determines as to when and how various tasks are to be performed by different nursing units. It brings efficiency, reduces wastage, and avoids needless efforts in various units.

Principles of Planning

The following list shows the principles of planning:
1. **The principle of meaningful objectives:** Planning should be done by clearly defined objectives. It is a means of achieving objectives. Hence objectives should be explicit, specific, and measurable. These should be formulated in light of the strengths and weaknesses of the organization and also keeping in mind other internal and external environmental variables that may influence in achieving those objectives.

2. **The principle of primacy:** All managerial activities after planning are executed. It provides the basis for organizing, staffing, directing, coordinating, and controlling and flows through all of them. It is the lifeblood for all functions of management.
3. **The principle of planning premises:** Planning premises are the anticipated environment in which the plans are expected to operate. These are also known as conditions that will affect an organization. The planner must keep in mind the premises of the organization while formulating objectives and planning the future course of action. Premises include assumptions and framework that is to work on in the future.
4. **The principle of alternatives:** The principle of alternative means developing many alternatives and then selecting the best one that would help in achieving predetermined goals. It is also known as the principle of rational process. The planner needs sound judgment and objective thinking while planning. He or she needs to have knowledge and ability to analyze alternatives. Various alternatives are developed, and pros and cons of each alternative in light of objectives, cost, and output are considered.
5. **The principle of timing and continuity:** Planning should be done quite ahead, and the action plans on time before execution are developed. It should be an ongoing process of making modification and reexamining new situations.
6. **The principle of flexibility:** Planning should be flexible. It should provide a way to reduce the risk involved in the future due to uncertainties. There should be a scope for readjustment to modify the plan according to the new situations.
7. **The principle of communication:** The principle of communication means that all people working in the organization must know the expectation and work from them. People of all levels must be aware of objectives and goals, policies, programs, and rules they are going to follow to achieve the said goals.
8. **The principle of adequate control techniques:** The principle of adequate control techniques states that there should be the provision of sufficient performance standards with time dimensions. Evaluation should be done for people who are working at all levels for their performance according to laid down standards. Planning must incorporate control techniques and code of conduct for corrective measures to achieve the goals of the organization successfully.
9. **The principle of participation:** There should be reasonable participation in planning and making managerial decisions. It is a bottom-to-top approach in management. It is the best technique to ensure cooperation and gain confidence and maximum contribution from employees toward various action plans.
10. **The principle of competitive action plans:** The principle of competitive action plans or strategies states that all plans must develop keeping in mind the actions and plans framed by competitors in similar situations. To strive to make the number one organization, one must know who the competitors are and what are their strategies and one should try to plan one step.
11. **The principle of economy:** According to this principle, the planner must do cost-and-benefit analysis of every planning process. The total cost of planning must be less than the added advantage of planning regarding money and another cost. The most economical plan was selected as possible with the maximum output.

Importance of Planning

The list below shows the importance of planning:
- It provides a blueprint to guide and support the management of the organization
- All staff working in the organization must be aware of its vision, mission, and objectives
- It focusses on organizational goals
- It facilitates quality of services and a means to monitor and evaluate services given
- It promotes creativity and innovation
- It secures economy in operations through proper allocation of resources to various operations
- It sets priorities according to the resources available
- It facilitates decision-making
- It establishes benchmarks for appraisal of actual performance
- It reduces uncertainty and overcomes threats
- It achieves coordination among all departments
- It helps to manage the crisis.

PLANNING PROCESS

The planning process varies from organization to organization because of their different sizes and complexities. The process of planning comprises the following steps **(Fig. 12.7)**:

1. **Perception of opportunities and gathering information:** Before carrying out the actual planning, one needs to explore and gather the relevant and related information regarding threats and possible opportunities, strengths, and weaknesses of the organization. Information gathered should be accurate, precise, and up to date as based on estimation. Evaluate all the pros and cons of possible new opportunities. It is the preliminary step before the formulation of objectives.
2. **Establishing objectives:** Frame objectives by the availability of opportunities and resources. Objectives form the core to the planning process. It aids the staff to understand the expectation of the organization. Objectives are the endpoints of any organization translated into the departmental objective. These departmental objectives then serve as the means of accomplishing the overall objective of the organization.
3. **Developing premises (forecast future):** Premises are the expected environmental or external and internal

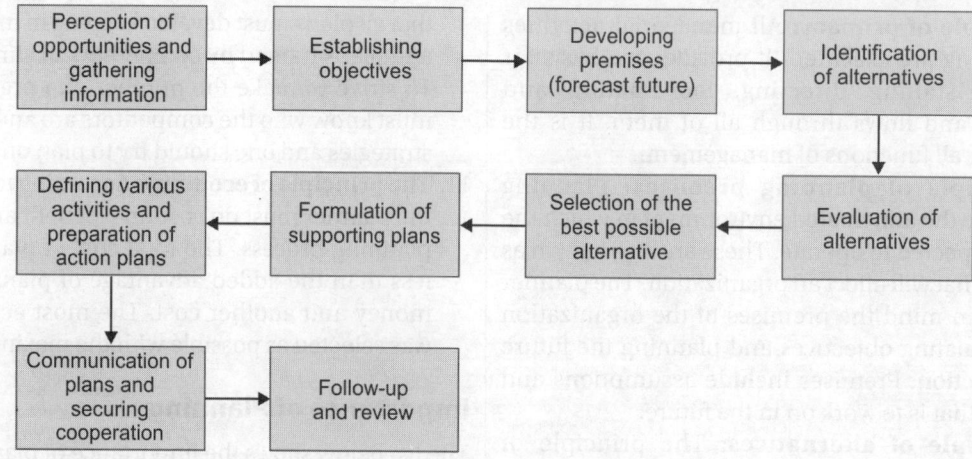

Fig. 12.7: Steps of the planning process.

conditions to undertake planning activities. These are an asset of forecasts regarding these conditions or factors, and the success of planning depends on the accuracy of these forecasts.

4. **Identification of alternatives:** After determining the various planning assumptions, the next step is to work to find out the maximum alternatives based on the empirical evidence or experiences or intuitions. Then a short listing of the alternatives is done for the detailed analysis.
5. **Evaluation of alternatives:** In this step, an attempt has been made to evaluate the selected alternatives per the criteria required for achieving particular objectives. All the merits and demerits of the alternatives are listed and compared with the criteria laid down,
6. **Selection of the best possible alternatives:** After evaluating all the short-listed alternatives, the most appropriate alternative is taken up. It is the actual stage of decision-making in the process of planning.
7. **Developing subsidiary plans:** After selecting the best plan, various derivative plans such as policies, procedures, schedules, methods, and budgets are put into practice. These supportive plans are the subsidiary plans formulated for various units, sections, and activities in the light of the master plan to help the organization to achieve its objectives in a unified manner.
8. **Defining various activities and preparation of action plans:** Related activities according to plans are developed and defined. Time plans using various managerial techniques such as Programme Evaluation and Review Technique are developed. These planning and control techniques are important to minimize the time and cost and for ensuring the completion of projects.
9. **Communication of plans and securing cooperation:** Supportive plans properly to the lower levels in the organization are communicated. All staff should be aware of the plans, its scope, and benefits. The participation of the staff at this stage helps them to boost their morale to implement the plans effectively to the best of their skills and abilities.
10. **Follow-up and review:** After implementation of the plan, it is essential to follow it up to remove difficulties at every step of implementation. If needed, plans may even be modified or revised to achieve the indented goal.

TYPES OF PLANNING

It can be classified based on the period involved, the approach used, and the degree of formalization (**Fig. 12.8**).
1. **Long-term and short-term planning:** The nature of planning classified according to the time involved in preparing plans. It is of two types—long-term and short-term. Long-term planning takes more time compared to short-term planning. Long-term planning usually takes a period of 3–5 years. Functional planning is long-term and requires to consider many external threats. Short-term planning is brief and takes mostly 1 year, and many short-term plans are derived from a long-term plan, which may be monthly, half-yearly, and so on.
2. **Proactive and reactive planning:** Proactive planning, as the name indicates, is the planning in anticipation.

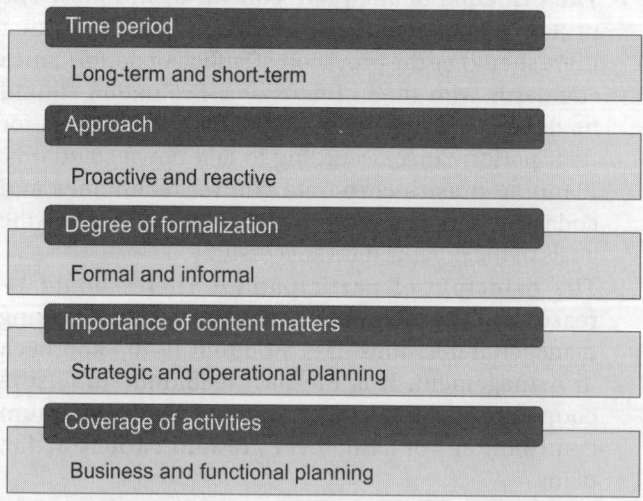

Fig. 12.8: Dimension-wise classification of planning.

The suitable courses of action according to expected changes in the relevant environment are designed. The reactive planning is the planning done after the environmental changes take place.
3. **Formal and informal planning:** Based on the degree of formalization, planning is of two types—formal and informal. Formal planning is a systematic evaluation of external and internal variables. Planning is systematically and carries formal steps. Informal planning is by managers' own experiences and intuitions. While preparing plans, the degree of formalization based on the type of activities was estimated.
4. **Strategic and operational planning:** Strategic planning takes a long period for planning. The period of planning is from one year to twenty years or more. It sets plans to meet specific goals, aims, and objectives in the light of available resources. These are flexible and may modify according to changes that occur. In contrast, operational planning takes a short period for planning and is meant to implement according to the plan.
5. **Management (corporate) and functional planning:** Planning done at the higher level of management is termed management or corporate planning. It usually covers all the planning activities of the organization. In this type of planning, managers prepare plans with long-term objectives. In contrast, the functional planning is at the functional level by each department, e.g. personnel department and accounts department. It derives from management planning and should contribute to it.

ADVANTAGES OF PLANNING

The advantages of planning are as follows:
1. **Clarity of objectives:** It must be clear, comprehensive, measurable, and defined qualitatively and quantitatively.
2. **Better utilization of resources:** Planning ensures better utilization of resources and thus increases efficiency.
3. **Helps in coordination:** Planning is regarded as a prime function of management as it covers all other functions of management. Since it is a step-to-step systematic approach, it helps in coordination to carry out all activities in harmony.
4. **Reduces uncertainties:** Planning is always done considering various threats and opportunities available from the external environment, strengths, and weaknesses of the organization. It helps to reduce many uncertainties.
5. **Encourages creative thinking:** Planning is a thinking process. Management tries to develop realistic plans. It requires and creative thinking and foresightedness while planning.
6. **Provides reasonable flexibility:** There is always a scope of flexibility in planning to make the required modification and adjustment in between without affecting its main objectives.
7. **Facilitates decision-making:** Decision-making is the core of planning. During the planning process, the best course of action among various courses of action was selected. Planning provides guidelines for decision-making and prevents ambiguity.
8. **Promotes efficiency:** Planning is a process of selecting the best alternative based on the cost–benefit analysis, finance, and rational reasoning. Thus planning helps to minimize the cost regarding time and other resources and promotes efficiency in the organization.
9. **Facilitates control:** Planning helps in controlling performance by setting performance standards. It involves designing various control and corrective measures. Thus planning facilitates effective control to achieve desired results.
10. **Facilitates delegation:** According to the predetermined goals, each department and individual are made accountable for their work to achieve desired goals. This delegation of authority facilitates through the planning process.

LIMITATIONS OF PLANNING

The following list explains the limitations of planning:
1. **Restricts creativity:** Planning involves deciding in advance and planning of all activities. Thus there is a very little scope or no scope for making the major modification. This nature of planning discourages individuals to take initiatives and freedom.
2. **Rigidity:** Planning is a predetermined development to achieve the desired objectives. Hence these should have stability. It may leave no room for individuals to use their experiences and ability, resulting in rigidity in planning.
3. **Uncertainty:** There are certain unforeseen internal and external factors such as economic, social, political, legal, and international climate that may act as a limitation on the planning process.
4. **Lack of reliable facts:** It is always not possible to get authentic information and facts relating to the future, and sometimes the planner may not supply accurate information. Then it becomes very difficult for management to draw accurate premises and predict the plan of actions.
5. **Time-consuming and expensive process:** Planning is time consuming. It takes a series of steps and actions on various operations. The collection of data itself is time consuming and expensive. Many operations are delayed due to poor planning, and sometimes urgent actions carry out without planning.
6. **Resistance to change:** It is very difficult to change the mindset of people; they do not want to adopt a change.

This type of attitude of people becomes a limitation to planning.
7. **Fast-changing conditions:** Planning is done keeping in mind unforeseen conditions. Therefore strategic plans are flexible and require modifications per need.
8. **Government policies:** There are no fixed policies of government. These are revised time to time per requirement. Revisions in health policies change from time to time and reflect on planning.
9. **Advancement in technology:** In the modern technology world, technology changes occur so fast that may upset planning.

CHAPTER HIGHLIGHTS

- Planning is a major function of management and concerned with answers about why, what, how, when, and by whom.
- Planning is a continuous process of thinking in advance for the future to achieve the organizational goals.
- Planning is goal oriented, an intellectual process, and includes forecasting and decision-making for the future.
- Six P's, i.e. purpose, philosophy, promise, policies, plans, and priorities, are required for planning.
- Planning is principle based and comprises various steps from the perception of opportunities to follow up and review.
- Planning has both advantages and limitations. It must be implemented effectively to get better results.

REVIEW QUESTIONS

I. Essay Type Questions
1. Define planning. Discuss its main characteristics.
2. Describe various steps of the planning process.
3. Explain the principles of planning in detail.
4. Discuss the objectives of planning.
5. Why is planning basically to all managerial functions? Explain.

II. Short Notes
1. Importance of planning
2. Nature of planning
3. Long-term and short-term planning
4. Types of planning
5. Advantages and limitations of planning

III. Multiple Choice Questions
1. Planning involves:
    a. Future course of action
    b. Review of past experiences
    c. Analysis of policies
    d. Unnecessary exercise on limiting factors
2. Planning is helpful in:
    a. Reducing inefficiency
    b. Better utilization of resources
    c. Improving employees' morale
    d. Exploring changing conditions
3. Planning provides:
    a. Information to managers
    b. Basis for future policy formulation
    c. Guidance to plan programs
    d. Purpose and direction to all persons
4. Planning is basic to other managerial functions because:
    a. It provides a framework for an entire organization to operate
    b. It requires forecasting and decision-making for future
    c. It follows other functions of management
    d. It involves vision and foresightedness to decide actions in future
5. Planning is extended throughout the organization and required at all levels at all times and hence it is referred to a planning function known as:
    a. Continuity   b. Pervasive
    c. Dynamic   d. Realistic
6. The promise is a process of:
    a. Setting objectives and detailed course of actions
    b. Providing statements of beliefs and values
    c. Careful understanding of the purpose of an organization
    d. Assessing the strong and week points of an organization
7. The choice of appropriate means of achieving stated objectives is known as:
    a. Rationality   b. Strategic
    c. Pervasiveness   d. Dynamic
8. Use of appropriate control measures and proper utilization of resources leads to organizational:
    a. Efficiency
    b. Coordination
    c. Effectiveness
    d. Creativity
9. Which principle of planning suggests anticipating environmental threats and opportunities to plan activities?
    a. The principle of primacy
    b. The principle of alternative
    c. The principle of flexibility
    d. The principle of planning premises
10. Which of the following type is strategic planning?
    a. Operational planning
    b. Short-term planning
    c. Long-term planning
    d. Functional planning

Answer Keys

1. a   2. b   3. d   4. c   5. b   6. d   7. a
8. c   9. d   10. c

SUGGESTED READING

1. American College of Hospital Administrators. The Evolving of the Hospital Chief Executive Officer. Chicago: The American College of Hospital Administrators; 1984.
2. Arnold J. The seven building blocks to better decisions. New York: Amazon; 1978.
3. Awani A. Project management techniques. New York: Petrocelli Books; 1983.
4. Beinstock E. Creative problem solving (Cassette Recording). Stamford: Waldentapes; 1984.
5. Bransford J, Stein B. The IDEAL problem solver. New York: W. H. Freeman; 1984.
6. Drucker PF. An introductory view of management. New York: Harper's College Press; 1977.
7. Hasting JEF, Mindell WR, Browne JW, Barnsley JM. Canadian health administrator study. Can J Public Health. 1981;72(1):1-6.
8. Higgins JM. The Management Challenge: An Introduction to Management. New York: Macmillan; 1991.
9. Hoyt P. An International approach to Problem Solving for Better Health nursing (PSBHN). Journal Compilation© 2007 International Council of Nurses; 2007:100-106.
10. Huitt, W. Problem-solving and decision making: consideration of individual differences using the Myers-Briggs type indicator. J Psychol Type. 1992;24:33-44.
11. Rakich JS, Krigline AB. Problem-solving in health services organizations. Hosp Top. 1996;74(2):21-27.
12. Jonathon S Rakich, Beaufort B, Longest Jr, Kurt Darr. Managing Health Services Organizations. 3rd ed. Baltimore, Mariland: Health Professions Press, Inc., 1996.
13. Smith BH, Barnett S, Collado D, et al. Resources for health: problem-solving for better health. World Health Forum. 1994;15:9-15.
14. Victor H Vroom, Arthur G Jago. The New Leadership: Managing Participation in Organizations. 1st ed. New Jersey: Prentice Hall, Inc., 1988.

13 CHAPTER

Mission, Philosophy and Objectives

CHAPTER OUTLINE

- Mission and Purpose
  - Definitions
  - Features
  - Formulation of Mission
  - Mission Statement
- Philosophy
  - Meaning
  - Definitions of Philosophy
  - Definitions of Nursing Philosophy
  - Philosophy of Nursing
- Objectives
  - Definitions
  - Importance of Objectives
  - Nature/Characteristics of Objectives
  - Guidelines for Setting Objectives
  - Basis for Setting Objectives
  - Classification of Nursing Objectives
  - Objectives of Hospital Nursing Services

LEARNING OUTCOMES

After completion of this chapter, the learner will be able to:
- Describe mission and its elements
- Formulate mission statements
- Describe the characteristics of mission
- Appreciate the concept of philosophy
- Describe the concept and nature of objectives
- Discuss the importance of developing objectives
- Explain the features of nursing objectives
- Enumerate basis in developing objectives of nursing service
- Develop guidelines for setting objectives
- Enlist significant nursing objectives' service administration

KEY TERMS

Mission, purpose, philosophy, goals, objectives, policies, nursing service

INTRODUCTION

As we know planning is the first step in all processes of management and the continuous intellectual process of determining philosophy, objectives, policies, procedures and programs and rules, projects, and procedures. It includes various activities to achieve the future targets. All these form a hierarchical model for planning.

MISSION AND PURPOSE

The word "mission" is obtained from Latin, meaning the "act of sending" members abroad. The terms "mission" and "purpose" are used interchangeably, though these terms have different concepts. Mission tells about the purpose and existence of an organization. It sometimes is used as a model of organization's future. The mission of the organization reflects the contribution it will make to the country, while purpose always indicates the ways to make the contribution.

Definitions

Definitions of mission are listed below:
- A mission is the highest level description of why the organization exists and what it aims to achieve. It describes the principal means by which the organization seeks to accomplish its goals.
- Mission identifies the primary function of an enterprise or any part of it. It outlines the organization's plans to be accomplished and aims and tasks for its existence.

Features

A mission's characteristics are as follows:
- Mission describes the purpose of the organization.
- It defines the beneficiaries and processes.

- It answers questions such as "what are we in this organization?" Or "Why do we exist?"
- It acts like a general and comprehensive philosophy for organizational existence.
- It is a source of vision and foundation for priorities, strategies, plans, and work assignment.
  It is a starting point for planning the managerial activities and structure.
- It distinguishes the organization from others that are working toward a similar vision.
- It informs the desired level of performance.
- In the statement form and addresses, the following questions are listed:
  - Need your organization
  - Uniqueness of organization
  - Beneficiaries of services.

Formulation of Mission

An organization's mission consists of its desire, belief, and assumption, keeping in mind the elements of the mission. Per the requirement of the organization, its mission can be refined, but it should reflect the same set of features. The underlying philosophy of the organization and the visionary long-term concept of organization is the basis to formulate a mission. The objectives and purpose of the organization form the base to develop long-term ideas **(Fig. 13.1)**.

Mission Statement

A mission statement is a short and written statement reflecting the objective and operational purpose of the organization. An organization's mission links various activities to be carried out according to the needs of the society and country. Mission statements incorporate the culture of the organization.

The mission of nursing services also describes what it should be and what it will be. The purpose of nursing is to render the best possible nursing care to patients, and the promotion of self-care is one aspect of nursing care. Thus, the definition of nursing and self-care can be included in the mission statement.

- **Elements of the mission statement**
  - *Purpose:* The main component of a mission is "purpose." A mission statement must incorporate the object or the goal of the organization, i.e. "what an organization wants to achieve?" It should also indicate the objectives of the organization.
  - *Activities:* Organizational goals are achieved through various activities. The programs and procedures enumerate these activities. The statement outlines multiple actions/events to accomplish their purpose.
  - *Values:* Values are the beliefs of people working for the organization, namely commitment to excellent services, innovation, diversity, teamwork, leadership, continuous learning, competence, creativity, respect, compassion, honesty, integrity, and so on. Values inspire people to work hard and be loyal to their work. The mission statement must reflect values for members of the organization.
- **Prerequisites of a mission statement**
  Defined goals, the values, preplanned strategies, type of services, clients, and satisfaction of stakeholders are the prerequisites to form a mission statement of an organization.
- **Characteristics of mission statements**
  - Mission should be written in a statement form.
  - Statements should be specific, short, precise, and self-explanatory.
    - Personnel working in the organization must be aware of it.
    - The statement must convey its meaning.
    - The mission must be measurable and achievable.
    - It should be dynamic, flexible, action oriented, and objective based.
    - A mission statement must reflect organizational ethics, principles, and standards.
    - It should express the vision and values of the organization.
    - The statement must be consumer and stakeholder oriented.
    - It is future oriented and should be designed to last for 5 or more years.
    - It must act as a guiding force to provide a sense of direction.
    - It must be a blueprint to formulate organizational strategies.
    - It should provide an overall umbrella under which all functions of the organization will take place.
    - It should be distinctive and should uniquely describe organization purpose.
    - It should be so alive that everyone knows its existence.

PHILOSOPHY

Meaning

The word "philosophy," meaning "love of wisdom," is derived from two Greek words: "phileo" means "love" and "Sophia" means "wisdom." It refers to love and wisdom.

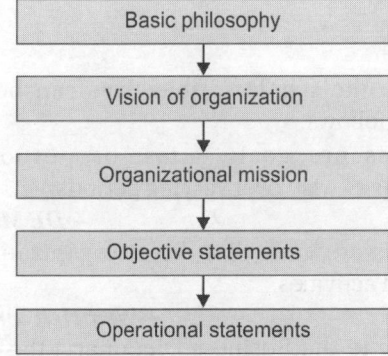

Fig. 13.1: Mission formulation.

Its origin is also from a Sanskrit word: "Irish" means "to see," i.e. "darshan," which means "knowledge of reality." According to the Webster dictionary, philosophy is the most fundamental belief, attitude, and concepts of an individual. It is an attitude toward life and practice.

Philosophy has assumptions and beliefs to view the world. Decision makers of the organization create assumptions and expectations to formulate the mission and vision of the organization. Purpose or mission of the organization must reflect these assumptions and opinions. Philosophy of a person represents unobstructed views of the world and the person's view regarding specific goals and activities.

The statement of philosophy is abstract and contains value statements about the human being as clients, patients, and staff. It states the work performed by nursing personnel, nursing as a profession, and education of competence.

Definitions of Philosophy

The term "philosophy" has been defined differently by various scholars:

- Philosophy signifies "wisdom that would influence the conduct of life." —*John Dewey*
- Philosophy is the logical reasoning of the nature of reality. —*Dr Radhakrishnan*
- Philosophy is "methodical training" or "Sadhana." —*Dr Baldev Upadhyaya*
- Philosophy is a search for self-understanding and a general understanding of values and reality. It studies the concepts that form the thought processes, presumptions, morality, reason, and purpose.

Definitions of Nursing Philosophy

Nursing philosophy can be explained as follows:

- Nursing philosophy is a statement having universal assumptions, beliefs, and principles. —*Reed, 1995*
- Nursing philosophy is a conceptual model. It provides a frame of reference to nurses and guides them to think, observe, interpret, and practice. It should include ideals about a person, environment, health and illness, and nurse. —*Seedhouse, 2000*
- Nursing management philosophy can refer to the belief system of a profession that can provide perspectives to the management of nursing services and nursing education and can become a base for defining the vision of nursing service organization and nursing educational institutions.

Philosophy of Nursing

Nursing is an art and science to improve the overall health of patients. Philosophy of nursing services is influenced by the social philosophy of country, national health philosophy, philosophy of health and health policies, state health policy, and organizational philosophy. Philosophy of nursing service states that:

We work to achieve the goals of the department of nursing services and patient care. Nursing management works to create an environment, which promotes decision-making, supports participative management, and fosters innovation. Staff provides quality, cost-effective care in an environment recognized for excellence in clinical practice and achievements in education, management, and research.

a. **Bases of nursing philosophy:** Nursing philosophy has a distinctive contribution to the development of nursing theories. According to Griffin, four concerns form the bases in formulating the nursing philosophy:
   1. Concept of caring
   2. Importance of assumptions
   3. Ethical implications for applying the nursing process
   4. Nursing theory.

b. **Characteristics of nursing philosophy**
   - Nursing philosophy should be in a written format.
   - Philosophy must be developed by involving caregivers and consumers.
   - It should reflect the meaning of the clinical practice of nursing.
   - Philosophy must include the responsibilities of the nurse.
   - It should consist of both external and internal forces such as humanity, society, health, nursing, nursing process and self-care relevant to the community, law, personnel, clients, material resources, research, education, and family.
   - Nursing philosophy must in line with its organization.
   - It should give direction to achieve the mission.

OBJECTIVES

If you don't know where you're going, then sure as anything you won't get there.

Objectives are vital in management. Identifying and developing the objectives of an organization is the first step in the planning process. It has an inherent power within itself to direct and stimulate action. It is essential to establish common goals, so that all efforts must work toward the known ultimate achievements. Objectives are crucial to management, especially important in a dynamic, high-tech, and changing environment.

Definitions

According to the scholars, objectives can be defined differently as follows:

- Objectives are goals, aims, or purposes that organizations wish over varying periods. —*DE McFarland*
- Objectives are ends that direct organizational and individual activities. —*Weihrich and Koontz*
- According to the Business Dictionary, the objective is achievable within set time by utilizing available

resources. Objectives frame mission, purpose, policies, and standards of the organization, which are the means of planning short-term and long-term activities.

From the above definitions, we can describe objectives as *goals*, i.e. expected and anticipated results to direct all resources. It defines "what to achieve" and "to what extent." It has a *definite scope* and tells us where we to go and how to reach there? Hence, these objectives act as a *guide* to performing actions.

Importance of Objectives

Objectives are important for planning, implementing, and evaluating all management activities. Planning cannot initiate without objectives. Objectives provide specific direction to the managers to carry on events and to measure the outcome of those planned activities of the organization (Fig. 13.2).

Management process starts with planning, and formulation of objectives initiates the planning process. Based on the objectives, managers can implement, monitor, and measure the performance of employees per the plan. Based on the degree of performance, remedial actions are taken by the managers to correct the deficiencies.

Nature/Characteristics of Objectives

The 12 major characteristics of objectives are listed subsequently (Box 13.1):

1. **Objectives are to be in hierarchy:** The objectives are to be in hierarchical order. To formulate objectives, managers use a top-down or bottom-up approach. Managers follow a combination of both approaches to formulate objectives since the approaches have their own merits and demerits.

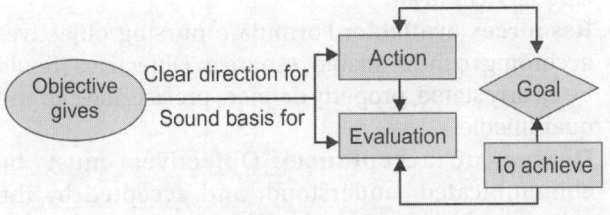

Fig. 13.2: Importance of objectives.

Box 13.1: Characteristics of Objectives.
1. Follows hierarchy
2. Have multiplicity
3. Have time limit
4. Interrelated and interdependent
5. Have different priorities
6. Realistic and operational
7. General and specific
8. Short-term and long-term
9. Tangible and intangible
10. Means of control
11. Measureable and achievable
12. Flexible

2. **Objectives can be multiple:** An organization may have various objectives. The type and number of targets vary according to the goal of a particular department. Managers of different levels also have different purposes. The activities for each department and each level vary according to the objectives. Managers may delegate few activities to the immediate subordinates to obtain better results.
3. **Objectives have a time limit:** The objectives are to be framed keeping in mind the time limit. Each objective should mention the time to achieve the predetermined quantitative and qualitative performance goals.
4. **Objectives are interrelated and interdependent:** All the objectives are interrelated but relate to each other per the management functions.
5. **Objectives have different priorities:** The success of an organization depends on a rational approach to objectives and the determination of priorities. Prioritize objectives according to its importance.
6. **Objectives should be realistic and operational:** Formulate practical and functional objectives according to the available resources as only practical purposes can convert into actual performance.
7. **Objectives should be general and specific:** Formulate both general and specific objectives. General objectives must specify the outcome of the department in general, and specific objectives are for a particular project, department, or work.
8. **Objectives may be short-term and long-term:** The project may be of short or long duration. Therefore, it is necessary to frame the objectives accordingly. Short-term objectives are output oriented, whereas long-term objectives have a provision of organizational expansion.
9. **Objectives are tangible and intangible:** Tangible objectives measure the quantity and invisible objectives qualitatively. The performance, morale, social responsibility-based objectives are qualitative and are converted into quantitative terms.
10. **Objectives are essential means of control:** Objectives may act as a measuring tool for all activities. According to the objectives, the performance standards are to be set, so that employees can be evaluated. Therefore, objectives serve as a means of control.
11. **Objectives are measurable and achievable:** Formulate objectives in such a manner that it will be easy to measure the results.
12. **Objectives must be flexible:** Objectives should be flexible and adaptable according to the changing conditions and demand. There should be a provision to modify and to make it more practicable.

Features of Nursing Objectives (Fig. 13.3)

The following lists the features of nursing objectives:
- Nursing objectives should be clear, specific, and defined.
- These should be the philosophy of nation, state, and organization.

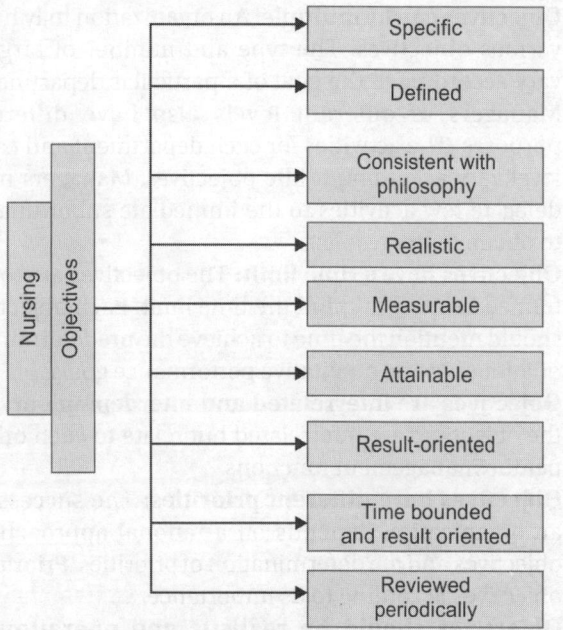

Fig. 13.3: Features of nursing objectives.

- These should be realistic and practical, measurable, attainable, and achievable.
- These should be action and result oriented and time bound.
- Objectives should be reviewed periodically.

Guidelines for Setting Objectives

All the organizations need to formulate general and specific objectives according to the need of an organization. Formulating objectives involves a continuous process of research and decision-making. Following points should be kept in mind while setting objectives:

a. **Classify objectives:** Objectives of the overall organization are classified according to their level, importance, and type, which can be primary, secondary, departmental, and individual objectives. Objectives should be specific to achieve the overall or the main organizational goals.
b. **Determine the area of objectives:** After classifying primary objectives into subobjectives, the next step is to determine specific areas to achieve those objectives. The organization has functional and technical departments or sections. Each area or department should have to set its objectives. These objectives should be inconsistent with the overall organizational objective. Setting objectives area-wise helps in proper planning and control.
c. **Coordinate objectives area-wise:** Objectives of each department should be in coordination to achieve a common goal. Consider the key factors of the organization while developing departmental objectives, which are finance, material supply, etc.
d. **State objectives clearly and precisely and in quantifiable terms:** Define all objectives clearly. It should indicate the expectation of the organization and should provide direction to management.
e. **Express objectives in quantitative and qualitative terms:** Objectives are both tangible and intangible and can be expressed in quantitative and qualitative terms, respectively. These objectives have some assumptions. Hence, it is necessary to identify and interpret the underlined assumptions. Objectives are to be communicated in quantifiable terms.
f. **Formulate realistic and attainable objectives:** The objective should be realistic and attainable and set by including all the available resources.
g. **Formulate general and specific objectives:** Objectives must be stated in broad and particular terms.
h. **Keep a scope of objectives for flexibility:** Objectives must be flexible to be modified per requirement.

Basis for Setting Objectives

a. **National health policy:** The national health policy is formulated based on the diverse health needs of the people. Democratic and scientific techniques must be used to find out the actual health needs and problems of people. The nurse administrator needs to involve and plan for the nursing services (**Fig. 13.4**).
b. **Needs of the population:** Formulate nursing objectives based on the health needs of the community, so that they improve the health status of the people at large, ensuring a basic level of preventive, promotive, curative, and rehabilitative health services to all people. Objectives should be inconsistent with the overall health objectives.
c. **Priority areas for improvement of nursing services:** Nursing objectives should be according to the rural and urban population, the weaker, or neglected section of the society, considering a minimum level of nursing care services to all.
d. **Resources available:** Formulate nursing objectives according to the available resources. Objectives should be clearly stated, properly defined, precise, logical, and quantifiable.
e. **Degree of acceptance:** Objectives must be communicated, understood, and accepted by the management, caretakers, and beneficiaries.
f. **Philosophy of nursing services:** Objectives will have to be set according to the philosophy of nursing services. Philosophy of nursing services is influenced by the philosophy of the organization, nation, and health.
g. **Approval from administrators:** Objectives of the nursing services are framed immediately after obtaining permission from the institutional head, and the written format of the permission obtained should be available.

Classification of Nursing Objectives

Nursing objectives are classified based on various levels and are listed below:

Chapter 13: Mission, Philosophy and Objectives

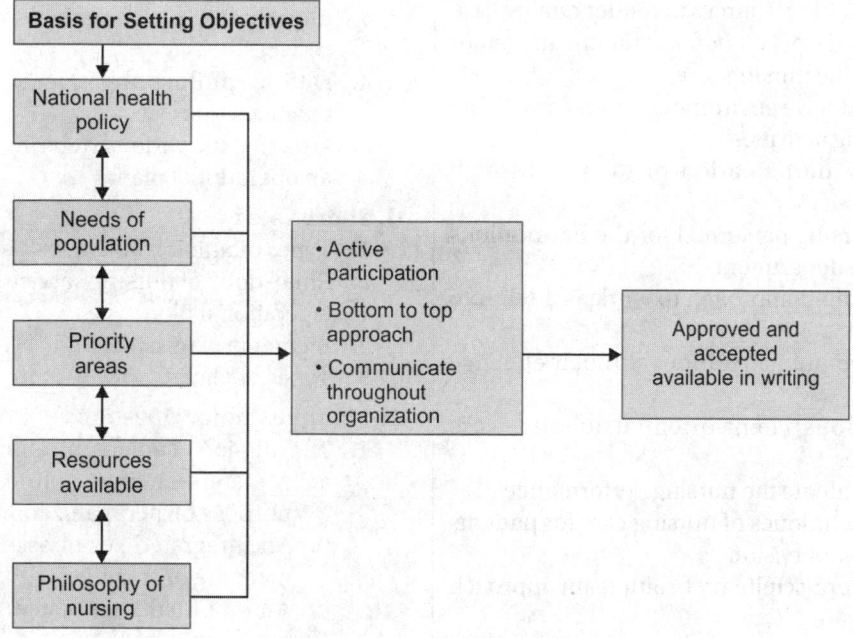

Fig. 13.4: Basis for setting objectives of nursing services.

a. **According to levels**
  1. *Organizational objectives:* These refers to the overall nursing organization objectives.
  2. *Departmental objectives:* These are related to various departments of the nursing organization.
  3. *Group objectives:* These refer to multiple groups formed in the nursing organization.
  4. *Unit objectives:* Unit objectives are particularly for nursing units.
  5. *Individual objectives:* These are nurse employee-oriented objectives.

b. **According to the purpose/objective**
  1. *Profit based:* These objectives are the owner based, where the profit or money return is the primary purpose of the organization. Mostly private-sector organizations frame such objectives.
  2. *Personal based:* Personal objectives relate to economic, social, psychological, and satisfaction of employees.
  3. *Social based:* These objectives are of public interests and relate to the social welfare of the public.
  4. *Service based:* Service-based objectives are clients' or customer' interests.

Objectives of Hospital Nursing Services

The aim of the nursing organization is also service based. The main goal of nursing services is providing the best possible quality nursing services and are of two types: primary and subsidiary objectives **(Fig. 13.5)**:

a. **Primary objectives:** The primary objectives of hospital services are to provide curative services by ensuring patient care to indoor patients.
b. **Subsidiary objectives:** These objectives are managerial and professional activities based.

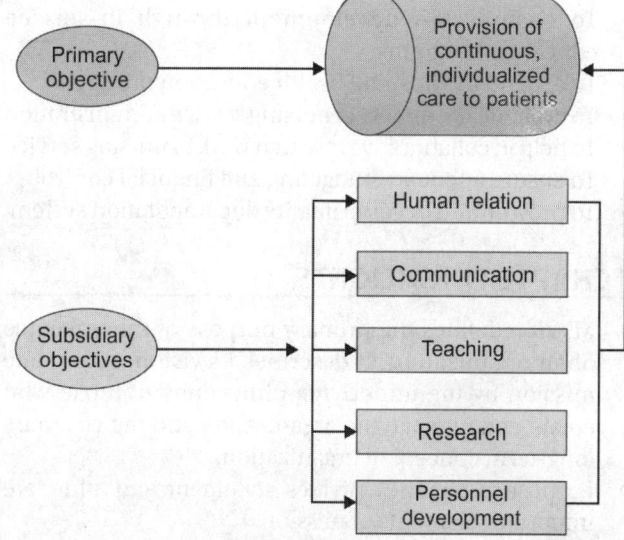

Fig. 13.5: Types of service objectives.

The overall goal of the nursing service administration is to provide efficient and effective care to the clients. Following are the objectives of hospital nursing services:

- To plan, deliver, and ensure the highest quality of nursing care to the clients whether in a hospital or community
- To utilize the conceptual framework as the basis for all nursing services
- To implement variety, cost-effective care to all customers/clients strategies
- To ensure middle management accountability for the quality and appropriateness of nursing activities
- To visualize properly organized nursing component at the operational level

- To utilize the available resources to render quality care
- To plan the time and work plans for optimum utilization of the staff to provide nursing care
- To promote a conducive environment to staff involving in decision-making activities
- To ensure active participation of nurses through teamwork
- To coordinate nursing personnel for the harmonious functioning of the department
- To have an integrated approach to work as a team to provide care
- To promote active public relations through effective communication
- To evaluate various client-oriented nursing care delivery modalities
- To analyze and evaluate the nursing performance
- To improve the techniques of nursing care for patients through efficient supervision
- To expand the interdisciplinary health team approach to assess patient care
- To develop and implement nursing practice standards
- To provide training to the nursing students and auxiliary workers
- To ensure staff development through in-service education programs
- To expand the hospital health education programs
- To evaluate the quality of nursing service administration
- To help in collaborative research work in nursing service
- To ensure adequate budgeting and financial control
- To provide and develop quality documentation system.

CHAPTER HIGHLIGHTS

- Mission defines the primary purpose of the existence of an organization. It describes its vision. Formulate mission by the underlying philosophy of those who create and manage the organization and the visionary long-term concept of organization.
- Purpose statement, activities' statement, and values are important elements of mission.
- Philosophy is an integrated set of assumptions and beliefs regarding the purpose of activities. Nursing philosophy describes the belief system of the profession. It provides direction for practice and research.
- A managerial objective is an intended goal that prescribes limited scope and suggests a direction to the planning efforts of a manager.

REVIEW QUESTIONS

I. Essay Type Questions
1. Define mission and purpose. Describe its characteristics in detail.
2. Explain the meaning of "objective." Describe the steps involved in formulating managerial objectives.
3. Enumerate the objectives of hospital nursing services.
4. Define philosophy. Describe its basis and characteristics.
5. Describe the various steps involved in developing an operational plan.

II. Short Notes
1. Types of nursing objectives
2. Philosophy of nursing service
3. Operational plan
4. Elements of mission
5. Types of plans

III. Multiple Choice Questions
1. The mission of an organization is:
   a. A statement that defines the fundamental purpose of an organization
   b. An integrated set of assumptions about the meaning of activities
   c. An intended goal that suggests direction for planning
   d. A commitment of resources to a proposed project
2. A search for self and general understanding of value and reality refers to:
   a. Objective   b. Mission
   c. Purpose   d. Philosophy
3. Type of objectives that can be expressed in quantitative terms is:
   a. Rational   b. Intangible
   c. Tangible   d. Operational
4. SMART acronym is related to:
   a. Mission   b. Objective
   c. Philosophy   d. Plan
5. A designated plan or course of actions to be taken in a specific situation is known as:
   a. Strategy   b. Policy
   c. Protocol   d. Procedure
6. Norms that are related to human behavior and spell out specific required actions are:
   a. Standards   b. Objectives
   c. Policies   d. Rules
7. An authoritative statement that describes the acceptable level of performance is:
   a. Goal   b. Objective
   c. Standard   d. Mission
8. A detailed standard plan that includes various activities related to legal formalities, technical skills, and resource management is known as:
   a. Budget   b. Rule
   c. Plan   d. Protocol
9. Which plan provides guidelines for managerial decisions and is used over a period of time again and again?
   a. Standing plan b. Operational plan
   c. Strategic plan d. Long-range plan

10. A written blueprint of events and responsibilities that details actions to be taken to achieve the intended goal refers to:
    a. Short-term plan   b. Program plan
    c. Operational plan   d. Functional plan

Answer Keys

1. a 2. d 3. c 4. b 5. b 6. d 7. c
8. d 9. a 10. c

SUGGESTED READING

1. Andrews KR. The Concept of Corporate Strategy. Homewood, IL: Johns Irwin; 1971. p. 28.
2. Anne P. Griffin B.A. (Ed.).Philosophy and nursing. Journal of Advanced Nursing1980; 5 (3):261-72.
3. Bradford RW, Duncan JP, Tarcy B. Simplified Strategic Planning: A No-nonsense Guide for Busy People who Want Results Fast! Worcester, Massachusetts: Chandler House Press, 2000.
4. Business operational plan. [online] Available from http://www.businessdictionary.com/definition/objective.html.
5. Gillies DA Nursing Management: A System Approach. 2nd ed. Tokyo: WB Saunders Co., 1989.
6. Griffin AP (Ed). Philosophy and nursing. J Adv Nurs. 1980;5(3):261-72.
7. Hill C, Jones G. Strategic Management. New York, NY: Houghton Mifflin Company; 2008. p. 11.
8. Niu TC. The philosophy of nursing management: a conceptual analysis. Hu Li Za Zhi. 2005;52(5):5-9.
9. Podolak I. A comprehensive philosophy for nursing: the total approach. Can J Nurs Adm. 1995;8(4):23-41.
10. Vati J. Organisation and administration of nursing services in district hospitals of North India. PhD Unpublished Theses, Panjab University, India; 1992.
11. Weihrich H, Koontz H. Management—A Global Perspective. New York: McGraw-Hill, Inc.; 1993.
12. What is a plan? [online]. Available from http://www.thefreedictionary.com/plan. [Accessed on 18.12.2018].

14 CHAPTER

Strategic Planning, Operating Plans and Planning New Venture

CHAPTER OUTLINE

- ⊃ Strategic Planning
  - ✦ Defining Strategy
  - ✦ Defining Strategic Planning
  - ✦ Purposes of Strategic Planning
  - ✦ Importance of Strategic Planning
  - ✦ Principles of Strategic Planning
  - ✦ Strategic Planning Process
- ⊃ Operating Plan
  - ✦ Types of Plans
- ✦ Strategic Plan
- ✦ Operational Plan
- ✦ Management Plan
- ⊃ Planning New Venture
  - ✦ Concept of a New Venture
  - ✦ A Venture-Building Process
  - ✦ Factors Determining the Need for a New Venture
  - ✦ Steps for Planning a New Venture

LEARNING OUTCOMES

After completion of this chapter, the learner will be able to:
- Understand strategy and strategic planning
- Describe the various types and ways of developing strategies
- Enumerate the steps involved in strategic planning
- Describe the guiding principles of strategic planning
- Describe the different types of plans
- Explain in detail strategic, operational, and management plans
- Differentiate between a strategic plan and an operational plan
- Describe the phases and steps of starting a new venture

KEY TERMS

Strategy, strategic planning, strategic plan, operational plan, management plan, a new venture

INTRODUCTION

Each organization involves in decision-making to meet the long-term and short-term goals. These decisions generate imperative, functional, and management plans, which are important to formulate policy, procedure, methods, rules, projects, and standards. Strategic planning is essential to manage the organization effectively and also to start up a new venture.

STRATEGIC PLANNING

Defining Strategy

The term "strategy" came from the Greek word "strategikos." "Strategos" means "leader or commander of an army," "stratos" means army host and "agos" means leader chief. Thus, the word strategy means the art of general action. It is used in military science and later in management. Strategy is an approach to meet particular aims, taking into account internal and external factors. These include a set of actions required to achieve the predetermined goals. It is a broad and high-level approach and covers 3–5 years. It determines the long-term goals and objectives of an organization, which can be attained by selecting a course of action with the available resources.

The three types of strategies are organizational, programmatic, and functional. The organizational strategy outlines the actions for the development of the organization; programmatic approach deals with the methods of developing, managing, and implementing programs; and functional strategies concern with managing administration to improve efficiency and effectiveness of the organization.

Chapter 14: Strategic Planning, Operating Plans and Planning New Venture

Defining Strategic Planning

- It is a process of determining the organizational strategy, directions, and decision-making to allocate resources, considering the external and internal factors. It focuses on the strengths and opportunities of an organization and directs the workforce to attain its objectives.
- It is a decision-making process to answer the questions raised in the planning process, to make choices, and to select the best option to achieve goals.
- Strategic planning in nursing is a systematic approach and cooperative effort between the nursing department and the organization to decide to promote and improve nursing practice.
- Strategic planning is a mental process as it requires critical thinking and decision-making in every stage of development of a strategic plan.
- Strategic planning is an architecture process that provides an overview of different plans and its areas in different time periods, such as the type of plan, the duration of each plan, the time taken for preparing a plan, the completion period, the frequency of updating a plan, responsibilities, and the way different plans fit together **(Fig. 14.1)**.
- Strategic planning is a social process as it is carried out in consultation and coordination with all involved in planning. It also includes all the employees of the organization.

Purposes of Strategic Planning

- To utilize available resources
- To manage the performance of the department
- To acquire and develop new practices
- To improve the goals, values, and communication
- To bring changes in operations, management, and organization.

Importance of Strategic Planning

Strategic planning is useful to improve the nursing management in the following ways:
- It provides accountability and monitors performance.
- It helps in setting a planning program that requires department and unit planning.
- It integrates strategic planning with operational and financial plans.
- It concentrates more on strategic issues.
- It improves knowledge and skill in strategic planning.
- It enhances coordination among nursing managers and organization administrator.
- It allows better execution of plans.
- It is more realistic and rational.
- It anticipates the future.
- It develops an annual budget.
- It focuses on quality outputs to improve performance and care.
- It assists in benchmarking and performance monitoring.

Principles of Strategic Planning

1. **The principle of action:** Successful strategic planning should lead to action.
2. **The principle of vision:** It should build a value-based shared vision.
3. **The principle of participation:** It should be an inclusive and participatory process.

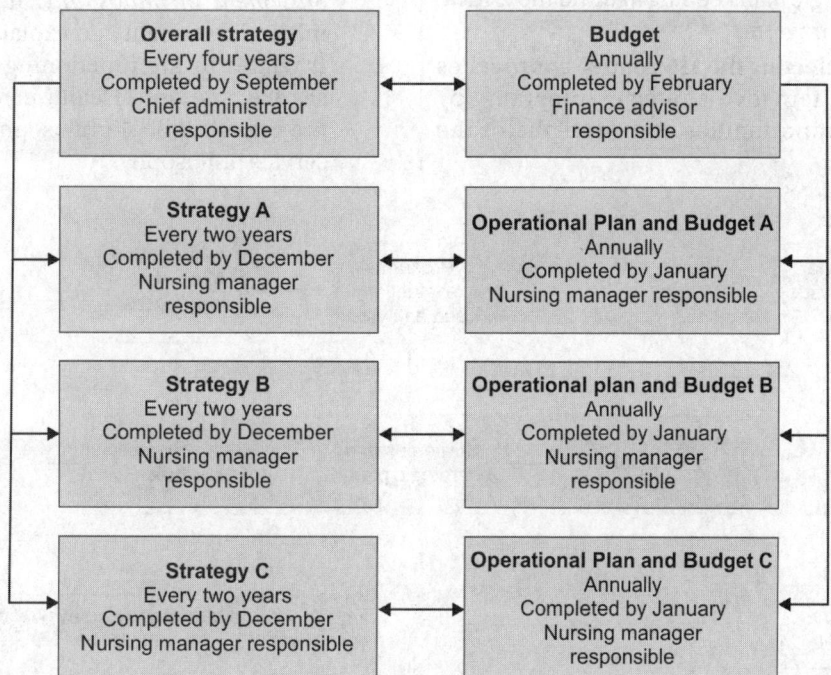

Fig. 14.1: Strategic planning as an architecture process.

4. **The principle of accountability:** It should accept liability to the society.
5. **The principle of sensitivity:** It should be externally focused and sensitive to the organization's environment.

Strategic Planning Process

Strategic planning is a rational and scientific approach and requires intuitions. A series of steps is involved in planning a strategy **(Fig. 14.2)**.

1. **Need identification and situation analysis**
   - Identify specific critical issues in light of the mission and vision of the organization; a vision statement will help provide an idea for strategic planning
   - Gather information regarding the perception of stakeholder about the organization and define the previously applied strategies
   - Analyze critical areas by using Strength, Weakness, Opportunity, Threat—SWOT
   - Analyze the available resources and estimate the requirement to operate the program based on objectives and outcome regarding the benefit to clients.
2. **Developing strategies, goals, and objectives**
   Outline the organization's strategic directions: The general strategies, long-range goals, and specific objectives of its response to identify critical issues and situation analysis.
3. **Developing a strategic plan and getting ready**
   Be ready with the following tasks to build a work plan:
   - Constitute the planning committee
   - Clarify the roles of all those involved in planning
   - Develop an organizational profile
   - Find out the management structure
   - Prepare a strategic plan keeping in mind the critical issues of each program.
4. **Identifying and selecting the alternative approaches**
   - Identify the alternative strategies/programs by utilizing the opportunities and strengths of the organization
   - Evaluate programs through cost-benefit analysis based on the database
   - Analyze programs through competitive analysis and with previously implied strategies
   - Select the best approach to implement.
5. **Implementing and reviewing the plan**
   - Implement the best strategy for the organization
   - Monitor and evaluate it per performance indicators
   - Review periodically for its effectiveness.

OPERATING PLAN

A plan is a scheme, program, or method worked out beforehand for the accomplishment of an objective. It is also a commitment of resources to a proposed or tentative project or course of action to achieve specific results.

Types of Plans

There are several types of plans: both major and minor. It is easy to understand when the procedures are classified into two: hierarchical and management point of view.

1. **Hierarchical point of view**
   The hierarchical view forms part of the management activity and is interlinked within the hierarchy. Plans of higher level are derivatives of the lower level of plans **(Fig. 14.3)**.
   a. *Purposes or mission:* All organizations have an object or a reason for existence. The reason for existence expresses a mission.
   b. *Philosophy:* It outlines the organization plans to attain its goals and functions. Based on organizational existence, philosophies can be general and comprehensive.
   c. *Statement of philosophy:* It has the purpose or mission statement and explains beliefs and values. It relates to the functioning of the organization, service, and unit. Health-care organizations have the organizational philosophy and also a nursing service philosophy.

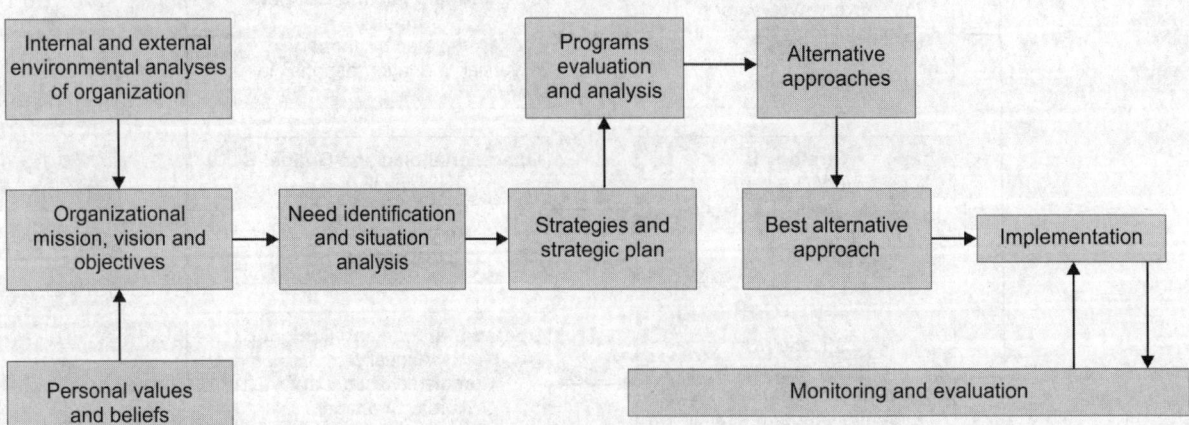

Fig. 14.2: Strategic planning process.

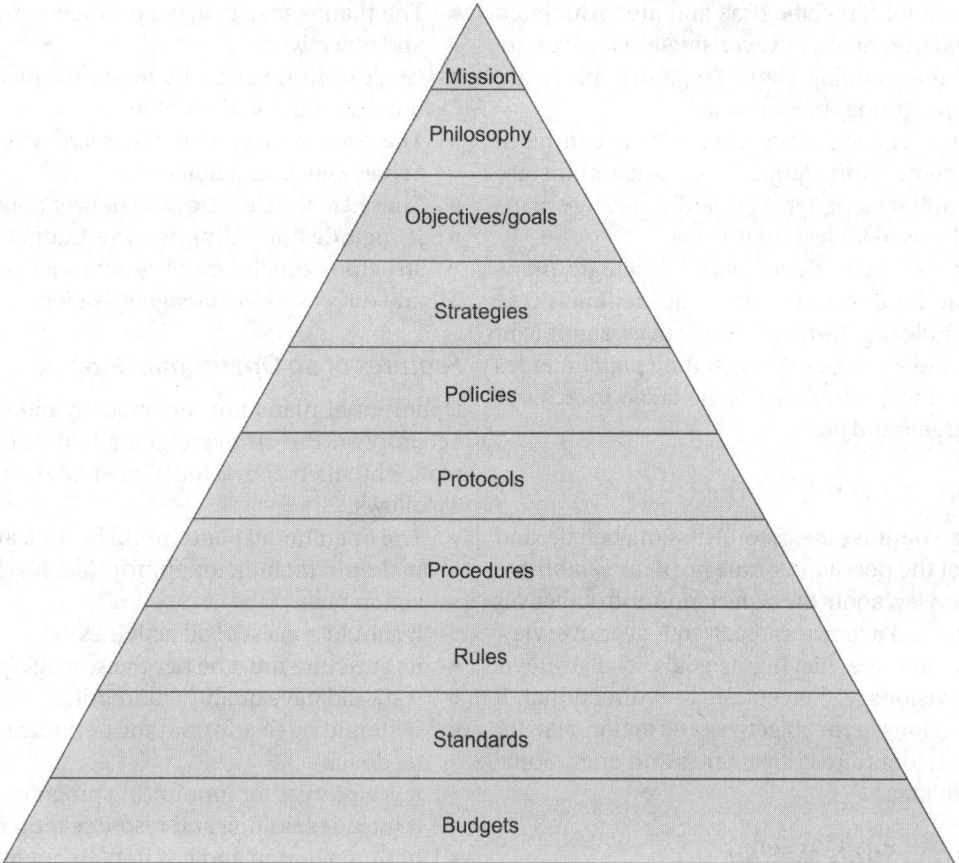

Fig. 14.3: Types of plans.

d. *Objectives or goals:* Health institute objectives are the basic plan of the hospital. A nursing department may also have its objectives and goals.
e. *Strategies:* Strategies are the action plans obtained based on the long-term objectives of an organization. Strategies form a framework to guide in thinking and action. It helps in analyzing the different aspects of goals.
f. *Policies:* A policy is a designated plan or course of action to be taken in a specific situation. Policies are general statements that guide or channel thinking in decision-making. Policies define an area to make a decision. The decision must be inconsistent with an objective. Written procedures are in the policy manual that should be available in each department.
g. *Protocols:* A protocol is a detailed standard plan for patient care, such as a protocol related to disaster management in the emergency area. It would include various activities related to legal formalities, technical skills, and other resources management.
h. *Procedures:* Procedures are the plans that establish a required method of handling future activities. They are chronological sequences of required actions. Procedures specify a particular nursing activity often described in some steps or processes.
i. *Rules:* Rules spell out specific required actions or nonaction, allowing no discretion. These are the code of conduct or norms. It relates to human behavior and does not lay down any specific sequence of action. The prime aim of developing rules is to maintain discipline, and there should be a penalty for violation. Hence, rules are authoritative. Rules identify specific desired outcomes for each day of hospitalization and actions to achieve the result.
j. *Standards of nursing practice:* These are authoritative statements that describe a normal or acceptable level of professional nursing performance. The rules of practice, therefore, define professional practice. Indian Nursing Council devised general standards and guidelines for nursing practice.
k. *Budgets:* It is a statement of expected results expressed in numerical terms. Budget is a fundamental planning instrument for health agencies.

2. **A management point of view**
   a. *Standing and single-use plans:* Standing plans are used again and again. They provide guidelines for managerial decisions. These plans ensure quick decisions and actions whenever needs arise. Mission, objectives, strategies, policies, procedures, methods, and rules are standing used ideas. Single-use plans are used to handle new or unique problems. These

are relevant for a specific time and are formulated when used next time. However, single-use plans are a part of the standing plans. Single-use plans are projects, programs, and budgets.
  b. *Short-range or long-range plans:* Plans can be of long range or short range. Long-range plans are strategic and set long-term goals. Short-range plans are usually used for less than 1 year.
  c. *Strategic and operational plans:* Strategic plans define the long-term course of an action. These plans include organizational objectives, significant policies, and strategies. An operating plan includes events and responsibilities to be taken to achieve the set targets and goals.

Strategic Plan

The strategic plan outlines the vision, mission, beliefs, and values that direct the decisions. Strategic plans establish a clear and realistic view about the expectation and objectives of the organization to achieve and a 3- to 5-year overview of how it will set about achieving its goals. The strategic plan is concise, visionary, conceptual, and directional. It is concerned with long-term objectives and action plan for a long duration. It identifies critical areas and operational programs of each area.

Characteristic of a Strategic Plan

- A strategic plan is a blueprint to take decisions.
- It provides a platform for more detailed planning.
- It relates to the mid term.
- It should be simple, logical, practical, and in written form.
- It focuses on matters of strategic importance.
- The plan should separate from day-to-day work.
- It should be complete and integrated.
- The plan should distinguish between the cause and effect.
- It should stimulate change and become a building block for the next plan.
- The plan should be realistic, critical, and attainable.

Operational Plan

Operational plans are single-use, short-term plans derived from the strategic plan to accomplish the goals and objectives of the organization. An organization should have operating plans for each primary organizational unit, which correspond to its fiscal year. It links the strategic plan by delivering organizational activities and the resources required to provide them. These plans usually establish the activities and budgets for each part of the organization.

Concept and Meaning

- An operating plan includes the actions to achieve the set objectives.
- The plan is a step-by-step process of achieving goals and objectives.
- Goals of strategic and operational plans are the same, but they differ in their objectives.
- These are management plans and written blueprints to achieve goals and objectives.
- These are the directions to deliver managed services.
- It includes planning for the budget, organizational structure, quality monitoring process, new programs, and directions to managers/leaders.

Features of an Operational Plan

Operational plans are the specific action plans used to accomplish the strategic goals laid out in the strategic plan. The main characteristics of an operational plan are as follows:

- The operational plan should have clear objectives.
- It should include an appropriate level of the detailed action plan.
- It should consist of all activities.
- Its structure must be per the strategic plan.
- It should have quality standards.
- It should have a format for periodical evaluation and feedback.
- It is a process for monitoring progress.
- It includes staffing and resource requirements.
- It is time bound and has implementation timetables.

Purposes of Operational Plan

- To specify activities and procedures
- To set a time frame for achieving the objectives
- To allocate responsibilities to staff involved in a particular business
- To prepare the team for taking up responsibility
- To specify the records to be kept and the policies needed
- To give freedom to each group to plan its own goals and objectives with departmental and institutional goals.

Formulation of Operational Plans

Members responsible for the implementation of activities should prepare operational plans. They must formulate an effective practical/action plan by using the **six W's method**, i.e. want, why, what, when, who, and what if.

1. **Recognize the need for the operational plan:** The first step in formulating operational plan is to create an awareness of the expectations and requirements of the organization. The expectations should be made obsessive because that will lead to commitment. Before venturing on an operational plan, it is a must to evaluate the pros and cons of each alternative.
2. **Collection of necessary information and facts:** Gather detailed information related to various activities and programs, including the time required for each action. However, the information should be accurate.

3. **Laying down the objectives:** Objectives are the results and used to direct the efforts of the workforce to attain predetermined goals. Formulate specific, measurable, attainable, realistic, and time-bound objectives. The purpose of the goals are to be kept in mind.
4. **Determine the knowledge, attitudinal behavior, skills, and habits level of employees:** Determine the knowledge, attitudinal behavior, skills, and habits (KASH) required to achieve the objectives. Refer to current organizational KASH inventory to find out the current level of employees and raise their level to the expected standard.
5. **Selection of team:** The range of the group is an essential step in formulating an operational plan. Select a team and team up with the staffs who have similar goals and objectives in the organization.
6. **Prepare time frame:** Make a definitive time frame to achieve objectives, which will in turn help in utilizing time, money, and effort more effectively.
7. **Develop alternative action plans:** Be ready with alternative action plans. The planner must study all plans and select the best one by looking at all the pros and cons.
8. **Evaluation of the operational plan:** Prepare a checklist to evaluate the prepared operational plan. It is assessed based on various parameters given below:
   - Staff responsible for implementation should be committed to the program
   - Operational plan should fit the strategic plan
   - Objectives, actions, and outcome measures should be specified
   - It should have a clear implementation time frame
   - Responsibilities of every event must be defined and allocated clearly
   - There should be an explicit process for monitoring progress.
9. **Determine secondary plans:** After the formulation of the operational plan, prepare supportive plans. All secondary plans should reflect a part of the main operational plan.
10. **Plan for implementation:** Implementation is the last step in planning an operational plan. Operationalize the developed strategy to achieve the organizational objectives. Prepare a schedule and implement policies, procedures, and standards.

Strategic Plan Vs Operational Plan

Operational planning is a part of strategic planning. Operational planning should align with the operation plan and generally forms a basis for operational decisions to address short-term planning. Operational plan differs from the strategic plan with regard to the need, time frame, integration, input, output, planning approach, forecasting, supply and demand requirement, etc. **(Table 14.1)**.

TABLE 14.1: Difference between staffing operational and strategic plan.

	Operational plan	Strategic plan
Need	Accurately forecast recruitment and staff development needs	Develop strategies for long term
Time frame	Planning usually 12 months with a quarterly focus—matches the yearly business plan	Usually 3 years or longer—matches the organizational strategic plan
Integrated with	Annual or quarterly financial/budgeting process	Strategic planning process
Input	Mostly internal data, some management decisions	Internal and external factors, business strategies, global trends, etc.
Output	Staffing plans, skill gaps	Human resource/people strategies
Management approach	Different models	Uses future techniques based on today's approach
Forecasting	Key focus	The only part of the process—forecasting is too limited with regard to time line and scope to be the core of the process
Segmentation – focus	Internal demand	Internal and external demand and supply
Ability	Assesses individual ability	Assesses group-level capability
Focus	Operational management—line and bottom-up managers	Strategic management—executive and board
Aligns with	Management plan	Strategic plan
Terms used	"Predict," "calculate"	"Explore," "design"

Management Plan

A management plan is a framework of day-to-day and long-term strategy of an organization. It depicts the managerial functional and operating areas, methods of doing work, managing staff, finance, coordinating, directing, and various systems to accomplish the goals and objectives of an organization. The management plan should be inconsistent with organizational mission and philosophy.

The purpose of management plans varies according to the mission, philosophy, goals, and objectives of the organization. It also depends upon the authority and accountability of the decision made by the management team, resources available, and the nature of work in the organization.

Importance of Management Plan

1. To make everyone clear about their position in the organization, i.e. to whom to report, who will report, and job responsibilities.
2. To assign reasonable duties on an equitable basis.

3. To create accountability among management team toward their job.
4. To keep everyone on schedule to accomplish objectives.
5. To define the role of the organization about its mission and vision.
6. To run an organization smooth to achieve its goal by utilizing available resources.
7. To improve work efficiency.

Steps in Developing a Management Plan

1. **Identify the need for a management plan:** The first step in formulating management plan is to know the expectations and requirements of the organization. Make expectations obsessive because that will lead to commitment. Before venturing on a management plan, evaluate the pros and cons of each alternative.
2. **Gather necessary information and facts:** Gather detailed information related to management structure, management members, their responsibilities, organization chart defining responsibilities and ownership, authority at different level of management, departments, policies, and programs. However, the information should be accurate.
3. **Develop objectives:** Formulate specific, measurable, attainable, realistic, and time-bound targets for management plans with regard to the purpose and goals of the organization.
4. **Prepare an outline/rough draft of the management plan:** The outline of management plan must include management structure, management team members, their abilities, their job responsibilities, authority and ownership, need for an expert/consultant, different departments, policies and procedures of each department, and a planned schedule.
   Decide the type of management approach for developing a management plan, i.e. a top-down approach, democratic, collaborative, or collective approach. Define the responsibilities and accountability for each management team member. Prepare a schedule for each managerial function or activity. Prepare an evaluation checklist to assess the effectiveness of the plan.
5. **Develop policies and standard operating procedure:** Prepare policies and procedures for each area. Select one of the approaches as mentioned above to plan department-wise management activity. Ensure the policies and procedures must commensurate with the mission and philosophy of the organization.
6. **Revise and refine the plan:** Prepare a final draft of the plan and check its format and areas. Get it validated by experts/consultants. Seek approval from the competent authority. Implement as a pilot project. Evaluate it by using an assessment checklist. Get feedback from employees, by self-assessment, and through organizational audits. Modify per suggestions. Refine and make it ready for implementation.

PLANNING NEW VENTURE

Concept of a New Venture

A new venture is a new activity or business that involves risks and uncertainties in operationalizing. It is a plan of action that needs strategic and business planning. It provides an opportunity to set up a venture/business by innovative business and management ideas. It is a sort of competition that offers an excellent chance to formulate a creative plan to start a new venture. It may be a joint or business venture.

A Venture-Building Process

The main focus of the venture-building process is on delivering the annual operating plan. Management of a new high-growth business is centered on a client-driven idea or a technology. The venture-building process has four phases: startup, initial growth, rapid growth, and continuous growth. At the time of startup, it is necessary to create a business model and a business plan, build a management team, and develop product/strategy that should be different from the competitive world. Raise venture capital. During initial and rapid growth, one has to continuously monitor the implementation of operative and strategic plans and the progress of the new venture to achieve its goals. Continuous growth is essential for the survival of a business/venture.

Factors Determining the Need for a New Venture

According to Gartner (1985), four factors determine the need for creating a new venture **(Fig. 14.4)**:
1. Personal characteristics of a person including motive, attitude, desire, and capability of a person to carry out the decision to start a new venture.
2. Environmental factors including external surroundings and socioeconomic factors.
3. A business policy framework that can affect decisions before, during, and after starting a new venture.
4. Type of venture, the entrepreneurship process, leadership qualities and skills, and risk-taking behavior.

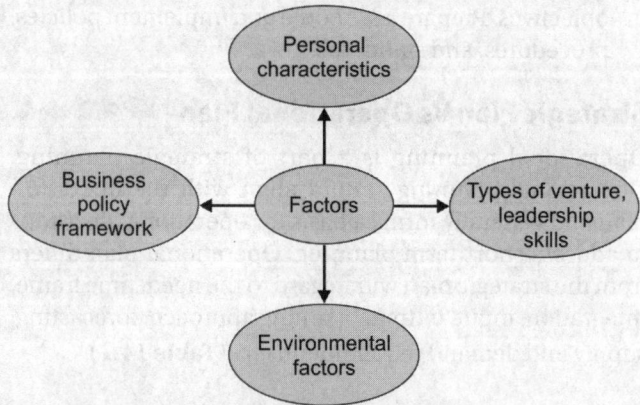

Fig. 14.4: Factors affecting the plan of a new venture.

Steps for Planning a New Venture

a. **Preplanning stage**
  - Assess motivation and attitude for planning a new venture and taking the risk of uncertainty and failure of a new venture
  - Plan the investment based on experience, expertise, and interest
  - Plan work schedule legally and systematically
  - Find the sources of finance and conditions
  - Plan the requirements and formalities to start venture/business
  - Plan market, operational, and financial model for the venture.

b. **Identify the demand of the decided venture**
  - Assess the value of the new business and requirement of clients for the product/service
  - Define clear goals and assess strengths and weaknesses
  - Define the objective of starting a new venture.

c. **Evaluate the feasibility of the new venture**
  To begin a new venture, assess the feasibility and potentials with regard to its demand, productivity, availability, better competitor, market value, financial risk, backup monetary, profit margin, management skills, and capability instead of taking a chance and dealing with the worst. Seek expert advice from team members, marketing experts, lawyers, and financial advisors.

d. **List down the requirements**
  - Legal formalities, filing the name of the business, address of office and attorney in case of partnership project
  - Consider legal, accounting and tax, insurance, and professional banking needs
  - Permissions, licenses, rules, and regulations applicable to the new venture
  - Types of records for tax purposes, management, and control, and plan documentation systems
  - Registration, select mailing address, and telephone number
  - Finalize the location of the business office and its design layout and furnishing.

e. **Develop a business and budget plan**
  - Develop a strategic and operational plan
  - Ensure that the program fulfilled all the requirements
  - Mention about the venture, its clients, and methods of promotion and planned cost for the initial stage
  - Outline the framework of venture.

f. **Plan the financial request/loan**
  Find the sources of finance apart from the personal investment that has to be at least 25–30%. Open a separate business account.

g. **Make a final check of the requirements**
  Check for the completion of all the formalities, plans, finance, permission, contract, fees, etc. to start a new venture. Prepare a checklist.

CHAPTER HIGHLIGHTS

- Strategy determines the long-term goals and objectives of an organization, which are attained by selecting a course of action with the available resources.
- Strategic planning is a process of defining the organizational strategy and directions and making decisions to allocate resources, considering the external and internal factors. A series of steps are involved in planning a strategy.
- A plan is a scheme, program, or method worked out beforehand for the accomplishment of an objective. Plans are classified according to the hierarchy and management point of view.
- Strategic plan outlines the vision, mission, beliefs, and values that direct the decisions. Operational plans are single-use, short-term plans derived from the strategic plan. A management plan is a framework of day-to-day and long-term plan of managerial functional and operating areas.
- A new venture is a new business involving risks and uncertainties and is a plan of action that needs strategic and business planning. Many steps are involved in planning a new venture.

REVIEW QUESTIONS

I. Essay Type Questions
1. Define strategy. Describe the strategic planning process.
2. Describe the purposes and importance of strategic planning.
3. Discuss the different types of operating plans.
4. Enumerate the features of the operational plan and describe the process of formulating an operational plan.
5. Explain the steps involved in planning a new venture.

II. Short Notes
1. Strategic plan
2. Development of management plan
3. Operational plan
4. Venture-building process
5. Strategic plan Vs. operational plan.

III. Multiple Choice Questions
1. The action plan based on long-term objectives of an organization refers to:
   a. Strategy
   b. Operational plan
   c. Management plan
   d. Business plan
2. A detailed standard plan that specifies various activities, technical skills, legal formalities, and other resource management is:
   a. Policy   b. Protocol
   c. Procedure   d. Rules

3. A single-use plan is a type of plan that:
   a. Includes events and responsibilities to achieve the organizational objectives
   b. Provides guidelines for management actions to be used again and again
   c. Includes organizational objectives, major policies, and strategies
   d. Handles new and unique problems in management
4. A plan that outlines vision, mission, beliefs, and values to direct decisions refers to:
   a. Long-term plan
   b. Short-term plan
   c. Strategic plan
   d. Management plan
5. A designated plan or course of action taken in a specific situation is known as:
   a. Policy
   b. Strategy
   c. Protocol
   d. Procedure
6. Which plan provides guidelines for managerial decisions and is used again and again?
   a. Operational plan
   b. Standing plan
   c. Strategic plan
   d. Long-range plan
7. A written blueprint of events and responsibilities that details actions to be taken to achieve the intended goal refers to:
   a. Short-term plan
   b. Program plan
   c. Operational plan
   d. Functional plan

Answer Keys

1. a   2. b   3. d   4. c   5. a   6. b   7. c

SUGGESTED READING

1. Available from http://www.newventure.nl/resources/uploads/files/starting-up%20versie%203.pdf.
2. Available from http://www.newventuredesign.com/packages.html.
3. Bradford RW, Tarcy B, Duncan JP. Simplified Strategic Planning. Chandler House; 2000.
4. Burkhart PL, Reuss S. Successful Strategic Planning: A Guide for Nonprofit Agencies And Organizations. Newbury Park, CA: Sage Publications; 1993.
5. Business operational plan. [online] Available from http://www.businessdictionary.com/definition/objective.html.
6. Griffin AP (Ed.). Philosophy and nursing. J Adv Nurs. 1980;5(3):261-72.
7. Niu TC. The philosophy of nursing management: a conceptual analysis. Hu Li Za Zhi. 2005;52(5):5-9.
8. Podolak I. A comprehensive philosophy for nursing: the total approach. Can J Nurs Adm. 1995;8(4):23-41.
9. Rousell L, Russel C. Management and Leadership for Nurse Administrators. Jones & Bartlett Publishers; 2006. pp. 225-35.
10. Watson, J. Nursing: Human Sciences and Human Care. New York: National League for Nursing; 1988.
11. What is a plan? [online] Available from http://www.thefreedictionary.com/plan.

15 CHAPTER

Innovation in Nursing and Planning for Change

CHAPTER OUTLINE

- Innovation in Nursing
    - Defining Innovation
    - Need for Innovation
    - Characteristics of Innovation
    - Components of Innovation
    - Stages of Innovative Process
    - Types of Innovations
    - Barriers to Innovations
    - Innovative Nursing Strategies
- Planning for Change
    - Concept of Change Management
    - Areas of Planned Change
    - Aims and Objectives of Planned Change
    - Factors Affecting Change
    - Principles of Change Management
    - Change Management Model/Approaches
    - Strategies for Change
    - Process of Planning Change
    - Role of a Nurse Manager in Change Management

LEARNING OUTCOMES

After completion of this chapter, the learner will be able to:
- Understand the concept and need for innovation
- Describe the components of innovation and the various stages of the innovative process
- Enumerate different types of innovations and barriers to innovations
- Highlight innovative nursing strategies
- Understand the concept of change management
- Identify areas and objectives of planned change
- Evaluate factors affecting change
- Apply principles and approaches to change management
- Enumerate strategy and process for change
- Recognize the role of a nurse manager in change management

KEY TERMS
Innovation, innovative process, innovative nursing strategies, change management

INTRODUCTION

The advancement of technology and increased health needs of the population lead to immense possibilities for the broader scope to adapt and implement new ideas and practices in nursing education and training. A challenge for nurses is to play a constructive role in improving educational opportunities and providing quality care.

Planning for change is a compelling way to build a working philosophy for action. Planned change is a conscious, deliberate, and collaborative effort to improve the operation of a human system. In this high-tech world, managing change has become a matter of systematic inquiry. Therefore, a nurse administrator must think and plan for quality changes in the nursing services to keep pace with the fast-changing technology. There is a need for change at both organizational and individual levels.

INNOVATION IN NURSING

Defining Innovation

The word "innovation" is derived from the Latin word "in + novare" means "to make new." From a regulatory perspective, it means "to change into something new" but not concerning with making it better. It is an idea-generating process that creates new or something significantly different from others to improve the services and products of novelty.

It is a systematic, dynamic, and continuous process that requires communication to identify "best practices"

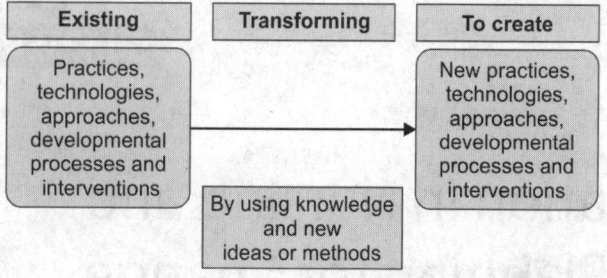

Fig. 15.1: Concept of innovation.

to share with others, collaboration with regulatory bodies, and partnership with practitioners to enhance clinical experiences. It is a process of transforming the existing services and also involves ways of doing things, approaches, technologies, and various developmental processes or interventions to create new ones by using the knowledge and innovative ideas. Successful innovation depends upon human creativity, culture, and skills and talents nurtured and developed through education **(Fig. 15.1)**.

Need for Innovation

Change is necessary for the following:
- Continuous improvement in nursing
- Fulfilling the growing demand for health services
- Rendering holistic and high-quality care
- Advancement in communication, education, and technology
- Compensating shortage of workforce
- Replacing traditional methods of teaching and practices
- Adapting change and facing competitions with other organizations
- Coping with the changing needs of clients
- Maximizing globalization sharing
- Solving work-related problems.

I: **Nursing Education:** In nursing education, innovation requires conceptualization and implementing new approaches in the teaching–learning process to attain excellence in nursing practice and to develop risk-taking, creative, and distinctive culture within nursing education. Hence, the faculty has to think differently about curriculum, instructional methods for theory and clinical teaching, and clinical experience. Many queries need to be resolved, such as the aim of teaching–learning, methods of education, the content matter, and the teachers and sources for teachings. We need to generate creative ideas to find ways to prepare nurses to deliver safe and effective care and for new teaching strategies that can be used to optimize clinical learning in the present health-care system.

Innovation is required in all aspects of the teaching–learning process, which include curriculum, instructional methods, teaching–learning experiences, learning environment, characteristics of educator/resources, and evaluation methods **(Fig. 15.2)**.

The learning environment must include the resources that the educators can use to teach learners. *Resources*

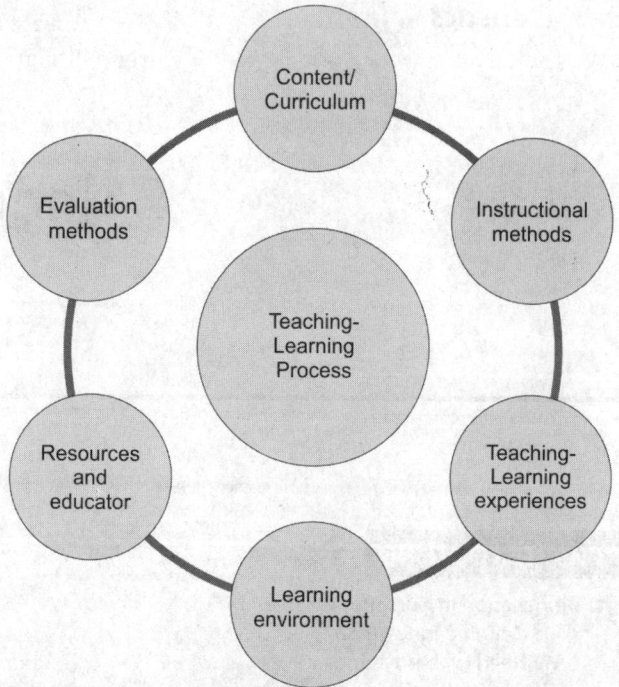

Fig. 15.2: Areas of generating ideas in the teaching–learning process.

refer to digital resources and technology that facilitate infrastructure and learning space. It is also necessary to conceptualize the elements of pedagogic core and competencies such as digital and media literacy, teamwork and collaboration, capacity for problem solving, reflective critical thinking, and clinical and social competence of learners. The *learners* may be regular, online, or distant learners. The instruction methods must be student centered and concept based, rather than teacher-centered content driven to have the skill for learning. The educator must be professional, experts, peer teachers, and distant teachers.

The organization dynamic needs regrouping of educators and learners, rescheduling of learning time, and changing pedagogic approaches. The educators need to focus on team teaching and teamwork. However, the learners may opt to learn in a small group of varying size. Along with academic curriculum, flexible timetables and provision of cocurricular activities are essential. The *curriculum* needs evidence, value, problem, competency, and inquiry-based learning. Formative, summative, continuous, comprehensive evaluation, and self-assessment methods are used to measure performance. The curriculum should also have a clinical orientation with sustainability, interdisciplinary, intercultural and place for language.

II: **Nursing Practice:** To improve quality nursing care, a need for successful and sustained innovation is required in nursing practice. The nurse managers need to create an organizational culture and working environment for the nurses to generate and evaluate ideas and make a link with external partners in developing innovative, client-focused strategies.

Characteristics of Innovation

Innovation is creativity characterized by originality and expressiveness enhanced by building an environment of trust, interpersonal relationship, and a spirit of cooperation. The main features of innovation are as listed subsequently:

1. **Relatively superior:** With regard to its utility and outcome, the innovation must be superior to the existing one. It must focus on the needs and satisfaction of the client and be cost-effective.
2. **Compatibility:** The new ideas must be compatible with the existing values, norms, skills and practices, and cost. It must also fit with the needs, experiences, and benefits of clients.
3. **Complexity:** Innovations if challenging in understanding and sophisticated to practice may lose its adaptability. Therefore, innovation must satisfy the needs of the client.
4. **Trialability:** Creative ideas/products and processes need to be tested for its efficiency and effectiveness, generating positive effects and reducing the chances of adaptability.
5. **Observable and measurable:** Creative ideas must be able to observe and measure their outcomes without any adverse effects. The effectiveness of an innovation must be checked.

Components of Innovation

Innovation has main three elements: innovation, individual/team creativity, and environment. All these three components are interdependent of creating and implementing changes in an organization.

1. **Innovation:** Changes can be accounted for by implementing new ideas or creating new technology, tools or products, policies, services, procedures, or devices. Clients should adapt and customize an innovation based on their individual need.
2. **Individuals/innovators:** Individuals/innovators comprise individuals or groups of people who solve the problems or create well-accepted technology, tools, products, or intervention of novelty. The innovator must be sensitive to each opportunity. The we-feeling among the team members allow free communication and exchange of ideas from different perspectives.
3. **Environment:** Environmental–structural support is critical to give shape to innovation. It constitutes the culture, physical, social, and psychological and organizational atmosphere essential to facilitate and support creative ideas. It provides an opportunity for individuals to test and implement innovation. The nature of tasks and goals poses a challenge to take a risk and motivate the individuals to think and try to solve the problems. The favorable and positive attitude of the supervisor is critical for the development and implementation of creative ideas.

Stages of Innovation Process

The seven stages of innovation process (**Fig. 15.3**) are listed subsequently:

Stage 1: Idea generation: In the idea generation stage, the individual or team generates creative ideas, which in turn originates from creativity and by analyzing and evaluating the existing services, practices, and approaches. It also arises from other sources such as feedback from clients; suggestions from the users (health-care workers); feedback from the community, competitors, partners, team members; and from basic research. This stage will provide an opportunity to look for new ideas in different perspectives, thereby selecting the best one. The generated design must meet the criteria of the existing practices, policies, and plans.

Stage 2: Critical examination and advocacy: In this stage, it is necessary to assess each idea critically to understand its potential benefits and risks, negative effects, cost, resources required, and compatibility with the criteria; evaluate each idea for its acceptance by the client, market value, and technology required to have an operational plan to make a decision; compare its benefits and risks with the existing practices; and find the gap. The new idea must fill the gap. After analyzing the idea critically, it should be communicated and discussed and suggestions are to be sought from the team members and other members of the organization, which will help in refining the idea. This comprises the idea acceptance stage.

Stage 3: Experimentation: Validation and testing: This stage involves validation and trial, wherein the ideas are converted into a prototype and then tested for its suitability and feasibility by conducting a study on clients. If it is suitable and feasible for the organization, then move on to the next stage. Experimentation is a continuous process, and new ideas are generated during this phase.

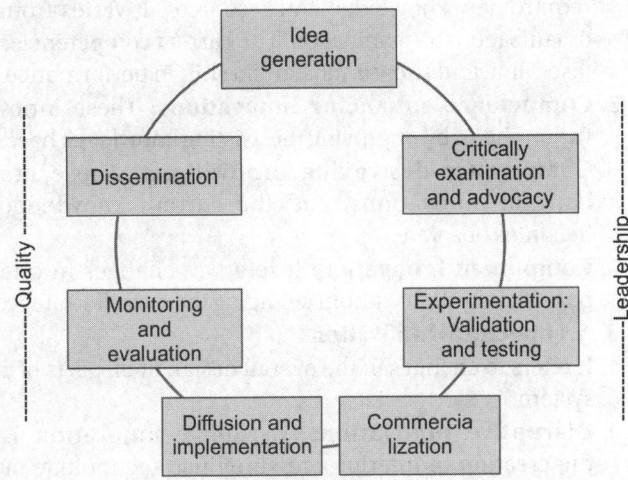

Fig. 15.3: Stages of the innovation process.

Stage 4: Commercialization: In this stage, try to convince the target audience that this method is useful to implement. Make them aware of their potential benefits and effectiveness and demonstrate the interest of innovation and how to use.

Stage 5: Diffusion and implementation: Diffusion is a stage when the organization accepts the new method and communicates the specific information about the innovative method before its implementation.

Stage 6: Monitoring and evaluating: Monitor the new method during the implementation phase and evaluate it by measuring its outcome/performance. In case of any deficiency, modify and replan, which will help in refining the new method. The new method must meet its characteristics, i.e. compatibility, trialability, and relatively superior to the existing one.

Stage 7: Dissemination: After refining the new method, it is necessary to disseminate it across disciplines for implementation and then obtain feedback from users, clients, and organizations. The innovation is concerned with quality; hence, the whole process requires leadership.

Types of Innovations

The list below shows the nine different types of innovations:
1. **Process innovations:** Process innovations are the novelties within services, interventions, approaches, etc.
2. **Product innovations:** These innovations concern products, tools, and standard procedures required to carry out the processes.
3. **Incremental innovations:** Incremental innovations create new practices by minor modification in the existing methods, knowledge, and resources. It enhances competency on a small scale and considers lifeblood of innovation.
4. **Radical innovations:** Radical innovations are significant changes in the existing practices and require new knowledge and resources. It varies from organization to organization. The current competencies lose value and show a substantial shift in performance.
5. **Competence-enhancing innovations:** These innovations build by improving the existing knowledge base.
6. **Competence-destroying innovations:** These are harmful innovations, and the current knowledge becomes obsolete.
7. **Component innovation:** It refers to changes in one part of the system without changing the overall strategy.
8. **Architectural innovation**
   It refers to changes in the overall design or all parts of a system.
9. **Disruptive innovation:** Disruptive innovation is the creation of inferior and simplified technology or product, which results in a change in the regulation and standards. The organization follows low-cost innovative models and economically coherent network.

Barrier to Innovations

The two barriers to innovation are barriers related to education and practitioners. The following shows further subdivisions of each barrier:
1. **Barriers related to education**
   - Traditional and comfortable pedagogy
   - Fear of mistakes
   - Students deficient in clinical experience
   - Lack of organizational support
   - Incompetent nurse educators
   - Lack of in-service training
   - Limited exposure of student nurses in the clinical areas
   - Fearing liability to practice by student nurses
   - Noncooperation between educators and practitioners
   - Insufficient preparation of the student for problem-solving and caring patients.
2. **Barriers related to practitioners**
   - Lack of nursing policies and standard operative procedures
   - Lack of uniformity in practice
   - Incompetent nurse practitioners
   - Lack of support for nurses in practice areas
   - Nurses' role conflict and undefined job descriptions
   - Lack of workforce
   - Dissatisfaction and lack of motivation among nurses.

Innovative Nursing Strategies

I: *Nursing Education:* Nursing education comprises nine strategies, which are listed below:
1. **Simulation and virtual simulations:** It is an education strategy or teaching–learning method with a competency assessment tool to improve the students' competence and to achieve quality patient care. Anticipating a real situation with guided experiences, it is useful in preparing new students for clinical placement and also used as a complement to clinical experience. However, its limitations are that it is costly, requires technical assistance, and faculty development. Simulations are of many types, namely, Personal Computer (PC)-based simulation, virtual patient simulation, task trainer, etc.
2. **Personal digital assistants:** The students can use personal digital assistants (PDAs) for recording and evaluating. These are useful for assessing, calculating the dose and growth charts, and for many other guidelines.
3. **Distance and online education:** Universities are providing distance education programs and online courses in nursing.
4. **New degree and certificate courses:** Many new diplomas, degrees and specialty courses are available for the nurses, e.g. geriatric nursing, disaster nursing, forensic nursing, independent nursing practitioner, advance nursing practice, etc.

5. **Videoconferencing and Web-based learning:** These are useful to link educator and the learners for discussion and evaluation.
6. **Microteaching:** It is an innovative and controlled method to equip teachers with the teaching skills. It is a highly individualized teacher training technique to improve their teaching skills. It promotes real-time teaching experiences and aids in providing confidence, feedback, and reinforcement.
7. **E-learning and computer-assisted learning:** E-learning is a self-directed active learning method. The computer-assisted learning is one of the innovative teaching–learning approaches and is also an effective and interactive teaching and learning tool in combination with audio and visual data (multimedia).
8. **Problem-based learning:** It is one of the innovative, student-centered, self-directed, project-oriented, and individual or group/team-based instructional methods of teaching, whose central focus of learning is "problem."
9. **Objective structured clinical examination:** The Objective Structured Clinical Examination (OSCE) is a structured way of assessing the students' clinical competencies.

II: *Nursing Practice:* Nursing practice also consists of nine subtypes that are listed subsequently:

1. **Health information technology:** Electronic health record (EHR) is a documentation tool used to enhance patient safety in medication, to evaluate the quality of care, to maximize efficiency, and measure staffing in clinical settings.
2. **Mobile technologies:** These are useful in improving communication with the clients, such as reminding the follow-up visits, for medication, etc.
3. **Bar coding and incidence reporting system:** Bar coding is matching drugs to patients by using bar codes on both the medications and patients' arm bracelets. The incidence reporting system is useful for immediately reporting the adverse events due to the use of medical devices.
4. **Automated dispensing machines:** This technology distributes medication doses.
5. **Virtual nurse avatars:** These are computer software that provide care to patients and are also useful in taking a health history, assessing health status, and for exhibiting interactive behavior.
6. **Telenursing/Telehealth:** Telenursing is the use of technology to deliver nursing care and conduct nursing practice. Nurses provide telenursing, but telemedicine may be more appropriate, as the success of this modality requires multiple partners.
7. **Wireless and handheld technologies:** It includes PDAs for patient tracking, medical reference, and drug dosage.
8. **Knowledge management and generation:** Information and Communication Technology (ICT) has various approaches to knowledge generation and nursing research. For example, International Council of Nursing started an electronic International Nursing Partnership Database Project to document and share ongoing and new international partnerships as a tool to encourage similar initiatives and aid in planning new ventures.
9. **Knowledge-based systems:** The Internet offers a vast amount of information of variable quality and computer-based education for patients/clients and staff.

PLANNING FOR CHANGE

Concept of Change Management

Change

The word "change" in the Sanskrit language is "vishwa." Etymologically it comes from the root word "vish" meaning spreading, especially that which is never the same at two different points of time. It is not an occurrence but a way of survival. To change means to alter, to become changed, or to transform. Change refers to an alteration in the physical, biological, or social system of an individual or the organization to cope with internal and external environmental factors.

Change Management

Change management is a structured approach to modify/transition individuals, teams, and organizations as a whole from current status to the desired future status. It also tries to improve the ability of the organization to adjust to the changes. It focuses on values, cost, quality, and schedule. There is a shift in behaviors and attitudes of people to adapt and adjust to future changes. An organization needs a planned transition, not merely in response to some event or problem. In project management, change management usually concerns technical or specification point of view.

Planned Change

Planned change is a systematic and organized evidence-based change. It involves deliberate designing and implementing of a new policy based on changed operating philosophy, climate, and style, which are all done in a systematic and organized way. Planned change always prepares the organization for new goals or directions, enabling it to face challenges for its betterment and to facilitate the process in a better manner. It consists of planning and diagnosing the organization's problems and solving and revising the philosophy, goals, policies, and strategies per the gathered information. Planned change uses a humanistic approach and applies principles of behavioral science and open-system theory to solve the problems

Areas of Planned Change

Planned change attempts to cover all areas of the organization when viewed as a multivariate system. It

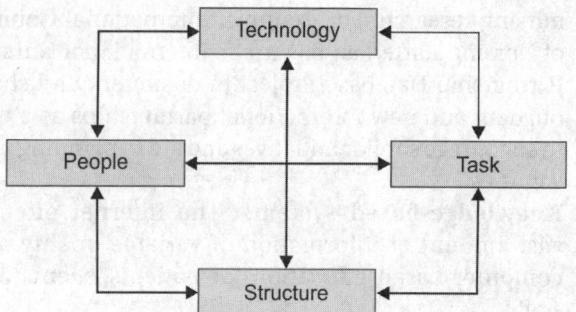

Fig. 15.4: Areas of planned changes.

includes changes in technology, task, structure, and people. The difference in one area affects the other areas (**Fig. 15.4**).

1. **Change in management technology:** To improve efficiency, coordination, and communication and relationship, the shift in management technology is a must. For example, by using modern technology data processing, decision-making and problem-solving can improve the efficiency, flowchart analysis can be used for better coordination, and democratic and participative type of supervisors can be replaced by supervisors with different leadership style to improve the relationship.
2. **Change in tasks:** Technical task can be improved by designing and simplifying the procedures, using high-tech equipment, and enhancing their competencies and skills. Various motivational techniques such as assigning additional responsibilities, recognition for good work, advancement, etc., can enhance motivation.
3. **Change in structure:** The difference in the structure area can improve relationships, formal communication and interaction, work assignment, and authority structure, which can be achieved by replacing the key personnel, modifying the cadre for a better career, and providing better administrative guidance.
4. **People-related changes:** The changes among employees in their behavior, attitude, and skill and knowledge can bring a drastic change in organizational performance, leading to its achievement of goals. Sociopsychological factors such as motivation, positive attitude, and high morale do matters in the performance of the employees, which is turn made possible by formal and informal training and other development methods. The most challenging task in planning a move in the organization is to bring the desired changes in behavior, attitude, belief, and values among employees.

Changes must take place at individual and organizational level. At the individual level, subjective changes include behavior regarding their attitude, belief, and values, which are necessary to bring changes in work culture. At the organizational level, the technological and operation management and financial consultations are essential to improve the economic, financial, and technical aspects of the organization. At the micro level, the improvement involves leadership development, group dynamics, and work design. The macro-level changes are strategic, organizational design, and international relations. The changes at the organizational systems and processes are a more holistic approach involving individuals and cultural transformation.

Aims and Objectives of Planned Change

The main objective of the planned change is to modify and reinforce strategies, structure, and processes (interventions), which lead to organizational effectiveness.

- To bring overall development of the organization both at the micro and macro level
- To bring stability and certainty in the organization
- To improve work culture by applying behavioral theories
- To adapt to changes in the environment for its existence
- To improve the capability of the organization to solve problems
- To cope with external environment threats
- To increase the effectiveness of the organization through planned intervention
- To develop self-renewing capability through a collaborative approach
- To bring useful changes in the organizational structure, technology, task, and among people to adopt
- To compete with other similar organizations nationally and internationally.

Factors Affecting Change

I: At management level

1. **Vision:** A clear vision to accomplish the first essential element for implementing change, at the micro or macro level.
2. **Values and beliefs:** Values and beliefs determine one's ability to accomplish the vision.
3. **Mission:** A mission statement determines the existence of a group.
4. **Goals and objectives:** Goals can be achieved through objectives. An aim is a short-term, practical target related to a goal. Objectives are specific, measurable, attainable, realistic, and time-bound goals.
5. **Organizational structure and work culture:** Organization may choose any combination of the models: team model, whole-group model, or hierarchical model.
6. **External and internal environment:** It is to highlight the internal and external factors that can support or harm an organization.
7. **Strategic plans:** Outlines that need to be met to achieve the objectives.
8. **Financial plan:** It is established by the goals and objectives of the group.

9. **Communications plan:** It is a strategy or plan to establish a better communication system at different levels for the organization.
10. **Evaluation plan:** It includes outcomes, indicators, and measures.

II: At individual level
1. Competency and skill
2. Positive attitude
3. Highly motivated to work
4. High morale

Principles of Change Management
1. Understanding the current situation of the organization and diagnosing the problems.
2. Planning out a target, time, and the reason for the change and also the methodology for change.
3. Planning development in appropriate achievable and measurable stages.
4. Communicating, involving people and facilitating the changes openly.
5. Seeking support from people to change environment, processes, culture, relationships, and behaviors, whether personal or organizational.

Change Management Model/Approaches
Various models and approaches are available in the literature for effective management and leading change. Lewin's change model based on its theory is the most preferred in planning for a change in the organization.

I: *Lewin's Change Model*
Lewin's field theory is a basis for the process of planned change. Planned change occurs in a planned manner, not spontaneously. Lewin's theory has field and force concepts. A field is viewed as a system. If a change occurs in one part of the system, it affects the whole system. Force gives direction and strength to move. According to Lewin, due to internal and external factors, a disruption occurs in the balance of forces; and planned change would stabilize and bring those forces to the desired equilibrium. Lewin proposes a "force field analysis" diagram to identify and analyze resisting (restraining forces) and promoting (driving forces) change **(Fig. 15.5)**.

Based on the theory, Kurt Lewin developed a change model consisting of three phases with a "top-down" perspective **(Fig. 15.6)**
1. **Unfreezing phase:** It is the first stage in the process of planned change. The old ideas and methods including internal and external factors are to be identified in the organization, so that rooms are made for newer purposes and transformation. Information is collected to diagnosis the problems. Finally, the individuals involved are informed of the need for change, and they should also agree that change is needed.
2. **Changing phase:** During this phase, define, learn and implement new ideas and processes. The role of a change

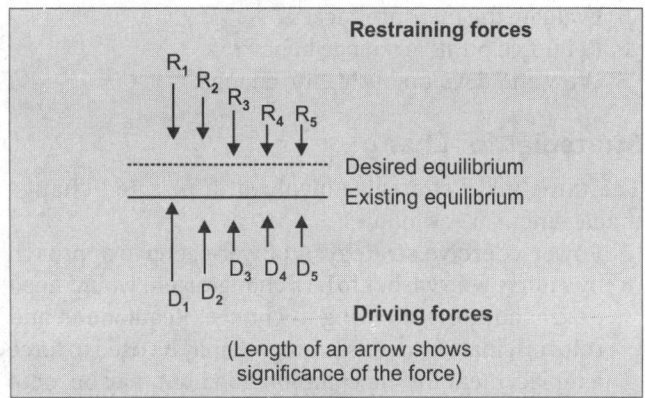

Fig. 15.5: Lewin's force field analysis.

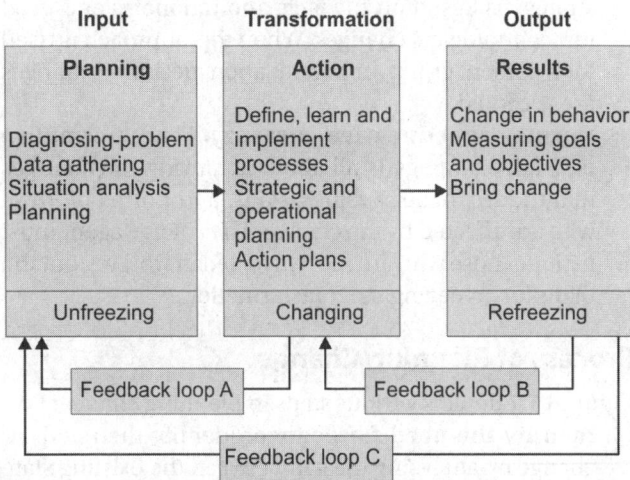

Fig. 15.6: Lewin's change model.

agent is to convince the people to adopt the change and overcome their frustrations. The change agent should anticipate and expect the difference and recognize that change takes place gradually. The change agent must identify the driving and restraining forces to determine the best plan for implementing change. Therefore, it is necessary to carefully plan to make changes in an organized way before implementation. It is imperative to apply many behavioral science approaches to bring about the desired change.
3. **Refreezing phase:** This phase comprises standardized and accepted changes. It is also referred to as a stabilization phase. After successful stabilization, the replacement must integrate into the system. Evaluate the new behavior after applying the planned change and reinforce, if required.

II: *An Iceberg Approach*
The following are the steps involved in the iceberg approach:
1. **I**dentify the need
2. **C**ommunicate objectives and processes
3. **E**ngage each person to participate
4. **B**uild change in communities: Informal, cohorts, and support groups

5. Evaluate the measure success
6. Reinforce positive change behaviors
7. Grow and develop during the change.

Strategies for Change

The three main strategies involved in planned change management are as follows:
1. **Power-coercive strategy:** A power-coercive approach by a nurse who wishes to be a change agent would need official authority to bring in change. Regulations and rules originate from this strategy. It may be used to force a replacement for the common good but may become very costly and fail due to the resistance.
2. **Empirical–rational strategy:** The empirical–rational strategy is based on the facts and rationales and used for technological changes. When this approach is used for a person, group, or organization, desirable changes are accepted.
3. **Normative educative strategy:** The normative educative strategy is all about achieving the changes in attitudes, beliefs, values, skills, and norms of those who are affected by the change. The change agent must include those who are most involved in working out the plans for achieving the transformation.

Process of Planning Change

Figure 15.7 depicts various steps in planning change:
1. **Identify the need for change:** Identify the need for change by analyzing the gap between the existing state and the desired future state. It should be a continuous process. The difference in any aspect requires a change in other aspects of the organization. Gather information from existing feedback and control data. Assess the internal and external factors of an organization that needs to be replaced.

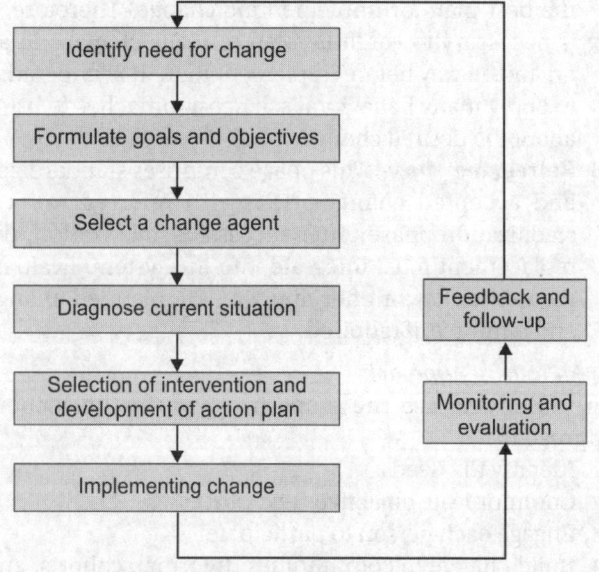

Fig. 15.7: Steps in the planned change process.

2. **Formulate goals and objectives:** After getting information and diagnosing the problems, formulate the goals of change. Evaluate opportunities and identify areas for change. Usually, organization structure, technology, and people need change. The nature and size of the area depending on the type and severity of the problem identified any difference in the evident gap.
3. **Select a change agent:** Assign responsibility to a change agent, that is, a person who has the leadership capabilities, communication abilities, creative and decision-making skills to solve problems. The change agent must be open-minded, willing to take risks, flexible, and supportive of initiating changes. The agent should be trustworthy, unbiased, and have a positive attitude and also welcome resistance toward the change.
4. **Diagnose the current situation:** Gather information to assess the situation. Consider both external and internal factors for the organization as a whole, that is, both for organizational development and for individuals with a commitment for action through planned change. Evaluate existing practices, processes, cultural norms, and performance matrices; the behavior of managers and employees; and communication process that may need modification. Identify both restraining and driving forces. Driving forces influence organizational change. Hence, it is necessary to find strategies to convert restringing forces into driving forces, so that the employees accept the change.
5. **Selection of interventions and development of the action plan:** Change is a complex, continuous, and challenging process. Change can be brought about only through proper planning and anticipating problems. Adequate preparation can overcome many challenges associated with change management.
   a. *Plan for a change in organizational structure:*
      - The design solution, the period of the change
      - Resources and support
      - Develop new processes, systems, and organizational structure
      - Implementation solution in the organization.
   b. *Plan for managing change in general:*
      - Define and implement new values, attitudes, norms, and behaviors within an organization and overcome resistance to change
      - Build consensus among employees on specific reforms designed to meet their needs better
      - Plan, test, implement, and evaluate all aspects of change
      - Develop a checklist to monitor and assess the planned change.
   c. *Anticipate reaction and resistance to change:* Both managers and employees react to any change. Attitudes are necessary to determine the response to change. The three types of alternative reactions to change are resistance, indifference, and acceptance. Resistance to change is average but has to be

handled carefully. Resistance to change includes both individual and organizational factors.

The individual's-related factors include problems of adjustment, insecurity, fear of unknown, defensiveness, group norms, lack of trust, comfort with the contemporary style of doing things, lack of information, or understanding about change. The organizational and administrative factors include organizational structure itself and resource constraints, poor timings of the change, a poorly planned proposal for the change, and improper pacing of the change.

    d. *Prepare for people to change and minimize resistance:*
- Create awareness among people regarding the need for change and provide change details
- Develop a trusting relationship through open communication
- Listen to their viewpoints, fears, and the losses they perceive
- Prepare to participate and support the change
- Allow questions and suggestions
- Demonstrate commitment to the change
- Reinforce to keep the change in place.

6. **Implementation:** The implementation of planned change involves carrying out and monitoring activities per plans by utilizing resources.
7. **Monitoring and evaluation:** During this stage, monitor and evaluate the situation for its progression by using evaluation and monitoring checklist. Ensure that the change is achieving the goals within the allocated time and resources. Is the anticipated change occurring? Are the participants showing hope and satisfaction with the change?
8. **Feedback and follow-up:** Get inputs and do a follow-up to ensure that the change program is progressing in the right direction or requires modifications. In case of any problem, replan and make necessary modifications and reframe strategies immediately to achieve the goal. Prepare a process report that will provide a reference for the future.

Role of a Nurse Manager in Change Management

As a change agent, the role of a nurse manager is very challenging to establish new routines by replacing old ones to bring a change. A nurse manager is expected to perform various roles including the followings:

1. Making staff understand the need for the change
2. Encouraging them to identify the areas for changes
3. Motivating them to take part in the change process
4. Inviting suggestions for planning and implementing change
5. Respecting the staff's ideas and opinions
6. Counseling staff who resist the change
7. Restoring accountability in the change process
8. Being flexible and robust to take a risk in change management
9. Being a catalyst and seeking support from the staff during implementation
10. Rewarding the team for bringing the successful changes.

CHAPTER HIGHLIGHTS

- Innovation is an idea-generating process, which creates new or something significantly different from others and depends upon human creativity, knowledge, and skills and talents.
- Innovation requires in all aspects of the teaching-learning process and nursing practice.
- Innovation itself, individual/team creativity, and environment are three components of change.
- Change management is a structured approach to modify individuals, teams, and organization as a whole from current status to the desired future status.
- Planned change is a systematic and organized evidence-based change and always prepares the organization for new goals or a new direction. It attempts to cover all areas of the organization, including technology, task, structure, and people.
- Lewin's change model gives direction for change management in the organization. It has three phases, namely unfreezing, changing, and refreezing phase.
- The role of a nurse manager as a change agent is very challenging to establish new routines by replacing the traditional methods.

REVIEW QUESTIONS

I. Essay Type Questions
1. Define the term "innovation." Explain its components in detail.
2. Describe the stages of innovative process in detail.
3. Enumerate the characteristics of innovation and discuss its need in nursing.
4. Enlist the objectives of planned change and discuss the factors affecting change.
5. Describe the process of planning change.

II. Short Notes
1. Barriers to innovations in nursing
2. Principles of change management
3. Role of a nurse manager in change management
4. Lewin's change model
5. Innovative nursing strategies

III. Multiple Choice Questions
1. A process that depends upon creativity, knowledge, and skill refers to:
   a. Change management
   b. Conceptualization
   c. Innovation
   d. Planned change

2. The new idea that is in harmony with the existing values, norms, and practices refers to:
   a. Compatibility   b. Mission
   c. Philosophy   d. Purpose
3. Which of the innovation is created by doing minor modification to the existing one?
   a. Radical   b. Incremental
   c. Component   d. Process
4. Which strategy nursing students use for recording and evaluation purpose?
   a. Web-based learning
   b. Robots
   c. Personal digital assistant
   d. Simulation
5. Virtual avatar is:
   a. A computer software that provides care to patients
   b. A documentation tool that enhances a patient's safety
   c. An individual-based instructional method of teaching
   d. A self-directed active learning method
6. Which area of planned change in the organization takes place by modifying the cadre and providing better administrative guidance?
   a. Change in management technology
   b. Change in structure
   c. Change in tasks
   d. Change in people
7. Which type of plan includes outcomes, indicators, and measures?
   a. Financial plan
   b. Communication plan
   c. Evaluation plan
   d. Strategic plan
8. Which phase in Lewin's change model makes institutionalized and accepted changes?
   a. Iceberg   b. Changing
   c. Unfreezing   d. Refreezing
9. Which strategy aims to achieve the change in attitude, beliefs, values, and skills among individuals in the organization?
   a. Normative educative
   b. Power coercive
   c. Empirical–rational
   d. Rational educative
10. Which area of planned change requires improvement at micro level of the organization?
    a. Strategy, organizational design, and international relation
    b. Behavior, attitude, and skill of individuals
    c. Leadership development, group dynamics, and work design
    d. Technology, data processing, and decision-making

Answer Keys

1. d   2. a   3. b   4. c   5. a   6. b   7. c.
8. d   9. a   10. c

SUGGESTED READING

1. Burns N, Grove SK. The Practice of Nursing Research, Conduct, Critique, and Utilization. Philadelphia: WB Saunders; 1997.
2. Clark DL. Leadership-change. [Online] Available from: http://www.nwlink.com/~donclark/leader/leadchg.html
3. Five top innovations in nursing education. [Online] Available from: https://www.nursingjobs.com/five-top-innovations-in-nursing-education/
4. Innovation in nursing: a concept analysis. [Online] Available from https://www.omicsonline.org/open-access/innovation-in-nursing-a-concept-analysis-jcphn-1000108.php?aid=66689. [Accessed on 17.01.2019].
5. Innovation in nursing practice: a means of tackling the global challenges facing nurses, midwives and nurse leaders, and managers in the future. [Online] Available from https://onlinelibrary.wiley.com/doi/pdf/10.1111/j.1365-2834.2011.01241.x. [Accessed on 17.01.2019].
6. Lewin K. Field Theory in Social Science. New York: Harper and Row; 1951.
7. Robbins SP, DeCenzo DA. Fundamentals of Management, 3rd edition. Upper Saddle River: Prentice-Hall; 2001.
8. Warren NAM, Ruddle K, Moore K. From organizational development to change management: the emergence of a new profession. J Appl Behav Sci. 1999;35(3):273-86.
9. Welch LB. Planned change in nursing: the theory. Nurs Clin North Am. 1979;14(2):307-21.

16. Program Evaluation Review Technique, Activity Plan, Management by Objectives, and Benchmarking

CHAPTER OUTLINE

- Program Evaluation Review Technique (PERT)
  - Defining PERT
  - Purposes of PERT
  - Features of PERT
  - Operational-Definitions
  - Steps Involved in PERT
  - Advantages
  - Limitations
- Activity Plan (Gantt Chart)
  - What is the Action Plan (Gantt Chart)
  - Purposes of Gantt Chart
  - Features of Gantt Chart
  - Construction of Gantt Chart
  - Uses of Gantt Chart
  - Advantages
- Management by Objectives (MBO)
  - Defining MBO
  - Objectives of MBO
  - Features of MBO
  - Steps in the MBO Process
  - Advantages of MBO
  - Limitations of MBO
  - Implications of MBO in Nursing
- Benchmarking
  - Definitions
  - Aim of Benchmarking
  - Characteristics of Benchmarking
  - Principles of Benchmarking
  - Benefits of Benchmarking
  - Typology of Benchmarking
  - Benchmarking Process

LEARNING OUTCOMES

After completion of this chapter, the learner will be able to:
- Understand program evaluation and review technique (PERT)
- Identify purposes of PERT
- Explain the steps of PERT and its applications in planning and controlling
- Understand the concept of an action plan (Gantt chart)
- Enumerate advantages of Gantt chart
- Understand management by objectives (MBO)
- Describe the process of MBO
- Enumerate advantages and limitations of MBO
- Define benchmarking and highlight its aims and objectives
- Enumerate characteristics and principles of benchmarking
- Appreciate benefits of benchmarking
- Classify benchmarking and discuss benchmarking process

KEY TERMS

Time-event network analysis, program evaluation and review technique (PERT), logistics, activity plan (Gantt chart), management by objectives, benchmarking

INTRODUCTION

Currently, as healthcare is the fastest-growing category of private consumption, hospitals require sufficient resources. It is, therefore, necessary to plan for continuous quality improvement through network analysis by utilizing excellent resources.

A manager uses some tools and techniques to exercise control. One of the methods of planning and control (logistics) is time-event network analysis, which is a realistic plan to depict events and activities to accomplish the objectives. Program evaluation and review technique, Gantt charts, milestone budgeting, and critical path method are the types of time-event network analysis. We will limit our discussion to PERT, Gantt chart, MBO, and benchmarking, which are vital to ensure uniform, high-quality health services.

PROGRAM EVALUATION AND REVIEW TECHNIQUE

Defining PERT

Program evaluation and review technique is a refined version of the original Gantt chart. It is the most advanced and recent technique for logistics (planning, scheduling, and controlling) of program/project-type activities. This technique has replaced the traditional flowchart method for budgeting activities about time.

PERT is a model to analyze and represent the tasks/events involved in the completion of a given program. Booz Allen Hamilton, Inc. developed PERT in 1958. PERT is a refined milestone budgeting. Milestones are identifiable and controllable pieces of a task and form. A PERT/time-event network is a network of many signs and time showing to complete each sign.

Purposes of PERT

- To minimize time and cost for completing a program
- To minimize idle resources
- To improve communication and coordination among different management levels
- To identify issues and obstacles
- To monitor the work progress
- To complete the project so as to minimize time.

Features of PERT

- PERT is a task-oriented technique.
- It may contain hundreds or thousands of events.
- It identifies events (tasks/activities).
- The graph shows the relationship between events.
- It identifies critical activities.
- It specifies the time required to complete each identified event/task/activity.
- It calculates the minimum time for project completion.
- It allows uncertainty in the duration of tasks/activities.
- It includes uncertainty in scheduling time estimates measured by three parameters:
  1. Time estimation based on the assumption that everything will go per plan (optimistic time)
  2. An estimate of time based on whether the time manager thinks that it is necessary to complete the task (most likely time)
  3. An estimate of time based on the assumption that some problem may occur (pessimistic time).

Operational Definitions

- **Program:** A program comprises many tasks/events.
- **Activity:** An activity designates a task or a subproject of the total project. It is an action that goes on between the event with which an operation begins and the event with which it concludes.
- **Event:** An event is "to start," "to finish," "to order," and "to receive." Usually, it terminates one activity and simultaneously represents the beginning of another event.
- **A PERT event:** A PERT event represents the beginning or completion of a task or more tasks.
- **A predecessor event:** An event that comes immediately before another event.
- **A successor event:** An event that occurs quickly after another event.
- **A PERT activity:** It refers to a task that requires a fixed schedule and resources to carry out.
- Critical path: A complete path to finish a program from start to reach the final point. It is the total scheduled time to carry out all activities.
- **Critical activity:** An activity that has no slack time.
- **Slack:** A time is taken to complete an event either on schedule (zero slack), ahead of schedule (positive slack), or behind schedule (negative slack).
- **Expected time of activity (T_E):** A predicted time required to complete a given task, based on the assumption that everything will go per plan.
- **Expected time:** It is the average time needed for a task if repeated.

Steps Involved in PERT

1. Define the objectives of the program/project.
2. Identify and list down both critical and noncritical activities of the project.
3. Arrange all activities in a technological sequence.
4. Locate both predecessor and successor events in sequential order.
5. Estimate the time to complete each activity. It includes elapsed time (days, weeks, and months), "optimistic" time (O) showing the least time of activity, "pessimistic" time (P) indicating the maximum time of activity, and "most likely" time (M) that lies between the two.
6. Calculate T_E (expected time of activity)
   Expected time of activity $(T_E) = (O+4M+P) \div 6$
   where
   O denotes "optimistic" time (time estimation based on the assumption that everything will go per plan)
   P denotes "pessimistic" time (an estimate of time based on the assumption that some problem may encounter, excluding major catastrophes)
   M denotes the "most likely" time (an estimate of time based on whether manager thinks that it is necessary to complete the task).
7. Estimate the shape of the probability distribution for the expected time for each activity. This distribution is described as variance ($\sigma^2 t_e$). Calculate variance using the following formula:
   $$\sigma^2 t_e = (b-a/\sigma)^2$$
   $$SD = \sqrt{\sigma^2 t_e}$$
8. Prepare or draw a draft of the network diagram that should show the relationship between the activities and the events **(Fig. 16.1)** using the arrow diagram, which represents the logical sequence in which the vents must

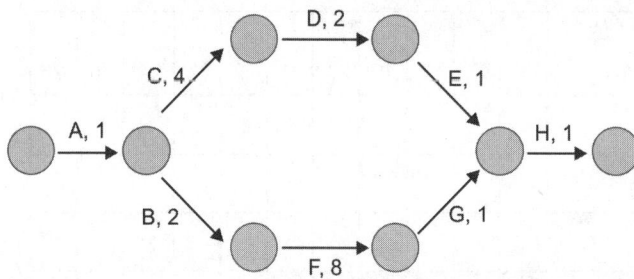

Fig. 16.1: PERT flowchart.

Note:
- The CIRCLE (NODE) indicates the starting and finishing time of the task.
- Each ARROW represents the task-time consuming element.
- Alphabets indicate different TASK and time required to carry out the activity by NUMBERS.

take place. Numbers on the arrow depict the elapsed time estimate.

9. Identify critical path and amount and location of float by subjecting this network to mathematical analysis. Revise the relationship and make changes, if required. Perform another accurate analysis. Steps 1–6 are the line manager's functions, and steps 7–9 are the staff functions for which one needs to have experts in this field.
10. Determine critical path: A complete path to finish a program from start to reach a final point. It is the total scheduled time without any or the least slack time to perform all activities. The events and the time of each event determine the critical path. In **Figure 16.1**, the critical path denotes from A to G with a scheduled time of 12 months.

Advantages

- It is simple, comprehensive, and the most accessible tool for organizational planning and management development, acquisition and installation of a system, and development of projects and programs.
- It is an essential means to improve communication and coordination among different management levels.
- It is a helpful technique to identify various issues and problems during the process.
- It provides grounds for monitoring the continuous and timely progress of the project.
- It provides a base for evaluation and control system.

Limitations

1. There is a chance to omit the necessary step at the time of project planning.
2. Uncertainty is attached to the time estimate.
3. Amount of resources available is a significant restriction.
4. All activities may not be progressing on schedule.
5. Lack of trained staff to adopt PERT/CPM techniques.

ACTIVITY PLAN (GANTT CHART)

What is an Activity Plan (Gantt Chart)?

An activity plan (Gantt chart) is a traditional method of planning that depicts the sequence of tasks to be completed within the set time frame. It is a simple graphical representation of various activities performed in the stipulated time framework or against the progression of time in the form of a bar diagram. It was developed by Henry Gantt, a mechanical engineer, in 1910. It shows time relationships between the "events" of a program; these events are goal oriented.

The Gantt chart is a tool to assess the progress of the program. It shows the relationship between tasks and time duration in the bar diagram to accomplish a plan. Gantt chart can be used in many software tools for project management planning and other activities, for example, one can prepare Gantt charts in Excel program.

Purposes of Gantt Chart

1. To plan and provide a visual graphical illustration of schedule tasks/activities.
2. To track specific critical activity to observe carefully.
3. To monitor and control program activities.
4. For logistics of a project or program.

Features of Gantt Chart

- It gives a graphical illustration of a schedule.
- It is a time-oriented activity plan depicted in the graphical chart.
- It visualizes all activities of the project and total time of the project.
- It represents each event in a bar.
- Each bar represents the time duration of that activity.
- Length of the bar also depicts its starting time and ending time.
- Each event in a bar corresponds to other activity.

Construction of Gantt Chart

A Gantt chart (**Fig. 16.2**) has the following:
- A horizontal line (X-axis) is the time scale over which to complete a program. The length of each task/event bar corresponds to the duration of the task/event. Specify period in days, weeks or months, years, etc.
- A vertical axis/line depicts different activities of the project, e.g. A, B, C, D. List the tasks sequentially/chronologically.
- The event/taskbar depicts the starting time and finishing time of that event/task.
- One event/taskbar describes relationship with another event/taskbars for its starting and ending time, e.g. Task "D" will begin after completing Task "C"; Task "B" will start after 2 weeks of Task "A"; and "C" will start after 4 weeks of Task "A" and after 2 weeks of Task "A" and so on.
- Some tasks are independent, e.g. Task "A" will start at the beginning of a project.

Uses of Gantt Chart

- To represent time and type of task of the project
- To plan and schedule projects

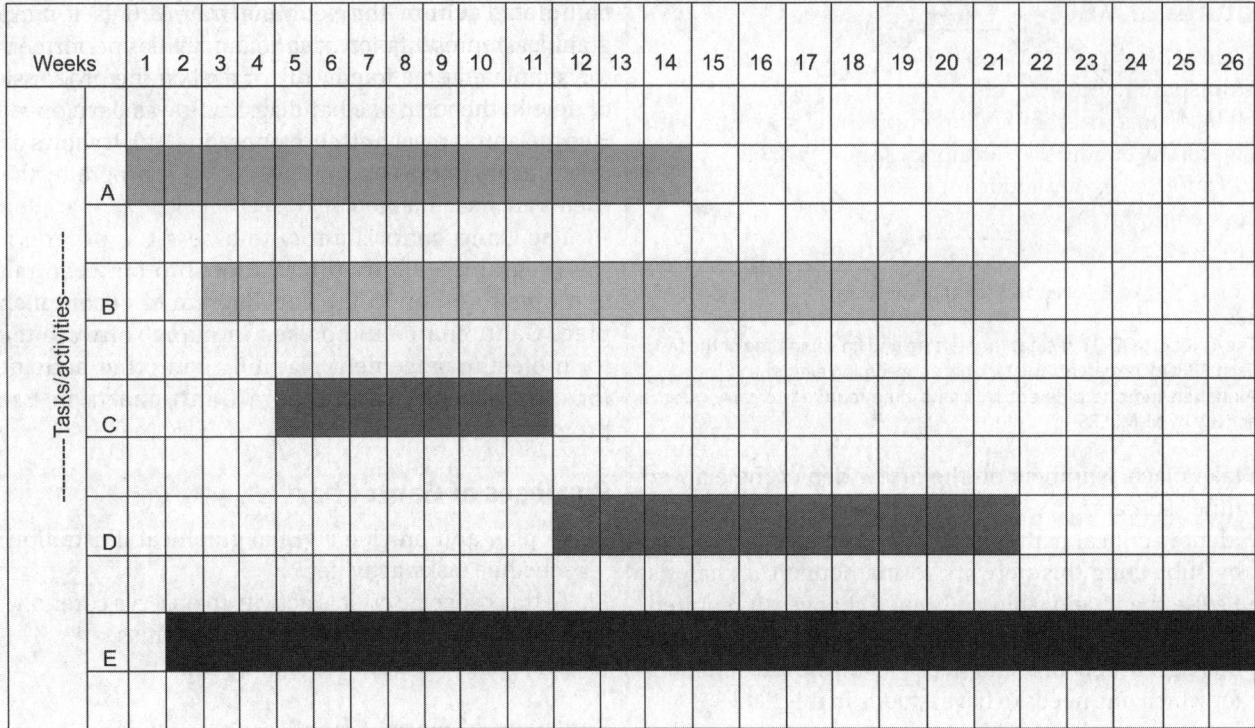

Fig. 16.2: Gantt chart.

- To depict a sequence of the functions
- To monitor the functioning of the project
- To take immediate remedial action if delays.

Advantages

The merits of Gantt chart are as follows:
1. It is simple and easy to use.
2. It represents activities on a scale.
3. It expresses time of each event explicitly.
4. It is easy to understand the starting and completion time of each operation.
5. It makes easy to calculate the total time of the program.
6. It assists in planning, monitoring, and controlling program activities.
7. It depicts a deadline for each action.

MANAGEMENT BY OBJECTIVES

Management by Objectives (MBO) is a boon for healthcare administration and has its implication in nursing. Peter Drucker was the pioneer of introducing the concept of MBO in 1954. George Odiorne, Dale D, McCaskey, and others also contributed to MBO

Defining MBO

- MBO is a process whereby the top and subordinate managers of an organization jointly identify its common goals, determine each significant area of responsibilities regarding the results expected of an individual.
—*Odiorne*

- MBO is a management system that has many management-related activities organized systematically and collaboratively to achieve organizational objectives efficiently and effectively.
—*Heinz Weihrichs and Hernold Koontz*

- MBO is a collective endeavor to create an environment to provide each one with the optimum opportunity to realize his or her full potential. It makes each employee a manager of his or her particular work.
—*George Terry*

Objectives of MBO

The main aim of MBO is helped managers and supervisors to make the most effective use of the human resources such that each member, as a part of a team, creates a maximum contribution to the organizational performance and profitability. The objectives are as follows:
- To identify and define goals and objectives
- To develop strategic and operational plans
- To assign roles, tasks, and responsibilities from managers to employees level
- To ensure proper communication and coordination among employees
- To empower employees to participate in decision-making at the individual level during the whole process
- To direct employees for their actions and guide them to give their level best to achieve goals and objectives
- To set objective-based standards to measure performance
- To facilitate work efficiency in the organization.

Features of MBO

1. The MBO is result oriented, focused on objectives and transparency at all levels.
2. It leads to a well-defined organizational structure with hierarchy and lines of authority.
3. It emphasizes all significant priority areas, appropriate systems, and procedures.
4. Managers and employees anticipate in setting objectives and reviewing performance.
5. It provides an opportunity for subordinates to participate in planning and implementing the program.
6. It believes in role clarity and accountability at different levels.

Steps in the MBO Process

MBO is essentially a philosophy of management, based on identifying the purpose, objectives, strategy, desired results, and evaluating performance in achieving goals. It is a continuous process and has a series of activities (**Fig. 16.3**).

1. **Defining organizational goals and objectives:** The first step in MBO is to define organizational goals based on the mission and purpose of the organization and develop aims and objectives for both short- and long-term organizational, departmental, unit objectives under given appropriate planning premises by analysis and judgment.
2. **Identifying key result areas:** Key result areas (KRAs) indicate the priority areas for organizational performance. It also shows current strengths, weaknesses, opportunities, and threats of the organization and the perspective for the future.
3. **Clarifying organizational roles:** According to goals and subgoals, it defines the role and responsibility of each department/unit manager. Hence, each coordinating manager's contribution is to achieve the organizational goal.
4. **Setting subordinates objectives:** After setting the goals and objectives, identifying KRAs, and clarifying each manager's role in KRAs, the top-level managers work with employees to set and define employees' objectives at par with organizational goals within the specified period and available resources. They along with subordinates develop a strategic and operational plan for each department.
5. **Measuring and monitoring progress:** During this stage of MBO, each departmental manager implements operational plans in their respective departments, and the employees perform their defined roles and responsibility accordingly. The managers monitor actual performance and achievement of each employee against set objectives using the management information system. The senior managers conduct periodic meetings with subordinate managers to discuss the work progress and implementation of the plans.
6. **Continuous tracking and providing feedback:** Providing feedback is a constant process. Managers give ongoing feedback to employees about their performance against set objectives. It is a way of monitoring the employees' performance and guiding them to correct their actions.
7. **Performance evaluation:** Review the performance of employees within the organization regularly and organization as a whole at the end of an operating cycle.
8. **Reevaluating the process:** Reevaluate the whole process, replan, and develop an improvement plan if required (**Fig. 16.4**).

Advantages of MBO

1. It is a goal- and result-oriented process.
2. It identifies structure, strategies, and practice-related problems.
3. It can manage the decentralized operation.
4. It emphasizes in development and utilization of human resources.
5. It exercises participatory management for organizational development.
6. All the superiors and subordinates work together with a team spirit.
7. It coordinates the activities of different units and departments.

Limitations of MBO

- Developing objectives is a difficult task.
- The process of MBO is time consuming.

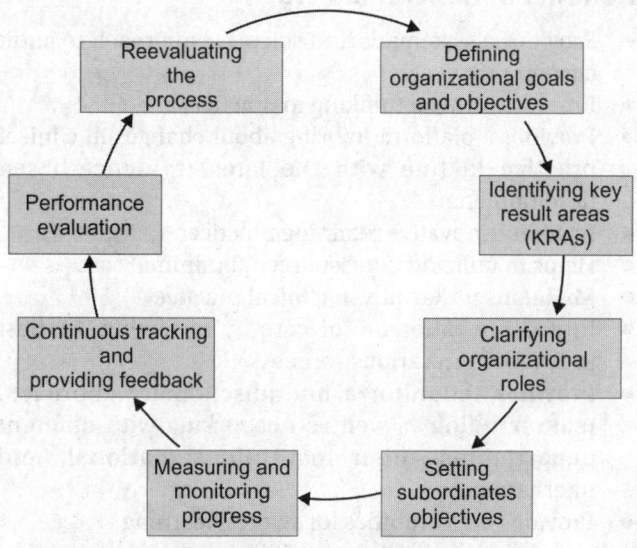

Fig. 16.3: Steps in the process of MBO.

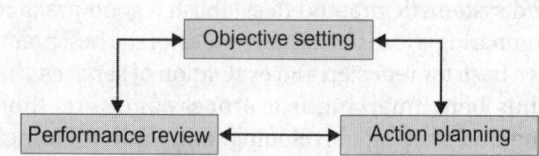

Fig. 16.4: Reevaluation in the MBO process.

- There is a lack of cooperation between management and employees.
- It needs competent and trained managers.
- It lacks flexibility in the revision of objectives.
- It focusses on goal setting and results rather than implementation.
- There is no room for considering external factors.

Implications of MBO in Nursing

MBO is not only essential and useful for business managers but is equally important to nursing administrators to improve the efficiency of nursing personnel. MBO based on Taylorist principles applies in the nursing managerial process. The implementations of MBO are as follows:
- It measures performance.
- It correlates individual performance to organizational goals.
- It clarifies the job responsibilities expected from employees.
- It fosters the increasing competence and growth of the subordinates.
- It provides data to estimate remuneration and promotion.
- It stimulates the subordinate's motivation.
- It helps in organizational work control and integrating the activities.

BENCHMARKING

Benchmarking is a dynamic and continuous process to find out, communicate, and put in action the best practices to attain excellence in performance. It is a constant process of achieving the benchmark. Different authors have been given different viewpoints and viewed differently by a different organization. It has its origin from industry late in the 1970s as an approach to measuring quality, continuously improving performance to become the best performer. JCAHO originated the concept of benchmarking in the 1990s. According to the dictionary, it is considered as a standard to measure something.

Definitions

- According to David Kearns (1980s) and Camp RC (1989 and 1990), benchmarking is a continuous process of comparing products, services, and practices with competitors to be the best in that field. Cook (1995) views benchmarking as a process for improving practices in the organization.
- Vlasceanu et al. (2007) and Department of Health and Social Care, UK (2010) considered it as a standardized and systematic method to establish a good practice by comparing with external references for the best practices as a base for redesign and evaluation of services.

Thus benchmarking is a process and a method of finding out, sharing, developing, and implementing the excellent practices to attain performance of the highest level of client satisfaction.

Aims and Purposes of Benchmarking

- To ensure uniform, high-quality health services
- To search benchmark standards
- To find out benchmark gaps
- To close the benchmark gaps
- To establish benchmark practices
- To bring benchmarking as a component of the management process.

Characteristics of Benchmarking

- It is externally focused and competitive.
- It acts as a standard to compare services and methods within and outside the organization.
- It provides scope for networking to share and compare evidence-based best practices.
- It is viewed regarding performance comparison, searching for the best practices, and continuous improvement.
- It requires the assessment of own and partner organization's performance.
- It is goal oriented to improve practices and provide world-class best services.
- Practices should lead to the performance improvement.
- It is not constant but goes on changing; it needs continuous analysis, comparison, and upgrading to achieve a standard of excellence.
- It is an ongoing process, searching for the best practices of the services, work processes, support facilities, and various strategies.
- It meets the clients' requirements.

Principles of Benchmarking

- Maintain quality and standard of practices
- Client satisfaction
- Continuous improvement in performance.

Benefits of Benchmarking

- Provides a systematic and scientific approach to audit current practices
- Promotes critical thinking to practice
- Provides a platform to bring about changes in clinical practice in line with the latest evidence-based developments
- Ensures innovative retaining practices
- Helps in utilizing the resources at minimal cost
- Maintains uniformity in clinical practice
- Provides a rationale for care by reviewing the best practices from various sources
- Provides scope for a multidisciplinary approach, team building as well as networking with different departments, other institutions, national, and international
- Provides opportunities for sharing learning
- Enhances a sense of responsibility and desire to achieve excellence in service

- Maintains quality and go for continuous improvement in practice
- Helps in fulfilling clients' requirements and satisfaction.

Typology of Benchmarking

There are different forms of benchmarking depending upon (1) the type of partners, (2) nature of the object of study, and (3) purpose of the partnership **(Fig. 16.5)**.

I. According to the type of partners

Benchmarking process, according to the kind of partners, is classified into five categories: (1) internal, (2) external, (3) competitive, (4) functional, and (5) generic.

1. **Internal benchmarking:** It is a process of analyzing, sharing, and comparing the best practices of similar operation among different departments of the same organization. Any department has better performance indicators that will help another department to find the gap and where to improve. Internal benchmarking helps the organization/department to examine itself; provides a baseline for comparison with others to gather information to see the difference or deficiency; and offers an opportunity to share information.
2. **External benchmarking:** It is comparing practices with other organization (1) to find out new ideas, methods, procedures, and services; (2) to monitor continuously improving performance; (3) to identify strengths, weaknesses, opportunities, and threats in systems, practices; (4) and then to find out their ways and means of achieving best performance.
3. **Competitive benchmarking:** This is the approach for a competition of practices with direct competitors in the health market. Purposes of the competition are: (1) to show improvement in the quality of services, (2) to bring out the changes in input, process, and outcome; and (3) to exchange information with the partners to know their progress status.
4. **Functional benchmarking:** This is the approach of comparing practices not only with direct competitors in the health market but also to compare business performance with the best performer by examining evidence and try to seek world-class excellence.
5. **Generic benchmarking:** Comparison should be done with other organizations having the same type of work processes and modification should be done per the standard set by those organizations.

II. According to the type of objective of benchmarking

Benchmarking process, according to its goal, is classified into five categories: (1) process, (2) service (product), (3) strategic, (4) future, and (5) performance benchmarking.

1. **Process benchmarking:** This is a process to find and analyze the cause how to achieve excellent performance by comparing practices and operation.
2. **Service (product) benchmarking:** This is used to compare the functions of the organization.
3. **Strategic (management) benchmarking:** This is a process to compare organization structure and managerial functions.
4. **Future benchmarking:** This is concerned with forward looking to have the best practices with innovative ideas, improvement in knowledge, and practices.
5. **Performance benchmarking:** This is concerned with comparing the performance of the organization with other organizations.

III. According to the purpose of the partnership

Benchmarking process, according to the purpose of the partnership, is classified into two main categories: (1) competitive and (2) collaborative.

1. **Competitive benchmarking:** The primary purpose of partnership in competitive benchmarking is to be the best among all health organizations.
2. **Collaborative benchmarking:** The goal of collaborative benchmarking is inculcate learning environment and to share knowledge with other partner organizations.

Benchmarking Process

As we know, benchmarking is a continuous process for users to adapt, adopt, and improve the approach. For planning and implementing improvements, it uses the following procedures:

PDSA Approach

PDSA is an acronym for four main activities (plan, do, study, and act; **Fig. 16.6**).

1. **Plan:** Plan phase focuses on decisions related to the identification and selection of area (process/function) for benchmarking, benchmark indicators, and benchmarking study, determining data collection methods.
2. **Do:** Doing self-study regarding the selected areas, performance indicators, documenting practices, and collecting data from benchmarking partner.
3. **Study:** Observe gap analysis by comparing the findings of an owner and benchmarking partner either positive or negative, and future project performance. Communicate results and develop functional goals.
4. **Act:** Develop an action plan based on the functional goals and implement strategies to improve negative gaps and

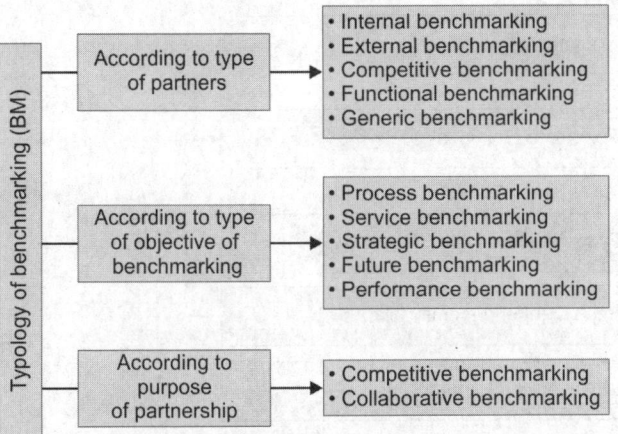

Fig. 16.5: Typology of benchmarking.

maintaining positive ones after performing an action plan, monitor results, and reassess benchmarking.

Phases of the Benchmarking Process

According to Camp (1995), benchmarking process comprises four stages: (1) planning, (2) analysis, (3) integration, and (4) action, which also fit in PDSA cycle for the quality measurement **(Fig. 16.6)**.

Phase I: Planning Phase

The planning phase includes all the activities that a manager will undertake to start the process of benchmarking until the data collection. It has three steps as follows:

Identify areas of benchmarking: The first step in planning benchmarking is to identify an area of practice for benchmarking through the need assessment. The main areas for benchmarking include services, work practices, support facilities, organizational performance, and strategies of the organization. Prioritize the fields according to requirements. Develop purpose, long-term, and short-term objectives for each area. Identify criteria to measure and level of change required in each practice area.

Identify benchmarking partner: After identifying the benchmarking areas, it is essential to find out the competitor partner or the organization. A partner who can openly exchange information for learning and sharing in the areas of interest identify competitive partner from various sources such as the library, internet, web page, annual reports, and so on. There are specific criteria such as location, size of the organization, similarities in services, technology, management style, culture, and accessibility, which should be kept in mind while selecting the partner.

Data collection procedure: Develop a plan for gathering information regarding the best practices of a competitor. Determine the best practices from various sources, both internal and external, e.g. available evidence by reviewing literature, practice guidelines, professional consensus, and others. Prepare preliminary survey form covering the areas of interest and sent to contact persons of the organization or gather information through personal interviews. One can plan a site visit to collect required data through observation. Write a summary of the received information. Plan and develop scoring methods using Likert's scale.

Phase II: Analysis Phase

During the analysis phase, the data collected are analyzed and compared with the set criteria to find out the gap. Based on that difference or deficiencies, future planning can be done to achieve the expected performance.

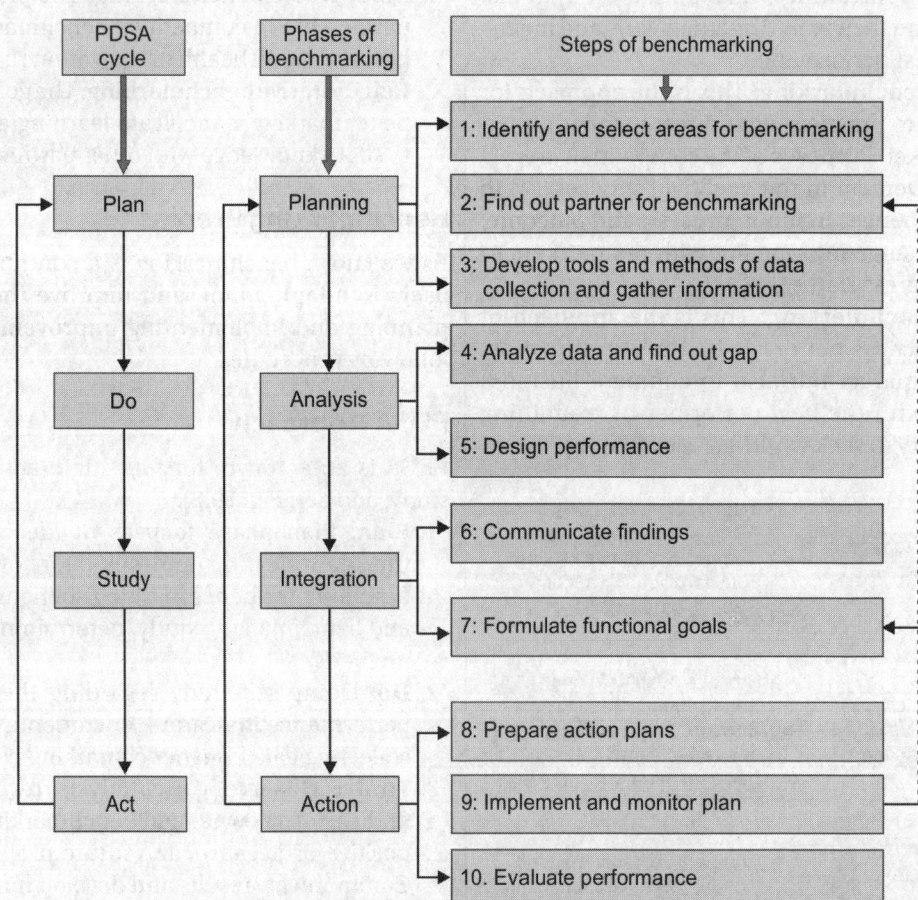

Fig. 16.6: Phases and steps of benchmarking.

Analyze the gap: Analyze the data gathered and found out the results of the benchmark organization on areas of interest regarding its performance and customers' satisfaction. Compare practices of benchmark organization with the current methods of your organization. Find out the gap regarding cost, resources required, quality, and ease of use. The specific performance gap is in quantitative terms.

Project future performance: After finding out the gap in practices performance, plan to make changes for the future. Propose modifications in the current practices within a specific period. Develop the performance measurement criteria to compare the results after the implementation of proposed changes.

Phase III: Integration Phase

During the integration phase, communicate the results to the team members and management. Goals are revised keeping in mind the modification to be incorporated. It has two significant steps, as discussed below:

Communicate results: Prepare a report and future planning. Communicate to all concerned staff about the proposed modification required in the current practices. Motivate them to adopt those changes, and make them understand the importance of changes in the current methods of different areas.

Develop functional goals: After communicating the plan to all concerned, revise the goals. Develop goals in measurable terms. Formulate realistic standards for each identified area. Seek approval from management. Management commitment and support are essential at this stage to bring about required changes in practices.

Phase IV: Action Phase

During this phase, develop an action plan; take approval from the management, before it is implemented to close the gap. Measure performance and proceed appropriate remedial actions. The practices are evaluated periodically to sustain benchmarking in the organization.

Develop an action plan: Determine priorities in work practices to be implemented and develop outcome-oriented performance criteria to close the gap. Prepare an activity schedule. Break down all tasks into various steps and list down in sequence. Plan out resources required for each function. Get approval from management before implementing the action plan. Select appropriate staff; assign them responsibilities and deadlines to accomplish a particular task. Offer training to the selected team for the assigned job. Communicate them about the changes in the current practices. The team should also show commitment, motivation, and dedication on their part.

Executing and monitor plans: After getting approval from the management, implement the action plan with trained staff. Monitor performance of team recruited for the job. Develop timeline charts to monitor and control execution.

Any variance if observed should be corrected immediately. Provide feedback. Retain the most successful operations and eliminate the least successful services.

Reassess benchmarks: Reassess benchmarks to identify areas of improved practice. Evaluate benchmarking or "the best from the best" practices regarding performance and customers' satisfaction continuously and periodically. Changes should be made accordingly to sustain benchmarking to adopt best practices.

Phase V: Maturity Phase

Realization regarding the importance of change in benchmarking becomes a critical component of the management process. Identify the performance gap and try to integrate the excellent services into the process.

CHAPTER HIGHLIGHTS

- PERT is a technique for the planning and scheduling project. It is an event-oriented technique.
- The critical path is a complete path to finish a program from start to reach a final point. It is the total scheduled time to carry out all activities.
- Activity plan depicts the sequence of tasks to be completed within the set time frame.
- A Gantt chart is a simple graphical table depicts various activities performed in the stipulated time framework in the form of a bar diagram.
- MBO is a process whereby the top and subordinate managers of an organization jointly identify its common goals, define each significant area of responsibilities regarding the results expected of an individual.
- Benchmarking is a dynamic and continuous process to find out, communicate, and put in action the best practices to attain excellence in performance, and classified according to the type of partners, the objective of benchmarking, and purpose of the partnership.

REVIEW QUESTIONS

I. Essay Type Questions
1. What do you mean by the term PERT? Discuss its features.
2. Describe essential steps of PERT process.
3. Define the Gantt chart. Describe how to construct a Gantt chart.
4. What do you mean by benchmarking? Write the process of benchmarking in detail.
5. Describe the steps of MBO.

II. Short Notes
1. Advantages of PERT
2. Benefits of benchmarking
3. Purposes and uses of Gantt chart
4. Activity planning
5. Objectives of MBO

III. Multiple Choice Questions

1. Who develops program evaluation and review technique?
   a. Camp
   b. Kearns
   c. Hamilton, Inc
   d. Kozak
2. Which technique is event oriented in network analysis?
   a. CPM
   b. Benchmarking
   c. Gantt
   d. PERT
3. In PERT, when the time is estimated based on assumptions that some problem may encounter during the process is known as:
   a. Pessimistic
   b. Most likely
   c. Optimistic
   d. Elapsed
4. A point that represents the beginning or completion of a task or more tasks is known as:
   a. Activity
   b. PERT activity
   c. Event
   d. PERT event
5. A complete path to finish a program from start to reach a final point on is:
   a. A time-event network
   b. A critical path
   c. A PERT event
   d. A milestone bridging
6. What does the "CIRCLE" in PERT flowchart indicate?
   a. Beginning and ends of task
   b. Task-time consuming the element
   c. Duration of task
   d. Elapsed time required completing the task
7. When does the Gantt chart develop as a planning tool?
   a. 1905
   b. 1910
   c. 1915
   d. 1920
8. A benchmarking that analyze, share, and compare practices of similar operations among departments of the organization is known as:
   a. Functional benchmarking
   b. Process benchmarking
   c. Internal benchmarking
   d. Competitive benchmarking
9. In which of the following statements, process benchmarking is concerning to achieve the excellent performance:
   a. Comparing, analyzing performance level, and finding a gap
   b. Comparison of practices with direct competitors
   c. Comparing and analyzing the cause
   d. Comparison of practices with other organizations
10. A process of creating an environment to provide each one with the optimum opportunity to realize his or her full potential and a particular work refers to:
    a. PERT
    b. Benchmarking
    c. CPM
    d. MBO

Answer Keys

1. c   2. d   3. a   4. d   5. b   6. a   7. b
8. c   9. c   10. d

SUGGESTED READING

1. Arthur A, Thomson, Jr, Strictland AJ, et al. (Eds). Readings in Strategic Management, 5th edition. Chicago Irwin; 1995.
2. Available from: http://www.scholarshipeasy.com/tags/critical-path-method-CPM-pert.html. [Accessed on 20.01.2019].
3. Burke CJ. 10 steps to best practices are benchmarking. Quality Digest. 1996;23-28.
4. Druker P. Management, Tasks, Responsibilities, and Practices. New York: Harper & Row; 1974.
5. Essence of care 2010-GOV.UK. [Online] https://www.gov.uk/government/publications/essence-of-care-2010 accessed on 07.01.2020.
6. Gantt chart. Available from: http://www.ganttchart.com/. [Accessed on 21.01.2019].
7. Krajewski LJ, Ritzman LP. Operations Management: Strategy, and Analysis, 5th edition. Indian Reprint. Addison Wesley (Pearson Education); 2002.
8. Levinson H. Management by whose objectives? Adapted by Elaine L. La Monica. J Nurs Admin. 1980;10:23-30.
9. Miglore RH, Gunn BJ. Strategic planning/management by objectives. Hosp Top. 1995;73:26-32.
10. Odiorne G. Management by Objectives: A System of Managerial Leadership. New York: Pitman; 1965.
11. O'Rourke L, Santalucia P, Papson A, et al. Handbook on Applying Environmental Benchmarking in Freight Transportation-NCFRP Report 21. Washington DC; 2012.
12. Stroud, JD. Understanding the purpose and use of benchmarking. Six Sigma. [Online] Available from: http://www.isixsigma/understanding-purpose-use-benchmarking/. [Accessed on 20.01.2019].
13. Weihrichs H, Koontz H. Management. New York: McGraw-Hill; 1993.
14. West JD, Ferdinand KL. A Management Guide to PERT/CPM, 2nd edition. Prentice-Hall, NJ: Englewood Cliffs; 1977.

SECTION 4

Fundamentals of Organization, Planning and Organizing Hospital Nursing and Ancillary Services

17. Organization and Organization Structure
18. Organizational Climate and Organizational Effectiveness
19. Planning of Hospitals and Patient Care Units
20. Ward Management and Methods of Patient Assignment
21. Planning and Organizing Ancillary Services
22. Planning for Emergency and Disaster Management

17 CHAPTER

Organization and Organization Structure

CHAPTER OUTLINE

- Basics of Organization
  - Concept of Organization
  - Defining Organization
  - Characteristics of Organization
  - Principles of Organization
  - Objectives of Organization
- The Formal and Informal Organization
- Organization Theories
- Minimum Requirements for an Organization
- Organization Structure
  - Basic Parts of an Organization Structure
  - Features of an Organization Structure
  - Organization Charts
- Types of Organization
  - Line Organization
  - Functional Organization
  - Line and Staff Organization
  - Committee Form of Organization

LEARNING OUTCOMES

After completion of this chapter, the learner will be able to:
- Understand the fundamentals of organization
- Differentiate formal with informal organizations
- Describe organizational theories
- Enumerate minimum requirement of an organization
- Discuss organization structure
- Describe different types of organizations

KEY TERMS

Organization, formal and informal organization, organization charts, organization theories, organization structure, line, staff, committee

INTRODUCTION

An organization is one of the important elements of the management process and next to planning. It is like a nucleus of a cell around which the human efforts revolve to achieve the objectives. A sound organization essentially conducts all managerial activities efficiently and effectively. The success of the management is determined by its sound organization.

BASICS OF ORGANIZATION

Concept of Organization

The organization is the act of organizing or the state of being organized. It refers to an organized structure as a whole. It is a functional group working together for achieving everyday purposes/objectives. According to Urwick, it is the act of designing and building the administrative structure, and sometimes it is the structure itself. The classics have used the term organization in the form of organizing which is a part of the management process.

1. **Organization as a structure**
   The organization is a structure that describes the relationships among individuals and positions that they hold. According to Wheeler, the organization is the structural framework of the duties and responsibilities of personnel in performing various functions within the enterprise. Organization chart reveals a formal relationship among the employees and clarifies the authority and responsibilities of each position either horizontally or vertically. Horizontally, it has various departments; vertically, it creates a hierarchy of

superiors and subordinates. It has a pyramid shape and acts as a framework to facilitate managerial actions.

In a static sense, the organization is a structure operated by a group of individuals to work together to achieve a common goal. Structure denotes an established pattern of relationships among the parts of the organization. Thus organization structure provides a framework in which people can work happily to bring out a productive outcome.

2. **Organization as a group of people**
   Organization refers to different groups created either formally or informally. It is composed of people who interact among themselves to achieve some common objectives. It is the rational coordination of the activities of some people for the achievement of some common purpose or goal, through the division of labor and functions and a hierarchy of authority and responsibility.

3. **The organization has both structure and human being**
   The organization, as the structure of the relationship, is a vehicle to attain the predetermined goals. It has both structure and human being. As the organization is the systematic bringing together interdependent parts to form a unified whole to exercise authority, coordinate, and control to achieve a given purpose. The interdependent parts are the people who need direction and motivation to work.

4. **The organization as a process**
   The organization is a dynamic process and managerial activity. It is a management tool for the effective pursuit of a common goal. It is a process that defines responsibilities, delegates' authority, and coordinate activities among the employees. It involves the following:
   - Identifying various activities and dividing the work
   - Grouping the activities into workable units/departments
   - Defining, assigning and delegating responsibilities and authority (centralization/decentralization)
   - Defining hierarchy and relationship between superiors and subordinates
   - Developing a system of coordination to integrate the activities.

5. **Organization as a system**
   The organization is a system comprised many interrelated subsystems. It has an identifiable boundary that distinguishes it from the macro environment. The boundary defines the domain of the system that can be open or closed. The social system has open boundaries, whereas physical and mechanical systems have closed boundaries. Within microenvironment, all subsystems interrelate with each other. A system is a whole, a set of connected things or parts. Each system consists of five elements: (1) input, (2) process, (3) output, (4) controls (monitoring), and (5) feedback **(Fig. 17.1)**.
   - *Inputs* include various resources required to carry out various activities to attain organizational objectives.

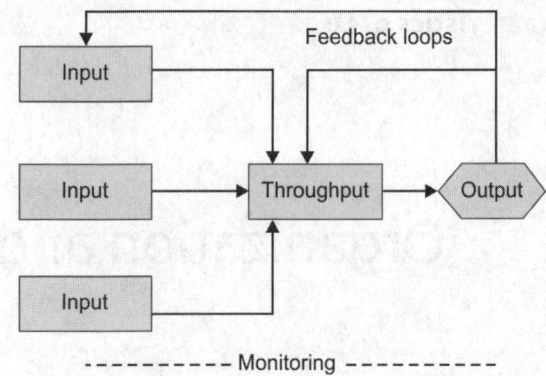

Fig. 17.1: Organization as a system.

- *Throughput* is a process that includes a series of activities to implement a specific action plan. It is an implementation phase where activities of people aligned, moved along, and carefully coordinated to achieve the goals set for the system.
- *Outputs* are the results of the implemented plan in the system. It is in the form of product or services delivered to the clients. **The outcome** is the benefit that clients get after the action plan, e.g. enhanced quality of life for patients.
- *Feedback* is responses of employees who implement plans, customers/clients using the products and services regarding the result or outcome.

Defining Organization

Many authors defined the term "Organization" various ways as given below:
- An organization constitutes an identifiable group of people contributing their efforts towards the attainment of goals.

  —*Mc Farland*
- The organization comprises a group of people cooperating under the leadership for the accomplishment of a common end.

  —*RC Davis*
- Organization refers to a grouping of activities necessary to attain objectives of an enterprise and assigning each group to a manager with authority, essential to supervise it.

  —*Koontz and O' Donnell*
- The organization is the formal structure of power through which work subdivisions are arranged, defined, and coordinated for the defined objectives.

  —*Luther Gulick*
- The organization is a process of purposive and systematic assigning functions, duties, and responsibilities among members of a team. It describes the roles of each member of an enterprise expected to perform.

  —*Dale Yoder*
- According to George R Terry "Organization is the establishment of the productive behavioral relationship among the selected work persons and workplaces for the group to work together efficiently."

Chapter 17: Organization and Organization Structure

Characteristics of Organization

Some characteristics of organization are listed below:
1. **Organizing is an essential function of management:** In any organization, organizing is a primary function of management to achieve its goals. These functions are planning, staffing, directing, and controlling.
2. **The organization has common goals and objectives:** The organization has common goals and objectives that help to divide operations into suitable jobs, authority, and responsibility.
3. **The organization creates a structure of relationships:** The managerial structural link in the organization refers to a formal organization. The organization includes a social relationship that formed an informal organization. Both formal and intimate relationships are essential to achieve the goals of the organization.
4. **The organization is a process:** It is a process whereby some activities take place systematically to achieve a common goal. It is a process of purposive and systematic assigning functions, duties, and responsibilities among the members of a team.

Principles of Organization

An organization constitutes a group of people cooperating and contributing their efforts towards the attainment of goals. It creates a structure of relationships and provides a framework for the performance of managerial activities. There are principles of organization, which are essential to apply for the success of an organization.

1. **Principle of objectives:** According to this principle, sharing goals and objectives are essential for an active organization. The organization must develop its goals and objectives according to its philosophy and purpose.
2. **Principle of specialization:** Specialization means dividing the tasks according to the skill and qualification of the individuals. It is one of the features of the line organization. Divide the whole activities of the organization and assign according to specialization to get the best from the individuals.
3. **Principle of coordination:** It means that the organization must observe the coordination of activities of different departments to achieve a common organizational goal.
4. **Principle of authority and responsibility:** This principle of the organization refers that the power must flow from top to bottom in the line structure. The superior must delegate the duties to an immediate subordinate with or without accountability depending on the situation.
5. **Principle of defining authority:** It means that the management in the organization must determine the power and responsibilities of managers of every level and to heads of departments. There should be clarity in the relationship among all departments.
6. **Principle of the span of control:** According to this principle, the management must assign a proportionate number of persons under a supervisor to control their work. It accounts for a maximum number of subordinates supervised by a superior for adequate control.
7. **Principle of balance:** It helps an organization to follow a proper and equal distribution of work policy among all individuals.
8. **Principle of uniformity:** The organization must observe the consistency of workload in all the departments. Each department must have a separate head to avoid confusion and conflict.
9. **Principle of flexibility and continuity:** The organization must continually evaluate its function and modify according to the situation. The organization structure should be flexible to adapt to changing conditions and permit expansion or replacement without any severe disruption. There should be an in-built arrangement to facilitate the growth and development of an organization.
10. **Principle of unity of command:** The organization should follow unity of command from top to bottom. An individual must report and accountable to only one head to avoid confusion and conflict.
11. **Principle of exception:** It means that the top management must concentrate only policy and planning functions and must assign/delegate the rest of supervisory duties to lower-level management. It will improve organizational efficiency and development.
12. **Principle of simplicity:** The structure of the organization must be simple. Everyone from managerial to operational level must be clear about their authority, responsibilities, and assignments. It will help in the successful operation of an organization.
13. **Principle of efficiency:** It means that ability is vital in the organization. The organization must prepare goal-oriented policies, standards, and procedures to run all the activities smoothly to achieve its goals and objectives within the set time.
14. **Scalar principle:** This principle suggests that as far as possible, the chain of authority should be short without interruption. The power must descend from top to lower level.

Objectives of Organization

The list below provides the objectives of organization:
1. To facilitate all managerial functions.
2. To provide a framework for the performance of managerial activities. It helps the administrators to create structure and effective utilization of various resources to produce the desired services.
3. To define the authority and responsibility of each category and reduce conflict over the use of authority.
4. To lead specialization as it divides the work according to qualification, experience, and specialty.
5. To have a formal line of communication for the coordination of the activities with inter and intradepartments.

6. To ensure to place every employee on the job according to their capability to utilize in a better way.
7. To create a team that represents reasonable, unified efforts towards a single shared objective.
8. To direct human efforts to achieve the set objectives as acts as an essential tool and essential vehicle.
9. To help the employees to discharge their job duties and avoid the duplication of effort through well-defined job descriptions.
10. To facilitate growth and expansion by encouraging employees to think and give innovative ideas to bring an effective change.
11. To provide a broader scope to introduce new methods and technology.

THE FORMAL AND INFORMAL ORGANIZATION

The organization structure is a basic framework that deals with human beings. Two types of relationships formal and informal exist in the organization. Both formal and informal organizations are essential for the effective functioning of the organization.

Formal Organization

Formal organizations refer to the organization structure designed to achieve its objectives. It is structured, stable, and static. It has defined hierarchical levels and relationships, authority, responsibility and accountability, and channels of control and coordination.

Features of Formal Organization

The following lists the features of formal organization:
- It is official and consciously designed, and follows the division of work principle.
- It has a well-defined organizational structure with an established line of authority and responsibility.
- Its structure is stable and very rigid.
- It reveals a span of control, lines of communication and command, and control.
- It has functional processes to achieve the organizational goals.

Advantages of Formal Organization

The following shows the advantages of formal orgnization:
- It provides the basic structure showing division of work and responsibilities.
- It has clearly defined goals and objectives.
- It gives a well-defined hierarchical structure.
- It has organizational plans and policies.
- It promotes discipline in the organization.
- It encourages to adopt new practices.

Disadvantages of Formal Organization

The following shows the disadvantages of formal organization:
- It has a lack of flexibility.
- It does not allow long-term planning.
- It lacks the scope of creativity.

Informal Organization

Informal organization refers to social groups having relationships among its employees. They develop a relationship with personal attitudes, likes and dislikes, feelings, emotions, prejudices, cultures, norms, rather than work consideration. It influences the functioning of the organization by exchange and dissemination of information in the organization. Informal organization originates from the formal organization.

Features of Informal Organization

The features of informal organization are as follows:
1. The groups form spontaneously and constantly.
2. The relationship created by trust and exchange of information.
3. It is dynamic and responsive and treats the individual as human beings.
4. Personal attitudes, emotions, likes, dislikes, and other social factors are the base for interaction.
5. It has an informal communication network or a grapevine.
6. Its focus is on individual and group goal.
7. It helps to improve motivation among employees.

Advantages of Informal Organization

The list below provides the advantages of informal organization:
- It inculcates cultural and social norms.
- It provides social status and satisfaction.
- It helps to have social control by regulating behavior.
- It encourages effective communication among employees.
- It fills gaps of formal structures and widens the effective span of control.

Disadvantages of Informal Organization

The list below provides the disadvantages of informal organization:
- The employees may show resistance to change.
- There is the possibility of role conflict.
- It provides room for rumors and conformity.

Formal Versus Informal Organizations

Both organizations differ by their structure, focus, concerns, nature, and formation, the source of power, size, and communication **(Table 17.1)**.
1. **Structure:** The formal organization has a well-defined structure with legal authority relationships. The informal organization has no clear cut structure and developed spontaneously with personal and social relations among employees.

Chapter 17: Organization and Organization Structure

TABLE 17.1: Difference between formal and informal organization.

Basis	Formal	Informal
Structure	Well structured	Not defined
Focus	Position	People (employees)
Major concerns	Authority and responsibility	Power and politics
Purpose	To achieve organizational goals and objectives	Individual and group goals based on social needs
Nature	Official	Unofficial
Formation	Planned and deliberate	Developed spontaneously among people associated with each other
Source of power	Delegated	Given by group
Rigidity	Based on rigid rules and regulations and follows a strict structure	Based on social relations, thus loosely structured
Interdependence	Exist independently	Dependent on people working in a formal organization
Size	Tends to large	Tends to small
Tenure	Stable, permanent, and predictable	Unstable, continually changing, and unpredictable
Communication	Follows official formal channel	Social and grapevine
Leadership	Superior are the leaders by position	Group members select leader
Source of control	Rewards and penalties	Sanctions
Flow of authority	From top to bottom	No fixed line of authority follows leaders instructions
Rules	Well defined and violation leads to penalties	As per social norms
Human behavior	Does not take care of human sentiments	It is by attitudes, likes, and dislikes of members
Presentation	Depicted in organizational charts	Not shown in organizational charts

2. **Focus:** The formal organization focuses on different levels/positions in the hierarchy. The informal organization is employees focused.
3. **Major concerns:** Authority and responsibility are the significant concerns informal organization while power and politics are the concern of the informal organization.
4. **Purpose:** The formal organization is to achieve organizational goals and objectives; the informal organization satisfies the social needs of the employees.
5. **Nature:** The formal organization is official and consciously designed, but the informal organization formed spontaneously thus unofficial.
6. **Formation:** The formal organization is static and stable. Informal relations existence automatically by likes and dislikes in the informal organization.
7. **Source of power:** In the formal organization, power flows from the top to down levels in the organization. The members of the informal groups within the organization have informal group power.
8. **Rigidity:** The formal organization observes rigid procedures and policies, rules, regulations, and delegation. But the informal organization follows social relation, social norms, and the conduct of individuals within the organization. It is highly flexible and continually changing.
9. **Interdependence:** Formal organization can work independently. But informal organization depends on people working in the formal organization.
10. **Size and tenure:** Formal organization is large, stable and impersonal in conduct; the informal organization depends on rumors and communication is, like grapevine, small and unstable.
11. **Communication:** There are fixed lines of communication in the formal organization. The informal organization has informal channels of communication which are flexible and very fast.
12. **Leadership:** Superiors by position, exercise power, and leadership in the formal organization. In the informal organization the members select leader.
13. **Source of control:** In the formal organization, the discipline maintains through rules and regulations and takes disciplinary actions as per rules. The informal organization follows group norms.

ORGANIZATION THEORIES

There are three organization theories: (1) classic, (2) neoclassic, and (3) modern theories.

Classical Theory of Organization

Classic theory of organization is a structural theory considering the organization as a close system. The organization is a machine, and individuals working in the organization are its components. Its major concepts are structural related.

Major Concepts

1. The organization is like a machine, and human beings are its essential components.
2. Human beings are necessary for effective working of an organization.
3. It includes thoughts of scientific and administrative management.
4. Scientific management is concerning with the task performance by the lower-level employees to achieve the goals.
5. The emphasis is for identifying and grouping of activities according to specialization lead to departmentation.
6. Division of work, departmentation, coordinated effort, and human are its main features.
7. There is no room for the sociopsychological and motivation aspects of human behavior.
8. It is a task-oriented structural theory of organization.

Criticism

- The classical theory believes in the line and staff structure.
- It emphasizes the decision-making process.
- It ignores the sociopsychological behavior of individuals.
- Environment influences organization and vice versa but has no interaction.

Neoclassic Theory of Organization

The neoclassic theory of organization believes in a humanistic approach. According to this theory, the organization is a social system and the individuals are essential assets for the effective functioning of the organization.

Major Concepts

1. The organization being a social system must have an informal organization within a formal organization.
2. Human behavior is essential and viewed regarding social factors to influence work.
3. Sociopsychological variables such as attitudes, emotions, interests, needs, norms of conduct affect the motivation and morale of individuals towards the accomplishment of objectives.
4. Teamwork and motivated individuals are essential for higher productivity.
5. Individual and organizational goals must conform.
6. Reward as discipline and control measure.
7. Communication is critical to the functioning of the organization and the individuals.

Merits

- It develops the concept of informal organization.
- It emphasizes the role of human approach in organizational functioning.

Criticism

- No consideration for the structural aspect of the organization.
- The individuals may have conflicting interests, attitudes, and so on.
- The organization structure format may not apply to all the organizations.
- It lacks a unified approach and only focuses on the humanistic, behavioral approach.

Modern Theory of Organization

Modern theory has a conceptual and analytical base. The concepts derived from empirical research and integrated into a different situation in the organization. It is the combination of system and contingency approaches.

By the system approach, the organization can study its totality. Internal and external factors influence the organization. It has subsystems—each subsystem has its processes, roles, structure, and norms of conduct. There are mainly five subsystems: technical, supportive, functional, adaptive, and managerial. The system approach suggested the model of organization structure without considering external and internal factors.

The contingency approach suggested the design of the structure of the organization according to the situation and factors that influence the function of an organization. It emphasizes to consider factors such as environment, technology, size, and type of activities nod people while deciding a structure of the organization.

MINIMUM REQUIREMENTS FOR AN ORGANIZATION

An active organization must fix up the duties and responsibilities of all employees and certain degree and type of authority power of all managerial levels' personnel. It must ensure proper supervision and control, effective communication channel, and facilitates expansion and development of the organization. An effective organization has the following minimum requirements.

1. **Well-defined organizational set up:** The organization must have a well-defined organizational setup. It must have credibility and reputation within the profession/business. The top management must be competent and dynamic. They should know interest and know all aspects of organizing and managing the activities of the organization. They should possess leadership and entrepreneurship qualities.
2. **Legal requirements:** The organization must fulfill the legal requirements of registration and other formalities to set up. It must be a registered legal entity.
3. **Clear vision and mission:** The organization must have a clear vision, mission, and philosophy.
4. **Defined goals, objectives, and policies:** The management must be clear about the organizational goals and objectives. The organizational policies must aim to achieve the goals and define clearly, and all managers at different levels must know about the procedures. The management must set the priority areas as per its requirement.
5. **Organization structure:** The organization must have a defined structure. The essentials should be remembered while developing and planning to create an organizational structure. It must depict a line of communication, a line of authority and responsibility, and superior-subordinate relationships very clearly.
6. **Strategic and operational plans:** An effective organization must have strategic and operational plans, systems, processes, and other requirements of quality assurance. These are essential for the successful functioning of an enterprise.
7. **Standards, protocols, and guidelines:** Each department must maintain the minimum standards and should have well-defined protocols and instructions for each activity.

8. **Defined resource parameters:** It must be defined that minimum resources should be available as per the norms for a particular organization. These must be defined clearly. There should be adequate funding sources, facilities, and staff.
9. **Adequate supervision and control system:** There should be effective supervision and control systems to operationalize and monitoring different plans and procedures. The management must define the realistic span of control. There should be a well-defined performance appraisal system, and every employee must be aware of it.
10. **Coordination and cooperation:** The entire department must coordinate and cooperate for the attainment of objectives. The employees must have a positive attitude, high morale, and motivation towards work.
11. **Effective management of personnel:** The successful organizations have adequate personnel policies to recruit, select, place, develop, and retain them in the organization. The organization must have various motivational strategies, occupational health safety measures, security, and other benefits policies to manage the employees of all level. They are the asset and lifeblood of the organization. They need to handle and control carefully.
12. **Organization development and expansion:** Competent staff should manage and support their regular activities. They should commit and information regarding future programs for the development and maintenance of standards. The organization must have the flexibility to cope up and update the process as per the changing environment. It must attain certification, accreditation and facilitate auditing for its improvement and progression.

ORGANIZATION STRUCTURE

Organization structure refers to the formally established pattern of relationship among the various parts of any organization; whereas "formal" means deliberately, specified and adopted and does not evolve at its own; and "established" means the relationship when spelled out and accepted by everyone. It is the framework of the organization to carry out the whole management process. O'Neill et al. (2001) viewed structure as the degree of centralization of decision-making, formalization of rules, authority, and communication. It includes standardization of work processes skills and control of the output.

The structure is the foundation of the whole superstructure of management. It binds managers and employees to work together to attain common objectives. The organization needs to establish a proper organizational structure for its efficient functioning.

Basic Parts of Organization Structure

There are five essential parts of the organization structure—(1) strategic apex, (2) middle line, (3) operating core, (4) technostructure, and (5) supporting staff. Strategic apex, middle line, and operating core are in a single line of hierarchical authority and the functional levels in the organization.

- Strategic apex comprises the people with overall responsibilities for the organization, that is, board, chief executive and other top-level managers. They are concerned with setting goals, plan, and policies, develop strategies to implement programs, and accomplish goals.
- The middle line is the linking between the strategic apex and the operating core. The chain runs from superior managers down to first-line supervisors.
- The operating core consists of all those who perform the necessary work related to production or services. It is the heart of the organization that is a concern with the output. It secures the input for service.
- Technostructure and supporting staff are in the right and left of the middle line who assist people of the strategic apex and middle line in carrying out all activities and advising management.

Features of an Organization Structure

The following is the list of features of an organization structure:
1. The organization must possess a clearly defined line of authority that flows from top to the bottom level.
2. The delegation of authority must go with assigned responsibility.
3. The organization must have less managerial levels to avoid delay in decision-making.
4. The supervisor must have a manageable person under supervision.
5. The structure must be simple to avoid confusion and flexible to cope up with changing needs and have scope for expansion.

Organization Charts

An organization chart is a simple diagrammatic method of describing an organization structure. Daniel C. McCallum was the first who introduced organization chart in 1855. This chart is like a blueprint of a building. It indicates departments, formal relationship, and relative ranks of its positions, a chain of command, and communication. It is the link between departments by authority and responsibility. The organization charts usually have boxes with titles which represent various positions or levels in the organization; the distance of the box from the top indicates its place in the hierarchy and lines joining the different ranks represent the formal reporting relationship between superiors and subordinates.

Features of Organization Chart

The features of organization chart are as follows:
- It has a diagrammatical presentation.
- It represents the formal organization structure.

- It shows the lines of authority and a formal relationship in the organization.
- It indicates the channel of communication and department linkages.

Advantages of Organization Chart

The list below shows the advantages of organization chart:
1. It brings clarity about organization structure both to the employees and outsiders.
2. It serves as a quick method of visualizing an organization.
3. It is useful in familiarizing and training new employees.
4. It provides particular departmental information to use in planning and budgeting purposes.
5. It provides an effective way to communicate organizational and employee's information.
6. It is an invaluable management tool, allows to organize the teams with clear responsibilities, titles, and lines of authority.

Limitations of Organization Chart

Organization chart also has some limitations, which are as follows:
1. It provides a static structure of the organization.
2. It lacks in giving details of organization structure.
3. It limits to show only formal relationships and channels of communication.
4. It requires in revealing social relations and the managerial styles.
5. It leads to rank consciousness among the staff and destroys team spirit.

Types of Organization Chart

There are different ways of presenting organization in charts such as hierarchical, matrix, flat, horizontal, and circular charts.
1. **Hierarchical** charts indicate the formal structure of an organization. The vertically placed boxes represent the ranks; horizontally placed boxes represent the departments or level. The boxes may vary in size; the top position managers may have a big size box than their subordinates. The same levels generally have boxes of similar size. Laterally placed boxes indicate a relationship between departments on the same level of hierarchy in the organization.
2. **Matrix** chart depicts the same level employees in a group reporting to their respective manager. It has two axes representing two chains of command. The vertical axis represents functional/hierarchy structure; the horizontal axis represents the group of people of different technical departments.
3. **The flat** chart has few or no horizontal layers/lines. It may depict only top- and lower-level managers applicable only in small or individual unit organizations.
4. **Horizontal chart** has a pyramid shape, that is, narrow at the top and broad at the bottom.
5. **Circular chart** depicts top management at the center of the circle and other management levels in concentric circles.

TYPES OF ORGANIZATION

There are various types of formal organizational structures. Each organization has to create its organizational structure. The form of organization mainly depends on the activities of organization, size, and competence of personnel and philosophy of the organization. The essential types of organization are line organization, functional, line and staff organization, and committee form of organization.

Line Organization

The line organization is the oldest form of administrative organization. It originated from the Roman army and later adopted by armies of all over the world. The authority flows from top to bottom. The responsibility flows in an upward direction. It is also known as a scalar/vertical and departmental organization. The top management always takes significant decisions.

It is of two types—pure and departmental line organization. In genuine line organization, all employees of the same level do a similar kind of functions and division supervises and controls the functions (Fig. 17.2). In the departmental line organization, the organization divided into departments, and each department have different features. The whole organization is under the control of one administrator. Each department has its separate head that gets order and reports to the organization administrator.

Features of the Line Organization

Line organization has the following features:
- It is the simplest form of organization.
- Authority flows from top to bottom level of organization.
- Line of responsibility and accountability flows in the opposite direction, but equally direct manner.
- It strictly observes the principles of unity of command, unity of direction, order, and discipline.

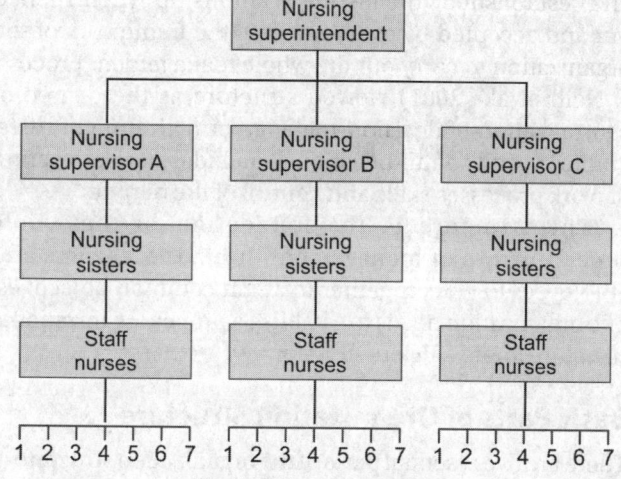

Fig. 17.2: Line organization.

- The top administrator takes major decisions.
- A two-way communication flows from top to bottom and bottom to top.
- It ensures effective communication and stability of the organization.

Merits of the Line Organization

Line organization has the following advantages:
1. It is a simple and old form of administration.
2. There is a direct superior–subordinate relationship and the command flows from top to bottom.
3. Each employee takes orders from and accountable to only one superior.
4. It provides clear-cut authority and responsibility for each position.
5. There is coordination between the top authority and bottom line authority.
6. It facilitates prompt decision-making at every level due to fixed duty.
7. It is economical by not appointing experts.
8. It brings talented persons in the organization.
9. It provides scope for staff development.

Demerits of the Line Organization

The disadvantages of the line organization are as follows:
1. Lack of specialization due to a scalar chain from top to bottom
2. Top executives are overburden by decision-making and supervisory duties
3. Lack of feedback and delay in communication
4. Lack of decision by middle and lower level
5. Lack of coordination and cooperation among departments
6. Chances of misusing authority positions by autocratic managers
7. Limited scope for managerial growth.

Functional Organization

The functional organization emerges from the idea that the organization must perform certain functions and follows the principle of total specialization and total division of work. The organization has technical departments, according to specialty. Every functional department is responsible for the performance of that function for the organization as a whole. For example, the personnel department will look after the recruitment, selection, training, wage payment, and so on.

Characteristics of Functional Organization

The following is the list of characteristics of functional organization:
- The work is as per specialization and performed by specialists.
- The head of each functional department is a technical specialist.
- It has functional authority relationships and limited span of management.
- There are a clear-cut line and staff division.

Merits of Functional Organization

The following list shows the merits of functional organization structure:
1. **Facilitates specialization:** Functional organization facilitates a high degree of specialization by division of work. Every functional in-charge is an expert in its areas and in a better position to guide and help the staff at the operational level.
2. **High morale and sense of belongingness among staff:** The personnel becomes expert in their areas. They have high confidence, and it gives them a sense of belongingness.
3. **Promotes professional and career development:** Functional organization provides enormous scope for the development of the employees. There is the provision of in-depth training and skill development and career paths within functions.
4. **Effective coordination:** There is one specialist head that supervises and control all the activities. It facilitates effective coordination within the function.
5. **Flexibility:** Being the decision-making rests with the functional head, there is a scope of flexibility and opportunity to bring changes for the betterment of the organization.
6. **Adequate supervision and control:** This type of organization facilitates effective control being one functional head and due to specialization; they concentrate on the specific technical area and also keep adequate supervision on their subordinates.
7. **A higher degree of the span of control:** The manager can effectively manage a large number of subordinates due to uniformity in activities.
8. **Order and clarity:** Functional organization brings clarity in their functions; better supervision and thus maintain the quality of work.
9. **Accountability:** Increased individual accountability towards the work brings efficiency.
10. **Less workload:** Each functional head looks after its area; thus there is less burden on the top-level administrator.
11. **Increases efficiency:** Greater efficiency can achieve if every functional unit is performing a limited number of functions.

Demerits of Functional Organization Structure

The following list is the demerits of functional organization structure:
1. **Multiple commands:** Unity of command is absent in the technical organization as each staff at lower level gets orders and instructions from several persons in a team.
2. **Conflict and confusion:** As there is too much emphasis on specialization and performance, each department

starts working independently. Moreover, the functional system is quite complicated to put into operation, primarily when it is carried out at low levels.

3. **Lack of responsiveness:** It lacks responsiveness necessary to cope up with new and rapidly changing work environment.
4. **Delays in decision-making:** Taking decisions by multidepartment delays in decision-making.
5. **Interdepartmental confusion:** Functional organization has specialization as the function is a base for dividing the work. There is an overlapping of authority and shared responsibility. It creates interdepartmental confusion that affects organizational efficiency.
6. **Narrow perspective:** A functional head tends to create boundaries around her/him and does only for the department rather than for the organization as a whole.
7. **Poor communication and coordination:** The departmental heads may lack the coordination to take decisions to solve the problem of a particular department.
8. **Weak disciplinary control:** Owing to the lack of unity of command, one person gets an order from more than one person. Thus, disciplinary authority becomes weak.
9. **Expensive:** Functional organization is very costly because of many functional expert heads of departments.
10. **Divided responsibility:** In a functional organization, responsibility is challenging to fix on a particular person instead assigning responsibility to individuals.
11. **Overspecialization:** The employees of functional departments become overspecialized; they become self-centered, narrow viewpoints, and lose the whole system perspective.
12. **Slow innovation:** Loss of clear responsibility drives a gradual change in response to the environmental changes.

Line and Staff Organization

Line and staff organization is a complex organization and a modified line organization. As the name indicates, it has both types of managers—the line and staff. The line managers have the authority and power of command. The authority flows from top to bottom level. He takes a decision and responsible execution of plans and policies to achieve the objectives. The staff officers are specialist who is experts in their fields and attached to line managers to advise in their specialization (**Fig. 17.3**).

There are mainly three types of staff: personal, specialists, and general staff. The individual staff such as a personal assistant or Private Secretary is attached to line managers. The specialists are technical staff who serve line managers and other staff in planning, organizing, and coordinating their work, e.g. legal advisor, administrative officer, and so on. The general team is attached to the key executives such as deputy manager/Director, Assistant, or Additional managers to assist executives. They have the same background as executives.

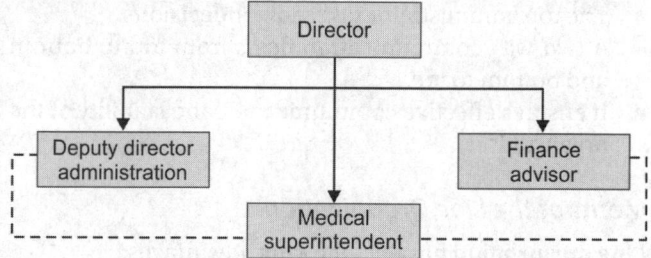

Fig. 17.3: The line and staff organization.

Characteristics of Line and Staff Organization

Line and staff organization has the following characteristics:
- It is more complex having both line and staff functions.
- It has both divisions of work and specialization that improve organizational efficiency.
- It has planning and execution aspects of administration.
- The staff provides guidance and advice to line executives.
- Planning is staff function, and execution is a line function.
- The line executive has the power of command; staff officers lack such authority.
- It improves efficiency.

Merits of Line and Staff Organization

Line and staff organization has the following advantages:
1. **Specialization:** Line managers get the benefits of specialized knowledge of the staff at every level.
2. **Less workload:** Top managers have less work due to staff officers.
3. **Better decision-making:** Staff officers help the line executives to make better decisions.
4. **Clearly defined functions:** Line and staff have two different types of service. The staff has an advisory role, whereas the line has execution functions.
5. **Flexibility:** Staff is more flexible than the line organization.
6. **Opportunity for advancement:** This form of the organization provides better opportunities for improvement to employees.
7. **Undivided responsibility:** Everybody inline structure has accountability for their work.
8. **Unity of command:** Line managers have unity of command, and the staff provides specialist advice and guidance to line managers.

Demerits of Line and Staff Organization

The disadvantages of line and staff organization are as follows:
1. **Lack of understanding:** Conflicts between line managers and staff specialists are quite common in this type of organization. The line managers have a lack of interest in seeking advice from experts; staff managers feel that the line managers lack the knowledge of new ideas. There is a shifting of responsibility.
2. **Dependency:** Line managers are more dependent on staff for seeking advice, planning, and development.

3. **Delay in decision-making:** Line executives consult staff experts before finalizing the choices that may delay in taking decisions.
4. **Lack of coordination:** There are chances of lack of coordination between line and staff managers due to unclear and overlapping of roles.
5. **Lack of accountability:** Since the power of command remains with the line executive, the staff is not accountable for the work.
6. **Expensive:** Line and staff organization is costly as the line executives are supported by highly paid staff executives who are experts, which adds the expense of the organization.
7. **Complexity:** The organization complicated due to dual authority. There is a division of functions, but line executives are dependent on staff officers for finalizing any decisions.

Table 17.2 depicts the comparison between the line, functional, and line and staff organization

Committee Form of Organization

A committee is a form of a formal group. According to the dictionary, a meaning committee is a group of people officially delegated to perform a function. According to LM Prasad, a committee is a group of persons appointed to discuss and deal matters brought before it. Gillies stated that a committee is a group of employees engaged in some aspect of management functions. A committee is a group of persons to whom, as a group, some matter is committed. It involves group decision making (Koontz).

The committees usually have elected and coopted or nominated members of the organization. Size of the committee depends on the nature of the committee; often, it has 6–8 members. The members may be elected for 1–5 years, depending on the quality of the committee or maybe for a short period until the completion of the task.

Purposes of Committees

The following list shows the purposes of committees:
1. To make the decisions about different managerial functions
2. To seek opinions regarding various organizational programs
3. To coordinate the activities of different departments
4. To seek advice from the specialists.

Types of Committees

Committee has the following types:
1. **Line and advisory committee:** The committees constituted for taking different managerial decisions are line committees such as planning committee, finance committee, etc. The staff committees are advisory and constituted to seek suggestion by line management. Line management takes the final decision.
2. **Formal and informal committees:** The committees as a part of an organization with specifically delegated duties and authority are formal. The informal committees are not part of the organizational committees but mostly formed to take decisions on some urgent and immediate problem.
3. **Permanent and temporary committees:** The formal committees are permanent and organizational constituted. The interim committees are of short duration constituted for the specific purpose.

Advantages of Committees

The merits of committees are as follows:
1. **Pooling of opinions:** The committee is helpful to pool knowledge from experts of a different background. Decisions come through group deliberation and judgment.
2. **Broader perspective:** The committees decide on the more comprehensive view of the organization as decisions are group's opinions, not an individual's choice.
3. **Better coordination:** The committees provide an opportunity to conclude by coordinating and cooperating with different experts.
4. **Democratic approach:** The committees provide an opportunity for each member to participate.
5. **Better communication:** The committee meetings provide a platform to exchange idea face to face.

TABLE 17.2: Comparison of line, functional and line and staff organization.

Basis	Line organization	Functional organization	Line and staff organization
Top administration	Only line executives	Functional experts	Line and staff
Authority	Follows the principle of scalar chain flows from top to bottom	The flow of authority is diagonal and restricted, over the functions	The staff has advisory; Authority vested with line
Specialization	Managers are generalists	Specialist in their respective fields	Specialist in different fields
Simplicity	The simplest form	The most complex structure	Relatively more complex
Unity of command	Observes unity of command principle	Not followed	Notes to some extent
Discipline	Strict	Loose discipline	More or less strict
Executives workload	Overburdened	Evenly divided	Shared by staff
Decision making	Without delay	May get delayed	Often gets delayed
Economy	Highly economical	Expensive	Slightly costlier
Suitability	For small-scale organization	Large scale	Medium scale

6. **Motivation:** The group members feel motivated as getting recognition by participating in decision making.
7. **Administrative training:** The meetings provide a platform for its members to learn the value of interaction, interpersonal relation, and group dynamics.
8. **Avoidance of action:** It is management tactile to form a committee when to avoid or delay to decide in certain situations.

Disadvantages of Committees

The following list shows the disadvantages of committees:
1. **Delay in execution:** The committee delays to reach a conclusion for collective effort and group decision.
2. **Ineffective decision:** The group decision sometimes wrong due to the incompetence of members/chairperson or matters decided in a hurry.
3. **Indecision:** The committee meetings may end with indecisive results due to its divided responsibility. All members may not participate actively; few may be passive.
4. **Expensive:** The committee meetings are costly regarding time and money. The committee needs to spend on all administrative expenses for conducting meetings.
5. **Misusing committee:** Sometimes the administrators try to make decisions of their matters under the umbrella of the committee, thus abusing the committee.

How to Make Committees Effective?

Following are the ways to make the committees productive and successful:
1. **Size of the committee:** Decide the adequate size of the committee members; neither too small nor too large.
2. **Clear purpose and role of the committee:** Define the purpose and function of the committee clearly; spell out responsibilities. Appoint a committee if the problem is of three or four departments, or group consensus is required, or to decide one best alternative.
3. **Effective executives and members:** Select the chairperson, vice chairperson, and convener by knowledge, experience, organizing human relation capabilities. Select members showing interest and take initiatives and participate in meetings. They should be representatives of their field.
4. **Define committee meetings procedures:** Define the process of conducting committee meetings, documentation, and meeting minutes.
5. **Well-informed members:** Inform members about the venue, date, day, time, and agenda well in advance. Inform about TA/DA, accommodation, and other details as well.
6. **Proper briefing:** Inform members about the agenda and background papers of the meeting so that they come prepared with the solutions.

Guidelines for Conducting a Committee Meeting

To conduct a committee meeting, the guidelines listed below should be followed:
1. The convener must fix the date, time, and venue with the consultation of chairperson for the meeting. He should prepare agenda items and ensures the availability of the place and budget. Inform all the members at least three days in advance and reminds one day before the meeting.
2. The convener should keep the minutes of all previous meetings. The chairperson and members must be on schedule on the day of the meeting.
3. The chairperson should ensure the minimum quorum to start the meeting and await 10–15 minutes; postpone the meeting if one-third members are not present.
4. The chairperson should declare the meeting open and confirm the previous meeting minutes at least by two members.
5. The members should ensure the cordial and informal atmosphere during the meeting. The chairperson should sportingly conduct the meeting without interruption, attend with respect, and give the opportunity to participate with all the members. He should welcome their criticisms and comments and try to reach in conclusion.
6. The chairperson should summarize the highlights of the meeting at the end, thank everyone for their contribution, and ask the date for the next meeting before adjourning the meeting.
7. The convener must maintain an attendance record of meeting and writes meeting minutes.

CHAPTER HIGHLIGHTS

- The organization is viewed differently by different theorists. It is a structure which describes the relationships of individuals of different levels; a group of people created formally or informally.
- It is a dynamic process and managerial activity, and a system comprised many interrelated subsystems.
- Formal and informal relationships exist in the organization. The formal organization has defined the structure, and informal organization refers to social groups having relationships among employees and originates from the formal organization.
- Classic, neoclassic, and modern theories viewed the organization from different perspectives. The contemporary theory has a combination of system and contingency approach based on empirical research.
- There are different types of formal organizations such as line, functional, line and staff organization, and committee form of organization.

REVIEW QUESTIONS

I. Essay Type Questions
1. Define the term "Organization." Describe various concepts of organization.
2. Discuss the principles of organization and its application in nursing management.
3. Describe the formal organization. Distinguish between formal and informal organization.
4. Describe the minimum requirement for an organization briefly.
5. What are the different types of organization? Explain line and staff organization in detail.

II. Short Notes
1. Organization as a system
2. Organization theories
3. Essential parts of organization
4. Organization chart
5. Committee form of organization

III. Multiple Choice Questions
1. Which concept of the organization describes the relationship among individuals and the positions they hold?
    a. Organization as a system
    b. Organization as a process
    c. Organization as a group of people
    d. Organization as a structure
2. The principle of specialization means:
    a. Division of labor according to skill and qualification
    b. Coordinating the activities of different departments
    c. Defining the goals and objectives of the organization
    d. Delegating responsibilities
3. In which direction, the authority flows in the line organization?
    a. Vertical to horizontal
    b. Horizontal to vertical
    c. From top to bottom
    d. From bottom to top
4. Which principle of organization is concerning with assigning a proportionate number of persons under a supervisor?
    a. Principle of balance
    b. Principle of span of control
    c. Principle of defining authority
    d. Principle of unity of command
5. An organization that defines hierarchical relationships, authority and responsibilities is a:
    a. Formal organization
    b. Informal organization
    c. Line organization
    d. Functional organization
6. The classical theorists view organization as:
    a. A social system and individuals as important assets
    b. A machine and human beings its components
    c. A structural design influenced by situation
    d. A system in totality
7. Which basic part of the organization assist and advice executives in managerial functions?
    a. Strategic apex
    b. Middle line
    c. Operating core
    d. Techno-structural staff
8. What does an organization chart indicate?
    a. A social relationship and managerial style
    b. A large number of employees
    c. A formal relationship and channel of communication
    d. All details of organization structure
9. Which type of chart depicts the same level of employees in a group reporting to their respective managers?
    a. Hierarchical chart   b. Matrix chart
    c. Horizontal chart   d. Circular chart
10. Which type of committee is a part of an organization with specifically delegated duties and authority?
    a. Line   b. Advisory
    c. Formal   d. Ad hoc

Answer Keys
1. d   2. a   3. c   4. b   5. a   6. b   7. d
8. c   9. b   10. c

SUGGESTED READING

1. Beechy P, Biester D. Restructuring group meetings for effectiveness. J Nurs Admin. 1986;13(1):20-24.
2. Dubois HF, Fattore G. Definitions and typologies in public administration research: the case of decentralization. Int J Public Admin. 2009;32(8):704-727.
3. George R Terry. Principles of Management. Homewood, IL, Richard D. Irwin; 1988.
4. O'Donnell C. Ground rules for using committees. Manag Rev. 1961:63-67.
5. Prasad LM. Principles and Practice of Management. New Delhi: Sultan Chand & Sons Publishers; 2001. pp. 356-64.
6. Qadiri GJ, Tabish A. Chairing committees. Hosp Admin. 1995;XXXII(1&2):47-54.
7. Weihrichs H, Koontz H. Management. New York, NY: McGraw-Hill; 1994.

18 CHAPTER

Organizational Climate and Organizational Effectiveness

CHAPTER OUTLINE

- Organizational Climate
  - Meaning and Definitions
  - Importance of Sound Organizational Climate
  - Approaches to Organizational Climate
  - Good or Bad Organizational Climate
  - Characteristics of Organizational Climate
  - Organizational Climate versus Organizational Culture
  - Factors Affecting Organizational Climate
  - Types of Organizational Climate
  - Need for Measuring Organizational Climate
  - Methods of Measuring Organizational Climate
  - Means of Developing a Sound Organizational Climate
- Organizational Effectiveness
  - Concept of Organizational Effectiveness
  - Definitions
  - Characteristics of Organizational Effectiveness
  - Approaches to Organizational Effectiveness
  - Factors Affecting Organizational Effectiveness
  - Methods of Improving Organizational Effectiveness

LEARNING OUTCOMES

After completion of this chapter, the learner will be able to:
- Understand the concept of organizational climate (OC)
- Discuss factors affecting organizational climate (OC)
- Describe the dimensions of organizational climate (OC)
- Appreciate the importance organizational climate (OC)
- Understand the ways to develop a sound organizational climate (OC)

KEY TERMS

Organizational climate, organizational effectiveness, organization culture

INTRODUCTION

The effectiveness of any organization depends on its work climate. The work climate is the quality of the internal environment of the organization, which influences the behavior of employees, group, and organization system. Organization climate is a measure of the collective perception of the employees for their organization. Developing a productive environment is a crucial component for any organization seeking to increase its efficiency to achieve the organizational goals.

ORGANIZATIONAL CLIMATE

The organizational climate first described as a social climate in the article by Lewin in 1930s concerning leadership styles. Fleishman (1939) described it as a leading climate and developed behavioral leadership scales. Argyris was the first to introduce the concept of Organizational Climate in 1958. He defined climate regarding formal organizational policies, employee needs, values, and personalities. Later on, many theorists and scholars have worked on it and tried to find out its role, importance, and impact on the organization.

Meaning and Definitions

Organizational climate refers to the perception, feeling, and attitudes of employees towards its elements and works environment; the way they participate, interact, behave, and value the organization. The work climate includes norms, values, expectations, policies, and procedures that influence individual and group behavior. It also consists of a set of attributes such as loyalty, autonomy, trust, cohesiveness, support, recognition, innovation, and fairness. It is more of a psychological climate based on policies and procedures, feedback, and also the behavior of supervisors and coworkers within the informal organization. In the context of an organization, it is difficult to observe and measure as it is continually changing according to the situation.

- Georgopoulos described organizational Climate (OC) as a normative structure of attitudes and behavioral standards of employees, which help them to interpret the situations and direct to perform.
- Forehand & Gilmer viewed OC as a set of developed characteristics of an organization that influence the behavior of the people. It describes and differentiates the organization from other organization.
- Likert (1967) described OC as a psychological, multidimensional, and complex phenomenon that affects the organizational performance regarding values, performance, turnover, absenteeism, and tenure of employees.
- Campbell et al. (1970) defined OC as a set of attributes of a particular organization that may be induced by the organization, deals with its members and its environment. It takes the form of attitudes and expectancies that describe the organization.
- According to Nicholson and Miljus (1992), OC serves as a measure of individuals' perception of an organization. It includes leadership styles, decision-making power, challenging jobs, job satisfaction, benefits, personnel policies, right working conditions, and creation of suitable career ladder for academics.

Importance of Sound Organizational Climate

A sound OC is essential for the following:
- To achieve organizational goals and objectives
- To improve the work performance
- To utilize the maximum potential of the employees
- To bring out work efficiency by improving job satisfaction
- To reduce absenteeism, stress, negligence errors, and accidents.

Approaches to Organizational Climate

Organization climate is viewed differently by different authors.
1. **The structural approach:** According to this approach, the organization climate originates from the organizational structure. The organization climate results from the individual's perception regarding organization structure as per their experiences in the organization. The type of organization structure influences the perception of individuals. But this approach is not free from criticism; there can be different workgroup climates in one organization, and there is a lack of evidence to support the individuals' reactions to a situation.
2. **The perceptual approach:** The individuals are the basis for the organizational climate. They interpret and react according to the conditions provided by the organization. It refers to the collective perception, feeling, and attitude of individuals towards the organizational requirements as a result of activities, interactions, and reactions within the organization.
3. **The interactive approach:** The individual interaction with organizational members regarding conditions provided by the organization create an organizational climate. The communication is central to form organization climate. The interactive approach is the combination of structural and perceptual approach and consensus of group members based on the individuals' perception of the structure of the organization. This approach includes understanding and interpretation of the organization's members. The values, beliefs, and attitudes of group members also influence the OC.
4. **Cultural approach:** The culture is also the predictor of organizational climate. In an organization, the culture group interacts and shares their common abstract values, attitudes, and beliefs regarding conditions of the organization. The culture reflects the group dynamics-norms, values, myths, ideologies, and symbols. Thus organization forms a part of organizational culture.

Good or Bad Organizational Climate

If the OC is pleasant, the employees feel respected, supportive, entrepreneurship, and innovative. The organization has full support and cooperation, successful management practices, knowledge management, organizational learning, and employee readiness to change, collective learning, and openness. The employees have job satisfaction, perform better, and take the risk. They have faith in management, have open communication, and free to work that help in their development.

In a bad OC, the employees feel fear, crisis, anxiety, aggression, burnout, and frustrations. There are high absenteeism, poor performance, frequent negligence errors, accidents, and stagnation.

Characteristics of Organizational Climate

Characteristics of OC are given below:
1. **General perception:** Organization climate is the result of the widespread expression of individuals towards the conditions, processes, and system of organization.
2. **Abstract and intangible concept:** Organization climate is a very complex phenomenon; it influences with attitude and values of the individuals apart from the organization internal environment. It makes it abstract and challenging to measure. However, there are quantitative methods to study its nature to make it more observable and reality-based.
3. **Unique and distinct identity:** The type of OC differs in the organization to organization. It is not the same for all organizations. Also, it keeps changing according to

the situation in the organization. It provides a distinct identity to each organization.

4. **Enduring quality:** Organization climate represents a relatively constant internal environment of the organization. It overgrows over time and changes rapidly.
5. **Multidimensional concept:** Organization climate has multidimensional thoughts. It has its origin from structural, perception, interaction, and related cultural ideas.

Organizational Climate versus Organizational Culture

Both the terms are interchangeable in the organization differ in many aspects. Both are related concepts and originated as a part of the organization. The organizational climate is more expressive, observable, and socially constructed dimension, whereas the organization culture is a hidden and unspoken component of organization and influences the attitudes and human behavior. Organizational climate and culture differs in its origin, focus, nature, and its characteristics **(Table 18.1)**.

Factors Affecting Organizational Climate

The OC is influenced by the following factors:
1. **Organization orientation:** The mission, goals and objectives, strategies, and structure of the organization affect the organizational climate. It should not be too rigid and too flexible. It must address the needs and interest of the employees. The degree and type of authority and responsibilities, the delegation also do affect the behavior and perceptions of members of the organization and collectively the organizational climate.

TABLE 18.1: Difference between organizational climate and organization culture

Criterion	Organization Climate	Organization Culture
Origin	Social psychology	Anthropology
Focus	Individuals' perception and knowledge used to interpret the characteristics of the internal organizational environment	Analyzing the structure of myths, ideologies, practices leading to group norms, values and meaning
Characteristic	Relatively constant forms quickly and changes rapidly	Highly consistent, forms slowly and painful to change
Individual response	At the personal conscious level, visible, communicative and based on reality	At the preconscious level, forms attitude and value which are hidden, invisible based on assumptions
Basis	On individuals characteristics and perception	On collective characteristics
Method of study its nature	Quantitatively	Qualitatively

2. **Organizational values and norms:** The organizational policies and standards if implemented strictly or not directed towards the behavior of employees, do affect the organizational climate. It should be framed considering the value system and must be flexible. It should also include loyalty and conformity.
3. **Organizational control system:** Organizational control identifies how a flexible and rigid rules and regulation of the organization affect the behavior of the individuals working in the organization. The organization characterized by achievement rather than control by strict rules and regulations.
4. **Autonomy:** Feeling of individuals towards their responsibilities and freedom to make decisions, and participation in managerial function affect their behavior. There should be sufficient autonomy to work and exercise authority to lead effectively.
5. **Communication:** The flow, channel, and the type of communication system are determinants of organizational climate. In a proper communication system, the subordinates can express their ideas and can give their suggestion without any fear.
6. **Risk and risk taking:** Perception of individuals to make initiatives, challenges, and risk without fear in the organization affect the organization climate.
7. **Management support:** It is the degree of encouragement and support provided by the supervisors and higher authority in the work setting that affect the organizational climate.
8. **Leadership style:** The leadership behavior, lines of communication, and decision-making affect the perception of employees towards the organization.
9. **Employee–employer relationship:** The relationship between employee and employer has an impact on employees' motivational level that affects the organizational climate.
10. **Concern for the employees:** The perception of individuals how much the management show concern regarding their work profile, health, and safety by providing safety measures and physical facilities.
11. **Reward and punishment:** The reward and punishment system of the organization affect the motivational and satisfaction level of individuals and thereby changing the organizational climate.
12. **Trust on management:** Perception of individuals regarding the trust they have in control regarding their work and welfare.
13. **Scope for development:** It depends on the individuals' perception regarding the opportunities provided by the organization to grow, training, and career development.
14. **Work environment:** The physical, social, and psychological context of the organization and the perception of individuals towards it is also the determinant of organizational climate.
15. **Transformation practices:** The changing practices due to globalization, high competition, and changing technology affect the organizational climate.

Types of Organizational Climate

1. **According to level**
   1. *Organizational climate:* The climate created by manipulating the characteristics of the organization is the organizational climate. The established organization is the motivational force to modify the group behavior. It is an organizational level in totality. The environment differs from one organization to another, therefore, uses to determine the climate differences between organizations.
   2. *Group climate:* The organization has different groups for various practices and procedures. Each group has a group climate. Therefore, the organization may have many subclimates. These subclimates are relevant to the group situation rather than individual characteristics. It describes subclimates in the same organization.
   3. *Psychological climate:* Each is unique and reacts differently in different situations. The perception of each affects the environment. The climate forms due to individual characteristics, which include attitudes, feelings, values, norms, interaction, support, and satisfaction referred to psychological climate.
2. **According to orientation**
   1. *People-oriented OC:* The atmosphere concluded due to perception and interpretation of the people towards the organization. It includes norms, value, characteristics of individuals who create the organizational climate. The culture of an organization creates the environment perceived by the people, the group resulting in organizational climate.
   2. *Rule-oriented OC:* The OC created as a result of strict rule and regulations, defined procedures and strategies of the organization is a control-oriented OC.
   3. *Innovation-oriented OC:* The innovation-oriented atmosphere created as a result of the organizational focus on its development and competitions. The people are free to try new ideas and able to take risks.
   4. *Goal-oriented OC:* As the name indicates, the main focus of the organization is to achieve the goal. The environment created to meet the defined goals and objectives perceived by the individuals, the group, and the results in a goal-oriented OC.

Need for Measuring Organizational Climate

The organizational performance and climate are directly and nearly correlated with each other. Organizational climate influences employees' performance based on their motivation and satisfaction level. The specific purposes of measuring the OC are as follows:
- To find out the degree and level of OC
- To find out the various factors affecting OC
- To analyze positive and negative factors contributing to OC
- To plan out the strategies to improve OC
- To reorganize practices for the development of the organization
- To enhance employees' commitment, satisfaction, and motivation
- To create a high performing OC.

Methods of Measuring Organizational Climate

There are mainly four methods of measuring OC: (1) observation, (2) perceptual, (3) field studies, and (4) experimental studies.

The observation- and perception-related studies are the primary method of measuring OC. The observation studies are conducted to gather objective information regarding the properties of the organization. The descriptive studies are conducted to collect the subjective data on perceptions of organizational members regarding OC.

The other two methods are field studies and experimental studies. The primary purpose of conducting field studies is to gather information regarding the daily activities of the OC. The data are collected through observation, presentations, interviews, conferences, reviewing diaries, memos, emails, and so on. The comparative and longitudinal studies can provide information regarding variations of the organizational properties.

Means of Developing a Sound Organizational Climate

The following means are essential for developing a sound OC:

1. **Organization purpose:** Define mission, goals, strategies based on individual needs. Seek employees' participation in developing goals and objectives and policy. Make them aware of the operational plans and their outcomes.
2. **Organizational values:** To improve the OC, it is essential to reorganize policies, procedures, and rules regarding value structure and must implement flexible.
3. **Active communication system**: Two-way communications is vital to maintain a healthy relationship between employees and employers/supervisors. It encourages their level of confidence and teaches positive feelings.
4. **Concern for the people:** Good management creates a life-giving force to the organization with effective utilization of resources. The organization must provide physical facilities and have policies concerning their welfare, safety, and development.
5. **Balancing work and life:** There should be flexible working hours, leaves, and other benefits for the employees to balance their personal life and work. It will improve their satisfaction level.
6. **Recognition and career development plans:** The organization must give recognition to employees for their excellent performance and plan for a career ladder.

7. **Problem-solving and conflict management:** It works most constructively for both organizations as well as the employees. The employees feel contented and give their best. Sound control is the art of solving the problems and conflict so constructively to push the employees to get to work and deal with them.
8. **Flexibility in risk-taking:** The organization must create such a work environment that provides flexibility and opportunity for employees to favor risk-taking by exchanging knowledge and ideas.
9. **Participation:** It is a handy tool to develop a healthy OC and job satisfaction. More satisfied employees possess some personality characteristics that are likely to be reflected in excellent work performance, self-efficacy, and locus of control.
10. **Cooperation:** An atmosphere of collaboration opens access among group members and individual creative motivation to exchange knowledge with group members resulting in more productivity.
11. **Performance evaluation:** The organization must evaluate employees through self-evaluation and evaluation from immediate supervisors combining both subjective and objective criteria.
12. **Motivational and value-related strategies:** The organization must plan and implement reward and punishment strategies to motivate individuals. To teach positive values among employees, use the following methods:
    - Provide free communication
    - Use consensus agreement and compromise approach
    - Encourage competence and creative ideas
    - Encourage emotional expressive and task-oriented environment
    - Involve emotionally
    - Accept responsibilities
    - Encourage and motivate to work.

ORGANIZATIONAL EFFECTIVENESS

Organizational effectiveness is the center of excellence in organizations. No organization can survive in this competitive world without its efficacy. It is the degree to which the organization realizes its goals. An organization can mobilize its power for action-producing and adaptation. Organizational effectiveness is a significant indicator of its survival to show the direction, position, and future of the organization.

Concept of Organizational Effectiveness

Organizational effectiveness is concerning with achieving its goal within the available resources and means. It reflects how well an organization accomplishes the purposes for which it exists. Efficiency or effectiveness is a broad concept which includes both internal and external environment, including organizational environmental interface and employees; whereas efficacy is a narrow concept that considers only internal factors to achieve the desired outcome. Organizational effectiveness represents a desirable attribute in an organization considering internal and external factors.

Definitions

The organizational effectiveness is defined as follows:
- Richard et al. (2009) defined organizational effectiveness as organizational performance regarding internal performance outcomes associated with effective operations and other external measures, including economic valuation.
- According to Silver and Sherman, organizational effectiveness is the extent of growth and profit by utilizing defined and finite resources without disturbing its internal resources.
- Houck Levis viewed organizational effectiveness as a tool to accomplish the quality task to achieve organizational goal; whereas according to Mondy et al. (1990), it is the degree to which an organization produces the intended output.
- Oguntimehin (2001) referred to the organizational effectiveness as the ability of the organization to produce the desired results. It is the process of meeting organizational objectives and expectations of society.

Characteristics of Organizational Effectiveness

The following is the list of characteristics of OE:
1. Organizational effectiveness is goal-oriented, aiming at the achievement of goals and sustainability of the organization.
2. It has short-term, intermediate, and long-term objectives to achieve its immediate and future goals.
3. It is multidimensional; both internal and external environmental factors influence organizational performance.
4. It focuses on cost-effectiveness and quality services.
5. The clients' satisfaction and quality services are the prime responsibilities.
6. It is the collective effort of the organization, group, and individuals.
7. It is a tool to measure the performance of individuals, groups, and organization.
8. It concerns all the systems, processes, outcome, and organizational climate of the organization.

Approaches to Organizational Effectiveness

There are mainly three approaches to conceptualize the term organization effectiveness.
1. **Goal approach:** According to this approach, goal attainment is the criterion to determine organizational effectiveness. An organization can identify goals and find out means by defining its activities to achieve its goals. In this context, effectiveness refers to maximizing output by providing quality services. It will help to improve the morale of employees and maximize

production. Many organizational factors such as quality, efficiency, confidence, motivation, satisfaction, and turn over, and absenteeism can measure organizational effectiveness. The indicator of measuring organization effectiveness is measured by comparing the activities accomplished with planned ones.

2. **Functional approach:** In the technical approach, the social consequences of its activities are the determinants to measure the OE. It is concerning with the level of fulfilling the needs of the clients through planned activities of the organization.

3. **System-resource approach:** The system resource approach focuses on processes and various resources as inputs to produce the intended outcome within the environment. It also analyzes the capability of decision-makers to distribute resources among various subsystems as per need efficiently. It defines the organization as a network of interrelated subsystems.

None of these approaches give specific concept of organizational effectiveness. The operative goals can be a base to measure organizational effectiveness. It includes managerial effectiveness, which determines the behavior of managers. Organization effectiveness is a strategy to achieve goals and sustain organizational performance.

Factors Affecting Organizational Effectiveness

Various determinants of organizational effectiveness are managerial characteristics, organizational characteristics, environmental characteristics, and employee characteristics.

1. **Managerial characteristics**
   1. *Formalization:* Organizational effectiveness depends on the number of written policies, practices, principles, procedures, and rules to achieve the immediate and long-term goals of the organization and managing relations among employees. The vision, mission, strategies, goals, and objectives affect the organization.
   2. *Standards:* The standards are the directive to attain predetermined objectives and sustainability of the organization. The employees must be aware of the structural, process, and outcome rules of the organization.
   3. *Autonomy:* The degree of freedom to make decisions, and participation in managerial function help to determine the objectives achieved by the organization. There should be sufficient autonomy to work and exercise authority to lead effectively.
   4. *Communication:* The flow, channel, and type of communication system are determinants of organizational effectiveness. In a proper communication system, the subordinates can express their ideas and can give their suggestion without any fear.
   5. *Leadership style:* The leadership behavior, lines of communication, and decision-making affect the functioning of the organization.
   6. *Human resource management:* The way of attracting, retaining, motivating, and utilizing human resources affect the overall operations of the organization.
   7. *Rewards and recognition:* The awards and punishment policy affect the performance of employees. It will boost employees' morale and enable them to improve the quality and quantity of work.
   8. *Promotion policies:* The career ladder and promotional avenues in the organization affect the employees' performance.
   9. *Effective interaction:* The relationship between employee and employer or employee and employee has an impact on the performance of employees.
   10. *Managing conflicts and disputes:* The participation of employees in resolving problems, negotiations, and collective bargaining have an impact on their performance.

2. **Organizational characteristics**
   1. *Structural design:* It defines the formal division, grouping, and coordination of the job tasks within the organization. The vital elements such as the division of work, a line of authority, and so on to determine the organizational effectiveness.
   2. *Output variables:* The output variables such as profit, loss, costs, and type of services provided also reflect the achievement of the organization.
   3. *Size:* It refers to the personnel available to the organization, the organizational inputs or outputs, and the resources. The effectiveness and efficiency of an organization are dependent on the size of the organization.
   4. *Organizational climate:* The organizational environment and performance are interrelated. Organizational climate influences employees to perform their best. The degree of recognition and appreciation, promotion, working conditions, participation, security measures, welfare facilities, and grievance handling, and more affect the OC.

3. **Environmental characteristics**
   1. *Internal:* Supply of human resources, raw material, budget, and others affects the external environment.
   2. *Complexity:* It includes a range of operative activities of the organizations.
   3. *Public opinion:* It refers to the public regarding the function of the organization. They view the organization regarding the type and quality of services provided and the cost of services.

4. **Employee characteristics**
   1. *Individual goals:* The personal goals are essential to achieve the organizational objectives.
   2. *Competence:* Competent and skilled person can lead the organization. They can suggest and try the innovative idea to modify the methods to meet the expected goals.
   3. *Satisfaction and motivation:* Motivated employees have high zeal and enthusiasm to perform better to

achieve their respective organizational goals. Their job satisfaction regarding the nature of the job, pay, promotion, behavior of coworkers, supervisors. leadership style, welfare facilities, job security, and many more affects work performance.
4. *Attitudes:* The employees with a positive attitude can influence job behavior as well as the effectiveness of the organizational goal.
5. *Group norms and values:* Group norms and values have an impact on the performance of employees by influencing their attitude and behavior towards work.
6. *Perception:* The level positive or negative attitude of individuals towards organization affects their performance.
7. *Commitment:* The degree of dedication and loyalty towards the organization reflects in their performance. The employees committed towards the job perform better to achieve organizational goals.

Methods of Improving Organizational Effectiveness

Various methods at individual, group, and organization level can be used to improve the organizational performance effectiveness as given below:

1. **Effectiveness-oriented policies, procedure, and structure:** Make sure that current systems, practices must base on the needs and capabilities of employees. Ensure the working relationship between departments.
2. **Clarity about the organizational goal:** The vision and goals of the organization should be definite. All the members of the organization must understand their operational objectives, performance standards, and their responsibilities to achieve those objectives and goals. The aims of the organization must aim at promoting operational efficiency and productivity of employees for performance improvement.
3. **Promoting responsibility and accountability:** The immediate supervisors must create a sense of responsibility and liability towards the work performance among their subordinates. They must delegate the task appropriately; provide sufficient resources and adequate working conditions. They must guide and give freedom to work.
4. **Specialization and proper work division:** The organization must have a right number of levels and adequate span of control to have effective communication and must provide a certain degree of autonomy in decision-making in their working and taking initiatives.
5. **Focus on organizational strategies:** The strategies must focus on quality services based on clients' needs, cost-effective, and provided up to their satisfaction. There should be a healthy relationship between clients and service providers.
6. **Engage the workforce:** Utilize the maximum potentials of the workforce. Involve them in designing and implementing new innovative strategies to improve organizational performance. Build trust and show concern. Make them familiar with the approach and their role in organizational development. Focus to departmental improvement through set standards of procedures and activities.
7. **Training and development strategies:** The organization must identify skills and deficient areas of the employees. Each employee must undergo induction training and need-based staff and development skill training programs. Develop a career ladder for individuals to progress by identifying individual goals. The competent and motivated workforce contributes maximum effort to bring work efficiency.
8. **Improved leadership practices:** Encourage managers to have two-way communications with their subordinates. They must communicate the principles and goals; interact and discuss with them the departmental performance target, progress, and day-to-day problems. Create a team spirit among members and provide an opportunity to participate in decision-making. Exhibit participative and democratic leadership style.
9. **Use of motivational strategies:** Value each and recognize their contribution to the development and achievement of the organization. They play an essential role in OE and sustainability. Plan various need-based financial and nonfinancial motivational strategies such as promotions, balancing work and life, leaves, flexible working hours, work from home, occupational health and safety, security, and other social benefits.
10. **Create a positive work culture:** The organization must set and implement well-defined reward and punishment policy, recruitment and training, and other related policies to create a work culture of honesty and transparency.
11. **Use of technology:** The purpose of advanced technology in providing services also plays an essential role in improving organizational effectiveness. Make use of appropriate technology and innovative ideas which help to reduce the cost, save time, improve work efficiency, and provide quality service.
12. **Systematic performance evaluation:** Plan out innovative performance approach to measure and evaluate individual performances individually or in a group. Use operative system indicators. Detect and correct the deficiencies through training and development. At the organizational level, use organizational effectiveness approach to measure its performance. It concerns to top management level personnel. Use strategies indicators based on effective communication and delivery of services throughout the organization.

CHAPTER HIGHLIGHTS

- Organizational climate(OC) refers to the perception, feeling, and attitudes of employees towards its elements and works environment.

- It is an input of various approaches such as structural, perceptual, interactive, and cultural approaches.
- As compared to organization culture, OC is a broad concept and socially constructed.
- Both internal and external environmental factors and practices affect the OC.
- Organizational climate exists at the individual, group, and organizational level. It is either rule-oriented or people and innovation-oriented.
- Organizational effectiveness is concerning with achieving its goals within the available resources and means. It is the process of meeting organizational objectives and expectations of society.
- It has various approaches, such as goals, functional, and system-resource approaches.
- Managerial, organizational, environmental, and employees related factors affect the performance of an organization.
- Various methods at a different level can use OE to improve organizational performance.

REVIEW QUESTIONS

I. Essay Type Questions
1. Define organization climate. Describe various factors affecting organizational climate.
2. Discuss different types of organizational climates.
3. Describe various methods of developing a sound organizational climate.
4. Define organizational effectiveness. Discuss its characteristics and approaches.
5. Describe various methods of improving organizational effectiveness.

II. Short Notes
1. Good and bad organizational climate
2. Characteristics of organizational climate
3. Distinguish between organization climate and organization culture
4. Factors affecting organizational effectiveness
5. The concept of organizational effectiveness

III. Multiple Choice Questions
1. The perception, feeling, and attitude of employees towards its elements and work environment refers to:
    a. Organizational climate
    b. Organizational effectiveness
    c. Organizational culture
    d. Organizational group climate
2. Which type of organizational climate created as a result of the organization focus on its development and competitions?
    a. People oriented
    b. Goal oriented
    c. Innovative oriented
    d. Rule oriented
3. The organizational culture is:
    a. Focused on individual perception regarding internal environment of organization
    b. A hidden, unspoken component influences attitude and behavior
    c. Originated from social psychology
    d. Measured through quantitative methods
4. The climate that forms due to individual characteristics such as attitude, feeling, and so on is:
    a. Organizational climate
    b. Group climate
    c. Innovative climate
    d. Psychological climate
5. Which type of study is appropriate to use to gather information regarding daily activities of an organization?
    a. Observational study
    b. Experimental study
    c. Field study
    d. Descriptive study

Answer Keys

1. a   2. c   3. b   4. d   5. c

SUGGESTED READING

1. Argyris C. Some problems in conceptualizing organizational climate: A case study of a bank. Adm Sci Quart. 1958;2:501-520.
2. Available from: http://shodhganga.inflibnet.ac.in/bitstream/10603/43845/5/05_chapter1.pdf. [Accessed on 17.2.2019].
3. Available from: http://www.yourarticlelibrary.com/organization/organisational-climate-meaning-characteristics-and-factors/53226. [Accessed on 15.2.2019].
4. Available from: https://www.brighthub.com/office/human-resources/articles/112905.aspx. [Accessed on 22.2.2019].
5. Available from: https://www.business.com/articles/6-steps-to-improve-organization-performance-2/. [Accessed on 17.2.2019].
6. Available from: https://www.researchgate.net/publication/50350185_Assessing_operational_effectiveness_in_healthcare_organizations_A_systematic_approach. [Accessed on 18.2.2019].
7. Baron R. Behaviour in Organizations. Newton: Allyn and Bacon; 1996.
8. Boro L, Thompson S, Patton C. Organizational Behaviour. London: Routledge; 2001.
9. Campbell JR, Dunnett MD, Lawler EE et al. Managerial Behavior, Performance, and Effectiveness. New York: McGraw-Hill; 1970.
10. Georgopoulos B. Normative structure variables and organizational behavior. Hum Relat.1965;18:115-170.
11. Mondy RW, et al. Management and Organization Behavior. Boston: Allyn and Bacon Publishers; 1990.

CHAPTER 19

Planning of Hospitals and Patient Care Units

CHAPTER OUTLINE

- Hospital
  - Definitions of a Hospital
  - Characteristics of a Hospital
  - Types of Hospitals
  - Functions of Hospitals
  - Hospital Services
- Planning of Hospital
  - Factors Influencing Hospital Planning
  - Principles of Hospital Planning
  - General Features of Hospital Plan
  - Process/Steps of Hospital Planning
- Planning of Patient Care Unit (PCU)
  - Introduction
  - Meaning of PCU
  - Functional Goals of PCU
  - Objectives of PCU
  - Types of PCUS
  - Components of the PCU
  - Principles of Planning the PCU
  - Advantages of Proper Planning
  - Factors Consideration for Planning
  - Prerequisite for Planning (PCU)
  - Consideration for Planning the Patient Care Unit

LEARNING OUTCOMES

After completion of this chapter, the learner will be able to:
- Understand the concept and meaning of hospital
- Describe different types of hospital
- Discuss the characteristics and functions of the hospital
- Enumerate factors affecting hospital planning
- Explain the process of hospital planning
- Describe different types of patient care units (PCUs)
- Enlist principles of planning PCUs
- Describe the essential components of the PCUs

KEY TERMS
Hospital, hospital planning, hospital services, patient care unit, Nightingale ward, Rigs ward

INTRODUCTION

The word "hospital" has its origin from the Latin word *hospes* means an apartment for strangers or guests. The term "hospital" has been referring to an institution for the aged and infirm along with to take care of sick and wounded patients. Hospitals were the temples of God during the Roman and Greek periods. In the beginning, charity institutions were set up to take care of the poor only, but later on, these institutions gradually turned to serve all sections of society. Today, the hospitals are considered to provide treatment to sick and also to trained medical and other health professionals.

In India hospitals date back to Buddha period, followed by Asoka in 273–232 BC. Hospitals were also set up in the sixth century during the Sushruta period and in 200 AD during the Charaka period. East India Company in 1664 opened the first hospital at Chennai in India for treating wounded soldiers and in 1668 for civilians. The modern system of medicine came up in the late 18th century. First medical college with systematic medical training was opened in Kolkata (in 1835), Mumbai (in 1845), and Chennai (in 1850). Later on, many hospitals and dispensaries at tehsil and district levels were set up for treating the army as well as civil population.

After independence, modernized research and referred hospital were set up. At present hospitals are formal institutions for patient care, a place where patients come for treatment and care for their illnesses.

Definitions of a Hospital

A hospital can be defined in various ways:
- According to the American Heritage Dictionary, the hospital is an institution that renders services to

patients suffering from medical, surgical, or psychiatric problems.
- WHO defines a hospital as a health organization to provide diagnostic, curative, preventive, and rehabilitative services to the population at large. It is a training and research center for health professionals.
- Hospital is a type of health-care institution, which has an organized medical and other staff, and inpatient facilities, and delivers services throughout the day and year. It offers a range of acute, convalescence, and terminal care, using diagnostic and curative services.

Characteristics of a Hospital

The characteristics of hospital are given below:
- Hospital is a highly sophisticated organization, deals with acute, emergency, life-threatening illnesses that need immediate and prompt treatment.
- It is an open system that interacts with its internal and external environments.
- The internal environment comprises specialized professional, technical, supportive, and auxiliary services, such as medical, surgical, nursing, dietary, and laboratory are needed at all times to fulfill the needs of patients.
- It requires services of unskilled, semiskilled, and highly skilled persons.
- It runs round the clock providing indoor and outdoor health-care services.
- A hospital system should be dynamic and in equilibrium with the broader social network.
- It is a part of the national health-care system.
- Clients with varied demographics and different social and cultural backgrounds seek and utilize its services.

Types of Hospitals

Hospitals are classified on the basis of the following criteria (Fig. 19.1):

1. **According to the system of medicine:** Hospitals can classify according to the system of medicine, e.g., allopathic, Ayurvedic, Homeopathic, Unani, Siddha, and Nature Cure.
2. **According to ownership:** Hospitals, according to ownership, are divided into two major categories: public and private.
   a. **Government/public hospitals:** The government runs public hospitals that are of three types: central government hospitals, state government, and local self-government hospitals.
      - *Central government hospitals*: These hospitals are governed and funded by the central government or maybe autonomous such as railways hospitals, defense, AIIMS, and PGIMER.
      - *State government hospitals*: Hospitals under the State government are local hospitals or district hospitals, community health center (CHC), or general hospitals.
      - *Local self-government hospitals*: Municipalities or corporation run these hospitals such as BMC hospital.
   b. **Private hospitals:** Trust, religious bodies, private limited companies, private hospitals, run these hospitals. Hospitals registered under Society Act.
      - *Voluntary/trust hospitals*: These types of the hospital are owned and managed by trustees, for example, Jaslok hospital.
      - *Charitable hospitals*: These types of the hospital are owned and controlled by religious bodies or order such as CMC hospitals.
      - *Corporate hospitals*: Limited companies own and operate these types of hospitals. Apollo hospitals (40 hospitals) are a corporate chain of hospitals. Max Healthcare (10 hospitals),

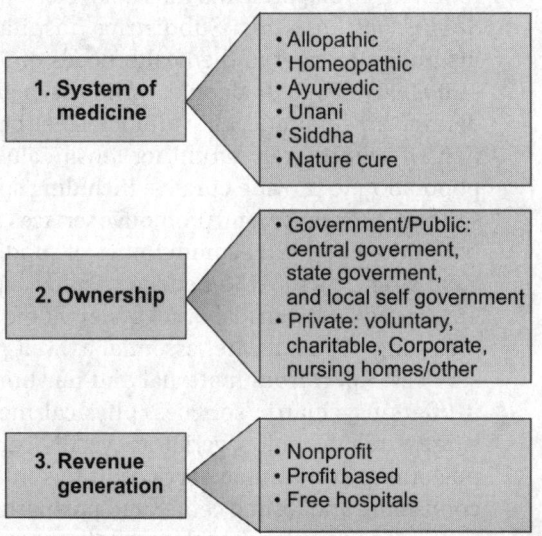
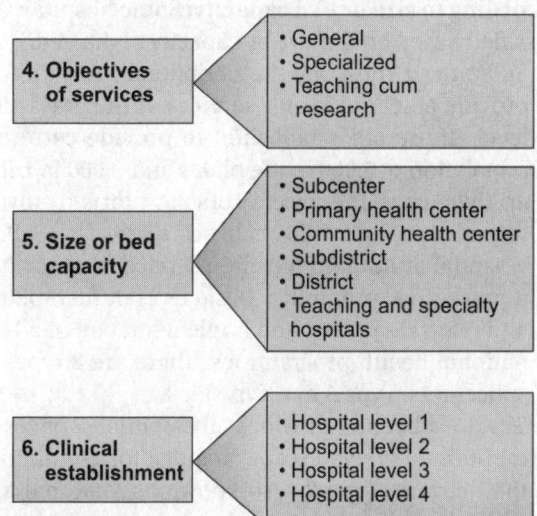

Fig. 19.1: Types of hospitals.

which is run by the public limited company. Columbia Asia (8 hospitals) is a private health-care company with chains of hospitals. Fortis hospitals are 50 hospitals, chain of super-specialty hospitals.
- *Nursing homes or other private hospitals*: These are the recognized institutions or clinical establishments that provide medical services and facilities of any system requiring diagnosis, treatment, and care owned and run by any person or body of persons.

3. **Based on revenue generation:** Hospitals are further subdivided into the following types:
   a. *Nonprofit hospitals:* Hospitals run by a voluntary organization for nonprofit basis.
   b. *For-profit hospitals:* Hospitals run by private health-care companies and corporations for-profit basis.
   c. *Free hospitals:* Free types of hospitals provide health services for free of cost.

4. **According to the objective of services offered by the hospital:** Hospitals are also further subgrouped into the listed types based on the services offered by the hospital:
   a. *General hospitals:* These are the hospitals that provide indoor and outdoor medical services requiring diagnosis, treatment, and care for types of patients and may have some specialized units staffed with skilled professionals.
   b. *Specialized hospitals:* The hospitals that render services and facilities to particular conditions, e.g. a pediatric hospital, mental hospital, maternity, and orthopedic hospitals, are termed as specialized hospitals.
   c. *Teaching cum research hospitals:* The hospitals provide indoor and outdoor patient care services of any system of medicine with the attached medical institute. Research hospitals have a research facility. Teaching hospitals have the facility of research and teaching.

5. **According to size or bed capacity:** Some hospitals are classified based on the size or capacity of the bed:
   a. *Subcenters:* These are the peripheral institution to provide essential health services at the grass-root level. These are established to provide care to a population of 5,000 in the plains and 3,000 in tribal and hilly areas. The objective of subcenter is to provide reproductive and child health-care services. It offers essential or minimum certain services that include a preventive, promotive, basic level of therapeutic and referral services, and implementation of all the national health programmes. There are 2 types of subcenters: Type A and Type B.
   Type A subcenter provides all essential services as mentioned above except facilities for conducting the delivery. *Type B*, also known as Maternal and Child Health (MCH) service center, contains all necessary functions as specified including facilities for conducting transportation and newborn care. Though the facilities for performing home deliveries are available in subcenters, the focus is on institutional deliveries. It has four to five rooms; one waiting room, one labor room (with one delivery table and facility for newborn care), one bedroom with a capacity of two to four beds, one store, one place for clinic/office.
   b. *Primary health center:* Primary health center (PHC) is the institution to cater to the health needs of the rural population of 30,000 in plains, and 20,000 people in tribal, hilly, and challenging areas. It is a referral unit for six subcenters. It provides services to sick who directly report, and subcenters refer patients. It has six indoor beds. There are two types of PHCs: Type A and Type B. Type A PHC have a load of fewer than 20 deliveries, and Type B has a capacity of more than 20 births. It provides all essential or minimum assured services.
   c. *Community health center:* It offers secondary level expert/specialist health-care services to a population of approximately 80,000 in tribal/hilly/desert areas and 1,20,000 populations residing in plain areas. It is the first referral unit of 30-bedded to provide medical, surgical, obstetrics, and gynecology, pediatrics, dental, and AYUSH services. The objective of CHC is to provide routine and emergency services related to medicine, surgery, maternal health, newborn care, family planning, and implementation of other national health programmes, school health, and adolescence health. It also has a facility for blood storage apart from diagnostic facilities. It has separate wards for male and females with a well-equipped nursing station, independent examination, and dressing table, ancillary room, operation theater/labor room. There are support services as Central Sterile Services Department (CSSD), laundry, emergency services, water supply, emergency lighting, and telephone facilities, record room, waste disposal, and mortuary, etc.
   d. *Subdistrict hospitals:* Subdistrict hospital is an institution to cater to the health needs of 5–6 lakh (1,00,000–5,00,000) people, which is below the district hospital and above block-level hospital/CHC. It is the first referral unit for Tehsil/Taluk/Block population to provide curative including specialist services, preventive, and promotive services to cover both urban and rural communities of subdivision/subdistrict. It is 100–150-bedded hospital to provide emergency obstetrical and gynecological care including neonatal care; essential as well popular services. Apart from maternal and newborn care, it offers psychiatric services, physical medicine, surgery, rehabilitation, geriatric, eye, ENT, accident, poisoning, and trauma services. It has integrated counseling and testing center and postpartum unit to provide secondary health care both specialist and referral services. There are two types of hospitals:

category I have 31–50 beds and category II have 51–100 beds.
   e. *District hospitals:* District hospital is a secondary referral level hospital to provide comprehensive secondary health services both specialist and referral services to urban and rural people at the district level (bed strength of district hospital varies from district to district depending on size, terrain, and population; usually districts have more than 75 beds and a maximum of 500 beds. Based on the size of the hospital, district hospitals are categorized into Grade I (500 beds), Grade II (400 beds), Grade III (300 beds), Grade IV (200 beds), and Grade V (100 beds). Apart from essential and desirable services (superspecialty), it provides newborn special, psychiatric, physical medicine and rehabilitation, accident and trauma, dialysis, and antiretroviral therapy (ART). It also has education and training facilities for primary health-care providers.
   f. *Teaching and specialty hospitals:* Teaching and specialty hospitals attached to state medical colleges provide tertiary level health-care services. These hospitals provide referral services and support to secondary level care hospitals; as well it should have access to the training of medical and other paramedical students, workforce development, and research at the state level.
6. **According to the clinical establishment (central government) rules 2012**: They are also classified per central government rules:
a. **Hospital-level 1:** This type of hospital has not more than 30-bed strength to cater primary health-care services to the people by trained and qualified staff. It provides all outdoor and emergency services including general medicine, first aid, maternal, newborn, pediatrics, and minor surgeries.
b. **Hospital-level 2:** This type of hospital is usually a general hospital providing secondary and multispecialty health-care services by several trained professional medical and paramedical staff. It has an additional facility for surgeries and anesthesia. Apart from care, it has other support systems such as pharmacy, laboratory, and diagnostic facilities.
c. **Hospital-level 3:** This type of hospital provides multispecialty care having different departments including the intensive care unit and dental department. It also has an additional facility of tertiary care with other support systems such as pharmacy, laboratory, and diagnostic and imaging facilities.
d. **Hospital-level 4:** All services are provided by level 3 hospital having attached teaching institute. This type of hospital provides tertiary care services and other support systems.

Functions of Hospitals

Functions of hospitals vary according to the type of hospital. Hospitals usually meet the health needs of the people. It has many features within and outside the hospital. The main functions of hospitals are to provide:
1. **Curative services:** Hospitals through its emergency and outdoor patient department offer services to the people who seek assistance during sickness for early diagnosis and appropriate treatment.
2. **Diagnostic services:** Hospital has various types of laboratory facilities for diagnosing multiple ailments. Different medical procedures are carried out in the hospital.
3. **Emergency and disaster management services:** Hospital is a center for providing all types of emergency services, first aid and manages any disasters at the time of any emergency occur to the people at anytime and anywhere.
4. **Specialized medical services:** Hospital provides specialized services as per the patient's need, e.g. medical, surgical, neurological, nephrology, oncology, mental health, geriatric care, and many more.
5. **Maternal and child health services:** Hospital has the facility for providing care to antenatal, intranatal, and postnatal care services. Each hospital has a separate labor room to conduct normal and abnormal deliveries and facilities to give immediate care to the newborn.
6. **Rehabilitative services:** Hospital provides physical, mental, and social rehabilitation to both in or outpatients through physiotherapy department and occupational therapy department by a trained physiotherapist.
7. **Social services:** Hospital has the provision to provide social services and help the patients through Red Cross or other societies. A social worker is appointed for this purpose.
8. **Guidance and counseling services:** Many general and teaching hospitals provide guidance and counseling services to children and parents and marriage counseling.
9. **Preventive services**: Hospital has the facilities of antenatal services to prevent any obstetric complications and includes immunization facilities, monitor growth, and development of children; prevention of prolonged illnesses, control of infectious diseases, etc.
10. **Community services:** Usually general hospitals have its community department that takes care of the health needs of the adopted community. Many governments and private-aided projects are initiated to prevent and promote the health of people. Many health camps, healthy meals, blood donation camps, eye camps, orthopedic camps, etc. are organized by related departments.
11. **Education and training:** Hospital is also a center of providing education and training to medical undergraduates, graduates, specialists, postgraduates, nurses and midwives, medical social workers, health workers, and other paramedical personnel. Hospital organizes various orientation programs, skill training, management, and continuing education programs for hospital health professionals.

12. **Research activities:** Hospital provides a platform for the health professionals to conduct various types of research studies and clinical trial under ethical consideration to improve the care of patients; hospital practices and administration; to provide innovative, evidence-based care.
13. **Infection control and biomedical waste management:** Each hospital should have infection control and biomedical waste management policy and programme. All personnel should comply guidelines given under "Biomedical Management and Handling Rules, 1998" to prevent the chances of cross-infection and hospital-acquired infection (HAI) to patients, staff or the general public, to minimize the environmental pollution as well as improve the standard of hygiene and sanitation in the hospital.
14. **Implementation of national health programmes:** Hospital plays a vital role to implement various national health programmes to achieve health for all community people.
15. **Hospital information system services:** Hospital has the facility to receive, process, and store information/data from every department, section, activity, and present information to all users working in the hospital. It is a valuable aid in the education and training of health professionals.
16. **Logistic support services:** Hospital provides other support services such as pharmacy, dietary, laundry, housekeeping, engineering, medical record, security, fire safety, mortuary, and outreach services.
17. **Information and health education:** Hospital provides information about its available services, before availing services; health professional before starting briefs about treatment, disease/diagnosis, possible causes, investigations required, treatment procedures, after effects and potential complications, chances of recovery and cost of treatment, etc. The hospital also provides brochures, pamphlets, booklets about the hospital, and health aspects in OPDs/wards/every patient waiting area. The information may be disseminated through audio-visual aids in the waiting areas, departments, or the display board around corridors to convey health message to patients and the public. Use a public address system for announcing the vital message especially to the relatives of patients undergoing operations waiting outside operation theaters.
18. **Telecommunication services:** Many large and research hospitals are providing telecommunication services including teaching, and health information to the community, and health personnel through telephone, mobile, broadcasting, and satellite.
19. **Safeguard the rights of consumers and health professionals:** Hospital has the plan to safeguard the interests of sick and suffering of patients. The program must address legal and ethical rights and also protect the rights of health-care workers. **Figure 19.2** depicts the services provided by the hospital.

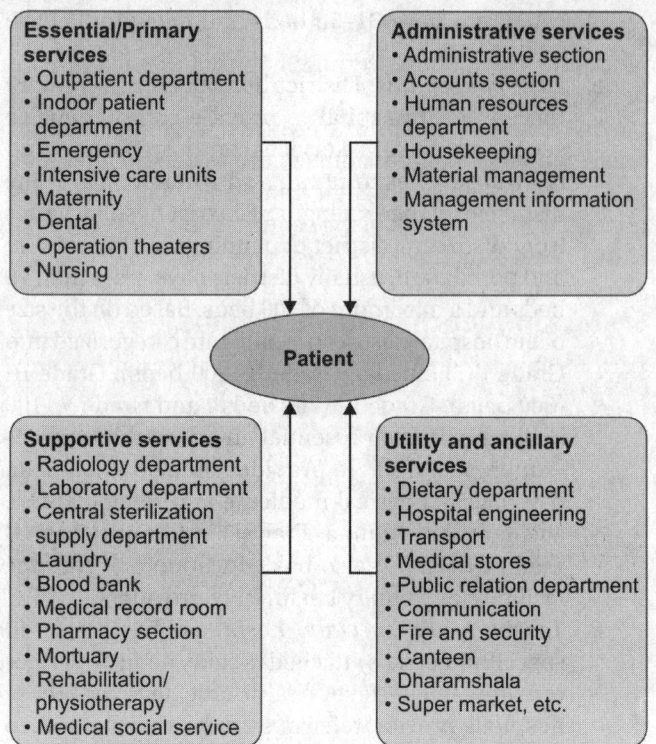

Fig. 19.2: Services provided by the hospital.

PLANNING OF HOSPITAL

Introduction

Planning is the first step in managerial decision-making. The plan is a process by which a manager develops a framework for the allocation of resources. The health-care institution has its philosophy and broad objectives for providing services for comprehensive healthcare, training, and research. A proper planning enables the management to translate these broad ends to specific goals and to work out ways and means to meet these objectives and decide on how best to match the available resources of men, money, supplies and equipment, time, and space.

The concern of hospital planning is the quality of medical care and the improvement of its standards. A successful plan is a key to finding and acting on opportunities within external constraints and uncertainties of hospitals. To plan a new hospital and its extension is not only a job for an architect, but the administrator also plays an essential role in guiding. It is the first requirement to decide the function of the hospital, the type of patient to be treated, and locality of patients. Hospitals have been changing in shape, size, and services to adapt themselves to the advancements in the medical field and socioeconomic changes around them.

The planning at the Central government is at the macro level. At this level, it provides direction and broad guidelines for the State and regions to follow. On the other hand, we have departmental planning within health organizations where the staff works out a program of activities for the forthcoming period, including those resources they may need and the results they hope to achieve. Between the two extremes, there are many levels. There are the state, district, block and down and governing board of the health-care organization.

An efficient hospital requires a well-balanced organization for compassionate care within an adequate technical and environmental framework. This basis has remained vital throughout the centuries, although patterns of diagnostics, therapeutics, and care have changed.

Factors Influencing Hospital Planning

Various factors given below have impact on hospital planning:

1. **Modular construction:** More efficient forms of development are required to keep pace with the health-care modernization process and for better quality outcomes in lesser time. The use of this type of structure is directly influenced by the patient's requirements for speed of development and the addition of new departments.
2. **Flexibility in designing:** The hospital design should be flexible as to continually adapt the changing needs coming mainly from technological development and new medical practices.
3. **Ownership:** Ownership helps in determining the objectives, profit, power, properties, tax, funding, size, structure, and quality of services.
4. **Disease profile:** The planning must suit the upcoming diseases, changes in the disease patterns and nutrition-related conditions predominated, to one where non communicable and lifestyle-related diseases, accidents, and injuries are the significant causes of morbidity and mortality.
5. **Technology advancement:** Electronic health records, computerized physician order entries, biometric identifications of the patient are some of the new trends emerging in information technology. Technology will enable revenue cycle management. Providing the facility for nanotechnology should be taken into consideration for the near future. Nano, a Greek word meaning dwarf (one billionth of a meter in length), is finding its way into multiple applications. Also, microsensor monitoring healing process decreases postoperative hospitalization and the waiting time for transplant devices too.
6. **Services utilization:** In ambulatory surgical or diagnostic centers, many new medical technologies allow many procedures that were previously performed only in the hospital.
7. **Hospital asepsis:** Consider location and type of construction material to maintain asepsis in a hospital. The design of the hospital must support handwashing by way of placement of sinks and autodisinfectant dispensers.
8. **Patient safety:** Patients are always the main focus in a hospital; protection of the patients is the primary rule. Planning and designing must provide a safe, comfortable, and healthy environment for the patient. The consumers are increasingly demanding convenient, reliable, and timely services offered in a caring, safe, and high-quality environment. There should be restricted exits and at least two exits. Ensure the security of persons and property.
9. **Social and political changes:** Patient safety concerns have both social and political overtones. Many Western countries have passed legislation on same, and India will also follow suit. Consumer Protection Act is already in place. Computerized physician order entry (CPOE), automation of pharmaceutical dispensing, and evidence-based hospital referral have emerged as solutions to these concerns.
10. **Consumers' needs:** Consumers' consideration is another important issue to recall during hospital planning. The hospital must serve the needs of the community. The plan must do the need assessment and demographic survey to initiate a project of planning hospital.
11. **Cost:** Consider both capital and recurring costs of the hospital in establishing the hospitals.
12. **Physical facilities:** Consider the design and shape of the hospital at the time of planning. Plan all physical facilities as per norms. Provide enough spaces and circulation routes for the patients for transferring from one place to another and for doing other activities. There should be proper lightening, ventilation, privacy, water supply, waste disposal, sanitation, housekeeping, fire protection, signage, parking facilities, zoning, and functionally related to each other.

Principles of Hospital Planning

Following are the guiding principles of hospital planning (Fig. 19.3):

General Principles

1. **The principle of quality-centered care:** Hospital must ensure the quality of the patient's care. There should be an accreditation committee, patient safety committee, quality assurance and training unit, laid down standards and indicators, standard operating procedures for each department. The policy must include incidence reporting, client survey, nursing audit.
2. **The principle of service utilization:** Ensure proper use of resources through analysis of vital statistics such as

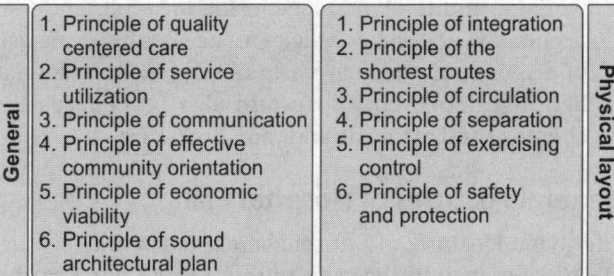

Fig. 19.3: Principles of hospital planning.

bed count, hospital census, the average length of stay, bed occupancy rates, etc.

3. **The principle of communication:** To keep the information confidential, the hospital information system must have good security practices, safekeeping of information, back up, and safeguarding of passwords.
4. **The principle of effective community orientation:** There should be an excellent public relationship between the governing body and local community leaders. The hospital must cater to the diverse needs of the community. The community must know various programs and services provided by the hospital through a public information system.
5. **The principle of economic viability:** Governance must ensure that they have a financial position through sponsorship, contributions, and other funding agencies to run the hospital. It should also be ensured that they can hire skilled personnel and purchase high-quality equipment to provide services.
6. **The principle of sound architectural plans:** Have a competent and experienced architect who should be expert in hospital designing and construction. The architect plays a vital role in selecting the site suitable for building a hospital, advising the size of the hospital, and interior designing.

Principles Related to Hospital Building Layout

1. **The principle of integration:** Integrate all departments in the hospital.
2. **The principle of the shortest routes:** Traffic routes must be kept short for the health personnel and patients.
3. **The principle of circulation:** There should be proper space for patients' movement, staff movement, supply delivery, disposal of used goods, laundry service, food service, and other domestic services.
4. **The principle of separation:** This principle advocates that there should be a separation of different activities, that is, a separation of clean and dirty operations in the departments. Patients' utility room and collection of soiled linen should be at another corner of the department.
5. **The principle of exercising control:** There should be control over patients' corridors, visitors' entering and leaving units, and for the staff working in the hospital.
6. **The principle of safety and protection:** There should be the provision of security of the patients, health workers, and the workplace in the hospital. Endorse occupation and safety policies for acute injury, safe use of disposal, biomedical waste management, essential lighting, floors, corridors, and also procedures for chemical and cytotoxic and radiation safety.

General Features of Hospital Plan

The general features of a hospital are listed below:
1. Allow maximum light and breeze to all parts of the building.
2. Windows should be screed to keep out mosquitoes and flies.
3. There should be four separate entrances in the hospital, namely main hospital entrance, outpatient entrance, emergency, and service entrance.
4. Service entrance must be adjacent to the kitchen and stores.
5. Main entrance and lobby must be attractive and designed properly.
6. The traffic pattern for patient, staff, and visitors within the building and within and between departments should be such that should eliminate congestion.
7. The separate public corridor from patient and staff corridor.
8. Outpatient departments should route from registration and medical record room.
9. In-patient departments should route from admitting offices.
10. Visitors' routes should be controlled carefully.
11. There should be proper signage system.
12. Floors should be constructed from a maintenance point of view.
13. Walls must be smooth, straight, and of sufficient heights.
14. The provision of stairways and elevators as well as locating a maximum concentration of traffic should be there in a hospital.
15. Fire safety provision must be in the hospital.

Process/Steps of Hospital Planning

Planning of a hospital is a complex process and requires a long-term plan. Following steps can be undertaken whether doing the planning for a big or small hospital, by and large, proceeded through the following stages (**Fig. 19.4**):

Stage 1: Master Planning

This stage, also known as "bricks-and-mortar" planning, is related to the design and construction of physical facilities. It should also define the institutional role and future programs.
1. **Constitution of the planning committee:** A hospital planning committee should constitute hospital administrator, specialists from various clinical areas, engineers from a civil and electrical branch, senior architect, nursing advisor, and a representative from the local body. The committee is formulated to find out the demographic pattern and site selection and to assess the needs of the community.
2. **Outlines of functions:** It includes the assessment of needs, which are to be served, estimating the number of beds, size of departments and their workload, staff and accommodation, the nature of site area, access, and planning position.
3. **Preliminary survey/feasibility study:** An initial survey is done to check the feasibility of establishing a hospital. It is essential to get the basic idea of what is to be done

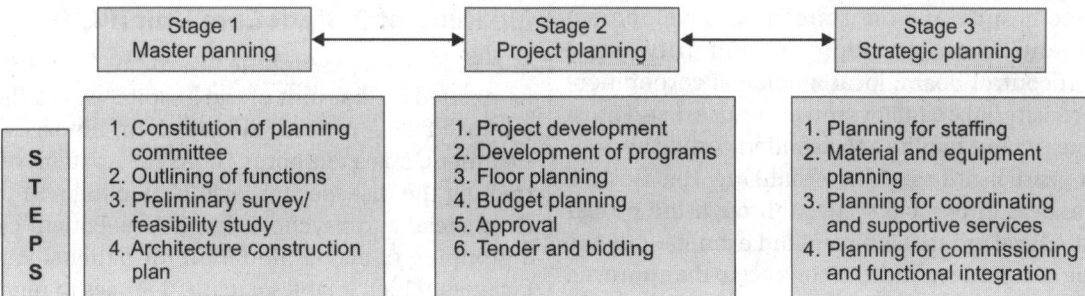

Fig. 19.4: Process/Steps in hospital planning.

based on the needs of the community. The members of the planning committee conduct a preliminary survey to gather the following information:

i. *Demographic data:* It includes the size of the community, character, type of population residing in that locality, socioeconomic status and source of income, affordability, beliefs, attitudes, practices, cultures of people, present health-care facilities, and number of population to be covered.
ii. A study of health needs and liabilities of the service area.
iii. *Geographical data:* It includes location or site selection, land area according to the size of the hospital to be planned, approachability, suitability for construction, provision for drainage, and water supply.
iv. *Environmental data:* It includes area-facing sunlight, noise, smoke, climate, and traffic should be appropriate for the hospital.
v. *Electricity and water supply:* During the survey, consider the availability of three-phase electricity supply with an appropriate load, a facility for installing generators. There should be adequate 24 hours water supply and proper sewerage system, and sewerage treatment plant, and a suitable nearby facility for biomedical waste management.
vi. *Communication, transport, and other facility:* There should be adequate telephone exchange facilities. There should also be nearby public (train/bus) and private proper available transport facility available for the patients. There should be a provision of other facilities such as nearby sarai, canteen, bank, and supermarkets.

4. **Architecture construction plan:** The architect should plan the design and get approved a blueprint of construction by town planning/local authority. A design must possess functional areas, floors, facilities for all departments and other facilities such as electricity and air conditioning plant, lifts, fire safety, and water supply. Consult with members of the planning committee for the final construction plan.

Stage 2: Project/Institutional Planning

This stage was for the planning of programs and departments of the hospital. There was an expansion of existing applications on the one hand and exploring new types of health-care services on the other besides setting annual and long-term objectives for them. Thus the budgeting was tied to these objectives.

1. **Preparation of project proposal:** Prepare a plan to establish a hospital. It must have mission, philosophy, objectives, need, and justification for undertaking the project. It must mention or include size, shape, location, and type of the hospital, type of services to be provided, and cost both capital and recurring of the project, etc.
2. **Development of the program:** A written plan should include:
    - A statement of mission and philosophy, objective
    - Organization structure and organization chart
    - Administrative policies, rules, and regulation, organization of internal functions
    - Service rules, standing orders, recruitment policies, job descriptions, remuneration policies, employees benefits, policies, standard operative procedures, and procedure manuals
    - Orientation programs, performance evaluation
    - Grievances policies and disciplinary action procedures
    - Signage system, disaster plan, and public relation
    - Admission and discharge policies, among other rules
    - Insurances, schedules of rates, methods of maintaining vital statistics banking, audit, hospital budget, etc.

   Under operational policies, develop plans regarding the location of departments, movements of staff, and equipment, etc.
3. **Floor planning:** Floor planning should consist of ward units, diagnostic X-ray department, physiotherapy, and technical department, kitchen, OPDs, CSSD, pathology department, administrative department, record room, maternity department, emergency, pediatric ward, laundry, operation theaters, ancillary services, dispensary, mortuary, etc.
4. **Budget planning:** Estimate the cost needed at the early stage and must be realistic. Make full provision for contingencies. Prepare both capital and recurrent budgets.
5. **Project and budget approval:** Get approval from the administrative body and finance committee, from the

government such as from state/rural development department/urban development authority, state pollution control board, local municipal corporation, and electricity/Jal board for land clearance. Land must be registered and require a registration certificate.
6. **Tender and bidding:** After finalizing the design, invite tenders in two bid systems through the proper method. These are then opened and examined by the planning committee. Offer the contract to the approved construction agency.

Stage 3: Strategic Planning

Strategic planning is the planning of resources such as staffing, materials, equipment, furniture, machinery, and other supplies. Do planning during the construction period.
1. **Staffing:** Planning for human resources such as doctors, nurses, paramedical, technicians, technical staff, supportive staff, sanitation staff, administrative staff, clerical, and for coordinating services such as receptionists, clerks, accountants, and cashier. The essential requirement must be planned and calculated per the norms and policies.
2. **Material and equipment planning:** Material and equipment planning includes the plan for heavy machinery/monitors, equipment, articles, linen, drugs, and disposables, transport, stationeries, reagents, furniture, etc. Quantity and quality must be decided, considering the personal preferences of users so far these should be compatible with the standardization and per norms. Design and color should fit with the surroundings. Ensure proper procedures to procure.
3. **Planning for coordinating and supportive services:** Do prepare for all coordinating and supportive services such as dietary, CSSD, linen, and labs services.
4. **Planning for commissioning and functional integration:** It should start after the construction is over. Commissioning means bringing the building into operational order. Install materials such as air conditioning, lifts, equipment; recruitment of staff, advertisement, publicity, and date of inauguration. Test all the elements and make functional. Various planning tools such as Programme Evaluation and Review Technique (PERT) and/or Critical Path Method (CPM) can be used to monitor the progress of the project.

PLANNING OF PATIENT CARE UNIT (PCU)

Introduction

The most basic management function is planning. The essential stages of planning are analysis, implementation, and evaluation. It is choosing between alternatives, in the highest form of decision-making, is an exercise at maximizing available resources. It is a multidisciplinary approach. A specialized planning unit at a high level of government prepares the developmental program. A hospital planning team takes part in planning and discusses the outline of the proposed group.

Meaning of Patient Care Unit (PCU)

The PCU is also called the "ward," or "nursing unit" can be defined as that unit of the hospital where the patients admitted and nursed during their illnesses for their treatment. It is a temporary home of a patient not only for treating the diseases but also protecting and promoting their social and psychological needs. Patient care unit is a grouping of accommodation for patients with service facilities, which enables a team of nurses to render care to inpatients under the best possible conditions. It is a part of a hospital designed in a particular manner to provide care to the specific types of patients.

Patient care unit refers to an area in a hospital or any health setting where patients of similar needs are grouped to facilitate health-care delivery by health-care professionals, including nurses. It includes patients' beds, nursing station, service area, storage area, work area, and a clean area.

Functional Goals of PCU

The PCUs should be designed to serve practical goals. An ideal PCU must:
- Result in building at the lowest possible capital cost
- Provide for the best possible physical facilities
- Enhance the nurse–patient interaction
- Be operated at the lowest possible cost
- Provide the most desirable patient environment
- Result in inefficient operation of the unit and ability of nurses
- Provide a friendly environment for nursing and medical staff
- Provide the highest level of satisfaction for nursing and medical staff
- Provision of the needs of the visitors
- Regulate the highest quality of communication and information system.

Objectives of Patient Care Unit

The objectives of PCU are to:
1. Provide a safe, comfortable, pleasant environment for the patients and staff
2. Make available required facilities to carry out all the activities
3. Provide enough space to carry out various activities
4. Give attention to the economy of attendance and ease of supervision
5. Meet the functional requirement and thus enhance administrative efficiency and economy
6. Satisfy practical needs necessarily those of patients and nursing staff
7. Achieve the role of the nursing unit through better handling of material and other resources.

Types of PCUs

There are various types of the patients care units/wards designs as follows:

1. **Open ward:** Open wards were meant for visibility of the patients at all times, cross ventilation and for the economy as well as for construction and maintenance. The disadvantages of this type of PCU/ward were lack of privacy, difficulty in controlling noise, and climatic conditions apart from a higher risk of hospital cross infections.
2. **Nightingale ward:** Nightingale ward is a traditional type of PCU based on the ward concept established by Florence Nightingale. It was a unit of 30–40 or more patients, with its kitchen and arrangement for all stores and supplies. It was an example of the rectangular design of PCUs. The beds of patients are in rows; the toilets and bathrooms are at one end, and the nurses' table, doctor's room, and other technical facilities are at the other end of the ward. It lacks patients' privacy, a not-so-quiet ward atmosphere and danger of cross infection. It is the best design in case of an acute shortage of nurses and limited professional knowledge of nurses.
3. **Rigs ward design:** Rig pattern type/ward design is an improvement over the pavilion type regarding the provision of privacy and comfort for the patients. Practicing aseptic techniques of the department is easy. Rig ward is another example of rectangular wards. It has small cubicles with beds in parallel to the longitudinal wall. This type of design is useful for learning purposes. But challenging to observe and communicate with patients. There is a considerable distance from the nursing station to the patient's bed **(Fig. 19.5)**.
4. **Single corridor design wards:** These are rectangular wards with a single corridor aimed to reduce travel distance from the nursing station to patients' beds. These are of different shapes like H shape, T shape, Y shape; E shape designed to reduce cost and provides several facilities **(Fig. 19.6)**.
5. **Double corridor/cross design wards:** Double corridor design of wards further reduce the travel distance of nurses from the nursing station to patients' beds. It saves nursing time and facilitates patient segregation. The nursing station and other facilities like utilities and supply rooms, treatment and procedure rooms, doctors' room, etc. are positioned in the center of the ward. It may create ventilation and lighting problems. Patient rooms are outside the track **(Fig. 19.6)**.
6. **Circular design:** In the circular design of wards nursing station is in the center aiming to keep a check on all the patients by nurses and doctors. The patients' beds are very close to the nursing station. The main disadvantages of this type of wards are difficulty in expansion and lack of indirect observation of all patients at one time.
7. **Square design:** Square type of PCUs are better for nurses of varying degrees of skills and training background, shortage of financial resources and to meet the most vigorous functional requirements for some time to come.

Components of the PCU

Components of the PCU are given below:
1. **Patient areas/rooms:** These rooms comprise private, semiprivate or general wards. These rooms provide a safe and esthetically pleasing treatment area conducive for a speedy recovery. It must contain space for equipment, staff, and various needs of the patients. Bed strength is the criteria to plan space.
2. **Nursing station:** The nurse control station provides workspace for the nursing staff. The location and design of nursing stations are such that the nurse can observe patient rooms and direct the traffic entering and leaving the unit and at the same time carry on nursing care and safety of the patients' activities. It must enhance nurse–patient interaction and reduces the nurses' fatigue factor by minimizing to and fro movement between the patient's bed and treatment room, nursing station, storeroom, etc.
3. **Service/work area:** The function of service/work area is related to handling material required for patient care to meet the social and physical needs of the patients and specific needs of the staff.

Principles of Planning the PCU

A patient/nursing care unit in a hospital has been called by the planner as the greatest common measure (GCM), regarding cost. The principles of planning a nursing unit are as follows:
1. The nursing unit should suit the cultural background of the community
2. Minimize nurses fatigue factor
3. Sound planning should provide a safe environment for patients and staffs to:
   - Prevent chances for cross infections. Cross infection may be due to overcrowding, poor ventilation, and inadequate sterilization

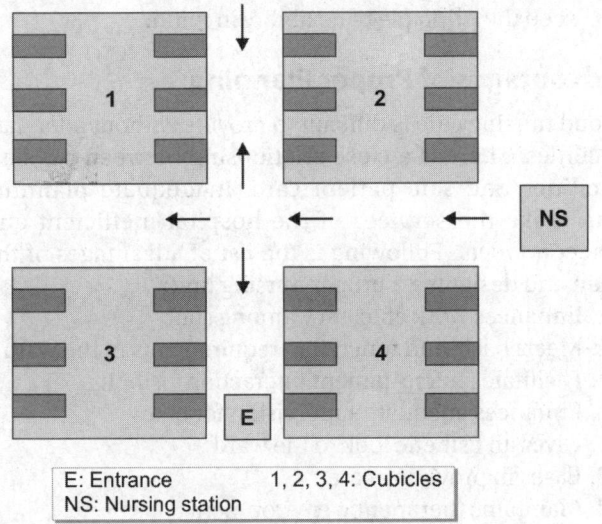

E: Entrance 1, 2, 3, 4: Cubicles
NS: Nursing station

Fig. 19.5: Rigs ward design.

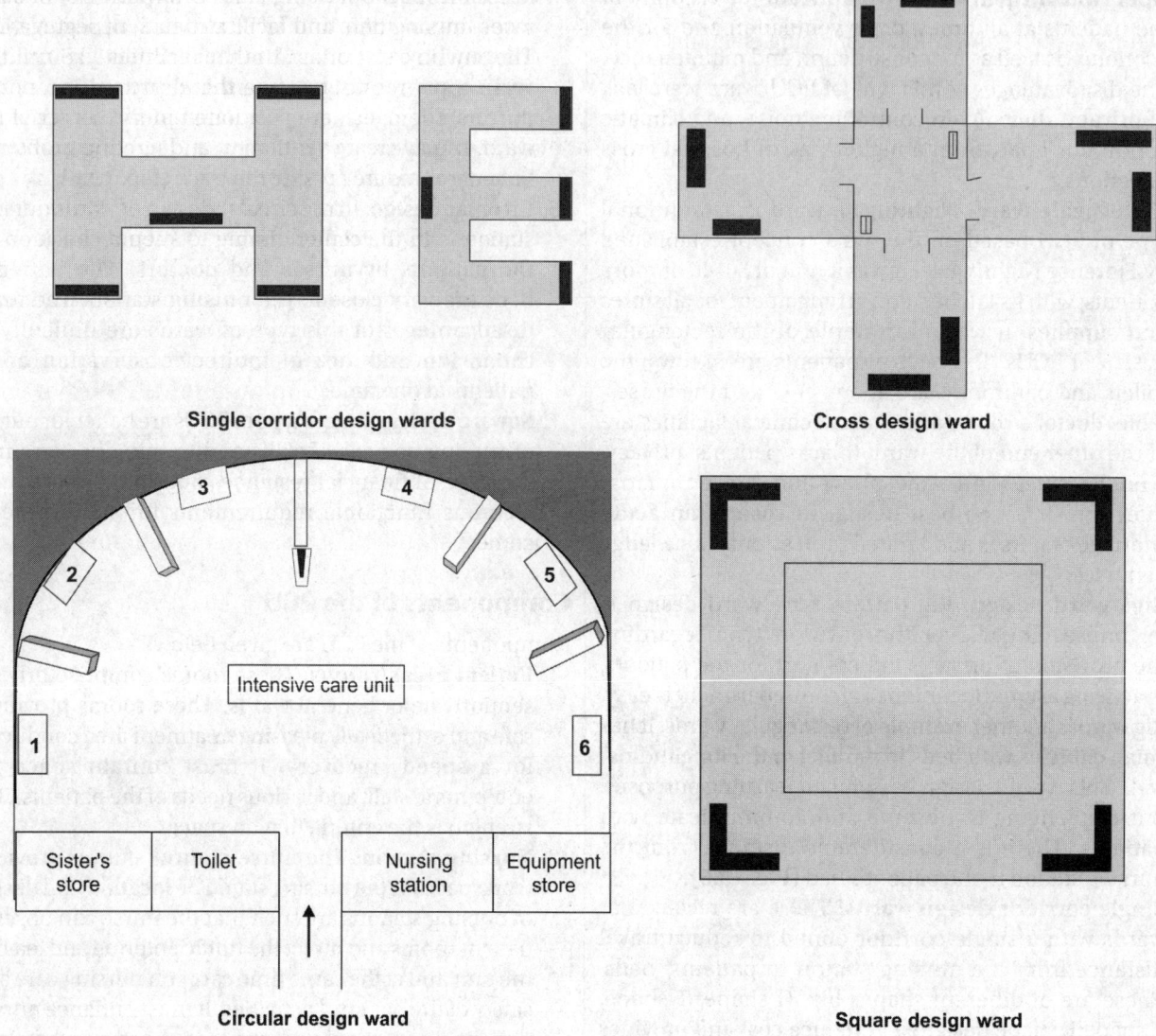

Fig. 19.6: Different designs of the wards.

- Prevent chances for accidents; accidents may be due to uneven or slippery floors, poor lighting, and high beds, etc.
- Prevent chances for a fire that may be due to short circuits, faulty electric equipment
- Prevent chances for negligence and nursing errors due to poor lighting.

4. Sound planning must provide a pleasant environment for patients and staff by:
   - Preventing opportunities for noise due to noisy plumbing, the proximity of ward to kitchen or sluice room, etc.
   - Lack of privacy for patients who may be due to nonavailability of screen, bed curtains, or inadequate toilet facilities
   - Dull surroundings may be due to a poor choice of color, high windows, etc.

5. Sound planning must promote efficiency and ease of work of the staff

6. Maintain the principle of observability
7. Plan according to the number of sanctioned nurses
8. Keep the principle of flexibility in mind.

Advantages of Proper Planning

Good nursing care is difficult to provide without adequate facilities. There is a close relationship between physical facilities and safe patient care. Inadequate planning can make the services of the hospital inefficient and uneconomical. Following is the list of advantages of the plan and designing a proper nursing unit:

1. Enhances work efficiency among staff
2. Meets basic and functional requirements of the ward
3. Facilitates nurse–patient interaction visibility
4. Enhances adequate supervision for care
5. Gives an esthetic look to the ward
6. Eases in providing care
7. Maintains therapeutic environment
8. Reduces fatigue among staff.

Factors Consideration for Planning

For planning a type of ward, the following elements must consider:
1. Age of patients of admission
2. Nature of illness and treatment required
3. The degree of physical and mental capabilities of patients
4. Availability of centralized services
5. Need to provide facilities for clinical teaching.

Prerequisite for Planning the PCU

The prerequisites for planning the PCU are as follows:
- Efficiency and cost-effectiveness
- Flexibility and expandability
- Therapeutic environment
- Cleanliness and sanitation
- Esthetic
- Safety and security.

Consideration for Planning the Patient Care Unit

The following criteria should be taken into account for planning the PCU:

Location

- Patient care units have a close relationship with the operating room, pharmacy, central stores, laboratories, and the kitchen. They are highly dependent on vertical transportation and efficient communication system. Therefore, the plan should favor the location of PCUs from these departments in the hospital.
- Separate critical areas like operation theaters, intensive care units from general traffic and avoid air movements from areas like laboratories and infectious disease wards toward critical areas.
- Keep isolation wards out of circulation from infectious causes.

Design: Size and Configuration

- Decide the size of PCUs and the distribution of beds during the planning stage. Whether or not the unit should be a single ward providing one clinical specialty/general medicine under one consultant.
- Consider the cost of construction of the unit, staffing requirements, and the distance between the nursing station, the patient rooms, and the supply points.
- Avoid any duplication of facilities and equipment.
- The size of the PCUs varies; these may be very small or very large. Both are uneconomical. The minimal units are more expensive to build and maintain. The large units are unsatisfactory from the service point of view and facilities need in duplicate. The size is between 20 and 40 beds. Each PCU has its specific requirements and possibilities.

- Calculate the optimum size of the general PCU according to the number of patients and nurse-in-charge who can manage the unit efficiently. Since the nursing service operates on three shifts to cover 24-hour period, consider other parameters like activities of the unit, bed utilization, and degree of acuity of patients' illness for considering the adequate size of a nursing unit.
- Consider appropriate possible configuration such as round, square, straight, oval, circular, H shape, T shape, or Y shape as discussed above at the time of planning. These can be with a single corridor or double doors.
- The design should support the concept of zoning (protective, clean, aseptic/sterile, and disposable/dirty) and ventilation standards.
- Provision of washbasins within patient care areas and nursing station to facilitate handwashing practices.
- Provision of separate staircases and lifts for removal of garbage and infectious waste removal from wards and departments.
- Provision of isolation unit within PCUs.

Physical Layout Classification

I. **Four-group classification:** Primary, auxiliary, sanitary, and ancillary **(Fig. 19.7)**.
   1. *Primary area/accommodation:* Primary area of the PCU comprises bed accommodation (patient rooms), nursing station, and treatment room.
   2. *Auxiliary area/accommodation:* Auxiliary area includes doctors' room, nurses' room, stores, and clean utility.
   3. *Sanitary area/accommodation:* It consists of a toilet block, dirty utility, and safai karamchari closet.
   4. *Ancillary area/accommodation:* The ancillary area has ward pantry, day room, conference/seminar room, and stretcher trolley bay.

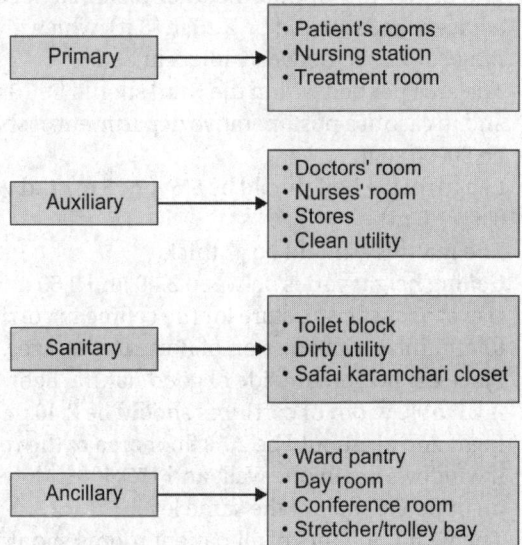

Fig.19.7: Physical layout of a patient care unit.

II. **Three-group classification:**
1. *Accommodation for patients:* These accommodations include patients' rooms, general plan, and ancillary accommodation.
2. *Accommodation for staff:* It includes offices (sisters' office, doctors' room), clinical areas (treatment area, dressing room, investigating/test room, clean utility room, dirty utility room, and sluice room), storage room (storeroom for linen and drugs; store for bulky equipment; space for parking wheelchairs, trolley, and stretcher; and cleaner's room), and domestic area like kitchen.
3. *Accommodation for visitors:* It includeswaiting room (lobby or entrance hall), accommodation for relatives of a seriously ill patient like cloakroom.

We will explain in detail the critical areas of PCU:
1. **Patient rooms:** The hospitals adopt different types of floor plans. Selection of floor plan depends on suitability and prevailing trends and consultation of the architect. There are multiple types of floor plans according to the kind of PCUs. Within ward, the program mostly adopted for grouping of patients into six-bed and four-bed rooms, rooms with two beds and with one bed for the patients who are acutely ill and require segregation from other standard patients' room. The nursing station, doctors' room, treatment room, nurses' office should be in the center. This type of arrangement has the particular advantage in the deployment of nurses and permit flexibility to use the beds. The unit must have the following criteria:
   - The minimum floor space between beds should be 7.0 m^2 physically per bed.
   - The suggested maximum floor space for a single-bedroom is 14.00 m^2 and for the two-bedroom is 21.00 m^2.
   - Beds must arrange in such a manner to allow maximum privacy.
   - The center to minimum center distance between adjacent beds should be 2.25 m (8 ft), which gives a range of 1.25 m between adjacent beds.
   - The area per bed within the ward should be 70 sq ft, and in case of a postoperative department, it should be 80–90 sq ft.
   - Length of the bed should be 6'6" (2.15 m) and width 3'3" (1.0 m).
   - The mattress should be 4" thick.
   - Ceiling height varies between 3.00 and 3.60 m.
   - Use of acoustic structure for the ceiling in corridors to minimize transmission of noise in passages.
   - Place the bed on the side of good natural light.
   - A suitable width of corridors should be 2.40 m.
   - Light and air should be 20% floor area of the rooms if windows are in one wall, and 15% if windows are on opposite walls at the same level.
   - The width of doors of all patient rooms should not be less than 1.20 m.
   - There should be moveable bedside lockers, stool/chair, and built-in cupboards.
   - No patient room should be 90' from the nurses' station.
2. **Nurses' station:** Nurses' station is the nerve of the unit. It should be close to the patients' beds but in the center to view the entire unit and adequate functioning of the unit. It should have glass on three sides to facilitate continuous observe the patients. It should be open to the corridor side with a counter which acts a barrier and as a desk. The adequate size of nurses' station should not be < 60 sq ft. The nurses' room should be 120 sq ft. The following facilities are as follows:
   - Nurses' station must have the sister's room with attached WC
   - A table for preparation of medicine and injection trays, etc.
   - Sufficient space for working
   - Cupboards for storage of digs, dressings, and instruments
   - A small separate room adjacent to the nurses' station for medical store
   - A closet for narcotics and dangerous drugs, and medical cupboard
   - A refrigerator for the storage of medicines
   - Call system panel
   - Wall clock and bulletin board
   - Telephone, paging, and intercommunication systems
   - A chart desk/rack with chart holders
   - Storage for stationery, forms, etc.
   - Handwashing facilities, etc.
   - Nurse lavatory and clockroom of approximate size of 60 sq ft
   - Ward furniture must be comfortable to move from one place to other, easy to maintain, durable, and well designed.
3. **Treatment room:** One can plan to have treatment and dressing room in one place with a facility of a sterilizer and sink. There should be one treatment cum dressing room for 25–30 beds. It must be close to the nurses' station for easy access.
4. **Isolation room:** Any patient's room can convert into the isolation unit to protect patients and staff from infections. In most cases, there is a provision of a separate isolation room with one bed. The room has a sink and bedpan washing facility for barrier nursing outside the door of the room.
5. **Doctor's office:** Plan a separate room for the use of doctor for examination of patients and consultations in one side of the PCU. It can serve as a conference/seminar room. There should be an examination table, desk, chair, and a washbasin.
6. **Stores:** The units sent weekly requirements of clothes, bedsheets, and other linen to central stores and kept near the ward for daily use. The size may be about 80

sq ft. There should be a special arrangement for the delivery of material to the department.
7. **Clean utility room:** The clean utility room is for sterilizing instrument, packing surgical dressing drums, and for setting treatment trolleys and trays. Plan a separate room of the size of 100–120 sq ft located near to treatment to keep the things for storage purpose.
8. **Dirty utility room:** The dirty utility room is also known as a sluice room. This room is required for emptying and cleaning of bedpans, urinals, and sputum mugs and for the temporary storage of stool and urine specimens. The size of a room ranges 100–120 sq ft. There should be one urinal per 16 beds.
9. **WCs and bathrooms:** Sufficient WCs and bath closets should be in each PCU. There should be one WC for 6–8 beds and one bathroom for 8–16 beds. Apart from the toilets and bathroom provided in a single-bed and two-bed rooms, there should be a lavatory block. WCs and bathrooms should be clean and well maintained.
10. **Washbasin/water closets:** The washbasins should be at appropriate places at the height of 91.5 cm at the basin rim. There should be one washbasin for 8–10 beds. The cubicle with four and six beds must have a separate washbasin. It should be 7 cm deep and of 80 cm height for patients with a wheelchair.
11. **Safai karamchari closet:** There should be as luice room for safai karamchari to keep things for cleansing purposes. The recommended space for sluice room is 120 sq ft.
12. **Sanitary unit:** If there is no facility for sluice room or janitor room separately, combine both with water closets and bathrooms. The size of the sanitary unit should be 300–350 sq ft for a PCU of 20–30 beds. There should be an additional arrangement for collection of soiled linen.
13. **Ward pantry:** In most of the hospitals, the dietary service is centralized. The centralized kitchen distributes main meals to patients. But there should be a separate provision or a small kitchen/pantry facility in the ward for receiving, warming, and distributing meals. There should be a wash-up room with a large sink and drainboard for cleansing food tray/plates and utensils. The size of the room should not be less than 12 m^2 (100 sq ft). If combined with the ward kitchen, it should not be less than 25 m^2.
14. **Dayroom:** Day room is a place to relax and meet visitors. The day room location is at the end of the ward, away from all the activities. Provide a common day room for adjoining wards.
15. **Conference/seminar room:** There should be an examination table, desk, chair, and a washbasin in the conference/seminar room.
16. **Stretcher, trolley bay:** Each PCU should have recessed space for storing stretchers, trolleys, and wheelchairs. Space for the stretcher is 21 sq ft, and total store space is 200 sq ft.
17. **Circulation/movements in the unit:** Keep circulation and movements as low as possible. There should be 4 ft space between the beds. The corridor width should be more than 8 ft. The corridors should be well lit and ventilated. The overall proportion of circulation space shall not exceed 20% of the total floor area of the ward unit.
18. **Engineering services:** Ensure safety and comfort, ease of maintenance, and without interruptions to the services and disturbances to the working of the hospital wards during construction.
    a. *Water supply:* There should be minimum of 300 L water/bed/day round the clock. There should be a provision of hot and cold water supply.
    b. *Electrical installations:* Electricity control board in a unit should be near the nurses' station and adequately protected from unauthorized interferences and at the same time easily accessible from the corridor. Conceal conduct and cables, service duct being practicable.
    c. *Ward ventilation:* Most of the hospitals depend on natural ventilation as on windows and fans. Natural ventilation is also more acceptable for the patients. Ventilation of lavatories and kitchen should be by the extraction method and patients room by the input method if mechanical ventilation is essential. Mechanical ventilation is costly and requires the installation of plant and ducting sufficient to extract 10 air changes/hour.
    d. *Ward heating and lighting:* Lighting has to be adequate to carry out routine tasks. An illumination level of 150–300 lux is normal to works and 20 lux per sq ft in treatment rooms. For patients, a level of illumination of 100 lux is satisfactory. The service room needs brighter illumination of about 200 lux, and general lighting is about 100 lux. Usually, it is advisable to use filament lighting for general lighting purposes in the hospital. The room temperature should be 65°F. Provision of inner healing is preferred; otherwise, heaters can use to maintain temperature.
    e. *Patient call bell system:* There should be a provision of call bell near the bedside of the patient to call nurses on duty. There is also a telephone facility in the nurse's station, doctor's room, and sister's room for internal and external calls.
19. **Miscellaneous services:** There are many miscellaneous services as follows:
    - *Fire protection:* Materials used to construct should be incombustible and fire resistant.
    - *Fire alarm:* There should be a manually operated fire alarm in each PCU.
    - *Fly proofing:* Lavatory and wards should provide fly proof wire gauze.
    - *Noise control device:* Noise is a health hazard; consult engineers at the time of planning to make

provision of minimizing noise at the time of construction.
- *Visitor waiting unit:* Provide a visitor room for waiting.
- *Safai karamchari retiring room:* There can be the provision of a retiring room for safai karamcharies.
- *Arrangement for piped oxygen and suction, etc.:* Arrangement can be made to have piped oxygen and suction to units supplied from the central manifold room. These pipes run near the ceiling, with the outlet mounted at common points on the walls next to patient beds.

CHAPTER HIGHLIGHTS

- Hospital is an institution, which provides services such as medical, surgical, or psychiatric care and treatment for the sick or the injured.
- The type of hospital is according to the system of medicine, ownership, size or number of beds, clinical orientation, specialization, client-group services, cost, and diverse ways.
- The essential functions of hospitals are to provide therapeutic, diagnostic, emergency and disaster, medical and specialized, maternity and child health, preventive, promotive, and rehabilitative services. It also offers other services such as administrative, supportive, and utility and ancillary services.
- Hospital planning is by general and building layout related principles. Master planning, project planning, and strategic planning are carried out in the planning of hospital.
- Patient care unit is a part of hospital designing. It is an area in a hospital or any health-care setting where patients of similar needs are grouped to facilitate health-care delivery by health-care professionals including nurses.
- There are different types of PCUs labeled as an open ward, nightingale, rigs, single door, double door, circular, square-designed units.

REVIEW QUESTIONS

I. Essay Type Questions
1. Define hospital. Describe different types of hospitals.
2. Enumerate functions of a hospital.
3. Describe various steps required in planning a hospital.
4. Define the patient care unit. Discuss the principles of planning a patient care unit.
5. Describe various components of patient care unit.

II. Short Notes
1. Principles of hospital planning
2. Types of patient care units
3. Services provided by the hospital
4. Features of a hospital plan
5. Highlights of the nursing station

III. Multiple Choice Questions
1. The hospitals run by corporation or municipalities are:
    a. Voluntary hospitals
    b. Local self-government hospitals
    c. Corporate hospitals
    d. General hospitals
2. Which type of hospital provides basic primary health-care services to a population of 5,000 people?
    a. Subdistrict hospital
    b. Community health center
    c. Primary health center
    d. Subcenter
3. A type of hospital (under central government rule, 2012) that provides secondary and multispecialty health-care services by trained professional medical and paramedical staff:
    a. Hospital level 1
    b. Hospital level 2
    c. Hospital level 3
    d. Hospital level 4
4. Which principle of hospital planning advocates that there should be proper space for patients' movement, staff movement, supply delivery, disposal, laundry, food, and other domestic services?
    a. Principle of circulation
    b. Principle of integration
    c. Principle of separation
    d. Principle of safety
5. The type of ward that is divided into small cubicles and beds are arranged parallel to longitudinal wall is called:
    a. Open ward   b. Nightingale ward
    c. Rigs ward   d. Square ward
6. The common size of a patient care unit is between:
    a. 20–40 beds   b. 30–50 beds
    c. 40–60 beds   d. 50–60 beds
7. The minimum distance between adjacent beds should be:
    a. 2.25 m   b. 2.00 m
    c. 1.75 m   d. 1.25 m
8. The recommended space for sluice room in the ward should be in the range of:
    a. 60 sq ft   b. 120 sq ft
    c. 80 sq ft   d. 240 sq ft
9. The minimum size of nurses' station should be:
    a. 30 sq ft   b. 40 sq ft
    c. 50 sq ft   d. 60 sq ft
10. What should be the minimum area per bed within the ward?
    a. 50 sq ft   b. 60 sq ft
    c. 70 sq ft   d. 80 sq ft

Answer Keys
1. b   2. d   3. b   4. a   5. c   6. a   7. d
8. b   9. d   10. c

SUGGESTED READING

1. Barrett J. Ward Management and Teaching, 4th edition. New Delhi: Konark Publisher; 2003.
2. Home - Bureau of Indian Standards. https://bis.gov.in/index.php/laboratorys/laboratory-services-overview/. [Accessed on 07.01.2020].
3. Clinical establishment. [Online] Available from: http://clinicalestablishments.nic.in/WriteReadData/437.pdf. [Accessed on 19.01.2019].
4. Francis CM, de Souza MC. Hospital Administration. New Delhi: Jaypee Brothers; 2000.
5. Gandhi N. 10-Steps in Hospital Planning-Projects to "Go Live." 2015 March 9. [Online] Available from: https://www.linkdin.com/pulse/10steps-hospital-planning-projects-go-live-nitiraj-gandhi. [Accessed on 19.01.2019].
6. Goel SL, Kumar R (Eds). Hospital Supportive Services: Hospital Administration in the 21st Century. New Delhi: Deep & Deep Publication; 2002.
7. Indian Railway Medical services. [Online] Available from: https://en.wikipedia.org/wiki/Indian_Railway_Medical_Services. [Accessed on 20.01.2019].
8. Sharma MP, Sadana BL, Kaur H. Public Administration in Theory and Practice, 7th edition. Delhi: Kitab Mahal; 2010.
9. Stewart M, Brown JB, Donner A, et al. The impact of patient-centered care on patient outcomes. J Fam Pract. 2000: 796-804.
10. Tabish SA. Hospital and Health Services Administration: Principles and Practice. New Delhi: Oxford University Press; 2005.

20 CHAPTER

Ward Management and Methods of Patient Assignment

CHAPTER OUTLINE
- Ward Management
  - Concept of Ward Management
  - Objectives of Ward Management
  - Principles of Ward Management
  - Functions of the Ward Sister
  - Components of Ward Management
  - Factors Involved in Good Ward Management
- Methods of Patient Assignment
  - Meaning and Definitions
  - Purposes of Patient Assignment
  - Principles of Assignment
  - Factors Influencing Patient Assignment
  - Methods of Patient Assignment

LEARNING OUTCOMES

After completion of this chapter, the learner will be able to:
- Understand the concept of ward management
- Enumerate objectives of ward management
- Describe principles of ward management
- Discuss components of ward management
- Identify factors of proper ward management
- Understand the concept of patient assignment
- Discuss methods of patients' allocation

KEY TERMS

Ward management, ward sister, policies, patient assignment

INTRODUCTION

Ward management is managing the work of a ward that involves planning, organizing, directing and controlling the staff, material and support services of the unit to achieve the best patient care. A head nurse must have a skill in directing the ward activity and should think of professional coworkers, auxiliary staff and patients. The assignment of nursing staff is a primary activity of health-care systems to achieve its goals.

WARD MANAGEMENT

Concept of Ward Management

Ward is a place or a nursing/patient care unit for the treatment of admitted patients. It is also a block, which forms a division in a hospital, that is shared by patients who need similar kinds of care. Number and types of wards depend upon the type of hospital like district hospital, general hospital, referred hospital, specialized hospitals and (maybe) private voluntary aided or government hospitals. Mostly, there are two types of wards, viz. general and special wards, e.g. the intensive care units (ICUs), pediatric ward, and psychiatric ward. The head nurse is in charge of a nursing unit.

Management is a process that involves planning, organizing, directing and controlling resources to achieve desired goals. Resources include man, money, material, and methods. It is also an activity that involves getting the work done through others by directing their efforts, decision-making and interpersonal relationship (IPR). Management as a group has the responsibility of managing the unit/organization. Good governance can get things done through their staff skillfully and efficiently and adapt the principles of administration to fulfill the needs and requirements of the situation in which it is operating.

All the departments of a hospital, including all wards, are involved in caring for the sick and injured, promoting health, preventing diseases, education, teaching and research. As the ward/nursing unit is the place for patients to stay, it becomes the center for coordinating all efforts to help him or her.

Objectives of Ward Management

The objectives of ward management are to:
- Make sure that the highest possible quality of patient care is provided

- Provide a clean, safe, comfortable and free from infection, accident, and hazards environment
- Help staff in achieving the highest level of work satisfaction
- Ensure all the facilities are available to meet the needs of patients and their attendants
- Direct and supervise staff working under a head nurse
- Coordinate and communicate with team members.

Principles of Ward Management

The principles of ward management are as follows:
1. Identify the staff of the ward as their most significant asset
2. Recognize the value and importance of each person associated and inspire them for their best thinking and performance
3. Approach every task in an organized, conscious manner to achieve the outcome
4. Establish definite short-term and long-range objectives to ensure more significant accomplishment
5. Secure full attainment of goals through general understanding and acceptance of them by others
6. Utilize resources carefully to achieve the most significant possible benefit
7. Keep individual faculty of the team well-adjusted by ensuring that each one knows what he or she is supposed to do, how well, with what authority and what type of work relationship he or she has with others
8. Concentrate on individual improvement through regular review of performance and potential
9. Provide an opportunity for assistance and guidance in self-development as a fundamental of institutional growth
10. Maintain adequate and timely incentives and rewards for an increase in human efforts
11. Supply work satisfaction for those who perform their work and those who are served by it
12. Be flexible to meet the changing conditions and emergencies.

Functions of the Ward Sister

A ward sister is the head of a nursing unit/ward. He or she performs various activities toward the unit/ward management, these include to:
1. Formulate and implement ward policies, rules and regulations and procedures and methods in multiple areas to achieve the ward's objectives
2. Assist the nursing supervisor, nursing superintendent and matrons by periodical submission of the daily evening and night reports and other information
3. Give assignments to staff and decide to delegate duties
4. Manage nursing and other staff working under him or her
5. Direct all staff for their activities
6. Conduct ward rounds
7. Efficiently manage and maintain material, supply, drugs and equipment
8. Establish and keep records and reports
9. Ensure a therapeutic environment
10. Appraise staff for their performance
11. Have an excellent public relation.

Components of Ward Management

Ward management mainly includes five elements, viz. the management of patient care, personnel, supplies, equipment and environment and the interpretation of policies and procedures (**Fig. 20.1**).

Management of Patient Care

The management of patient care includes all activities necessary to provide nursing care. These are:
1. **Admission and orientation of the patient:** At the time of entry, nurses orient patients and their relatives in the following areas:
   - The hospital as a whole and the unit or ward
   - The routines of the hospital and department like doctor's visiting time, round time, visitor's time, time for meals and so on
   - Rules and regulation about patients and his or her relatives
   - Staff and other patients and his or her relatives
   - Ward equipment for patient
   - Ward procedures
2. **Assessment of the needs of the patients and planning care:** After admission and orientation, the patient is assessed to identify his or her needs. The nurse makes every opportunity to gather information for making a correct nursing diagnosis and planning a nursing intervention. The plan is made known to all team members to provide continuity of care. The critical aspect of planning should include:
   - Establishing a patent airway and ensuring the patient is breathing normally
   - Checking vital signs, such as temperature, blood pressure and pulse, and respiration for adequate circulation and tissue perfusion

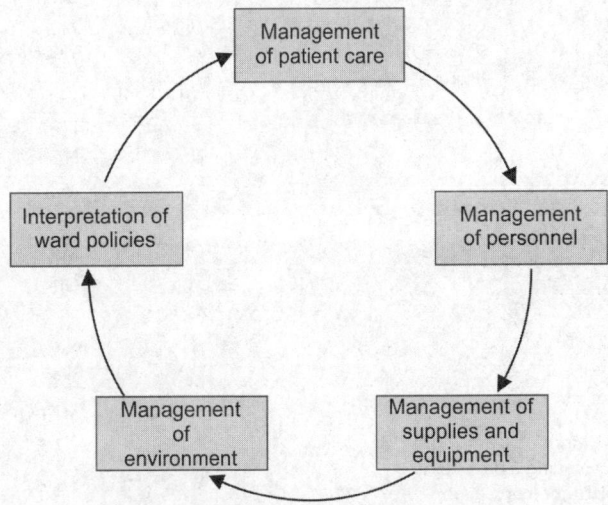

Fig. 20.1: Components of ward management.

- Providing comfortable positioning and well-being of the patient
- Providing psychological support and meeting spiritual needs
- Preventing the development of further complications
- Carrying out medical treatment and helping the physician in carrying out procedures and preparing equipment, trolleys and trays for assisting them in carrying out various diagnostic tests and therapeutic procedures
- Ensuring and supporting activities of daily living, such as smooth care, daily bath, feeding, changing clothes, elimination and so on
- Administering medicines and other treatment as and when required
- Monitoring the patients continuously for his or her health status by checking temperature, vitals, intake and output, skin color, the integrity of the skin and so on
- Facilitating rehabilitation of the patient
- Ensuring the safety of the patient.

3. **Prioritize nursing care:** Prioritize the patient's needs while preparing nursing care plan. Give priority to meet physiological needs and then the other requirements of the patients. The life-threatening crises are the priority in nursing care.
4. **Planned and incidental teaching:** The planned and accidental teachings/health education should be organized for patients and their relatives about maintaining and improving health and about the treatment and follow-up.
5. **Supervision of patient care:** Ward sister must supervise patient care provided by nurses. She can monitor it directly through observation or by asking the patients by doing independent patients' round. It can also be done during handing and taking at the time of shift change over. She can conduct the supervisory round for evaluating the condition of a patient's room, his or her safety, working conditions, dietary services and other services concerning the patient.
6. **Planning a program for the improvement of patient care:** Involve entire nursing staff to prepare a standard for care of patients. Educate and train staff for providing progressive quality patient care. Supervise them and evaluate based on the accepted level of attention to be given.
7. **Preparing patients for discharge:** Ensure that all instructions are carried out after discharge to the patient. Give directions and health education regarding medication, personal hygiene, activity and rest, diet and elimination, avoidance of infections, mental health and other teachings related to a healthy lifestyle.
8. **Assignment of personnel for patient care:** Head nurse assigns the patient care to the nurses working under her. There are different methods of allocating nursing care, viz. the functional method, patient care method and nursing-team method of assignment. The head nurse assigns patients according to the unit, qualification and experiences of the staff.
9. **Planning time schedules and work schedules:** The head nurse prepares time schedules and work schedules to carry out various activities in the wards **(Table 20.1)**.

The purposes of preparing schedule are to:
- Provide adequate nursing care 24 hours each day
- Ensure the best possible experience for each person
- Promote good IPR and satisfaction among the staff.

Time schedules prepared weekly or monthly should indicate the following:

TABLE 20.1: A sample of weekly time schedule.

Name	Designation	Mon	Tue	Wed	Thu	Fri	Sat	Sun
A	Head nurse	M	M	M	N	Off	E	M
B	Staff nurse	M	Off	M	M	M	M	M
C	"	M	M	Off	M	M	M	M
D	"	M	M	M	M	M	M	Off
E	"	Off	E	E	E	E	E	E
F	"	E	E	E	E	E	Off	E
G	"	N	N	N	Off	N	N	N
H	"	M	M	M	N	Off	E	M
I	Reliever	E	M	M	M	M	M	M
J	Orderly	Off	M	M	M	M	M	M
K	"	M	Off	M	M	M	M	M
L	"	E	E	Off	E	E	E	E
M	"	N	N	N	Off	N	N	N
N	"	M	M	E	N	Off	A reliever in another ward	
M: Morning 8 am–2 pm E: Evening 2 pm–8 pm N: Night 8 pm–8 am		SN + O 4 + 2 2 + 1 1 + 1	SN + O 4 + 2 2 + 1 1 + 1	SN + O 4 + 2 2 + 1 1 + 1	SN + O 4 + 2 2 + 1 1 + 1	SN + O 4 + 2 2 + 1 1 + 1	SN + O 4 + 2 2 + 1 1 + 1	SN + O 3 + 2 2 + 1 1 + 1

1. Names of all staff members with their designations
2. Hours of duty and days of leave against the name, every day from Monday to Sunday
3. Reliever nurses, their names, and designation.
4. Number of nurses for each shift at the bottom of the schedule
5. Total of nurses in each shift at the bottom of the plan

The head nurse must prepare a master rotation plan for a month will help to adjust the days off and rotation of nurses. Work schedule outlines the essential duties of staff, which may be prepared daily, weekly, monthly, and yearly. **Box 20.1** depicts a sample of the weekly work schedule for the head nurse.

10. **Ward rounds:** The head nurse makes rounds to supervise the nurses on duty and for evaluation purposes. There are different types of ward rounds, such as wards rounds with the doctors, nursing/medical superintendent and staff nurses and students and independent rounds. The purposes of ward rounds are to:
    - Observe the physical and mental condition and progress in the health condition of the patients
    - See the work of the staff
    - Make a specific observation of the patients and give reports to the doctors
    - Introduce the patients to the team and staff to patient
    - Check any preventable conditions present in the patients, such as bedsores, foot drops, and so on
    - Test if the emergency equipment are kept in order
    - Observe the cleanliness of the ward
    - Take over and hand over the duties at the change of shift
    - Expedite the work left undone
    - Do prior preparation for rounds, as well as prepare and keep ready all the things that are likely to be ask for during the round
    - Take immediate, prompt action after the round to carry out the instructions given during the rounds.

11. **Reports and records:** Concise and complete reports are essential in ward management. Reporting is one method of communicating information about the patient's condition, including his treatment and day-to-day progress. These can be oral and written. A full report needs to be made at the time of shift change. The essential reports in the ward situations are the 24-hour report, census report, birth and death reports, anecdotal reports and accidental reports.

> **Box 20.1:** Sample of the weekly work schedule of a head nurse.
> - Planning working hours and duty assignment for staff, students, and others
> - Indenting new supplies in the ward
> - Checking general cleanliness of the department
> - Arranging ward teaching program for faculty and students
> - Arranging for the ward conferences
> - Sending breakage, losses, and getting them replaced
> - Evaluating the week's schedule
> - Supervision of performance of the evening and night staff

12. **Management of emergencies:** The head nurse makes sure that all nursing staff is prepared to meet any crisis. They need to keep the unit ready at all the times, and all resuscitation equipment should be in working order so that timely assistance and treatment can be given to save the patients. The nurses must follow the standing order and policies of the hospital to resuscitate the patient while waiting for the doctor's arrival.

13. **Patient education:** The patient teaching should be started with the admission of the patient and continue throughout his or her stay in the ward and even after discharge. It is a regular feature of the rehabilitation program. Teachings can be formal or incidental and given individually or in a group. Various types of printing material such as leaflets, pamphlets, booklets, guidelines on related aspects of the disease must be distributed to patients and their relatives to educate them.

    The health teaching should be only about one subject at a time, concise and straightforward. Content must be in a logical sequence; start from simple to complex and from known to unknown facts. Whenever possible, simple audiovisual aids should be used.

14. **Appraisal of nursing services:** It is essential to have periodical evaluation of nursing services in terms of physical facilities, equipment and supplies, staffing, nursing techniques, nursing procedures, quality of care, patients' satisfaction, satisfaction of staff working in the ward, lower accidents and complication rates and meeting of objectives and policies of the department and hospital.

Management of Personnel

A. Management of nursing staff

The components are as follows (Fig. 20.2):

1. **The orientation of the new personnel:** It is essential to plan an orientation program for the new staff. The

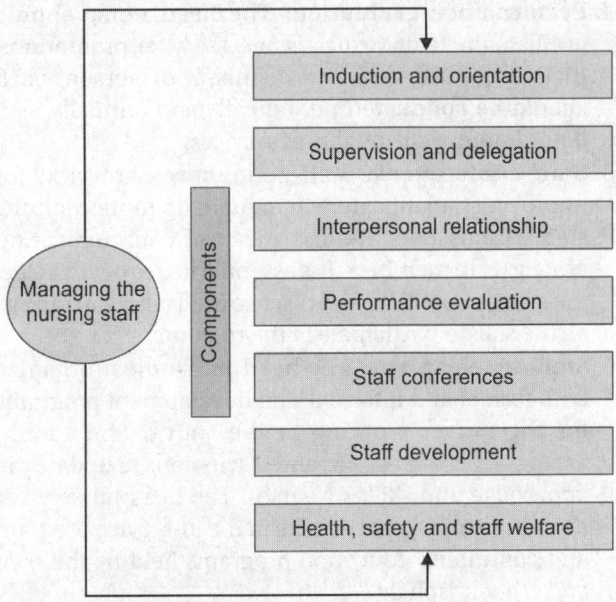

Fig. 20.2: Components of nursing staff management.

program should include the direction of the hospital and every department, and it must explain about the organization of the hospital, line of authority, channel of communication and hospital and ward policies.

The new personnel should be introduced to the ward. He or she must be allowed to either spend a few days in the department without any assignment to observe the functioning of the ward or assist other personnel for few a days, or be given a small task of caring for uncomplicated patients. The new staff must be acquainted with the ward routines.

2. **Supervision and delegation of responsibility:** The head nurse must use the democratic way of guiding, as it pays attention to the staff and work. When assigning duties, the head nurse must keep the following points in mind:
   - Ensure that the team must be aware of the work assigned to her.
   - Give orientation and explicit instruction for the assigned work.
   - Delegate responsibility with authority.
   - Specify the duties, responsibilities.
   - Consider each staff as an individual and give assignment based on their professional qualification, experience, personal qualities and technical competence.
   - Consider total workload and equally assign it to everyone.
   - Everyone must be supervised and guided; new staff may require more supervision and guidance.
   - Make plans flexible.

3. **Establishing an interpersonal relationship:** Head nurse has the responsibility to develop and maintain good IPR with the team in her ward. A positive, warm and friendly attitude of nurses will help to establish good interpersonal therapeutic relationship with the patients and employees.

4. **Performance evaluation:** The head nurse should evaluate the team, which is necessary for promotions, incentives, transfers and dismissal of personnel. It should be conducted periodically and annually as it helps improve the quality of services.

5. **Staff conferences:** Staff conferences are vital for improving patient care and to build up morale among staff. Discussions are also mean of communication among team members. It is essential to frequently select the appropriate time and place to hold talks. Encourage all the staff to participate in the rotation.

6. **Staff development:** The head nurse must organize both formal and informal staff development programs for the nurses working in the wards. She should arrange teaching rounds and discussions to update the knowledge and skills of nurses. The head nurse gives an opportunity to participate in the in-service program and continuing education programs held by the own and other hospitals.

7. **Health, safety and welfare of the staff:** Educate the nurses about the principles of health and hygiene. Provide a healthy environment in the ward. There should be a provision of welfare service for the nurses, such as social and recreational facilities, counseling, retirement plans and provision of restrooms, canteen and living facilities.

B. Responsibility toward Class IV employees:
Depute a fixed number of officials, including Class IV and *safai karamchari*, to the ward. The head nurse has the following responsibilities toward the Class IV employees:
1. Prepares duty schedule and keeps a record of their off days
2. Adjusts casual leaves, compensatory leaves and earned leaves
3. Forwards late attendance and absenteeism to the sanitary inspector
4. Requests for a substitute against absentees
5. Fills annual confidence report and forwards it to a sanitary inspector.

Management of Supplies and Equipment

The head nurse ensures proper utilization of the supplies and equipment by the staff. She applies the principles of material management while managing the supplies and equipment.

She must maintain an adequate supply of material at hand at all times. These should be in good and working conditions. Keep all articles and equipment ready for use and readily available. Keep the items and supplies under lock and key. Regularly check and maintain inventory up to date. Educate the staff to use the material properly and replace it in the same places after use. Ensure that there should not be any wastage and misuse of documents. Follow hospital policies regarding indenting and maintaining supplies and equipment.

Management of Environment

Head nurse must make sure that the environment is safe and comfortable for the patients and staff working in the ward. It includes:
1. Regulation of atmospheric temperature, humidity and ventilation
2. Adequate lighting
3. Prevention of noise
4. Safe water supply
5. Elimination of unpleasant odors
6. Safe disposal of excreta
7. Dust control
8. Free from insects and pest
9. Protection from all types of injuries
10. Protection from radiation
11. Provide adequate privacy
12. Restriction of visitors
13. Prevention of infection.

Integrating Ward Policies

Ward policies are the policies formulated for the better management of the ward. The procedure is a course of action adopted and followed by an organization. It provides a framework within which all activities are to be organized to achieve the desired goal. These are the guidelines for operations. Ward policies help ward sisters to manage the functioning of ward smoothly and efficiently to improve and provide better patient care. The head nurse must contribute to formulating and implementing ward policies. These policies are related to patients, various aspects of ward management and staff working in the ward.

A. Policies related to patients and patient care

1. **Admission policy:** On admission, the patients admitted through either outpatient departments (OPDs) or emergency or transferred from other wards, must have admission or transfer files along with all required documents, such as the admission order, medical unit in-charge, investigations, admission fees receipts, and so on. The admitting nursing staff must ensure all the records are in place and order. Every patient must be entered in the census book. He or she must be welcomed in the ward.
2. **Orientation policy:** After the admission process, the patients must be oriented. He or she must be assigned the allotted bed. In addition, the patient and his or her relatives must be explained the rules and regulations of the hospital and ward. The following necessary instructions must be given:
   - Personal hygiene-related articles, such as toothbrush, toothpaste, comb, towel, glass, spoon, and so on, require to be with the patient.
   - No valuables must be kept in the ward, and the patient should keep only needed belongings.
   - No personal furniture allowed for use in the unit.
   - Only one relative/no relative is asked to stay with the patient.
   - Just one visiting pass is permitted.
   - Services available for keeping articles, if the clock room is available.
   - The timing for doctors' visiting.
   - Renewal of admission and other charges.
   - Maintenance of cleanliness of the ward.
   - Health teaching timings and so on.
3. **Visiting hour policy:** Policy for visitors provides schedules and additional information related to visiting relatives or significant ones during the stay of the patient. It informs about the visiting morning and evening hours, e.g. morning 6 am to 7 am and evening from 4 pm to 6 pm in winter and 5 pm to 7 pm in summer. It tells about the number of relatives who can stay with a dependent patient. The timings are flexible and liable to change as per the hospital policy. The visiting relatives or significant ones must be instructed about the restriction of visitors in the hospital from prevention of infection point of view.
4. **Diet policy:** Diet policy contains information to be given regarding hospital diet, including:
   - The supply of food from the hospital or provision made for the patient
   - The charges of diet
   - The timing of distributing food; breakfast, lunch, evening tea, and dinner
   - Type of diet available.
5. **Policy regarding sample collection:** Inform the patients regarding the system related to specimen collection, including:
   - The doctor draws all the samples.
   - The samples are sent to the respective labs in the morning by the ward attendant.
   - Labs send the reports to the ward itself.
6. **Preoperative and postoperative policy:** This policy is regarding the preoperative preparation one day before surgery and day of surgery and about postoperative period. Concerning unit doctor will give instructions regarding one day before surgery preparation, consent, fasting, premedication and time to send to the operation theater (OT). The staff on duty will carry out all the directions. The patient is shipped with the files and received back from the OT.
7. **Transfer policy:** Entry into the census book on the transfer of a patient in another ward is made.
8. **Discharge policy:** The patient is prepared for discharge. The consulting doctor writes all the discharge notes. Patients are discharged from the hospital after clearing their dues. The patient/relatives are told where to deposit fees. All the instructions regarding follow up, home care and treatment to the patients are explained.
9. **Leave against medical advice and discharge on request:** The relatives of the patient may take the patient home with permission if prognosis of patient is poor. Then they can request the doctor to discharge the patient after completing all the formalities.
10. **Last office policy:** After the body is packed, it may be sent to mortuary along with the death certificate and handed over after the autopsy, if required. Otherwise, the body is handed over directly to the relatives after getting dues cleared.
11. **For absconding patients:** If the patient runs away from the hospital without paying any dues, inform the medical superintendent through proper channel. Inform the security officer also.
12. **Policy for medicolegal cases**
    The policy for medicolegal cases is as follows:
    - Send police information to all medicolegal cases
    - Keep all the belongings of the patient under lock and key after listing and handing over to the police or any other responsible authority
    - Inform the unit medical officer
    - On the death of the medico legal case, send for autopsy and do not hand over the body to relatives directly.

B. Policies related to the ward management

The policies related to the ward management are given below:

1. **Central sterile supply:** The policy related to the sterilized articles and materials to the wards. The district and general hospitals have the plan to have a separate central sterile supply department. Each nursing unit receives a sterile supply of dressing material from the department and other equipment/sets in an exchange with nonsterile/used sets. Whereas, in a few hospitals, the dressing material is prepared by the nurses and sent in dressing drums for autoclaving from the main OT.

2. **Indent policy:** The indent policy also varies from hospital to hospital. In some hospitals, the indents are sent to respective stores for different supplies, such as drugs, bandages, solutions, and so on, on two solid days in a week/weekly/monthly. They get the monthly indents from the sanitary store, surgical store, stationery store, and so on This policy includes:
   - *Equipment and supply policy:* Equipment must be kept carefully in order, and the staffs on duty are accountable for any loss. The ward sister maintains a stock book.
   - *For condemnation:* All nonfunctional and worn-out equipment must be carefully stored and entered in the condemnation book by the sister in-charge. The condemnation objects are condemned by the condemnation committee once in a year with proper procedure.
   - *Maintenance of equipment:* All equipment must be checked daily and repaired timely.

3. **Records and report policy:** Generally, the records of patients include his or her file, treatment chart, vital signs, particular diet chart, nurses' notes, intake output chart and other charts required as per the type of ward, diagnosis and severity of illness. Drug book is maintained to record the medicine received and consumed each day by the ward sister/ward aide. It is essential to maintain a stock book for recording equipment and supplies.

4. **Census policy:** Census is an important document to have hospital statistics. It is prepared from 12 MN to 12 MN next day during nighttime by the night staff in each ward. The night nurse has to send report to the night supervisors' office. The supervisor should get the census report from all departments. Census shows the total number of patients admitted, discharged, transfer, LAMA/absconded, births and deaths, and so on

5. **Drug policy:** The medicine is supplied free of cost from the hospital to the patients. The nurses send the requisition as per the requirement of the ward to the medicine/drug store and get the medicine from the store. In case, the medication is not available in the store, all concerned personnel are intimated and the patients and their relatives are asked to purchase from the market.

The nurses need to keep emergency drugs and dangerous drugs under lock and key. They must use refrigerators to store medicines under a low degree temperature. A drug book is maintained to record the balance of receiving and consuming the drugs in the ward by the ward sister in-charge.

6. **Linen policy:** Each ward should have a standard supply of linen, according to the number and type of patients. Each patient should have three sets of clothes, including bed sheets, pillow covers, kurtas, pajamas, and so on A person assigned by the linen bank collects dirty/soiled linen daily or fixed days of the week and receives a replacement of clean linen from that department. He or she maintains an accurate stock of linen and sends a list of a shortage of linen to the medical superintendent through nursing superintendent/matron.

   In a few hospitals, the soiled linen from the ward is collected by nursing orderly daily. In addition, in exchange for it, washed linen is received from the linen store on a fixed day of a week. Linen store in-charge nurse keeps the record of linen both soiled/clean linen and in the store and supplied to each ward.

7. **Sanitation policy:** The *safaikaramcharis* are responsible for the sanitation of the ward. The ward sister supervises and directs them for cleaning and provides them with hygiene-related material and supplies.

8. **Hand washing policy:** Each ward must have a handwashing policy in writing for all the staff and patients. In addition, providing handwashing facilities for the patients and staff is crucial. All teams, including doctors and nurses, must be aware of the plan for the type of hand washings and disinfectant to be used.

9. **Policy for prevention of infection:** Hospital infection control and prevention plan must be prepared and implemented in each ward.

10. **Waste management policy:** Waste management policy concerns the biomedical waste management, including segregation, collection and disposal of different types of biomedical waste. All must follow it.

11. **Ward round policy:** There are various types of rounds, such as the doctors' round, administrative round, teaching round, handing and taking round, and so on. There should be a clear-cut policy for each type of round, when to conduct, how to perform, after round instructions follow up, and so on.

12. **Standard operative procedures:** Each ward must have a manual of standard operative procedures. All the staff must follow those standards to render patient care.

C. Policies related to staff

Some of the staff-related policies are as follows:

1. **Policy on orientation for new team:** Newly joined team should be made familiar with the general plans of the hospital and ward routines.

2. **Policies for time schedules and assignment of staff:** There should be a duty roster/time plan of staff according to the hospital policy. The ward sister

Chapter 20: Ward Management and Methods of Patient Assignment

must plan duty timings and days off and assignment according to the hospital policy.

3. **Leave policy:** Casual leave and other leaves are given as per hospital policy/government rules but planned in such a way that the patient care should not suffer.
4. **Discipline policy:** Discipline policy is related to maintaining the discipline in the ward. It is similar to preserving punctuality and maintaining a quiet and calm atmosphere in the ward. There should be a proper bed-to-bed handing and taking over during a change of shift without disturbing the patients.
5. **Supervision and appraisal:** The ward sister must have a policy regarding the method of supervising and appraising the staff. She sends the annual confidential report every year. It should provide reliable tools to evaluate the performance of the team.
6. **Policy for staff development:** There should be a provision of informal and formal staff developmental education programs in the ward. Each ward must have a policy regarding the timings and frequency of conducting staff conferences and teaching rounds in the wards.

D. Policies for the medical staff

The policies for the medical staff include:
1. The staff nurse, who is the mediator between doctors and patients, should have thorough knowledge about the health status of patients, including their treatment, investigations, diet, and so on.
2. The ward sister or senior staff should accompany medical staff during rounds.
3. A doctor must first write all instructions on the treatment chart and order/instruction book.
4. One doctor is always on duty during day and night. During an emergency, the staff must inform the senior doctor, if the junior doctor is not available.

Factors Involved in Good Ward Management

The factors involving good ward management are as follows:
1. A planned program/work schedule for each day's work
2. Beginning the day on time
3. Preventing interruptions
4. Establishment of ward routines and policies
5. Use of the democratic method in establishing ward policies
6. Orientation to newly joined staff
7. Maintaining a safe and healthy work environment
8. Provision of adequate supplies and equipment for efficient work
9. Clear cut doctors' and nurses' instructions
10. Accurate reports and records
11. Keeping high morale and IPR among staff
12. Delegation of responsibility
13. Proper schedule plans
14. Good teaching and supervision
15. Periodical evaluation of the team
16. Staff development programs
17. Social gatherings.

METHODS OF PATIENT ASSIGNMENT

Meaning and Definitions

The patient assignment is delegating or assigning duties to the trained nurses for the care of a group of patients admitted to the unit. The terms nursing assignment patterns, nursing assignment systems and organization mode of nursing care synonymously refer to the methods of patient assignment.

The method of patient assignment is a process or system by which the nurses deliver the care to the assigned patients. The nurses are responsible and accountable for the care of patients. Methods used to assign number and type of patients depend on the policies and practices of the hospital, nursing department and other factors, such as clinical decision-making, work allocation, communication and management and coordination.

Purposes of Patient Assignment

The purposes and elements of patient assignment are to:
1. Provide nursing care to patients in an efficient and effective manner
2. Describe a structure to the organization nursing workload
3. Identify the types of health-care personnel in providing nursing care
4. Define the boundaries for the distribution of work and delegation of authority.

Principles of Assignment

The principles of assignments are as follows:
1. Assigning of the task of patient care by the head nurse
2. Following departmental policy/guidelines
3. Considering patient's needs, unit activities and geographical location of the unit
4. Assigning equal and balanced workload among staff on duty and rotation
5. Considering capabilities, experience and interest of nursing staff
6. Assuring continuity of care and selecting the method well in advance
7. Documenting and making everyone familiar.

Factors Influencing Patient Assignment

The factors influencing the assignment of patients include the following:
1. **Availability of nursing workforce:** The availability is one of the predictors to choose the mode of patient assignment. The institutions usually select the process of assigning patients according to the availability of nurses.
2. **Organizational complexity:** The decision to select a method of patient assignment depends on the nature or

complexity of the organization. The patients admitted to referral hospitals require a different type of care as compared with patients of the district or general hospitals.

3. **The severity of illness:** The severity of the disease of patients and the amount of nursing care required by the patient is an essential factor in determining the method of patient assignment. The method is based on the patients' needs, use of technology and amount of interdisciplinary support.
4. **Patient characteristics:** It includes age, length of stay, the stability of condition, the variability of care, uncertainty, the predictability of care and cure at the time of admission, care complexity of patient, needs for learning, and so on.
5. **The physical design of the unit:** The design of the nursing unit where the patient stays is a criterion to decide the method of patient assignment. The patients who require continuous mentoring and observation require different ways of assignment than the patient who don't need continuous mentoring and observation. Nursing units designed in circles, squares or rectangles with central or decentralized medication and supply services may require different configurations of staff to provide observation and care safely. The smaller sections of the area may require more staff.
6. **Nursing resources:** It includes the percentage of qualified personnel and ancillary staff, the ratio of patients and nurses, experience, education levels, competence, additional training and motivation.
7. **Organization support:** It includes the presence of a physician in the nursing ward, communication between nurses and physicians, the documentation process, rounds, shift reports, supportive services, laboratory services and nursing ward design.
8. **The financial health of the institution:** Sometimes, it is an essential variable to consider while selecting the method of patient assignment for delivering care to the patients.
9. **Recommendation of the accrediting body:** The advice of accreditation and licensing bodies determine the staffing and method of assignment to meet the quality of care standards.

Methods of Patient Assignment

There are different methods of patient assigning for nursing care, viz. the functional approach and patient care approach. The use of these approaches depends upon the way of nursing care delivery the system approaches. The head nurse assigns patients depending on the availability of nursing staff, the types of units and the qualifications and experiences of the staff.

In the functional approach of assignment, the head nurse divides the nursing acre activities of a particular shift among nursing staff on duty. For example, one nurse may take temperatures and vitals of all patients in the ward; other staff may administer medicines and injections to all patients. In patient care approach of assignment, nurses are assigned a group of patients for complete patient care regardless of their qualifications and experiences. The head nurse needs critical analysis in terms of workload and type of patients before assigning patients. There can be a mixed approach by using combination of these two approaches. The method of patient assignment depends upon nursing care delivery system as given below:

Private Duty Nursing

This nursing care delivery system was popular as *case nursing*. Private duty nursing is one nurse caring for one client. According to this system, the private duty nurse is responsible for one patient who is responsible for providing total patient care.

Advantages

The advantages of private duty nursing are that it:
1. Is based on the need of the patient
2. Focuses on the therapeutic nurse–client relationship
3. Increases nurse and client satisfaction with care delivery.

Disadvantages

The disadvantages of private duty nursing are that it:
1. Is a costly model
2. Offers low efficiency
3. Lacks job security and job mobility.

Case Method

The case method of patient assignment is a patient-care method. The head nurse assigns a group of patients to nurses on duty irrespective of their qualifications and experiences. The nurses are responsible for the total care of the assigned patients during their duty hours **(Fig. 20.3)**.

Mostly, the nursing units with acutely ill patients who require constant observation and monitoring, such as intensive care, hospice care and home health-care units, follow this method. The head nurse analyzes the workload and type of patients before assigning them. This method does not apply to hospitals having less number of nurses.

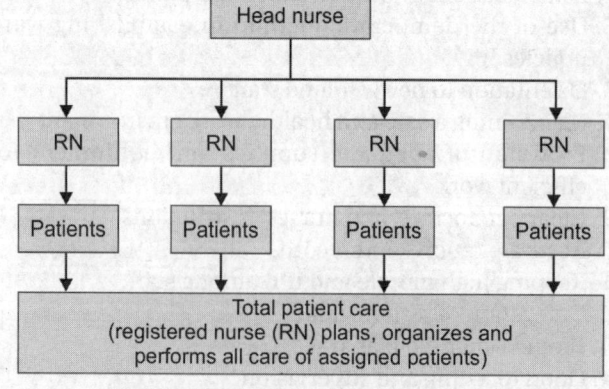

Fig. 20.3: Case method of patient assignment.

Chapter 20: Ward Management and Methods of Patient Assignment

Advantages
The advantages of the case method are that it:
1. Is a holistic method of rendering nursing care
2. Provides the patients individualized nursing care based on their needs
3. Gives the nurses a clear ideal about their responsibilities and accountability
4. Keeps the nurses accountable for the care
5. Offers nurses the satisfaction of providing total patient care.

Disadvantages
The disadvantages of the case method are that it:
1. Lacks communication among team members
2. Lacks continuity of care
3. Has a care approach that may differ from staff to staff
4. Is expensive as it requires sufficient nurses.

Functional Method

The functional method of patient assignment is efficient. It aims to get the maximum amount of task at the least cost of time and staff. This method developed in response to the increased demand for hospital nursing in the late 1800s due to the acute shortage of nurses. This method is also familiar as "work assignment by functions or tasks" **(Fig. 20.4)**.

Patient assignment method
The functional method is a task-oriented method of assigning patients in which individual nurses perform specific assigned tasks. The head nurse is responsible for both administrative and clinical functions, such as taking orders, contacting physicians for patient needs, assisting personnel in an emergency, adjusting staffing schedules and evaluating or orienting staff. She makes clinical decisions and collects all pertinent information about the patients.

The head nurse, based on task analysis in a particular shift, divides the work among nurses on duty. For example, she assigns a task of taking temperatures and vital signs of all unit patients to one nurse; to change dressings and carry out instruction for all unit patients to another nurse and so on. One nurse aid is assigned to make beds for all ambulatory patients and assist in mobility-impaired patients to move in bed. The clerk attends telephones, recording admission and discharge, preparing a diet sheet, and so on.

Advantages
The advantages of the patient assignment method are that it:
1. Emphasizes the concept of specialization and division of labor
2. Requires less number of nurses to render care to a large number of patients
3. Is a quite economical and efficient way of doing the work
4. Carries out some activities within a limited period of time
5. Makes the nurses competent to carry out the assigned tasks repeatedly
6. Helps establish managerial control over the planning and executing the job
7. Is appropriate for handling emergencies
8. Ensures nurses have less confusion over the assignment
9. Requires minimum articles and equipment for care.

Disadvantages
The disadvantages of the patient assignment method are that it:
1. Is task focused and not patient focused
2. Makes care more mechanical than humanistic
3. Requires some nurses to look after one patient through different activities
4. Causes communication barriers among various persons
5. No nurse is responsible for the overall responsibility of the patient
6. Neglects the holistic approach and individual needs of the patient
7. Makes the nurses task-oriented rather than patient oriented.

Team Method

The concept of team nursing was introduced in the early 1950s in response to the dissatisfaction of nurses with the functional method of assignment. The team method of allocation is a care model that utilizes a team of personnel comprising of professional, technical and nurse aids to deliver nursing care led by a nurse leader. He or she assigns the work/patient according to expertise of each staff to meet the nursing needs of a group of patients **(Fig. 20.5)**:

Patient assignment method
In the nursing team method, the head nurse delegates clinical decisions to several team leaders to work together to achieve a common goal. A group of team nurses works together, in a coordinated and collaborative way to carry out individualized patient care. The head nurse assigns a few patients and team members. The team leader assigns the individual patient assignment to a team according to the diagnosis of the patient. All the staff of that team works under the supervision of one nurse called the team leader.

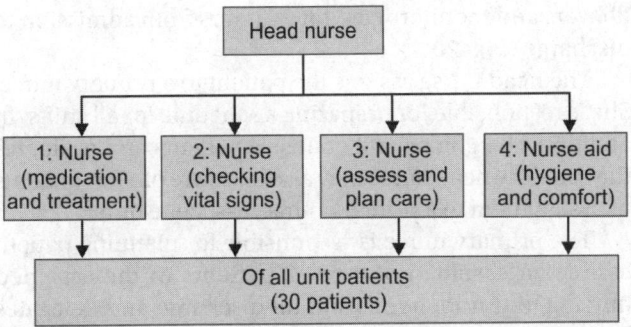

Fig. 20.4: Functional method of patient assignment (for 30-bedded medical wards).

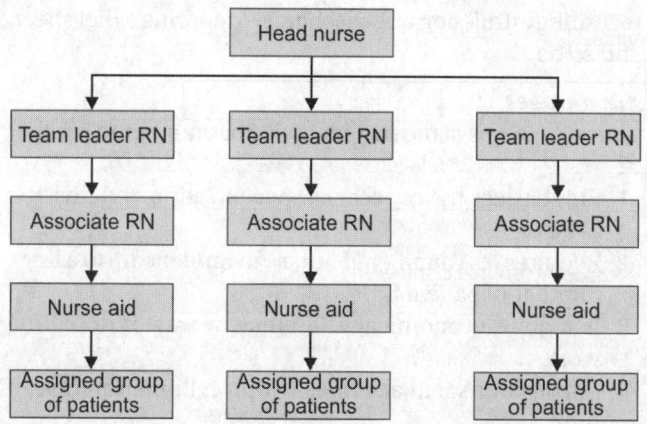

Fig. 20.5: Team method of patient assignment.

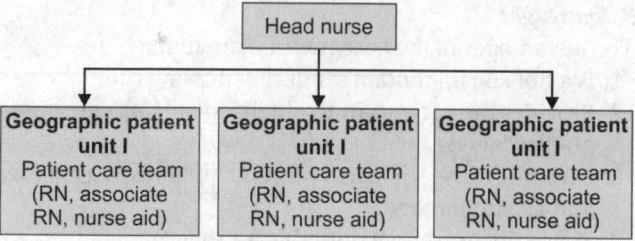

Fig. 20.6: Modular method of patient assignment.

Planning, coordination, communication, monitoring and evaluation are critical factors for the success of the team method assignment. The team leader plans and assigns nursing care to each team member.

The team method of assignment is the assignment of a group of patients to a small group of personnel to work under a team leader. Each team member assigns care for assigned patients. For example, the team leader administers medications and monitors intravenous (IV) fluid therapy of all patients. A professional nurse takes care of seriously ill patients and so on. This method is just a modification of the functional approach.

Advantages

The advantages of this method are that it:
1. Offers comprehensive care from all expertise
2. Ensures the integration of nursing personnel with varying skills into a team
3. Focuses on patients' needs than on staff members' needs
4. Enhances communication and coordination
5. Offers cohesive participation by the team members in decision-making
6. Fosters a sense of contribution via the team
7. Improves patient care by using diverse skills
8. Economizes time and efforts.

Disadvantages

The disadvantages of this method are as follows:
1. There is a possibility of in-continuity of care due to a change in the leaders, team members and patient assignments.
2. None is accountable for total patient care.
3. There is role confusion and resentment against team leaders.
4. It requires knowledgeable and skilled team leader with leadership qualities.
5. It needs more staff.

Modular Nursing

The modular nursing method has a combination of functional and team nursing methods with some modifications. It aims to provide bedside competent nursing care (**Fig. 20.6**).

Patient assignment method

It has a unit-based modular committee to form some modules. Each module consists of a group of nurses comprising of technical and nurse aides, professional nurses and two to three nonprofessional members and a group of patients. Patients are grouped by floor plan clustering or based on the severity of their illnesses. Usually, open design wards are preferred to practice this system. The nurse/patient assignment is standardized. The nurse has a wide range of responsibilities, including guiding and teaching nonprofessional staff. Modular care planning rounds occur regularly.

Advantages

The advantages of the modular method of patient assignment are as follows:
1. It improves the continuity of care.
2. Modular nurses are more involved in planning and coordinating care.
3. It provides effective coordination and communication.

Disadvantages

The disadvantages of the modular method of patient assignment are as follows:
1. It increases the costs to manage each module.
2. Long corridors or rooms are not conducive to modular nursing.

Primary Nursing Method

The primary nursing method of patient assignment developed in the late 1960s or early 1970s in response to the lack of autonomy to the professional nurses and declining of quality patient care. One primary nurse has the assignment of all assigned patients to whom she/he plans, delivers and monitors care for 24 hours from admission to discharge (**Fig. 20.7**)

The head nurse assigns the patient to a primary nurse. She is responsible for preparing a schedule for all shifts. In addition, she guides and counsels patients and evaluates the care. The head nurse may also take care of a few patients or assign them to a primary nurse/associate nurse.

The primary nurse is responsible for planning patient care for a caseload of 8 to 12 patients of the assigned nursing unit from admission till discharge and delegates her responsibility to an associate nurse in case of the day off. He or she is accountable for the planning, coordinating,

Chapter 20: Ward Management and Methods of Patient Assignment

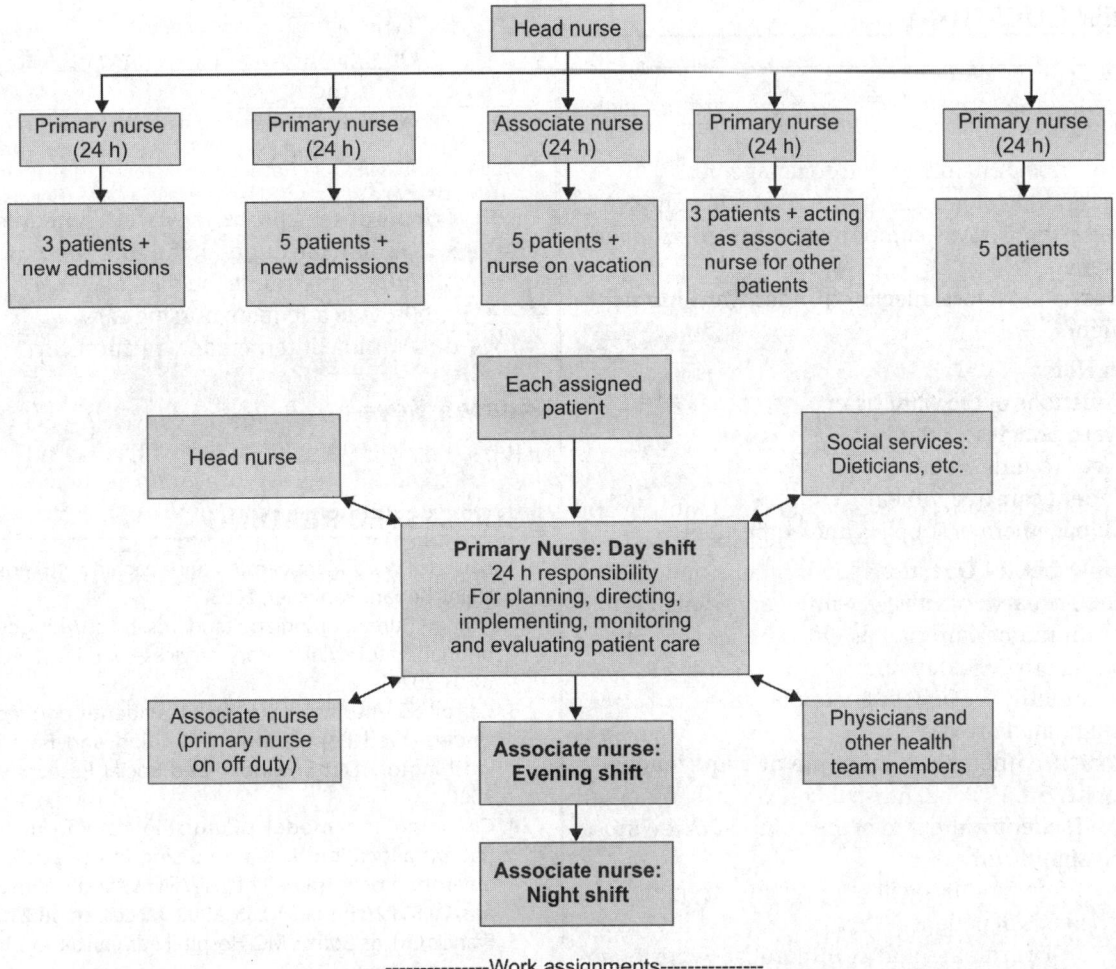

Fig. 20.7: Primary method of patient assignment.

monitoring and continuity of care of the assigned patients. In addition, he or she collaborates with the medical, head nurse and higher authority and team members. Other staff, nurse aids and clerical staff assist him or her. He/she has accountability for the care of patients and can take independent decisions.

Advantages
The advantages of the primary nursing method are that it:
1. Ensures quality, holistic and continuity of patient care
2. Establishes a therapeutic relationship with the patient
3. Enhances patient safety and reduces negligence, errors, infections, and so on
4. Encourages collaborative relationships and team spirit
5. Makes professional nurses feel responsible, free to work and satisfaction
6. Gives the nurses the autonomy to make decisions independently
7. Helps to reduce nurses attrition and turnover.

Disadvantages
The disadvantages of the primary nursing method are that it:
1. Requires a high degree of responsibility for 24 hours that may create burnout may threaten poorly prepared nurses
2. Is expensive and requires sufficient nurses to render care.

CHAPTER HIGHLIGHTS

- Ward is a place or a nursing/patient care unit for the treatment of admitted patients.
- Ward management is managing the work of ward that involves planning, organizing, directing and controlling staff, material and support services about the department to achieve the best patient care.
- A head nurse plays a vital role in directing the ward activity and thinking of professional coworkers, auxiliary staff and patients.
- The prime objective of ward management is to ensure the highest possible quality of patient care.
- The essential principle of ward management is to identify the staff of the ward as it's the most significant asset.
- The main components of ward management are managing patient care, personnel, supplies and equipment and the integration of ward policies.
- The case methods, functional approach, team method, modular method and primary nursing methods are the most common methods of patient assignment.

REVIEW QUESTIONS

I. Essay Type Questions
1. Define the term "ward." Describe ward management.
2. Describe principles of ward management.
3. Enumerate objectives of ward management.
4. Describe various components of ward management.
5. Describe factors affecting proper ward management.

II. Short Notes
1. Functions of the ward sister
2. Ward policies
3. Ward rounds
4. Patient care assignment
5. Management of supplies and equipment

III. Multiple Choice Questions
1. The primary objective of ward management is to:
    a. Conduct ward rounds
    b. Improve quality care
    c. Identify the needs of patients
    d. Evaluate staff
2. Which is the prime principle of ward management?
    a. To identify the staff of the ward as it's the most significant asset
    b. To ensure all facilities available to meet the needs of patients
    c. To coordinate and communicate with team members
    d. To have an excellent public relation
3. A method of assignment that needs critical thinking in analyzing and planning individualized patient care is:
    a. Individual method
    b. Patient care method
    c. Functional method
    d. Nursing team method
4. Which is the best option out of given factors that should keep in mind while assigning the work to staff?
    A. Availability of staff,
    B. Type of unit,
    C. Qualification and experience of staff:
        a. A and B
        b. B and C
        c. A, B and C
        d. A
5. The purpose of preparing a work schedule is to:
    a. Outline the duties of the staff
    b. Adjust and rotate the days off
    c. Provide adequate nursing care
    d. Promote interpersonal relationship

Answer Keys
1. b   2. b   3. d   4. c   5. a

SUGGESTED READING

1. Barrett J. Ward Management and Teaching, 4th edition. New Delhi: Konark Publisher; 2003.
2. Home - Bureau of Indian Standards. https://bis.gov.in/index.php/laboratorys/laboratory-services-overview/. [Accessed on 07.01.2020].
3. Carroll SS, Alturas A, Stepnick L. Patient-Centered Care for Underserved Populations: Definition and Best Practices. Washington, DC: Economic and Social Research Institute; 2006.
4. Changing the model of nursing care from individual patient allocation to team nursing in the acute inpatient environment. [Online] https://www.tandfonline.com/doi/abs/10.5172/conu.2010.35.2.202. [Accessed on 25.01.2019].
5. Francis CM, de Souza, MC. Hospital Administration. New Delhi: Jaypee Brothers; 2000.
6. Goddard HA. Principles of Administration Applied to Nursing Service, 5th edition. Geneva: WHO; 1979.
7. Perceptions of a Primary Nursing Care Model in a Pediatric Hematology/Oncology Unit. [Online] Available from https://journals.sagepub.com/doi/full/10.1177/1043454216631472. [Accessed on 25.01.2019].
8. Stewart M, Brown JB, Donner A, et al. The impact of patient-centered care on patient outcomes. J Fam Pract. 2000; 796-804.
9. [PDF]Team Assignment Method in Improving Nurse Performance in ... https://download.atlantis-press.com › article. [Accessed on 07.01.2020].
10. Tiedeman ME, Lookinland S. Traditional models of care delivery. What have we learned? J Nurs Adm. 2004;34(6): 291-97.

21 Planning and Organizing Ancillary Services

CHAPTER OUTLINE
- Planning and Organizing CSSD Services
- Planning and Organizing Laundry Services
- Planning and Organizing Dietary Services/Kitchen
- Planning and Organizing Laboratory Services

LEARNING OUTCOMES
After completion of this chapter, the learner will be able to:
- Understand the concept of planning and organizing ancillary services
- Frame objectives and scope of organizing ancillary services
- Discuss the physical layout and workflow of different ancillary services
- Describe staffing and other aspects of organizing ancillary services

KEY TERMS
Planning, Central Sterile Supply Department, laundry, kitchen, laboratory services

INTRODUCTION

The ancillary services are an essential part of the hospital. Its proper functioning contributes to the success of providing quality patient care. The critical hospital ancillary services include the Central Sterile Supply Department (CSSD), laundry, kitchen, laboratory services, radiology, operation theater, and so on. Each department has its particular norms for planning and organizing its services.

PLANNING AND ORGANIZING CENTRAL STERILE SUPPLY DEPARTMENT SERVICES

A Central Sterile Supply Department (CSSD) is an independent service department that supplies sterile articles and materials to all departments of the hospital, outpatient departments, and other general and individual departments. It is also known as Central Sterile Services Department.

Aims and Scope

To provide sterile equipment available for the use of caring patients through various activities such as receiving, cleaning, assembling, packing, disinfecting, sterilizing, storing, and distributing sterile supplies as per hospital protocol. The CSSD has a significant role in preventing hospital-acquired infection by supplying adequate sterile supplies.

Objectives

The objectives of the CSSD services are to:
1. Provide a source of sterile equipment and material.
2. Receive and supply sterile articles, equipment, and other materials.
3. Ensure proper sterilization process, procedures according to the type of articles, equipment, and other materials.
4. Monitor and enforce controls to prevent hospital cross-infection.
5. Organize and maintain efficient services.

Space Requirement

The space requirement for planning CSSD depends on the size of the hospital, average number, type of surgical procedures, and beds. According to Bhattacharya, the space requirement to plan CSSD is as follows:

75–99 beds	10 sq ft/bed
100–149 beds	9 sq ft/bed
150–199 beds	8½ sq ft/bed
200–249 beds	8 sq ft/bed
250–299 beds	7½ sq ft/bed
≥300	7 sq ft/bed

Location

The location of CSSD should be close to the emergency department, Trauma center, operation theaters (OT), and wards. It is preferred to construct in the ground floor near to OT to easy access for transportation. It should have the provision of proper ventilation, light, and supply of both cold and hot water, compressed air, and electrical supply.

Physical Layout and Workflow

The physical design of CSSD has unidirectional flow. The articles/material must move in one direction throughout the process. Mainly it has three zones: (1) soiled/protective, (2) clean, and (3) sterile zones. The protective zone includes receiving counter area, cleaning, washing, drying area, assembling, and packing areas. The clean zone includes autoclaving area, and a sterile zone consists of a sterile storage room, and counters for issuing supplies. The CSSD has four functional sections: (1) procedure sets, (2) dressing sets, (3) vial, and (4) autoclave section. The areas of the workflow must start with:

1. **Area for receiving used supplies/equipment/articles:** The CSSD receives unsterile/dirty material/items from all departments during receiving timings of the hospital at reception/receiving area. As per Indian hospital guidelines, there is no restriction of schedules for receiving and issuing of items in CSSD. The CSSD assistant segregates the articles, checks for any damage, and maintains records. The standard items received from various departments are syringes, needles, procedure sets, gloves, rubber wares, IV fluids, bowels, treatment trays, instruments, linen, dressing drums, infusion fluids for renal dialysis, etc.
2. **Unsterile bulk storage:** This area is meant to store the clean receipt of material/items, and gauze and cotton received from bulk/main stores.
3. **Cleaning, washing, and drying area:** After segregation, cleaning and laundry of used equipment, rubber, and plastic articles are done either manually or by using machines and dryers. The instruments used in HIV/Hepatitis B patients must be socked in 1% sodium hypochlorite solution for 3 days in CSSD.
    - Sorting area: A table space is provided next to the washing area for sorting and space.
    - Drying area: The drying area has a provision of a table space and wires for hanging gloves.
4. **Assembling and packing/preparation area:** It includes checking of breakable articles and instruments for its sharpness and breakage, and gathering of equipment after cleaning, washing, and drying.
5. **Glove processing area:** This area has a table space for gloves processing.
6. **Gauze cutting area:** This area has a table space for cutting gauze.
7. **Packing area:** This area has a table space for packing. All the packs are getting ready after labeling and by pasting autoclave indicator before sterilization.
8. **Area for storage of pack sets before sterilization:** This is a presterilization storage area to keep unsterile items before sterilization.
9. **Area for sterilization:** This is the area allocated for sterilization of packs by using different autoclaves. Different types of autoclaves are placed in this area. At the end of the sterilization process, all packages are removed from autoclaves and checked to confirm adequate sterilization through autoclave indicators.
10. **Sterile storage area:** This is the area to store sterile items and the packs not issued on the same day. The torn, open, and wet packs are sent for sterilization again.
11. **Counter for issuing supplies:** This area is for issuing sterile supplies. The sterile items/packs/instruments are either issued to departments during fixed timings or distributed to different departments after entry of items in the dispatch/issuing register.
12. **Changing room with toilets for staff:** There should be a provision of changing room with toilets for staff working in the CSSD.
13. **Supervisors' room:** There should be a provision of office for supervisor/in-charge of the department.

Staffing

Central Sterile Supply Department must staff with the adequately qualified superintendent in-charge and a supervisor who is the chief of the department. There should be trained CSSD attendants, technicians, storekeeper, and *safaikaramcharies*. The recommended staffing for CSSD in a 500-bedded hospital is five technicians, four technical assistance, four nursing aides, and four CSSD attendants. The staffing strength also depends on workload, method of collection, and delivery of items, and hospital policy. The staff must undergo regular refresher courses. They should adhere to wear personal protective clothes and immunized for hepatitis B and tetanus.

Monitoring

There should be monitoring standard operating protocols in CSSD to ensure quality standards. There should be a record of temperature, pressure, and time of each cycle as per recommendation. There should be the use of mechanical, chemical, biological quality indicators for adequate sterilization process and adherence of the CSSD policy and regulations. CSSD must have regular internal and external audits, and supervision for quality assurance.

Record Keeping

Central Sterile Supply Department should have proper record system for maintaining the record of all items received including date, time, and type of instruments, packs, name of department, and signature of obtaining a person. There must be a record of quality indicator tests and culture reports. A logbook registers for the details of equipment as per warranty. There should be annual maintenance of autoclaves, gas sterilization machines, and of minor machinery.

Biomedical Waste Management

There should be a policy for biomedical waste management generated during the process of cleaning, disinfection, and sterilization process as per its guidelines. There should be color-coding bins available in the department.

PLANNING AND ORGANIZING LAUNDRY SERVICES

Linen and laundry department is an important support service area and essential component of the hospital. It provides clean and safe linen to different departments of the hospital and thus contributing towards the infection control practices of the hospital. It may be a part of a hospital in the house or outsourced, on rental or contractual depending on the decision of management.

Aims and Scope

To provide clean and safe linen required for the patients and the use of caring patients. It includes various activities such as procuring/receiving, segregating, disinfecting, washing, cleaning, drying, ironing, and distributing clean linen as per hospital protocol. The laundry has a significant role in preventing hospital-acquired infection by supplying an adequate linen supplies. Its importance in this regard realized in the 12th century AD. Florence Nightingale contributed to organize these services in 1854. The hospital laundry services require special attention as linen is soiled with various body fluids and also infected needs to be segregated and disinfected before washing and drying.

Objectives

1. Provide a source of an adequate supply of clean and safe linen to indoor and outdoor patient departments.
2. Receive and supply fresh and safe linen regularly and timely to patients and staff.
3. Ensure proper laundry process, procedures according to the type of linen.
4. Monitor and enforce controls to prevent hospital cross-infection.
5. Organize and maintain efficient laundry services of the hospital services.

Types of Hospital Laundry

The linen may be infected, soiled, foul, and radioactive in use. According to the category of linen, it is of four types:
1. **The linen of general use**: This type of linen is used only for general purpose such as curtains, and table cloths used in the hospital.
2. **Linen used for patients**: The linen used by the patients during their stay in the hospital.
3. **Ward linen**: This linen used as bed clothing for the patients such as bed sheets and pillow covers.
4. **Linen used in special departments/procedures**: The linen used in OTs, labor room, etc., and used by the staff working in these departments.

Quantification of Hospital Laundry

There should be a minimum of six sets of linen per bed.

Location

The location of the department should be within the premises of the hospital, usually on the ground floor. It should have easy access to user areas, near to CSSD, dietary services, garage, and maintenance department. There should be a provision of a separate entrance and exit with a unidirectional flow of linen.

Design

The laundry department may be straight, U-shaped or gravitational designs. Usually, in high building, the gravitational design is preferred.

Space and Engineering Requirement

The space requirement for planning laundry services depends on size and type of hospital, average number, and type of surgical procedures, weather conditions, and types of consumers. The estimated laundry workload as a rule of thumb is 3.5 kg/bed/day as per Indian Standards. The minimum space requirement is 10 sq ft/bed or 10 sq ft/2.5 kg of linen. The minimum space requirement for planning the laundry department of 300-bedded hospitals is 3,240 sq ft, 600-bedded hospitals is 4,068 sq ft, and 500–600-bedded hospital is 5,800 sq ft.

The floor should be smooth, washable, and nonslippery. The walls must be hard, soft, and washable. The ceiling must be high enough, and there should be a minimum 10 and maximum 20 air changes during hot weather. There should be proper lighting at least 300 lux in working areas, and temperature should be 20–30°C with humidity 30–50%.

Water requirement for the linen department is 30 L/kg of linen for hot water and 10 L/kg of linen for cold water. As a rule of thumb, the laundry process requires approximate 100 L/bed/day water. There should be boiler supplying steam, water softening plant, and a 400 volts three-phase connection with backup supply.

Physical Layout and Workflow

There are four major functional areas: (1) reception and sorting area, (2) processing area, (3) clean storage area, and (4) tailoring area. There should be separate collecting/receiving areas for soiled and fresh linen. There should also be the provision of negative air pressure in dirty linen areas and positive air pressure/flow from clean area to

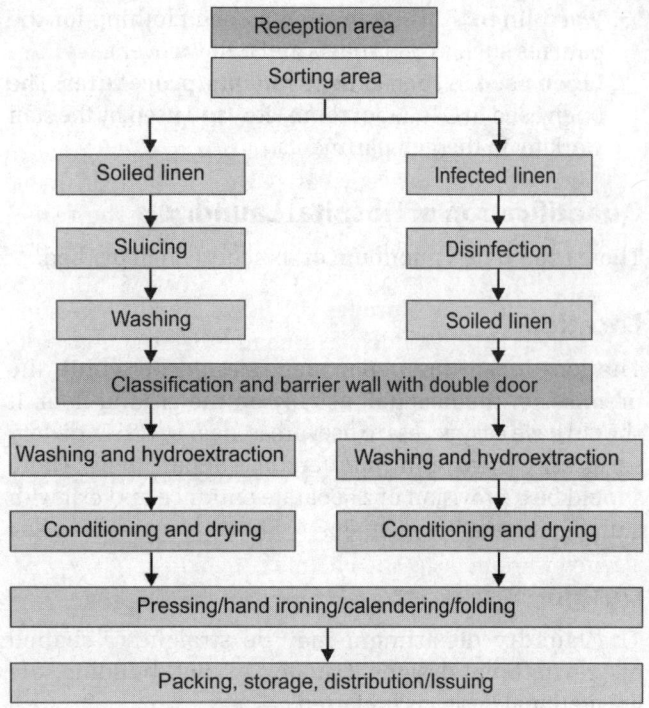

Fig. 21.1: Physical layout and workflow of laundry.

soiled linen area to outside vent. **Figure 21.1** depicts the workflow areas.

Equipment

There should be washing machine for 30-bed line/load and 60 pillow covers/load, water extractor with a capacity of 8-bed sheet/load and 30 pillow covers/load, flatwork iron (calendering), hand iron box, and sewing machine.

Staffing

The department must staff with a chief manager (a chemical engineer), laundry superintendent, and technical staff including operators and tailor, and supporting staff.

Linen Identification

There should be a system of identifying linen by using barcoding or transducers for linen flow control, management system, preventing pilfering, etc.

Monitoring and Control

There should be monitoring standard operating protocols in the department to ensure quality standards. The department should keep a record of the use of washing formula as per recommendation. There should be the use of mechanical, chemical, biological quality indicators for the adequate cleaning process and adherence of policy and regulations. The department must have regular internal and external audits and supervision for quality assurance. The department should maintain a proper record system of all items received including date, time, and type of linen, name of department, and signature of acquiring a person.

There must be a record of quality indicator tests and culture reports.

Biomedical Waste Management

There should be a policy for biomedical waste management generated during the process of sluicing, washing, disinfection, drying, ironing, calendering as per its guidelines.

There should be color coding for sorting and transporting dirty and contaminated linen. Use of white fabric bag for soiled linen, clear white bag firstly for fouled linen, double bag using the inner water-soluble bag and then in a red plaster bag labeled with yellow marking as "infected linen." Use a white bag with a prominent orange strip for heat liable linen. There should be the use of detergent mechanical movement for the removal of dust.

PLANNING AND ORGANIZING DIETARY SERVICES/KITCHEN

The department of dietetics in the hospital is vital that carries multiple responsibilities related to patients' daily intake of nutrition. It supplies diet to indoor patients. Its main aim is to provide clean, hygienic, and nutritious food to patients as per their calorie requirements. It can be a division of hospital or by outsourcing.

Objectives

The department of dietetics has the objectives to:
1. Provide hygienic, balanced and therapeutic diet to indoor patients
2. Provide counseling and advice to patients suffering from different diseases
3. Educate patients as per their requirement for the dietary needs and diet preparation
4. Supply special diets to indoor, diet clinics and private patients
5. Guide and supervise staff working in the department
6. Provide training to dietetic interns, nursing staff, and other staff working in the department
7. Develop policies regarding diets, administrative staff, food safety and food quality
8. Organize orientation programs to kitchen staff on food safety and personal hygiene and nutrition awareness programs to the community.

Functions

The main functions of this department are administrative, educative, and therapeutic.
1. The administrative function includes planning and management of hospital diets that include devising of infrastructure, formulation of policies about indents, selection, procurement, storage, preparation, and distribution of foods in consultation with medical superintendent. It includes establishment and accounts, record maintaining, menu planning, diet

monitoring and evaluation, budget planning, quality control, organization, and staffing. It also includes other functions such as general supervision of staff, housekeeping, and sanitation, and condemnation of equipment.
2. The clinical functions include planning of therapeutic diets, food processing, production, and presentation of menus. It also includes providing dietary advice and counseling to indoor and outdoor patients attending the specialized clinics.
3. The educative functions include demonstrating cooking sessions to hospital and kitchen staff, and follow up the chart, training to dietetic interns, and nursing staff.

Types of Hospital Diets

There are different types of foods prepared in dietetic department according to the kind of patients such as balanced diet, liquid diet, semisolid diet, low-fat diet, cardiac diet, renal diet, high-protein diet, diabetic diet, high carbohydrate, low-protein diet, salt-restricted, bland diet, fat-free diet, Ryles tube diet, postoperative high carbohydrate, formula, and jejunostomy feed.

Bases for Planning

The dietary services planning is according to the number of hospital beds, type of patients, number of meals to be served per day, policies for serving visitors, students, staff, and kind of dietary services, purchasing strategies, type of food to be served, and turnover of the patients.

Location

Its location must be on the ground floor with easy access to the transportation of food to nursing units. Its location is close to material management departments/stores. The cafeteria and dining room must be near to the food preparation area.

Space Requirement

The space required for a 500-bedded hospital is 15 sq ft/bed, and for up to 200 beds, it should be 20 sq ft/bed.

Physical Layout and Workflow

It is divided into four major functional areas:(1) receiving supplies area, (2) storage and refrigeration room, (3) prepreparation, and (4) cooking area. It also has facilities of serving room, food delivery/tray assembly room, special diet kitchen, dishwashing and pot washing area, garbage disposal facilities, housekeeping facilities, and LPG bank for cooking. There should be the provision of food service manager office, office space for chief dietitian, and other staff, dining hall with adequate facilities, and cafeteria/coffee shop.
1. **Dietary procurement:** Dietary procurement for the hospital is estimated based on the actual consumption of raw material forecasting for the next full financial year. The purchase committee approves the procurement procedure and requirements for the purchase—the purchased items categorized into perishable and nonperishable items. Perishable items such as milk, curd, fruits, and vegetables are procured on a daily, biweekly, and triweekly basis, whereas nonperishable items on a monthly or bimonthly basis. The rest of the ration is purchased by floating yearly tenders and entering the lowest quotations.
2. **Inspection and storage:** The items are inspected and verified by the dietician in-charge before entering in the stock books. Some of the perishable items stored in the cold room/refrigeration room. Stock books for each item are maintained separately.
3. **Prepreparation and preparation:** Food items are issued daily. There should be a separate prepreparation area for sorting, peeling, slicing, and chopping. Each item should be washed before cooking.
4. **Equipment accessories:** There are separate stores for different types of equipment accessories. Service items can be purchased annually.
5. **Accounts and records:** There are essential records that are maintained by the dietary department such as daily diet requisition, master diet chart, daily expense book, ration store register, general stock register (deadstock), imprested accounts register, and standard diet schedules, etc.

The sister-in-charge/ward aide daily prepares the diet list of indoor patients and sends it to the dietetic department. The meal services may be fully centralized or decentralized based on the hospital policy. Usually, in general wards, tea and breakfast services are decentralized where the ward staff collects and distributes the same under the supervision of ward sister. Lunch and dinner services are centralized. The kitchen staff carries the cooked food in food trolleys and distributes the food in the individual trays of patients. The dishes are washed in the ward by the attendants. In the private departments, it is usually centralized, and private wards have its pantry. From there, the food served to individual patients. The used trays are collected, washed, and sterilized after each meal. **Figure 21.2** depicts the workflow of the kitchen.

Staffing

For 500-bedded hospitals, there should be 1 dietician who should be assisted by 5 assistant dieticians, 1 steward, 2 storekeepers; 1 for ration and other general storekeeper, 1 clerk, 2 head cooks, and 2 therapeutic cooks, 10 cooks, 28 bearers, 8 masalchi, 2 store attendants, and 2 safai karamcharies. **Figure 21.3** depicts the organization chart of a tertiary hospital.

Monitoring and Control

There should be monitoring standard operating protocols in the department to ensure quality standards. The cleanliness, hygiene, and sanitation of all the areas must

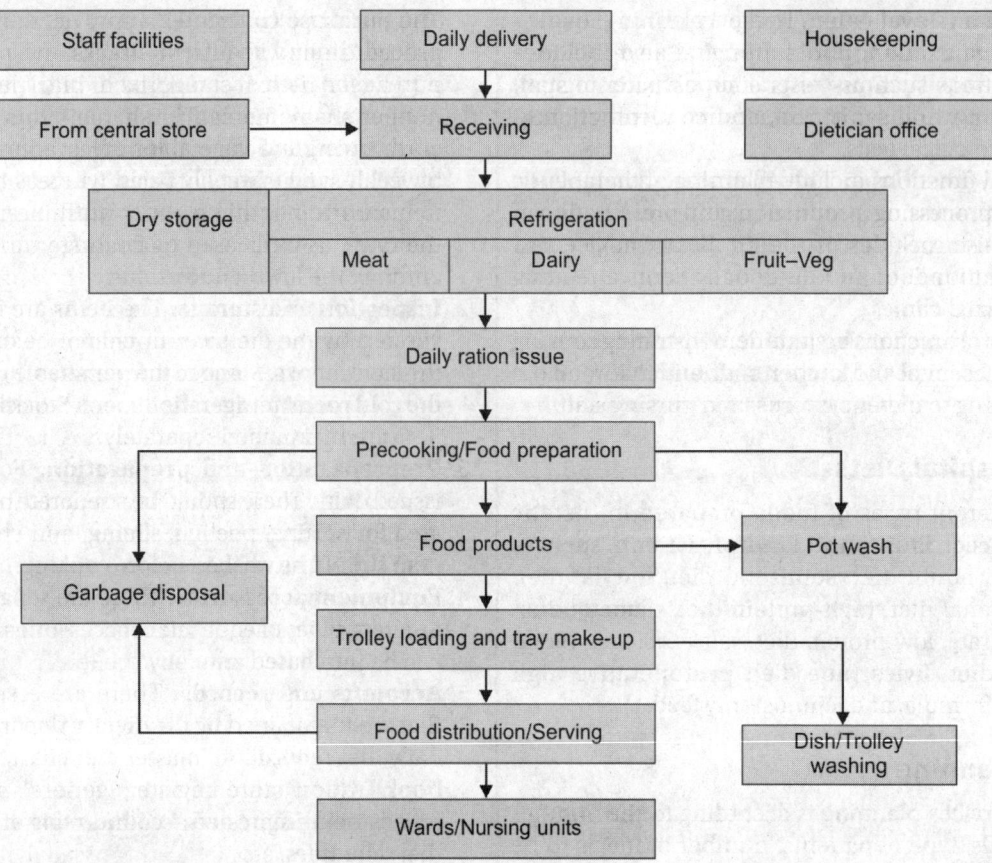

Fig. 21.2: Dietary service workflow.

be monitored daily. The dietician must monitor the diet quantity and quality. Ensure that the hygienic measures are in practice during the preparation and distribution of diets. There should be a policy for a periodic checkup for the staff working in the kitchen. The orientation programs regarding food safety and personal hygiene for the kitchen staff must conduct regularly.

PLANNING AND ORGANIZING LABORATORY SERVICES

The laboratory services in the hospital are an essential part of the hospital. Different types of laboratories perform specific lab tests to help medical staff in making and confirming the diagnosis. It has a significant role in the treatment and prevention of diseases. The tests performed by the labs are of routine and specialized levels.

Classification of Labs

1. **According to the tests performed by labs:** These are hematology and blood banking, microbiology and serology, clinical pathology, clinical biochemistry, histopathology, cytology, molecular biology, and molecular pathology, etc.
2. **According to the levels of labs:** Based on the health-care facility, there are four types of labs:

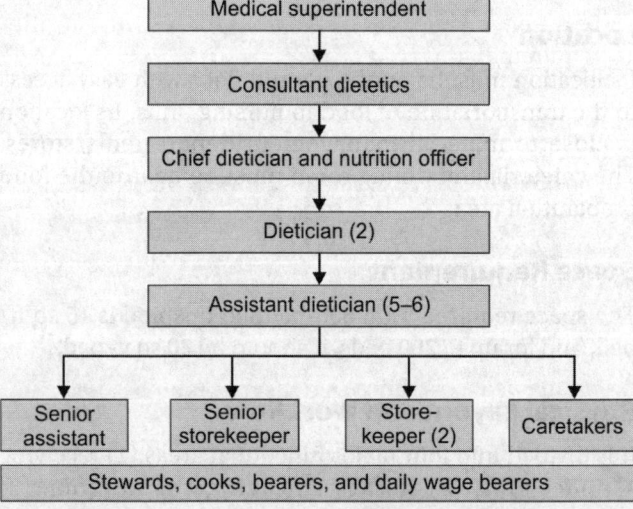

Fig. 21.3: Organization chart of dietary department in a tertiary hospital.

a. **Primary-level labs:** These are routine or simple labs at primary and urban health centers. These labs perform hematological, urine examination, microscopy tests for detecting malarial parasites, and sputum for acid-fast bacilli and have a cold chain system. In community health centers, additional criteria such as reproductive tract infections/sexually transmitted infections, screening for G6PD, typhoid, etc. are performed.

b. **Secondary-level labs:** These types of labs are available at the district hospital level. These labs perform various tests such as pathological, clinical pathology, biochemistry, serology, and microbiological tests.
c. **Tertiary-level labs:** These labs are available in teaching and nonteaching large hospitals. These labs perform sophisticated diagnostics and investigations. These labs usually receive referral specimens.
d. **Reference/research/specific disease reference labs:** These types of labs operationalize in medical colleges, research institutes, and private institutes. These are of high-standard labs.

Principles of Planning Labs

1. The labs' design is based on their functions, processes, and sequence.
2. Integrate various services within access, keep travel time short.
3. It should be approachable to OPD and IPD, mostly on the ground floor.
4. The sample collection centers must be at central points; ICU, OPD, and emergency.
5. There should be a single window for report collection and should have provision to intimate abnormal results to consultants.
6. There should be unidirectional flow of activities: preanalysis and postanalysis to promote efficacy, flexibility, and veracity and also to have a boundary between clean and dirty areas based on sterility requirement.
7. There should be a scope for future expansion.
8. Use appropriate material for building the labs.
9. The labs must be free from biological hazards, and have the fire and electrical safety.
10. There should be intra- and extramural communication.

Location

The labs must locate on the ground floor for easy access to outpatient, emergency, and inpatient departments. It should be near to surgical, intensive care, radiology, and obstetrical departments.

Space Requirement

For Primary Health Center (PHC) having lab load 10–20 patients, the minimum area is 10 m² with a total area of 13.46 sq m; for Community health center (CHC) with lab load 30–50 patients, the minimum space required is 90 m², and for district hospital of 100–500 bed capacity, it should be 150 m² with lab load 100 collections.

Workflow and Physical Layout

1. **Workflow:** The workflow must follow a unidirectional path to have infection control and work efficiency. Usually, there are three paths: (1) sample path, (2) reagent path, and (3) report path. The personnel must go along with all three tracks.
   a. *Sample path:* It should be in black lines. This path has areas for sampling/registration, room for receiving/collection of samples; accession (a record of all specimens obtained by the lab for analysis, preparing, analyzing with washing and autoclave room, a facility for sample storage and sample disposal. The labs must have the provision of cold, hot, distilled and deionized water in individual sections, and uninterrupted power supply.
   b. *Reagent path:* The red line denotes the reagent path. This path has area/facilities for receiving, storage, indenting, using, and disposal of reagent and materials.
   c. *Report path:* The blue line denotes the report path. This path follows in pathology, microbiology, and biochemistry labs; it has the provision of offices and reporting window.
2. **Corridors:** The inside lab corridor must be minimum 2,550 mm without any obstruction in the passageway and the passage of exit.
3. **Ceilings:** The minimum heights of the roof should be 3,000 mm.
4. **Doors:** The minimum width of entries should be 1,200 mm in all analytic areas with double shutters. There should be panels for indicating preanalytic and analytic domains.
5. **Entry to lab:** There should be a lobby at each exit point to have demarcation between lab and nonlab space and to have hygienic, safe, and secure lab spaces. There should also be the facility for hand washing and coat pegs for hangings lab-protective clothing and space for storing dirty protective clothing in the lobby.
6. **Workbenches:** The area for analytic and the testing sample should be 10 ft × 20 ft with workbenches 750 mm long and 720 mm high. It should have the provision of safe cable management and minimum counter-to-counter clearance should be 2,150 mm. There should be enough space at the back for the equipment and air circulation.
7. **Other facilities:** Other facilities include a separate room for reporting and recording, facility of cleaning glassware, sterilizers, and waste disposal facilities for disposing of liquid reagents, by-products, and waste. There should be adequate ventilation with mechanical ventilation systems, climate control, and lighting arrangement. It should be equipped with hand washing, eating, storing food, etc. facilities. The labs must have adequate communication facilities, facilities for transportation of samples, etc. There should also be a room for a meeting, doctors' rooms, and administrative offices. There should be a staff room with adequate facilities.

Staffing

The labs must have Head of the department who should be in-charge of the lab and have administrative control. The requirement of staffing depends on the level of the facility. Roles and responsibilities must be defined. The department must conduct training programs for the staff and evaluate them annually based on performance.

Safety and Infection Control

There should be a documentation of lab safety policies and procedures. The labs must have general safety and must adhere to bio-safety precautions as per the level of Biosafety Laboratories (BSL1, BSL2, BSL3, and BSL4). The staff must follow safe, hygienic practices such as hand washing, wearing protective clothing, gloves, eye protection, etc.

There should be proper segregation, storage, transport, and disinfection as per Biomedical Waste Management Rules 2016, and first aid rooms with lifesaving drugs. The lab must equip with decontamination of lab wastes such as autoclaves, chemical disinfectants, etc. Label all biohazards material with the biohazards symbol. The fire/emergency exits must consider in planning that must lead to open space. The fire extinguishers and fire blankets should be available. The staff must be aware of their ethical responsibilities and follow a moral code of conduct.

Security

For security purpose, the location of the lab must be in a secure area. Only the authorized personnel have access to the lab.

Monitoring and Quality Control

1. **For equipment:** There should be a list of consumable and nonconsumable items, and these should be suitable located, in functional order with warranty cards, periodically inspected for cleaning and maintenance. The labs must have standing operative procedures and logbooks for equipment. Equipment must be verified for its reliability and should have checked through both internal and external quality audits. The labs must have calibration certificates for all analytical equipment by National Accreditation Board of Testing and Calibration Laboratories (NABL), which is ISO 15189;2007 standard in India.
2. **For reagent and material:** There should be a standard for analysis. The reagent must have batchwise records in ledger for its quality. These should be defined in the SOP for quality, storing for reagents, chemicals, and consumables under appropriate temperature conditions. The reagent needs checking for its quality validation before using. All reagents in use must have labels with date, concentration, and name of the manufacturer, expiry date, storage conditions, and warning. For microbiological labs, check the potency of each antibiotic sensitivity disc at least weekly, all strips against reference strains, quality, and pH of media. Check the culture media for sterility before issuing to the patients and water quality for its grade and presence of interference elements according to the Bureau of Indian Standards.

CHAPTER HIGHLIGHTS

- Ancillary or support services are essential for the adequate functioning of the hospital and play a crucial role in the treatment of patients.
- The CSSD supplies sterile articles and materials to all departments of the hospital, OPDs, and other general and specialized departments.
- The laundry department provides clean and safe linen to different departments of the hospital.
- The dietetics department supplies a healthy and therapeutic diet to indoor patients. Apart from this function, it is a center for providing counseling and advice to the patients through its clinics, and also provides training to the students of other disciplines.
- Laboratory services carry out the significant responsibilities to help medical staff in making and confirming the diagnosis.
- All supporting departments should have their norms for planning and organizing their services. All have to follow standard operative procedures to provide quality services.

REVIEW QUESTIONS

I. Essay Type Questions
1. Describe the planning and organization of the Central Sterile Supply Department (CSSD).
2. Enumerate the aims and objectives of Linen and Laundry department. Discuss its monitoring and control function.
3. Explain the workflow of the dietary department in detail.
4. What are the different types of laboratory services? What points you will keep in mind while planning quality laboratory services?

II. Short Notes
1. Aims and objectives of CSSD
2. The workflow of laundry services
3. Types and quantification of hospital laundry
4. Workflow and physical layout of the laboratory

III. Multiple Choice Questions
1. The space requirement to plan CSSD for 300-bedded hospital is:
   a. 7 sq ft/bed   b. 8 sq ft/bed
   c. 9 sq ft/bed   d. 10 sq ft/bed
2. The main function of preparation area in CSSD is to:
   a. Segregate clean and infected article
   b. Check breakage and assembling equipment
   c. Store clean received material
   d. Label all the packs
3. Mechanical, chemical, and biological indicators are to:
   a. Monitor standard operative procedures

b. Have regular internal and external audits
c. Have a record of the use of washing formula
d. Check sterilization for its adequacy

4. How must many sets of linen be in a hospital laundry?
   a. 5
   b. 6
   c. 7
   d. 8

5. How much laundry workload is estimated as a rule of thumb as per Indian Standard?
   a. 4.5 kg
   b. 3.5 kg
   c. 2.5 kg
   d. 1.5 kg

6. What is the minimum space requirement for planning hospital laundry in a 300 bedded hospital?
   a. 3,240 Sq ft
   b. 3,580 sq ft
   c. 4,068 sq ft
   d. 5,800 sq ft

7. What is the minimum space requirement for planning hospital dietary services in a 500-bedded hospital?
   a. 10 sq ft
   b. 12 sq ft
   c. 15 sq ft
   d. 20 sq ft

8. Which level of health-care facility is restricted to perform pathological, biochemistry, serological, and bacteriological lab tests?
   a. Primary level
   b. Secondary level
   c. Tertiary level
   d. Reference level

9. What is the minimum space requirement for planning hospital laboratory services with lab load of 10–12 patients?
   a. 150 m^2
   b. 90 m^2
   c. 50 m^2
   d. 10 m^2

10. Which path in the workflow of labs denoted by black lines?
    a. Reagent path
    b. Report path
    c. Sample path
    d. Exit path

Answer Keys

1. a.   2. b.   3. d   4. b   5. c   6. a   7. c
8. b   9. d   10. c

SUGGESTED READING

1. Banu A, Subhas GT. Central Sterile Supply Department – Need Of The Hour. [Online] Available from http://jphmr.com/wp-content/uploads/2013/11/Article-14.pdf. [Accessed on 07.05.2019].
2. Singh S, et al. Int J Community Med Public Health. 2019 Mar;6(3):1264-68.[Online] Available from http://www.ijcmph.com https://www.ijcmph.com/index.php/ijcmph/article/view/4287/2873. [Accessed on 09.05.2019].
3. Central Sterile Supply Department (CSSD). Ministry of Health and ... [Online] Available from https://rmlh.nic.in/Index1.aspx?lid=1297&lsid=1762&pid=17&lev=3&langid=1. [Accessed on 07.05.2019].
4. Srikar K, Sharma S, Ghosh SS. Quality Assurance Hospital Linen and Laundry Services. [Online] Available from https://www.ijsr.net/archive/v6i3/ART20171405.pdf. [Accessed on 05.05.2019].
5. Department of health & family welfare government of Orissa. Study on improvement of dietary services and management in medical college hospitals and selected DHHS of Department of Health & Family Welfare, Government of Orissa. [Online] Available from http://www.nrhmorissa.gov.in/writereaddata/Upload/Documents/STUDY%20ON%20IMPROVEMENT%20OF%20DIETARY%20SERVICES%20AND.pdf. [Accessed on 18.05.2019].
6. Dietary Services. [Online] Available from http://www.neigrihms.gov.in/dietary.html. [Accessed on 18.05.2019].
7. Guideline Document for Design of BSL 2 Labs (District Hospitals, CHC, AND PHC) Level. [Online] Available from http://www.naco.gov.in/sites/default/files/1Guideline%20doc%20design%20of%20BSL2%20labs(dist, hosp,chc&phc)%20level.pdf. [Accessed on 19.05.2019].
8. Guidelines for Good Clinical Laboratory Practices – ICMR. [Online] Available from https://icmr.nic.in/sites/default/files/guidelines/GCLP.pdf. [Accessed on 19.05.2019].

CHAPTER 22

Planning for Emergency and Disaster Management

CHAPTER OUTLINE

- Emergency and Disaster Management
  - Defining Disaster
  - Types of Disasters
  - Factors Contributing to the Risk of Disaster
  - Defining Emergency and Disaster Management
  - Objectives of Disaster Management
  - Principles of Disaster Management
  - Disaster Management Cycle
  - Disaster Management-related Processes
- Planning For Emergency and Disaster Management
  - Types of Emergency and Disaster Planning
  - Planning at the National Level
  - Planning at State Level
  - Planning at District and Local Level
  - Planning at the Hospital Level

LEARNING OUTCOMES

After completion of this chapter, the learner will be able to:
- Understand the concept of emergency and disaster
- Explain emergency and disaster management
- Enumerate objectives of disaster management
- Describe principles of emergency and disaster management
- Discuss the components of disaster management
- Describe the planning of crisis and disaster management at different levels

KEY TERMS

Emergency, disaster, emergency and disaster management, risks, hazards, vulnerability, preparedness, mitigation

INTRODUCTION

Emergency and disaster planning are a coordinating and collective effort to plan various activities systematically to manage future unforeseen events and disasters. India is prone to have disasters of varying intensity of natural, human made, and combinations of both. It is due to changing geographical conditions, extreme climatic variation, increased urbanization and industrialization, enhanced technology, and social reasons. According to government statistics, India is affected by more than 50% geographic areas with the different magnitudes of earthquakes, by more than 40% land with floods and river erosion, about 75% coastline with cyclones and tsunami, over 65% cultivated land with droughts, and hilly areas with landslides. All these disasters have severe effects on its population, economy, and development.

EMERGENCY AND DISASTER MANAGEMENT

Emergency and disaster both are unforeseen, unknown events of the unpredictable cause, type, date, time, and extent of the damage. An "emergency" is an event, a local incident characterized by impacts that local responders can handle by utilizing available resources.

Disaster, on the other hand, has a high magnitude of emergency, causes severe disruption of life, health, and other losses. Moreover, it is beyond the capacity of local responders to respond against the disaster. They need external assistance to handle the casualties. Disaster may be a catastrophe if the magnitude of the event is so severe that need international aid on the district, state, and national response. These are unpredictable, unfamiliar, uncertain, urgent, and speedy and pose a threat to life, material, economy, and environment.

Defining Disaster

United Nations International Strategy for Disaster Reduction (UNISDR) outlines disaster like a severe event that affects the functioning of the community at large and has a high impact on their life, property, assets, economy,

Chapter 22: Planning for Emergency and Disaster Management

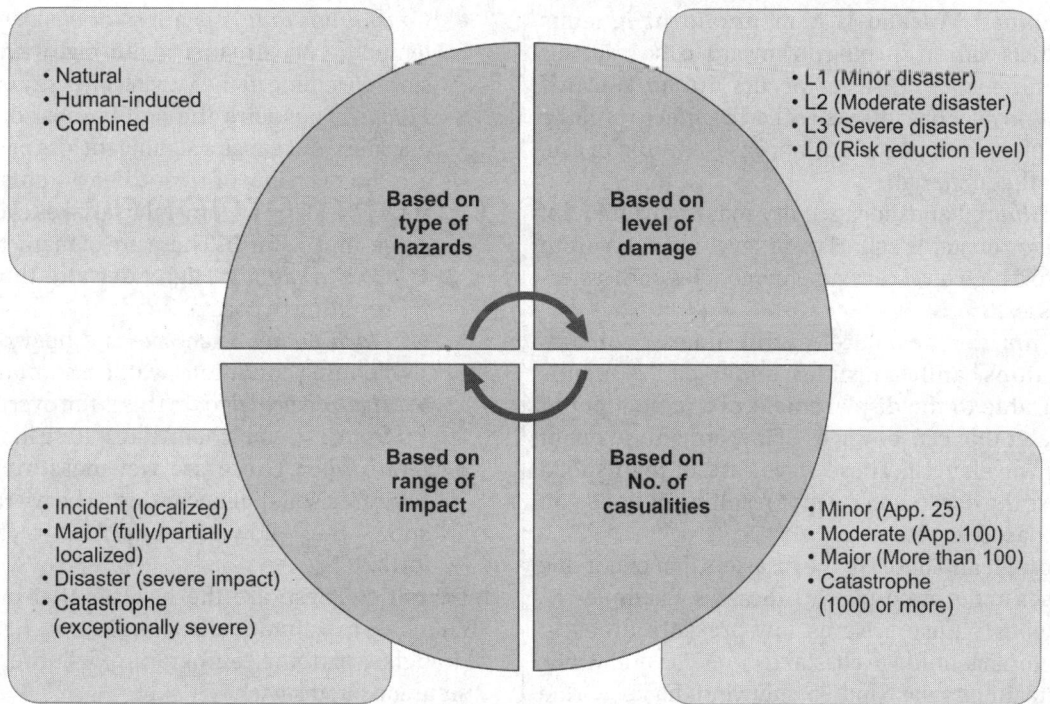

Fig. 22.1: Classification of disasters.

and environment. The intensity of occurrence is so high that it requires external resources to cope up with the losses.

Disaster Management Act (2005) describes the disaster as a mishap, calamity, catastrophe, or grave occurrence resulting from any cause either natural, human made, or due to negligence, which causes a significant loss of life, suffering, property, or to the environment. The magnitude of occurrence is such that need assistance from outside sources to cope up.

Disaster is an occurrence arising with little or no warning, which causes severe disruption of life, losses, injury to a large number of people resulting from human made or natural that causes destruction and devastation that is beyond the capacity of the affected community. It leaves high human mortality, and morbidity leads to epidemics, including injury, psychological impact, destruction, damages, loss of assets, property, animals' mortality and morbidity, loss of employment, and so forth.

Types of Disasters

There are different ways to classify disasters. Classification is according to the kind of hazards, level of damage, the number of casualties involved, and the range of impact **(Fig. 22.1)**.

According to the Type of Hazards

Generally, disasters are of two types: Natural and human induced. Emergencies or disasters can arise due to a combination of two kinds of risks or secondary disasters that occur after primary disasters.

Natural disasters

A natural disaster is the consequence of natural hazard that affects the significant loss of life, destruction of property,

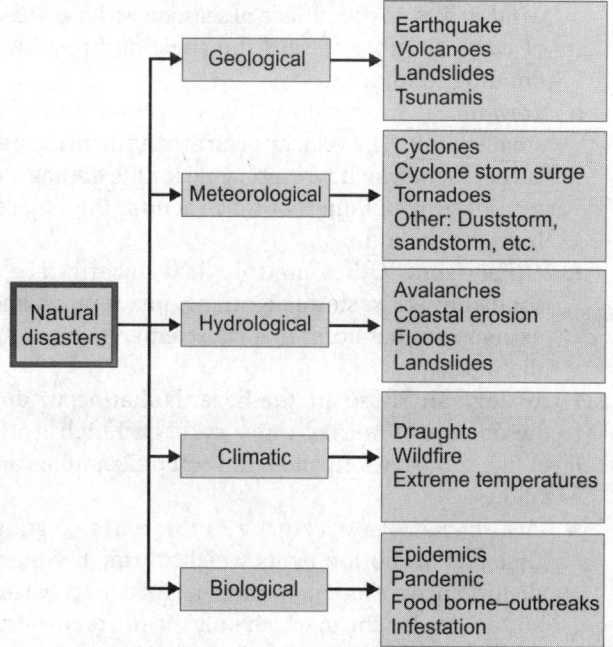

Fig. 22.2: Types of natural disasters.

economic, and to the environment. There are mainly five hazards resulting in disasters **(Fig. 22.2)**:

a. **Geological:** These types of hazards/risks occur due to geological processes of the earth. Examples are earthquakes, volcanoes, landslides and tsunamis.
   - *Earthquakes:* These results due to interaction at the edge of high plates of the ground. These are of varying intensity and trigger shaking of the earth. Earthquakes thus cause the collapse of buildings, landslides, liquefaction, and surface displacement resulting in losses.

- *Volcanoes:* Volcano is a mountain of igneous products with an opening downward to the reservoir of molten rock. Disaster occurs due to volcanic eruption near or at the vent of earth surface resulting flowing of lava, poisonous hot gases, fleeing of ash, and other material.
- *Landslides:* Landslides are dry mass movement of loose or unstable soil. Hazard level may vary from low to a high level causing emergencies or disasters of losses.
- *Tsunamis:* These are earthquakes, volcano eruptions, and landslides undersea. Tsunamis occur due to the displacement of a large amount of water that causes waves of low amplitude but of long wavelength. These waves are of high speed across the ocean and steeper resulting in floods on the coastal lands.

b. **Meteorological:** These are the disasters that occur due to changes in the atmospheric processes. Examples:
- *Cyclones:* These arise as low-pressure areas in equatorial latitude in coastal regions. Several winds flow in the circular band. Speedy winds highest in the center and lowest in the periphery cause cyclones.
- *Cyclone storm surge:* It occurs when the high-speed wind strikes on the surface of sea cause a large mass of water to move toward the coast and resulting flooding conditions.
- *Tornadoes:* A tornado is like a cyclone but of a smaller scale. The velocity of air arising in the center is very high, which is responsible for the damage. It may destroy buildings or may vacuum the objects from the ground.
- *Other types:* Other metrological hazards are a sandstorm, dust storm, lightning, heavy rains, and extreme temperatures that cause emergencies and disasters.

c. **Hydrological:** These are the hazards that occur due to the change of normal water cycle and high water level due to heavy rain and wind setup. Examples are as follows:
- *Avalanches:* An avalanche is the mass of snow that sets in motion by its weight through violent disturbances of its equilibrium. It is of two types: the surface avalanche in which only the top is covering of snow slips and another the ground avalanche in which the whole mass of snow slides. These are of many kinds:
  ♦ *Powder snow avalanche*: It usually occurs due to a strong wind or other disturbances in the winter season, after a fresh fall of snow.
  ♦ *Fresh wet snow avalanche*: It moves a little slower than powder snow.
  ♦ *Wet snow avalanche*: It is mainly during the spring season. It flows slowly with a great force.
  ♦ *Snow slab avalanche*: It occurs due to a compressed layer of snow.
  ♦ *Sea or river avalanche*: It happens by the movement of glaciers.
- *Coastal erosion:* It is a loss of coastal area either temporary or permanent due to high waves, wind, and storm resulting in the varying intensity of disasters.
- *Floods:* These are the commonest of all-natural disasters and cause a significant loss of life. Reasons are the overflow of rivers, heavy rains, melting of snow, breaking of dams, glacial lakes cyclonic storm surge, and so forth. These are of many types:
  ♦ *Coastal floods*: High tides and thunderstorm, resulting in coastal flooding.
  ♦ *Flash floods*: Excessive and heavy rains cause flooding conditions within a short period.
  ♦ *Hydrological floods*: This is the overflow of water from a stream channel resulting in flooding.
- *Landslides:* These are wet mass movements of saturated soil that occur due to heavy rain or heavy snow—these flow as debris, mud, rockfall, and so forth.

d. **Climatic:** These are the hazards that occur due to changes in climatically conditions. Examples are draughts, extreme temperature, wildfire, emergency situations or disaster.

e. **Biological:** These are the hazards that occur due to exposure to pathogenic and nonpathogenic microorganisms and vectors. Examples are epidemics, pandemics, foodborne outbreaks, and infestations due to flies, fleas, and rodents, which cause emergencies or disasters.

Human-induced disasters

Human-induced disasters are due to rapid urbanization, transition in cultural practices, industrialization, development in high-risk areas, the vulnerability of population environmental degradation, lack of knowledge-led disasters of many kinds. Human actions, negligence, or involving the failure of the system is resulting in human-induced disasters. These are as follows:

a. **Technological disasters:** These disasters are due to failure of technology: Examples are industrial hazards, fires, chemical, biological, radiological, and nuclear hazards, power interruptions, water supply disruption, transportation incidents/accidents during the air, road, rail, water transport, air pollution, structural collapses, food or water contamination, and hazards.

b. **Societal disasters:** Societal disasters are the result of sociological problems, such as criminal acts, stampedes, demonstrations, mass gathering events, displaced populations, and terrorists' activities, riots, and war.

According to the Level of Damage

Depending on the level of damage, and capacity of authorities to deal with the disaster, the High Power Committee on Disaster Management classifies disasters into various levels:

- **Level-L0 disaster:** It denotes planning stage or normal time that can be utilized for risk reduction and response activities including monitoring, documentation, prevention, mitigation, and preparation, training, etc.

- **Level-L1 disaster:** Level-L1 disaster is a minor disaster as it involves a minimal level of damage. The district can cope up emergency within its capacity and available resources without any assistance and mobilization of resources.
- **Level-L2 disasters:** Level-L2 disasters are moderate disasters as they have a modest impact on life and economy and require assistance and mobilization of resources at the state level to handle an emergency.
- **Level-L3 disasters:** Level-L3 disasters are severe. These are substantial scale disasters and pose severe losses to life, economy, and environment. State and district level authorities are unable to cope up within its capacity and resources. It needs central assistance immediately.

According to Victims Involved

According to the victim involved, emergency or disasters are of four kinds:
1. **Minor disaster:** It means approximate 25 casualties.
2. **Moderate disaster:** It affects approximately 100 victims.
3. **Major disasters:** It includes more than 100 victims.
4. **Catastrophic disaster:** When some losses reach up to 1,000 or more.

According to the Range of Impacts

1. **Incidents:** In incidents, the effect is much localized and requires only local resources without involving the public to handle. Only standard operative procedures (SOPs) are activated during the response period and have no challenge to recovery.
2. **Major incidents:** Major incident is an emergency that has fully or partially localized impact of the event and may require assistance from nearby areas and public participation. SOPs and emergency plans may be activated and have minor challenges to recovery.
3. **Disasters:** Disaster is a situation that has a severe impact in term of losses and requires assistance/resources from state and national level and full public participation and support in response. Disaster and emergency plans are in action in response. There are significant challenges to recovery and possibly phase-wise recovery and reconstruction.
4. **Catastrophes:** A type of disaster that is exceptionally severe regarding physical and social losses damages requires assistance and coordination with national and international resources. Both disaster and emergency plans are in action during the response period. The public is extensively participated during that time and poses massive challenges and has long-term consequences of the disaster.

Factors Contributing to the Risk of Disaster

Main four factors are contributing to the risk of disaster:
1. **Hazards:** Hazards, as discussed above, are natural and human induced or a combination of both. These are the trigger agents that initiate mishaps.
2. **Location:** These are disaster-prone areas. The community at seaside and hilly areas is at risk; earthquake-prone regions are likely to have disasters.
3. **Exposure:** The degree of impact due to hazards on infrastructure, transportation, life, network, etc.
4. **Vulnerability:** Vulnerability is the extent of damage to society, structure, and system, which are due to external events or hazards. It depends on underlying causes such as poverty, limited access to resources, economic policies, and illness and disabilities; lack of local institutions; lack of training and skill on disaster management; population expansion; environment degradation; and unsafe conditions such as dangerous buildings, dangerous location, low level of income, poor public actions, and so on. The level of vulnerability and hazards predict the magnitude of the disaster.

Defining Emergency and Disaster Management

Emergency and disaster management is a continuous and collaborative performance-based approach that involves planning, before, during, and after an emergency or disaster takes place. It is a process of planning and taking appropriate measures to reduce or prevent the possible risks, to provide timely help to victims, and to fasten recovery during postdisaster.

According to UNISDR (2015), disaster management is the process of organizing, planning, and applying all measures of preparation, responding, and initiating recovery from disaster. It is an integrating process that requires collective efforts to carry out all operational activities related to disaster management. It covers all aspects of disaster management including prevention, reduction of risks, control of risk, preparedness for disaster, the response on the disaster, and recovery after disasters per government policy and administrative decisions.

Objectives of Disaster Management

The main objectives of disaster management are as follows:
1. To prevent the risk of occurring any disaster
2. To reduce the risk of catastrophe, its intensity, and after effects
3. To train the workforce both officials, stakeholders, and community per guidelines to manage disaster
4. To prepare them to take protective measures in any event
5. To receive appropriate actions in an emergency or disaster situation
6. To assess the severity or consequences of the calamity
7. To evacuate, rescue, and provide relief to the victims
8. To rehabilitate the victims.

Principles of Disaster Management

The following principles are important in disaster management:
1. Prevention of disasters
2. Minimization of causalities

3. Prevention of further causalities
4. Prompt action
5. Rescue the victims
6. Immediate first aid
7. Evacuate the site
8. Provide care and refer
9. Rehabilitate
10. Reconstruction and recovery
11. Capacity building
12. Knowledge management, research, and development.

Disaster Management Cycle

Disaster management is a continuous process, in general, that involves mainly two stages with corresponding activities **(Fig. 22.3)**: Predisaster and postdisaster.

Predisaster Phase

a. **Prevention:** It includes all the measures to prevent the effects of hazards, unsafe conditions as a preventive measure to reduce losses in future disasters. These measures include:
- Developing plans at the national and state level
- Assessing and analyzing the risks by using various methods
- Educating the community through community awareness programmes and developing skills
- Following warning signals.

b. **Mitigation:** It includes all the measures to reduce hazards or to limit the effects of risks. These measures include as follows:
- Taking appropriate measures such as environmental friendly measures to save or restore the ecological system and adaptation to change the climate
- Probing the cause and lapses that occur in past disasters.

c. **Preparedness:** It includes all the protective and proactive measures before the mishap takes place with the aim to:
- Minimize loss of life, disruption of essential services, and damage to the structure
- Maximize immediate response from government, community, and individuals on disaster
- Prepare to everyone to cope up with calamities.

During this period, the protective and proactive measures include:
- Developing an emergency action or response plan
- Planning for an effective warning system
- Maintaining inventories to cope up with calamity
- Provision of training and practical session such as simulations, mock drill, and knowledge management of workforce
- Use of communication and information technology, connectivity at the site for control
- Preparing to establish an emergency control room
- Medical preparedness for mass casualty management
- Preparing, response plan, and standard operating procedures per guidelines.

Postdisaster Phase

a. **Response:** It includes all the measures during or immediately before the disaster. It deals with at the site action. Take immediate and adequate steps to deal with any emergency. It needs a caring approach with activation of the disaster management plan, including standard operating procedures (SOPs). Response team includes various forces such as police, fire, medical, and so forth. Multiple aspects of SOPs are as follows:
- Search and rescue operation
- Need assessments
- Medical assistance and managing mass casualties
- Evacuating area
- Restoration of essential and communication services at the site
- Therapeutic response, first aid, triage, transportation, and referral
- Provision of food, drinking water, sanitation, and clothing.

b. **Relief and rehabilitation:** Relief is providing immediate and adequate care per the minimum standard. It includes restoring conditions at the maximum level, e.g.:
- The setting of relief camps, which have the provision of drinking water, bathing, and sanitation facilities; essential health services; and food through community kitchen
- Provision of relief supplies per SOPs
- Reviewing standards of relief
- Rehabilitating/restoration of essential services to affected families per government norms
- Provision of temporary livelihood and shelters per local needs.

c. **Reconstruction and recovery:** This phase requires a comprehensive approach. It includes action on providing essential services, temporary shelters, the phase-wise rebuilding of houses, seeking the consultation of architects and engineers for designing homes in higher risk areas.

During the recovery phase, the focus is on improving the livelihood system of affected families, their education, health, caring elderly, women, and children, providing health and sanitation facilities, etc.

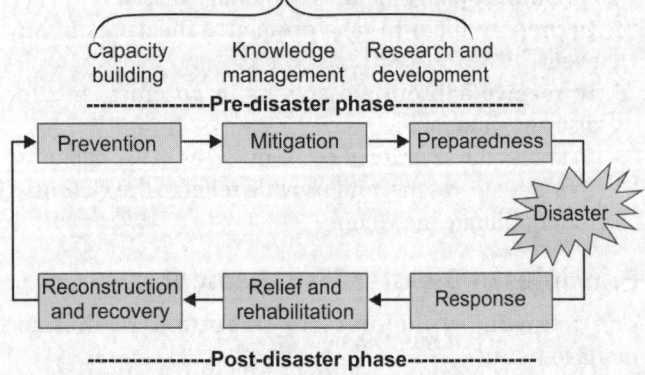

Fig. 22.3: Disaster mangement cycle.

Disaster Management (DM)–Related Processes

Capacity building, knowledge management, and research and development are a continuous process throughout disaster management.

1. **Capacity building:** Different institutions and management system are involved in capacity building to prevent, reduce, and handle a disaster. It needs adequate resources to manage an emergency. Capacity development has various activities such as awareness generation, education, training, and research development. It includes multiple activities:
   - Identification of institution who can impart knowledge on disaster management
   - Finding out traditional and global best practices and technology on DM
   - Involving official at national, state, and district level including local bodies, educational institutes of school, graduate, and postgraduate degree
   - Developing skills of officials, functionaries, trainers, community leaders, and professionals
   - Focusing on practical/exercises, simulations, and mock drill to build expertise on various aspects of DM
   - Implementing multiple programs such as awareness, sensitization, orientation, and skill training programs on DM for community and community leaders
   - Implementing disaster management-oriented curricula in all educational institutions
   - Organizing training programs for artisans and other groups such as social workers and counselors
   - Licensing and certification to qualified professionals in DM.
2. **Knowledge management:** Knowledge management requires techno and organizational approach. It focuses on utilizing services from technical institutes, academic, and training institutes, using information and communication technology, online disaster response networking, online knowledge networking, documentation of best practices and technology, and research on disaster management.
3. **Research and development:** Research and development is a relief-oriented approach. Focus areas are gathering information on types and intensity of hazards, both natural and human-induced disasters, disaster risk reduction especially on climatic changes and global warming, simulation studies on specific topics, based on short- and long-term consequences. It requires collaboration with different partners, institutions, and departments.

PLANNING FOR EMERGENCY AND DISASTER MANAGEMENT

Disaster is a multidisciplinary and multilevel process that needs careful planning involving various levels and departments. Plan as we know is the first step in management decisions. It is the process of developing a framework for allocation of resources to ensure the availability and ways of effective utilization of resources to meet specific objectives. There are different types of planning done at different levels and at various stages of disaster management to achieve its goals. These include development planning, strategic, preparedness, and contingency, and operation planning.

Emergency planning is a systematic and participatory process of preparing for the future to prevent major incidents, calamities, and disasters. Emergency and disaster planning are a coordinated, collaborative, and cooperative process, which is prepared to match the specific needs with available resources. It provides guidelines to manage unforeseen impacts successfully and usually based on policy and a national plan. The emergency or disaster plan is a living document and a blueprint for achieving the events. It is a framework to take actions at the time of an emergency or disaster.

Types of Emergency and Disaster Planning

There are different types of planning at different levels and for various stages of DM. These are as follows:

1. **Development planning:** It is carried out at the national level.
2. **Strategic plan:** Plan to outline the direction of an organization.
3. **Preparedness planning:** Planning concerning with mobilization of resources.
4. **Contingency/pre-emergency plan:** A plan to implement at the time of the event.
5. **Response planning:** Planning concerning to action following a disaster.
6. **Operational strategy:** A detailed action plan on disaster management.

Emergency and disaster planning involve hierarchical divisions at government setup. These are at the national, state, district, and local level.

Planning at the National Level

At the national level, the national executive committee, headed by Union Home Secretary and secretaries of other departments including National Disaster Management Authority (NDMA), formulates a national plan, development plan, and response plan for disaster management. NDMA is an apex body and an institutional framework under the Disaster Management Act (2005) headed by Prime Minister. The main functions are as follows:
- To formulate plans, policies, and guidelines
- To coordinate with the state and other departments
- To ensure an immediate and effective response to disasters
- To take the necessary measure of prevention, reduction, and preparation for the disaster
- To assist in building capacities
- To check funds for mitigation and preparedness measures

- To make emergency procurement at the time of relief and rescue
- To have control over national institutes of DM, National Disaster Response Force (NDRF) (armed forces, central paramilitary forces, state police forces, civil defense, home guard, state response forces, NCC, NSS)
- To be responsible for all kinds of emergencies and disasters involving security forces, intelligence agencies, law, and order situations.

There are other committees to oversee different aspects of DM such as cabinet committee on Natural Calamities, Cabinet Committee on Security, and High-Level Committee in catastrophes situation.

Planning at State Level

At state level, State Disaster Management Authority (SDMA), headed by the Chief Minister of the state, formulates a plan on disaster management based on guidelines of NDMA and National Disaster Plan. It coordinates with NDMA to implement the state plan. The Executive Committee at state level is headed by Chief Secretary who assists SDMA to perform all its functions. The functions are as follows:

- To prepare the State Emergency and Disaster Plan per NDMA guidelines and national plan and getting approval for the same from SDMA
- To coordinate and implement the plan
- To recommend funds for mitigation and preparedness measures
- To review developmental policies with different departments.

Planning at District and Local Level

Collector/District Commissioner/District Magistrate of the District prepares and implements the district disaster plan along with an elected representative of the local authority as a co-chairperson. It also coordinates with NDMA and SDMA related to disaster management and ensures its program per national and state policy. Local bodies play an essential part by controlling and managing civic services and provide capacity building for their officials and employees. These bodies also carry out all activities at different stages of a disaster. Disaster management at the district level is carried out in two steps: prehospital management and emergency hospital management.

Prehospital management includes the following:
- Triaging and first aid on site.
- First aid post either located in an existing health-care facility or through mobile hospital team, who will rush to the site to give immediate treatment to the casualties and refer patients, requires immediate hospitalization after providing first aid.
- Posting of the medical team comprising volunteer doctors and nurses in these first-aid post with necessary equipment and supplies.
- Transportation of casualties improvized ambulances from site to first-aid posts and hospital.
- Provision of mobile surgical units through networking with defense or railway hospitals to the site.

Planning at the hospital level discusses the emergency hospital organization.

Planning at the Hospital Level

Hospital has a vital role in saving the lives, preventing morbidity and mortality, preventing outbreaks of infectious diseases by providing 24-hour emergency services. Any emergency or disaster causes mass casualty incidents (MCIs) or the disaster for the hospitals. There is a need to have an adequate facility and an organized system to provide the best care within the limit time.

Disaster or Mass Casualty Incidence

Disaster or MCI is an unmanageable situation when the resources of the hospitals are beyond its standard capacity, and the hospital needs additional contingency measures to control the event or to provide emergency medical care. The bases to calculate the usual position of a hospital:

a. **Hospital treatment capacity:** A hospital capacity to treat casualties in 1 hour, which is 3% of the total number of beds.
b. **Hospital surgical capacity:** A hospital capacity to operate severely injured patients in 12 hours, which is number of operation theaters × 7 × 0.25 operations/12.

Ways to calculate the mass casualty emergencies
World Health Organization categorizes MCI as:
1. **According to casualties and considering the availability of workforce resources:**
   a. **Category 1:** If 30 patients with single or any emergency coming to the hospital.
   b. **Category 2:** If the number of patients with a single or any emergency varies from 30 to 50.
   c. **Category 3:** If the number of patients with a single or any emergency exceeds from 50.
2. **According to the severity of casualties:**
   a. **Category A:** If critically sick patients coming to the hospital.
   b. **Category B:** If severe patients coming to the hospital.
   c. **Category C:** If wounded but walking patients coming to the hospital.
3. **According to the contingency plan**
   a. **Class A:** Patients require treatment without disturbing the routine work of the hospital.
   b. **Class B:** Patients need treatment with the minimum disturbing everyday work of the hospital.
   c. **Class C:** Patients need treatment with the maximum disturbing routine work of the hospital.

Importance of Hospital Disaster Management Planning

- To provide the best possible immediate care in an organized and systematical way

- To prevent confusion and chaos during the response phase of disaster management
- To reduce morbidity and death rate.

Aims and Objectives of Hospital Disaster Management Planning

1. To prepare policies regarding response to both internal and external disasters
2. To develop different types of plans to manage emergency
3. To identify the roles and responsibilities of concerning personnel
4. To trained and educate the workforce to deal with disaster-related activities
5. To plan communication and network system
6. To develop standard operative procedures
7. To prepare and make provision of adequate supply and medical equipment
8. To build infrastructure to accommodate all types of patients.
   a. *For external disaster*
      1. To control and refer the patients to other facilities if required
      2. To mobilize the resources
      3. To provide adequate supply and medical equipment
      4. To integrate services with another department.
   b. *For internal disaster*
      1. To save the life of maximum patients, property, and environment
      2. To activate all preparedness measures
      3. To render care in an organized way
      4. To seek help from others
      5. To provide adequate supply and medical equipment.

Bases for Hospital Disaster Management Planning

Prepare plans according to
- MCI categorization
- Available workforce resources
- Available medical equipment and supply
- Type of disaster, internal or external.

Principles of Hospital Disaster Management Planning

1. **The principle of predictability:** The plan must indicate all stages and all aspects of disaster management.
2. **The principle of simplicity:** The plan must be simple to understand and operate.
3. **The principle of flexibility:** The program must be able to adjust the resources according to nature and kind of disaster.
4. **The principle of conciseness:** Every concerned person must be clear to their role and responsibility.
5. **The principle of comprehensive:** It means that the plan must indicate the proper networking and communication system.
6. **The principle of adaptability:** Plan must incorporate standard operative procedures for all disaster management-related activities.
7. **The principle of anticipation:** Plan must anticipate any disaster and catastrophic conditions.
8. **The principle of integration:** Prepare plan keeping in mind district/state/national guidelines.

Phases of Hospital Disaster Management Planning

There are mainly three phases of planning hospital disaster management: predisaster phase, disaster phase, and postdisaster phase **(Fig. 22.4)**:

A. Predisaster phase

1. **Planning phase:** Planning phase comprises the following steps:
   a. *Formulation of the hospital disaster and emergency management committee:* This is the first step to develop a disaster management plan. At the district hospital, Civil Surgeon/Medical Superintendent formulates a disaster management committee comprising heads of different departments; emergency, clinical, ancillary, nursing superintendent, store officers, engineering department, public relation, security officer, sanitation department, dietary, and social welfare.
   b. *Formulation of objectives of disaster management:* Have a meeting and develop general and specific goals phase wise.
   c. *Designing an incident command/control system (ICS):* It is a system to control and command

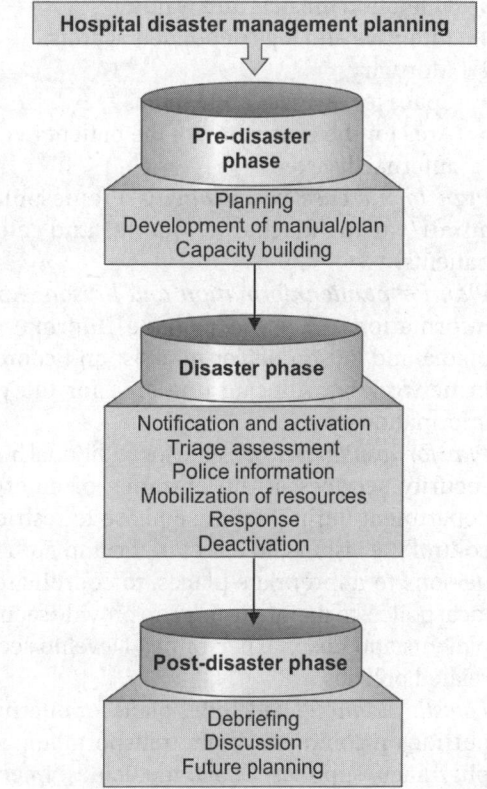

Fig. 22.4: Phases of hospital disaster management planning.

for personnel, equipment and supplies, and communication during the disaster event. It includes flexible organization structure, response to the specific disaster, response checklist, accountability, documentation, a common language of catastrophe, and effective emergency planning during an accident. Incident commander is the chief of the ICS, who has overall responsibility of managing the situation, and also prepares goals of that emergency. Usually, a senior medical officer of the emergency department is the incidence commander.

d. *Preparing job cards:* Prepare job responsibilities for each position. These are kept safe and coded.

e. *Hospital activation areas planning:* Plan and allocate different zones/areas in disaster/emergency plan.
- Incident command center, which should be near to emergency.
- Communication center with paging and telephone facilities.
- Security center/police chowki, near to the emergency department. Inform the police immediately being medicolegal cases.
- Reception and triage desk area for receiving and sorting victims.
- Area for decontamination in case of infectious outbreaks.
- Resuscitation and cardiac monitoring area.
- Area for minor treatment.
- Emergency department.
- Operation theaters and wards.
- Intensive and high dependency units.
- Mortuary.
- Space for relatives and media.
- Area for the evacuation of the patient in case of internal disaster.

f. *Plan to increase bed capacity:* Frame policy to admit/vacate/discharge stable and elective patients.

g. *Plan for public information and liaison:* Appoint information officer to provide information to media and liaison officer to assist and coordinate in networking. Allocate one area for the public information center.

h. *Plan for hospital security:* Plan for additional hospital security services at the entrance of emergency department during response phase to restrict and control the visitors, to direct traffic and authorized persons to appropriate places, to coordinate with local police, to maintain order, to provide security to patients and hospital personnel. Develop security-related policies.

i. *Logistic planning:* It includes plans for internal and outside on communication; transportation; stores, pharmacy, supplies, CSSD, medicines, injections, infusions, blood, and so forth; medical staff, nursing superintendent, ancillary staff, volunteers and for on-call duty, volunteers; and financial planning.

j. *Operations planning:* It includes planning for the activation of:
- Medical and ancillary staff in different identified activation areas such as:
  o Reception and triage area: The team comprises registration officer, triage medical and nursing staff, number of medical doctors in the emergency room, attendant, and security staff.
  o Triage is a method of categorizing patients according to the severity of their condition. Patients of *Category I* are those patients who need treatment without any delay; they are evident for a life-threatening emergency. *Category II* patients require treatment within 10 minutes of arrival; they are severe and potential for a life-threatening emergency. *Category III* patients need emergency care, but there is no possibility of a life-threatening emergency. They can be treated first come first.
  o Triage criteria to assign codes to the patients. These codes are assigning according to the conditions of patients. These are priority one-red code, for patients requiring immediate resuscitation; priority two-yellow code, for patients having potentially life-threatening injuries; priority three-green code, for walking wounded patients; and priority four-black/white, for dead patients.
  o Activate other areas such as decontamination, emergency, operation theaters, intensive and high dependency units, and minor treatment.
- Nursing staff: It includes the involvement of nursing superintendent, deputy nursing superintendent, and other administrative staff for activation.
- Essential ancillary services such as blood bank, radiology department, labs, and pharmacy.
- Mortuary and forensic medicine services.
- Activation of additional ancillary services such as dietary, sanitation, laundry, and CSSD supply, and other essential services such as water supply, light, and power, provision of generation at an emergency time in all identified activation areas.

k. Evacuation plan for internal disaster.

2. **Development of disaster manual/plan:** A disaster manual/plan must include all activities related to disaster management. It should be a tested and written document. The disaster management committee prepares it in consultation with an emergency, clinical, and nonclinical departments based on national, state,

Chapter 22: Planning for Emergency and Disaster Management

and district disaster management plan and policy. It is flexible to modify per the situation. It includes the following:
- Incident command system plan
- Incident control room location
- List of all medical, ancillary, and other staff with their names, addresses, contact numbers, according to their position in the hierarchy of ICS
- Alert/activation codes
- Response team formation and their job responsibilities
- Responsibilities of departments during on and off activation period
- Job cards with codes
- Detailing of identified disaster activation areas
- Action plans
- Standard operative procedures, standing orders, and protocols
- Detailing the mobilization of resources
- Inventory planning
- Criteria for hospital triage
- Communication and information system
- Reporting and documentation system
- Networking and information regarding nearby health facilities
- Pre- and postdisaster transportation
- Security and police network
- Evacuation and discharge details
- Medicolegal formalities; valuables, belongings, and clothing of unknown patients.
Disposal of dead bodies including details of mortuary and forensic medicine services.

3. **Planning for capacity building**
   - Plan orientation programs to those staff who will participate in implementing a preparedness action plan on disaster management. Give them proper training about the disaster plan, their roles, and specific skills required at the time of disaster event. Emphasize coordination, back up a communication system, and ways of getting equipment and supplies during mass casualties' management.
   - All administrators and heads of departments must attend these disaster training programs. They can undergo training for trainers.
   - Plan for regular disaster drill sessions on disaster preparedness and evacuation plan and tabletop drill exercises for working and communication during a disaster for administrators and managers.
   - Planning for continuing education programs on first aid and triage.

B. Disaster phase

1. **Notification and activation planning:** Activation phase is the phase of alerting the disaster management committee, staff, and other parties regarding the disaster.
   - For internal disaster, security staff should notify the administrator and employees to their supervisors. The nursing superintendent should also get information regarding this. The incident commander will take the lead to coordinate all activities of disaster management per plan.
   - For external disaster, emergency department gets a notification via telephone, EMS, through local disaster management authority, media, public, or police. In the district hospital, CMO/medical superintendent will inform the hospital administrator to activate the emergency response plan. Gather information regarding the nature and magnitude of the disaster, number of casualties, location, time of the mishap, and the expected time of receiving victims in the hospital. The incident commander comes in action on getting the alert, and he or she is free to direct and coordinate all disaster-related activities.
   - For mass casualty, put all identified areas such as administration, emergency department; nursing, security, and trauma units on altering by using yellow-plan code through emergency paging system repeated at a regular interval of time. Emergency operation-theaters are also put on alert if required. After identifying the need for staff requirement, alter the other departments.

2. **Triage assessment:** Track all disaster-related victims. Assess all received patients for triage, initiate care, and prioritize them. Tie disaster tags and bracelets to the patients to have their identification. After assessing the condition of patients, discharge those who do not require observation after providing treatment and first aid; refer them to outpatient departments or transfer to intensive care units, or keep under observation, or patients may require psychiatric consultation. Follow the guidelines of the disaster plan.

3. **Police information and security services:** Give information to police being medicolegal cases. Security staff will restrict the access to an emergency as far as possible; direct the relatives, hospital staff, and record entry of each staff member.

4. **Mobilization of resources:** After notification and activation of the emergency plan, mobilize various resources. Follow the guidelines of the disaster plan.

5. **Response/operation phase**
   - Activate operation planning per the disaster plan.
   - Incident staff will ensure and supervise enough staff for an emergency operation.
   - The operations head takes the responsibility of patient care activities and supervises the medical care, surgical, critical care, labs, radiology, pharmacy, mortuary, and other psychological and social work services.
   - The head of logistics will supervise and take the responsibility of communication system, transportation, dietary, stores, sanitation, public works water, and power supply.
   - The head of planning will be responsible for making an arrangement of the workforce and making immediate and extended duty rosters.

- The public relation officer will ensure the dissemination of accurate and timely information to the hospital, relatives, public, and media.
- The liaison officer will be responsible for making a close link with police, ambulance services, defense medical hospitals, railway hospitals, and other hospitals, blood banks or other ancillary services within the network.
- The security and fire officers will alert all security staff and arrange to post them in the emergency department.
- The finance officer will activate an emergency fund for emergency purchasing.

6. **Deactivation phase:** After assessing the situation, and completing all disaster operations, the incident commander and other hospital administrators deactivate the disaster phase. Notify the staff through yellow code all clear and by repeatedly announcing at regular interval of time for at least 30 minutes.

C. Postdisaster phase

It is a debriefing phase or the last step in hospital disaster (MCI) management. After the declaration of deactivating stage, the disaster committee critically reviews and discusses the performance. The incident commander presents the report. Based on the critical analysis, committee incorporate given suggestions in future planning.

CHAPTER HIGHLIGHTS

- An "emergency" is an event, characterized by impacts that local responders can handle by utilizing available resources. Disaster is a severe event that affects the functioning of the community at large and has a high impact on losses and requires external resources to cope up with the injuries.
- A natural disaster is due to geological, metrological, hydrological, climatic, and biological hazards. The human-induced disasters are consequences of human actions, negligence, or failure of the system is resulting in human-induced disasters.
- Emergency and disaster management (DM) is a continuous process of planning and taking appropriate measures to reduce the possible risks, to provide timely help to victims, and to fasten recovery during postdisaster.
- DM cycle involves mainly two stages predisaster and postdisaster. Predisaster phase comprises prevention, mitigation, and preparedness phases and postdisaster phase has a response, relief and rehabilitation, and reconstruction and recovery phases.
- Disaster planning is a coordinating and collective effort to plan various activities systematically to manage future unforeseen events and disasters. Planning is done at national, the state, and district level.
- Disaster or mass casualty incident (MCI) in the hospital is an unmanageable situation when the resources of the hospitals are beyond its standard capacity. World Health Organization categorizes MCI as Category 1/2/3 or Category A/B/C or Class A/B/C.
- There are mainly three phases of planning hospital disaster management: Predisaster phase, disaster phase, and postdisaster phase.
- Predisaster phase comprises the planning phase, development of the manual/plan, and capacity building phase.
- Disaster phase initiated with notification and activation phase, triage assessment, police information, mobilization of resources, and response and deactivation phases.
- The postdisaster phase starts with debriefing and further planning based on the critical review of performance during the disaster phase.

REVIEW QUESTIONS

I. Essay Type Questions
1. What do mean by the term "disaster?" Describe different types of disasters.
2. Define emergency and disaster management. Enumerate its objectives.
3. Explain in detail the disaster management cycle.
4. Discuss principles of hospital disaster management planning.
5. Describe various phases of emergency and disaster management.

II. Short Notes
1. Factors contributing to the risk of disaster
2. Emergency preparedness
3. Disaster management-related processes
4. Disaster planning at different levels
5. Mass casualty incident

III. Multiple Choice Questions
1. An event, a local incident, characterized by impacts that local respondents can handle by utilizing their resources is:
   a. Emergency   b. Disaster
   c. Tsunami   d. Catastrophe
2. A type of disaster that affects approximately 100 victims is:
   a. Minor disaster   b. Catastrophic
   c. Major disaster   d. Moderate disaster
3. The vulnerability is one of the factors for the risk of the disaster that refers to:
   a. A trigger agent that initiates mishap
   b. The disaster-prone area likely to have a disaster
   c. The degree of impact due to any hazard on life
   d. The extent to which society structure likely to damage due to an external event
4. Which phase of disaster management deals with all measures that limit the effect of risks?
   a. Prevention   b. Mitigation
   c. Preparedness   d. Response

Chapter 22: Planning for Emergency and Disaster Management

5. The awareness generation in disaster management is a part of:
   a. Knowledge management
   b. Research and development
   c. Capacity building
   d. Prevention
6. Which type of plan outlines the direction of an organization?
   a. Response plan
   b. Operation plan
   c. Strategic plan
   d. Contingency plan
7. What is the criterion to calculate the standard capacity of a given hospital?
   a. Treating casualties
   b. Number of casualties
   c. Severity of casualties
   d. Contingent plan
8. Under which category/class, the patients will fall who are getting treatment without interfering routine work the hospital during disaster management?
   a. Category A   b. Category 2
   c. Class A   d. Class C
9. Which principle of hospital disaster management states that all team members must be clear to their roles and responsibility?
   a. Principle of adaptability
   b. Principle of conciseness
   c. Principle of comprehensive
   d. Principle of integration
10. Which type of planning deals with communication, transportation, stores, pharmacy during disaster management?
    a. Activation planning
    b. Operation planning
    c. Security planning
    d. Logistic planning

Answer Keys

1. a	2. d	3. d	4. b	5. c	6. c	7. a
8. c	9. b	10. d				

SUGGESTED READING

1. Available from https://www.ncbi.nlm.nih.gov/pubmed/25215145. [Accessed October 2018].
2. Guidelines for Hospital Emergency Preparedness Planning. [Online] Available from http://asdma.gov.in/pdf/publication/undp/guidelines_hospital_emergency.pdf. [Accessed March 2019].
3. Hazard, Risk, and Vulnerability. [Online] Available from https://ndma.gov.in/en/vulnerability-profile.html. [Accessed March 2019].
4. National Disaster Management Plan (NDMP). May 2016. [Online] Available from https://ndma.gov.in/images/policyplan/dmplan/National%20Disaster%20Management%20Plan%20May%202016.pdf. [Accessed October 2018].
5. National Disaster Management Guidelines for Hospital Safety (Draft). December 2013. [Online] Available from https://ndma.gov.in/images/pdf/NDMAhospitalsafety.pdf. [Accessed October 2018].
6. National Policy on DM. [Online] Available from https://ndma.gov.in/en/national-policy.html. [Accessed October 2018].
7. Planning, Disaster Prevention, and Emergency Management. [Online] Available from http://apps.who.int/disasters/repo/5524.pdf. [Accessed October 2018].
8. Roy A, Sharma RK. Organization of emergency services. J Acad Hosp Adm. 1996;8(1):19-22.
9. The Nursing Journal of India. Disaster preparedness. Nurs J India. 2001;LXXXII(3):50.

SECTION 5

Human Resource Management and Staffing

23. Human Resource Management
24. Human Resource Management in Nursing Services
25. Fundamentals of Staffing: Staffing, Philosophy, Staffing Study and Norms
26. Nursing Activities, Patient Classification System, and Scheduling
27. Categories and Job Description
28. Personnel Policies
29. Staff Development and In-service Education
30. Career Planning, Development and Opportunities
31. Performance Appraisal
32. Discipline and Grievance Procedure
33. Stress Management
34. Occupational Health and Safety

23 CHAPTER

Human Resource Management

CHAPTER OUTLINE

- Human Resource Management
  - Definitions
  - Features
  - Scope
  - Objectives
  - Components of HRM
  - Functions of the HRM Department
- Recruitment
- Selection
- Deployment
- Retention
- Promotion
- Demotion
- Transfer
- Superannuation

LEARNING OUTCOMES

After completion of this chapter, the learner will be able to:
- Understand the concept of human resource management (HRM)
- Discuss the features, scope and objectives of HRM
- Understand the concept of recruitment and selection
- Define and describe the idea of deployment
- Identify strategies to retain employees
- Understand the concept of promotion, demotion and transfers
- Discuss promotion, demotion, and transfer policies
- Understand the concept and benefits of superannuation
- Describe different types of superannuation benefits

KEY TERMS

Human resource management, recruitment, selection, deployment, retention, promotion, promotion policy, transfers, transfer policy, superannuation

INTRODUCTION

Nurses form a significant component in the health sector. The contribution made by them determines the success of that organization. Organizations tend to be successful when their employees are satisfied and productive in performing their tasks of rendering patient care. It can be possible with competent personnel and HRM.

Personnel management concerns the "workforce" whereas HRM concerns "resource" management. However, recruitment, selection, deployment, retention, promotion, transfers and so on are the primary functions of both human resource (HR) and personnel management. HRM is mainly associated with identifying and developing persons, retaining suitable ones, creating work culture, conducting research and developing a communication system. The philosophy of HRM is to promote employees to meet individual goals and motivate them to help in achieving organizational goals.

HUMAN RESOURCE MANAGEMENT

Human resource (HR) is essential for the survival of any organization. One can develop and increase human resources to an unlimited level. The traditional concept of personnel management is replaced by HRM. The primary job of every manager is activating an HRM. Whereas, the personnel functions are the staff functions that are expected to be performed by staff mangers headed by personnel managers in most the organizations. From this point of view, HRM absorbs the personnel function in its refined form.

Definitions

Some of the definitions of HRM are as follows:
- HRM is a subsystem of the total management, mainly concerning managing people, individuals, and groups of people and their relationship.

- HRM is one of the managerial functions of the organization. It focuses on attracting, managing and guiding people working in the organization.
- It is the process of managing people and deals with personal and job-related issues of employees by using a strategic and comprehensive approach.
- It is the heart of an organization's workforce through which individuals working in the organization grow, develop, acquire knowledge and skills, and improve their talents and aptitudes. Both employees and employers work together to achieve a common goal of the organization.

Features

Some of the features of HRM are as follows:
- It is universal, needed in every organization.
- It is result oriented and aims to develop individuals.
- It focuses on the full utilization of the individuals' capacities.
- It deals with both personal and job-related problems of the employees.
- It concerns attracting, managing and guiding people.
- It orients, places and allocates the work to freshly joined people.
- It tries to produce competent and dedicated people to give maximum output.
- It maintains cordial relations among employees.

Scope

HRM has a wide scope. Its scope is as follows:
1. **Personnel management:** HRM is concerned with workforce planning, recruitment, selection, placement, transfer, promotion, training and development, remuneration, incentives, productivity, performance appraisal, developing new skills, disbursement of wages, incentives, allowances, travel policies and procedures, and so on.
2. **Employees' welfare:** It is concerned with working conditions and amenities, such as canteens, crèches, rest and housing, education, health and safety, recreation facilities and so on. Supervision, employee counseling, establishing harmonious relationships with employees, education and training are all included under HRM
3. **Employee–employer relations:** HRM also covers other issues like union–management relations, joint consultation, collective bargaining, grievance and disciplinary procedures, settlement of disputes and so on.

Objectives

The objectives of HRM are to:
- Maintain human relationships in the organization
- Attain the organizational goals
- Ensure effective utilization and maximum development of HRs
- Get better outcomes with better coordination
- Help in attaining maximum individual growth
- Recruit, select, develop, utilize and motivate the organization's HRs
- Satisfy the needs of employees
- Inculcate and maintain high morale among employees
- Develop and motivate employees to meet the objectives of the organization
- Improve job satisfaction and self-actualization among employees
- Build and maintain a quality of work life (QWL) of the employees
- Develop team spirit and teamwork among employees.

Components of HRM

Two significant elements of HRM are as follows:
1. **HR utilization:** It is concerned with recruitment, selection, placement, compensation and appraisal of HRs, more commonly termed as rational resource utilization.
2. **HR development:** This component is working with the existing HRs to improve their efficiency and effectiveness and design ways and means to enable the current employees to assume the new roles and functions.

Functions of the HRM Department

The following are the functions of the HRM department:
- Workforce planning
- Recruitment, selection and deployment
- Orientation and induction, training and development
- Staffing the organization
- Promotions and transfers
- Motivating, coaching, mentoring and counseling
- Appraisal of performance of employees
- Remuneration of employees
- Social security and welfare of employees
- Collective bargaining, contract negotiation and grievance handling
- Reviewing and auditing workforce management
- Potential appraisal
- Organization development (OD) and QWL.

RECRUITMENT

Recruitment and selection are the two primary functions of HRM. Recruitment is the first step toward creating competitive strength and a strategic advantage for the organization. It is a systematic process from sourcing the candidates to arrange and conduct interviews and requires a lot of resources and time.

Meaning and Definitions

According to William B Werther and K Devis, recruitment is the process to find out and attract capable applicants for the job. The process begins when recruits are sought and

Chapter 23: Human Resource Management

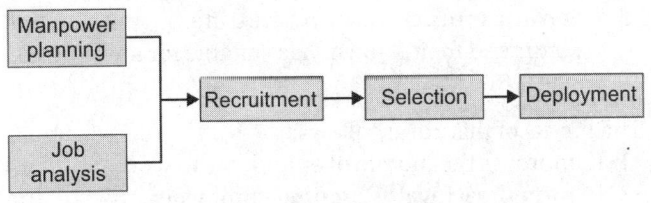

Fig. 23.1: Process of acquiring and placing HRs.

ends when their applications are submitted. Yoder refers to recruitment as the process to discover the sources of HRs to facilitate a valid selection of an efficient working force.

Flippo considered it the process of searching for prospective employees and stimulating them to apply for jobs in the organization. It is an actual process of finding and attracting capable applicants for employment. Recruitment is a process of discovering sources of HRs, using effective measures to attract them and facilitating valid selection to meet staffing requirements.

The recruitment process starts with initiating an employee by a manager for a particular job or an anticipated vacancy. In the process of acquiring and deploying, placing HRs in the organization, it falls in between different subprocesses, as shown in **Figure 23.1**.

Purposes and Importance

The purpose and importance of recruitment in HRM is to:
- Attract and encourage candidates to apply for the post in the organization
- Determine the present and future requirements of the organization
- Create a pool of candidates to enable the selection of best candidates for the organization
- Create a pool of candidates at low cost
- Identify and prepare potential applicants who will be appropriate candidates.

Recruitment Process

The recruitment process is a systematic procedure from searching for the candidates to arranging and conducting the interviews, and it requires a lot of resources and time. The process involves many activities **(Fig. 23.2)**.

1. **Identifying vacancies:** Identifying is the first step in the recruitment process. To identify jobs, the HRM department starts receiving requisitions for recruitment from different departments in the organization and their requirements. It includes the post to be filled, number of vacancies, duties to be performed and qualification with experience.
2. **Preparing recruitment specification:** The recruitment specification includes inventory for both job specification and personal specification. The job specification includes the main characteristics of the training, job background, primary responsibilities, job boundaries, expectations of the jobholders, and resources and constraints affecting the job.

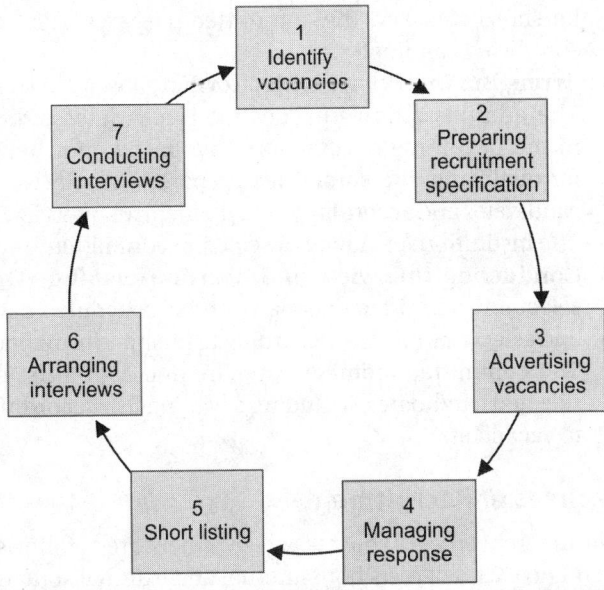

Fig. 23.2: Recruitment process.

The personal specification refers to individual requirements. It includes essential requirements like minimum qualification and work experience and desirable requirements like additional qualifications and personal qualities.

Personal attributes include:
a. *Physical specification:* It is the physical abilities and skills required for a particular job. These are physiological variables like vision, age, motor coordination and so on.
b. *Mental specification:* Mental specification of a person includes the intelligence quotient (IQ), memory, judgment, ability to plan, estimated reading, writing time and so on.
c. *Emotional and social specification:* These are personal characteristics, manners, emotional maturity and stability, aggressiveness or submission, extroversion, introversion, initiation, skills in dealing with others and the social adaptability of a person.
d. *Behavioral specification:* It is not formally listed out, but behavior specification needs to be kept in mind during the process of recruitment, selection and placement.

3. **Locating and developing sources for recruitment (advertising vacancies):** Finding sources for recruiting candidates is an essential step in recruitment. These include both internal and external sources. Method and material for advertisement are also decided and finalized during this stage of the recruitment process.
4. **Managing response:** Managing response refers to the way adopted to receive the applications and scrutinizing each application as per the requirement by the scrutiny committee.
5. **Shortlisting and identifying prospective candidates:** After the scrutiny, the eligible candidates need to

be shortlisted and the committee prepares a list of shortlisted candidates.
6. **Arranging interviews with shortlisted candidates:** The administration finalizes interview dates either in the beginning or after scrutiny. Based on criteria for qualifying, the committee prepares a merit list of candidates and according to it, calls them for interviews. The institution formulates a selection committee.
7. **Conducting interview and decision-making:** The selection committee interviews on the scheduled date and selects candidates according to their performance. The committee members prepare and sign a list of selected candidates, including a waiting list, according to vacancies.

Sources of Recruitment

The different types of sources of recruitment are as follows:
Figure 23.3 depicts both internal and external sources of recruitment:

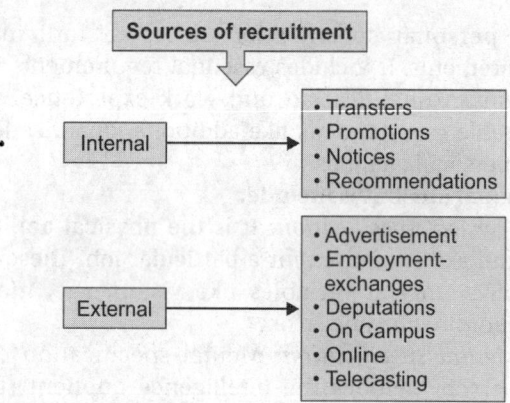

Fig. 23.3: Sources of recruitment.

Internal Sources

The internal resources of recruitment include candidates from within the organization and control by the organization. It invites candidates who are already on their payroll or those who were once on their payroll and planned to return or those who the organization would like to retire. The candidates may either transfer from other organizations or may apply for the promotional post. These are:
 a. **Transfers:** Transferring candidates are those who hold a similar type of job but shift from one unit to another. There are no drastic changes in their responsibilities, pay and status.
 b. **Promotions:** Promotional candidates are those who apply for the promotional post to attain a higher position to carry out more senior responsibilities, facilities, status and pay.
 c. **Notices:** It is another method to attract internal candidates by displaying advertisements on the notice board, circulating notes in the different departments or preparing a list of eligible candidates below the rank of the advertising post.
 d. **Recommendations:** Sometimes, employees recommend their known. It is suitable for lower posts.

Merits
The merits of this are as follows:
1. It improves the morale of employees to work.
2. It promotes loyalty among employees toward the organization.
3. It provides a better position to evaluate the performance of the present employee.
4. It is a cost-effective method of recruitment.
5. Candidates do not require induction or orientation training.
6. It is used to motivate employees.
7. It helps satisfy employees by keeping their aspirations high.
8. It ensures stability for the employees through continuity of employment.
9. It provides promotional avenues within the organization.
10. It establishes a better employer–employee relationship.
11. It creates a sense of security among employees.
12. Staff turnover may reduce using this source.

Drawbacks
The drawbacks of this are as follows:
1. It hampers new ideas and creativity.
2. It encourages favoritism.
3. A limited number of suitable candidates may be available.
4. Continuous promotions may not fit the required post.

External Sources

External resources of recruitment are candidates from outside the organization. To tap suitable, talented, experienced and knowledgeable candidates from an outside organization, an institute adopts the following sources:
 a. **Advertisement:** It is the most effective means or commonly used method to search for potential candidates from outside the health organizations for higher and skilled jobs. Advertisement is usually given in leading, local newspapers or in professional journals. Organizations also use their sites for vacant posts.
 Ernest Shackleton, the famous polar explorer, was the first person to insert an advertisement in a London newspaper in 1900. Speaking about the response to his ad, Shackleton said, "It was so overwhelming, it seemed that all the men in Great Britain were determined to accompany me." Advertisements can be made effective by the use of visuals, honing the headlines, developing a distinctive style and selecting the right medium.
 b. **Employment exchanges:** It is a good source of recruitment. In some cases, the employment exchange puts compulsory notifications of vacancies by law. There are two types of employment exchanges, namely, public and private employment exchanges. The government runs the public employment exchanges in all the districts. The employment seekers get

themselves registered with these exchanges. Private employment exchange provides employment services, particularly, for selecting the higher level and middle-level executives. In nursing, these types of agencies are hardly in practice.

c. **Deputation:** The employees of one organization are deputed from other organizations for filling required vacancies. Such employees are given a choice either to return to their original organization after a specific time or opt for the present organization.

d. **On-campus:** On-campus recruitment is a preliminary search of prospective employees through interviews on the campus. The suitable candidates are called for further meetings at particular places.

e. **Online:** Online recruitment is a quick method. The job seeking candidates apply online with all details. In less than a minute, the candidate can carry in his or her name and curriculum vitae (CV), much faster than with earlier systems. The recruiter reviews the CV and decides to go ahead. The candidate clicks on the interview zone and chooses the time and place for an interview. The system tells the recruiter details of the conversation. The candidate gets the reminder and can change time and place if necessary. The hiring manager can look at the candidate's profile online. More details can be built up about candidates with online tests. The selected candidate is introduced to a mentor.

f. **Telecasting:** It is the practice of telecasting vacant posts over media. TV (*Doordarshan* and another channel) is gaining importance these days. Programs like "Job Watch," "Youth Pulse" and "Employment News" over the TV have become quite popular in recruitment for various types of posts.

Merits

The merits of external sources are as follows:
1. Candidates with varied and broader skills are available.
2. External sources provide a more extensive choice of selection of candidates as a large number of applicants from outside the organization apply for the post.
3. It improves the overall working of an organization.
4. It creates a competitive spirit among the existing staff.
5. The external sources strengthen the diversity of talents in the organization.

Drawbacks

The drawbacks of external sources are as follows:
1. It takes a long time, first to notify the vacancies and then wait for applications to initiate the selection process.
2. It is a costly affair too.
3. The organization has to make more significant investments in their training and induction.
4. It may demoralize the existing employees to give their best performance.
5. It may deteriorate the employer–employee relationship.
6. It has limited scope for promotion as candidates apply for a fresh job.
7. There is higher staff turnover.

Internal Versus External Sources of Recruitment

Internal and external sources of recruitments differ in terms of their process, costs, choice of required candidates, scope and merit **(Table 23.1)**.

Recruitment Policy

All organizations should have a clear recruitment policy to fulfill their staffing requirements. The system should be clear and concise to recruit the best talent pool for the selection of the right candidates at the right place at the right time. It helps ensure a sound recruitment process. Recruitment policies provide a framework for the implementation of the recruitment program and specify the objectives of recruitment.

TABLE 23.1: Difference between internal and external sources of recruitment.

S. No	Internal sources	External sources
1.	It is a quick process	It is a lengthy procedure
2.	Recruiting cost is cheaper	The hiring cost is very high
3.	Candidates do not need induction or orientation training	Orientation and training can be lengthy and costly
4.	There is a limited choice of candidates	Selection of candidates is open
5.	There is a diminished scope of fresh talent	There is a scope to infuse fresh or new blood and new ideas in the organization
6.	The existing staff is motivated to improve their performance	The current team feels dissatisfied and demoralized
7.	Competitive spirit among existing staff if adopted a merit system for selection	Competitive spirit among existing staff with outside candidates
8.	Candidates of known skill, talent and knowledge are available	Candidates with varied skills, expertise and experience are available
9.	It provides promotional avenues within the organization	Limited scope for promotion, candidates apply for a fresh job
10.	Builds loyalty among employees toward the organization	Possibility of existing employees to broaden their personality with outside candidates
11.	Ensures the stability of employees through continuity of employment and reduces turnover	Possibility of frequent turnover and instability of employees
12.	It provides a better position to evaluate the performance of the present employee for the current post	The selection of candidates is through tests and interviews without any preconceived reservations
13.	The selected candidates get fixation of pay scale considering the existing one	The chosen candidates get the minimum pay scale of the post
14.	It creates a sense of security among employees	Existing employees may lose protection and may become disloyal to the organization
15.	Establishes a better employer–employee relationship	The employer–employee relationship may deteriorate

Components

Components of recruitment policy include:
  i. General recruitment policy and terms of the organization
  ii. Recruitment of temporary employees
  iii. Selection process
  iv. Job descriptions
  v. The general and desirable requirement for each post
  vi. The terms and conditions of the employment.

Characteristics

A recruitment policy should include the following characteristics:
- It has a basis for organizational needs.
- It should integrate employee needs with organizational needs.
- On hiring and employment, it should abide by government policy and legislation.
- Every applicant and employee must be treated equally.
- It should attract the best potential candidates.
- The number and criteria for the selection of committee members should be defined explicitly.
- Measures framed for selection should be fair enough.
- It must give appropriate weight to each test.
- Preference should be unbiased, transparent, task oriented, and merit based.
- The competent authority should chair and approve each selection.

Factors Affecting Recruitment Policy

The following factors affect recruitment policy:
- Type of organization
- Organizational objectives
- Personnel policies of the organization
- Preferred sources of recruitment
- The need for the organization
- Recruitment costs and financial implications.

SELECTION

Selection is an essential function of staffing, wherein one person gets selected for the said vacant post. It leads to the employment of personnel. Selection involves a series of steps to screen candidates for selecting the most suitable persons for vacant posts in the organization.

Definitions

Thomas S Stone defined selection as the process of choosing the fit candidates or rejecting the unfit candidates or a combination of both. According to Dharminder S et al., selection is a decision-making process in which the management decides certain norms and principles to adhere to the standards to discriminate between qualified and unqualified candidates. Yoder viewed it as the negative process of eliminating all those who appear uncompromising from all the candidates considered for possible employment.

Significance

The objective of the selection process is to achieve the best fit between the job requirements and jobholders. The importance of selecting the best fit or right kind of candidates for various posts is as follows:
- Proper selection and placement of nursing personnel lead to building up a suitable workforce.
- It helps to bring competent and skill nurses and thereby higher efficiency in providing the quality nursing care.
- Satisfied nurses with a positive attitude and good aptitude will initiate to fulfill the organizational goals.
- The morale of the satisfied nurses is often high.
- Low turnover and less absenteeism.
- It creates fewer occupational hazards and less negligence and errors.
- Selected nurses dedicate and contend toward their work and patients.
- Quality of organization usually depends on its staff.

Selection Process

The purpose of the selection process is choosing the right types of candidates to operate various positions in the organization. It is a process of determining suitability of candidates for the post. It comprises multiple activities that lead selection committee to choose from, the shortlisted candidates who best meet the stated selection criteria after a thorough explicit, transparent and legal screening process. The selection process has three stages, as discussed below:

Phases of the Selection Process

1. **Preselection:** The preselection stage is a part of recruitment. It involves defining the job and deciding what type of candidates are required. During this stage, all applications are checked and scrutinized. The candidates are shortlisted to invite for an interview.
2. **Interview:** The eligible candidates are notified and asked to face the selection committee for an interview. They have an interview for their ability as per the requirement of the said job.
3. **Assessment:** Sometimes the assessment follows an interview. In this stage, the candidates are assessed to predict how they are likely to behave in the future. For some posts, the institute may administer cognitive and psychometric tests before interview, and those who qualify, are called for an interview. The assessment report should end with a list of strengths and limitations, pointing to a final decision.

Steps in the Selection Procedure

Figure 23.4 depicts the general steps in selection procedures:

Chapter 23: Human Resource Management

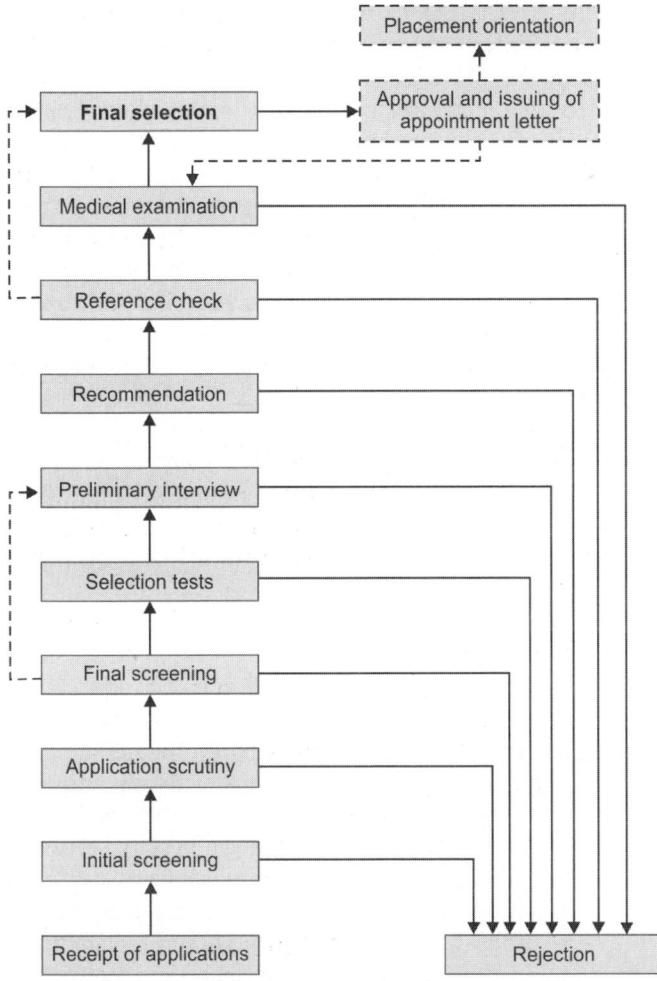

Fig. 23.4: Standard selection process.

The steps involved in the selection procedure are as follows:

1. **Receiving applications:** The process of selection start with the receiving, screening and scrutiny of applications. Application is a preliminary sorting device to provide information, which serves as a basis for an initial assessment of the candidate. Only the applications received on time are entertained.
2. **Initial screening and scrutiny of applications**
   a. **Initial screening:** It includes checking received applications with their supporting documents. The applications may be incomplete or without supporting documents. If the form is found to be deficient, it is likely to be rejected.
   b. **Applications scrutiny:** All complete applications forwarded to the scrutiny committee constituted by management. The examination of the application is essential to take out those applications, which do not fulfill essential requirements and qualifications for the said post. Some candidates may apply even when they do not possess the necessary element for the position. Scrutiny of applications is as follows:
      ♦ Check for completion of all the sections of the form and the vital requirements
      ♦ Look for any gap in the dates
      ♦ Look for any patterns (in job, interest education)
      ♦ Check carefully at the section on outside interests and career aspiration for preliminary clues to motivation, energy, and stability
      ♦ Do not take reports of health at face value.
   c. **Final screening:** The scrutiny committee again checks and verifies scrutinized applications. They prepare a list of eligible candidates as per the requirement of the said post. The committee may or may not inform the candidate of their rejected applications.
3. **Selection tests**
   a. *Selection by qualification and experience:* The eligible candidates are only to appear for interview. The selection committee will look for expected behavior and assess for their ability and knowledge based on set criteria.
   b. *Merit system:* It is also direct recruitment. The candidate is to appear for written selection tests, followed by interview/viva, and determine merit by performance test, qualification and experience.

The selection tests provide information about knowledge, skill, attitude, aptitude, interest, personality and so on of the candidates. These tests provide a basis for finding out the suitability of candidates and provide more objective criteria than any other method. Many studies have shown that modern psychological testing is one of the most valuable predictors of future job performance. Psychological tests are one of the most valid and cost-effective means for identifying the most suitable applicants for the job.

There are a variety of selection tests that are used in different organizations depending on their policy. A psychological test is a structured technique of testing behavior and to make inferences about the mental attributes. The test should be reliable, objective, standardized and consistent. The most common psychological tests are:

- *Achievement and aptitude tests:* These tests measure how much a person knows about a specific topic.
- *Intelligence tests:* These tests measure the intelligence of candidates or the essential ability of a candidate for understanding, assimilation and applying the knowledge.
- *Neuropsychological tests:* These tests measure the deficit in cognitive functioning (i.e., ability to think, speak, reason, etc.)
- *Functional tests:* These are to match candidates' interests with the interest of persons in known careers.
- *Personality tests:* These tests include personality, ability, aptitude and motivation scale. After conducting a test, an achievement score list of candidates prepared and displayed. Candidates who qualify minimum scores consider for an interview.

4. **Preliminary interview:** The preliminary interview is the core of the selection process. A selection or employment interview is fundamentally different from a clinical interview in terms of its aims, structure, rules and techniques. An interview should be structured, follow a logical sequence, with a purpose behind each question. The use of interviews is:
   - To observe the applicant for suitability both mentally and physically
   - To get an idea of general education, experience and training of the candidate
   - To test qualities and capabilities of the candidate (if selection test is not the criteria)

   The candidates called one by one by the selection board/committee as per the merit list and screened the candidates by a group/panel of interviewers for their qualities. The preparation of interview is essential to decide various aspects to be covered. An interview planned according to the type and nature of the said post. It will create confidence in the candidate, and they will feel ease. The questioning process usually started with broad open-ended questions, followed by probing questions, and finally narrowing down to closed questions by the interview panel. The interview should close at a friendly note. The candidate should not feel neglected.

   The interviewers assess the strengths and weaknesses of a candidate against the job criteria. It includes observations, impressions and information collected during the interview. It is either in narrative form, grading or rating form. It is better if each interviewer writes reasons with a particular evaluation and later based on discussion among interviewers.

5. **Recommendations and checking references:** Many organizations ask candidates to provide names of referees from whom the information about a candidate's ability and personality can find out. Before the final selection, employers usually make an investigation on these references supplied by candidate.

   Reference checks provided by an applicant are supposedly meant to test the bonafide of the candidate. These are important as 30% of applicants furnish incorrect data in their CVs. Most people bloat their salary and years of experience. Some organizations gave 90% weight-age to reference checks for top-level positions. However, sometimes it is found that the referee mentioned by the applicants is not very reliable, but that can be checked through networking.

6. **Medical examination:** The preemployment medical examination of a candidate is an essential step in the selection procedure. A medical board appointed by the organization certifies whether the candidate is physically and medically fit to join the duty. Usually, it is advised after issuing the appointment letter but before entering the job. Some organizations may require before the selection.

7. **The final selection, approval, and issuing of appointment letter:** After the candidate clears all the hurdles in the selection procedure, her or his name is recommended for selection by the selection committee and finally sent for approval to the competent authority. After getting approval, the selected candidates are informed by issuing an appointment letter to candidates and asked to join on duty within a specified period. The broad terms and conditions of employment, nature of the job, pay scale and so on are also an integral part of the appointment letter.

   The above steps in the selection procedure and order of measures vary from organization to organization and from job to job in the same organization.

8. **Placement and orientation:** After going through the lengthy procedure of recruitment and selection, the selection procedure is not complete. The placement and orientation of the employees are also essential steps as a part of the selection.
   a. *Placement:* Placement is said to be the process of fitting the selected persons at the right job or place. It is a process of assigning a specific job to each of the selected candidates. It involves assigning a particular rank and responsibility to an individual. It implies matching requirements of an appointment with the qualifications of the candidate. Proper placement of staff has many advantages as discussed below:
      - Avoids misfit between candidate and position.
      - Improves efficiency and inculcates high morale.
      - Increases employees satisfaction and motivation levels.
      - The employees dedicate and commit to work.
      - It helps to minimize error and negligence rates.
      - Reduces turnover and absenteeism.

      The candidates after joining placed on probation during the initial period from 6 months to 3 years. During this period, they are evaluated for their performance. If they complete this period successfully with excellent performance, become the permanent employees of the organization.
   b. *Orientation:* The selected candidates get copies of rules, regulations, procedures, job descriptions, and so on. They introduced the working and physical set up of organization. Generally, information provided during the orientation is regarding the type of organizational structure, departmental goals, organizational layout, general rules and regulations, standing orders, grievance system or procedure and so on.

      During orientation, employees are made aware of about mission and vision of the organization, nature of operation of the organization, policies and programs of the organization. The main aim of orientating is to build up confidence, morale and trust of the employee in the new organization. The nature of the orientation program

TABLE 23.2: Recruitment versus selection.

S. No.	Basis	Recruitment	Selection
1.	Meaning	It is a process of searching candidates and making them apply for the same	It is the process of selection of the right types of candidates and offering them jobs
2.	Objective	To attract a maximum number of candidates	To choose the best candidates
3.	Process	It is the process of creating an application post	It is a process of rejecting more candidates
4.	Approach	It is a positive approach	It is a negative approach
5.	Technique	It is a recruitment technique that does not require high skill	It is a selection technique that requires highly specialized skills
6.	Sequence	It precedes selection	It follows recruitment
7.	Economy	It is an economical method	It is an expensive method
8.	Period	Less time is required	More time is required
9.	Outcome	Application pool input for selection	Finalizing candidates and offering job

varies with the organizational size, that is, smaller the organization, the more informal is the orientation and more extensive the organization more formalized is the orientation program.

Recruitment Versus Selection

These are the two phases of the staffing process. Recruitment is the first phase envisages taking decisions on the choice of tapping the sources. Whereas selection is the second phase, which involves various activities to select suitable candidates only. There are differences and similarities in comparing both the processes.

Both processes require suitable candidates, and both are interrelated steps of workforce acquisition. However, recruitment differs with the selection process in terms of its concept, objective, method, approach, technique, sequence, cost, time to take process and outcome as depicted in **Table 23.2**.

DEPLOYMENT

Staff deployment is an essential function of HRM. It is an indicator of the performance of employees and the success of an organization.

Meaning and Definitions

Deployment is a process of moving or allocating an individual to a different function, use or position within the organization structure. Staff transferred from the activities which are of lesser priority or which have been rationalized, recognized or restructured, to areas of greater need.

Deployment is an organized practice or activity of moving their HRs to new work stations either within new departments, new stations, providing them with enhanced responsibilities and duties (Tubman, 2005). Mponda JM and Biwot GK refer it to the movement of staff from one's current assignment to another to the operational needs of the organization. ManagementMania.com describes staff deployment is a personnel activity to ensure that the labor of organization would be continuously in an optimal relation to the jobs and organization structure to match both number and qualification and personality structure of HRs to current organization structure and needs of an organization.

Staffing Versus Deployment

Staffing is a broader term than deployment and refers to a strategic or long-term staff planning. Staffing anticipates the plan, keeping in mind the future needs and situations of the organization. Deployment is a narrow concept aims to match number and qualification of employees. It also to ensure excellent staff available on duty at a given time.

Staff Allocation Versus Deployment

Staff Allocation or scheduling is the process of allotting or distributing staff available. In the nursing overall allocation of nursing personnel is decided by the administrator, or in other words, the administrator prepares a master rotation plan by allocating the number of staff for different units as a strategic planning/staffing process. Staff deployment is a part of staff allocation.

Placement Versus Deployment

Placement and deployment are interchangeable terms. Placement is assigning a unit or ward on the first joining of the candidate. Deployment is moving or shifting staff from the current place of work to others.

Transfers Versus Deployment

The transfer is a form of deployment. It is a movement of an employee from one job to another. It involves a change of employment without any significant increase in responsibilities or pay. It is used to fill the vacant post, correcting faulty selection and placement or as per the demand of employees. Deployment is shifting or movement of employees to optimize the number of staff in a particular shift/period or to cover a shortage in one specific department/unit.

Types of Deployment

Methods of deployment are not rigid; these vary from organization to organization, department to department.
1. **Interlocation deployment:** Interlocation deployment is shifting or reallocating staff from current main branches of the organization to relocation. It is also moving staff from the original location in new geographical areas as their workstations. It is applicable in those

organizations, having different branches/stations in the same city or the same country or different countries. For example, nurses may be deploying from current main command hospital to another hospital located near army areas. Interlocation deployment creates extra demand for employees to play new roles, motivation and requires positive viewing of the organization. It has both positive and negative effects on performance of employees. It provides an opportunity for employees to explore, learn and adapt to the new environment or may have consequences on employees.

2. **Interdepartmental deployment:** Interdepartmental deployment is shifting staff from the current department to another department, e.g. deploying nurses from the medical department to surgical department or from intensive care unit to the general patient care unit. Interdepartment deployment has more positive effects than adverse effects on performance of employees. It provides more opportunities to learn about the organization, its programs, activities and operations. They try to learn new ways and systems for doing work. It is getting re-employment taking place in the same organization.

3. **Intradepartmental deployment:** Intradepartmental deployment is shifting staff from the current unit to others within the same department. For example, deploying personnel from maternity ward to the Gynae ward under obstetrical and gynecological department. It has both positive and negative effects on the performance of employees. This type of deployment demands employees to learn different work formats, styles, ways of doing things, and personal and professional adjustments under the same medical team.

4. **Redesignation deployment:** Redesignation deployment is shifting to other workstations after redesignation from the current one. Redesignation deployment will be within the same position with fundamental shift of status, new job structure, social responsibilities, psychological makeup and physical set up. It has more benefits to employees than to the organization. Employees may get more recognition, achievement, growth and development prospects. On the other hand, more duties, different job structure may be the source of frustration, stress and fatigue.

5. **Short-term deployment:** Short-term deployment is a temporary placement of nurses in a ward or other unit for 12 hours or less (Matlakala, 2015). It applies within different nursing units or departments of a hospital to balance many nurses in a particular unit for a specific shift.

Short-term deployment is used to cover the shortage of nurses due to sickness, absenteeism and/or on leave. Nurses usually deployed where there is a shortage, especially during evening and night shifts by evening and night supervisors. Nurse supervisors deploy nurses from units where either the work is less or more staff is available during that shift. They also deploy relievers or on-call nurses, if possible, to the units, to cover staff shortage.

Advantages

Deployment provides an opportunity to:
1. Face new challenges and become more productive and innovative
2. Become more committed, loyal and satisfied to work in different settings
3. Develop positive attitudes toward different work format
4. Grow personally and professionally and to think in a creative way
5. Improve learning ability to work in various work cultures
6. Know more about the overall organization, its various activities and routines
7. Enhance organizing, communication and developmental skills
8. Develop mobile characteristics among employees irrespective of nature of work
9. Adjust physically, emotionally, psychologically and socially in a different environment
10. Develop a sense of new environment circumstances and new perspectives.

Disadvantages

The disadvantages of deployment are as follows:
1. Frustration and stress among employees
2. Poor performance, low level of initiative, and productivity
3. High turnover and absenteeism
4. A negative attitude toward administration and work
5. Intrapersonal conflicts, grievances, complaints and satisfaction problems
6. Emotional instability, role conflict, role ambiguity and emotional distress
7. Poor physical, emotional, psychological and social adjustment.

Effective Deployment Practices

Deployment plays a vital role in HR development. It is one of the functions of HRM. The utilization of HRs is a challenging task for managers. Performance is an indicator to measure the success of an organization. Performance is affected by many factors. Deployment practices and programs profoundly affect the performance of employees. Lack of familiarity with surroundings, limited orientation, schedule uncertainty, are causes of poor performances and hurdles in deployment practices. Therefore it is essential to have deployment practices. Critical ways of making deployment practices effective are as follows:
- The department should have written deployment policies, programs and guidelines covering deployment practices.
- Plan deployment practices carefully according to policies.

- Employees deployment manual should be made available indicating the role and responsibilities to perform in a particular unit.
- Conduct orientation programs regularly.
- Orientation and training programs related to unit activities before deploying.
- Staffing plans should include provision for deployment.
- Incorporate the deployment plan in a schedule plan.
- The department should have a contingency plan covering staff during leave and sickness, absenteeism.
- There should be a system of floating/on-call nurses.
- Provision of overtime/incentive for extra work.
- A policy covering lunch break, rest time, shifting time should be in staffing schedule.
- A policy covering lunch break, rest time, shifting time should be in staffing schedule.
- Prepare staffing schedule in consultation of staff, should be flexible.
- Peer support and supervisor support.

RETENTION

The organization attracts the most talented candidates and needs o to retain them for a longer-term. Keeping skilled resources is a challenging job in this competitive world.

Definitions

Mita et al. (2014) define employee retention as a technique adopted in the organization to maintain a productive workforce and to meet operational requirements. It is a process in which employees are encouraged to remain with the organization for a maximum period. - Bidisha and Mukulesh (2013). It is an activity of keeping or encouraging employees to stay in the organization for a maximum period. It is a method of taking measures to support the workforce to remain in the organization for the highest possible time duration.

Benefits

The benefits of retention are as follows:
1. Employee retention is cost-effective. It saves money and time spent on advertisement, recruitment, selection procedure, orientation and training of new employees.
2. It prevents loss of intellectual resources to go in the hands of competitors.
3. It helps to reduce turnover that may lead to more turnovers.
4. It aids in maintaining the goodwill of the organization by lowering the attrition rate.
5. It is helpful to regain efficiency by preventing loss of time and cost for appointing new candidates.

Determining Factors

The factors determining retention are as follows:
1. **Personal and professional growth:** Promotional avenues and career development determine the retention rate in an organization. There is a direct correlation between career development and retention. Organizations have promotional and career prospects, advance plans, and training programs so that the employees remain in the organization for an extended period.
2. **Remuneration and benefits:** Hike in pay, regular increments, benefits, leaves and other facilities are the motivational factors for employees to be in the organization for the highest possible time duration. Performance-based pay and wage rates facilitate retention and increase commitment among employees.
3. **Skill recognition and rewards:** Recognition for excellent performance is a motivational factor for job satisfaction and reduced turnover. Both monetary and nonmonetary rewards facilitate employee retention.
4. **Job security:** Job security is an essential determining factor in the retention of the workforce. It encourages employees to remain employed.
5. **Work-life balance:** The balance between personal and professional life affects employees to decide to remain in the organization. Flexible working time and schedule may help them to keep a balance of their work-life without disturbing official work. Employees have no intention to quit if they get possibility to fulfill responsibilities of family life. Offering emotional support by superiors is also reduces the attrition rate.
6. **Superiors' behavior:** Leadership styles of managers and superiors influence their workforce. Relationship with superiors, an attitude of superiors, fair and equal treatment and participative leadership style has a positive effect on employees' retention. There is a direct correlation between conservation and management behavior. Supportive and quality supervision by superiors makes subordinates to self-contented and committed toward work. It is considered as a contributory factor to retain employees.
7. **Work environment:** A favorable work environment is an essential factor in retaining employees. Flexibility in working hours, availability of resources, fun working and attractive working environment are ways to retain employees. The poor working environment is a source of occupational stress and stress creates job dissatisfaction. A flexible physical, psychological and social environment and adequate resources increase employee retention.
8. **Social support:** It refers to a satisfactory relationship of employees with team members and with superiors. The employees' professional relationships with each other and their superiors have a positive impact on retention. Unsatisfactory working relationships with superiors, coworkers, subordinates are the sources of stress and cause for low employee retention.
9. **Autonomy:** Autonomy in workload and work schedule decision-making is a determining factor for job satisfaction. Job satisfaction is an influencing factor for job retention.

10. **Training and career development opportunities:** Training and career development opportunities provided for employees increases their retention in the organization. Training and promotions increase loyalty and commitment among employees toward job and organization.

Strategies to Retain Employees

The organizational factors include work stress, relationship with team members, superior behavior, shift duty pattern, long working hours, job demand, too much workload, inadequate resources, role conflicts, role ambiguity, advanced technology, staff shortage, lack of task autonomy, unclear promotions prospects, poor working conditions, poor interpersonal relationship with supervisors, coworkers, subordinates, autocratic leadership style of superiors, poor career development opportunities and so on. Amongst factors related to employees' poor coping behavior, personality, indecisiveness is the significant predictors of job stress and job dissatisfaction. Therefore, it is essential for the organization to devise various methods to encourage and motivate employees to stay in the organization. Major strategies are **(Fig. 23.5)** as follows:

1. **Better retention policies:** An organization should have employee-oriented retention policies and procedures addressing to diverse needs of employees. Policies and procedures should encourage employees to remain employed. Efforts should be made to keep the workforce motivated. They should be satisfied with the working hours. There should be job security and resolution of employees' grievances.
2. **Induction and orientation training:** After a lengthy procedure of selection, the organization must initiate good policies to invest in the development of skills of employees by organizing planned induction and organization training programs. It is one of the most effective and significant tools in retaining them.

   These types of training help new candidates to adjust and adapt to a new environment. These training build confidence and maintain trust among employees. It also helps in maintaining good working relationship. The administrator introduces the new employees to policies, procedures and rules related to the work. The employees receive a full description of job. They learn work culture through induction training. In the first phase, induction training is delivered by in-service education unit, which supplies information regarding the organization and department. In the second phase, induction is done by supervisory managers who provide information related to the unit/ward.
3. **Job satisfaction:** Job satisfaction is one of the indicators of job retention. Employees who are satisfied with their jobs are found to remain in the organization. Job stress translates to a high attrition rate. Job satisfaction brings loyalty among employees. The organization should make an effort to motivate their workforce, so that have job satisfaction. Efforts should be made to keep workforce motivated. They should be satisfied with the working hours.
4. **Building trust and confidence:** Building trust in the workplace is possible through teamwork. Equal and fair treatment by superiors builds trust and confidence among employees. Job performance depends on loyalty to persons and related to their behavior and attitudes. Generate loyalty among employees.
5. **Empowerment:** Empowering each employee in the organization creates a sense of belongingness. Each employee must enjoy freedom in the job and ensure accountability.
6. **Building a relationship:** Develop healthy relationships with subordinates and create a family-like feeling within the organization. Motivate them and recognize their work.
7. **Recognition and reward:** Recognize the capability and potential of employees. Recognize their work and give rewards for excellent performance. Prioritize their recognition and help them to retain.
8. **Stress management:** The organization should plan stress management programs based on needs and stress levels. Stress management programs must organize at individual and organizational levels. At a corporate level, programs should direct toward strengthening social support to improve the individual-organization relationship and developmental programs to prevent job stress. Redesign job, define role and responsibilities, ensure appropriate workload, flexible working hours, participative management, effective communication, social interaction and establish work schedules are some of the measures that help to reduce job stress and increase job satisfaction among employees.
9. **Competitive compensation and benefits:** Salaries and compensation, increments, should be adequate as compared to other competitor organizations. Therefore, employees will not leave the organization. There should be a provision of benefits, leave and postretirement benefits. It is better to have performance-based rewards and promotions. Opportunities should be given to employees for their career development, to grow professionally and personally.

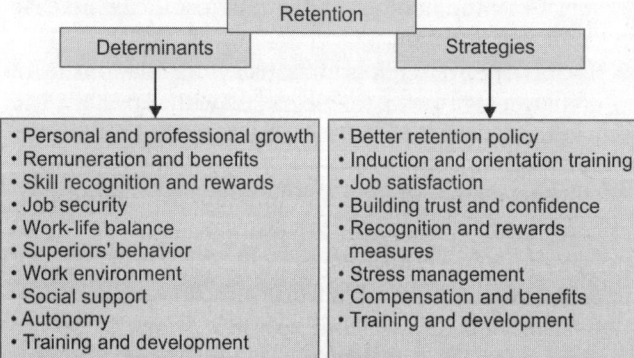

Fig. 23.5: Determinants and strategies of retention.

PROMOTION

Promotions and transfers are the most important source of recruitment within the organization. After the completion of selection procedure and placement, the employee needs to undergo adequate training, and as and when vacancies fall, he or she becomes ready for a higher position.

Meaning and Definitions

Promotion derived from the Latin word 'Promovers' meaning to move forward. The dictionary meaning is "to promote" as to evaluate, advance, contribute to growth or prosperity and progress from a given grade or class. Scott and Clothier refer to it as the transfer of an employee to a job that pays more money or carries higher status. It involves a change of one position to another better in terms of status and responsibilities (Flippo).

Promotion is a change within the organization to a higher position with greater responsibilities and used for more advanced skills than in the previous job. It usually involves higher status and increases in pay (Koontz O'Donnel). It is upward progress of an employee to a more senior job, which commands better pay/wages, better status/prestige, higher opportunities/challenges, responsibility, authority, better working environment, better hours of work and facilities and a higher rank.

Employer's point of view it means filling up more senior posts by the selection of the fittest person from within the organization. It leads to moving employees to a higher position with higher responsibilities, facilities, status and pay. It also means a change to a higher job accompanied by increased pay and privileges.

Purposes

The main purposes of promotion are to:
1. Motivate employees to a higher position
2. Attract and retain competent and most talented employees
3. Recognize and reward for better performance
4. Improve the efficiency and effectiveness of the organization
5. Fill more senior vacancies within the organization
6. Bring loyalty among employees toward the organization
7. Build morale and belongingness among employees
8. Facilitate employees to grow and develop
9. Provide job satisfaction to employees.

Importance

The importance of promotion is that it:
1. Motivates employees for considering within the organization
2. Leads to a chain of promotions at lower levels in the organization
3. Has a tremendous psychological impact on employees
4. Helps to retain employees already in the organization.

Types of Promotion

The different types of promotions are as follows:
1. **Limited promotion:** Limited promotion involves a movement of an employee toward a more responsible job with hike of the pay scale or senior scale withholding the same post. It is also the promotion of moving to a larger-scale without changing the job title.
2. **Dry promotion:** In dry promotion, the employees get a new and more extended job title without a hike in pay scale. The employee may get one or two increments as compensation.
3. **Horizontal promotion:** Horizontal promotions result in a change in designation, hike in pay and increased responsibilities in the same cadre.
4. **Vertical promotion:** A vertical promotion is a promotion as a result of a change in designation, hike in prestige and pay, with greater responsibilities and transformation of nature of the job.
5. **Time-bound promotion:** Time-bound promotion is a type of selection based on defined years of experience set for advancement to higher positions. The employees after attaining a fixed standard of expertise of the current post are eligible for the next promotion subject to the required conditions for the job, for example, minimum qualification, departmental exam or training. Neither seniority nor merit considered for this type of promotion.
6. **Temporary promotion:** As the name indicates, employees are promoted temporarily to a higher post if vacancies fall. This type of promotion is also called a promotion on an Adhoc basis. There is no guarantee that the candidates promoted permanently. It may automatically convert into permanent if the service is satisfactory during that period.
7. **Up and out promotion:** An up and out promotion is a type of promotion that results in a change in designation, hike in prestige and pays, with greater responsibilities by seeking a job elsewhere, outside the organization.

Basis of Promotion

The basis of promotion are as follows:

Seniority

The term 'seniority' means 'the length of service' or 'years of service.' According to rank, between two employees of the same cadre, the one who has been long in the service should be promoted.

Advantages of promotion on seniority

The advantages of promotion on seniority are as follows:
1. It is a simple system to understand and execute.
2. It is the cheapest system of recruitment.
3. It improves employee-employer relations by recognizing their services.

4. It meets the senior employees' desire for respect.
5. Talents of existing staff can be used to an optimum level.
6. It maintains discipline and respect for seniority.
7. It creates safety and security among employees.
8. It reduces the retention rate.
9. It provides very little room for favoritism.
10. Patronizes employee's service to the organization.

Disadvantages of promotion on seniority

The disadvantages of promotion on seniority are as follows:
1. All employees irrespective of their capabilities are fit for promotion.
2. Ignores the ability of employees.
3. Encourages lethargy and inefficiency.
4. No value for talents and efficient employees.
5. Leads chances of stagnation.
6. May deteriorate work efficiency.
7. Competent young employees may get frustrated.
8. Such a policy makes it difficult to attract capable persons.
9. Capable employees may leave the organization.

Merit System

The merit system is just opposite to the principle of seniority. The merit system attracts talented and intelligent persons within an organization and has objectivity in selection.

Methods of testing merit

a. **Written tests:** Applicants are evaluated based on written examination. These tests may be in competitive or departmental exams to test the cognitive behavior of candidates. These are also called promotional analysis.
b. **Discretion of the head of the department:** Sometimes, the merit of promotion is to the judgment of the head of the department, who is the best judge to know the performance of employees while working with them.
c. **Service record and efficiency rating:** Employees can promote based on their annual confidential record (ACR). ACR is a valuable tool to evaluate the performance of employees. It is filled by the next superior and forwarded by the head of the department. This record can be used as a valuable aid to consider for promotion.

Advantages of a merit system

The advantages of the merit system are it:
1. Is a logical and scientific system
2. Encourages capable and young employees to fill the post
3. Recognizes and rewards employees for their competence
4. Generates loyalty among competent workforce
5. Ensures the competent employees will stay in the organization
6. Improves efficiency in work by retaining qualified persons

Disadvantages of a merit system

The advantages of the merit system are as follows:
1. There are chances of favoritism.
2. It leads to resentment among senior employees.

Seniority Cum Merit System

Seniority, cum merit system, combines both seniority and merit basis for the promotion of employees. The merit has more weight along with seniority. It has benefits of both methods; the organization will be able to retain capable persons and seniority.

Promotion based on Selection

Promotion based on selection is a type of promotion where employees promoted after they undergo a thorough selection procedure. The selection procedure includes conducting tests and screening. The screening is done by a constituted scrutiny committee, which checks records, merit, qualifications, experience and other achievements of employees. The eligible candidates face interviews before a final selection.

Promotion Policy

Clear-cut promotion policy is essential in excellent organizations. The management and employees must frame the criteria for promoting employees. The salient features of a sound promotion policy are as follows:

Features of promotional policy

The features of a promotional policy are as follows:
- There should be a policy statement
- It is a fair and impartial and planned activity
- It includes the criteria for the promotion
- It specifies the promotional routes for different cadres
- It has a provision for training and development of existing employees considering promotion
- It maintains records of employee's performance properly to use at the time of promotion
- It communicates the promotional policy to the employees.

DEMOTION

Meaning and Definitions

Demotion means to go backward. It is the reverse of promotion. It is the lowering of rank and status and reduction in salary and responsibilities. Demotion is the assignment of an individual to a job of lower position and pay usually involves a lower level of responsibilities.

Demotion is a shift from the current position to a position having fewer responsibilities (Dale Yoder). It refers to a movement of employees from higher-order to immediate lower-order, whereby a reduction in pay or responsibilities. It implies lowering down of status, salary and duties of an employee. Demotion is a downgrading process when the employee suffers from emotional and financial loss in terms of rank, power, status, pay and so on.

Thus, demotion is concerned with lower job level or status, decreased salary and fall in job authority. It is considered negative employment.

Causes of Demotion

Some of the causes of demotion are as follows:
1. **Performance-related issues:** Poor employee's performance may be one of the reasons for demotion. New employees who lack the skill and not able to adjust to any change in technology, method and practices in their new position are likely to be demoted in the previous post.
2. **Inadequacy of knowledge:** Those employees unable to perform and unable to meet the requirement of the job may demote.
3. **Misconduct and negligence:** Demotion becomes necessary in case of employee misconduct and violets rule and regulation and commit serious negligence in their part of work. An employer may award demotion as a consequence of disciplinary action.
4. **Organizational restructuring:** When some jobs are abolished or eliminated due to restructuring of organization with merging of sections, the employee is asked to accept lower jobs.
5. **Promotion by default:** It means that employees are promoted wrongly, may be reverted to their original positions.
6. **Employees' request:** It means that employees refuse a higher position posted in different places or due to personal and family reasons such as to keep a balance between personal and professional life, want to reduce their workload and responsibilities accept a lower position.

Types of Demotions

The two types of demotions are:
1. **Compulsory demotion:** Compulsory demotions are the demotions caused due to performance-related issues, misconduct, negligence, inadequate knowledge of employees, restructuring of the organization or promotion by default.
2. **Voluntary demotions:** Voluntary demotions are demotions on the request of employees to lower down workload or other family reasons such as to keep a balance between personal and professional life or want to change position.

Method of Handling Demotion

Some of the methods for handling demotion are as follows:
1. Make sure that demotion does not violate rules of demotion policy of the organization.
2. Discuss with employees and respect during a discussion.
3. Communicate to an employee about demotion with reasons for the demotion.
4. Give a rationale to take up this action instead of termination.
5. Help the employee to respond positively.
6. Clearly explain a new position after demotion. Tell about new roles, responsibilities, the date of joining, to whom to report and about the payment if it is compensation with a low salary.
7. Be prepared for cross-questions from an employee.
8. Be ready to handle the emotional moments or adverse reactions from an employee.
9. Make communication or transition plan, if an employee is positive. Maintain the dignity of employees and set time for joining and department.
10. Inform only to the concerned supervisors without giving details of demotions.

Demotion Policy

The organizations must have a clear-cut demotion policy. Both the management and employees must be clear about the demotion criteria. The salient features of a sound demotion policy are as follows:
1. There should be clear cut and defined rules under which circumstances, employees may be demoted.
2. There should be a provision for the employee to represent the case to top management.
3. There should be a provision of investigation for the cause of demotion. It should be evidence-based, and a competent authority or a committee must investigate.
4. There should be a provision for reviewing the situation thoroughly.
5. An award of demotion must accompany with authentic and supportive documents.
6. Communicate the employee the ground for demotion.

TRANSFER

The transfer is the movement of an employee without involving any change in responsibilities or pay or any compensation. It initiated by an employee or organization. It may be temporary or permanent.

Definitions

The transfer is a change in the job within the organization where the new job is substantially equal to the previous one in terms of pay, status and responsibilities (Chhabra TN). Yoder et al. refer to it as a lateral shift causing movement of individuals from one position to another. It is the movement of an employee include a promotion, demotion or no change in job status. Marquis and Huston (2009) considered it is reassignment to another job within the organization.

Purposes of Transfer

The purposes of transfer could be to:
- Meet an organizational need that may arise due to shortage of staff in another department, change in

technology, change in the workload, change in work schedule, transfer policy of the institute.
- Fulfill employees' needs that may be due to their problem, dislike of present superior, lack of opportunities for advancement in the current department.
- Utilize employees in a better way either to transfer the capable employees or the one who is not performing well in that situation.
- Make employees more versatile.
- Provide relief to an overburdened employee.
- Use as a remedial measure to rectify situations arising due to specific reasons.
- Use as a correcting measure or as a punishment.

Benefits of Transfer

Some of the benefits of transfer are that it:
- Increases the work output and effectiveness of the organization being feel valued
- Improves the skill of employees as it keeps employees morale high
- Provides excellent job satisfaction, as they will like the job
- Helps to place the right employees at the right place
- Increases motivation to work is the work of their choice
- Improves superior-subordinates relationships
- Helps the employers for future promotion
- Meets employees personal needs; thus helps in retaining them
- Avoids monotony
- Is a remedy for faulty selection and placement
- Stabilizes the fluctuating workload.

Types of Transfer

The different types of transfer are given below:
1. **Production transfer:** It is the transferring of the employees from the surplus department to the department of having a shortage of HRs to balance.
2. **Shift transfers:** Shift transfers refer to transferring employees from one shift to another to fulfill a personal request of the employee or to rotate to give regular duties to all.
3. **Replacement transfers:** Replacement transfers resulted when employees are replaced by other employees to relieve or to give relief to old employees from the heavy pressure of work.
4. **Remedial transfer:** Remedial transfers are made to rectify mistakes in selection and placement.
5. **Versatility transfer:** A versatile transfer is moving employees from one job to others, making them all-rounder. This type of transfer is also known as rotation.
6. **Panel transfer:** Panel transfer is disciplinary action or consequences of misconduct to punish employees.
7. **Mutual transfer:** It is transferring employees after completion of the stipulated length of service at their present place of posting only with the employees of having similar training mutually.
8. **Lateral transfer:** Lateral transfer is moving staff from one unit to another to the same position with a similar scope of responsibilities.
9. **Downward transfer:** When employees take positions below their present level within an organization is downward transfers.
10. **Inappropriate transfer:** It is a type of transfer when problematic employees are transferred from one department to solve unit personnel problem to another unsuspected department.

Transfer Policies

The features of sound transfer policy are as follows:
- The transfer policy should be based on specific principles and should not differentiate among employees.
- There should be proper criteria to be laid down for transfers.
- The responsibility for initiating and approving transfers' decisions should be clearly defined and adequately located.
- Decide the area or unit within for transfers.
- The policy should specify the reason for transfer.
- It should prescribe the bases for transfers.
- It should determine the consequences of transfers on seniority and payroll.
- It should work in writing.
- It should be clearly defined either temporary or permanent.
- The employees should be communicated or clear about the transfer policy.

SUPERANNUATION

Meaning

Superannuation is the retirement benefit, a regular payment to an employee who is retired from work. Employers set the retirement benefit or superannuation funds and link either government or other nongovernment institutions with insurance companies.

The employer contributes on the employee's behalf to the group superannuation policy. Usually, a company/organization pays 15% of basic wages as a contribution. At the time of retirement, employee is eligible for 1/3 of contribution fund (tax-free) and rest is the Annuity Fund or pension, which is taxable as per individual tax bracket according to the option chosen by employer. These options for annuity fund are as follows:
1. Pension payable for life or Pension with Return of Corpus (ROC).
2. Joint life pension with/without ROC.
3. Joint life 50% pension to the spouse.
4. It is increasing pension at a rate of 3% p.a.

Benefits of Superannuation Scheme

The benefits of the superannuation scheme to the top employers are as follows:

1. Supports employment policies
2. Attracts and retains vital talented employees
3. Reduces turn over
4. Provides tax benefits to employees.

The benefits of the superannuation scheme to the employees are as follows:
1. Fixed income (pension) on retirement
2. Free from market risks
3. The recipient for contribution and pension
4. Long-term tax savings
5. Tax-free interest
6. Contributions not treated as income.

Types of Superannuation Benefits

The two types of superannuation benefits are as follows:
1. **Defined benefit:** An employee already knows the retirement or pension benefits and fixes it. Therefore, the employer has a risk of limited benefit and calculated based on a formula linked to salary, years of service.
2. **Defined contribution:** The contributions by employers are only known and fixed, but end benefits of retirement are not guaranteed and employees may not aware of the exact monetary gain he or she will get on retirement.

Superannuation Benefits to Government Retirees

The superannuation benefits to government retirees are as follows:
1. **Pension:** The minimum eligibility to receive a superannuation pension is at least ten years of qualifying service and calculated concerning average emoluments. Pension is payable up to including the date of death. According to the sixth pay commission, there is a provision of an additional hike of basic pension for old pensioners attaining the age of 80, 85, 90, 95, and 100 years.
2. **Commutation of pension:** There is a provision to commute pension, not exceeding 40% of it, into a lump sum payment with effect from 1.1.1996 for a Central Government servant. He or she will get a monthly pension after deducting the commuted portion up to 15 years from the commutation date of the pension. In addition, calculate other benefits such as Dearness Relief based on the original pension.
3. **Death/retirement gratuity:** A government servant who has a minimum of five years qualifying service is eligible to get the retirement benefit of one-time retirement gratuity. Whereas there is also a provision of getting death gratuity.
4. **Service gratuity:** A government servant who has less than ten years of service qualifying years is entitled to get service gratuity and not the pension.
5. **General provident fund and incentives:** All permanent employees, temporary employees after one year of service, all re-employed pensioners are eligible to subscribe to general provident fund and has the right to receive the amount that may stand to his or her credit or in case death; his or her nominee has the right to get the funds.
6. **Deposit-linked insurance revised scheme:** Under the GPF rules, the person is entitled to get the amount standing to the credit of the subscriber on the death, to be paid an additional amount during the three years immediately preceding the end of the subscriber with the condition.
7. **Contributory provident fund:** According to Contributory Provident Fund Rules (India), 1962 applies to every nonpensionable servant of the Government has the right to receive the amount that may stand to his creditor in case death; his or her nominee has the right to get the funds.
8. **Leave encashment:** It is not superannuation/pensionary benefit, but the government servant under the CCS (leave) Rules is appropriate to get encashment of leaves (earned leave/half pay leaves) standing at the credit to a maximum of 300 days on his or her retirement. On delayed leave encashment, there is no provision for payment of interest.
9. **Central government employees group insurance scheme:** The central government credits a portion of monthly contributions paid while the employee is in service in a saving fund with interest. The employee gets the amount credited in his or her account on retirement. It covers benefits to the family on the subscriber's death. There is no provision of paying interest on delayed payments under this scheme.

CHAPTER HIGHLIGHTS

- HRM is a comprehensive approach to manage people and workplace culture and the environment.
- Recruitment is a process to search and attract capable applicants for employment. Selection is a process of screening candidates for selection of the most suitable persons.
- Deployment is a process of allocating an employee to a different function, use or position within the organization structure. Interlocation, interdepartment, intradepartment, redesignation and short-term are examples of deployment.
- Employee retention is an activity of keeping and encouraging employees to remain in the organization for a maximum period. Promotion is filling up higher posts carrying a higher salary, status and higher responsibilities by fitting a suitable person from within the organization.
- Demotion is a shift of an employee to a job of lower rank and pay usually involving a lower level of responsibilities. A transfer is moving an employee without requiring any change in duties or pay or any compensation.
- Superannuation is the retirement benefit, a regular payment to an employee who is retired from work. The benefits of superannuation schemes are for both employers and employees.

REVIEW QUESTIONS

I. Essay Type Questions
1. Define recruitment. Describe in detail various sources of recruitment.
2. What is meant by selection? Explain various steps involved in the selection procedure.
3. Define promotion. Differentiate between promotion by seniority and promotion by merit.
4. What do you mean by employee retention? Describe essential strategies used to retain employees in the organization.

II. Short Notes
1. Recruitment process
2. Human resource management
3. Types of deployment
4. Superannuation

III. Multiple Choice Questions
1. Human resource management, according to personnel management point of view, is mainly concerned with:
   a. Working conditions
   b. Manpower planning
   c. Union management relation
   d. Supervision and counseling
2. A process of finding and attracting capable candidates for employment is known as:
   a. Promotion   b. Deployment
   c. Selection   d. Recruitment
3. The selection process is to:
   a. Help in locating candidates
   b. Prepare employees for training
   c. Determine the suitability of candidates
   d. Assign a specific job to a candidate
4. Intelligence tools measure:
   a. Training and development expertise of candidates
   b. Ability to understand, assimilate and apply knowledge
   c. Personality traits of candidates
   d. A deficit in cognitive functioning
5. A deployment that demands employees to learn different work format, styles and ways of doing things is:
   a. Intradepartment
   b. Interdepartment
   c. Interlocation
   d. Short-term deployment
6. Retention is a technique adopted by an organization to:
   a. Shift their human resources to a different function, use or position
   b. Decide certain norms and principles to adhere
   c. Maintain an effective workforce and to meet the operational requirement
   d. Fit selected candidates at the right job
7. Limited promotion is a type of promotion that involves a movement of employees with increased responsibilities with a:
   a. Hike of pay without a change in designation
   b. New job title without an increase in the pay scale
   c. Change in designation, hike in pay in the same cadre within the organization
   d. Change in designation, hike in pay and change in nature of the job in different cadre
8. Selection after defined years of experience set for promotion refers to:
   a. Seniority cum merit
   b. Promotion based on selection
   c. Promotion on seniority
   d. Time-bound promotion
9. Transfer involves:
   a. A change in designation with high pay and greater responsibilities
   b. A shift to a position with decreased responsibilities and rank
   c. A change of job without any significant increase in responsibilities or income
   d. A shift to other workstation after redesignation and new job structure
10. A government servant who has a minimum of 5 years of qualifying service is entitled to get the onetime benefit of:
    a. Service gratuity   b. Pension
    c. Provident fund   d. Retirement gratuity

Answer Keys

1. b   2. d   3. c   4. b   5. a   6. c   7. a
8. d   9. c   10. d

SUGGESTED READINGS

1. Adams O. Management of human resources in health care: The Canadian experience. Health Econ. 1992;1:131-43.
2. Bano R. Check your references. Hindustan Times: Career Guide, 13th October 2004;1(124):1.
3. Budget 2016: Tax exemption raised to Rs 1.5 lakh under a superannuation fund. [Online] Available from http://economictimes.indiatimes.com/articleshow/51194384.cms?utm_source=contentofinterest&utm_medium=text&utm_campaign=cppst. [Accessed April 2019].
4. GOI. Pensioner' Portal. [Online] Available from http://pensionersportal.gov.in/retire-benefit.asp. [Accessed April 2019].
5. Goddard HA. Principles of administration applied to nursing services. WHO Publication & Distribution; 1992.
6. Koontz H, Weihrichs H. Essentials of management: An international perspective, 1st edition. New Delhi: Tata McGraw Hill Publishers; 2001.
7. Koontz H, Weihrichs H. Management: A global perspective, 1st edition. New Delhi: Tata McGraw Hill Publishers; 2007.
8. Kossivi, B., Xu, M. and Kalgora, B. Study on determining factors of employee retention. Open J Soc Sci. 2016 May;4:261-8.

[Online] Available from https://pdfs.semanticscholar.org/1d6e/719e080e19d47301b6303a5fc1a4849ac7ea.pdf.
9. Mathimaran KB, Kumar, AA. Employee Retention Strategies– An empirical research. In: Balaji K, Ananda A. Glob J Manag Bus Res: E-Marketing. 2017;17(1):17-22. [Online] Available from https://globaljournals.org/GJMBR_Volume17/3-Employee-Retentio n-Strategies.pdf.
10. Matlakala MC. The view of intensive care nurses regarding short term deployment. Curationis. 2015;38(1):Art.#1418, 5 pages. [Online] Available from https://curationis.org.za/index.php/curationis/article/view/1478/1770#1 (Accessed March 2018).
11. Monappa A, Saiyadain M. Personnel Management. New Delhi: Tata McGraw Hill; 1996.
12. Perrodin MC. Supervision of nursing service personnel. The MacMillan Co; 1964.
13. Peter S. How nurses can influence policy. Nurs Times. 1997;93:35-6.
14. Rao VSP. Human resource management, 2nd edition. New Delhi: Excel Books Publishers; 2001.
15. Sinha D, Shukla SS. [Online] Available from jepr.org/doc/V2-IS1_Jan13/ij4.pdf. [Accessed May 2019].
16. Taylor MS, Bergmann TS. Organizational recruitment activities and applicants' reactions at different stages of the recruitment process. Pers Psychol. 1987;40:261-85.
17. Yoder D. Personnel management and industrial relations. New Delhi: Prentice-Hall; 1990.

24 CHAPTER

Human Resource Management in Nursing Services

CHAPTER OUTLINE

- Human Resource Management in Hospital Nursing Services
  - Objectives of HRM in Hospital Nursing Service
  - Organization of Hospital Nursing Services
  - Recruitment, Selection, and Placement of Nursing Personnel
  - Deployment and Promotion of Nursing Personnel
- Human Resource Management in Community Nursing Services
  - Objectives of HRM in Community Nursing Services
  - Health Infrastructure: Rural Health Care
  - Recruitment, Selection and Placement of Community Health Workers/Nursing Personnel in Rural Health Care Sector
  - Recruitment, Selection and Placement of Community Health Nursing Personnel in Primary Health Center, Community Health Centre, and District level
  - Health Infrastructure: Urban Health Care
  - Recruitment, Selection and Placement of Community Health Workers/Nursing Personnel in Urban Health Care Sector
  - Recruitment, Selection and Placement of Community Health Nursing Personnel in Urban Primary Health Center

LEARNING OUTCOMES

After completion of this chapter, the learner will be able to:
- Review the concept of human resource management (HRM)
- Enumerate objectives of HRM in nursing services
- Describe the principles of HRM applicable in nursing services
- Discuss the process of recruitment and selection for various posts in nursing services
- Describe multiple ways of deploying nurses in hospital and community setup
- Identify strategies to retain employees in nursing services
- Appraise different methods of promotions in nursing

KEY TERMS

Nursing service, human resource management, recruitment, selection, retention, development, superannuation

INTRODUCTION

Nursing service is an essential component of the healthcare delivery system. Nurses form the largest group in the health sector, who provide patient care in the hospital and look after family health care in the community in various capacities. Nurses assist the individual sick or well, families, and communities of all age-groups irrespective of caste, creed, and religion.

Human resource management (HRM) is an essential function of nursing services. In nursing, HRM is mainly concerned with managing nursing personnel, individual nurses, and a group of nurses and their relationship. Though nurse administrators/managers are not managing staffing functions independently, they are active members of the health team and various committees in carrying out recruitment, selection, deployment, retention, promotion, and transfers. As a human resource manager, they help in identifying and developing nurses, retaining them, creating work culture, conducting research, and establishing a communication system.

HUMAN RESOURCE MANAGEMENT IN HOSPITAL NURSING SERVICES

The nursing service department is one of the essential departments of any hospital. The working nurses are the vital human resource asset for all hospitals. Management of these resources is, in fact, a challenging job for a nurse manager. Nurses working in various capacities aim to render nursing service directly or indirectly to the individual patient and to assist in the recovery of patients. In the overall administration of nursing service, whether national, state, or local level, nurse managers have the responsibility of acquiring, utilizing, improving, and retaining the nursing workforce to maintain the necessary level of efficiency.

Objectives of HRM in Hospital Nursing Service

In the context of hospital nursing service, the main goals of HRM are as follows:

- To develop personnel policies for the nursing service department
- To prepare job descriptions for hospital nurses at different levels
- To establish nursing manuals, protocols, and standard operative procedures/activities
- To frame performance appraisal methods for nurses
- To forecast the requirement of hospital nurses at various levels
- To appraise the authority with the current strength of nurses
- To calculate the vacant posts of nurses
- To attract talented nursing personnel
- To recruit and select nurses for the vacant positions
- To determine the training and development needs of nursing services
- To train and deploy nurses in various nursing units
- To prepare the duty roster and work schedule
- To supervise and evaluate nurses for their performance
- To use the existing nursing workforce optimally
- To motivate and develop nurses
- To develop health and safety management practices for nurses
- To provide therapeutic and infection-free working facilities for nurses
- To promote good working relationship and team spirit
- To maintain discipline among nurses and manage their grievances
- To promote welfare, career development, and research activities
- To retain the nursing talents.

Organization of Hospital Nursing Services

The nursing service department in the hospital is not functioning in isolation; it is a part of an administrative set of the overall hospital organization. The head of the nursing department is the nursing director/chief nursing officer (CNO)/nursing superintendent (NS)/matron, depending on the type of hospital. The head is directly under the control of a medical administrator (medical superintendent/chief medical officer) and has the overall responsibility of organizing the nursing services. Under the head, various categories of nursing personnel (human resources) are working to meet the objective of the hospital organization. **Figure 24.1** depicts the different types of nursing personnel working in government hospitals.

Recruitment, Selection, and Placement of Nursing Personnel

Recruitment and selection are the main functions of HRM. Nurse administration in the nursing service department plays an important role. Recruitment is the first step and a systematic procedure to attract the capable, eligible, and suitable candidates for the organization. The selection process follows hiring.

The recruitment process usually includes the method of identifying vacancy positions, notification and advertisement for the post, scrutiny of applications, short listing of eligible candidates, conducting interviews, selecting, and appointing candidates. The process of recruitment attracts the candidates from both internal, i.e. who are already in the organization, and external sources, the candidates who are outside the organization, to fill the posts. The internal source of recruitment is usually for the promotional job, whereas the external sources are to attract the candidates for direct recruitment.

The method and mechanisms of recruitment, selection, and placement vary from state to state and also in central and referral and autonomous institutes. However, in general, at the state level, usually, the Staff Selection Commission does the recruitment of nursing personnel, and the respective director health directorate is responsible for recruiting the nursing personnel.

The nursing administrator initiates the process of recruitment and apprises medical administrators to fill the job in the department. The medical administrator sends the case to the authority for approval and the recruitment cell for further proceedings per the policy of the institute.

Staff Nurses

The staff nurses designated as "sister grade II" or "nursing officer" in many hospitals is the first level nurses who enter as professional nurses in the hospital. They are responsible for the total patient care and other activities assigned to them per their job description. The number of staff nurses required in the hospital is calculated based on the hospital norms, size of the hospital, type of hospital, budget allocation, and approval of the authority.

A. Recruitment process

Notifying and advertising the post: Notification for the job includes details about the said post, pay scale, essential eligible criteria, group, age limit, number of vacancies and reservation, the selection, and general terms and conditions for the post. The candidates come to know about the vacancy position through a notification on the Web sites of the institution/department and advertisement in the leading newspapers. Job criteria are according to the recruitment rules of the institution.

- **Name of hospital/institute:** Specify

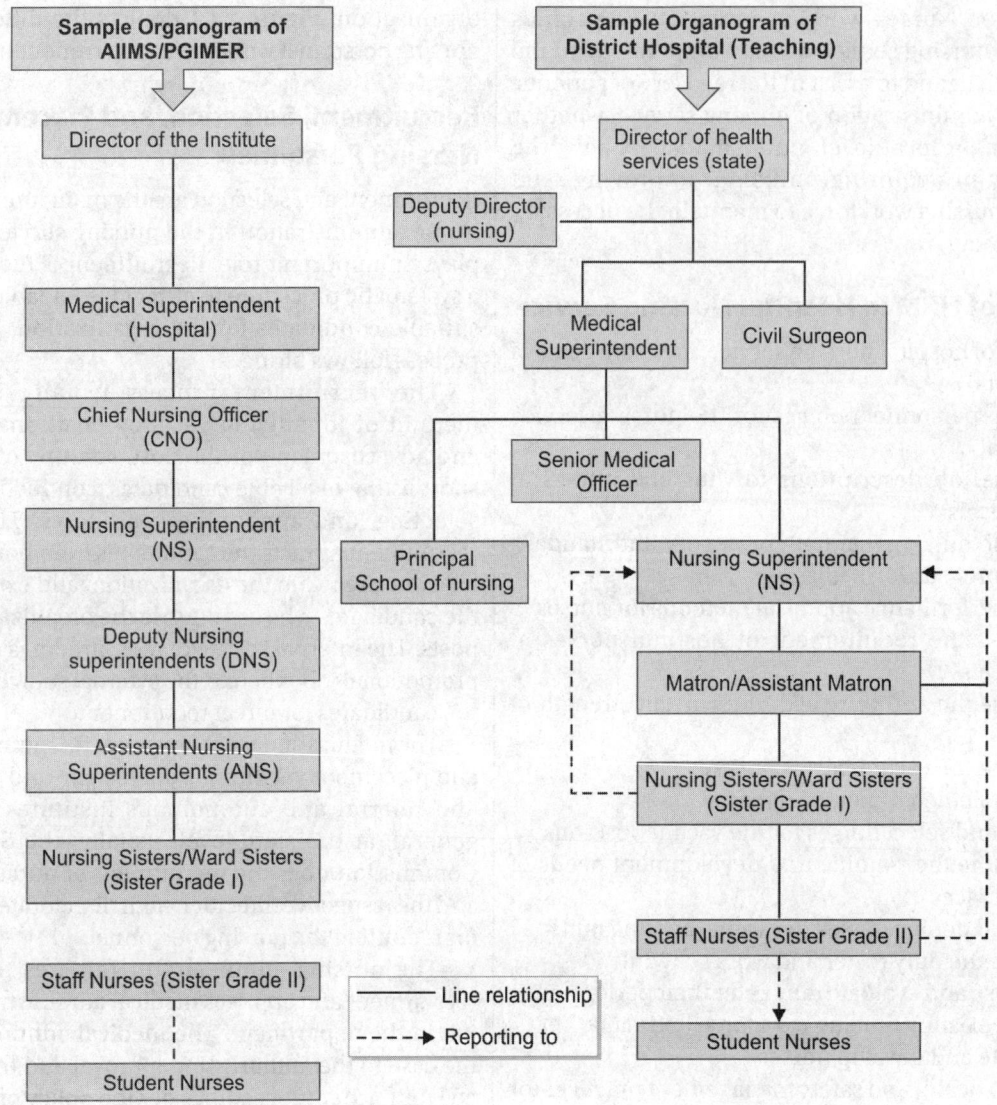

Fig. 24.1: Sample organogram of hospital nursing services.

- **Title of the post:** Staff Nurse/Nursing Officer /Sister Grade I
- **No. of posts vacant and reservation:** Specify vacant positions in the general category and another category (OBC, SC, ST) per the norms
- **Classification of the job:** Group "B"
- **Mode of recruitment:** 100% by Direct Recruitment
- **Pay scale:** Pay scale is as recommended by the Pay Commission (fall under level 07 in pay matrix of the Seventh Pay Commission, i.e. 9,300–34,800 grade pay Rs. 4,600)
- **Age limit:** Not exceeding 35 years (per government rules). In some hospitals, it is 18–30 years, but in some state hospitals, it is 18–40 years. Most of the hospitals relax age for reserved categories SC, ST, OBC, widows, and dependents of ex-servicemen with ethical conduct, for physically disabled candidates per the rule/policy/norms, and for government/departmental candidates up to 5 years. The government also has a special provision to those candidates who live near the country's borders.
- **Essential eligibility criteria:**
  BSc (Nursing)
  OR
  BSc (Post-Basic) Nursing from a recognized university
  Registered as "A Grade" Nurse and Midwife (RNRM) with State Nursing Council
  OR
  General Nursing and Midwifery (GNM) from recognized Board or Council
  Registered as "A Grade" Nurse and Midwife with State Nursing Council
  Experience: Per requirement of the hospital after completion of GNM
- **Period of probation:** 2 years.

B. Mode for applying the post

The method of recruitment for the position of staff nurse is a direct recruitment. The eligible candidates are to apply online in the institutional website or per instructions given in the advertisement by submitting an application through registered post, speed post, or by any other method. The

general guidelines for the candidates to use online are listed as follows:
- The candidate must be eligible for the said post.
- They must apply on or before the closing date of application.
- The candidate should register online on stipulated date and time.
- The candidate must fill all the columns carefully and should be visible, including photograph, signature, and thumb impression.
- The candidate is to pay prescribed application fees through any mode such as through net banking and credit card; and the application fee is nonrefundable.
- Check the date for the age limit for general, and the reserved category must be an upper limit, as mentioned.
- The candidates applying under any reserved category are to submit caste certificate as proof on a prescribed format duly issued from competent authority and disability proof document should be of competent medical authority per the notification of government.
- The eligible candidate will appear for the written test on the scheduled time and date, and venue.
- After the scrutiny of the application, the candidates can download their admit card from the site and required to bring the card at the time of the written test.
- The candidate is not allowed to take any electronic and communication devices inside the hall.

C. Selection procedure

The selection process for the post of staff nurse is through a written test of eligible candidates and interview of short-listed qualifying candidates.

a. **Written test:** The candidates for the said post (under direct recruitment) are to undergo a written examination. The written test usually is of 1 or 2 hours' duration containing about 100–150 multiple-choice questions with or without negative marking. (The weight for negative marking for wrong answers may be ¼, ½, or ¾ depending on the discretion of the authority.) There is also a mention of minimum qualifying marks.
b. **Final merit list:** The committee prepares a merit list per the marks obtained by the candidates and criteria laid down by the institute and displayed on the website. Qualified candidates are to appear for an interview.
c. **Preliminary interview:** The interview is the core of the selection process. The eligible candidates, who are to appear for the interview, are to bring their documents/original certificate along with photocopies to submit. The board of selection committee conducts the interview. The candidates per merit list appear for the interview. The selection committee verifies the required documents/certificates of successful candidates.
d. **The final selection list:** After conducting the interview, the selection board prepares a definitive list of selected candidates.
e. **Physical/medical fitness:** The selected candidates need to undergo physical fitness examination from the competent appointed medical/board before issuing an appointment letter.
f. **Approval:** The appropriate approves the selection list of the candidates.
g. **Appointing candidates:** The head of the institution offers appointment letters to selected candidates and medically fit candidates for the post of staff nurse. The appointment letter has the following information:
   - Employment conditions
   - Probation period and its termination
   - Service conditions
   - Hours of work, shift duty pattern
   - Salary and allowances
   - Leave and medical facilities
   - Uniform
   - Job description.

The committee prepares a selection list of eligible candidates and intimates the candidates. The head of the institution offers appointment letters to the selected candidates before placement. The appointment letter contains information regarding the nature of the job, service conditions, probation period (if any), and hours of work, leave and medical facilities, and to whom they will report.

D. Placement

On completion of all the formalities, the selected candidates are placed on their jobs initially on a probation period. The staff nurses report to the CNO/NS in the office wearing the proper uniform. They, on their first entry, take Florence Nightingale Oath and complete all formalities of joining. Nursing superintendent assigns the place of duty per departmental policy/requirement, where they report to nursing sister.

During the probation period, they are observed and evaluated for their performance. On successful completion of the probation period, they become permanent employees of the institution.

E. Orientation

After the selection and placement of candidates, they are made familiar with the hospital and with their job requirements. Nursing superintendent/deputy NS (DNS) (in-service education) organizes orientation or an induction training program for a week or a month to freshly joined staff. It is a formal and planned activity to introduce selected candidates about policies, rules and regulations, standing operative procedures, organization layout, etc.

Nursing Sister/Sister Grade I

The nursing sister/ward sister is designated as "sister grade I" in many hospitals and is the first supervisory-level nurses who are in charge of a nursing unit. They manage the work of the nursing unit and ensure the care of patients provided by staff nurses. They also carry out other supervisory and managerial activities assigned to them per their job description. The number of nursing sisters required in the hospital is calculated based on hospital norms, size of the hospital and type of hospital, budget allocation, and approval of the authority. The selection of nursing sisters is by promotion.

A. Recruitment details
The following is the job details for the post of nursing sister/ward sister/sister grade I:
- **Title of the post:** Nursing sister/ward sister/sister grade I
- **No. of posts vacant and reservation:** Specify vacant positions of the general category and another category (OBC, SC, ST)
- **Classification of the job:** Group "B"
- **Mode of recruitment:** 100% by promotion (seniority cum fitness)
- **Method of recruitment:** Internal recruitment
- **Pay scale:** As recommended by the Pay Commission (fall under level 08 in pay matrix of Seventh Pay Commission, i.e. 9,300–34,800 grade pay Rs. 4,800) for the central government employees
- **Age limit:** Not applicable
- **Essential eligibility criteria:** Educational qualification
  - BSc (Nursing)/BSc (Hons.) Nursing/BSc (Post-Basic) nursing recognized from university or institution/Diploma in GNM from recognized Board or Council
  - Registered as "A Grade" Nurse and Midwife with State Nursing Council
  - Regular 5 years' experience as a staff nurse/sister grade II
- **Period of probation:** 1 year.

B. Selection/promotion procedure
The method of recruitment for the post of nursing sister/ward sister/sister grade I is by internal recruitment and by promotion. The bases for selection or promotion of these posts are as follows:

a. **Experience/seniority:** After the probation period, each hospital prepares a seniority list and revises every year. The length of service is the base to prepare a seniority list. The revised list is circulated to keep staff nurses informed.

b. **Qualification:** The staff nurses, who acquire higher qualification than the minimum for the post, get the benefit for the promotion.

c. **Annual confidential report:** It is also a practice to fill the annual confidential report of staff nurses, either by nursing sister who submits it to the NS through proper channel or directly by NS/matron, and send to medical superintendent. Annual Confidential Report (ACR) is performance based and one of the essential criteria to consider at the time of promotion. The authority may decide the minimum level of ACR as a benchmark for the promotion.

d. **Medical fitness:** The candidates must be medically fit for the post.

e. **Recommendation of departmental promotion committee (DPC):** There are government hospitals/institutions that constitute DPC for promotion. At the institutional level, DPC comprises director/medical superintendent/deputy medical superintendent (nominated by the director of the institute) as a chairman, CNO; NS/matron; one representative of SC/ST (nominated); one representative of minority communities (appointed), deputy director; senior professor as members.

The committee prepares a selection list of eligible candidates and intimates the candidates. The head of the institution offers appointment letters to the selected candidates before placement. The appointment letter contains information regarding the nature of the job, service conditions, probation period (if any), and hours of work, leave and medical facilities, and to whom they will report.

C. Placement
On completion of all the formalities, the selected candidates are placed on their jobs initially on a probation period. The staff nurses report to CNO/NS in the office, wearing the uniform of nursing sister. NS assigns the place of duty.

During the probation period, they are observed and evaluated for their performance. Once the staff completes the probation period successfully, the staff will become permanent employees of this cadre in the institution.

D. Orientation
NS/DNS (in-service education) organizes orientation or an induction training program on ward management for a week. It is a formal and planned activity to introduce selected candidates for nursing ward management.

Assistant NS (ANS)

Assistant NS (assistant matron) is responsible for nursing services administration of a department/a block of two or two wards (either inpatient or outpatient/operation theaters, obstetrics units) managed by ward supervisors/nursing sisters. They carry out other supervisory, managerial, education, and teaching activities assigned to them per their job description. The number of ANS required in the hospital is calculated based on hospital norms, size of the hospital, and type of hospital, budget allocation, and approval of the authority. The selection of ANS is by the promotion.

A. Recruitment details
The following is the job detail for the recruitment process:
- **Title of the post:** ANS
- **No. of posts vacant and reservation:** Specify vacant positions of general category and another category (OBC, SC, ST)
- **Classification of the job:** Group "A"
- **Mode of recruitment:** 100% by promotion (merit cum seniority)
- **Method of recruitment:** Internal recruitment

- **Pay scale:** Mention pay scale as recommended by the Pay Commission (fall under level 09 in the pay matrix of Seventh Pay commission, i.e. 15,600–39,100 grade pay Rs. 5,400)
- **Age limit:** Not applicable
- **Essential eligibility criteria:**
    - Registered as "A Grade" Nurse and Midwife with State Nursing Council
    - BSc (Nursing)/BSc (Hons.) Nursing/Post-Basic BSc Nursing from a recognized university or institute OR
    - General Nursing and Midwifery from recognized Board or Council with Certificate in Education and Administration
    - Regular 3/5 years' experience as a sister grade I (experience period vary from hospital to hospital).

B. Selection/promotion procedure

The method of recruitment for the said post is by internal recruitment and selected by promotion. The bases for the promotion of these posts are as follows:

a. **Experience/seniority:** After the probation period, each hospital prepares a seniority list of nursing sisters and revises every year. The length of service is the base to make a seniority list. The revised list is circulated among all nursing sisters to keep them informed about their seniority position.
b. **Qualification:** The nursing sisters, who acquire higher qualification than the minimum for the post, get the benefit for the promotion.
c. **Annual confidential report:** ANS/NS fills the annual confidential report of nursing of ANS and sends it to the medical superintendent. ACR is one of the essential criteria to consider at the time of promotion. The authority may decide the minimum level of ACR as a benchmark for the promotion of ANS.
d. **Medical fitness:** The candidates must be medically fit for the post.
e. **Recommendation of DPC:** There are government hospitals/institutions that constitute DPC for promotion. At the institutional level, DPC comprises director/medical superintendent/deputy medical superintendent (nominated by the director of the institute) as a chairman, CNO; NS/matron; one representative of SC/ST (nominated); one nominated representative of minority communities, deputy director; senior professor as members.

The committee prepares a selection list of eligible candidates and intimates the candidates. The head of the institution offers appointment letters to the selected candidates, indicating the joining period. The appointment letter indicates the nature of the job, service conditions, and hours of work, leave and medical facilities, and to whom they will report.

C. Placement

On completion of all the formalities, the selected candidates are placed on their jobs initially on a probation period. The ANS report to CNO/NS in the office wearing the uniform of ANS. NS assigns the place of duty per policy or requirement.

Deputy Nursing Superintendent/Matron

Deputy NS assists in the administration of nursing services. She/he carries out managerial, education, teaching, and general duties. The number of DNS required in the hospital is calculated based on hospital norms, size of the hospital, and type of hospital, budget allocation, and approval of the authority. The selection of DNS is by promotion.

A. Recruitment details

The recruitment process for this post is as follows:
- **Title of the post:** DNS
- **No. of posts vacant and reservation:** Specify vacant positions of general category and another category (OBC, SC, ST)
- **Classification of the job:** Group "A"
- **Mode of recruitment:** 100% by promotion (merit cum seniority)
- **Method of recruitment:** Internal recruitment
- **Pay Scale:** Pay scale as recommended by the Public Service Pay Commission (fall under level 09 in the pay matrix of the Seventh Pay Commission, i.e. 15,600–39,100 grade pay Rs. 5,400)
- **Age limit:** Not applicable
- **Essential eligibility criteria:**
    - Registered as "A Grade" Nurse and Midwife with State Nursing Council
    - BSc (Nursing)/BSc (Hons.) Nursing/Post-Basic BSc Nursing from a recognized university or institute OR
    - General Nursing and Midwifery from recognized Board or Council with Certificate in Education and Administration
    - Regular 5 years of experience as a sister grade I/ANS (experience period vary from hospital to hospital).

B. Selection/promotion procedure

The method of recruitment for the said post is by internal recruitment and selected by promotion. The bases for the promotion of these posts are as follows:

a. **Experience/seniority:** Each hospital prepares a seniority list of sister grade I/ANS working in the institution, which is revised every year. The length of service of the required post is the base to prepare a seniority list. The revised list is circulated among all nursing sisters/ANS to keep them informed about their seniority position.
b. **Qualification:** The nursing sisters/ANS, who acquire higher qualification than the minimum for the post, get the benefit for the promotion.
c. **Annual confidential report:** NS fill the annual confidential report of DNS, who sends it to the medical superintendent. ACR is one of the necessary criteria to consider at the time of promotion. The authority may

decide the minimum level of ACR as a benchmark for the promotion of DNS.

d. **Medical fitness:** The candidates must be medically fit for the post.

e. **Recommendation of DPC:** There are government hospitals/institutions that constitute DPC for promotion. At the institutional level, DPC comprises director/medical superintendent/deputy medical superintendent (nominated by the director of the institute) as a chairman, CNO; NS/matron; one representative of SC/ST (nominated); one nominated representative of minority communities, deputy director; senior professor as members.

The committee prepares a selection list of eligible candidates and intimates the candidates. The head of the institution offers appointment letters to the selected candidates, indicating the joining period. The appointment letter indicates the nature of the job, service conditions, and hours of work, leave and medical facilities, and to whom they will report.

C. Placement

On completion of all the formalities, the selected candidates are initially on a probation period. The DNS report to CNO/NS in the office wearing the uniform of DNS. NS assigns the place of duty per policy or requirement.

Nursing Superintendent

In most of the hospitals, NS is the overall in charge of nursing services and is responsible to the medical superintendent. She/he plans to organize and carry out other managerial activities of nursing services. She/he assists and reports to CNO (if post exits) for all administrative actions.

A. Recruitment details

The recruitment process for this post is as follows:

- **Title of the post:** NS
- **No. of posts vacant and reservation:** Specify vacant position (either of general category or another category (OBC, SC, ST)
- **Classification of the job:** Group "A"
- **Mode of recruitment:** 100% by promotion (merit cum seniority) OR 50% by promotion and 50% by direct recruitment
- **Method of recruitment:** Internal recruitment if the post is by promotion and external recruitment if the post is by direct recruitment.
- **Promotion:** From the DNS grade with 3/5 years of regular experience (experience period varies from hospital to hospital)
- **Pay scale:** Mention pay scale as recommended by the Pay Commission (fall under level 10 in pay matrix of the Seventh Pay Commission, i.e. 15,600–39,100 grade pay Rs. 6,600)
- **Age limit:** Not applicable in case of a promotional post. For direct recruitment, the age limit is up to 40 years. Age limits may vary from hospital to hospital.

- **Essential eligibility criteria:**
  i. Registered as "A Grade" Nurse and Midwife with State Nursing Council
  ii. BSc (Nursing)/BSc (Hons.) In Nursing/Post-Basic BSc Nursing with 8 years of experience after a BSc Nursing, out of which 5 years of experience in teaching and administration from a large institution
  OR
  Matriculation or its equivalent qualification General Nursing and Midwifery from recognized Board or Council with Certificate in teaching and administration from the recognized institution, and 15 years of experience after GNM, including 5 years of experience in education and administration from a large institution.
  iii. MSc Nursing is desirable.

B. Selection/promotion procedure

- **Recruitment by promotion:** The bases for the selection are as follows:
  a. *Experience/seniority:* Each hospital prepares a seniority list of sister grade I/ANS working in the institution, which is revised every year. The length of service of the required post is the base to prepare a seniority list. The revised list is circulated among all nursing sisters/ANS to keep them informed about their seniority position.
  b. *Qualification:* The nursing sisters/ANS, who acquire higher qualification than the minimum for the post, get the benefit of the promotion.
  c. *Annual confidential report:* NS fills the annual confidential report of DNS and sends it to the medical superintendent. ACR is one of the necessary criteria to consider at the time of promotion. The authority may decide the minimum level of ACR as a benchmark for the promotion of NS.
  d. *Medical fitness:* The candidates must be medically fit for the post.
  e. *Recommendation of DPC:* There are government hospitals/institutions that constitute DPC for promotion. At the institutional level, DPC comprises director/medical superintendent/deputy medical superintendent (nominated by the director of the institute) as a chairman, CNO; NS/matron; one representative of SC/ST (nominated); one nominated representative of minority communities, deputy director; senior professor as members.

The committee prepares a selection list of eligible candidates and intimates the candidates. The head of the institution offers appointment letters to the selected candidates indicating the joining period. The appointment letter indicates the nature of the job, service conditions, and hours of work, leave and medical facilities, and to whom they will report.

- **Procedure for direct recruitment**
  A. *Mode for applying the post:* For the direct recruitment for the position of NS, the eligible candidates are to use either the online method in

Chapter 24: Human Resource Management in Nursing Services

the institutional website or the instruction given in the advertisement.

B. *Selection procedure:* The selection procedure for direct recruitment for the post of NS is the same as of the staff nurses, except no written test for the candidates applying for this job as follows:

a. **Preliminary interview:** The interview is the core of the selection process. The eligible candidates, who will be appearing in the interview, are to bring their documents/original certificate along with its photocopies to submit. The board of selection committee conducts the interview. The candidates per merit list appear for the interview. The selection committee verifies the required documents/certificates of successful candidates.

b. **The final selection list:** After undergoing an interview, the selection board prepares a definitive list of selected candidates.

c. **Physical/medical fitness:** The selected candidates need to undergo physical fitness examination from the competent appointed medical/board before issuing an appointment letter.

d. **Approval by the appropriate authority:** The appropriate approves the selection list of the candidates.

e. **Appointment of candidates:** The head of the institution offers an appointment letter to selected candidates and medically fit candidates for the post of staff nurse. The appointment letter has the following information:
   - Employment conditions
   - Probation period and its termination
   - Service conditions
   - Hours of work, shift duty pattern
   - Salary and allowances
   - Leave and medical facilities
   - Job description.

   The committee prepares a selection list of eligible candidates and intimates the candidates. The head of the institution offers appointment letters to the selected candidates, indicating the joining period.

f. **Joining:** After completing all the formalities of the job appointment, she/he submits a joining report to CNO/medical superintendent and takes charge of the nursing services.

Chief Nursing Officer

The CNO in the hospitals wherever applicable is in charge of the overall nursing services and is responsible to the medical superintendent. She/he plans to organize and carry out other managerial activities of nursing services.

A. **Recruitment details**

The recruitment process for this post is as follows:
- **Title of the post:** CNO
- **No. of posts vacant and reservation:** Specify vacant positions of general category and another category (OBC, SC, ST)
- **Classification of the job:** Group "A"
- **Pay scale:** Mention pay scale as recommended by the Pay Commission (fall under level 11 in the pay matrix of the Seventh Pay Commission, i.e. 15,600–39,100 grade pay Rs. 7,600)
- **Mode of recruitment:** 100% by promotion (merit cum seniority) failing which by deputation OR 100% by direct recruitment
- **Age limit:** Not applicable if the post is 100% by promotion; in 100% by direct recruitment, the age limit is 45 years
- **Essential eligibility criteria:**
  - *If the post is by promotion:* Five years of regular experience as NS (experience period vary from hospital to hospital)
  - *If the job is by direct recruitment:*
    - MSc Nursing from a recognized institution
    - Registered as "A Grade" Nurse and Midwife with State Nursing Council
    - 15 years of experience as ANS or 10 years of experience as DNS or 5 years of experience as NS from a large institution
- **Period of probation (if the post is by direct recruitment):** Two years.

B. *Selection procedure*

The procedure of selection for the said post is the same as followed to recruit, either by 100% promotion or by 100% direct recruitment for NS.

The committee prepares a selection list of eligible candidates and intimates the candidates. The head of the institution offers appointment letters to the selected candidates indicating the joining period.

C. *Joining*

After completing all the formalities of the job appointment, she/he submits a joining report to medical superintendent and takes charge of nursing services.

D. *Placement and deployment*

Placement is assigning a unit or ward on the first joining of the candidate. Deployment is moving or shifting staff from the current place of work to others. The transfer is a form of deployment.

Promotion of Nursing Personnel

The evidence revealed that there is a limited promotional avenue for nurses working in different hospitals. The study conducted in the 1990s also highlighted that all the nursing staff, including nurse administrators, supervisors, and bedside nurses, possessed minimum qualification for the general nursing post.

The duration of stagnation varies from more than 5–25 years, and seniority is linked with the promotion in district hospitals' nursing staff of North India (Vati J, 1990). In a referral hospital, the work experience of staff nurses ($n =$

353) ranged between 5 and 20 years and of nursing sisters (*n* = 100) ranged between 3 and 26 years, and administrators worked as nursing sisters for more than 18 years before getting the post of assistant matron or matron.

According to Earnest C, Kumari S, and Gupta JV, the recruitment of staff nurses, public health nurses, and the CNO was through direct selection and minimum qualification required is RNRM, BSc Nursing and MSc Nursing with 10 years of professional, teaching, and administrative experience, respectively. Thus, stagnating in one post of the nursing department at each level is common, and the extent of stagnation is more than sixfold from one post to the next promotion.

Bagga R, Jaiswal V, and Tiwari R, reported that a lack of opportunity for knowledge and skill upgradation, and a culture of supportive supervision but on-the-job learning is lacking. Stagnation is involved before each promotion to a higher post.

HUMAN RESOURCE MANAGEMENT IN COMMUNITY HEALTH NURSING SERVICES

Community health nursing has its primary focus on the health care of individuals, families at different settings such as medical and health centers. It is the outgrowth of personal services to mothers and children to prevent maternal and child morbidity and mortality, provide essential health services to the community, and establish referral linkages to hospitals and community as well.

There is no formal department of nursing in the community setup. However, the community health workers (CHWs) and nurses are working in different health facilities, various government health-related projects, and in a different setting to provide essential health care to the community at large. They are working as frontline agents, facilitators, motivators, counselors, and supervisors. The overall responsibility of the HRM of CHWs, including nurses, is of states, its Directorates of Health and Family Welfare, Ministry of Health and Family Welfare, Government of India under National Rural/Urban Health Mission, and Ministry of Women and Child Development.

Objectives of HRM in Community Nursing Services

In the context of community nursing service, the main goals of HRM are as follows:
- To strengthen the existing community workforce
- To prepare job descriptions of different level of CHWs/nurses
- To establish manuals, protocols, and standard operative procedures/activities
- To frame performance appraisal methods
- To forecast the requirement of CHWs/nurses at every level
- To appraise government with the current strength and vacant post of CHWs
- To attract voluntary personnel to serve the community
- To recruit and select CHWs on the contractual and regular bases
- To determine the training and development needs of community nursing services
- To train and deploy CHWs in various areas
- To plan and organize in-service education programs
- To assist them in conducting community surveys and for mapping
- To assign duties and areas
- Duty roster and work schedule
- To evaluate CHWs for their performance
- To utilize the existing workforce optimally
- To motivate and develop CHWs/nurses
- To build health and safety management practices
- To inculcate leadership, excellent working relationship, and team spirit
- To maintain discipline among them and manage their grievances
- To promote welfare, career development, and research activities
- To transfer and retain the CHWs/community nurses' talents.

Health Infrastucture: Rural Health Care

Primary health care or comprehensive health care is the main focus of public health. The basis for the primary health center (PHC) was laid down by Bhore Committee (1946), which later formed the base for national health policy with particular reference to rural health services. To implement the National Health Policy 2002 and to strengthen the rural health-care system, the government implemented a National Rural Health Mission (NRHM) (2005–2012) to provide integrated, comprehensive primary health care services to the rural population.

The rural health-care infrastructure/care facility is a three-tier system, and the health care is provided at subcenter, PHC, and community health center (CHC), so that essential services can reach the doorstep of the local people at the village level through CHWs and nurse midwives **(Fig. 24.2)**.

1. **At the village level:** At the village level, Accredited Social Health Activist (ASHA), auxiliary nurse midwife (ANM)/health worker (HW) female, and HW (male) are the CHWs providing services to a rural community. Anganwadi workers (AWWs) are the essential link between the rural poor and health workers under the Integrated Child Health Development Scheme (ICDS) launched on October 2, 1975, the world's most significant and unique program for early childhood development and to combat child hunger and malnutrition. ASHA and ANM, HW (male) work in coordination with AWW. Self-help groups also function to mobilize the community. Panchayat raj institutions/local elected bodies also assist in mobilizing the community for health initiative.
2. **At the subcenter level:** Each subcenter, which is within the radius of 2.54 km, is to provide mother and child

Chapter 24: Human Resource Management in Nursing Services

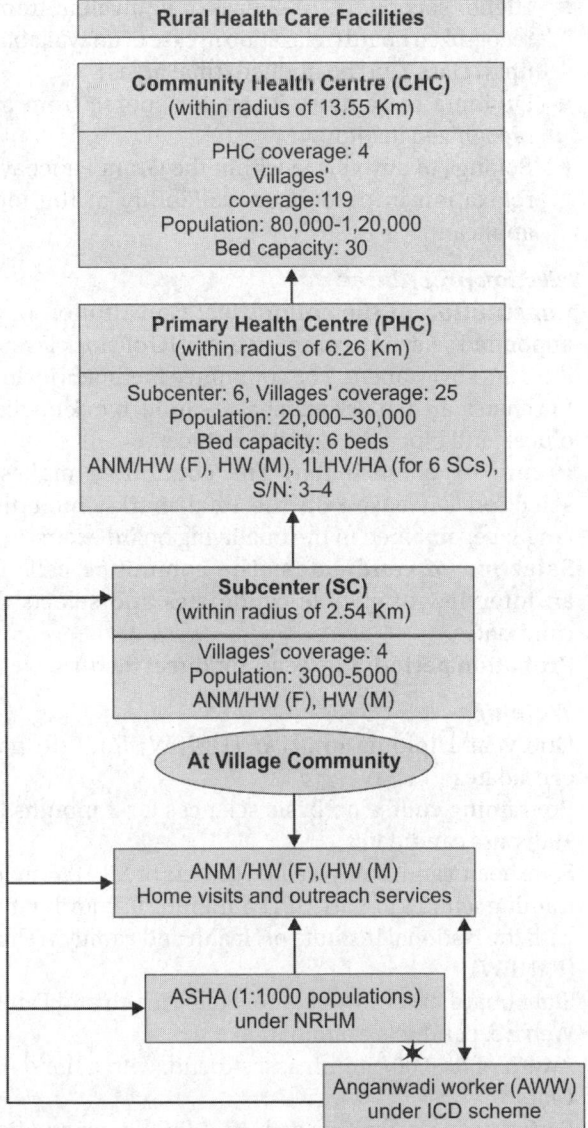

Fig. 24.2: Sample organogram of rural community health services facilities.

health-care services (including delivery facility with four to five rooms in type B subcenter), family planning, immunization, and other services under different programs to a population of 3,000–5,000 and to cover at least four villages. According to Indian Public Health Standard (2012), there is a requirement of one HW (male)/Multi purpose health workers and one ANM/HW (female) and an additional ANM/HW (female) on a contract basis to provide outreach services. It is recommended that one staff nurse (or ANM if S/N is not available in type B subcenter) conducts deliveries if the deliveries exceed 20 or more in a month.

3. **At the PHC level:** Each PHC, which is within a radius of 6.26 km, has the facility of four to six beds. It is a center to provide the preventive, promotive, Maternal and Child Health (MCH), curative, and other services to a rural population of 20,000–30,000, covering 25 villages or 6 subcenters. It is a referral unit of six subcenters and refers cases to the CHC. It varies from state to state.

It provides Out Patient Department (OPD), emergency, referral, and inpatient services. According to the Indian Public Health Standard, there is a requirement of one HW (female)/ANM for a subcenter of the area, one health assistant (male), one health assistant (female)/lady health visitor (LHV), and three to four staff nurses; and under NRHM, two additional staff nurses on a contract basis under the in charge of the medical officer.

4. **At CHC level:** Each CHC, which is within a radius of 13.55 km, is a functional 30-bedded rural hospital providing round-the-clock hospital services with specialist facilities. Each CHC covers 80,000–1,20,000 rural population. According to the norms, it should have 10 staff nurses (nurses and midwives) and one public health nurse under block medical officer or medical superintendent. At district hospitals, under the public health unit, there is a provision of one district public health officer

Recruitment, Selection, and Placement of CHWs/Nursing Personnel in Rural Health Care Sector

ASHA (Rural)

ASHA is a trained community-based link worker and acts as a bridge between the government functionaries and tribal and nontribal population who find it difficult to access the health services, which is under NRHM (2005–2012). Each village has one ASHA in the ratio of 1:1000 populations (relaxed in case of hilly and tribal areas). ASHA facilitator reinforces MCH services and immunization, promotes preventive services, institutional deliveries, and works in close coordination with AWWs. One ASHA facilitator supervises and guides 20 ASHA workers. In many states, ANM or other PHC staff supervises ASHA workers.

A. Recruitment
- **Title of post:** ASHA (rural)
- **Mode of recruitment:** 100% by direct recruitment
- **Salary:** Performance-based compensation (for an average performance: Rs. 1,000/month) for specific activities and services
- **Method of recruitment:** External recruitment
- **Age limit:** 25–45 years
- **Essential eligibility criteria:** Educational qualification
  - Up to eighth class
  - Belongs to the same village
  - Married, widowed, or divorced.

B. Selection procedure
- The community selects rural ASHA from within the community through Gram Sabha
- She reports and is accountable to the panchayat.

C. Training
- Induction training for 23 days in five rounds throughout a year with first exposure of 7 days by the ASHA trainers

- Periodic re-training once for 2 days in every alternate month (12 days/year)
- Work with AWW, HW (female), HW (male), traditional/skilled birth attendant, self-help group members
- Program-wise training.

Anganwadi Workers

An AWW is a health worker chosen from the community, who has to undergo 4 months of training in health, nutrition, and childcare. The AWW is in charge of an anganwadi center covering 1,000 rural population. ICDS anganwadi supervisor (Mukhyasevika) supervises about 25 AWWs. Four Mukhyasevikas are under the Child Development Project Officer (CDPO) at the block level.

The anganwadi center provides supplementary nutrition, nonformal preschool education, nutrition and health education, immunization, health checkup, and referral services. Along with ASHA and ANMs, the AWWs are the link between community and health services and all other services.

A. Recruitment and selection
Essential eligibility criteria
- Middle class
- Age: 21–45 years.

B. Training
- Initial 3 months of training
- Regular on-the-job 7 days of refresher courses.

There were trained local dais (traditional birth attendants) trained under the local Dais Scheme. Each dai is under the supervision of the village health guide/health worker females or ANM/health assistant (female) or LHV.

Multipurpose Health Worker (Male) (Rural)

Multiple health workers (MPHWs)/HWs (male) are functionaries at the subcenter level to provide preventive and promotive health-care services under MPHWs schemes since 1974. Each MPHW/HW (male) covers 3,000–5,000 rural population. His primary role is in communicable diseases control programmes mainly including malaria, tuberculosis, leprosy, kala-azar, waterborne diseases, and environmental sanitation apart from health education, detection of diseases, control of epidemic diseases, safe drinking water, school health, etc. in subcenters of high-focus districts at least for 3 years. He also helps ANM in MCH and other activities performed by her.

A. Recruitment
- **Title of the post:** Multipurpose health worker/HW (male)
- **Mode of recruitment:** 100% by direct recruitment
- **Method of recruitment:** External recruitment
- **Age limit:** 18–27 years, relaxation to candidates belonging to SC/OBC/ST/another category and departmental candidates or per rule
- **Essential eligibility criteria:** Educational qualification
  - Higher secondary/10+2 pass or equivalent from a recognized board (relaxation in case of unavailability up to class X in the notified tribal areas)
  - Diploma in sanitary inspector course from any recognized institution
  - Belongs to any village within the Gram Panchayat, relaxation in case of unavailability of the local applicant.

B. Selection procedure
- **Constitution of the committee:** Constitution of an appointed selection committee at PHC of block level by the state government. The committee members include the chairman of block panchayat samiti, block medical officer, and block development officer.
- **Preparing a merit list:** The committee makes a selection list based on the total marks, including language, obtained in the qualifying board exam.
- **Selection of candidates:** The committee calls for an interview of eligible candidates and selects the candidates.
- **Probation period:** Two years for direct recruits.

C. Training
- One year Diploma in MPW (DMPW) for 12th pass candidates
- Pretraining course on basic sciences for 3 months for 10th pass candidates
- State health and family welfare centers or MPHW (male) training schools impart MPHW training in coordination with the National Institute of Health and Family Welfare (NIHFW)
- State board, under Director of State Health and Family Welfare, conducts examination
- Award of Rs. 500/month as a stipend, with a bond of 5 years
- Performance evaluation at the training center and field level
- By 2010, they get only short-term training for 3–6 days under the Reproductive and Child Health (RCH) program.

Auxiliary Nurse Midwife/HW (Female) (Rural)

Auxiliary nurse midwife is the village-level health worker introduced in the 1960s and as a part of the health-care system in the 1970s. She was redesignated as MPHW (female). Since 2005, ANMs are the critical health workers under NRHM. They are posted in subcenters covering 3,000–5,000 rural populations of four villages. Her role is to carry out various activities related to national programs, including MCH, family planning, medical termination of pregnancy, nutrition, a universal program on immunization, communicable and noncommunicable diseases, maintaining records and reporting, treatment of minor ailments, and conducting the house-to-house survey. She also acts as a facilitator of ASHA workers. Out of two available ANMs in a subcenter, one performs field duties and the other visits homes. Health assistant (female)/LHV supervises ANMs but reports to the medical officer in charge of PHC.

A. Recruitment
- **Title of the post:** ANM/HW (female)
- **Class:** "C" under the General Central Service Group
- **Mode of recruitment:** 100% by direct recruitment
- **Method of recruitment:** External recruitment/through employment exchange
- **Age limit:** 18–27 years, relaxation to candidates belonging to SC/OBC/ST/another category or department candidates up to 40 years or per government rules (age limit based on the closing date of receiving applications)
- **Essential eligibility criteria:** Educational qualification
  - The candidate must have passed higher secondary/10+2 or its equivalent from a recognized university or board
    OR
    DMPW (female)/ANM certificate from recognized board or nursing council
  - Registration with State Nursing Council as ANM/HW (female) both in nursing and midwifery
- **Salary/Level in pay matrix:** Level 2 per 7th CPC. The contractual ANMs get a consolidated salary. The regular staff salary is per the State Public Service Commission.

B. Selection procedure
The health directorate constitutes a selection committee for selection of females health workers (FHWs)/ANMs, comprising additional director as a chairman and other members including an administrative officer, chief medical officer, and representative of ST/SC.
- Method of applying for the post and submitting application fee: Online through specified NRHM Web site and application fees through bank challan or submission of application by registered post, speed post, courier services, or any other mode on or before the closing date.
- Scrutiny of applications and preparation of eligible candidates: Make a list of qualified candidates.
- Selection process: Written exam and personal interview.
- Preparation of a merit list: The committee prepares a merit list based on written tests, and only qualifying candidates are allowed to take up the skill test. Qualified candidates need to also appear for a personal interview.
- Selection procedure: Merit cum interview.

Health Assistant

Health assistant (female)/LHV (rural)
LHV/health assistant (female) serves a population of 30,000 and 20,000 in hilly and tribal areas, respectively, under the MPHW scheme to cover six subcenters. She supervises and guides the work of ANMs of each subcenter and is responsible for the maintenance of equipment and supplies of subcenters and maintains records and reports. She is also involved in conducting training for dias and ASHA, with the help of ANM, and assists Medical Officer (MO) in conducting various training programs for health personnel.

A. Recruitment
- **Title of the post:** Health Assistant/Supervisor (female)/LHV
- **Mode of recruitment:** By promotion/failing which direct recruitment or (50–50%)
- **Group:** "C" (General Central Service)
- **Method of recruitment:** Direct/departmental recruitment
- **Essential eligibility criteria:** Educational qualification
  - Candidate must have passed higher secondary/10+2 or its equivalent from recognized university or board
  - Diploma (2 years) in ANM certificate from a recognized board or nursing council without or with 2–5 years' experience for direct recruitment
  - Experience of 5 years as ANM/HW (female) for promotional posts as ANM/HW (female) in any state or central organization
  - Registration with Nursing Council as ANM/HW (female) or both
  - A 6-month certificate course of health visitor from a recognized rural health training institute
  - Age: for nonselection posts: 18–27 years.
- **Desirable:**
  - A 6-month certificate course of health visitor from a recognized rural health training institute after ANM. OR
  - Diploma in GNM with 1-year experience and registered with the State Nursing Council.
- **Salary:** Level-5 in the pay matrix (Rs. 29,200–92,300) for central employees
  Per the Sixth Pay Commission: 10,300–34,800+4,200 grade pay
- **Period of probation:** Two years for direct recruits.

B. Promotion
From the post of HW (female)/ANM after 8 years of regular experience.

C. Selection procedure
- **For direct recruits:** Through selection commission/appropriate authority
- **For promotional recruits:** Through the DPC.

Health assistant (male) (rural)
Health assistant (male) serves populations of 30,000 and 20,000 in hilly and tribal areas, respectively, under the MPHW scheme to cover six subcenters. He supervises and guides the work of HW (male) of each subcenter. He is responsible for the maintenance of equipment and supplies of subcenters and also maintains records and reports. He is involved in the malaria program, nutrition, communicable, and noncommunicable diseases programs, and environmental sanitation.

A. Recruitment
- **Title of the post:** Health Assistant (male)
- **Class:** Group "C" under the General Central Service
- **Salary:** Level-5 in the pay matrix (Rs. 29,200–92,300/-) per CPC
  (10,300–34,800+4,200 grade pay) per the Sixth CPC
- **Mode of recruitment:** By promotion/direct recruitment
- **Method of recruitment:** Internal recruitment/employment exchange
- **Essential eligibility criteria:** Educational qualification
  - The candidate must have passed higher secondary/10+2 or its equivalent from a recognized university or board
  - Diploma in sanitary inspector course from any recognized institution
  - Experience of 5 years as an HW (male) in any state/central government organization
  - Relaxation in education qualification, experience, and age for SC/ST/OBC per government rules
- **Age limit:** 18–27 years (relaxation for a departmental candidate is up to 40 years)
- **Probation period:** Two years for direct recruits.

B. Promotion
From HW (male) after 8 years of regular experience in the grade.

C. Selection procedure
- **For direct recruits:** Through selection commission/appropriate authority
- **For promotional recruits:** Through the DPC.

Recruitment, Selection and Placement of Community Health Nursing Personnel in Primary Health Centre, Community Health Centre, and District Level

Staff Nurse

Staff nurses are posted in PHCs and CHCs to provide clinic preventive and curative services. They work in shift duties and report to medical in charge of respective health centers.

A. Recruitment
- **Title of the post:** Staff Nurse
- **Class:** Group "C" under the General Central Service
- **Salary:** 10,300–34,800+4,600 grade pay per the Sixth CPC
- **Mode of recruitment:** Direct recruitment/by promotion from among ANM with GNM diploma
- **Method of recruitment:** External sources/internal recruitment
- **Essential eligibility criteria:** Educational qualification
  - The candidate must have passed higher secondary/10+2 or its equivalent from recognized university or board
  - Diploma in GNM from any recognized university or institution
  - Registered nurse and midwife with State Nursing Council
  - Experience of 5 years as an ANM
- **Age limit:** 17–35 years for direct recruits.

B. Selection procedure
- Through the DPC
- By seniority cum merit

Public Health Nurse

Per the Indian Public Health Standards (2012), public health nurse is a nurse midwife. She provides preventive and promotive services, monitors, and supervises the work of health supervisors/LHVs and health workers/ANMs in the field.

A. Recruitment
- **Title of the post:** Public Health Nurse
- **Class:** Group "C" under the General Central Service
- **Salary:** 10,300–34,800+4,800 grade pay per the Sixth CPC
- **Mode of recruitment:** By promotion from the post of LHV
- **Method of recruitment:** Internal recruitment/external sources
- **Essential eligibility criteria:** Educational qualification
  - The candidate must have passed higher secondary/10+2 or its equivalent from recognized university or board
  - Diploma in GNM from any recognized university or institution
  - Registered nurse and midwife with State Nursing Council
  - Experience of 10 years as an LHV
- **Age limit:** For direct recruits: up to 35 years.

B. Selection procedure
- Through the DPC
- By seniority cum merit

C. Placement
CHC and Public Health Unit of the district hospitals and also created in referred hospitals for OPDs.

District Public Health Nurse Officer

A. Recruitment
- **Title of the post:** District Public Health Nurse Officer
- **Class:** Group "B" under the General Central Service
- **Salary:** 15,600–39,100+5,400 grade pay per the Sixth CPC
- **Mode of recruitment:** 100% by promotion among PHN or LHV with a BSc (Nursing) degree as an essential qualification provided no suitable candidates
- **Method of recruitment:** Internal recruitment
- **Essential eligibility criteria:** Educational qualification
  - BSc (Nursing) degree from any recognized university or institution
  - Registered Nurse and Midwife with State Nursing Council

- Three years of regular experience as PHN or 7 years of experience as LHV.

B. Selection procedure
- **For promotional recruits:** Through the DPC
- **Method:** Seniority cum merit.

C. Placement
- District level.

Health Infrastructure: Urban Health Care

In continuation with NRHM under National Health Mission (NHM), the government approved National Urban Health Mission (NUHM) on May 1, 2013, to provide comprehensive services to urban poor. The areas covered under NURM are town panchayat, notified area committee, municipalities, and municipal corporations. The city included are seven megacities, 40 million plus cities, 552 cities with a population of 1 to 10 lakh, and 604 cities with a population between 50,000 and 1 lakh. It provides services to a poor resident of listed and nonlisting slum areas and vulnerable people, especially to homeless, ragpickers, commercial sex workers, and so on.

Its institutional model is at national, state, district/city, and at the community level. It has close coordination with national disease control programmes, the Ministry of Health and Welfare Departments, and schemes run by other ministries. The urban health-care facilities under this mission are through home visits, outreach services, urban PHCs (outpatient departments), and the urban CHC level (Fig. 24.3).

1. **Community level:** At the urban community level, ASHA, Mahila Arogya Samiti (MAS), ANM female/HW female are the community health works providing services to the urban community.
2. **Urban PHC level (U-PHC):** The U-PHC caters to the needs of 50,000–60,000 urban population including a slum population of 20,000–30,000. Its location is near the slum area of ½ km radius. It provides services through OPDs, which runs for eight hours in two shifts from 8 PM to 12 PM and 4 PM to 8 PM with flexible timings according to need. It has three staff nurses, one LHV, three to five FHW/ANMs, and other staff under MO I/C. FHW/ANM provide services to 10,000–12,000 slum/vulnerable urban population.
3. **Urban CHC level (U-CHC):** Each U-CHC covers a population of 2.5 lakhs (5 lakh for metros). It has 30- to 50-bedded inpatient facilities (100-bedded facilities in metros). It provides curative and MCH services, including institutional deliveries, specialties services, and diagnostic facilities.

Recruitment, Selection, and Placement of CHWs/Nursing Personnel in Urban Health Care Sector

URBAN-ASHA

Urban ASHA is an essential link between urban communities through MAS. U-ASHA is a trained

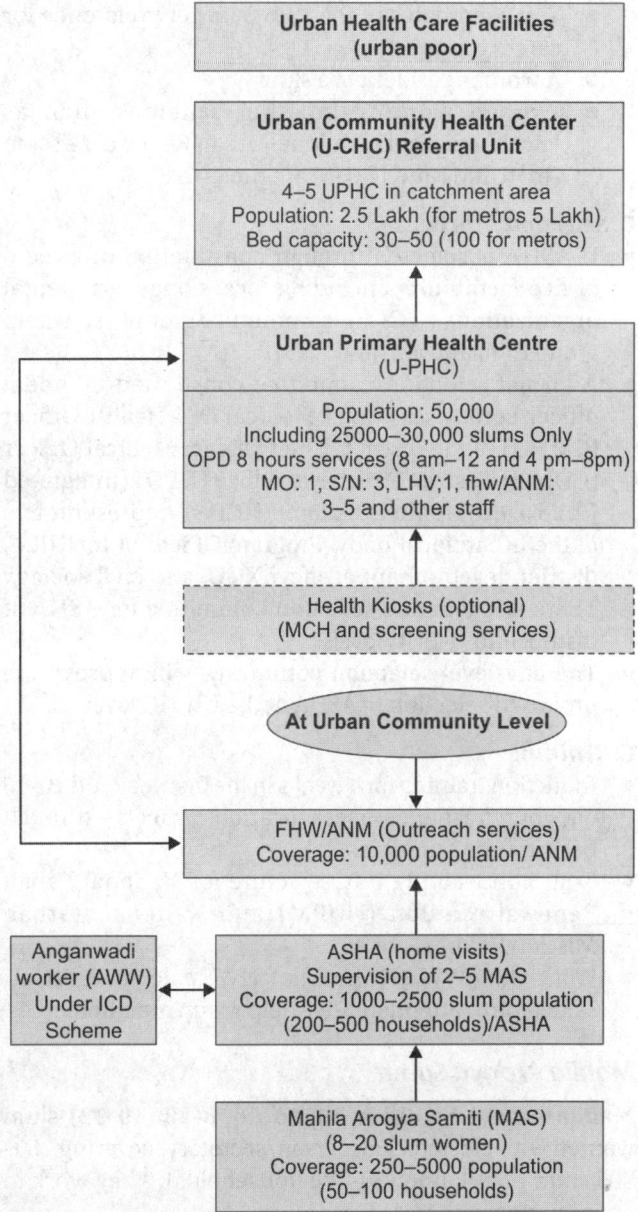

Fig. 24.3: Sample organogram of urban community health services facilities.

community-based link worker and acts as a bridge between the Government functionaries and various support systems in the community. Each U-ASHA covers 1,000–2,500 slum/vulnerable urban population and visits 200–500 households. She supervises two to five MAS in her assigned area, reinforces MCH services and immunization, promotes preventive services, and works in close coordination with AWWs.

A. Recruitment
- **Title of post:** U-ASHA
- **Mode of recruitment:** 100% by direct recruitment
- **Salary:** Performance-based compensation for specific activities and services
- **Age limit:** 25–45 years
- **Essential eligibility criteria:** Educational qualification
  - Up to class 10th (relaxation, if a suitable candidate is not available)

- The candidates of the 12th pass get preference for career purpose
- A woman resident of a slum
- Women working in other schemes such as Jawaharlal Nehru National Urban Renewal Mission (JnNURM) and NRHM are preferred.

B. Selection procedure
- U-ASHA is selected through consultation of a team of five facilitators, including local nongovernmental organizations (NGOs), community groups, self-help groups, anganwadi, and ANM.
- A formal selection committee constituted by nodal officer comprises Chief Medical and Health Officer (CMHO) of the district/ Chief District Medical Officer (CDMO)-District Panchayat Office (DPO) (Integrated Child Development Scheme (ICDS), representative of the urban local body, Program Officer of JnNURM, district development agency, NGO, and civil society. There is a separate selection committee for ASHA at district and U-PHC levels.
- The city-level selection committee will approve the proposed selection of ASHA at the U-PHC level.

C. Training
- Induction training for 4 weeks in the first year and 10–15 days of refresher courses on various aspects—through basic training modules
- Common training infrastructure for National Urban Renewal Mission (NURM) and National Rurban Mission (NRuM)
- Work with AWW, HW (female), HW (male), traditional/skilled birth attendant, self-help group members.

Mahila Arogya Samiti

Mahila Arogya Samiti is a group of 8–20 (10–12) slum women with elected chairperson/secretary, covering 250–500 slum population (50–100 households). They work in coordination with U-ASHA.

A. Method of MAS promotion
- ASHA forms a team at the slum level with the help of NGO, ANM, or AWW
- Several meetings with slum women with a team
- Identifying 10–12 active, interested, and dedicated women for 50–100 households
- Meeting with identified women
- Formation and nomination of office bearers
  - Chairperson unanimously elected by the group
  - Member secretary (ASHA)
- **Age limit:** No barrier.

B. Training
Quarterly orientation programs or meetings.

Auxiliary Nurse Midwife

Urban ANM is the urban community-level health worker under NURM. ANMs provide outreach services. Each Urban ANM covers 10,000 population. Those posted in U-PHC offers outreach services in the assigned urban slum area through organizing urban health and nutrition days and special outreach sessions. She is supposed to organize these outreach sessions monthly and weekly, respectively, at anganwadi center and schools in coordination with ASHA and MAS. She will do monthly health checkups at anganwadi center, with the assistance of ANM, ASHA, and AWW. She reports to the MO I/C of U-PHC. Her leading role in U-PHC involves mapping and vulnerability assessment, linking with urban local bodies, home visiting, supervision of ASHA and MCH, preventing and managing communicable and noncommunicable diseases, maintaining records and reporting, etc.

A. Recruitment
- **Title of the post: U-ANM**
- **Class:** "C" under the General Central Service Group
- **Mode of recruitment:** 100% by direct recruitment
- **Method of recruitment:** External recruitment/through employment exchange
- **Age limit:** 18–27 years, relaxation to candidates belonging to SC/OBC/ST/another category or department candidates up to 40 years or per the government rules (age limit based on the closing date of receiving applications)
- **Essential eligibility criteria:** Educational qualification
  - The candidate must have passed higher secondary/10+2 or its equivalent from a recognized university or board
    OR
    DMPW (female)/ANM certificate from a recognized board or Nursing Council
  - Registration with State Nursing Council as ANM/HW (female) both in nursing and in midwifery
- **Salary/level in pay matrix:** Level 2 per the Seventh CPC. The contractual ANMs get a consolidated salary. The regular staff salary is per the State Public Service Commission.

B. Selection procedure
The health directorate constitutes a selection committee for selection of FHW/ANMs, comprising additional director as a chairman and other members including an administrative officer, chief medical officer, and representative of ST/SC
- **Method of applying the post and submitting application fee:** Online through specified NRHM Website and application fees through bank challan or submission of application by registered post, speed post, courier services, or any other mode on or before the closing date.
- **Scrutiny of applications and preparation of eligible candidates:** Make a list of qualified candidates.
- **Selection process:** Written exam and personal interview
- **Preparation of a merit list:** The committee prepares a merit list based on written tests, and only qualifying

candidates are to appear for the skill test. Qualified candidates are called for the personal interview.
- **Selection procedure:** Candidate's selection is by merit cum personal interview.

Recruitment, Selection and Placement of Community Health Nursing Personnel in Urban Primary Health Center

Urban-LHV/Public Health Nurse

Each LHV/health assistant (female) serves an urban population of 50,000 including 25,000–30,000 slums at U-PHC. She supervises and guides the work of ANMs and ASHA workers. She also involved in conducting training of dias and ASHA with the help of ANM and assists MO in doing various training programs of health personnel. At PHC, she provides comprehensive preventive and promotive services of all communicable and noncommunicable diseases at OPDs. She operates at the block level.

A. Recruitment
- **Title of the post:** LHV/Public Health Nurse
- **Mode of recruitment:** By promotion/failing which direct recruitment or (50–50%)
- **Group:** "C" (General Central Service)
- **Method of recruitment:** Direct/departmental recruitment
- **Essential eligibility criteria:** Educational qualification
    - Candidate must have passed higher secondary/10+2 or its equivalent from recognized university or board
    - Diploma (2 years) in ANM certificate from a recognized board or nursing council with 2–5 years' experience and basic computer course
    - Registered with State Nursing Council as ANM
    OR
    BSc Nursing with 1 year experience with State department, RNRM with State Nursing Council
    OR
    Diploma in GNM and 2 years' experience RNRM with State Nursing Council
    - Age: Upper limit 45 years
- **Salary:** Per rule, in some states salary is Rs. 12,000/month.

B. Selection process
Per requirement. Walk in interview, merit cum interview.

Staff Nurse
Staff nurses are posted in PHCs and CHCs to provide clinic preventive and curative services. They work in shift duties in UCHC and do preventive and promotive services at U-PHC OPDs and report to medical in charge of respective health centers. Recruitment and selection are the same as for the rural PHC or rural CHC as a regular or on a contract basis.

CHAPTER HIGHLIGHTS
- HRM in nursing is mainly concerning managing nursing personnel, individual nurses, and a group of nurses and their relationship.
- The head of the nursing department is the Nursing Director/CNO/NS/Matron, depending on the type of hospital.
- The method and mechanisms of recruitment, selection, and placement vary from state to state and also in central and referral and autonomous institutes.
- The nursing administrator initiates the process of recruitment and apprises medical administrators to fill the job in the department.
- There is no formal department of nursing in the community setup. Nurses are working as frontline agents, facilitators, motivators, counselors, and supervisors.
- The rural health-care infrastructure/care facility is a three-tier system and provides health care at subcenter, PHC, and a CHC.
- In continuation with NRHM under NHM, the government approved NUHM on May 1, 2013, to provide comprehensive services to urban poor.

REVIEW QUESTIONS

I. Essay Type Questions
1. Describe the organization of hospital nursing services.
2. Explain the recruitment and selection procedures of hospital nurses.
3. Discuss the human resource management of community health nursing services.
4. Describe the deployment and transfer of hospital nursing personnel.

II. Short Notes
1. Objectives of human resource management
2. Superannuation applicable for nurses
3. Methods of deploying nurses
4. Method of promotion in nursing

III. Multiple Choice Questions
1. Who is responsible for recruiting nursing personnel at the state level?
    a. Director of health services
    b. The Staff Selection Commission
    c. Medical Superintendent
    d. Nursing Superintendent
2. The age limit for the post of staff nurse per government rule is:
    a. Up to 35 years   b. 18–30
    c. 18–45   d. 8–50
3. What is the selection procedure for the post of nursing sister?
    a. Internal recruitment

b. By promotion
c. Both internal recruitment and by promotion
d. Direct recruitment

4. Which committee laid down the basis for the primary health care?
   a. Mudaliar Committee
   b. Kartar Singh Committee
   c. Bhore Committee
   d. Jungalwalla Committee

5. Who is the essential link between rural poor and health-care services under ICDS?
   a. ANM
   b. MPHW
   c. ASHA
   d. AWW

Answer Keys

1. b   2. a   3. c   4. c   5. d

SUGGESTED READING

1. [PDF]Lady Health Visitor/Health Supervisor (Female), Group ... https://mohfw.gov.in › files › Meta Data for Documents_001 (1)_Part1. [Accessed January 2020].
2. Available from http://nhm.gov.in/images/pdf/NUHM/Implementation_Framework_NUHM.pdf. [Accessed November 2018].
3. Available from https://www.ncbi.nlm.nih.gov/pubmed/21554067. [Accessed November 2018].
4. Earnest C, Kumari S, Gupta JV. Stagnation among the nursing personnel working at Nehru hospital PGI Chandigarh- A perspective study up to May 1993. Hospital Administration1996; XXXIII (1&2): 83-94.
5. Indian Public Health Standards. IPHS Revised Guidelines 2012. [online] Available from https://nhm.gov.in/index1.php?lang=1&level=2&sublinkid=971&lid=154. [Accessed January 2020].
6. Ministry of Health and Family Welfare Government of India. National Rural Health Mission: framework for implementation; 2013.
7. National ASHA Mentoring Group. (online) Available from https://nhm.gov.in/index1.php?lang=1&level=2&sublinkid=178&lid=251. [Accessed January 2020].
8. National Health Mission. ASHA Training Module. [online] Available from http://www.nhm.gov.in/images/pdf/communitisation/asha/book-no-1.pdf. [Accessed March 2019].
9. Role of Directorates in Promoting Nursing and Midwifery ... https://www.ncbi.nlm.nih.gov › pmc › articles › PMC4389509
10. Scott K, Javadi D, Gergen J, et al. India's Auxiliary Nurse-Midwife, Anganwadi Worker, Accredited Social Health Activist, Multipurpose Worker, and Lady Health Visitor Programs. [online] Available from https://www.chwcentral.org/blog/indias-auxiliary-nurse-midwife-anganwadi-worker-accredited-social-health-activist-multipurpose. [Accessed March 2019].
11. Vati J. Organisation and administration of nursing services in district hospitals of North India. Unpublished Ph.D. Thesis. Faculty of Medical Sciences, Panjab University, Chandigarh,India; 1990.

25 Fundamentals of Staffing: Staffing, Philosophy, Staffing Study, and Norms

CHAPTER OUTLINE

- Staffing
  - Meaning and Definitions
  - Nature of Staffing
  - Features of Staffing
  - Need and Importance of Staffing
  - Staffing Process
  - Factors Affecting the Demand for Staffing
- Philosophy of Staffing
- Staffing Study/Estimation of Nursing Staff Requirement
  - Method Study/Work Sampling Study
  - Timed-task/Activity Study Method
  - Workload Measurement Studies
  - Regression Analysis Studies
- Staffing Norms and Normative Approaches
  - Staffing Norms
  - Norms-related Approaches

LEARNING OUTCOMES

After completion of this chapter, the learner will be able to:
- Understand the concept and nature of staffing
- Discuss the features, need, and importance of staffing
- Describe the philosophy and principles of staffing
- Enumerate the factors influencing staffing
- Discuss the analysis of staffing
- Enlist staffing norms and related approaches

KEY TERMS

Staffing, philosophy, staffing process, staffing study, staffing norms, strategies

INTRODUCTION

The most distinct and essential component of any healthy organization is the staff, not its physical facilities, buildings, equipment or the sophistication of computer services, high-tech machines, or streamlined procedures.

If the right kind of employees is not employed, it will result in the wastage of equipment, time, efforts, and energy; and even the software becomes defective. The services provided would be of low quality to achieve organizational goals. Therefore, it is essential that not only the right type of nursing personnel are employed but also they should be given adequate training, so that the wastage is minimum; moreover, the skilled staff needs to be retained and motivated to discharge their services to the fullest. All these can only be possible with an efficient and effective staffing system.

STAFFING

Meaning and Definitions

Staffing is the process that ensures that an organization has qualified staff at various levels of management to meet the short-term and long-term requirements. Staffing involves operating the organization structure through proper and effective selection, appraisal, and development of the personnel to fulfill the roles assigned to the employers/workforce. McFarland defines staffing as the function by which managers build an organization through recruitment, selection, and development of individuals as capable employees.

According to Koontz et al., the managerial functions of staffing are filling positions in the organizational structure through identifying workforce requirements, inventorying the people available, recruitment, selection, placement, promotion, appraisal, compensation, and training of the needed people. Staffing pertains to recruitment, selection, development, and payment of subordinates (Theo Haimann). Luther Gullick viewed staffing as the whole personnel function of bringing in and training the staff and maintaining favorable work conditions.

According to the American Nurses Association, safe staffing is an appropriate level of registered nurses (RNs) to always meet the needs to care for the patient. The term "staffing" is the process of procuring, developing, employing, appraising, rewarding, and retaining the nursing personnel at various levels, so that the right type of nursing personnel are available at the right positions and at the right time in the nursing organization. It is the process through which nursing personnel is made available for rendering care to patients.

Nature of Staffing

Staffing is an integral part of human resource management. It facilitates procurement and placing the right staff on the right job. The staffing functions are as follows:
- Staffing is team centered.
- It is applicable to all types of organizations.
- It is concerned with all categories of personnel from top to operational level.
- It is an essential function of management; like management, it also needs planning, organizing, directing, coordinating, and controlling features.
- Manager at each level is engaged in performing the staffing function.
- Staffing is a continuous activity as the manager is to guide and train the subordinates and also evaluate their performance.
- Staffing helps in placing the right person at the right job.
- Staffing is concerned with training and development of human resources.
- Each manager is required to have social relation skills to perform staffing functions.

Features of Staffing

Some of the features of staffing are as follows:
1. Staffing is the management of workforce or human resource.
2. Staffing function is related to the employment of nursing personnel of all types.
3. It includes a variety of activities to get the right kind of nurses on the right job, at the right time.
4. It is concerned with filling various positions or jobs in the nursing organization with suitable nursing personnel.
5. It is every nurse manager's job.

Need and Importance of Staffing

Following are the needs and importance of staffing:
1. **Staffing as a critical function of management:** Staffing is one of the vital features of control because it deals with human beings. They are the most valuable asset for an organization. The organization recruits and places the right type of personnel at the right time to carry out various activities to accomplish its goals.
2. **Staffing helps to build a sound human organization:** Staffing is concerned with finding the right type of person who is qualified and competent to place, train, and develop to achieve the objectives of the organization. Thus, staffing helps in building a sound human organization.
3. **Staffing ensures maximum output:** By appointing and placing appropriate person, maximum output can be ensured at minimum cost, time, and effort. It provides a positive impact on continuity and quality of care by the nurses.
4. **Staffing provides job satisfaction:** Staffing by way of assigning the appropriate jobs to the most suited person who will be capable and has the potential to perform helps them to ensure job satisfaction.
5. **Staffing reduces stress:** Through staffing, there will be a division of work. Every person is accountable for assigned work. The cordial relationship between supervisors motivates the staff to perform more efficiently and effectively.
6. **Staffing helps in reducing absenteeism and turnover rates:** There is a provision of providing incentives, both monetary and nonmonetary, to motivate staff to work. Nonmonetary incentives are the factors that give the satisfaction of doing something worthy. It can be in the form of recognition given for their excellent performance and ethical behavior and allow them to participate in decision-making, etc. It helps in reducing absenteeism and sustaining them.
7. **Staffing provides benefits to consumers:** Staffing offers benefits to customers. Through safe staffing, i.e. by appointing and developing competent staff to provide care reduces the incidence of adverse events and thus lowers morbidity and mortality. Studies have revealed low nurse staffing is associated with an increased risk of death (Kendall-Raynor 2017). Care through the competent staff provides satisfaction to clients and thus shortens the hospital stay.
8. **Staffing prepares for future challenges:** Through staffing, managers forecast staff requirements for the future and plan, train, and develop people accordingly. The managers enable them to grow so that they can take up future responsibilities. In this way, staffing helps and prepares the organization to face future challenges.

Staffing Process

Staffing involves implementing a planned program with and through qualified individuals having organizational goals. Components/steps/functions of staffing process are as listed below **(Fig. 25.1)**:
1. **Workforce planning:** It is the first step in staffing and is concerned with determining the number and type of nursing staff required for different types of hospitals.
2. **Job analysis:** Job analysis is a vital component/step for finalizing job specification and job description and thereby helps in developing the recruitment policies.
3. **Recruitment:** Recruitment refers to the identification of sources of nursing workforce and the efforts taken to secure or attract applicants for various job positions.

Chapter 25: Fundamentals of Staffing: Staffing, Philosophy, Staffing Study, and Norms

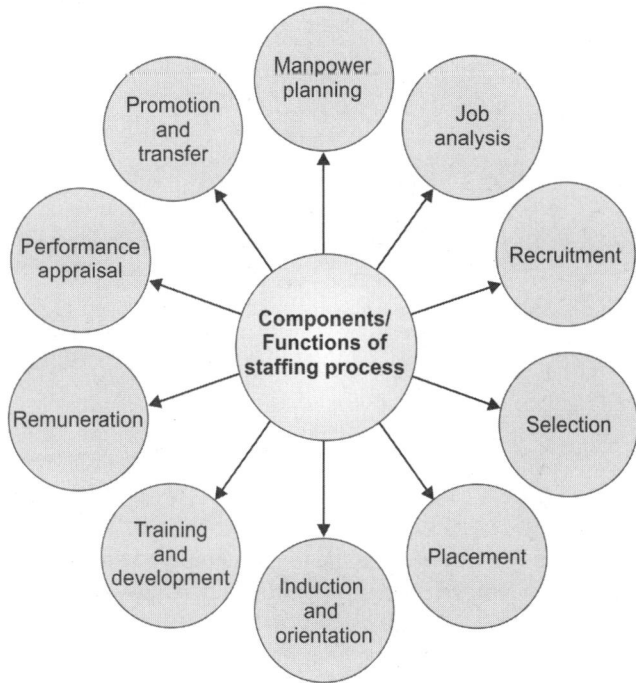

Fig. 25.1: Components of the staffing process.

4. **Selection:** Selection is the process of choosing and appointing the right candidates for the job in nursing. It includes receiving and screening applications, employment tests, interviews, and medical examination of the candidate.
5. **Placement:** Placement ensures the right staff in an assigned unit or hospital per the capability of team.
6. **Induction and orientation:** Induction is the process of orienting a new employee about the organization and the job. Newly recruited staff is informed about working hours, the procedure for availing leaves, safety precautions, uniform attire, legal and ethical responsibilities, perks, salary, etc.
7. **Training and development:** Training is essential to update the skills and knowledge of the staff. Training can be on the job and off the job.
8. **Remuneration:** Remuneration is a kind of compensation provided monetarily to the employees for their work performances. This is decided according to the nature of job—skilled or unskilled, physical or mental, etc. Remuneration forms an essential monetary incentive for the employees.
9. **Performance appraisal:** The performance appraisal function of staffing guides the staff per performance. The transfers and promotions are decided based on the performance of the employee.
10. **Promotion and transfer:** Promotion is a nonmonetary incentive to shift employees to a higher job demanding more responsibilities.

Factors Affecting the Demand for Staffing

Following are the factors affecting the need for staffing:
1. **Advancement in knowledge and technology:** There is a need to appoint the right type of personnel to use the latest technology and also the obligation to update their knowledge from time to time. It requires a plan for training and development programs.
2. **Specialization:** Being the specialty or super specialty in the profession, it is essential to find suitable personnel to fill various positions.
3. **The increasing size of health organizations:** Due to the demand for health services, the bed strength in the hospitals is increasing. The demand for staff also increases accordingly.
4. **Awareness of health and consumer's rights:** Competent and qualified staff demand is due to the knowledge about health and rights among clients.
5. **Shortage of staff:** The management is required to determine the workforce requirement well in advance and to develop the existing one for filling the future vacancies at the top levels because of staff shortage.
6. **Emphasis on human relation:** The behavior of individuals has become very complicated. That is why management of the social aspect of the organization has become critical. The staff should be motivated and learning environment or culture should also be created for them, so that they can contribute maximum toward organizational objectives. By performing staffing functions effectively, the management can plan and implement various strategies to increase the morale of the employees.
7. **The occurrence of major crises:** Significant crisis of diseases, such as AIDs, SARS, and potential flu outbreak, etc., which leads to nursing shortages and increasing health-care costs.

Factors Influencing Staffing Demand

For Community Health Nursing Services

The factors influencing the community health nursing services are as follows (**Fig. 25.2**):
1. **Demographic factors:** Size of population, distribution, density, growth rate, age and structure determine the amount and type of health services required for a defined geographical area. Accordingly, there is a need for appropriate staff to provide services to the community.
2. **Economic factors:** Since price is a mediating variable, if the demand exceeds the supply, the price will increase and there is a positive correlation between disposable income and the need for health care. Whereas in the government sector, where price variable is absent, the waiting time for services and other such variables will tend to replace the price as the mediator between supply and demand. Staff required is also estimated per the budget sanctioned.
3. **Social and cultural factors:** These factors play an essential role in staffing requirements, as health consciousness is directly proportional to demand services.
4. **Health status:** It varies inversely with demand. If community health status is functional, it requires

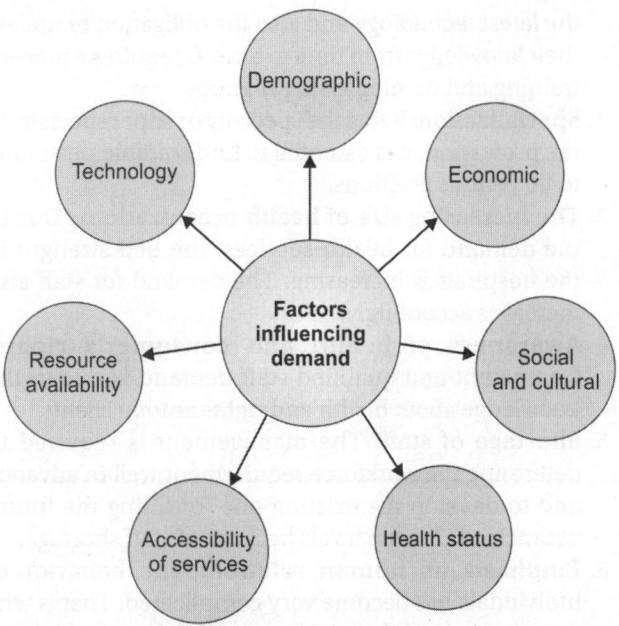

Fig. 25.2: Factors influencing staffing for community health services.

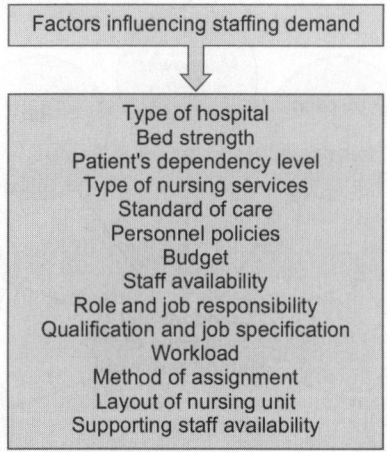

Fig. 25.3: Factors influencing staffing demand.

less staff; and if health status is poor, directing more services, thereby requiring more workforce.
5. **Accessibility of health services:** Easy accessibility of health services is directly proportional to the demand for services and required proportionate staff in health consciousness or awareness and demand more health services and thereby staff requirement is also increased.
6. **Resource availability:** This is another factor used as a predictor to forecast staff requirements.
7. **Health-care technology:** With the advancement of health-care technology, there is a need for staff requirements.

For Hospital Nursing Services

Some factors that are related to the staffing of nursing services are as follows (Fig. 25.3):
1. **Type of hospital:** Type of hospital, either teaching or nonteaching, determines the number of personnel required. A teaching hospital requires more staff as compared to nonteaching team due to the nature and quantity of workload.
2. **Bed strength:** The number of patients under care represents the major work assignment of the nurses, and it is one of the most significant bases for estimating the number of staff required.
3. **Patients' dependency on nursing care:** Patients who are acutely ill required more staff as compared to the patients who are moderately ill or mildly ill. The patients who are independent need lesser care, and, therefore, a need for less staff.
4. **Types of nursing services:** Staff pattern depends on the types of services. Careful evaluation of patients' needs takes more time and requires more skill than gross nursing procedures. The department of specialized services requires more staff than general care departments. It is the responsibility of the nurse to provide emotional support and comprehensive nursing care to the patients.
5. **Standard of care:** The hospital policies and standard of care reflect the kind and amount of nursing care. After establishing rules, it is an administrator's responsibility to determine what services and staff are implicit in them and make provision for necessary services to attain the goal.
6. **Personnel policies:** The recruitment and retention depend to a considerable degree on the personnel policies. Salary and security, hours of work, sick leave, and vacations are apparent factors, but other aspects of personnel management are greatly influenced by the morale of staff. These include working environments, feeling of mutual respect between staff at all levels and recognition of work accomplishment. Honest and regular evaluations of work performance, in-service education, and planned relief of staff to ensure patient care, when workloads become too heavy, are of real importance in staffing patterns.
7. **Budget:** The amount of money available for personnel is one of the most definite elements of the staffing pattern. The organization adjusts in case of a meager budget to employ the number and kinds of staff necessary to carry out the program. It may be possible to care for fewer patients, providing less comprehensive care, or employ less qualified personnel to provide care.
8. **Availability of trained staff:** The availability of trained personnel is another predictor of staffing requirements.
9. **Role and responsibilities of nurses:** One of the duties of a profession is to define its purpose or function to distinguish from other occupations. Since nurses are carrying out nursing and nonnursing duties, definitely extra nurses are required to compensate.
10. **Qualification and job specification:** The qualification and job specification of the personnel predicts staffing pattern. Staff qualifications refer to the preparation considered necessary for personnel to meet the level of responsibility inherent to each position. It includes

educational background and specific types of work experience. Job specification classifies the level of responsibility of each post and is supported by a description of particular activities involved in the job together with the qualifications required of the staff for the position.

11. **Workload:** The units having more workload, for example, surgical unit, medical unit, require more staff. Even shift wise, more nurses are needed in the morning than in the evening and night shifts. It also depends on the nature of work in a particular nursing unit.
12. **Method of assignment:** Staffing pattern varies with the type of assignment of the staff. The patients' assignments require more staff than the functional assignment.
13. **The layout of the nursing unit:** The design of the unit influences staffing patterns. There is a need for less supervision of staff in open wards as compared to a closed department having different units.
14. **Availability of supporting staff:** Ancillary staff is of great assistance. Nursing orderlies are helping staff in different types of work. If they are be available, nursing time can be saved to carry out those activities and hence requires less staff.

PHILOSOPHY OF STAFFING

Nurse administrators of a hospital nursing department should adopt the following staffing philosophy. Nurse administrators believe that:
- It is possible to match employees' competency to patient care needs in a manner that optimizes job satisfaction and care quality.
- The professional nurses require to carry out the technical and humanistic care needs of critically ill patients.
- A professional and technical nurse can provide health teaching and fulfill the rehabilitation needs of chronically ill patients.
- Use patient assessment, workload, and job analysis to determine the number of personnel in each category to be assigned to care for patients of each type (such as coronary care, renal failure, chronic arthritis, paraplegia, cancer, etc.).
- The nursing heads and staff of the hospital develop a master staffing plan and policies
- Accommodate the units' workload and workflow by calculating the staffing plan details such as shift duty rotation plan, the number of staff assigned on holidays, and the number of employees assigned to each shift.

STAFFING STUDY/ESTIMATION OF NURSING STAFF REQUIREMENT

Staffing study is a systematic, planned, and logical process or activity of gathering information and facts about issues related to staffing, its components including methods of

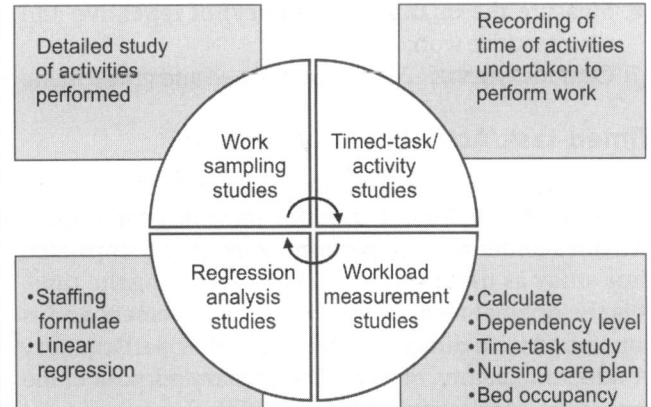

Fig. 25.4: Types of staffing studies to estimate staffing demand.

estimating staff requirement, patient classification, type of nursing activities, time required to carry out nursing activities, nursing time available, methods of calculating nursing workload, job satisfaction, nursing acuity, scheduling, etc. It is a continuous process involving all steps as followed in conducting research studies. It includes the assessment phase, planning phase, implementation phase, and evaluation phase.

1. **Assessment phase:** The assessment phase involves various steps, namely (1) identifying staffing issue, (2) formulating study questions and objectives of conducting the study, (3) formulating hypothesis and assumptions, delimitation, (4) defining terms, and (5) identifying determinants/variables.
2. **Planning phase:** Planning phase includes various steps such as (1) selecting methodology including sample and sampling techniques and (2) selecting and developing tools and methods of data collection.
3. **Implementation phase:** The implementation phase includes collecting and organizing data.
4. **Evaluation phase:** Evaluation phase includes analysis and interpretation of data, communication, and dissemination of findings, and utilizing results.

Staffing studies to estimate staff requirements are presented in **Figure 25.4**.

Method Study/Work Sampling Study

Method study is also known as a work sampling study. Work study is a detailed study of all activities performed by a person. In addition, observational or activity analysis studies analyze the type of operations performed by nurses of different categories. The methodology used to conduct method study in nursing is as listed below:

1. Select the work/procedure/nursing intervention to be measured
2. Make a list of all activities of the work by reviewing the literature and observing.
3. Breakdown work into steps
4. Examine the steps critically
5. Get it validated from experts

6. Measure the quantity (frequency) of repetitive and nonrepetitive work
7. Compile types of activities performed and group them.

Timed-task/Activity Study Method

Timed-task or time and motion study is a work measurement technique used for recording the time of activities undertaken to perform work. It is a stopwatch time study as using stopwatch is for recording the time. It is the original technique of work measurement and is concerned with direct observation, either participatory or nonparticipatory, of work. The primary purpose of the time study is to determine the time utilized/required to be taken to complete a particular activity. The time study is to determine repetitive work.

The three essentials for conducting time study are as follows: (1) an accurate specification of the work and the method by which it is to be carried out including the details of the equipment used, (2) a system of recording observed actual time taken by staff to do particular activity, and (3) a clear concept of what an average staff can do.

In nursing, based on time study, the hours of work required to meet the patients' caring needs in different categories are calculated. Calculate the average number of nursing hours needed for each category or the standard number of nursing hours for various nursing activities or combinations of these two. The methodology used for the time/activity study is as follows:

Methodology

1. **Identification of ward/unit:** Identify work stations/ward or nursing unit where nurses are working.
2. **Prepare a list of nursing activities:** Prepare a list of nursing care activities from the literature review, review of nursing charts and other documents of patients.
3. **Grouping of activities:** Classify activities by reviewing literature or according to priority. Many studies conducted abroad and in India analyzed the activities of nursing personnel to determine the proportion of time spent by professional nurses with patients and work activities required for their care. These activities have been categorized differently by different researchers and the time taken to carry out activities also differs in different wards.
Nursing activities in one of the World Health Organization (WHO) study by Derbyshire were described and grouped under nine categories according to their sphere of action. There are nine groups, namely patient care primary, patient care complex, administration, education, clerical, housekeeping, maintenance, off-station and nonproductive. Each group activity is further subdivided and described for more precise analysis (Annexure 1 of Chapter 26).
4. **Determine bed occupancy in percentage:** Develop a daily patient census record sheet. Calculate the rate of bed occupancy by dividing the total number of patients who occupied beds during a period of data collection (N) to total beds available during that period (A):

Bed occupancy (%) =
$$\frac{\text{Total number of patient beds occupied during a particular period }(N)}{\text{Total beds available during that period }(A)} \times 100$$

5. **Measure the time required for each nursing activity:** Plan and use either participatory or nonparticipatory observation technique to measure time taken/required to perform a particular activity by selected nurses. Use a stopwatch to record time. Decide the number of observations to make to get the average time for each nursing activity.
   a. Calculate the average time spent in an hour by nurses on various activities by dividing a total number of observations by a number of observations made in 1 hour. The formula applied is:

   $$= \frac{\text{Total number of observations}}{\text{Number of observations in 1 hour}}$$

   Calculate the total time available on various activities on all study days by adding the time spent in hours on all study days.
   b. Find out the average number of daily patients by dividing the number of patient during period of study by study days

   $$= \frac{\text{Total number of patients during the study period}}{\text{Number of study days}}$$

   c. Calculate the time spent by nurses in minutes, by multiplying the total hours spent by nurses for various activities by 60
   = Total hours spent by nurses on various activities × 60
   d. Calculate average time available daily by dividing total minutes spent by the number of days the study was carried out

   $$= \frac{\text{Total minutes spent}}{\text{Number of study days}}$$

   e. Calculate the average time available per day per patient by dividing the average amount of time available daily in minutes by an average number of patients:

   $$= \frac{\text{Total average amount of time available daily in minutes}}{\text{The average number of patients}}$$

Workload Measurement Studies

Workload measurement studies in nursing based on (1) the dependency of ward patients on a certain amount of nursing care in order to perform basic activities of daily living, (2) recording and predicting nursing activities/nursing interventions for individual patients, (3) producing nursing care plans, and (4) bed occupancy or in combinations as

Chapter 25: Fundamentals of Staffing: Staffing, Philosophy, Staffing Study, and Norms

predictors to estimate the number of nurses required in a particular ward.

Hospital Systems Study Group (HSSG) project is one example to measure workload index (WLI) based on the dependency level of patients for the amount of care required. A study conducted on nursing manpower requirement for patients of neurosurgical unit of a referral hospital (Kaur et al. 2009) used dependency of ward patients to perform basic activities of daily living and work sampling and timed-task/activity study to calculate work index in order to estimate nursing manpower required for the unit. The methodology used for the study is as follows:

Methodology

1. Determine patient dependency category by selecting and using the appropriate patient classification tool
2. Obtain an average number of patient in each dependency category
3. Calculate the average time required for each nursing care activity (direct and indirect) in different dependency categories and miscellaneous/ward-related activities
4. Determine the frequency of all nursing activities per day in different dependency categories
5. Determine the total average time required (in minutes) for direct and indirect nursing activities per day in different dependency categories
6. Determine the WLI for any given shift/day:
   - Calculate ratio time (R) between different categories of patients by dividing the total averaging times by the smallest value (d/smallest value from any category)
   - Calculate WLI by multiplying ratio time with an average number of patients per day for different dependency category patients
   - Add up WLI of all different dependency category patients to obtain total WLI of a ward for a day/given shift
7. Convert WLI into staff requirement
   - Calculate total time (in a minute) required to carry out all types of nursing activities for the unit per week
   - Divide total time (in a minute) required to carry out all kinds of nursing activities for the unit per week by 2,400 (40 hours) minutes to obtain a total number of nurses needed
   - Add 30% of the total number of nurses as time out value (offs, leaves, etc.) in the calculated number of nurses required to obtain the entire nursing workforce needed for the unit.

Regression Analysis Studies

Various staffing formulas such as Trent-Senior-Gratton formula, Aberdeen formula, regression analysis methods are used to calculate the workload and to predict staffing requirements. Staffing formulas are statistical methods that aim to predict nurse workforce needs from the measures of activities as a proxy for the workload achieved. Various parameters such as available beds, length of stay and demographic features of the population are used to measure each activity.

STAFFING NORMS AND NORMATIVE APPROACHES

Staffing Norms

Norm is a standard model or pattern that guides, controls, and regulates individuals and communities. These standards or trends are related to staffing and used as measures for forecasting the nursing workforce. These are known as normative methods for calculating nurses required in various hospitals. For estimating the requirement of the nursing workforce, multiple committees, nursing council, associations are recommended, and revised staffing norms are defined from time to time for hospitals, communities, both rural and urban, and nursing institutions in India.

1. **According to the Bhore Committee (1946) report:** According to the Health Survey and Development Committee, that is, Bhore Committee, recommendations, human resources required per nurse population is *one nurse for 500 populations* (targeted for 30 years). The proposed remedy was to reach in due course of time an international standard of one nurse to 2½ beds.
2. **According to Shetty Committee (1954) and Mudaliar Committee (1959–1961) report:** With the initiation of Union Minister of Health, Government of India constituted a committee on May 19, 1954, to review conditions, compensations, etc. of the nursing profession. The recommendation regarding the hospital staffing is one nurse (also qualified in midwifery for women and maternity services), including students, to three patients in hospitals used for training of nurses and midwives excluding the teaching and administrative staff.

    Recommendations of staffing pattern have been endorsed by the Mudaliar Committee (1959–1961) for Auxillary Nurse Midwife (ANM) as ,one ANM for 5,000 population, and for hospitals as mentioned below:
    - One nurse including students: Three patients in teaching hospitals
    - One nurse including students: Five patients in nonteaching hospitals
    - One superintendent for nursing services in each state.
3. **According to the Central Council of Health meeting:** According to the Central Council of Health meeting held at Bombay on October 16–17, 1968, under the agenda No. 13, resolution (No.120) passed regarding nursing workforce that in conformity with the recommendation of Health Survey and Planning Committee and special

TABLE 25.1: Revised prescribed staffing norms for nursing services (teaching hospitals).

Nursing superintendent	One for every hospital with 150 beds
Deputy nursing superintendent	One for every hospital with 150 beds
Assistant nursing superintendent	Two for every hospital with 150 beds For every 50 additional beds, 1 assistant nursing superintendent

Departments	Staff nurse	Sister per shift	Departmental sisters/assistant nursing superintendent
Medical wards	1:3	1:25	One for three to four departments
Surgical wards	1:3	1:25	One for three to four departments
Orthopedic department	1:3	1:25	One for three to four departments
Pediatric ward	1:3	1:25	One for three to four departments
Gynecology ward	1:3	1:25	One for three to four departments
Maternity ward (including newborns)	1:3	1:25	One for three to four wards
Intensive care unit (24 hours)	1:1	One each shift	One Departmental Sisters/ANS for 3-4 units
Coronary care unit (24 hours)	1:1	One each shift	Clubbed together
Nephrology (24 hours)	1:1	One each shift	
Neurology and Neurosurgery (24 hours)	1:1	One each shift	
Special wards—eye, ENT, etc. (24 hours)	1:1	One each shift	Departmental sisters/ANS
Operation theater (24 hours)	Three for 24 hours per table	One each shift One each shift	One departmental sister/ANS for four to five operation theaters
Casualty and emergency unit	Two to three depending on the number of beds	-	One departmental sister/ANS

committees appointed by the Government of India is as given below:
- For teaching hospitals: One nurse (qualified nurse/midwife)—three patients.
- For nonteaching hospitals: One nurse (qualified nurse/midwife)—five patients.

For determining the nurse–patient ratio, nursing staff engaged in teaching and administration, etc. should not be taken into consideration.

4. **According to a Guide for Staffing Pattern:** According to a Guide for Staffing, staffing pattern recommended by the Government of India (1977) is as given below:
   - For 100 beds: 1 matron, 6 sisters and 25 staff nurses.
   - For 300 beds: 1 matron, 1 assistant matron, 17 nursing sisters, and 81 staff nurses.

5. **Recommendations of Indian Nursing Council:** Indian Nursing Council (INC) in 1965–1975 has also recommended staffing pattern for hospitals according to nurse–patient ratio is given below:

   For every 100 beds and to cover 24 hours, the staff should be in the proportion of one sister to 25 beds and one staff nurse to 3 beds in teaching hospitals and one staff nurse to 5 beds in nonteaching hospitals. In addition to the nursing superintendent, there should be one assistant when the bed strength is 150–400 and additional assistant when the bed strength is 401–700 and for every 300 beds over 700. There should be separate staff for special departments with a sister in-charge of operating room and a sister in-charge of casualty department. The outpatient department should have one sister in-charge and a minimum of one staff nurse for each outpatient clinic operated daily, with not less than a total of two in department.

   Table 25.1 shows a revised recommended staffing norms for teaching hospitals (1986) by INC.

TABLE 25.2: Staffing pattern for hospital nursing services per recommendations by the Bajaj Committee, 1987.

Categories	Basis for calculation
Nursing superintendent	1:200 beds
Deputy nursing superintendent	1:300 beds
Department nursing supervisor/sisters	7:1,000 + 1 additional 1,000 beds (991 × 7 + 991)
Ward nursing supervisors/sisters	8:200 + 30% leave reserve
Staff nurses for wards	1:3 (or 1:9 for each shift) + 30% leave reserve
For OPD, blood bank, X-ray, diabetic clinics, etc.	1:100 patients (1 bed: 50 patient) +30% leave reserve
For intensive care units (8 beds ICU/200beds)	1:1 (or 1:3 for each shift) + 30% leave reserve
For specialized departments and clinics such as OT, labor room	8:200 + 30% leave reserve

6. **According to the Bajaj Committee (1987) recommendation:** Table 25.2 presents the workforce requirement for nursing services according to a report of the Expert Committee on Health Manpower Planning, Production and Management, Ministry of Health and Family Welfare, Government of India, New Delhi.

7. **Recommendations of the Staff Inspection Unit (SIU):** Table 25.3 shows the norms according to the recommendations of the SIU, Department of Expenditure, 1992, staffing norms for nurses working in central government hospitals [seven hospitals: Safdarjang Hospital, Dr. Ram Manohar Lohia Hospital, Smt. Sucheta Kriplani Hospital, Kalawati Saran Hospital, all in Delhi; Central Institute of Psychiatry in Ranchi; Jawaharlal Institute of Postgraduate Medical Education and Research (JIPMER) in Pondicherry; and Central Leprosy Teaching and Research Institute (CLTRI), Chengalpattu (Tamil Nadu), all under the administrative control of the Ministry of Health and

TABLE 25.3: Norms for nurses in select central government hospitals.

Normal wards	One staff nurse/nursing sister for every six beds
Special wards Pediatric, burns/burns plastic, neurosurgery, cardiothoracic, neuromedicine, nursing homes, tetanus, spinal injury, emergency wards attached to the casualty	One staff nurse/nursing sister for every four beds
Nursery	One staff nurse/nursing sister for every two beds
ICU/CCU/ICCU, nephrology [Artificial Kidney unit (AKU), dialysis]	One staff nurse/nursing sister for every bed
Labor room	One staff nurse/nursing sister for every labor/table
Major operation theaters	Two staff nurse/nursing sister for every functional operational table including recovery room
Minor operation theaters	Two staff nurse/nursing sister for every functional operational table including recovery room

Casualty
a. Casualty main (attendance up to 100 patients per day)
   After that for every addl. attendance of 35 patients per day
b. Burns (attendance up to 15 patients per day)
   Thereafter for every addl. attendance of 10 patients per day
c. Orthopedics patients (attendance up to 45 patients per day)
   Then for every addl. presence of 15 patients per day
d. Gyne/obstetrics (attendance up to 40 patients per day)
   After that for every addl. attendance of 15 patients per day
	Three staff nurse/nursing sister for 24 hours, i.e. one per shift
	One staff nurse/nursing sister
	Three staff nurse/nursing sister for 24 hours, i.e. one per shift
	One staff nurse/nursing sister
	Three staff nurse/nursing sister for 24 hours, i.e. one per shift
	One staff nurse/nursing sister
	Three staff nurse/nursing sister for 24 hours, i.e. one per shift
	One staff nurse/nursing sister

Injection room outpatient department (OPD)
   Attendance up to 100 patients per day
   Attendance up to 120–220 patients per day
   Attendance up to 221–320 patients per day
   Attendance up to 321–420 patients per day
	One staff nurses
	Two staff nurses
	Three staff nurses
	Four staff nurses

OPD Blood bank, central sample collection center, cardiac lab, bronchoscopy lab, vaccination antirabies, preanesthetic, medical, surgical, dental, eye, ENT, neurology, psychiatry, and OPDS Gyne, family planning, immunization work, pediatric, orthopedic, skin, burns, microbiology infection control, V.D center, and chemotherapy OPDs Obstetric OPD	No. of staff nurse/nursing sister One in each OPD One in each OPD Two in each OPD Three

Note:
1. 10% leave reserve in case maternity leave, earned leave, and days off as nurses are entitled to 8 days off per month and three national holidays per year when doing three-shift duties) and 45% posts reserve, where 365 days in a year/24 hours services provided.
2. The post of nursing sister and staff nurses clubbed together. Both will perform nursing care work.
3. Thirty percent of posts sanctioned as nursing sister. The nursing sister to staff nurse ratio will be 1:3.6.
4. The ratio of assistant nursing superintendent to nursing sisters recommended as 1:4.5. They will work in shift duty.
5. The ratio of deputy nursing superintendent to assistant nursing superintendent is recommended as 1:7.
6. Nursing superintendent: 1 for 250 beds or more.
7. Chief nursing officer: 1 for 500 beds or more.

Family Welfare, Directorate General of Health Services (DGHS)].

8. **Recommendation per High Power Committee on Nursing (1987):** The High Power Committee on Nursing appointed by the Government of India, Ministry of Health and Family Welfare on July 29, 1989 (under the Chairmanship of Smt. Sarojini Vardappan) to review the roles, functions, status, preparation of nursing personnel, nursing services, and other issues related to the development of the profession and to make suitable recommendations to the government. Table 25.4 the shows norms proposed/recommended for nursing services.

TABLE 25.4: Norms proposed for nursing service in the hospital setting by the High Power Committee, 1987.

Nursing superintendent	1:200 beds (hospitals with 200 or more beds)
Deputy nursing superintendent	1: 300 beds
Assistant nursing superintendent	1: 150 (7:1,000 beds)
Ward sister/ward supervisor	1:25 beds + 30% leave reserve
Staff nurse for wards	1:3 (or 1:9 for each shift) + 30% leave reserve
Staff nurses for OPD and emergency, etc.	1 bed: 5 outpatients + 30% leave reserve
For ICU	1:1 (or 1:3 for each shift) + 30% leave reserve
For specialized departments such as operation theater, labor room, etc.	1: 25 + 30% leave reserve

Norms-related Approaches

Consensus Approaches/Delphi Method

It is a method of seeking expert opinions. A panel of experts (Delphi technique) is used to make assumptions on the time required to deliver specific health interventions, given specific technological resources, and at various levels of care, by different professional categories. Consensus approaches are overly subjective. These approaches attempt to take a critical and reflective view of nursing workload and use two methods to estimate staff requirement and also to develop norms as discussed below:

a. **Intuitive methods**: This method refers to as descriptive methodology (Halloran 1987) and a "professional judgment" method (Clay 1987). It is the first and oldest method and widely used to forecast nursing workforce. The intuition or subjective decisions are the basis to calculate appropriate numbers and mix of nursing personnel. This method is simple to use and is suitable for use in all specialties. It takes account of actual workload (planned and unplanned workload, ad hoc activity) during a specific period.

b. **Consultative method:** This method is known as the Telford–Brighton method, which is a mix of Telford and Brighton methods. Telford utilizes the professional views of nurses to determine the number of nurses required to staff a clinical area. Brighton method (Waite and Hirsch 1986) is the extensive work upon Telford method to prove the reliability of professional judgment. This method attempts to synthesize objective and subjective workload-related information to provide more accurate and realistic recommendations.

Staffing Normative Approach

Staffing normative approach is one of the "top-down management approaches." It involves the nationally recognized recommendations that are used as a basis to determine the level of staffing. It examines the relationship between the number of nurses and measure of activity or cost. It may be done based on the calculated health needs of a population or based on historic workforce. It primarily uses norms or recommended standards to plan nurse staffing.

The staffing norm is also known as the normative method. Staff requirement is calculated based on the standards recommended by professional bodies and the committees set for framing the staffing norms. The nurse–patient ratio or nurse–doctor ratio is the basis to formulate the criteria for hospital staffing. For community health services, the health workforce to population ratio is the base. For example, Bhore Committee recommended manpower required per nurse population ratio is 1 nurse for 500 people (targeted for 30 years). This approach of estimating the requirement of workforce is on population or current best region ratio or a reference country. This method is quick, easy to apply and understand but does not provide insights into staff utilization.

Advantages
- This method is relatively easy to use.
- It has consistency due to a lack of subjective measures.
- Consider factors influencing staffing.
- It helps in future planning.

Disadvantages
- It cannot be generalized to all settings.
- It needs the data on the current staffing level.
- It is tough to construct and operate.
- It is sensitive to the number and mix of patients.

Need-based Approach

This approach estimates the future requirements based on estimated health deficit of population as well as on the potential for addressing these deficits using a blend of different health-care human resources to provide the services in efficient ways. Health needs are the deficiencies in health that call for preventive, curative, rehabilitative, or eradication measures. People's needs present as demands. These are due to imbalances or maladjustments in physical, biological, psychological, and social environmental factors.

It projects age- and gender-specific "service needs" based on service norms and morbidity trends and converts projected service needs into workforce/person requirements **(Fig. 25.5)** using *productivity norms and professional judgment* with the following assumptions that:
- Identify and meet all health-care needs
- Identify and implement cost-effective methods to address the needs
- Utilize resources by needs.

Service Target-based Approach

The strategy needs service targets to estimate staff requirements. The experts set targets for the production and delivery of specific outcome-oriented health services. They convert these targets into workforce requirements using *staffing and productivity standards/norms* within a specified period. This approach is relatively easy and understandable.

CHAPTER HIGHLIGHTS

- Staffing defined as the process of procuring, developing, employing, appraising, remunerating and retaining the nursing personnel of various levels.
- Staffing functions/components include manpower planning, recruitment, selection, placement, induction and orientation, training and development, remuneration, performance appraisal, and promotion and transfers.
- Staff planning is the process of estimating the required health workforce to meet future health service requirements and the development of strategies to meet those requirements.

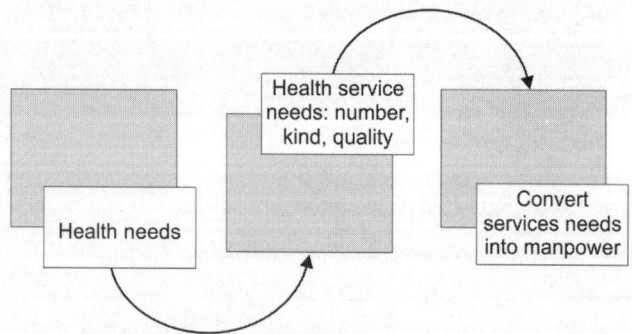

Fig. 25.5: Method of calculating workforce using the need-based approach.

- Staffing based on its philosophy indicates nurses' competency to patient care needs, their role toward critically and chronically ill patients, determining staff requirements and staffing plans.
- Many factors influence workforce planning of community and hospital nursing services. Many approaches such as need-based, utilization-based health workforce to population ratio, service target, normative methods, consensus and top-down and bottom-up approaches are in use to calculate nurses' requirements.
- Staffing study is a systematic and planned process or activity of gathering information and facts about issues related to staffing.
- Staffing norms are standards or patterns related to staffing and used as measures for forecasting the nursing workforce.

REVIEW QUESTIONS

I. Essay Type Questions
1. Define staffing. Describe its nature and importance.
2. Enlist norms-related approaches to estimate staff requirements. Describe any one of the approaches in detail.
3. Define the patient classification system. Describe the various methods of categorizing patients' acuity.
4. Define scheduling. Discuss the steps to be followed while preparing a schedule.
5. Describe the principles of staffing plan.

II. Short Notes
1. Philosophy of staffing
2. Factors affecting the need for safe staffing
3. Timed-task/activity study method
4. Staffing norms
5. Dependency acuity-quality method

III. Multiple Choice Questions
1. A management system built upon sound human organization is:
   a. Planning
   b. Coordination
   c. Staffing
   d. Communication
2. A process of choosing and appointing the right candidates for the right job refers to:
   a. Induction
   b. Recruitment
   c. Placement
   d. Selection
3. Staffing pattern is influenced by job specification because:
   a. It classifies the level of responsibility of each position supported by job description
   b. It is to meet a level of responsibility
   c. It depends on the nature of work
   d. It determines the number and kinds of staff required
4. Which type of staffing study requires an accurate specification of work and method, a system of recording time taken by staff to do a particular job/activity?
   a. Method study
   b. Work measurement study
   c. Activity study
   d. Workload measurement study
5. A formula of multiplying ratio time with the average number of patient per day for different dependency category patients is used to calculate:
   a. Average time spent/patient
   b. Workload index
   c. Patient dependency level
   d. Bed occupancy
6. Staffing norms per the recommendations of Indian Nursing Council to calculate the number of nursing sisters for a hospital is based on one of the following sister and patient ratio of:
   a. 1:10
   b. 1:15
   c. 1:20
   d. 1:25
7. According to the Bajaj Committee recommendations, what percentage is the provision of nurses against leave reserve?
   a. 10%
   b. 20%
   c. 30%
   d. 40%
8. Basic tasks such as hygiene, bathing, dressing, toileting, and eating are grouped under:
   a. Self-care deficit
   b. Activities of daily living
   c. Dependency level of patient
   d. Nursing care intensity
9. The patient classification system that comprises patient categorization, activity study, staffing situation, and quality of nursing care is known as:
   a. Hospital Systems Study Group (HSSG)
   b. Oulu Patient Classification system
   c. RAFELA Patient Classification System
   d. Zebra System of Patient Classification
10. How many days/weeks/months in advance a duty roster should be prepared and made available to staff?
    a. 7–10 days
    b. 2–4 weeks
    c. 3–4 months
    d. 4–6 months

Answer Keys
1. c 2. d 3. a 4. c 5. b 6. d 7. c
8. b 9. d 10. b

SUGGESTED READING
1. [PDF]Determining Hospital Workforce Requirements - World Health ... (online) Avaialble from https://www.who.int › hrh › HRDJ_3_3_05. [Accessed on 08.01.2020].
2. Anthony MK, Theresa S, Glick J, Duffy M, Paschall F. Leadership and nurse retention: the pivotal role of nurse managers. J Nurs Adm. 2005;35(3):146-55.
3. Available from https://rcni.com/nursing-standard/newsroom/news/low-nurse-staffing-levels-put-patients-greater-risk-of-death-study-warns-83841. [Accessed March, 2018].

4. Berkow S, Jaggi J, Fogelson R, et al. Fourteen unit attributes to guide staffing. J Nurs Adm. 2007;37(3):150-5.
5. Beyers M. Nurse executives' perspectives on succession planning. J Nurs Adm. 2006;36(6):304-12.
6. Blegen MA, Goode C J, Reed L. Nurse staffing and patient outcomes. Nurs Res. 1998;47(1):43-50.
7. Clay T. Nurses: power and politics. Heinemann Nursing, London, 1987. (Cross reference) (online) Available from https://www.academia.edu/10078940/Determining_nurse_staffing_levels_a_critical_review_of_the_literature. [Accessed on 08.01.2020].
8. Donald WS. Rational staffing of hospital nursing services by functional activity budgeting. Public Health Rep. 1976;91(2):119-21.
9. Halloran EJ, Variability in nurse staffing research. Journal of Nursing Administration 1987; 17: 26-32 (Cross reference) (online) Available from https://www.academia.edu/10078940/Determining_nurse_staffing_levels_a_critical_review_of_the_literature. [Accessed on 08.01.2020].
10. High Power Committee on Nursing and the Nursing Profession. [online] Available from http://www.communityhealth.in/~commun26/wiki/images/b/bd/High_Power_Committee_on_Nursing_and_Nursing_Profession_report_1989.PDF.pdf. [Accessed on 08.01.2020].
11. High Power Committee on Nursing in India. [online] Available from https://www.nursingpath.in/2013/04/high-power-committee-on-nursing-in-india.html. [Accessed on 08.01.2020].
12. ICN. Safe staffing saves lives. 2006. ICN. [Online] Available from www.icn.ch. [Accessed on March 2019].
13. Kaur R, Vati J, Chhabra R. An exploratory study on "nursing manpower" requirement for patients of a neurosurgical unit of Nehru Hospital, PGIMER, Chandigarh, 2008–2009. Unpublished Master's Thesis; 2009.
14. Kaur R, Vati J, Chhabra R. Exploratory study on "nursing manpower' requirement for patients of neurosurgical unit. Nursing & Midwifery Research Journal. April 2010;6(2): 58-70
15. Koontz H, Weihrich H. Essentials of Management: An International Perspective, 1st edition. New Delhi, India: Tata McGraw Hill Publishers; 2007.
16. Lanksbear AJ, Sheldon TA, Maynard A. Nurse staffing and health care outcomes: A systematic review of the international research evidence. Adv Nurs Sci. 2005;28(2):163-73.
17. Nurse Staffing - American Nurses Association, (online) Available from https://www.nursingworld.org › practice-policy › nurse-staffing. [Accessed on 08.01.2020].
18. Paetznick MA. Guide for staffing a hospital nursing service. Geneva: WHO Publication; No. 23; 1966.
19. Patient Classification Systems in Nursing: A Description and ... (online) Available from https://books.google.co.in › books. [Accessed on 08.01.2020].
20. Sharma NB, Vati J, Saini SK. A study on the utilization of morning duty hours and influencing environmental stimuli of the operational level nurses working in selected wards of Nehru hospital PGIMER, Chandigarh, 2001. Unpublished Master's Thesis; 2001.
21. Telford WA. A method of determining nursing establishments. East Birmingham Health District, Birmingham, 1979. (Cross reference) (online) Available from https://www.academia.edu/10078940/Determining_nurse_staffing_levels_a_critical_review_of_the_literature. [Accessed on 08.01.2020].
22. Vati J. Organisation and administration of nursing services in district hospitals of North India. Unpublished Ph.D. Thesis. Faculty of Medical Sciences, Panjab University, Chandigarh, India; 1990.
23. Waite R, Hirsch W. Not another dependency study. Senior Nurse 1986; 4(1): 29-32. (Cross reference) (online) Available from https://www.academia.edu/10078940/Determining_nurse_staffing_levels_a_critical_review_of_the_literature. [Accessed on 08.01.2020].

26. Nursing Activities, Patient Classification System, and Scheduling

CHAPTER OUTLINE

- Nursing Activities and and Activity-based Approaches
  - Nursing Activities
  - Activities-based Approaches/Methods
- Patient Classification System and Patient Dependency-related Approaches
  - Patient Classification System
  - Patient Dependency-related Approaches
- Scheduling
  - Definitions
  - Importance of Scheduling
  - Objectives
  - Principles of Scheduling
  - Type of Scheduling
  - Types of Scheduling Plans
  - Preparing a Time Schedule

LEARNING OUTCOMES

After completion of this chapter, the learner will be able to:
- Enlist the nursing activities and related approaches
- Discuss patients' classification system
- Describe scheduling, its objectives, and principles
- Appreciate the importance of scheduling
- Prepare time schedules

KEY TERMS

Nursing activities, patient classification system, scheduling

INTRODUCTION

Nursing is a unique profession as it addresses the responses of individuals and families to health promotions, health maintenance, and health problems. Nursing is an applied science and also an art, which provides skilled care for the sick in an appropriate relationship with the patient, family, and physician and with others who have related responsibilities.

According to Biddle, 1979, roles are sets of patterned behaviors unique to a given position, and position denotes status or place within a specified context such as a healthcare organization. These are sets of the contract between employees and employers. Professional nurses assume multiroles and have multiresponsibilities in different settings, different specialties, and indifferent diversity of nursing.

NURSING ACTIVITIES AND ACTIVITY-BASED APPROACHES

Nursing Activities

The literature revealed that various studies conducted on nursing activities from time to time. In most studies, the researchers used activity sampling and work measurement techniques. Most of these studies revealed that nurses render nursing care activities. **Table 26.1** shows the studies carried out on activities.

Kalara had classified nursing activities as patient care activities, nonproductive, and administrative activities that are carried out by nurses. A similar study by Ranga Idiculla had classified nursing activities as patient-centered activities and unit-centered activities. Ratni Thassu had discussed these activities as nursing activities and nonnursing activities. A similar classification of activity is documented by Raghava Rao, Dhaulta, Dube, and Joseph.

A WHO study conducted by Derbyshire described and grouped nursing activities under nine categories according to their sphere of action. There are nine groups, namely patient care, basic, patient care, complex, administration, education, clerical, housekeeping, maintenance, off-station, and nonproductive. Each group activity is further subdivided for a more precise analysis (Annexure 1). It revealed that more than 50% of the nursing care activities were the patient care complex. Patient care and basic,

TABLE 26.1: Studies carried out in India on nursing activities.

S. No.	Author, Year	Activities observed
1.	Kalara (1960)	Patient care, clerical activities, nonproductive, and administrative
2.	Idiculla (1966)	Patient-centered activities, unit centered, personnel centered other activities
3.	I Ranga (1966)	Patient care, clerical, housekeeping, nonproductive
4.	Darby Shire (1969)	The patient care, complex, a patient care, basic, maintaining supply and equipment, nonproductive activities, clerical, housekeeping, and administrative
5.	Ratni Thassu (1970) Raghva Rao (1973) Dhaulta (1975) Dube (1975), and Joseph (1982)	Nursing activities and nonnursing activities
6.	Chandrakanta (1973)	A patient care, essential nursing activities, nonessential activities, off station, and nonproductive activities
7.	Srinivasan (1982)	➤ A basic patient care, complex patient care, administration, clerical, housekeeping, maintaining supply, and equipment ➤ The off station, nonproductive
8.	Bobdey (1992)	➤ Productive activities ➤ Nonproductive activities
9.	Sharma (2001)	➤ A basic patient care, complex patient care, administration, clerical, housekeeping, maintaining supply and equipment ➤ The off station, nonproductive

were found to be carried out very less. However, other miscellaneous activities added up to almost half of the total activities carried out by nurses.

The activity sampling technique used by Bobdey in a 43-bedded subacute family ward of a large hospital showed that out of the 334 activities observed. Nursing activities classified under nonproductive and productive activities. It revealed that 78 (23.3%) activities were nonproductive, and 256 (76.7%) were productive. Out of the productive activities, 148 (43.3%) were on direct patient care, i.e. 46 (31.1%) on carrying out technical procedures, 36 (24.32%) for determining patient's needs, 20 (13.15%) for preparing patients for various procedures, and 15 (10.14%) for assisting in technical procedures.

Chandrakanta categorized observed nursing activities carried out by nurses as patient care activities, essential nursing activities, nonessential activities, off station, and nonproductive activities. Srinivasan had classified activities under the subheadings of basic patient care activities and complex patient care activities.

Another study conducted by Vati in four district hospitals of North India documented that more than 75% of bedside nurses perceived their activities as related to medical care as to nursing care of patients. She also expressed that nurses do patient care activities and nonnursing activities almost equally.

Sharma (2001) in her study classified nursing activities under headings of basic patient care, complex patient care, administration, clerical, housekeeping, maintaining supply and equipment, off station, and nonproductive.

Activity-based Approaches/Methods

Activity-based approaches are used to determine the type of activities performed by nurses, and the time required to carry out those activities to estimate nursing workforce requirement is as follows:

Timed-task/Activity Method

Time-task/activity method is one of the "Bottom-up" approaches to determine staffing levels or requirements from local, ward-level information. This approach is used to level and type of nursing intervention/activity as the method of measuring workload.

The time task/activity method is a nursing intervention method. It comprises some form of *work/activity sampling* and *time and motion studies*. The predictor of staffing requirements in this method is the frequency of the nursing interventions required by patients. Each patient's direct nursing care needs for the day observed and recorded on a developed checklist of nursing intervention sheet, and each nursing intervention is paired with a locally agreed time required for its completion. It added an allowance for related indirect care and rest time.

An example of this method is GRASP [Grace Reynolds Application of the Study of PETO (Poland, English, Thornton, and Owens) group] system. In this system, a nurse prepares a list of patient's needs and then weighted each item according to the timing of the required tasks. World Health Organization (WHO) also conducted an activity time study on nurses and developed a guide to the study of activities of health personnel.

The methodology used in various studies conducted on time required for multiple activities by nurses in different units (**Table 26.1** and timed-task/activity studies section) and used to calculate staff requirements in India.

Methodology
a. **Prepare a list of activities performed by nurses:** Develop a list of activities performed in a particular unit by reviewing literature, observing charts of patients, and getting experts' opinions. Use after validation.
b. **Study nursing activities:** Observe activities performed daily, weekly, and monthly by and record in a sheet developed for recording.
c. **Observe the time required for each activity:** Use observation technique to measure the time needed for each activity by using the stopwatch. Take many observations to calculate the average time for each nursing activity.
d. **Determine the frequency of each nursing activity:** Record frequency of each activity required by observing the patients during data collection, review of charts, and by getting experts' opinions.

e. **Calculate staffing requirement:** Calculate staffing requirement by the following steps given below:
- Compile the average time and standard deviation for each activity
- Multiply the frequency of each activity with the average time to get the normal time to perform various activities per day
- Calculate total normal time in minutes to complete all activities per week by multiplying total standard time with 40 hours per International Labour Organization (ILO) recommendation [Normal Time (NT)]
- Calculate standard time (ST) by adding 10% allowance time of NT in calculated NT
- Calculate the required nursing workforce by dividing ST by 40 hours and add 30% leave reserve per norms for staffing.

Strengths
- This approach is suitable to be developed for most areas.
- The standards are the part of quality, and the guidelines are specific for best practice according to specialty.
- It requires a calculator that automatically works out staffing needs based on workload entered into the system.
- This method can be developed into a multiprofessional and multidisciplinary workload as well.

Weaknesses
- This method is time consuming and expensive.
- Number of observations are required.
- It is a task-oriented approach.

Utilization-based Approach

A baseline for estimating future requirements is the quality, mix, and population distribution of the current level of healthcare resource utilization. The level of usage of the current workforce is expressed with future projections of the demographic profile of the population subgroup-specific rates of provider utilization with the following assumptions:
- If current level, mix, and distribution of health services are appropriate.
- Age- and sex-specific requirements remain constant in the future.
- Size and demographic profile of the population changes in ways predictable by observed trends in age- and sex-specific rates of mortality, fertility, and migration.

Nurses Per Occupied Bed Approach

An average nurse per occupied bed (NPOB) is another commonly used method of determining ward staffing.

Methodology

A: **Calculate the average number of working hours per week per nurse**

- *Step 1:* Find out the average number of days worked (working days) per year by the bedside nurse designated as a staff nurse.
  No. of average working days = 365 − average number of leave days*
- *Step 2:* Find out the number of available nurses per day throughout the year
  Number of available nurses per day throughout the year
  $$= \frac{\text{No. of average working days} \times \text{Number of bedside nurses in position in that unit}}{365}$$
- *Step 3:* Find out the number of nurses working in the morning, evening, and night duty
  Per policy of the hospital or arbitrary calculate the number of nurses in the ratio of 3:2:1 or 1:1:1 in the morning, evening, and night duty, respectively.
  If there is a fixed number of nurses posted in the evening and night duty, then:
  Number of nurses available in the morning shift = Total no. of nurses − Number of nurses in the evening and night duty or Divide number of nurses in the ratio of 3:2:1 or 1:1:1 (or as the hospital policy) in the morning, evening, and night shift respectively.
- *Step 4:* Find out the total available working hours per shift per year
  The working hours of the morning, evening, and night duty vary according to the hospital policy; it may be a straight shift of 8 hours or 6, 6, and 12 hours or split shift.
  Total available working hours in the morning shift in a year = Number of hours (duration) in the morning shift × Number of nurses available in the morning shift × 365
  ◆ Total available working hours in the evening shift in a year = Number of hours (duration) in the evening shift × Number of nurses available in the evening shift × 365
  ◆ Total available working hours in the night shift in a year = Number of hours (duration) in the night shift × Number of nurses available in the night shift × 365
- *Step 5:* Find out the total available working hours in a year
  Total available working hours in a year = Total available working hours in the morning shift in a year + total available working hours in the evening shift in a year + total available working hours in the night shift in a year
- *Step 6:* Find out the average number of working hours per week per nurse
  The average number of working hours per week per nurse
  $$= \frac{\text{Available working hours in a year}}{52 \times \text{Number of available nurses per day throughout the year}}$$

---
* Leave days include earned leaves, casual leaves, holidays if applicable, regular day offs

B: **Calculate nurse–patient ratio or number of patients per bedside nurse**

Follow 1, 2, and 3 steps as mentioned earlier.
- *Step 4:* Find out the nurse–patient ratio for each shift
  - Nurse patient ratio in the morning shift = No. of nurses in the morning shift: Total no. of patients
  - Nurse patient ratio in the evening shift = No. of nurses in the evening shift: Total no. of patients
  - Nurse patient ratio in the night shift = No. of nurses in the night shift: Total no. of patients

C: **Calculate the maximum nursing time available per patient per nurse per shift**

Follow all the steps of calculating the nurse–patient ratio and then calculate:

The maximum nursing time (in minutes) available per patient per nurse in the morning shift

$$= \frac{\text{Duration of the morning shift} \times 60}{\text{No. of patient per nurse in the morning shift}}$$

The maximum nursing time (in minutes) available per patient per nurse in the evening shift

$$= \frac{\text{Duration of the evening shift} \times 60}{\text{No. of patient per nurse in the evening shift}}$$

The maximum nursing time (in minutes) available per patient per nurse in the night shift

$$= \frac{\text{Duration of the evening shift} \times 60}{\text{No. of patient per nurse in the night shift}}$$

D: **Find out the desired number of nurses**

Calculate the desired number of nurses by abstracting available nurses from nurses required per norms or professional judgment method.

Strengths
- The NPOB method is useful for change in the ward bed complement.
- Applicable in all settings.
- A simple approach to demand-side workforce planning.
- It derives staffing and grade-mix formulas empirically.
- The data quickly be built into a computerized spreadsheet.

Weaknesses
- This method assumes that the base staffing data are rationally determined.
- Staffing formulas are insensitive to dependency changes.
- It is a costly affair to update formulas.
- It contains data such as bed occupancies, which is more error prone.

Adjusted Service-target Approach

This approach is an *activity method* to estimate the workforce required, especially for community health services. Various steps are undertaken to determine manpower requirement such as (1) identify service needs based on epidemiological and demographic profile and programmatic targets, (2) identify tasks and skills required to deliver interventions for specific programs, based on the functional job analysis, (3) estimate time required for each intervention by conducting time-motion studies or by getting expert opinion, and (4) translating time required into adjusted full-time equivalents, based on productivity.

PATIENT CLASSIFICATION SYSTEM AND PATIENT DEPENDENCY-RELATED APPROACHES

Patient Classification System

The patient classification system (PCS) is the method or system of grouping patients. These are used to measure nursing workload. Workload requirements are mainly dependent on the dependency of patients on a certain amount of care in performing basic activities of daily living (ADL). There are many ways of grouping patients admitted in hospital. According to the available literature, the patients' classification system is per their diagnosis, treatment, DGR, blood group, demographic factors, and also according to the nursing intensity or severity of diseases. Patient classification system is a method of categorizing patients admitted to the hospital on the specific criteria.

Definitions

According to Giovannetti (1979), patient classification is the categorization of patients according to the individual assessment of their nursing care requirements over a specified period. It is the identification and classification of patients into care groups or categories to measure or quantify nursing efforts required. Patient classification system is the patient acuity system used to manage workload and also to quantify patient care needs to estimate the number of staff required for each patient (Shaha, 1995).

Objectives of PCS

The list below shows the objectives of PCS:
1. To measure nursing efforts required to:
   - Calculate the workload and develop workload index: quantification of levels of care
   - Identify the needs of patients according to the severity of their illness
   - Calculate the number and level of staff required to meet the diverse needs of patients.
2. It is a tool to assign the daily float staff.
3. It helps to prepare a budget in long-term planning.
4. It is used for special management reports, quality assurance, and utilization review.
5. It is used to measure the efficiency of nurse managers in matching workload requirements on a daily, monthly, and annual basis.
6. It provides a rationale for nursing changes.

7. It is used to assess the quality and quantity of the care supplied and establish priorities for improvement.
8. To justify staffing ratio.

Characteristics of PCS

Following are the characteristics of PCS:
- PCS should be simple.
- It should be specific and need oriented.
- It should be auditable and individualized.
- It should be time bound.
- It should be reversible.

Methods of Categorizing Patients

The following methods are used to categorize the patients:

1. **Diagnosis-related group method**: The patients are classified based on the diagnosis of patients in diagnosis-related group (DRG) PCS. Cambell et al. (1997) and Neeleman et al. (2002) used this method to categorize patients for nurse staffing purposes.
2. **ADL method:** According to this method, patients are classified for their dependency level from the least (Group 1) to the most dependent (Group 4) on nurses for their ADL. Activities of daily living include bathing, dressing, getting in and out of bed or chair using the toilet, and eating. The hygiene, bathing, dressing, toileting, and feeding are the basic needs of each individual. There are many tools; rating scales are developed to measure the dependency level of patients based on ADLs.

    Katz's index is an example of categorizing patients. This scale has six activities—bathing, dressing, toileting, transferring, continence, and feeding. Assign one score for independency and 0 for dependency with a score range from 0 = low (patient very dependent) to 6 = high (patient independent).

    Manjit and Vati (2004) developed a self-care-deficit assessment scale related to ADL related to personal care is another example of categorizing the dependency level of all medical and surgical adult patients **(Table 26.2)**.

The scale has four activities of personal care, i.e. feeding, bathing, dressing, and toileting (defecation). These areas of personal care are the indicators of patients' classification for requiring care. Each area of care further comprises four determiners each to categorize patient's self-care deficit/degree of dependency for nursing care from 1 to 4. The patient may fall from 1 to 4 against each component; thus, total scores for all components range from 1 to 16. Based on the scores, the patient can categorize as follows:

Score 4:	Category 1	Independent/No self-care deficit
Scores 5–8:	Category 2	Mildly dependent/mild self-care deficit
Scores 9–12:	Category 3	Moderately dependent/moderate self-care deficit
Scores 13–16:	Category 4	Fully dependent/severe self-care deficit

3. **Nursing care intensity method:** Patient grouping is according to the amount of nursing care required based on the individual caring needs of the patients daily. Many scales are developed to quantify nursing care intensity (NCI) on selected parameters. Significant components of care to assess the amount of nursing care requirements are personal care, feeding, observation, ambulation, and others.

A sample of patient classification tool for neurosurgical patients developed (Kaur & Vati, 2009) based on K Hurst's adult and children ADL and critical care classification dependency tool. It has six components: level of consciousness, nutrition, and risk of developing bedsore, personal hygiene, elimination, and mobility **(Box 26.1)**.

These components of nursing care are the indicators of patients' classification for the requirement for nursing care. Each component of care further comprises four determiners each to categorize a patient's degree of dependency for nursing care from 1 to 4. The patient may fall from 1 to 4 against each component; thus, total scores

TABLE 26.2: Dependency/self-care-deficit assessment scale.

Area of care	Category 1	Category 2	Category 3	Category 4
Feeding	Patient feeds himself or herself independently or if provided articles for food	Can feed himself or herself but needs supervision during feeding	Needs help and assistance throughout the feeding	Nurse/relative administer feeding
Bathing	Takes a bath independently or if articles provided	Can wash some parts of the body but requires assistance for a complete bathing	Nurse/relative sponges the patient, but the patient follows the direction	No effort by the patient when the nurse/relative sponges the patient
Dressing	Patient dresses herself independently or if one provides clothes	Dresses herself but needs assistance	Nurse/relative dresses the patient with his or her cooperation	No efforts from the patient when nurse/relative dresses the patient
Toileting (defecation)	Uses the toilet, bedpan, commode, chair independently	Needs assistance in undressing and dressing for toileting	Needs continuous supervision and help during toileting	Nurse/relative does complete toileting care
Score interpretation	Score: 4 Independent/no self-care deficit	Score: 5–8 Mildly dependent/mild self-care deficit	Score: 9–12 Moderately dependent/moderate self-care deficit	Score: 13–16 Fully dependent/severe self-care deficit

> **Box 26.1:** Patient Classification Tool.
>
> (for neurosurgical adult patients)   Score
>
> **A. LEVEL OF CONSCIOUSNESS (LOC)** ☐
> 1. Patient responds spontaneously
> 2. The patient responds but takes a long time
> 3. The patient responds to painful stimuli
> 4. The patient does not respond at all
>
> **B. NUTRITION (N)** ☐
> 1. Patient feeds himself independently on serving a meal
> 2. The patient can feed himself but need supervision
> 3. Needs help and assistance to eat and drink
> 4. Dependent on care for eating and drinking (Ryle's tube feed/intravenous)
>
> **C. RISK OF DEVELOPING BEDSORE (BS)** ☐
> 1. Low-risk (ambulatory patient)
> 2. Moderate risk (need assistance in changing position)
> 3. High-risk (need every 2 hourly skincare)
> 4. Already having a bedsore
>
> **D. PERSONAL HYGIENE (PH)** ☐
> 1. The patient takes a bath independently
> 2. Needs assistance in taking a bath
> 3. Nurse/relative sponges the patient, but the patient follows directions (need one carer)
> 4. No efforts by the patient when the nurse sponges patient (need two carers)
>
> **E. ELIMINATION (E)** ☐
> 1. Uses the toilet, commode chair independently
> 2. Needs help in using the toilet
> 3. Need assistance in passing urine and stool in bed in the bedpan
> 4. Patient is incontinent / catheterized
>
> **F. MOBILITY (M)** ☐
> 1. The patient is independent—attendant present
> 2. Needs help to walk or move around
> 3. Two carers needed to help the patient walk or move around
> 4. The patient is immobile
>
> TOTAL SCORE _____ CATEGORY _____
> RATINGS
> Score < 7:   Category 1 Independent
> Scores 7–11:   Category 2 Between dependent and independent
> Scores 12–19:   Category 3 Dependent
> Score > 19:   Category 4 Fully dependent

components of nursing care are the indicators of patients' classification for the requirement for nursing care. Each element of care further comprises determiners to categorize the patient's degree of dependency for nursing care. After getting information, classify patients into four categories:

a. **Category 1 (self-care or minimum care):** The patient is physically capable of caring for himself but requires minimal support plus treatments or monitoring.
b. **Category 2 (average/moderate care):** The patient requires an average amount of nursing care and medical support.
c. **Category 3 (above average/maximum care):** Patient requires a higher than average amount of care, medical support, and use of special equipment.
d. **Category 4 (intensive care):** The patient requires very frequent to continuous intensive nursing care and close supervision by medical personnel with support from technical equipment.

Oulu Patient Classification

Oulu patient classification (OPC) was developed based on the HSSG patient classification in Finland. It has six subscales: (a) planning and coordination of nursing care; (b) breathing, blood circulation, and symptoms of the disease; (c) nutrition and medication; (d) personal hygiene and secretion; (e) activity, sleep, and rest; and (f) teaching, guidance, and follow-up care, emotional support. Each subarea is having one score and measured in 4 points as given below:

1. **Category A (=1 point):** Patient who manages relatively well on his or her own.
2. **Category B (=2 points):** Patient who requires nursing care occasionally.
3. **Category C (=3 points):** Patient who has repeated need for care.
4. **Category D (=4 points):** The care needs of the patient who cannot manage unaided at all.

The total score can vary between 6 and 24 points per patient. Calculate the Nursing Care Intensity (NCI) by adding scores of all patients. Divide the overall NCI score by the number of nurses to obtain NCI (OPC) per nurse. This tool further modified by using the "Professional Assessment of Optimal Nursing Care Intensity Level" (PAONCIL) scale.

RAFAELA Patient Classification

RAFAELA patient classification system is based on initials of the research team who developed the system (the names are not disclosed)
The system comprises of three measurement tools:
1. Oulu patient classification based on the individual caring needs of patients daily.
2. Daily data of nursing resources that include the number of nurses for one day (one nurse =8 hours/day).
3. Professional Assessment of Optimal Nursing Care Intensity Level (PAONCIL) scale: Assess the value of

for all components range from 1 to 24. Based on the scores, the patient can be categorizing as follows:

Score < 7:	Category 1	Independent
Scores 7–11:	Category 2	Between dependent and independent
Scores 12–19:	Category 3	Dependent
Score > 19:	Category 4	Fully dependent

Types of Patient Classification Systems

The list below shows the types of patient classification systems (PCSs):

Hospital Systems Study Group PCS

Canadian Hospital Systems Study Group (HSSG) PCS provides an objective method of daily categorizing of hospital patients. Classification of patients is based on the need of patients for nursing care. It comprises four major components, i.e. personal care, feeding, observation, and ambulation and the other two parts, i.e. regarding incontinence, and surgery if the need arises. These

the optimum nursing care intensity level of the ward by administering PAONCIL measurement to each nurse in every shift for 1 month to gather their opinion in three-point scale regarding workload as optimal (=0), above optimal (>0), and below optimal (<0). Calculate daily NCI value per nurse and compare it with the average NCI values of the same day. Calculate the optimal NCI per nurse of the ward by using linear regression analysis. Other information, such as length of stay, diagnosis, and Diagnosed Related Groups (DRGs).

Zebra System of Patient Classification

Levenstam and Berrgborn Engberg (1993, 2003) developed the zebra system of patient classification tool. It comprises four parts: the patient classification, the activity study as validation system, the staffing situation, and the quality of nursing care.

Patient classification encompasses four components: hygiene, nutrition, observation, mobilization, uncontrolled output (elimination), and specific need of care. Each has one to three determinators (A=minimal care, B=average care, C=intense care) to assess the dependency level and the level of direct care given. Assess patients for hygiene, observation, mobilization, and rest if the need arises.

Measure each combination of determinators in one to four categories of direct nursing care. Measure the total time of nursing care per patient and type of care required per patient by conducting time studies and using questionnaires. Calculate the workload and express under four categories and average time spent on that category.

Patient Dependency-related Approaches

Dependency-activity-quality (Acuity-quality) Method

An acuity-quality method is especially useful in nursing wards having fluctuation in bed occupancy and workload. The main aim of using this method is to balance the available nursing hours with the required hours and to staff the nursing wards during peak hours. It needs the data on:

1. **Patient dependency:** Grouping of patients in some ways according to the certain criteria.
2. **Nursing activity:** Pair dependency ratings with nursing and midwifery times for a patient in a dependency group, to work out the total amount of nursing time required to meet the demands of all patients in a nursing ward. Carry out activity sampling by splitting nursing time between patient care and other work.

Advantages

1. It is the most suitable method for use in inpatient areas where patient numbers and workload fluctuates.
2. Its utility is in adult and children inpatient settings including medical and surgical units.
3. The tool comprises three measures: patient dependency, activity, and quality.

4. Bed occupancy and actual patient dependency are significant to calculate staffing levels in Whole Time Equivalents (WTEs).

Weaknesses

1. The formula is more complex to construct and operate as compared to the professional judgment and NPOB staffing formulas.
2. One has to accept the daily direct care minutes for each dependency category. Otherwise, one can obtain local nursing activity values.
3. It requires computer software to enter data in spreadsheets and for calculations.

The Regression Method

The regression method aims to predict nurses' requirements according to the level of activity. These are two variables. The nurses' requirement depends on the level of activity required per patient and calculated using the regression method of statistics. The other independent variable may be bed occupancy, type of patients, type of hospital, etc.

Strengths

- The regression method is useful for situations where predictions are possible, such as the number of planned admissions.
- It helps managers to forecast and prepare for extra demands.
- It is easy to collect the data either from the same wards or other wards.
- It is a useful method with limited resources as compared to full dependency-activity quality or a timed-task/activity study.
- This method is more valid, reliable, and usable than the detailed and expensive acuity-quality and timed-task/activity methods.
- It is easy to test staffing recommendations for accuracy.

Weaknesses

- The knowledge and skills of a statistician will be needed to frame design, methodology, and type of data required to collect that should be the most appropriate data for the regression analysis.
- Data should be such that one can measure it on interval or ratio scales.

SCHEDULING

Nurses being an integral part of the health team have a significant contribution in providing the nursing care throughout 24 hours of a day. They need to work in shifts. The patterns of shift vary from one hospital to another, depending on the need of the institution. Usually, the hospitals follow three shifts, i.e. morning, evening, and night shifts. Staff scheduling is a challenging job for a nurse manager due to a shortage of nursing personnel and to have the unit productivity and nurses' morale high. It has become essential to create optimized schedules to keep nurses happy and content with their shift assignments.

Definition

Scheduling is one aspect of the staffing function. It is a roaster plan or time planning. It is an advanced pattern of on and off duty hours for nursing personnel in a particular unit, section, or division. It is a method of arranging the time for the staff to work.

- A schedule is a timetable showing planned work days and shifts for nursing personnel.
- Staff scheduling consists of assigning hours of work, place of work, and work role for a group of workers over weeks and months. It includes a length of shift and the type of rotation.
- A schedule/roster is a plan showing on and off duty periods for staff within a defined area, such as a nursing ward or community locality. Duty roasting is about matching staff to workload needs, and the plan should, therefore, reflect the peaks and troughs of expected workload, ensuring staff is available at the times they are required.

Importance of Scheduling

Scheduling and shift patterns are an extremely significant aspect of managing any team or department (Walker et al., 2006). According to Wells (2007), to adjust the "off duty" can be one of the most stressful and time-consuming tasks to a nurse manager. Adequate staffing in all shifts influences the quality of care of patients. Scheduling affects patient care and welfare of staff. Placing the right number of staff and skill mix at the correct times is vital to the smooth and safe running of a nursing ward or department.

Objectives

The objectives of scheduling are as follows:
- To ensure a safe and appropriate skill mix 24 hours a day and across all shifts to deliver a high standard of care
- To comply with good personnel practices
- To maintain morale high among staff.

Principles of Scheduling

Following are the principles of scheduling:
1. Scheduling must have a base on clear protocols (policy/rules).
2. The schedule should minimize variability in the ratio of staff size to workload at every level.
3. Make sure to staff each shift adequately; each shift requires the right number of nurses and nursing staff with the right combination of health-care skills.
4. It must ensure continuous coverage for patient care.
5. It should provide a means of making quick staffing adjustments during emergencies.
6. It should be prepared and available to staff 2/4 weeks in advance.
7. Distribute holidays evenly throughout the year.
8. There should be an even distribution of senior staff throughout the week and weekends.
9. Distribute holidays, vacation time, and days off equally among all employees in the interest of fairness.
10. There should be an equitable distribution of desirable and undesirable hours for staff satisfaction.
11. All wards to have a flow chart of how to cover the department if the staff goes off sick.
12. Nursing supervisor must keep clear records of the scheduling plan as it is a legal document showing when and who was working.
13. Review methods of rostering and shift patterns regularly.

Types of Scheduling

Scheduling is of two types, which are as follows:

Centralized Scheduling

In a centralized scheduling system, the nurse administrator prepares the schedule in her office and is responsible for scheduling both the staff members, who are permanently assigned to each unit and also required to make at the time of need in other units. Float (on-call) staff has to be there to fill in wherever there is a shortage.

Decentralized Scheduling

When the head nurse of each unit or supervisor of each section prepares time schedules for the nurses assigned to that unit that is independent of personnel schedules prepared by other head nurses. In this system, it is difficult to equalize staff across the unit, so the central nursing office provides and maintains a pool of "float" (on-call) personnel.

Types of Schedule Plans

A scheduled plan is also known as a rotation plan. These are of two types:

Master Schedule/Master Rotation Plan

A master plan for the nursing service of the hospital in totality depicts unit-wise/shift-wise and week/month-wise in case a centralized scheduling pattern (**Fig. 26.1**).

Figure 26.1 depicts a graphic presentation of the evening duty rotation plan of nurses working in a district hospital having 65 nurses' strength. Master rotation plan is prepared by head of nursing services for the nurses to work in all wards in such a way that to get an equal number of evening duties on rotation. Of 65, 60 nurses are assigned to do evening duties in the wards subsequently for consecutive 15 days with 2 or 3 days off (per hospital policy) in between, and during day offs, they are supposed to be relieved by evening reliever nurses. Thus each nurse will do 6.5 months evenings in 29 months of a year in the wards. Out of the rest, the head nurse assigns five nurses on rotation to evening duties in operation theatres. They assigned to do evening duties as one nurse for consecutive 15 days with two day offs. During days off, they are supposed to be relieved by day nurses.

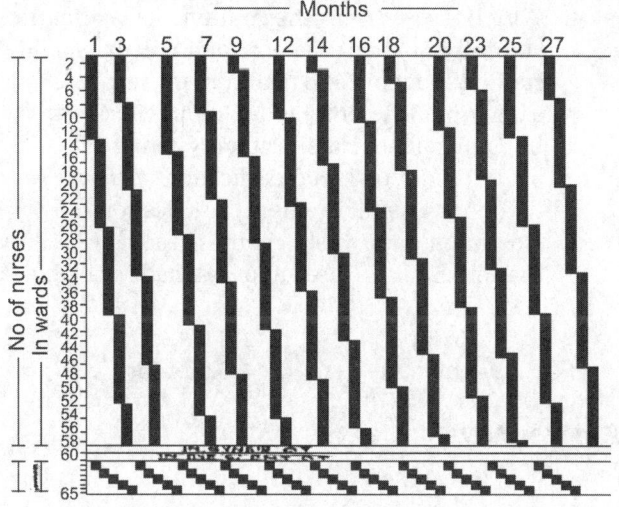

Fig. 26.1: A sample of evening master rotation plan.

In decentralized, the head nurse prepares ward-wise a master plan depicting the distribution of staff for each shift/day and week-wise.

Operational Plan

The operational plan is ward duty roaster or rotation plan. The head nurse prepares a rotation plan for the staff allocated to that particular ward as per shift duty pattern followed in the hospital.

Preparing Time Schedule

Prerequisite

The requirements for preparing time schedule are as follows:
1. Nurse supervisor should have protocols (rules/practices) about the minimum and the maximum number of staff, instruction to accommodate in the event of unplanned absences, how to maintain a record of scheduled plans, length of shifts, nature of individual's shift patterns, floating system, rest time, etc.
2. Have a list of different categories of nursing personnel, relieving nurses, floating nurses.
3. Make a list of offs, leaves, holidays, weekend, and consecutive working days.
4. Assessment of workload index during the morning, evening, and night duty, weekdays.

Steps for Preparing a Schedule

The following steps should be adhered when preparing a schedule:
- Prepare duty roaster well in advance preferably 2/4 weeks and notify staff.
- Distribute time throughout 24 hours keeping in mind nursing workload at different hours of the day, the experience of staff and nature of shift (straight or split shift).
- Plan days off in such a way that enough staff presents each day and during each period of the day.
- Consider request of staff for adjusting offs if feasible.
- The head nurse must plan a day off before and after evening and night shift.
- Distribute holidays, vacation time, and days off equally among all employees in the interest of fairness.
- Distribution desirable and undesirable hours equally among all staff.
- Place duties of senior staff evenly throughout the week and weekends.
- Have nurses on call in case emergency or during absenteeism of staff.
- Try to plan consecutive nights somewhat interrupted.

Role of a Nurse Manager/Supervisor in Preparing a Schedule

The list below shows the role of a nurse manager/supervisor in preparing a schedule:
- Identify staff skill and patient's needs.
- Investigate how holidays, sick leave, training days, vacation time, and other staff absences affect scheduling.
- Identify all of the ways that absences occur so that absence can be taken into account to formulate schedules. For example, make a list of holidays. Look as well into when nurses are unavailable because they are in training.
- Review scheduling processes with your staff.
- Ask each staff member to help you pinpoint critical problems in the scheduling system.
- Take significant issues into account when you optimize the nursing schedule.
- Optimize the scheduling process.
- Devise a procedure for reviewing and updating the master schedule, and all staff members must have access to this schedule.
- Provide flexibility. If nurses are permitted to swap shifts or relieve colleagues, provide guidelines for determining whether these work schedule changes are permissible.
- Establish a vacation-request procedure. Devise a system for deciding who gets vacation time during summer months and other times that are popular for vacations.
- Establish an employee backfill process. Establish a procedure for handling vacancies, planned as well as last minute.

CHAPTER HIGHLIGHTS

- The PCS is the method of grouping patients. Patients classified according to DRGs, ADL, or NCI method.
- Patient classification systems are based on either one or by combining more than one method of classifying patients. Important PCSs are HSSG, OPC, RAFAELA patient classification, and Zebra system of classification.

- Scheduling or time planning is an advance determination of the pattern of on and off duty hours for nursing personnel in a particular unit, section, or division. It is either centralized or decentralized.
- Nurse administrators or the head nurse prepares master rotation plan and ward rotation plan/duty roaster by keeping in mind its principles and follows various steps while preparing these schedules.

REVIEW QUESTIONS

I. Essay Type Questions
1. Enlist activity-based approaches for estimating staffing. Discuss anyone in detail.
2. Define the patient classification system. Describe various methods of categorizing patients.
3. Define scheduling. Discuss the role of a nurse manager in preparing a schedule.
4. Enlist patient-dependency approaches. Discuss any one in detail.

II. Short Notes
1. Time-task/activity study method
2. Dependency acuity-quality method
3. Types of scheduling
4. Oulu patient classification

III. Multiple Choice Questions
1. Which one of the activity related method comprises some form of work sampling and time and motion studies?
   a. Time-task method
   b. Utilization-based method
   c. Nurse per occupied bed method
   d. Adjusted service target method
2. Which one of the following methods of classifying patients based on their dependency level?
   a. DGR method
   b. ADL method
   c. Acuity method
   d. Katz's index
3. Under which grouping of the basic activities such as hygiene, bathing, dressing, toileting, and eating fall?
   a. Self-care deficit
   b. Nursing care intensity
   c. Activities of daily living
   d. Dependency level of patient
4. Which system of the patient classification comprises patient categorization, activity study, staffing situation, and quality of nursing care?
   a. Hospital Systems Study Group (HSSG)
   b. Oulu patient classification system
   c. RAFAELA patient classification system
   d. Zebra system of patient classification
5. How many days/weeks/months in advance, a duty roaster, should be prepared and made available to staff?
   a. 7–10 days   b. 2–4 weeks
   c. 3–4 months   d. 4–6 months

Answer Keys

1. a   2. b   3. c   4. d   5. b

SUGGESTED READING

1. Anthony MK, Theresa S, Glick J, Duffy M, Paschall F. Leadership and nurse retention, the pivotal role of nurse managers. JONA. 2005;35(3):146-55.
2. High Power Committee on Nursing and the nursing profession. [Online] Available from http://nrhm-mis.nic.in/ui/who/PDF/Report%20of%20the%20High%20Power%20Committee%20on%20Nursing%20and%20Nursing%20Profession%201989.pdf.
3. Kaur R, Vati J, Chhabra, R. An exploratory study on "Nursing Manpower" requirement for patients of a neurosurgical unit of Nehru Hospital, PGIMER, Chandigarh, 2008–2009. Unpublished Master's Thesis, 2009.
4. Koontz H, Weihrich H. Essentials of Management: An International Perspective, 1st edition. New Delhi: Tata McGraw Hill Publishers; 2007.
5. Lanksbear AJ, Sheldon TA, Maynard A. Nurse staffing and health care outcomes—A systematic review of the International research evidence. Adv Nurs Sci. 2005;28(2):163-73.
6. Paetznick MA. Guide for Staffing a Hospital Nursing Service. Geneva: WHO Publication, No. 23, 1966.
7. Sharma NB, Vati J, Saini SK. A study on the utilization of morning duty hours and influencing environmental stimuli of the operational level nurses working in selected wards of Nehru Hospital, PGIMER, Chandigarh, 2001. Unpublished Master's Thesis, 2001.
8. Staffing norms for hospitals. [Online] Available from http://www.citehr.com/103330-who-staffing-norms-hospitals.html.
9. Vati J. Organisation and administration of nursing services in district hospitals of North India. Unpublished Ph.D. in Nursing Thesis. Faculty of Medical Sciences, Panjab University, Chandigarh, India, 1990.

ANNEXURE

Who Grouping and Description of Nursing Activities

The nursing activities grouped according to their sphere of action. There are nine groups, namely
1. A patient care, basic
2. A patient care, complex
3. Administration
4. Education
5. Clerical
6. Housekeeping
7. Maintenance
8. Off-station
9. Nonproductive

These are subdivided for more precise analysis and described as follows:

1. Patient care, basic: Providing the care needed by patients to ensure their comfort and well-being for maintenance of health and prevention of infection, regardless of the patient's health status.

Code

11. Routine hygiene care
    - Washing and bathing
    - Haircare, nails care
    - Mouth care
12. The comfort of the patient in bed
    - Bedmaking
    - Tidying beds
    - Care of pressure areas
    - Use of comfort aids, e.g. bed cradles, backrests, air rings
13. Nutrition of the patient
    - Serving and distributing of food
    - Clearing away of trays and crockery
    - Feeding helpless patients
14. Care of body wastes
    - Giving bedpans and urinals
    - Disposal of products of elimination
    - Measuring urine, vomitus, sputum
    - Checking stools
15. Social aspects
    - Receiving patients and visitors
    - Assisting patients into wheelchairs or onto examination couches or trolleys
16. Simple health teaching about
    - Personal hygiene
    - Normal nutrition

2. Patient care, complex: Care given to the patient about his specific needs and health status

Code

21. Noting the patient's health status
    - Doing nursing rounds (at a change of shift)
    - Accompanying the doctor on rounds
    - Receiving or reading instructions on the patient's condition or treatment
22. Giving special care
    - To the patient who has vomited
    - To the patient who has collapsed
    - To the postoperative patient
23. Preparing for a procedure
    - Preparing the patient for
    - Examination
    - Laboratory test
    - Operation
    - Preparation and terminal care of supplies and equipment needed for examining and treatment of patients
24. Carrying out technical procedures
    - Those frequently performed, e.g. taking temperature, pulse, and respiration,
    - Giving medications via oral or injection
    - Those showed when specifically requested
25. The collection and examination of specimens
    - Blood
    - Stool
    - Urine
    - Gastric content
26. Assisting with technical procedures
    - Helping the doctor
    - Helping a nursing colleague
27. Health teaching about the necessary follow-up of
    - Patients with diabetes
    - Antenatal mothers
    - Postnatal mothers
    - Patients with special nutritional problems
28. Supportive care
    - Conversation with patients other than education
    - Listening to patients
    - Talking with relatives and friends about the patient's condition and issues
29. Charting
    - Recording temperature, pulse, and respiration rates
    - Recording blood pressure
    - Recording intake and output
    - Recording medications
    - Writing nurses' notes

3. Administration: Activities related to the directive process through which a unit or group functions code
31. The internal organization of the ward
    - Planning for staffing (weekly/monthly) schedules
    - Assignments, written or oral
    - Directing or instructing regarding the physician's orders

- Writing reports on the condition of patients
- Checking the patient's charts

32. Supervision of personnel
    - Participation in activities that are to improve nursing service and increase
    - The knowledge skill of the staff
    - Orientation
    - Teaching
    - Evaluation
    - Counseling and guidance
33. Assessment of nursing service
    - Checking to see that orders are carried out
    - Checking care given
    - Deciding where patients to place on the ward
34. Coordinating with other departments
    - With the director of nursing
    - With the medical superintendent
    - With departments having direct concern for patients
    - X-ray
    - Pharmacy
    - Laboratories
    - Kitchen
    - With departments concerned with the maintenance
    - Workshop
    - Laundry
    - Electrical department

4. Education
Activities that form a part of the education program for nursing students and in which other categories of worker are receiving instruction

Code
41. Activities involving the teachers
    - Discussion with other staff members about the nursing student's program
    - Observing and evaluating nursing student performance
    - Teaching, impromptu, and planned
42. Those activities of seeing the nursing student receiving instruction
43. Those activities of watching other categories of workers receiving education

5. Clerical:
Activities involving maintenance of records and reports and provision of tontine information

Code
51. Paperwork
    - Making out requisitions (indents) for supplies
    - Keeping patient's charts up to date, e.g. pasting the laboratory reports onto patient's records
    - Returning charts to the bedside
    - Filling in routine information on forms requesting treatment or investigation, e.g. X-ray, laboratory, physiotherapy
    - Ruling lines
    - Copying patient's names on to diet lists, medication lists, injection lists
    - Copying records from lists or books onto statistical sheets
    - Recording routine information in registers
52. Oral communication
    - Giving routine details on a patient to other departments
    - Providing routine information (e.g. on visiting hours, location of other departments) to patient's relatives and friends;
    - Contacting other agencies regarding the patient
    - Finding personnel on the unit.

6. Activities involving maintenance of a clean, safe, and comfortable environment

Code
61. Light housekeeping
    - Exchange of information about housekeeping activities
    - Dusting
    - Tidying cupboards
    - Changing curtains and screen covers
    - Moving furniture
    - Cleaning equipment after the discharge of patients
    - Washing dishes
    - Making unoccupied beds
    - Making a bed of ambulatory patients
62. Heavy housekeeping
    - Sweeping floors
    - Cleaning floors
    - Cleaning walls
    - Cleaning latrines
    - Sluicing soiled linen in units
    - Cleaning of such equipment as bedpans, sputum cups, urinals, wash-bowls
    - Collecting and emptying of buckets
    - Disposal of garbage

7. Maintaining supplies and equipment
Activities involving the replacement of equipment used and maintenance of supply for carrying out unit activities (other than writing indents).

Code
71. Preparing supplies needed for medical and nursing procedures
    - Making cotton swabs, gauze pieces, and gloves
    - Packing drums
    - Packing trays
    - Cleaning syringes
    - Obtaining and moving oxygen cylinders
72. Maintaining linen supplies
    - Clean
    - Soiled
73. Dispensing or receiving supplies for housekeeping activities

- Dusters
- Mops
- Cleaning aids
74. Condemning articles
75. Routine inventory
    - A change of shift©
    - As a part of the maintenance of ward supplies
76. Checking diets: Counting the amount sent from the kitchen
77. Checking drugs: When received from the pharmacy

8. **Off-station**

Activities that take the worker away from the unit but which have a definite relationship to the patient or the unit.

Code

81. Those activities relating to patients: Accompanying a patient to another department
82. Those activities relating to the unit in which the person is carrying messages, such as
    - Taking drums for sterilization; collecting drums from sterilization room
    - Making indents to various stores
    - Collecting clean linen
    - Taking soiled linen for exchange
    - Receiving tablets from the pharmacy
    - Taking specimens to the laboratory

9. **Nonproductive:** Those activities that do not directly benefit either the patient or the unit.

Code

91. Standby: Time spent waiting for the arrival of someone or something before being able to start purpose activity
92. Personal: All activities of a personal nature
93. Reporting on and off duty
94. Mealtime
95. Personal hygiene: When workers observed washing their hands after housekeeping activities

27 Categories and Job Description

CHAPTER OUTLINE

- Categories of Nursing Personnel
  - Hospital Nursing Services
  - Community Health Nursing
- Job Description
  - Defining Job Description
- Principles Applied in Preparing Job Description
- Job Descriptions of Hospital Nursing Personnel
- Job Descriptions of Community Health Nursing Personnel

LEARNING OUTCOMES

After completion of this chapter, the learner will be able to:
- Categorize nursing personnel working at different levels in hospitals and community
- Apply principles in preparing the job descriptions of nursing personnel
- Describe job descriptions of various categories of nursing personnel working in hospitals and community

KEY TERMS

Job description, nursing personnel, categories, hospital nursing services, community health nursing

INTRODUCTION

A nursing organization, like any other organization, viewed as a structure that provides a framework of duties and responsibilities of nursing personnel. It is also a group of nurses working together at different levels as a team to accomplish a single common objective of nursing services. It is a process or a system where nurses at different levels carry out many activities by utilizing various resources to ensure the best possible client care.

CATEGORIES OF NURSING PERSONNEL

Figure 27.1 depicts different categories of nursing personnel working in hospitals and community.

Hospital Nursing Services

Hospital nursing organization is like a pyramid, broad at the base, and tapering toward the top. The organization follows a line of hierarchy; each of the lower levels is immediately subordinate to the next higher one and so on the right up to the top. The superior–subordinate relationship through many levels of responsibility reaches from top to bottom in the nursing organization. Hence authority, command, and control descend from top to bottom. Based on the hierarchy, their position, and relative responsibilities, there are three categories/levels of nursing personnel: administrative, supervisory, and operational level **(Fig. 27.1)**.

Administrative Level

In a hospital setting, nursing personnel at the top or administrative level are concerned with formulating and executing policies, goals, objectives, and procedures for the nursing services. They plan and coordinate various executive and managerial activities. They give instructions to nurses at supervisory and operational levels.

Every teaching hospital with 150-bed strength should have one nursing superintendent (NS) assisted by one deputy nursing superintendent (DNS) and two assistant nursing superintendents (ANSs). The central government hospital and hospitals attached to autonomous Medical and Education Institutes have the post of chief nursing officer (CNO) in addition to NS, DNS, and ANS. In most district hospitals, matron is the head of the nursing department assisted by assistant matron to carry out administrative and managerial work. The head of the nursing department is directly responsible to the medical administrator in their respective hospitals.

Chapter 27: Categories and Job Description

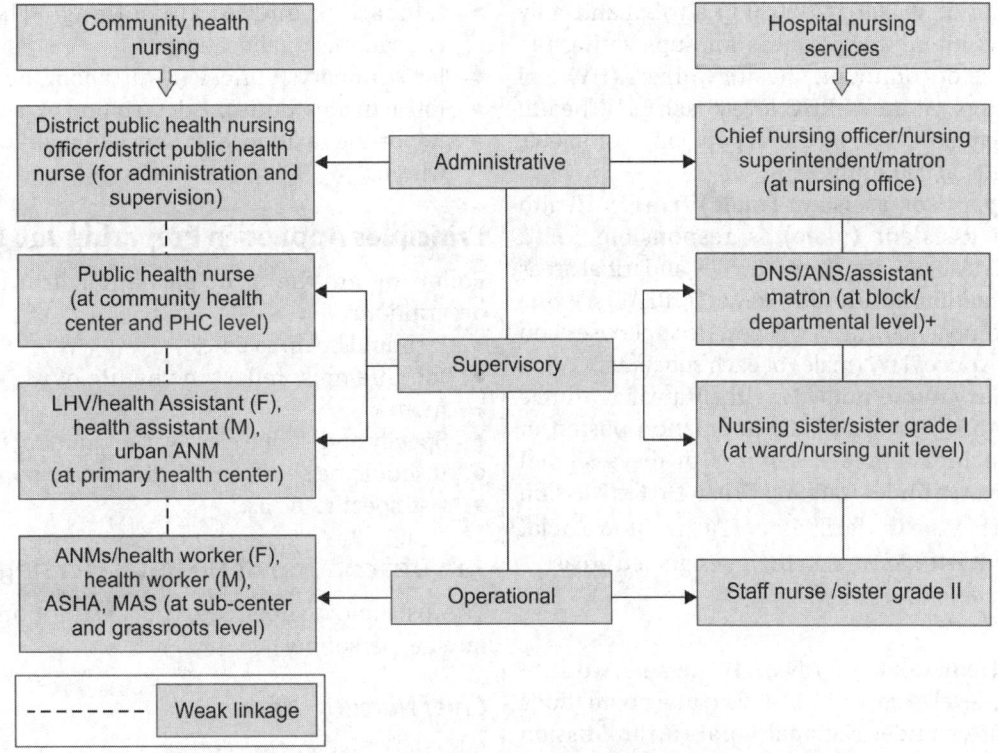

Fig. 27.1: Different categories of nursing personnel in hospitals and community.

Supervisory Level

The nursing personnel at the supervisory level concern with middle management of nursing services. They are the heads of either department or nursing unit/ward.

a. **Departmental wise:** Department wise, every teaching hospital should have departmental supervisor/sisters/Assistant Nursing Superintendents (ANSs) in the ratio of 1:3–4 wards/units and one ANS for four to five operation theaters, and one ANS separately for casualty and emergency unit to supervise nursing units/wards.

b. **Nursing unit/ward wise:** Ward/nursing unit wise, each teaching hospital should have ward sister/nursing sisters/sister Grade I in the ratio of 1:25 beds per shift and one per shift in Intensive Care Units (ICUs), special wards, Operation Theatres (OTs), casualty, and outpatient department (OPD).

The nurses at this level implement the departmental/ward policies and guidelines issued by nursing administrators at the top level. They concern with human resources and material management. They are engaged in staffing, supervision, appraising functions, and reporting and recording services.

Operational Level

Operation-level management comprises nurses at the operational category or first-line managers designated as staff nurses or sister Grade II. They work in different wards, nursing units, operation theaters, OPDs, and other units such as blood bank, infection control, and injection room. The job responsibilities vary according to the nature of work in a particular nursing unit.

Community Health Nursing

There is no formal hierarchy of nursing organizations in a community setting. However, various categories of nursing personnel are working at district, community health center (CHC), primary health centers (PHCs), family welfare, subcenters, and at periphery level to impart services to the community at large, at home, schools, industries, and nursing homes.

At District Level

District Public Health Nursing Officer

District Public Health Nursing Officer (DPHNO)/District Public Health Nurse (DPHN) is responsible for supervising activities related to health and family welfare in various public health programs in the district. The DPHNO is the senior position to DPHN, but they both had the same job profile. He or she is involved in managing including planning, organizing, and directing government-led national health programmes.

At PHC and CHC Level

1. **Public health nurse:** Public health nurse is the professional nursing personnel in the community, or public health is expected to render all services provided by the government and through its programs to the assigned community. They work at PHC and CHC of a district.

2. **Lady health visitor/health assistant (female supervisor):** Lady health visitors (LHVs) work as supervisors both at rural and at urban PHC level. At the R-PHC level, LHV is responsible for covering

a population of 30,000 or 20,000 in a tribal and hilly area. She is mainly responsible for supervising the performance of community health workers (HWs) of six subcenters. At the U-PHC level, each LHV/health assistant (female) serves an urban population of 50,000, including 25–30,000 slums.

3. **Health supervisor/assistant (male) (rural):** Health supervisor/assistant (male) is responsible for a population of 30,000 and 20,000 in hilly and tribal areas under the multipurpose health worker (MPHW) scheme to cover six subcenters or 25 villages. He supervises and guides the work of HW (male) of each subcenter.
4. **Ban-auxiliary nurse midwife:** Urban-auxiliary nurse midwife (ANM) covers 10,000 population posted in U-PHC provides outreach services in the assigned urban slum area under National Urban Health Mission (NUHM). They are the facilitator of Accredited Social Health Activists (ASHAs) in their designated areas.

At Subcenter Level

1. **ANM/HW (female):** Rural-ANM/HW (female) works at a subcenter level to cover 3,000–5,000 rural populations of four villages under National Rural Health Mission (NRHM).
2. **HW (male):** Multipurpose health workers/HW (male) works at the subcenter level to provide preventive and promotive healthcare, especially communicable and noncommunicable diseases-related services to 3,000–5,000 rural population.

At Village/Slum Level

Accredited Social Health Activist

Each village has one rural ASHA in the ratio of 1:1,000 populations (relaxed in case of hilly and tribal areas) under NRHM. One ASHA facilitator supervises and guides 20 ASHA workers. In many states, ANM or other PHC staff supervises ASHA workers. Each U-ASHA covers 1,000–2,500 slum/vulnerable urban population and visits 200–500 households. She supervises two to five Mahila Arogya Samiti (MAS) in her assigned area.

JOB DESCRIPTION

Jobs are essential for individuals as well as for the organization to accomplish its goals. There is flexibility in defining the role and is subject to change over some time due to advanced technology and competitive pressures. There may be the creation of new positions and change of cadre. Therefore the nurse administrators need to revise the job responsibilities for various categories of nursing personnel per hospital requirement.

Meaning of Job Description

The job description is communicating written statement of duties and responsibilities. It usually covers the following:
- Job title and location: The title of the job/designation, department, code number
- Education and qualifications: The minimum educational qualification
- Job summary: A brief write up about the job
- Job activities/duties: A description of tasks/duties
- Reporting relationship: Reporting and responsible for whom.

Principles Applied in Preparing Job Description

Following are the principles applied in preparing job description:
- It should be up to date.
- Job title must reflect the nature of work per requirement.
- Specify and define clearly the summary of duties.
- It should be short, descriptive, and complete.
- Use specific terms.

Job Description of Hospital Nursing Personnel

The list below shows the job descriptions of hospital nursing personnel:

Chief Nursing Officer

Job title: Chief nursing officer
Place of work: Nursing office
Responsible to: Medical superintendent (MS)/medical officer (MO)
Responsible for: Nursing Superintendent (NS)

Job Summary (Roles)

Chief nursing officer is overall incharge of nursing services and is responsible directly to the MS and indirectly to the director. His or her primary role is in planning, organizing, and implementing a high standard of nursing care. He or she involves organizing in-service education programs and conducting research projects. Chief nursing officer is responsible for overall administration and management of nursing services.

Duties and Responsibilities (Functions)

- Plans and estimates workforce, material, and the budget requirement for the nursing department
- Coordinates and controls nursing staff to accomplish organizational goals
- Formulates nursing policies, standard operative procedures, standards for nursing care
- Prepares nursing manuals, nursing procedure manuals, organization charts, job descriptions of nursing staff of all levels
- Participates in the recruitment of nursing staff
- Recommends the recruitment details to the authority from time to time
- Intimates vacancy position time to time
- Ensures adequate material resources for each nursing unit for the patient care
- Maintains records and reports and confidential files of nursing staff
- Plans staff development and in-service education program for nurses

- Be the mentor for nursing supervisors in carrying out their job efficiently
- Conducts meetings with nursing staff and participate in various hospital and other departmental meetings and conferences
- Coordinates and collaborates with another multidisciplinary team in the formulation of policies
- Approves prepared master rotation plan of nurse supervisors and nursing sisters
- Establishes and maintains a good professional interpersonal relationship with professional and nonprofessional agencies
- Uses a problem-solving approach to resolve any conflict or problem
- Conducts independent rounds and round with MS/director
- Participates in teaching and research
- Evaluates the performance of nursing staff periodically.

Nursing Superintendent

Job title: Nursing superintendent
Place of work: Nursing office
Responsible to: CNO/MS/MO
Responsible for: DNS/ANS/nursing sisters

Job Summary (Roles)
Nursing superintendent is responsible to CNO for all administrative activities. In the absence of CNO, as in most of the hospitals, he or she is overall in-charge of nursing services and is responsible to the MS. He or she plans to organize and carry out other managerial activities of nursing services with the assistance of DNS/ANS/nursing sisters.

Responsibilities (Functions)
a. **Nursing service-related activities**
   - Assists in the formulation of philosophy and policies of nursing services
   - Implements hospital policies and rules through various nursing units
   - Plans staffing and the material required for nursing services
   - Ensures the therapeutic environment and safe working conditions
   - Ensures quality and safe care rendered to patients in various nursing units
   - Conducts regular hospital and supervisory rounds
   - Accompanies CNO/Joint Medical Superintendent (JMS)/MS/MO during hospital and sanitation rounds
   - Prepares master rotation plan, schedule plan, and leave plan
   - Attends hospital and other meetings and conferences
   - Guides and counsels nursing staff
   - Visits nursing staff during their illness
   - Notifies Chief Nursing Officer (CNO) regarding any emergency or disaster
   - Solves the problems and complaints of nursing staff
   - Plans for the welfare of nursing staff, patients, and their relatives
   - Maintains good public relation
   - Initiates and conducts nursing research
   - Organizes student clinical experience and examinations.

b. **General and office duties**
   - Deals with general correspondence
   - Maintains annual confidence reports, cumulative, and health records
   - Prepares and submits annual reports of the nursing services
   - Sends hospital night, evening, morning, and other specific reports to Medical Superintendent (MS)/Medical Officer (MO)
   - Participates in professional and social activities
   - Carries out the duties as delegated by CNO/MS/MO.

Deputy Nursing Superintendent

Job title: Deputy nursing superintendent
Place of work: Nursing office
Responsible to: Immediate superior Nursing Superintendent (NS)/matron/CNO
Responsible for: ANS

Job Summary (Roles)
Deputy nursing superintendent is responsible for NS/CNO and assists him or her in nursing service administration. He or she has an indirect relationship with the hospital administrator or MS with whom he or she collaborates in the absence of NS or matron. He or she assists in the administration of nursing services. He or she carries out managerial, education, teaching, and general duties.

Responsibilities (Functions)
a. **Nursing service-related activities**
   - Assists in the formulation of the philosophy, mission, objectives, and policies of nursing services
   - Assists in recruitment and selection of nursing staff
   - Prepares master rotation plan of ANS and nursing sisters
   - Assists NS/CNO in allocating and deploying nursing staff in various nursing units and departments
   - Involves in keeping and maintaining records and reports of nursing services
   - Participates in planning new nursing units in the hospital
   - Takes regular hospital and patients rounds
   - Participates in various hospital committees
   - Keeps informing subordinate nursing staff about policies and standard operative procedures of the hospitals
   - Coordinates with NS and the nursing staff of the hospital
   - Maintains attendance, leave records, and cumulative records of nurses

- Keeps annual confidence reports and other documents of nursing staff
- Receives night reports from night supervisor and brief to NS/CNO
- Visits sick nurses in the hostel or the wards if admitted
- Conducts regular physical verification of stock maintained by nurses
- Initiates condemnation of worn-out articles and procurement of new items
- Attends emergency calls in rotation related to hostel or hospital.

b. **Education and teaching-related functions**
- Participates in planning orientation, skill training, and other staff development program for nurses
- Ensures clinical facilities for the nursing staff and nursing students
- Maintains discipline among nursing staff
- Guides and counsels nursing staff.

c. **General duties**
- Accompanies NS, MS, or any other special visitors for hospital rounds
- Organizes and participates in professional and social functions of the nursing staff
- Maintains good public relation
- Carries out duties as and when NS/CNO delegates
- DNS (nurse educator) and DNS (nurse epidemiologist) have different job responsibilities.

Assistant Nursing Superintendent (Assistant Matron)

Job title: Assistant nursing superintendent (assistant matron)
Place of work: Hospital (nursing office/nursing units)
Responsible for Immediate superior DNS/NS or matron
Responsible for: Nursing sisters/ward sisters and staff nurses.

Job Summary (Roles)

Assistant nursing superintendent (assistant matron) is accountable for nursing service administration either in the nursing office or in a department/a block of two/two wards or units (either inpatient or outpatient/operation theaters, obstetrics units) managed by ward supervisors or nursing sisters or for the supervision of nursing services and patient care of hospital. He or she has an indirect relationship with the hospital administrator or MS with whom he or she collaborates in the absence of an NS or matron. They carry out other supervisory, managerial, education, and teaching activities.

Responsibilities (Functions)

a. **Ward management activities**
- Organizes and plans nursing care activities of the department according to hospital policies
- Plans staffing pattern and allocates nursing staff in collaboration with nursing service administrator
- Plans the necessary requirement for the department
- Maintains discipline among nursing and other domestic staff
- Writes confidential reports after taking feedback from sister-in-charge of units
- Develops and maintains office records about the administration of his or her department
- Implements administrative policies
- Makes regular rounds of his or her department
- Communicates with patients' and their relatives during hospital rounds
- Ensures safety and cleanliness of the department
- Provides the general comfort of patients
- Receives reports from night superintendent
- Conducts and attends departmental and inter-departmental meetings and conferences from time to time
- Accompanies NS or MS during administrative and supervisory rounds
- Notifies any special incidence or emergency to the nursing administrator immediately
- Plans ward management with ward sisters
- Assists nursing sister in procuring and maintain records of equipment, supplies, and other materials
- Supervises proper utilization of staff and material in the department
- Acts as a public relation officer of department and deals with the problem faced by nursing sister especially with Class IV and patients' relatives by using problem-solving techniques
- Keeps NS informed about the requirement of the department.

b. **Supervisory activities**
- Establishes efficient admission and discharge policy in each ward
- Ensures quality nursing care and personal comfort
- Provides proper administration of medications, treatments, and diets
- Encourages accurate observation, critical thinking, recording and taking over charge, maintenance of intake and output chart, recording vital signs of seriously ill patients, etc.
- Ensures the smooth functioning of each ward through job assignments and allocation and by maintaining work culture.
- Ensures proper stock maintenance in each ward
- Provides a safe and clean environment.

c. **Education and teaching-related activities**
- Plans and organizes classes and clinical teachings for students and staff
- Plans and organizes in-service education and training programs to new staff and other staff of wards
- Counsels staff and students.

d. **General responsibilities**
- Participates in staff meetings
- Keeps environment stress free
- Attends meetings and participates in activities of professional organizations

- Carries out other duties assigned by nursing and medical administrators from time to time
- As a liaison officer between the nursing department and higher hospital authorities.

Nursing Sister/Ward Sister (Sister Grade I)

Job title: Nursing sister/ward sister (sister Grade I)
Place of work: Hospital
Responsible to: ANS/DNS/NS (matron)
Responsible for: Staff nurses and supporting staff

Job Summary (Roles)

The nursing sister/ward sister is designated as "sister Grade I" in many hospitals and is the first supervisory level nurses who are the in-charge of a nursing unit. He or she is responsible for the immediate superior nursing administrator. He or she is accountable for the nursing care management of a nursing unit/ward and assists sister Grade II (staff nurses) directly for nursing care. They manage the work of the nursing unit and ensure the care of patients provided by staff nurses. He or she also plays a role as an educator, supervisor, researcher, facilitator, counselor, and evaluator in an assigned unit. He or she is also expected to work in the morning, evening, and night shifts.

Responsibilities (Functions)

a. **Clinical activities**
   - Assesses environment, facilities of the assigned unit according to types of patients, and work
   - Attends report read by night staff nurse and takes the bed-to-bed patient round
   - Identifies patients' needs/problems
   - Assigns patients and other duties to staff nurses and other staff
   - Evaluates patient care given by staff nurses
   - Conducts teaching and sanitation rounds with nursing staff and nursing administrators and attends medical rounds with unit doctors and supervisory round with MS
   - Checks and carries out or delegates instructions given during rounds
   - Ensures proper admission and discharge of patients
   - Assists indirect care of patients when required
   - Ensures safety, comfort, and activities of daily living of all patients
   - Prepares diet list of patients daily and ensures all patients get proper diets/meals (normal or therapeutic).

b. **Supervisory activities**
   - Guides and supervises all staff nurses and students in rendering quality nursing care
   - Checks all patients' documents concerning patients maintained by staff nurses
   - Provides guidance and directly supervises nursing and nonnursing personnel in managing ward and in carrying out nursing routines
   - Supervises all staff in the following standard safety measures and following ward policies
   - Prepares and implements standard guidelines and procedure manual for supervision
   - Encourages teamwork, motivates staff, and maintains work culture and work environment.

c. **Administrative and ward management-related activities**
   - Prepares organization chart of the unit/ward; have a list of all staff working in the unit, their job descriptions, and orient staff about their job responsibilities
   - Keeps ward policies, rules, and regulations of the ward; implements ward policies and rules; orients all staff, patients, and relatives about rules and regulations of staff
   - Makes staff duty roaster for 24 hours/a week to meet the optimum nursing care requirement
   - Makes necessary changes in duty roaster and keep on-call staff in emergency
   - Keeps attendance record of all staff and sends monthly to the nursing office
   - Informs absenteeism or sickness of any staff of ward
   - Maintains discipline among staff and report any indiscipline or nuisance created by staff; investigates and reports to a higher authority and/or takes action according to rules
   - Uses a problem-solving approach to solve any managerial problem
   - Maintains a clean and safe environment, furnitures, equipment, articles, etc.
   - Keeps guidelines of standard safety measures, orients staff about these measures, and ensures that they are following
   - Maintains adequate linen and other supplies for each shift
   - Maintains linen stock, sends dirty or soiled linen for wash, and receives washed linen
   - Maintains proper record of materials, supplies, and equipment; consumption of drugs, supplies, and other materials
   - Keeps an up-to-date record of drugs including emergency drugs
   - Checks and manages all equipment periodically for its functioning
   - Initiates condemnation of nonfunctioning and damaged articles; sends articles for repair if not properly working
   - Checks daily availability and working condition of emergency and life-supporting equipment and supplies
   - Maintains inventories, reports, breakages, and losses
   - Assists in controlling visitors of patients as needed
   - Ensures that relatives of very sick patients are allowed to stay with patients when necessary
   - Informs and reports the nursing administrator about emergency

- Coordinates with the nursing administrator and staff nurses and with other departments
- Assists nursing administrator in planning staff and budget and also for disaster management
- Delegates responsibilities to the next senior staff in his or her absence
- Evaluates nursing and nonnursing activities
- Gets feedback from patients for improvement of care
- Participates in nursing audit
- Evaluates the performance of staff and sends an annual confidential report (ACR) to the nursing administrator considered for promotion
- Does self-evaluation.

d. **Education and teaching-related activities**
- Identifies learning needs of staff in the ward
- Plans conduct and recommend in-service education and skill training programs for all staff
- Encourages nurses to attend conferences and workshop and use of the library to keep up-to-date knowledge
- Conducts and facilitates clinical teaching and demonstrations for students and staff
- Keeps himself or herself in touch with the latest trends in nursing care and management
- Acquaints patients and their relatives with ward policies, rules, and regulations and assists them in adjusting in the hospital and ward routines.

e. **Research-related activities**
- Participates in research activities per the need to improve quality care
- Conducts research studies for evidence-based nursing practice.

f. **Reporting and recording-related activities**
- Maintains proper records and reports of all patients
- Ensures that all records of patients are written clearly and are complete
- Keeps up-to-date records of all inventories, confidential reports, and leave
- Ensures that all documents sent to the record section promptly.

g. **Communication and counseling-related activities**
- Maintains an excellent interpersonal relationship with staff and patients and their relatives
- Coordinates and cooperates with staff and other departments
- Guides and counsels staff and patients as required.

h. **Responsibilities of the evening nursing supervisor**
- Takes over from assistant matron/ANS and emergency ward sister/supervisor
- Reads out previous 24-hour report
- Takes a round of emergency unit and OPDs along with emergency sister-in-charge
- Takes a round of entire hospital and see staff members, VIPs, and acuity ill patients.

i. **Responsibilities of the night nursing supervisor**
- Takes over from evening nursing sister/supervisor and read evening report
- Takes a round of emergency unit and the entire hospital including operation theater and see staff members, VIPs, and acuity ill patients.

j. **Special activities of evening/night nursing supervisor**
- Plans priorities before starting round and inform sister-in-charge of the emergency department
- Guides staff regarding nursing care wherever required
- Listens to patients and relatives' problems and clear their doubts, fears, etc.
- Meets nurses, nursing students, residents in each ward, and listens and solves their problems
- Ensures cleanliness in each department
- Supervises and ensures the distribution of meals to all patients
- Writes evening/night report.

k. **Responsibilities of nursing sister/supervisor in emergency areas during evening and night shifts**
- Takes over from the morning sister and reads out the morning report
- Participates, assists, and guides all nursing staff regarding nursing care
- Goes for rounds with a consultant or administrative authority
- Ensures that CSSD articles and other supplies such as drugs and fluids are available and in stock
- Takes attendance and supervises work of Class IV employees
- Verifies the position of vacant beds in other wards and assists in transferring patients at the earliest
- Ensures files of discharge, death, and medicolegal cases must be submitted
- Writes evening/night reports.

Staff Nurse (Sister Grade II)

Job title: Staff nurse/sister Grade II
Place of work: Hospital
Reporting to: Nursing sister Grade I (ward sister)/assistant matron and matron
Responsible for: Nursing orderlies, coworkers

Job Summary (Roles)

Nursing sister Grade II is a first-level professional nurse who enters as professional nurses in the hospital works. He or she is under the immediate supervision of nursing sister Grade I (ward/nursing sister) in the assigned ward or nursing unit. He or she is responsible for providing direct or indirect nursing care to assigned patients applying nursing process during duty shifts. He or she assists in ward management and supervision, supervises nursing orderlies and other coworkers, and gives health education to patients/relatives.

The job responsibilities of staff nurses vary according to the nature of the work of that particular nursing unit. The job responsibilities of nurses working in operation theater differ from the nurses working in OPDs or blood banks or the injection rooms.

Responsibilities (Functions)

a. **Clinical activities**
   - Arrives on time and attends report read by night staff nurse
   - Takes over on arrival on duty and hands over after duty the charge of unit/bed-to-bed charge of patients assigned by sister Grade I (ward sister)
   - Identifies the needs of each patient after taking over
   - Does bed making or makes sure that bed is tidy and the patient is in a comfortable position
   - Maintains a therapeutic, clean, and safe environment for patients
   - Plans and provides basic care according to priority needs of patients and carries out assigned jobs
   - Maintains personal hygiene and comfort of patients
   - Maintains the intake and output of patients
   - Meets other activities of daily living of individual patients
   - Follows ward routines and standard safety measures while nursing patients
   - Carries out all patient-related basic and complex nursing care activities related to the patient, e.g. administration of medications, checking vital signs, tube feeding giving enema, stomach wash, bowel wash, nasogastric feeding, aspiration, dressing, intravenous (IV) infusion, etc.
   - Documents nursing care activities
   - Observes and records any significant change in the patient's health condition; takes necessary action and reports to concerned unit doctor/sister in-charge
   - Ensures the distribution of that normal or therapeutic diet to each patient
   - Keeps informed herself or himself about patients' diagnostic procedures and reports
   - Prepares patients for special diagnostic procedures if any and assists doctors to perform
   - Sends specimen with appropriate filled forms for tests to concerned laboratories
   - Assists doctors in physical examination, diagnosis, dressings, and treatment of patients
   - Coordinates with various members of the health-care team regarding patient care
   - Maintains interpersonal relationship with team members, patients, families, and community
   - Attends medical, supervisory, sanitary, and nursing rounds
   - Carries out and documents all the instructions or orders given by the unit doctor time to time
   - Carries out all formalities related to admission, discharge, or transfer of patients
   - Provides orientation to patients and their relatives regarding ward and ward policies such as visiting hours, visiting pass, etc.
   - Gives health education and follow-up instructions to patients and their significant ones.

b. **Ward management activities**
   - Hands over or takes over ward equipment and supplies (medicine, injections, linen, dressing material, etc.) and maintains inventory register daily
   - Keeps drugs in custody
   - Maintains drug consumption record register daily in each shift
   - Checks and keeps ready emergency trolley with medicines and other life-supporting articles and equipment for use
   - Follows ward policies and takes special attention to medical-legal cases, dead, and absconded patients
   - Creates a safe environment to prevent any accident and minimizes the noise in the ward
   - Ensures availability of filled oxygen cylinder, working suction machines, filled IV fluid bottles, and other resuscitation articles and materials, etc.
   - Follows himself or herself and instructs others to follow standard safety measures.

c. **Educational activities**
   - Participates in clinical teaching, both planned and incidental
   - Plans and provides health teachings to domestic staff, patients, and relatives
   - Takes an active part in teaching good health habits to patients and their relatives
   - Participates in-service education programs
   - Helps students and trainees in teaching-learning activities.

d. **Supervisory activities**
   - Supervises and guides junior nursing staff, nursing orderlies, nursing aids, and coworkers
   - Monitors patients and visitors for maintaining health promotion.

e. **Recording and reporting**
   - Reports critical condition or change/deterioration in the health condition of patients immediately in verbal and written
   - Reports any absenteeism of staff to concerned
   - Records and reports vital signs, nursing care, treatment, and medications correctly and promptly
   - Reports and records and losses, breakage and any incidence, occurred in the unit.

f. **Communication activities**
   - Maintains good interpersonal relationship with patients' relatives, supervisory staff, colleagues, coworkers, and other departmental staff
   - Provides psychological support to patients and relatives and manifests his or her interest in the spiritual welfare of patients
   - Orients patients and relatives about physical facilities, policies, rules, and regulations and routines of the hospital
   - Motivates patients and family through health-care teaching and continuing care directed toward an optimal level of health

- Participates in pre- and postconferences
- Reports any incidences to concerned staff.

g. **Research activities**
- Participates in research activities for the improvement of nursing care and implementing the nursing model
- Conducts research studies to establish an evidence-based nursing practice
- Participates in action-based surveys.

h. **Counseling-related activities**
- Counsels junior staff, students, and relatives when required.

i. **Evaluation-related activities**
- Does self-evaluation regularly
- Evaluates patients' health condition and nursing care
- Assists nursing sister in staff performance appraisal
- Takes part in students' performance evaluation.

Job Descriptions of Community Health Nursing Personnel

The list below shows the job descriptions of community health nursing personnel:

District Public Health Nursing Officer

Job title: District Public Health Nursing Officer
Place of work: At District Health Office
Responsible to: District Health Officer
Responsible for: Community staff at block and PHCs

Job Summary (Roles)

District Public Health Nursing Officer and DPHN is a supervisor of PHN staff in a district under directly under district health officer and indirectly to the nursing officer at the state level. They are responsible for planning, organizing, and supervising all the community health programs of that district. He or she participates in policy-making activities and evaluates the performance of community staff.

Responsibilities (Functions)

A. **Managerial and administrative activities**
- Participates in implementing all public health programs
- Takes the initiative in planning staff requirement and recommends to the district health officer
- Attends regular meetings at the district level.

B. **Supervision and guidance-related activities**
- Supervises each staff at block and PHC level on normal days and Mamta (Health and Nutrition) Day
- Guides HWs for planning and organizing their work
- Conducts regular meetings with them
- Carries out weekly field visits in subcenters and PHCs
- Checks registers such as home visits, eligible couples, family planning (FP), MCH, malaria, medical stock, birth and death registers, etc. to maintain at subcenters
- Fills up a supervisory checklist with details of the health center
- Checks are working conditions and sanitation of health centers
- Sends annual reports for all the visits with recommendations for improvement
- Listens and solves work-related and personal problems of HWs and discusses with MO of the PHC
- Guides and assists them in gathering and recording information, using records and writing reports.

C. **Teaching and education-related activities**
- Plans and organizes in-service and staff development programs, workshops, and seminars for the staff
- Encourages them and helps them to grow professionally.

D. **Service related**
- Participates in various national health programmes such as MCH and FP
- Participates in special health campaigns
- Monitors and evaluates the performance of staff working at the grassroot level
- Receives and compiles reports from block/PHCs and sends to state
- Makes entries in the registers and diaries
- Counsels mothers and families.

Public Health Nurse

Job title: Public health nursing
Place of work: At PHC and CHC
Responsible to: MO/MS
Responsible for: Health supervisors/LHVs, and HWs/ANMs

Job Summary (Roles)

Public health nurse is a nurse midwife. She provides preventive and promotive services, monitors, and supervises the work of health supervisors/LHVs, and HWs/ANMs in the field. She participates in the planning, execution, and evaluation of all programs run by PHC/CHC and gives suggestions related to community health nursing.

Responsibilities (Functions)

A. **Managerial and administrative activities**
- Participates in implementing all health programs at PHCs and CHCs
- Organizes MCH and FP clinics at the agency level
- Attends regular meetings at PHC/CHC level.

B. **Supervision and guidance**
- Supervises the work of all health assistants and HWs
- Guides them to plan and organizes work.

C. **Health counseling and teaching**
- Provides family health counseling
- Teaches them regarding family care
- Either renders direct care to nonhospitalized sick or teaches their caretakers about care.

D. **Environmental sanitation-related activities**
- Plans teaching program for the community to help them in controlling accidents, hazards at home, school, workplace, and prevention of infection.

E. **Subcenter action plan related**
- Estimates needs of beneficiaries at the community level
- Plans service requirement for meeting needs of MCH programmes
- Plans equipment and the material required for the community regarding MCH
- Makes provision of supply at PHC.

F. **Field and other activities**
- Regarding MCH: ensures enrollment of pregnant women, antenatal care (ANC) formalities and postnatal services and complete registers maintained by LHV/ANM/HW (female)
- Child health services: birth registers in MCH registers and immunization status
- Assesses and prepares an annual action plan and monthly advance field visit program
- Ensures adequate supply at PHC.

LHV/Health Assistant/Supervisor (Female)

Job title: Lady health visitor/health assistant/supervisor (female)
Place of work: At PHC
Responsible to: Medical officer
Responsible for: ANM, ASHA, TBA/MAS

Job Summary (Roles)

Lady health visitor/health assistant (F) are a supervisor for six subcenters and its HWs. She is posted at PHC level and is responsible for mainly MCH-related activities and the equipment and supplies and maintenance of proper records and reports of subcenters. She also conducts training of dais and ASHAs with the help of ANM and assists MO in conducting various training programs of health personnel, the professional supervisor/nurse in the community or public health.

Each LHV/health assistant (female) serves an urban population of 50,000, including 25–30,000 slums at U-PHC. She supervises and guides the work of ANMs and ASHA workers. She also involved in conducting training of dais and ASHA with the help of ANM and assists MO in doing various training programs of health personnel. At PHC, she provides comprehensive preventive and promotive services of all communicable and noncommunicable diseases at OPDs. She operates at the block level.

Responsibilities (Functions)

A. **Related to supervision and guidance**
- Supervises HWs at a peripheral level
- Assists ANM/HW (F) in planning and organizing various programs
- Guides them in proving their knowledge and skill in delivering healthcare
- Visits subcenters weekly to monitor and evaluates the work of ANMs
- Checks records and reports maintained by ANMs under various public health programs
- Supervises HW during planned home and field visiting
- Supervises referral of enrolled expecting mothers for Rapid Plasma Reagine (RPR) testing at PHCs.

B. **Coordinating activities**
- Coordinates her activities with activities of HWs
- Conducts regular meetings with male health assistants and another HW
- Attends meetings held at PHCs
- Assists and coordinates with MO for various programs
- Assists and guides ANM/HW (F) in organizing Mamta Day.

C. **Records and reporting**
- Checks and reviews record maintained by ANM, compiles, and submits to MO of PHC
- Prepares and submits a monthly report regarding the functioning of subcenters to MO.

D. **Equipment, supplies, and maintenance of subcenter-related activities**
- Checks store inventories at subcenters regularly
- Helps in procuring required supplies and equipment
- Checks various types of kits such as general kits, midwifery kits, and *dai* kits
- Supervises and inspects sanitation and cleanliness of subcenters.

E. **Training and education-related activities**
- Conducts training programs for ASHA/*dais*
- Assists MO in organizing training programs at the PHC level and FP camps.

F. **MCH and FP-related activities**
- Conducts weekly MCH and FP clinics at subcenters involving female HWs
- Performs deliveries at PHC, as and when required
- Checks various MCH and child health-related registers
- Motivates couples for FP
- Provides intrauterine contraceptive device (IUCD) services
- Involves female HWs in establishing female depot holders and providing training to them to distribute contraceptives
- Refers cases for Medical termination of pregnancy (MTP) to the approved centers.

G. **Activities related to health programs**
Universal immunization programme: Supervises and guides health works regarding immunization of mothers and infants. Organizes immunization camps and teaches HWs to maintain cold chain and storage of vaccines.
Nutrition: Provides treatment to malnourished infants and older children and refers to a serious one. Makes

provision and distributes iron and folic acid and vitamin A supplements.

School health: Assists MO in providing health services.

Acute respiratory infection: She makes the diagnosis of pneumonia and gives treatment per standing instruction to mild and moderate cases and refers to doubtful and severe cases.

Health education: Imparts health education by using various information and education technologies and methodologies on multiple topics such as nutrition and immunization, dental care, tuberculosis, noncommunicable diseases, etc. involving female HWs. She trains women leaders, organizes, and utilizes Mahila Mandal, teachers in organizing various programs in the community.

Primary medical care: Handles and gives treatment in minor ailments, ORS therapy, first aids in case of accidents and emergencies and refers for further treatment to the nearest PHC.

H. **Additional and individual responsibilities in endemic areas of Kala-azar, Japanese encephalitis**
Supervises female HWs in endemic areas of Kala-azar and Japanese encephalitis (JE) for doing their duties and verifies their visits to at least 10% of the houses in a village
- Checks their records for identifying cases
- Ensures complete treatment and coverage during the spray activities and search operation
- Conducts health education sessions through individual, group meetings, and mass communication.

Health Assistant/Supervisor (Male)

Job title: Health assistant/supervisor (male)
Place of work: At PHC
Responsible to: Medical officer
Responsible for: Male HWs

Job Summary (Roles)
The health assistant/supervisor male is a supervisor for six subcenters. He is posted at PHC level and supervises and guides HW (male) of each subcenter. He is involved in the malaria program, nutrition, communicable, and noncommunicable disease programs and environmental sanitation.

Responsibilities (Functions)
The male health assistant/supervisor performs all the activities involving male HWs related to supervision and guidance, coordinating, supplies and equipment, and maintenance of subcenters, records and reports, Universal Immunization Programme and family welfare as of LHV. In addition to these activities, he has other job responsibilities:

A. **Communicable diseases**
- Takes remedial measures during an outbreak of epidemics and necessary control measures during noticeable ailments and steps to control stray dogs by utilizing local authorities
- Provides treatment to leprosy cases and assesses their disability status
- Checks compliance of tuberculosis patients for Direct Observed treatment Shortcourse (DOTS) therapy.

B. **Noncommunicable diseases**
- Participates in health promotion and information education and communication activities to control noncommunicable diseases.

C. **Environmental sanitation**
- Joins in maintain community sanitation
- Makes provision of soakage pits, manure pits, compost pits, sanitary latrines, smokeless chullas, and safe water supply with the help of local authorities
- Encourages the community to have kitchen gardens
- Makes efforts to supervise the proper chlorination of water sources.

D. **Additional and specific responsibilities**
- Supervises male HWs in endemic areas of Kala-azar, JE, and lymphatic filariasis for doing their duties and verifies their visits to at least 10% of the houses in a village
- Checks their records for identifying cases and guidelines for drugs and its distribution
- Ensures complete treatment and coverage during the spray activities for Kala-azar and search operation
- Conducts health education sessions through individual, group meetings, and mass communication.

E. **Malaria**
- Supervises male HWs during visits for doing their duties per the schedule and verifies their visits to at least 100 of the houses in a village
- Draws blood and prepares thick and thin blood smear of cases with fever during visits
- Provides treatment for the positive cases of malaria
- Ensures insecticide spraying along with male HWs.

Auxiliary Nurse Midwife/Health Worker (Female)

Job title: Auxiliary nurse midwife/health worker female
Place of work: At subcenter
Responsible to: Medical officer
Responsible for: ASHA/Dais/Traditional Birth Attendant (TBA)

Job Summary (Roles)
Auxiliary nurse midwife/HW female is the village-level HW. She is posted in subcenter under NRHM and covering 3,000–5,000 rural populations of four villages. She performs various activities related to national programs, including MCH, FP, medical termination of pregnancy, nutrition, a universal program on immunization, communicable and noncommunicable diseases, maintaining records, reporting treatment of minor ailments, and conducting the house-to-house survey. She also acts as a facilitator of ASHA workers. Out of two available ANMs in subcenter, one performs field duties and home visits. Health assistant

(female)/LHV supervises ANMs, but they report to MO-in-charge of PHC.

Urban-ANM is the urban community-level HW under NURM. ANMs provide outreach services in the assigned urban slum area during urban health and nutrition days and special outreach sessions monthly and weekly, respectively, at Anganwadi center and schools in coordination with ASHA and MAS. She will do monthly health checkups at Anganwadi center with the assistance of ANM, ASHA, and Anganwadi Worker (AWW). She reports to MO I/C of U-PHC. Her leading role in U-PHC is in mapping and vulnerability assessment, links with urban local bodies, home visiting, supervision of ASHA, MCH, preventive and managing communicable and noncommunicable diseases, maintaining records and reporting, etc.

Responsibilities (Functions)
A. **Maternal and child health**
- Registers all pregnant cases. Ensures at least four visits by them; first visit within 12 weeks, second between 14 and 26 weeks, third between 28 and 34 weeks, and fourth between 36 weeks and term
- Tests urine and blood for hemoglobin
- Refers to PHC/CHC for blood testing for syphilis and grouping and abnormal cases to LHV/PHC
- Conducts deliveries at subcenter; supervises deliveries conducted by dais
- Refers to difficult deliveries and assist them in getting institutional care
- Identifies beneficiaries under Janani Suraksha Yojana and performs all formalities
- Prepares monthly work schedule of ASHAs during the meeting with them under Janani Suraksha Yojana (JSY) (every third Friday of the month) and conducts regular meetings with them per schedule
- Tracks all pregnancies and provides ANC and Post Natal Care (PNC) services and home visits per plan
- Initiates breastfeeding within 1 hour of birth of the baby and emphasizes exclusive breastfeeding at least for 6 months
- Provides treatment in diarrhea and acute respiratory infections and refers when required
- Teaches mothers regarding MCH care, FP, nutrition, immunization, etc.
- Assists MO/LHV in conducting ANC/PNC clinics at subcenter.

B. **FP and medical termination of pregnancy**
- Registers eligible couples; motivates them for FP
- Distributes contraceptives to the couples and assists them in utilizing FP services and performs Intra Uterine Contraceptive Devices (IUCD) insertion
- Helps in establishing female depot holders and trained them for distributing contraceptives
- Conducts Mahila Mandal meetings
- Identifies and refers to women requiring MTP and discourages unsafe abortion methods.

C. **Activities related to health programs**
Universal Immunization Programme
- Immunizes pregnant mothers and infants
- Maintains cold chain for carrying vaccines during fixed and outreach sessions
- Reports any adverse events after immunization immediately
- Prepares and submits monthly Universal Immunization Programme (UIP) report, weekly surveillance reports
- Follows biomedical waste management guidelines generated after vaccination
- Maintains tracking bags, village-wise record dropouts and left-outs, and any incidence of vaccine-associated complications
- Makes indents of vaccines and other supplies weekly
- Prepares work plan; estimates the number of beneficiaries and another requirement

Nutrition
- Assesses children under five for malnutrition and identify low birth weight cases, provides treatment to malnourished infants and older children, and refers serious one to PHC
- Makes provision and distributes iron and folic acid for pregnant and adolescent girls and vitamin A supplements to children
- Educates mothers about a balanced diet.

Communicable diseases
- Notifies MO and informs LHV/HW male regarding any cases of diarrhea, fever with rigor, rashes, tetanus, fever with jaundice, with unconsciousness and takes appropriate actions to prevent the spread of infections
- Provides ORS to all diarrheal cases; refers to all cases/suspected cases of blindness, cataract, dehydration, vomiting, and dysentery to PHC
- Counsels, screens, refers, and follow-up any HIV/Sexually Transmitted Infection (STI)/Reproductive Tract Infections (RTI) cases
- Maintains a record of leprosy at subcenters and treatment register at PHC. Educates them about leprosy and its treatment. Refers suspected cases and complicated ones to PHC. Gives treatment per guidelines and ensures compliance for taking medicines. Assists the cases with a disability to carry on their self-care activities
- Identifies any case of malaria, prepares blood smear slide for testing. Provides treatment to positive cases. Maintains a record of all cases and patients on antimalaria treatment
- Performs special duties per guidelines in endemic areas of filaria, Kala-azar, dengue/chikungunya, JE, and malaria.

Noncommunicable diseases
- Uses information, education, and communication technology and methods to impart health education

and make them aware of prevention, healthy lifestyle, and early detection of noncommunicable diseases, iodine deficiency, harmful effects of tobacco, and fluorosis at health centers, community, schools, etc.
- Prepares a survey list of all identified cases of visual and hearing impairment half-yearly/annually. Sensitizes ASHA/AWW and mobilizes the community for conducting screening camps
- Refers to cases of mental illnesses and epilepsy to district hospitals
- Emphasizes dental and oral care to all age groups and high-risk groups
- Forms and registers self-health-care group of elderly persons.

D. **Records and reports**
- Maintains all documents, including birth and death, concerning mothers, children, and eligible couples
- Registers pregnant women, infants under 1 year, children under 5 years of age, women aged 15–44 years, and adolescents
- Maintains records of the use of FP devices/methods
- Maintains a passive malaria surveillance register to record cases, blood slides prepared, positive cases, and cases under treatment
- Prepares and submits a weekly/monthly report to female health assistant.

E. **Primary medical care**
Handles and gives treatment in minor ailments, ORS, first aids in case of accidents and emergencies and refers for further treatment to the nearest PHC/CHC/hospital.

F. **Coordinating and team activities**
- Attends various meetings at PHC/CHC/community development block, with female health assistant
- Coordinates with male HWs/ASHA/health volunteer/dais and with all committees
- Holds meetings with ASHA as a facilitator and acts as a resource person to give training
- Plans and informs ASHA about outreach sessions and guides them to organize health days and maintains eligible couple register
- Takes help of ASHA for ANC and PNC and gives training in salt testing
- Prepares the village health plan with the help of team members to submit to block
- Maintains cleanliness of subcenter and follows guidelines to dispose of biomedical waste
- Plans and organizes and assists in organizing Village Health and Nutrition Day at Anganwadi centers
- Participates in health camps and campaigns.

G. **House-to-house survey**
- Conducts monthly/annually house-to-house survey.

Health Worker (Male)

Job title: Health worker male
Place of work: At subcenter
Responsible to: Medical officer

Job Summary (Roles)
Health worker male is a functionary at subcenter level to provide preventive and promotive health-care services. Each male HW covers a 3,000–5,000 rural population. His leading role is in infectious diseases control programmes including malaria, tuberculosis, leprosy, Kala-azar, waterborne disease, and environmental sanitation apart from health education, detection of diseases, control of epidemic diseases, safe drinking water, school health, etc. in subcenters of high focus districts at least for 3 years. He also helps ANM in MCH and other activities performed by her.

Responsibilities (Functions)
A. The male HW carries out all activities such as early detection and treatment, Information Education Communication (IEC)/Behaviour Change Communication (BCC), recording and reporting, meetings and discussion, team coordination, and referral services related to
- National Vector Borne Disease Control Programme (NVBDCP)
- Malaria; endemic areas of filaria, Kala-azar, acute encephalitis syndrome/JE, dengue/chikungunya
- National Leprosy Eradication Programme
- National Blindness Control Programme
- Revised National Tuberculosis Control Programme.

B. Activities related to Universal Immunization Programmes, Reproductive and Child Health Programme (RCH), Communicable Diseases, noncommunicable diseases are the same as of ANM/female HW.

C. **House-to-house survey**
- Conducts monthly/annually house-to-house survey.

D. **Environmental sanitation**
- Chlorination of public water sources
- Makes community aware of regarding safe drinking water, liquid and solid waste management, home cleanliness, use of sanitary latrines, and smokeless chullas, and also for personal hygiene
- Coordinates with village sanitation and nutrition committee.

E. **Primary medical care**
- Handles and gives treatment in minor ailments, ORS, first aids in case of accidents and emergencies and refers for further treatment to the nearest PHC/CHC/hospital.

F. **Health education**
- Educates and encourages community regarding the availability of health services including maternal and child health services
- Gives health education to mothers about a balanced diet.

G. **School health and nutrition**
- Assesses children under five for malnutrition and identifies low birth weight cases, provides treatment to malnourished infants and older

children, and refers to serious one to PHC. Refers to supplementary feeding to Anganwadi
- Visits all schools in the assigned area and educates them regarding personal hygiene, nutrition, safe drinking water, etc.

H. **Records and reporting**
- Performs mapping of his area and prepares maps and charts
- Maintains family and village records, tuberculosis and leprosy patients under treatment, passive surveillance record of malaria cases, cases of diarrhea, dysentery, fever, jaundice, etc. and assists ANM in maintaining eligible couple and MCH health register
- Prepares village health plan annually with the help of ANM and other team members and submit to block
- Prepares monthly report and sends to male HW
- Educates mothers about a balanced diet.

ASHA (Rural)

Job title: ASHA
Place of work: At village
Responsible to: Medical officer

Job Summary (Roles)
Accredited Social Health Activist is a trained community-based link worker and covers 1,000 populations (relaxed in case of hilly and tribal areas) of a village. She reinforces MCH services and immunization, promotes preventive services and institutional deliveries, and works in close coordination with Anganwadi workers. One ASHA facilitator supervises and guides 20 ASHA workers. In many states, ANM or other PHC staff supervises ASHA workers. Block community mobilizes and supervises ASHA facilitators at the block level.

Urban ASHA is an essential link between urban communities through MAS. U-ASHA is a trained community-based link worker and acts as a bridge between the government functionaries and various support systems in the community. Each U-ASHA covers 1,000–2,500 slum/vulnerable urban population and visits 200–500 households. She supervises two to five MAS in her assigned area, reinforces MCH services, immunization, promotes preventive services, and works in close coordination with Anganwadi workers.

Main Responsibilities (Functions)
A. **Maternal care**
- Ensures ANC and postpartum care and FP through home visits
- Counsels pregnant mothers and prepares a birth plan and encourages for safe delivery.

B. **Newborn and childcare**
- Regarding breastfeeding, keeping baby warm, management of low birth weight and preterm baby
- Identifying asphyxia and sepsis
- Home care in case of diarrhea, acute respiratory infection and fever, and referral
- Feeding and temperature management during illness
- Deworming and iron deficiency treatment
- Counseling regarding immunization and prevention of diseases.

C. **Nutrition**
- Counsels and helps mothers for exclusive breastfeeding, complementary feeding, and referral in cases of malnutrition.

D. **Infectious and noninfectious diseases**
- Identifies and refers the cases with malaria, leprosy, tuberculosis, and other infectious diseases and noncommunicable diseases
- Teaches and encourages to take protective and preventive measures in case of infection.

E. **Social mobilization**
- Plans and conducts meetings with MAS and women's groups
- Helps ANM to prepare community health plans and community to access available health services
- Makes the public aware of health facilities, their entitlement, on issues regarding violence against women and children.

Anganwadi Worker

Job title: Anganwadi worker
Place of work: At the Anganwadi center [under Integrated Child Development Services (ICDS)]
Responsible to: Anganwadi supervisor

Job Summary (Roles)
The AWW is an HW, chosen from the community, and they have to undergo 4 months of training in health, nutrition, and childcare. She is the in-charge of an Anganwadi center covering 1,000 rural population. ICDS Anganwadi supervisor (Mukhyasevika) supervises about 25 Anganwadi workers. Four Mukhyasevikas are under the Child Development Project Officer (CDPO) at the block level.

The Anganwadi center provides supplementary nutrition, nonformal preschool education, nutrition and health education, immunization, health checkup, and referral services. Along with ASHA and ANMs, the Anganwadi workers are the link between community and health services and all other services.

Main Responsibilities (Functions)
A. **Supplementary nutrition**
- Ensures supplementary nutrition in the form of a cooked meal or take-home ration to children under 6 years, pregnant and lactating mothers, additional food supplements to malnourished girls
- Distributes fefol supplements to adolescent girls.

B. **Growth monitoring**
- Takes the weight of children under the age of 5 years

- Monitors and maintains growth charts
- Identifies and refers severely malnourished children.

C. Preschool nonformal education
- Plays and other creative and stimulating activities for children between 3 and 6 years of age.

CHAPTER HIGHLIGHTS

- The nursing organization is a process or a system where nurses at different levels carry out activities by utilizing various resources to ensure the best possible client care.
- In hospital setup, there are three categories/levels of nursing personnel: administrative, supervisory, and operational level.
- Nursing personnel designated as NS/matron/CNO are at administrative level; at the supervisory level, DNS/ANS are supervisors at block/department, and nursing sister/sister Grade I is supervisor at ward/nursing unit level. The nursing personnel designated as staff nurse/sister Grade II are operational-level nurses.
- There is no formal hierarchy of nursing organizations in a community setting. At district level, DPHNO/DPHN is at the top level. Public health nurse works at the middle level at CHC; LHV/health assistant/supervisor (F), and health assistant/supervisor (M) at PHC. Whereas ANM, male HW at subcenter; and ASHA, MAS, health volunteers, dais at village/slum (grassroots) level.
- In a hospital setting, the nursing personnel working at administrative level are responsible for overall management of nursing services; supervisory is accountable for the management and supervision of their assigned areas.
- The operational-level nurses are responsible for the management of patient care and supervision of supportive staff and students in the hospitals.
- In a community setting, the nursing personnel at different levels are responsible for the supervisory and performing activities related to various programs, reproductive, maternal, newborn, child, and adolescent health programmes and National Disease Control Programmes under National Health Mission.

REVIEW QUESTIONS

I. Essay Type Questions
1. Enlist various categories of nursing personnel working at hospitals and community.
2. Describe different categories of nursing personnel in hospital nursing services.
3. Describe the job responsibilities of the NS.
4. Discuss in detail the nursing personnel working in different public health facilities.
5. Explain the role of Auxillary Nurse Midwife under the National Health Mission.

II. Short Notes
1. Role of health assistant (female) as a supervisor
2. The supervisory role of nursing sister of general ward
3. ASHA as a frontline health worker
4. Job responsibilities of male health worker
5. Functions of staff nurse

III. Multiple Choice Questions
1. What should be a nursing sister and patient ratio in a teaching hospital?
   a. 1:10
   b. 1:15
   c. 1:20
   d. 1:25
2. Who is the head of nursing services in most of the district hospitals?
   a. Matron
   b. Nursing superintendent
   c. Chief nursing officer
   d. Nursing sister
3. How many units/wards one assistant nursing superintendent is suppose to supervise?
   a. 1–2
   b. 3–4
   c. 4–5
   d. 5–6
4. Who supervises the work of ANMs?
   a. Female health assistant
   b. Male health assistant
   c. Public health nurse
   d. Block supervisor
5. What is the place of work of a male health worker?
   a. Community health center
   b. Primary health center
   c. Subcenter
   d. Village level
6. Who is directly responsible to medical administrator in a hospital nursing services?
   a. Staff nurse
   b. Nursing sister
   c. Deputy nursing superintendent
   d. Nursing superintendent
7. How many slum/vulnerable urban household, ASHA is to visit?
   a. 100–150
   b. 150–200
   c. 200–500
   d. 250–350
8. To whom lady health visitor is responsible?
   a. Block officer
   b. Medical officer
   c. PHN
   d. DPHNO
9. Which of the following outreach services ANM provides?
   a. Village Health and Nutrition Day (VHND)
   b. Special outreach sessions
   c. Both VHND and special outreach sessions
   d. None of the above-mentioned services
10. Which one of the following weeks would ANM advise a pregnant woman for second ANC visit?
    a. 6–12 weeks
    b. 14 and 26 weeks
    c. 20–30 weeks
    d. 26–34 weeks

Answer Keys

1. d 2. a 3. b 4. a 5. c 6. d 7. c
8. d 9. c 10. b

SUGGESTED READING

1. Balasco E, Black A. Advancing nursing practice: description, recognition, and reward. Nurs Admin Quarterly. 1988;12(2):52-62.
2. Brett J. How much is a nurse's job worth? Am J Nurs. 1983;83(6):877-80.
3. Carson KP, Stewart GL. Job analysis and sociotechnical approach to quality: A critical examination. J Quality Manag. 1996;1(1):49-65.
4. Cascio WF. Managing Human Resources. New York: McGraw-Hill, Inc.; 1992.
5. Cornelius EJ, Carron TJ, Collins MN. Job analysis models and job classification. Pers Psychol. 1979:693-708.
6. DeCenzo DA, Stephen PR. Human Resource Management. New York: John Wiley & Sons; 1999.
7. Dessler G. Human Resource Management. New Delhi: Prentice-Hall of India; 2004.
8. Disch J, Feldstein. An economic analysis of comparable worth. J Nurs Admin. 1986;16(6):21-31.
9. Gael S (Ed). The Job Analysis Handbook for Business. New York: John Wiley & Sons; 1988.
10. Gomez-Mejia LR David BB. Managing Human Resources. Upper Saddle River: Prentice-Hall, Inc.; 2001.
11. Lawler III, EE. From job-based to the competency-based organization. J Organ Behav. 1994;15(1):3-15 (first published online: 21st Nov 2006).
12. McCormick EJ. Job Analysis. New York: American Management Association; 1979.
13. Mridulal A, Premarajan KC, Kumar SG. Performance assessment of junior public health nurse in maternal and child health services in a district of Kerala, India. Int J Adv Med Health Res. (Serial online) 2015 (cited Dec 3, 2018);2:16-21. Available from http://www.ijamhrjournal.org/text.asp?2015/2/1/16/159121. [Accessed June 2019].
14. Nelson JB. The boundaryless organization: Implication for job analysis, recruitment, and selection. Human Res Plan. 1997;20(4):39-49.
15. Nolan P. Competencies drive decision making. Nurs Manag. 1998;29(3):27-9.
16. Roedel R, Nystrom P. Nursing jobs and satisfaction. Nurs Manag. 1988;19(2):34-8.
17. Schofield P. Improving the candidate job-match. Pers Manag. 1993;25(2):69.
18. Sharma B, Roy S, Mavalankar D, et al. (2010 Feb). Available from http://www.academia.edu/7966627/The_Role_of_the_District_Public_Health_Nurses_A_. [Accessed June 2019].
19. Van Cleve, Roy R. Job analysis for nurses and related health care professionals: A task inventory approach. Health Resources Administration (DHEW/PHS), Bethesda, MD: Div. of Regional Medical Programs; 1975. Available from http://www.eric.ed.gov/ERICWebPortal/search/detailmini.jsp?_nfpb=true&_&ERICExtSearch_SearchValue_0=ED141571&ERICExtSearch_SearchType_0=no&accno=ED141571. [Accessed June 2019].

28 Personnel Policies

CHAPTER OUTLINE

- Personnel Policies
  - Definition of Personnel Policies
  - Importance of Personnel Policies
  - Need for Personnel Policies
  - Types of Personnel Policies
  - Common Personnel Policies
  - Characteristics of Personnel Policies
- Organization of Personnel Policies
- Formulation of Personnel Policies

LEARNING OUTCOMES
After completion of this chapter, the learner will be able to:
- Understand the concept of personnel policies
- Justify the importance and need for personnel policies
- Describe various types of personnel policies
- Appreciate the features of planned personnel policies
- Discuss different areas of personnel policies
- Explain the procedure for developing personnel policies

KEY TERMS
Policy, personnel policies, appealed policy, imposed policy, implied policy

INTRODUCTION

Personnel policies are a set of statements that explain what the employer expects from its employees and what employees may expect from the employer. Policies offer guidelines for decision-making. Personnel policies are guidelines that an organization creates to manage their employees. The most written policies are general rules that apply to all employees rather than specific job requirements for the individual employee.

PERSONAL POLICIES

Definition of Personnel Policies

Some definitions of personnel policy are given below:
- Personnel policy is the body of principles, rules, and regulations establishing working conditions under which the employees who are working and governing the hospital in its relations with the employees are known as the personnel policy of the hospital.
- Personnel policies are the predetermined course of actions set up to guide the performance of the personnel. These are established to ensure that these functions contribute to the objectives of the personnel program and the entire organization.
- These are the statements of accepted personnel principles and the resulting course of administrative actions by which the specific organization determines the pattern of its employment conditions.

Importance of Personnel Policies

The list given below shows the importance of personnel policies:
- Concerned with the basic needs of the organization and the employees
- Ensures consistent treatment of all personnel throughout the organization
- Minimizes favoritism and discrimination
- Promotes stability
- Serve as a standard of performance
- Improves employee motivation and loyalty
- Helps people grow within the organization
- Establishes uniformity
- Reduces the incidence of inequities
- Promotes good public relations

Need for Personnel Policies

The following lists the need for personnel policies in nursing:
1. To ensure adequate nursing care through procurement, development, and retention of competent nursing personnel
2. To develop the competencies of nursing personnel by self and under supervision
3. To provide the impersonal, unemotional, and unbiased basis for supervising staff
4. To provide an opportunity for implementing principles of democracy
5. To prove a helpful guide for employees
6. To clarify the responsibilities of different personnel
7. To help in knowing the channel of communication
8. To have the provision for periodic evaluation and revision
9. To assist in outlining the procedures to be followed in the event of suggestions for improvement
10. To help in describing the procedures to be followed if major or minor disciplinary problem occurs.

Objectives of Personnel Policies

The list below shows the objectives of personnel policies:
1. To contribute to defining specific job and responsibilities of personnel
2. To utilize optimally human resources according to their capabilities selected for the job
3. To train and prepare competent staff according to their job specification
4. To provide an opportunity for each person for growth and development
5. To create a sound therapeutic and human relationship among personnel
6. To establish conditions for mutual interest and understanding
7. To avoid operational problems
8. To ensure employees to give fair wages and provide healthy working conditions
9. To provide security of a job to employees
10. To ensure fair and equal treatment to every employee.

Types of Personnel Policies

According to the Source

- **Originated policies:** These policies are related to managerial functions.
- **Appealed policies:** These policies are not part of general policies, but there is a scope to handle a particular situation.
- **Imposed policies:** These are the policies that are imposed by pressures, usually by associations.

According to Forms

- **Implied policies:** These are related to the behavior of employees, e.g. dress code.
- **Within policies:** These spell out the managerial thinking in writing.

According to Scope

- **General policies:** These are related to public administration about the personnel employed in the institute.
- **Specific policies:** These are the application of the general policies to specific situations, e.g. policies on terms and conditions of employment, housing, transport, uniform and allowances, training and development, and public relation.

Common Personnel Policies

Some of the common personnel policies are as follows:
- Recruitment and selection policy: It includes minimum eligibility criteria, qualification, experience, reservation, method of selection, wage, benefits, etc.
- Human resource planning strategy
- Hours of work and conditions of employment policy
- Wage and allowance policy
- Retention policy
- Promotion, demotion, termination, and superannuation policy
- Deployment, placement, allocation, and transfer policy
- Induction and orientation policy
- In-service and staff development policy
- The nursing shift scheduling policy
- Assignment and rotation policy
- Incentives and compensation policy
- Leave and absenteeism policy including maternity and paternity leave
- Public holidays and work days
- Uniform dress code policy
- Annual performance appraisal policy
- Staff welfare policy including gratuity and provident fund
- Discipline and grievance policy
- Personnel security policy
- The policy of prevention of harassment at work including sexual harassment.

Characteristics of Personnel Policies

The following lists the characteristics of personnel policies:
- Frame the personnel policies with the guidelines of respective government and concerned statutory bodies.
- It should be comprehensive, flexible, and easy to understand.
- These should have facts and evidence base.
- It includes information about workplace rules.
- It contains summaries of past experiences in the form of guidelines.
- It should also include a discussion of sensitive legal issues such as sexual harassment and employee safety regulations.
- Every employee must be aware of policies.
- The policies need to review during employee orientation and periodic training sessions.

- Employers should avoid making unconditional promises in their personnel policies.
- Policies need to be understood by both superiors and subordinates.

ORGANIZATION OF PERSONNEL POLICIES

The following list plays a main role in the organization of personnel policies:
1. Personnel policies often begin with a welcome.
2. Procedure for initiating new personnel policies and amending existing policies.
3. Operational definitions need to state clearly.
4. General statement of purpose of personnel policies in terms of patients, nursing service, hospital.
5. List of principles that are basic to organization, interpretation, and application of personnel policies.
6. State the brief history of the hospital values, vision objectives, and a description of its organizational structure.
7. General statement of the function of the personnel department if existing.
8. Details of organization—lines of authority, hierarchy, the channel of communication, etc.
9. Responsibilities of supervisors for personnel policies.
10. General policies regarding conditions of employment, job analysis, and descriptions.
11. Public policies covering salary and wage administration, work schedule, vacation, leaves, and absence.
12. General policies regarding employee's selection, recruitment, promotion, transfers, training, rating, and termination.
13. Public policies concerning employees' benefits and welfare program, safety conditions, and health services.
14. Procedure to be followed during grievances and problems.

FORMULATION OF PERSONNEL POLICIES

The personnel policy formulation is a five-step process (Fig. 28.1):
1. **Identification of need:** It is the first step in formulating the policies. Spell out the demand in the essential areas of personnel management.
2. **Collection of facts:** Gather the facts from various sources, e.g. from records, experiences, and philosophy.
3. **Finding out alternatives**: Based on the facts, find out the alternatives, and select the best from various options per the criteria or priorities of the organization. State the selected option in the form of policy.
4. **Approval of policy:** Get approval for the final stated policy from the appropriate authority and communicate throughout the organization.
5. **Evaluation of the policy:** Evaluate the policy after implementation, review it, and endorse modifications if required. Evaluate the personnel policies based on their outcome such as turnover, absenteeism, commitment, and cost-effectiveness.

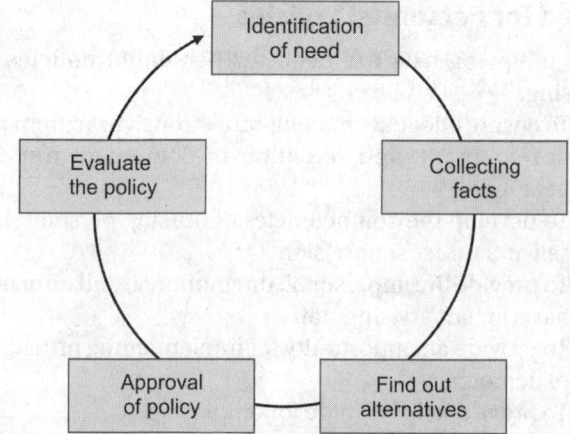

Fig. 28.1: Steps in the formulation of personnel policy.

CHAPTER HIGHLIGHTS

- Personnel policies are guidelines in an organization to manage its employees.
- These fulfill the basic need of the organization and employees and serve to have standard and uniformity.
- There are different types of personnel policies according to their sources, forms, and scope.
- Personnel policies include the rules enforced at the workplace about employees, their benefits, and also discussion on sensitive legal issues.
- There are five steps to formulate the policies.

REVIEW QUESTIONS

I. Essay Type Questions
1. What do you mean by personnel policy? Enumerate its characteristics.
2. Discuss the need and importance of personnel policies.
3. Describe the process of formulating policies.

II. Short Notes
1. Types of personnel policies
2. Organization of personnel policies
3. Features of personnel policies
4. Common types of personnel policies

III. Multiple Choice Questions
1. Which type of personnel policy is related to the behavior of employees?
    a. Appealed
    b. Implied
    c. Imposed
    d. Originated
2. Which type of policy is related to administration about employees?
    a. General   b. Specific
    c. Within   d. Imposed
3. The policy that is related to legal sensitive issues is:
    a. Annual confidential appraisal
    b. Discipline and grievance

c. Leave
d. Prevention of sexual harrassment
4. The recruitment policy includes:
   a. Human resource planning
   b. Staff welfare and benefits
   c. Eligibility and selection procedure
   d. Placement and transfer

Answer Keys

1. b   2. a   3. d   4. c

SUGGESTED READING

1. Bamberger P, Meshoularn T. Human Resource Strategy; Formulation, Implementation, and Impact. Thousand Oaks, CA: Sage; 2000.
2. Davar RS. Personnel Management and Industrial Relations. Vikas: New Delhi; 1988.
3. Dessler G. Human Resource Management. Prentice-Hall: New Delhi; 2003.
4. Harvey BH, Schultze JA, Rogers JF. Rewarding Employees for Not Using Sick Leave. PersAdm. 1983;55-59. Available from https://dpe.gov.in/dpe-guidelines/personnel-policies[Accessed April 2019].
5. ILO Nursing Personnel Convention No.149. World Health Organization. [Online] Available from https://www.who.int/hrh/nursing_midwifery/nursing_convention_C149.pdf [Accessed April 2019].
6. Matteson MT, Ivancevich JM. Controlling Work Stress: Effective Human Resource Management Strategies. San Francisco: Jossey-Bass Publishers; 1987.
7. Personnel Policies - HealthReach Community Health Centers. [Online] Available from http://www.healthreach.org/New_Hire/Forms/NewHirePacket/2017%20Personnel%20Policy%20book%20-%20print.pdf. [Accessed April 2019].
8. Policies & Procedures.Dress code –nursing personnel.[Online] Available fromhttps://www.saskatoonhealthregion.ca/about/NursingManual/1005.pdf[Accessed April 2019].
9. Storey J (Ed). New Perspectives on Human Resource Management. London: Routledge; 1989.
10. Mahoney T, and Deckop J. (1986). Evolution of Concept and Practice in Personnel Administration/Human Resource Management (PA/HRM). J Manag 1986;12: 223–41 (Cross refer.) available from (online) Search Results. Web results. Human Resource Management: Critical Perspectives on Business ... https://books.google.co.in › books. [Accessed January 2020].
11. Yoder Dale. Personnel Management and Industrial Relations. New Delhi: Prentice-Hall; 1990.

29 Staff Development and In-service Education

CHAPTER OUTLINE

- Staff Development
  - Concept and Meaning
  - Importance and Need of Staff Development
  - Philosophy of Staff Development
  - Goals and Objectives of Staff Development
  - Advantages of Staff Development
- Staff Development Models
- Staff Development Methods
- Staff Development Programs
- In-service Education
  - Definition
  - Objectives of In-service Education
  - Areas of In-service Education
  - Training and Development
  - Principles of Adult Learning
  - Planning and Organizing In-service Education/Training Programs

LEARNING OUTCOMES

After completion of this chapter, the learner will be able to:
- Understand the concept of staff development
- Appreciate importance and need for staff development
- Describe the philosophy of staff development
- Identify the goal and objectives of staff development
- Explain various models of staff development
- Discuss and implement multiple methods of staff development
- Describe various staff development programs
- Discuss various aspects of in-service education

KEY TERMS

Staff development, in-service education, staff development programs, on-the-job, off-the-job methods, adult learning

INTRODUCTION

For any organization to be active, adequate resources are needed, i.e. competent staff, adequate finance, material, techniques, and machines. It is more of a staff who should be well qualified than any other factors that determine the quality and quantity of performance. The development and success of the organization depend on their staff. Hence the staff development must plan for the employees.

STAFF DEVELOPMENT

Concept and Meaning

The concept and meaning of staff development are as follows:
- According to the medical dictionary, staff development is a process to assist employees in attaining skills and knowledge and gain levels of competence and to grow through orientation, in-service education, and continuing education and other programs.
- Staff development includes all the training and education undertaken by the employer to improve professional and personal knowledge, skill, and attitudes of employees. It is an application of individual efforts for raising the performance standards of high level and for improving attitudes and activities that enter into or influence their work and relation.
- Staff development also includes various types of activities; programs to develop, improve, and enhance skills; competencies; and overall performance of employees.
- Staff development is viewed as the process to provide opportunities for employees to improve their knowledge, skills, and performance to achieve the goals

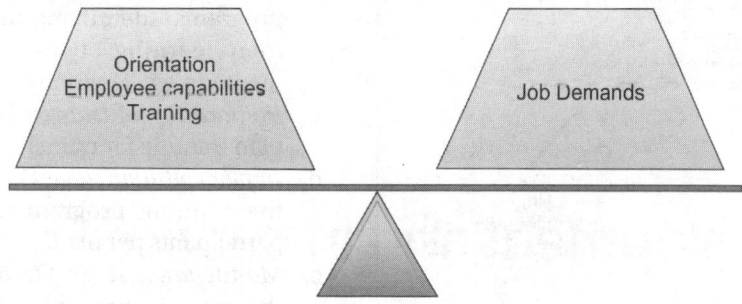

Fig. 29.1: The balance between employee capabilities and job demand.

of the organization in the interests and needs of the employees.
- Staff development is the process of improving the job-related knowledge, skills, or attitudes of employees. It focuses on enhancing the capabilities of employees for their professional and personal growth and advancement in the organization. The progress of technology and superspecialty, treatment modalities, and stagnation of all factors can cause imbalance, decrease, or mismatch the capabilities of nurse employees with their job demand. It is possible through staff education and development to balance the job demand and employees' capabilities **(Fig. 29.1)**.

Importance and Need of Staff Development

The following list shows the importance and need of staff development:
1. To update knowledge, skill, and practices with the advancement in the medical field
2. To cope up with rapid societal changes and improvements in health sciences
3. To fill the demand and interest of the public in health promotion
4. To fill the gap due to increased specialization and research among nursing personnel
5. To have a challenge in growing unionization and legislative control of nursing
6. To help nurses to be aware of unfamiliar practice roles and rules
7. To emphasize quality rather than quantity.

Philosophy of Staff Development

Philosophy of staff development in nursing should be consistent with the primary goal of health-care organizations to achieve a high quality of nursing care. Staff development aims in the overall development of all nurse employees for rendering nursing care. They should be able to apply knowledge in the actual work environment, and all the programs should be directed to have an impact on the learners, system, and the patient and his family.

The educational environment should be nonthreatening, with a dynamic, collaborative teaching-learning process, resulting in the cognitive, psychomotor, and affective behavior of the individual nursing personnel.

The newly joined employees should achieve an acceptable level of performance and should be utilized to provide a basis for accountability to the patients. It is a continuous process and involves meticulous and rigorous planning.

Goal and Objectives of Staff Development

The goal is of staff development is to see measurable improvements in staff performance and overall productivity in the medium- to long-term period. The objectives are as follows:
1. To improve the knowledge, competence, and attitude of the staff
2. To maximize potential and utilization of staff
3. To identify the training needs of staff
4. To assist new entrants in getting adjusted to a new environment, new roles, and responsibilities
5. To satisfy the interest of the staff in a particular area
6. To have competent and talented persons in the organization
7. To develop staff professionally and personally
8. To build sound and professional work culture
9. To reduce turnover and absenteeism
10. To fill the gap between senior and new staff and provide job satisfaction.

Advantages of Staff Development

Following are the advantages of staff development:
- To improve the knowledge, skill, and attitude of nurses
- To develop competent future nurse managers and administrators
- To develop a positive attitude and inculcate motivation among staff to work hard
- To prepare nurses to assume increased responsibilities
- To educate new nurses on workplace culture issues specific to that hospital
- To improve professional standards by keeping all nurses with updates.

STAFF DEVELOPMENT MODELS

1. **The RPTIM model:** The readiness, planning, trainers preparation, implementation, and maintenance (RPTIM) model for staff development is a research-based

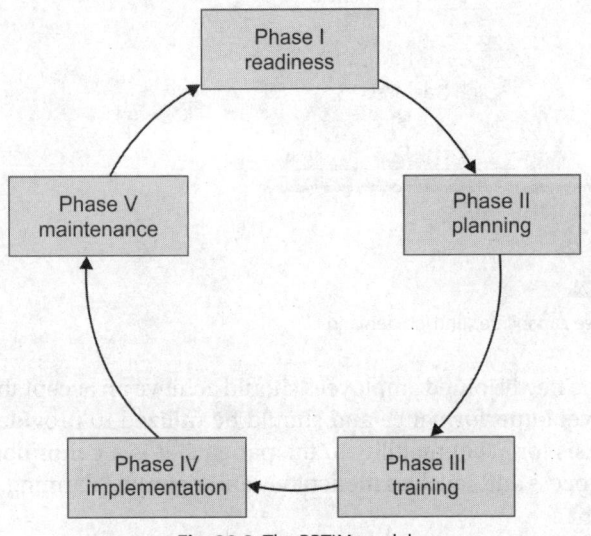

Fig. 29.2: The RPTIM model.

model, created by Woods, Thompson, and Russell in 1981. The model conceptualizes staff development into five stages **(Fig. 29.2)**:

a. *Readiness stage:* The readiness stage focuses on the development of a positive climate before planning the staff development activities. During this stage, gather the information regarding the current practices and identify the need for the specific staff to formulate goals for the staff development.

b. *Planning stage:* During this stage, initiate the planning of all activities of staff development programs. Identifying the needs of participants, their learning styles, specific objectives, and methodology of various staff development activities.

c. *Preparation of trainer:* During the training stage, plan training for trainers.

d. *Implementation stage:* During this stage, implement the training program on selected employees/participants per plan.

e. *Maintenance stage:* During this stage, determine the effectiveness of a program based on the performance of participants.

2. **Iowa professional development model:** Iowa's professional development model provides a roadmap to conduct a staff development program in nursing. It describes an action research process to study data, set goals, and make decisions about professional development. The model depicts the "cycle within the cycle" **(Fig. 29.3)**. It includes two components: planning and ongoing components.

    a. *The planning stage:* It includes the following activities:
    - Gathering and analyzing required information to identify and prioritize need and areas of staff development
    - Formulating goals and objectives for the program based on employees learning needs
    - Selecting and finalizing the content matter
    - Designing and completing the plan.

    b. *Implementation and evaluation:* This component includes the implementation of a training program and evaluation process. The evaluation

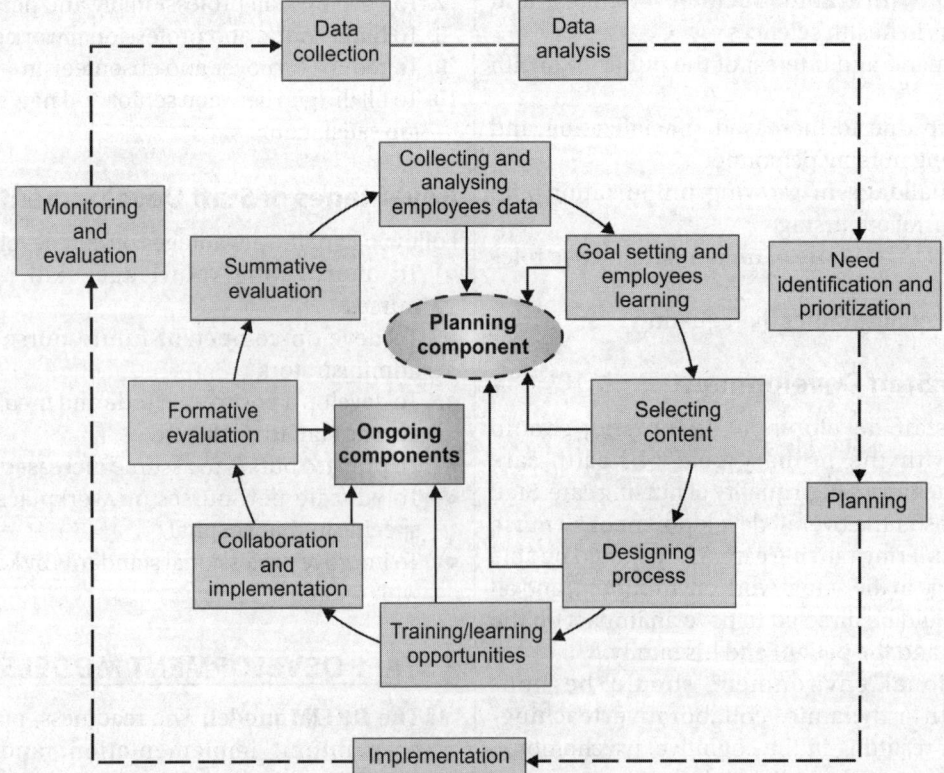

Fig. 29.3: Modified Iowa model.

process comprises carrying out the formative review, monitoring performance, and summative evaluation activities.

STAFF DEVELOPMENT METHODS

1. **On-the-job methods:** On-the-job methods, the employees receive training on-the-job at their workplace. These are simple, most commonly used, and cost-effective training methods. The employees get training on an individual basis aiming "learning by doing" under the actual working conditions. The success of this method of staff development depends on the competency of the trainer. Examples of such on-job training methods are job rotation, coaching, temporary promotions, etc.
2. **Off-the-job methods:** Off-the-job training methods or vestibule training are methods provided away from the actual working place preferably to newly joined employees. Examples of off-the-job methods are workshops, seminars, conferences, lectures, panel discussions, case study methods, demonstration, role-playing, etc. Other training techniques include individual assignments, printed materials, and practical manuals and also encourage self-learning.

STAFF DEVELOPMENT PROGRAMS

Staff development programs include various programs such as induction training, orientation, in-service education, leadership and management training, and continuing education programs.

Induction Training

Induction training is the process by which the new nurses' employees introduce to the organization. It is a brief standardized introduction about hospital philosophy, purpose, programs, policies and regulations. The employees get training for the first 2–3 days of employment. The main objective of induction training is to ensure new nurse employees to retain; to help in settling down quickly and happily to its role; and to identify them with institutional goals and programs.

Orientation

Orientation is the activity to introduce new nurse employees to organizations, tasks, superiors, and workgroups. The main objective of orientation is to acquaint nurses with relevant information. It also helps the staff to adjust to the environment and ensure a minimum level of competence within a given period.

The duration of orientation varies according to areas and usually has three-stage processes: orientation to the overall organization, orientation to the specific department, and orientation to the particular job. The information provided is of organization and personnel issues. The organizational information includes components like its history and philosophy and its mission, goals, objectives, organizational structure, etc. It also provides information regarding personnel policies, procedures, compensation issues, fringe benefits, physical facilities, etc.

The essential aspects of the orientation of the department include departmental functions, activities, policies, rules, and regulations; visiting the physical environment; and introduction to staff members of the department. Orientation to the job includes a detailed explanation of the situation based on the job description, responsibilities, records and reports, performance standards, supervision practices, instructions on the use of equipment, monitors, and information regarding supplies, materials, and routines. **Box 29.1** depicts the guidelines to organize the orientation program by Reed-Mendenhall and Millard (1980) and St John (1980).

In-service Education

In-service education includes all on-the-job instructions that are undertaken to enhance his or her work performance in the present job. The topic has full discussion separately.

Continuing Education

Continuing education is a form of education an individual undertakes after completing the necessary professional

Box 29.1: Guidelines to organize orientation program.

Orientation to the organization	
Organizational information	*Personnel information*
❖ History and philosophy of the organization	❖ Key policies and procedures
❖ Goals and priorities of the organization	❖ Compensation issues
❖ Scope and diversities of activities	❖ Fringe benefits
❖ Clients served	❖ Safety facilities
❖ Chain of command	❖ Physical facilities
❖ Facts about key personnel	❖ Leaves, etc.

Orientation to the department
❖ History of department
❖ Departmental role in the organization and relationship to other departments
❖ Departmental goals and priorities
❖ Activities and functions of the department
❖ Policies, procedure, rules, and regulations
❖ Visit the department and all units
❖ Introduction to the departmental supervisors and other superiors
❖ Introduction to clients

Orientation to the job
❖ Detailed about the job based on the job description
❖ Discussion of common problems and how to solve them
❖ Review of performance activities
❖ Nursing care standards
❖ Review of supervision practices
❖ Overview of records and reports
❖ Instruction regarding the use of equipment and monitors
❖ Information regarding supplies and materials
❖ Rotational plan, timings, offs, rest, leaves, etc.
❖ Legal and ethical responsibilities
❖ Staff development programs
❖ Safety
❖ Evaluation

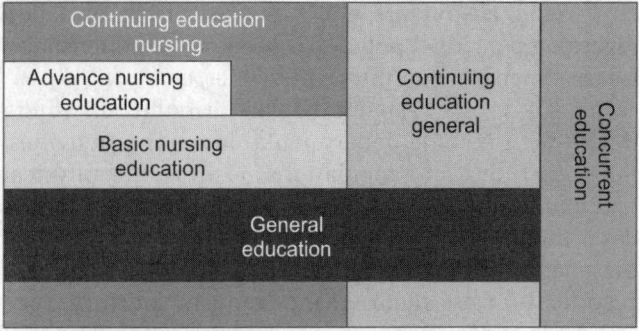

Fig. 29.4: A conceptual scheme of continuing education in nursing.

training to improve competency. It comprises planned learning experiences to develop and enhance knowledge, skills, and attitude of professional practice (WHO, 1980) **(Fig. 29.4)**.

Continuing Education Distinguishes from Academic Pursuits

In continuing education, there is no formal credit grant, and the acquisition of a higher degree is not the goal. Hence continuing education refers the structured nonacademic learning after completion of the basic program; systematic or structured experiences are designed to build upon preserved knowledge and skills; and to assist nursing personnel to gain new knowledge and skills, review and add to knowledge already acquired, investigate new approaches in nursing, and strengthen their clinical competencies.

Continuing Education is Different from In-service Training

Continuing education coordinates attendance at approved programs locally as well as in the state, helps in the presentation of an appropriately approved program within own facility, and furnishes opportunities for sharing with other staff.

Objectives of Continuing Education

The list below shows the objectives of continuing education:
- To bridge the gap between knowledge and demand for service.
- To improve learning, interpersonal skills, and practice.
- To balance employee's capabilities and job demands.
- To assist in career and personal development.

Benefits of Continuing Education

Owen et al. (1998) identified the following personal and professional interests of continuing education:
a. **Patient related:** It includes better patient care, more knowledge, skilled practitioner, and improved information outcomes.
b. **Personal:** It includes a sense of achievement, personal development in terms of confidence, assertiveness, creativeness, the mind of enquiring, and research-oriented outcomes.

TABLE 29.1: Outcomes for ongoing training.

Study conducted	Outcomes
Lathlean et al., 1986	Improve knowledge, interpersonal skills, personnel development (self-development), and career development
Bignell and Crolty, 1988	Improve care, professional development, educational development, and individual development
Barriball et al., 1992	Improve knowledge, skills, and attitude; improve practice; increase job satisfaction, better job retention, and career development
Nolan et al., 1995	Update knowledge, improve care, facilitate change, enhance the status of nursing, personal development, professional development, interpersonal benefits, and educational benefits
Wood, 1998	Individual-level: increase confidence, improve knowledge, increase self-awareness, increase professional awareness Patient care level: improve communication skills, enhance individualized care and research-centered practice

c. **Professional (individual):** The outcomes related to professionally developed individuals are toward increased career opportunities and lifelong learners and help employees to enhance their professional status and also recognition.
d. **Professional (interpersonal):** The staff develops interpersonal professionalism through the exchange of ideas and motivation and by improving interdisciplinary working.
e. **Organizational:** Continuing education also helps the organization to meet organizational objectives and enhance the motivation level of employees. The studies also highlighted the positive outcomes of continuing professional education **(Table 29.1)**.

Leadership and Management Training

The main objective of organizing leadership and management training programs is to equip the selected group of staff to fit them in the position of management and leadership. They are either at the supervisory level or managerial level. In some institutions, it is mandatory to undergo a management training program to apply for the supervisory or administrative posts.

IN-SERVICE EDUCATION

In-service education, as the name indicates, refers to all the programs organized in the institution and is intended to increase skills, competence, and work performance of employees in a particular area in the present job. The word "in-service" originated from Latin word *in*, within, *servus*, a slave, *educare*, to rear. In-service education may be a part of any program of staff development.

Definition

Hamelin defined in-service education as a planned educational activity organized by the employer to the employees to improve the knowledge and skills to accomplish the specific purpose of the organization.

Objectives of In-service Education

Employee Based
- Improve personal and professional growth
- Motivate them toward their work
- Improve work performance
- Able to acquire, maintain, and improve competencies
- Enhance skills, knowledge, and attitude toward work and work setting
- Able to provide quality nursing services to the patients
- Provide job satisfaction
- Improve communication skills
- Provide a platform for promotion.

Organization Based
- Improve the quality of patient care
- Decrease turnover of staff
- Better work effectiveness
- Meet both immediate and long-term goals.

Areas of In-Service Education

As a part of any program of staff development, it includes various areas such as orientation, skill training/technical training, leadership and management training, safety training, and continuing education on different aspects. The most common identified areas in nursing service are human relation in health care, management techniques for nursing administrators, and care in the emergency of all specialties for staff nurses and educational technology for nurse educators.

Training and Development

Training refers to learning experiences provided to improve performance on the present job. According to William G Torpey, it is the process of developing skills, habits, knowledge, and aptitude in employees to increase the effectiveness of employees in their present positions as well as prepare them for future posts.

The development consists of learning experiences unrelated to the job that may have some impact on the present position. Education is learning skills to improve the performance of a future career or enable the employees to accept new responsibilities or assignments on their current job.

Types of Development

Development is of two types, which are as follows:
a. **Personal development:** The personal development is concerning with the development of individuals in terms of their behavior, attitude, personality, and other personal qualities. Personal development affects the professional development of individuals. There are various ways of developing individuals personally, such as taking care of the health of staff, implementing stress management strategies, inculcating leadership qualities, developing reading habits, organizing social gatherings, informal meetings with the staff, counseling, etc.
b. **Professional development:** The professional development is concerning with the development of staff professionally. The staff must follow the professional code of ethics. There are various formal and informal methods to make staff professionally grow such as imparting in-service training programs per their learning needs, adequate supervisory ways to control them, and other communication and coordination methods.

Training versus Development

Training and development differ from each other based on its purpose, level of personnel involved (trainees), depth of knowledge imparted, an initiative in learning, the scope of education, goal, content, and time frame **(Table 29.2)**.

Benefits of Training

Training is beneficial to both the employers and the employees. The benefits of training in an organization are as follows:
- It increases productivity and efficiency among employees.
- It improves the performance level and helps them to achieve their career goals.

TABLE 29.2: Distinctions between training and development.

Basis	Training	Development
Purpose	It aims to maintain and improve job performance of personnel	It is designed to enhance the overall effectiveness of staff in their present position and to prepare them for greater responsibility when they get a promotion
Meant for	Training programs are designed and planned for personnel at operational level	Development programs are designed for middle level (supervisory) and managerial level personnel
Depth of knowledge imparted	It is related to specific job techniques and manual skills	It is similar to supervisory and management techniques, principles, concepts, and philosophy
Initiative in learning	The management takes effort to organize and conduct training programs	The management or individual itself takes the initiative
Scope of learning	Training is job focused	Development is management or career oriented and focused for current and future job
Goal	Fixed current skill deficit	Prepare for future work demands
Content	Specific job-related information	General knowledge
Time frame	It is a short-term process	It is a long-term process

- It leads to improvement of the quality and quantity of work output.
- It helps to keep employees informed about the latest development and rapid technological changes in care.
- It helps to make employees mobile, active, and versatile in their job.
- It helps in the full utilization of materials, supplies, and other equipment by the skilled employees.
- It helps in eliminating mistakes, errors, and reducing cost.
- It helps in improving the relationship among staff, with team members and management.
- It leads to high job satisfaction and lower turnover.

Principles of Adult Learning

As we know, in-service education or any training program is essential for job success. It is beneficial to both nursing staff and nursing organizations if nurse managers understand the principles behind the training process. Training efforts must follow certain principles of adult learning, conceptualized by Malcolm Knowles, an adult learning theorist. He used the term "andragogy" since adult learners have distinct and unique characteristics and need learner-centered teaching-learning methods. Following are the core principles of adult learning:

1. **Principle of self-directing:** Knowles, in his andragogical model, conceptualized that adults are autonomous and self-directing. Adults are experienced, mature, and self-governed and have achieved self-concept of being responsible for their own life; they have their own beliefs. They have self-pride and expect to be respected. They are goal oriented. Hence they need to know rationale, purpose, value, and aim of a training program and need to be taught by teaching methods that should acknowledge and respect their experiences, beliefs, knowledge, and ideas. They need to engage in the structure of their exposure to learn new skills.
2. **Principle of learning by doing:** Adults are practical oriented and can quickly grasp through getting a direct learning experience. Hence they need to be taught through practical oriented teaching-learning strategies requiring their active participation. Learning strategies must be a focus on teaching skills and should be goal oriented and problem centered.
3. **Principle of relevance:** Adults are relevancy oriented; they will be most interested in subjects that have immediate relevance to a job or personal life. Therefore the content of training programs must be related to their job, career oriented, and personal and professional development. Hence training programs must be selected according to the need of individuals, and material should be a plan and taught in such a way that they can immediately apply in their present job and personal life.
4. **Principle of motivation:** Motivation is another principle of adult learning. When the learner is motivated, he or she pays attention to what is being said, done, and presented. Many factors, such as the importance of the job, training, promotion, interest, relationship, cognitive interest, and external expectations, affect the motivation level of the learners. They learn more quickly and retain for a longer time if the material is essential and relevant to them and participate actively. Hence, the administrator must plan the content at the appropriate level of concern and difficulty level. Set a feeling for learning by providing an appropriate motivating learning environment.
5. **Principle of reinforcement:** According to this principle, punishment is less effective in learning than reward. To be effective, the trainer must reward desired behavior only as adults avoid certain practices that invite criticism and punishment. If he or she rewards poor performance, results may be disastrous; good performers may quit in frustration or may not improve.
6. **Principle of feedback:** Every learner wants to know the expectation from him or her and about his or her performance. They learn best if they get immediate feedback on how they are doing. Positive feedback is preferred to negative feedback when we want to change the behavior. The trainer must provide opportunities for learners to get feedback immediately after the training program and must discuss the right way of doing things so that those who were off the track can rectify quickly.
7. **Principle of spaced learning:** According to the principle of spaced learning, the practice session must spread over a while to better knowledge. Therefore it is better to plan an orientation program for a period of two or three days or a week. This type of incremental approach is best for skill acquisition to minimize physical fatigue that deters learning.
8. **Principle of whole learning:** Adult learners learn better if job information is explained as an entirely logical process so that they can bring life experiences and previous knowledge and can see how the various actions fit together into the whole or big picture. The learners can learn best if they relate new knowledge and information with previous experience and skill. The task if practices all at once rather than trying to master various components of the job at different intervals.
9. **Principle of active practice:** As we know, "Practice makes a man perfect." Give opportunity to the trainee to repeat the tasks to enhance learning. Therefore, give weight to the practical session and plan throughout the training period.
10. **Principle of orientation to learning:** Adults want to be engaged in problem-centered learning experiences rather content oriented. They learn best if teaching is related to the problem they face in personal and professional life and useful in tackling those problems. They are practical and want to be involved in the planning and evaluation of their instructions. Hence trainees must include application in each learning activity and plan content jointly to fit their needs.

Chapter 29: Staff Development and In-service Education

11. **Principle of readiness**: Readiness refers to the degree of willingness and eagerness of a learner to learn. If a learner is ready physically, mentally, and emotionally to learn, he or she will learn more quickly, effectively, and best as compared to situations when he or she is not willing and does not show eagerness and enthusiasm to learn. Readiness is also dependent on maturation and experience of the learner. Readiness prepares the learner for action. It is an essential factor in learning.
12. **Principle of collaboration and reciprocity**: Adults learn best through reflection on their own and others' experiences through discussion, sharing previous knowledge and skill. Therefore trainee must plan small group discussions and other interacting methods such as seminars, role plays, and quiz. Further, use a team approach to strengthen their self-pride and self-respect.

Planning and Organizing In-service Education/Training Programs

The success of the in-service education program depends on planning and conduction of program. Planning and organization of in-service education programs have four main phases: assessment phase, designing phase, implementation phase, and evaluation phase **(Fig. 29.5)**.

Assessment Phase

During this phase, determine organizational and its employees' needs and performance-deficit areas. Gather relevant information regarding participants' entry level; knowledge; skills and training desires; and expectations of the staff through organizational, operational, and personal analysis methods. The purpose of the organizational analysis is to identify the area for training; functional analysis is to identify possible content of practice, and personal review is to determine individual needs for the type of training. Conduct individual or group interviews with key supervisors, participants, records, observation, surveys, or tests to gather information.

The Designing and Preparation Phase

The next phase in a planning training program is to design programs and incorporate activities keeping in mind behaviorist, cognitive, and humanistic approaches based on theories. The behaviorist approach is useful in teaching psychomotor skills necessary to perform the task and correctly repeat the demonstration. The cognitive approach is helpful to recall and in the application of past experiences, whereas the humanistic approach is vital to building curiosity among nurse participants. The design document should have program background, target group (trainees), training climate, trainers, and performance objectives, training topics, and contents, methods, learning the outcome, budget, time targets, pre–post tests, and other requirements. Prepare a checklist that can ensure all the activities to be carried out during implementation **(Box 29.2)**.

> **Box 29.2:** A checklist for planning a training program.
>
> ❖ Formulate objective of the program based on the identified need
> ❖ Selection of planning team/expert
> ❖ Selection of coordinator
> ❖ Define participants: level, number, method of selection
> ❖ Decide place/venue
> ❖ Duration of course/time
> ❖ Learning experiences: time/duration of theory, practical
> ❖ Decide on topics/plan course/units/subunits/theory/practical; sequencing of content
> ❖ Decide methodology and audio-visual aids
> ❖ Select/plan clinical facilities
> ❖ Prepare clinical plan/schedule, staff assignment
> ❖ Prepare pre–post test evaluation performed based on objectives
> ❖ Check administrative details: permission/funds, etc.
> ❖ Prepare handouts if any
> ❖ Send letters, confirmations with experts, teachers, participants

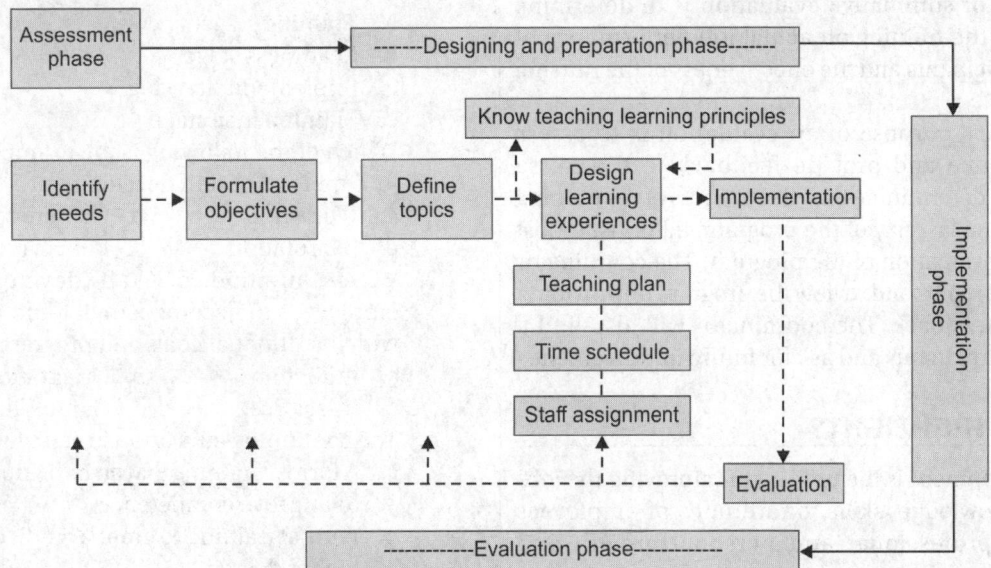

Fig. 29.5: Planning and organizing in-service education program.

Implementation Phase

Before actual conducting in-service education program, ensure completion of task analysis, specification of entry-level skills, development of instructional objectives, and identification of media and materials. This phase requires continual adjusting, redesigning, and refining. Preparation is the most important in the success of the training program. Good physical setup is prerequisite for an effective and successful training program. Prepare trainers mentally and keep ready all the material required well in advance. Review the objectives of the program and establish a rapport with the participants.

On an opening day, set the tone and establish an in-service education program as a community of learners, comfortable seating arrangement, music depending on the nature of the program, and the greeting of participants. The coordinator of the program will welcome the chief guest and introduce the program plan, objectives, methodology, and evaluation and will give a brief introduction of participants and organizers.

After introducing the session, the coordinator will administer the pretest, followed by the first session of the program. The program will carry on per plan. Keep in mind the principles of adult learning while conducting sessions. Arrange group photographs. On the last day, familiarize with the next day program and inform if any change. Each subsequent day reviews the previous lesson.

Evaluation and Follow-up Phase

This phase includes the enhancement and evaluation of training and development. The process of examining training program is training evaluation. It includes formative, process, and outcome evaluation. Plan the methods of formative evaluation before the implementation of a training program. Process evaluation is the evaluation of participants' satisfaction, knowledge, skills, and abilities to find out the effectiveness of training. The outcome or summative evaluation is to determine the impact of the training on actual job performance of the nurse participants and the effectiveness of the nursing organization.

The primary purpose of an evaluation is to assess the performance and provide feedback to the nurse participants in determining the effectiveness of the training program. On the last day of the program, administer post test and seek evaluation of the program. The coordinator will give a brief report and review the program by providing performance feedback. The coordinator will also find a report from participants and ask for future improvement.

CHAPTER HIGHLIGHTS

- Staff development is the process of improving the job-related knowledge, skills, or attitudes of employees for their professional and personal growth and advancement in the organization.
- Staff development aims in the overall development of all nurse employees for rendering nursing care.
- Staff development includes both on-the-job and off-the-job methods.
- Induction training, orientation, in-service education, leadership and management training, and continuing education programs are part of staff development programs.
- The training aims at maintaining and improving job performance of personnel, whereas development is concerning with overall growth and is career oriented and focused on current and future jobs.
- Adult learners need learner-centered teaching-learning methods and follow andragogy principles.

REVIEW QUESTIONS

I. Essay Type Questions
1. What do you mean by staff development? Discuss its importance.
2. Enumerate different types of staff development programs. Discuss orientation program in detail.
3. Define "in-service education." Discuss its objectives.
4. What are the benefits of training? Describe the principles of adult learning.
5. Describe the steps of planning and organizing in-service education.

II. Short Notes
1. Staff development models
2. Continuing education
3. Advantages of staff development
4. Training versus development
5. Philosophy of staff development

III. Multiple Choice Questions
1. Which stage focuses on the development of a positive climate to plan staff development in the RPTIM model?
    a. Training stage
    b. Readiness stage
    c. Implementation stage
    d. Maintenance stage
2. Which of the following is the example of "on-the-job" method of staff development?
    a. Workshop   b. Conference
    c. Job rotation   d. Role play
3. Which method of staff development help employees to become familiar and identify them with institutional goals and programs?
    a. Induction   b. Orientation
    c. In-service   d. Continuing
4. The continuing education in staff development is:
    a. A form of training that an individual undertakes to improve competence.
    b. Formal training to grant a credit of acquiring a higher degree

Chapter 29: Staff Development and In-service Education

c. A planned educational activity to achieve a specific purpose of the organization
d. A type of training to equip staff to fit in a position of management and leadership

5. Which one of the following programs is related to specific job techniques and manual skills?
    a. Continuing education
    b. Training
    c. Development
    d. Orientation
6. Which principle of adult learning conceptualizes that punishment is less effective in learning than reward?
    a. Principle of feedback
    b. Principle of motivation
    c. Principle of self-directing
    d. Principle of reinforcement
7. Which type of analysis designs to identify possible content of the training?
    a. Organizational analysis
    b. Personal analysis
    c. Operational analysis
    d. Performance analysis
8. The approach that is useful in teaching psychomotor skill is:
    a. Cognitive   b. Affective
    c. Humanistic   d. Behavioral

Answer Keys

1. b   2. c   3. a   4. a   5. b   6. d   7. c
8. d

SUGGESTED READING

1. Alspach JG. The Educational Process in Nursing Staff Development. St. Louis: Mosby; 1995.
2. Available from https://bbamantra.com/training-objectives-purpose-methods-hrm/. [Accessed July 2019].
3. Concepts of In-Service Education In Hospital Nursing (n.d.). [Online] Available from https://www.coursehero.com/file/p6jaag7/CONCEPTS-OF-IN-SERVICE-EDUCATION-In-hosp. [Accessed August 2019].
4. Elias S. Putting it all together: An integrated staff development program. In Caldwell S (Ed). Staff development: A handbook of effective practices. Oxford, OH: National Staff Development Council; 1989.
5. Fundamentals of Adult Learning. [Online] Available from http://sarahcordiner.com/the-8-fundamental-principles-of-adu/. [Accessed August 2019].
6. Furze G, Pearcey P. Continuing education in nursing: A review of the literature. J Adv Nurs. 1999;29(2):355-63.
7. Gaston C. Inservice education: Career development for South Australian nurses. Aust J Adv Nurs. 1989;6(4):5-9.
8. Glickman E. Developing teacher thought. J Staff Dev. 1986;7(1):6-21.
9. Gordon BN, Franklin EM. An orientation for inexperienced educators. Journal of Nursing Staff Development. 1993;9(2):75-7.
10. Griscti O, Jacono J. Effectiveness of continuing education programs in nursing: A literature review. J Adv Nurs. 2006;55(4):449-56.
11. In-Service Education |authorstream. (n.d.). [Online] Available from http://www.authorstream.com/Presentation/anitarobins-2292127-service-education/. [Accessed July 2019].
12. Joyce B, Weil M. Models of Teaching. Englewood Cliffs, NJ: Prentice-Hall; 1972.
13. Kearsley G. Andragogy (M Knowles). The Theory into Practice Data Base, 2010. Avaialble from http://tip.psychology.org. [Accessed August 2019].
14. Knowles MS. Andragogy in Action. San Francisco: Jossey-Bass; 1984.
15. Norushe TF, Van Rooyen D, Strumpher J. In-service education and training as experienced by registered nurses. Curationis. 2004;27(4):63-72.
16. Russell L. The Fundamental of Adult Learning. [Online] Available from tps://www.td.org/Publications/Newsletters/Links/2009/11/The-Fundamentals-of-Adult-Learning. [Accessed August 2019].
17. Sparks D, Loucks-Horsley S. Five models of staff development. J Staff Dev Fall. 1989;10(4). Online on Sunday, March 27, 2011.
18. Vati J, Walia I. Staff, and professional development methods: Facilities available and used by hospital nurses of north India. Nurs J India. 2001;92(2):38-40 (Abstract, Pub Med indexed for Medline). [Accessed August 2019].
19. Vesuwala S. Orientation. Nurs J India. 2000;91(10):225-6.
20. Wood I. The effects of continuing professional education on the clinical practice of nurses: A review of the literature. Int J Nurs Stud. 1998;35(3):125-31 (Abstract, Pub Med indexed for Medline). [Accessed August 2019].

30 CHAPTER

Career Planning, Development and Opportunities

CHAPTER OUTLINE

- Career Planning
  - Career: Concept and Features
  - Career Planning: Introduction
  - Objectives of Career Planning in Nursing
  - Importance of Career Planning in Nursing
  - Career Development
- Career Planning and Development
  - Career Planning and Development Process
  - Stages of Career Planning and Development
  - Career Planning and Development Responsibility
- High Power Committee Recommendations on Career Development-related Issues
- Nursing as a Career, Career Positions, and Opportunities in Nursing
- Nursing Career Development Opportunities and Practices

LEARNING OUTCOMES

After completion of this chapter, the learner will be able to:
- Understand the concept of career
- Enumerate the features of career
- Appreciate nursing as a career
- Define career planning and development
- Enlist objectives of career planning
- Recognize the importance of career planning
- List down the stages of career planning and development
- Explain the responsibility toward career planning and development at different levels
- Cite the recommendations of the High Power Committee of nursing with particular emphasis on career development
- Discuss present scenario of career positions and opportunities in nursing
- Describe evidence-based nursing career and development practices in India

KEY TERMS

Career, development, career planning, career and development planning, High Power Committee, career opportunities

INTRODUCTION

Career planning is an essential aspect of human resource management, especially in nursing to obtain maximum performance output from nursing personnel. It is necessary for the organization to grow and to accomplish nursing organizational goals. Nursing is an excellent career for men and women who wish to have long-term job security. There is a positive change in the nursing workforce over the past decades. The current information about the shortage of nurses shows the positive signs about those entering and working in the nursing profession.

CAREER PLANNING

Career: Concept and Features

The word "career" derives from the Middle French word *carriere*, and Late Latin word *carriria* (*via*) means "road." According to Webster Dictionary, career indicates "a field for or pursuit of consecutive progressive achievement especially in public, professional, or business life" (http://www.merriam-webster.com/dictionary/career) and it is a path or progress through life or history (http://www.thefreedictionary.com/career).

Career refers to a series of work-related activities that provide continuity, order, and meaning to a person's life (Schein, 1996) and have changes in values, attitudes, and motivation as the person grows older (Hall, 1976).

According to Arthur et al. (1989), career is "the evolving sequence of a person's work experiences over time," and career leads to an organized path by an individual in a lifetime.

Features of Career

- It is a lifelong process of a person.

- It is individualized. The individual has to set his or her own career goals and path.
- It includes a series of work activities and positions that bring continuity and order.
- It brings a sense of personal accomplishments and achievements.

Career Planning: Introduction

Career planning is an ongoing and lifelong process that can help to manage learning and development. It is a process of development of human resources to achieve maximum results. It is the process by which one selects career goals and path to achieve those goals.

In an organization, it means helping the employees to plan their career according to their capabilities and keeping in mind the organizational goals, thus synthesizing and harmonizing the organizational goals and employees' aspirations. It is the process of career movement from the entry of an individual to the point of retirement. It is the management technique to map the entire career of the employee in higher-skilled, supervisory, and managerial positions.

In an organization, the career plan is the career path/graph of different categories showing how they can advance up in the organization. Clark (1997) describes this process as "self-concept and identity formation."

Objectives of Career Planning in Nursing

1. To attract and secure the right person at the right time in the nursing organization
2. To provide career avenues to nurses to higher levels of responsibilities per their capability and interest
3. To improve the morale of the nurses to work by providing a career ladder
4. To get the maximum performance from them
5. To reduce the turnover and absenteeism
6. To provide individual guidance and encourage nurses to show their potentials
7. To achieve nursing organizational development.

Importance of Career Planning in Nursing

- To utilize the nursing staff reserve within the organization properly
- To ensure the performance of nursing staff at the satisfactory level through staff development
- To reduce the turnover for lack of promotional avenues
- To maintain and improve motivation and morale of employees
- It helps to make adjustments throughout the life.

Career Development

Career development is a dynamic process of understanding career preferences, identifying, obtaining, and developing appropriate skills and training for that career. It includes the personal actions taken by an individual to achieve a career plan.

Career development is a lifelong professional activity, which includes a series of activities carried out lifelong for developing one's career. It usually refers to developing one's career within an organization or different organizations or starting one's own business. It includes career planning. The first step is the first job, and then it involves training on new skills to cope up with workplace issues, moving to higher job responsibilities, status, salary structure, etc. However, it needs proper planning.

CAREER PLANNING AND DEVELOPMENT

Career Planning and Development Process

Career planning and development is a process of awareness of individuals about personal career-related attributes and lifelong progression that contribute to his or her career fulfillment. It is the process that adapts to the changes experienced by nurses as they build their professional knowledge, experience, and identity. It is in long-term career effectiveness. Career planning and development is an essential and necessary tool in the development of nurses as professionals and in retaining nurses in a facility.

Career planning and development is a process directly based on career goals and objectives set by an individual. To meet the goals, develop a career plan or map. It needs self-actualization and self-assessment of the interests and capabilities of the individuals.

The components of career plans include the following:
- A summary paragraph describing critical elements about oneself
- Resume (a brief about career, current and core information about demographic data, education, credentials, goals, relevant experience, and key achievements to identify critical professional expertise and knowledge)
- Curriculum vitae (detailed information about to date professional career), the portfolio (exhaustive collection of data focuses on career goals and objectives, annual work plan, annual performance appraisal, annual achievements, appreciations, etc.)
- Professional career development plan (includes professional goals, target time frame, strategies, or activities to reach goals or to achieve objectives).

Formulate alternative action plans and strategies for dealing with the match and mismatch with self-assessment and set a goal and according to the professional career development plan. If required, the nurse needs to undergo training to acquire the skills required for the option or career path chosen by him or her. Finally, after receiving the desired competency, he or she has to perform to achieve the goals and targets set by him or her and then review periodically **(Fig. 30.1)**.

Stages of Career Planning and Development

There are five stages of career planning and development: exploration, guidance from various sources, mid-career stage, late-career stage, and declining stage.

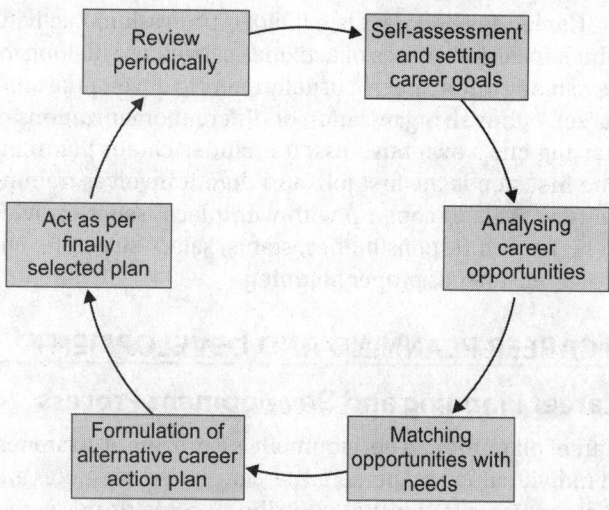

Fig. 30.1: Career planning process.

1. **Exploration stage:** This stage starts at the time of school or college education before joining for the profession or on or before completion of nursing education. There is no relevance to the nursing organization with this stage because this stage is before employment.
2. **Guidance from various sources:** The staff before joining the profession or job seek help from multiple sources, e.g. friends, relatives, seniors, teachers, and media, keeping in mind the aim of joining the profession.
3. **Mid-career stage:** This is a crucial stage after deciding and joining the first job. The staff will work very hard to perform well to get the promotion or change the position if not satisfied. Authority, reward, and incentives are highest at this stage.
4. **Late career stage:** This stage is pleasant to the senior staff who like to work with the past glory and help the juniors. Others may still struggle to achieve higher positions or go high up in their careers.
5. **Declining stage:** This career stage is usually on completion of career and advancing toward retirement. The achievers typically find it difficult to compromise to retire. Others may think of life after retirement.

Career Planning and Development Responsibility

The question arises who is responsible for career planning: Basically, career planning is an individual responsibility. The action for career development can be initiated both by individual and organization as well as a professional organization can play an essential role in developing a nursing career.

At Individual Level

Largely the outcome of the action is taken at a personal level. The nurses at the personal level can push their career through performance; improving qualification; identifying, obtaining, and developing appropriate and need-based skills and competencies in specialties and subspecialties; exposure; networking (professional and personal contacts); mentors; seniors, key subordinates based on their interest, preferences, and opportunities available and need of organization. Active and structured participation in self-discovery can assist them to reflect on their growing professional values and attitudes and to learn and refine skills that will allow them to successfully and confidently participate in a formidable work environment in the beginning and throughout stages of their career (Waddell, Bauer, 2005).

At the Organizational Level

Whereas the organization e.g., guide and direct the nurses to develop and utilize their knowledge, skill, qualification, and resources toward staff and organizational development. For nurse employees, the organization can plan through career counseling, workshops, assessment, etc.

Professional Organizations

The professional organizations, for example, the Trained Nurses Association of India (TNAI), Nursing Research Society of India (NRSI), and Society of Midwives, India (SOMI), are involved in developing leadership and professional skills, improving networking through organizing continuing education, conferences, workshop, etc., and thus increasing professional socialization.

HIGH POWER COMMITTEE RECOMMENDATIONS ON CAREER DEVELOPMENT-RELATED ISSUES

High Power Committee (HPC) on Nursing and Nursing professional (1988) recommended on the following career development-related issues of nurses:

Career Development

HPC recommended having the provision of deputation for higher studies after 5 years of regular course. There should be provisions for attending refresher courses and facilities for undergoing higher study on deputation.

Promotional Opportunities

HPC also recommended the promotion avenues for nurses. There is a need to have at least a degree in nursing for the supervisory post in nursing. It should apply all nursing and for all levels. Irrespective of the place of posting, the nursing staff must get at least three promotions during their service tenure and must keep in mind the selection through merit cum seniority at the middle level and open and on merit base for the managerial and administrative posts.

Continuing Education and Staff Development

There is a need to frame specific policies for deputing 5–10% of staff for higher studies by each state. There should be a provision for training reserve, deputation after 5 years for higher study, refresher courses, and a nursing Institute for Education, Research, and Training at the national level.

NURSING AS A CAREER, CAREER POSITIONS, AND OPPORTUNITIES IN NURSING

Nursing is a service to humanity. More a person is dedicated to this service: more significant will be the benefit rendered to the society. It was in 1860 when professional nursing established in the Nightingale School of Nursing. Since then, nursing is considered a vocation, an art, a science, and a profession. As a profession, nursing is comparatively new; it is developing and will develop trends in nursing training in the future. In India, nursing training is advanced from Auxiliary Nurse Midwife (ANM) to PhD in nursing, even fellowship as well.

"Nursing is not an honorable profession" was a firm belief in the past. The study conducted by Martin (1974) had shown that the Indian Christian girls did not like to join nursing as it required hard labor, and life was unprotected. Oommen (1978) had revealed that a much higher percentage of Christian girls were entering the profession as they wanted to become a nurse and had desired to help people.

Kakar et al. (1980 and 1981), in two separate studies, explored some of the critical factors considered by the nurses in deciding to join nursing as a profession. These were uniform, financial consideration, family opinion, intellectual satisfaction, the influence of friends, and easy job availability. A study conducted by Gupta (1983) on 32 BSc nursing students of a nursing college revealed that majority (93.75%) of the students opted for the nursing profession as a career to go abroad and out of the 68.28% wanted to go overseas to seek a job. The nonavailability of the seat in medical college was another factor considered by the girls to join the nursing profession as an alternative. At that time, there were fewer job prospects in India and was an eye-opener to the planners to bring about a change in the job and job career.

At present many girls are opting to nursing as a career as it has a wide variety of different positions. There are many job opportunities throughout the world. Most of these jobs have specializations that a nurse can opt and that give even more chances. Although nursing has not always been broad, nursing in the present day has many different positions that a person can fill and is an excellent example of how diverse this profession can be. Nursing is necessary in hospitals all over the world, and there had been a need for thousands of years. Per the specialty, it corresponds to the field of medicine.

A study conducted by Patidar et al. (2011) in selected five Punjab nursing colleges comprising General Nursing and Midwifery (GNM) ($n=225$), BSc ($n=1550$), and post-basic BSc Nursing ($n=150$) students revealed that 99.1% (525 of 530) of nursing students perceived that it is is a humanity profession, and there is personal growth in this profession (81.9%). As for the future career plan, two third of them planned to go abroad and prefer to join bedside nursing (<50%). More post-basic students wanted to join teaching institutions; only less than 50% had planned to go for higher studies. However, most of them were not interested in changing the profession. It means that there is an opportunity for graduate and diploma nurses in the country and abroad.

One of the critical reviews on nursing and midwifery in India (Bagga, 2012) revealed that a variety of positions exist in the current Indian scenario although there is the unequal geographical distribution of nursing institutions for ANM, GNM, and degree and postgraduate courses. The positions and grades per sixth pay commission and career opportunities in nursing in Indian scenario in clinical, public health, and nursing institutions are listed in **Table 30.1**.

ANM/Female Health Worker

After 10+2 with arts, one can opt for ANM training. In the first entry, she can join as ANM. The career opportunity is open for the post of Lady Health Visitor (LHV)/Female Health Supervisor following qualifying 6 months promotional training of LHV after 5 years of experience as ANM **(Fig. 30.2)** and also can undergo GNM training program.

TABLE 30.1: Distribution of nursing positions and their grade pay per Sixth Pay Commission.

Settings	Nursing positions	Grade pay
Community Health Nursing	Auxiliary Nurse Midwife (ANM) (multipurpose health worker [F]/health worker [M])	4,200
	Junior Public Health Nurse	4,800
	Lady Health Visitor/Female Health Supervisor	5,200
	District Public Health Nurse	5,400
	Chief of Public Health Nurse	6,600
Hospital Nursing Services	Staff Nurse	4,600
	Nursing Sister	4,800
	Assistant Nursing Superintendent	5,400
	Deputy Nursing Superintendent	6,600
	Nursing Superintendent	6,600
	Chief Nursing Officer	6,600
School of Nursing	Clinical Instructor	4,800
	Sister Tutor/Nurse Tutor	5,400
	Senior Sister Tutor/Nurse Tutor	6,600
	Vice Principal	6,600
	Principal	6,600
College of Nursing	Clinical Instructor	4,800
	Sister Tutor/Nurse Tutor	5,400
	Senior Sister Tutor/Nurse Tutor	6,600
	Vice Principal	6,600
	Professor	6,600
	Principal	8,700
Ministry	Assistant Director-General of Nursing Services (ADGNS)	6,600
	Nursing Advisor of Government of India (GOI)	8,700

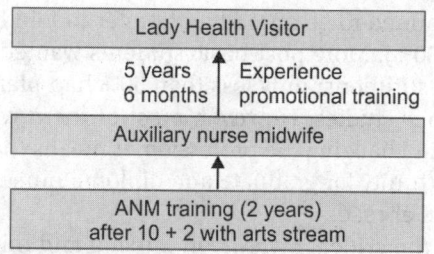

Fig. 30.2: Career opportunities with Auxiliary Nurse Midwife training.

GNM

The candidate should be with 10+2 Arts/Science examination OR 10+2 vocational ANM under CBSE board or other equivalent board from the school and should be recognized by Indian Nursing Council with 40% marks and should be registered as ANM with State Nursing Registration Council. After successful completion, they have the opportunity to work in a hospital setting as a staff nurse, and career opportunities are open for the promotion of higher post like a nursing sister or opt for the degree program.

The current Public Health Nurse Diploma Course is of the 10-month duration. The eligibility to get this diploma program is either GNM or 4 years of BSc Nursing with 5 years of work experience as a staff nurse in a clinical setup and 2 years of experience in public health. Public Health Nurses can work in nursing schools, hospitals, regional offices' district training teams (DTTs) or district panchayat. They get promotions to the post of District Public Health Nursing Officer after obtaining the diploma. Those who get appointed at the district panchayat are responsible for supervising the nursing workforce of their respective districts. They work as District Public Health Nurses.

BSc Nursing (4 Years) and Post-basic BSc Nursing

BSc Nursing (4 years) is a professionally oriented course after 10+2 with medical stream (Physics, Chemistry, and Biology) and English core/English elective with an aggregate of 45% marks from a recognized board or other equivalent board.

Post-basic BSc Nursing is of 2 years of university undergraduate program at post-basic level after Diploma in General Nursing and Midwifery training for the candidate passed Higher Secondary/Senior Secondary/Intermediate/10+2 or an equivalent examination recognized by the university. After successful completion, they have the opportunity to work in a hospital setting as a staff nurse. And career opportunities are open for the promotion of higher posts such as nursing sister, assistant nursing superintendent/assistant matron, deputy nursing superintendent, superintendent/matron, infection control nurse/epidemiologist or public health nurse in selected nursing units, CSSD supervisor, etc., in nursing institutes as clinical instructor/tutor, demonstrator after experience. In the community, she can opt for as Public Health Nurse after getting a diploma in Public Health and public health nurse officer after the experience. After graduate degree in nursing, the doors are open for a postgraduate degree in nursing.

MSc Nursing

Master's degree course is a 2-year postgraduate program for the registered nurse and midwife candidates with minimum qualification of passing BSc Nursing/BSc Hons. Nursing/Post-basic BSc Nursing with a minimum of 55% aggregate marks, having minimum 1 year of work experience after Basic BSc Nursing or prior or after Post-basic BSc Nursing. The career opportunities are open for the post of chief nursing officer in the hospital after obtaining a postgraduate nursing degree with required experience in administration and clinical and teaching. And, after the required experience, the opportunities are also open for the promotion of higher posts such as a lecturer, assistant professor, associate professor, professor, and principal and director, dean in nursing, nursing advisor, and assistant nursing advisor to Government of India. They can work in different research projects and can hold various positions in professional organizations such as TNAI, WHO, and regulatory bodies such as the Indian Nursing Council and so on. They can undergo higher studies such as PhD in nursing, MPhil, or for fellowships.

NURSING CAREER DEVELOPMENT OPPORTUNITIES AND PRACTICES

In a study conducted by Sonmez and Yildirim (2009) on 373 nurse managers in 200+ bed hospitals on the European side of Istanbul province, Turkey, data were collected with a 32-item survey form. The findings revealed that education programs were the most common technique used for career development for nurses.

The different practices found in public and private hospitals, but no effective career development practices identified, and the nurse managers did not have agreement on the subject of career development. However, the career development practices of private hospitals were more developed than public hospitals, and the nurse managers' perceptions about career development were different according to their management level, age group, and educational level ($p < 0.05$). Hospitals that provide an opportunity for horizontal and vertical promotion and have clear development policies will be successful hospitals that are preferred by high-quality nurses.

A research paper by Vati et al. (2001) revealed that although there was an opportunity for the nurses to attend conferences and workshops to undergo higher study in few states, yet only a few nurses had availed these facilities in district hospitals of north India. The majority of nursing staff at supervisory and administrative levels were without management training. The skill training program, conferences, and seminars were attended only by a few nurses. Their hospitals used other methods such as case discussion, supervisory rounds, and demonstrations as 15.5% nurses reported learning techniques. Professional career development through continuing scheme education programs and in-service education programs for the district hospitals' nursing staff was negligible. But presently, it is observed that the nurses are attending/organizing conferences, workshop, going for higher study to develop their career in North India.

The similar findings reported in a critical review on nursing and midwifery in India (Bagga et al. 2012) that there is a lack of opportunity for knowledge and skill upgradation and culture of supportive supervision and learning on the job is lacking. There is a stagnation in the promotion of higher posts.

The study conducted in the 1990s also highlighted that all the nursing staff, including nurse administrators, supervisors, and bedside nurses, possessed minimum qualification of General Nursing for the post. It is also highlighted that there was stagnation of more than 5 to 25 years for the higher post, and promotion is based on seniority of nursing staff in district hospitals' of North India (Vati, 1992). And in a referral hospital, the work experience of staff nurses ($n=353$) ranged between 5 and 20 years and of nursing sisters ($n=100$) ranged from 3 to 26 years, and administrators worked as nursing sisters for more than 18 years before getting the post of assistant matron or matron. The recruitment of staff nurses, public health nurses, and the chief nursing officer was through direct selection, and the minimum qualification required is RNRM, BSc Nursing, and MSc Nursing with 10 years of professional, teaching, and administrative experience, respectively. Thus the stagnation on one post of the nursing department at each level and the extent of stagnation are more than sixfolds as required for the next promotion (Earnest et al. 1996).

CHAPTER HIGHLIGHTS

- Career is a lifelong ongoing process that includes a series of work activities, positions that bring continuity, and order over a period that brings a sense of personal accomplishments and achievements.
- Career development is a dynamic process of developing one's career within an organization or different organizations or starting one's own business.
- Components of career plans are short profile, resume, and curriculum vitae, the portfolio, and career development plan.
- Career planning and development process include (1) self-assessment and setting career goals, (2) analyzing career opportunities, (3) matching opportunities with need and goals, (4) developing alternative career action plans, (5) taking action per finally selected plan, and (6) reviewing periodically with the achieved and acquired goal activities.
- Stages of career planning and development are exploration, guidance from various sources, mid-career stage, late-career stage, and declining stage.

- High Power Committee on Nursing and Nursing professional (1988) also recommended for the career development, promotions, and professional and staff development of nurses.
- Presently many girls are opting to nurse as a career compared to past. There is a wide variety of different positions and many job opportunities throughout the world in nursing.
- Evidence revealed that there is a variety of positions, and a good salary exists in the current Indian scenario although there is the unequal geographical distribution of nursing institutions.

REVIEW QUESTIONS

I. Essay Type Questions
1. Define "career" and "career planning." Discuss the need for proper career planning.
2. Distinguish between career planning and career development. Describe the responsibility of career planning at the individual level.
3. Describe various stages of career development.
4. Discuss the career options in nursing with examples.
5. Describe various career opportunities and practices in nursing.

II. Short Notes
1. Importance of career planning
2. Responsibility of career planning at an organizational level
3. Components of career plan
4. Features of career

III. Multiple Choice Questions
1. Which of the following is a lifelong activity that includes an understanding of career preferences and trying to gain skill and training for the career?
    a. Career development
    b. Career planning
    c. Career plan
    d. Career opportunity
2. Which of the following has detailed information about to date a professional career?
    a. Resume
    b. Career development plan
    c. Curriculum vitae
    d. Career strategy
3. Which of the following is the basis for career planning?
    a. Developing career plan
    b. Career goals and objectives
    c. Self-actualization
    d. Self-assessment
4. Career planning is a process of:
    a. Ensuring the performance of individuals through the development
    b. Adjusting to life for the career

c. Improving the morale of individuals to work for career ladder
d. Career movement from the entry to the point of the retirement of the individual

5. In which stage of career planning and development, the staff try to work hard to achieve reward and authority?
    a. Exploration
    b. Mid-career
    c. Late career
    d. Declining stage

Answer Keys

1. a   2. c   3. b   4. a   5. b

SUGGESTED READING

1. Alavi C, Cattoni J. Good nurse, bad nurse. J Adv Nurs. 1995;21:344-9.
2. Arthur MB, Hall DT, Lawrence BS (Eds). Handbook of Career Theory. Cambridge: Cambridge University Press; 1989.
3. Bagga R, et al. Study on Nursing and Midwifery in India—A Critical Review. National Institute of Health and Family Welfare and the World Health Organization, 22.11.2012.
4. Career | Definition of Career at Dictionary.com. https://www.dictionary.com › browse › career. [Accessed on Jan. 2020].
5. Carper B. Fundamental patterns of knowing in nursing. Adv Nurs Sci. 1997;1(1):13-23.
6. Clark PG. Values in health care professional socialization: Implications for geriatric education in interdisciplinary teamwork. Gerontologist. 1997;37:441-51.
7. Clements J, Parrinello K. Climbing higher. Nurs Manag. Dec 1998;29(12):41-5.
8. Collin A, Watts AG. The death and transfiguration of career- and career guidance? Br J Guid Couns. 1996;24:385-98.
9. Earnest C, Saini SK, Gupta JV. Stagnation among the nursing personnel working at Nehru Hospital, PGI, Chandigarh-a perspective study up to May 1993. Indian J Health Admin. 1996;33(1&2):83-94.
10. Gupta J. Nursing as a career to go abroad. Pratichaya. Chandigarh: College of Nursing, PGIMER; 1984.
11. Hall DT. Career in Organizations. Santa Monica, CA: Goodyear, 1976. Available from (online) Handbook of Organizational Politics - Page 284 - Google Books Result. https://books.google.co.in › books. [Accessed Jan. 2020].
12. Kakar DN, Dean M, Misra P, Chopr S. Nursing background: their role performance and future orientation—a sociological study. Nurs J India. 1981;72:70-3.
13. Kakar DN, Dean MA. Study of nursing student-background choices of profession and professional satisfaction. Nurs J India. 1980;71:30-3.
14. Oomme TK. Doctor and Nurses—A Study of Occupational Role Structure. New Delhi: The McMillan Co.; 1978.
15. Patidar AB, Kaur J, et al. Future nurses' perception towards profession: A cross-sectional survey in Punjab State. Nurs Midwifery Res J. 2011 October;7(4):175-85.
16. Schein EH. Career Anchors Revisited: Implications for Career Development in the 21st Century. The Academy of Management Executive (1993-2005) 1996; 10 (4): 80¨C88. Available from (Online)JSTOR, www.jstor.org/stable/4165355. Accessed 11 Jan. 2020.
17. Shermont H, Krepcio D, Murphy J. Career mapping: developing nurse leaders, reinvigorating careers. J Nurs Admin. 2009 October;39(10):432-7.
18. Sonmez B, Yildirim A. What are the career planning and development practices for nurses in hospitals? Is there a difference between private and public hospitals? J Clin Nurs. 2009 Dec;18(24):3461-71.
19. Vati J, Walia I. Staff and professional development methods: facilities available and used by nurses of north India. Nurs J India. 2001 Feb;92(2):38-40.
20. Vati J. Organization and Administration of Nursing Services in District Hospitals of North India. The unpublished thesis of Ph.D. (Nursing). Punjab University; 1990.
21. Waddell J, Bauer M. Career planning and development for students: Building a career in a professional practice discipline. Can J Career Dev. 2005;4(2):4-13.
22. Zimmer M.The rationale for a ladder for clinical advancement. J Nur Admin 1972;2(6):18-24. Available from (online) https://www.ncbi.nlm.nih.gov › pubmed. [Accessed Jan. 2020].

31 Performance Appraisal

CHAPTER OUTLINE

- Performance Appraisal
  - Definitions
  - Characteristics
  - Purposes
  - Principles
  - Consideration for Planning Performance Appraisal
- Approaches to Performance Appraisal
  - Traditional Approaches
  - Modern Approaches
- Performance Appraisal Process
- Methods of Performance Appraisal
  - Individual Methods
  - Multiple-person Evaluation Methods
  - Other Methods
- Guidelines for Effective Performance Appraisal

LEARNING OUTCOMES

After completion of this chapter, the learner will be able to:
- Define and understand the concept of performance appraisal
- State the essential characteristics of performance appraisal
- Enlist the purposes of performance appraisal
- Apply the principles used for performance appraisal
- Discuss the performance appraisal system
- Familiarize with various approaches to performance appraisal
- Elaborate steps of the performance appraisal process
- Explain in detail strategies and methods of performance appraisal
- Explain the 360° appraisal system
- Utilize guidelines to make performance appraisal effective
- Outline performance appraisal practices in nursing

KEY TERMS

Performance appraisal, appraisal approaches, 360° appraisal system, appraisal practices

INTRODUCTION

Performance appraisal has been an essential activity of managerial staffing, which is a primary key to managing itself. The other name of performance appraisal is evaluation. Evaluation is critical in any sphere of life, in education, in administration. As organization structure forms the anatomy, the management is the physiology and assessment is the Heel "Achilles" of the management, a vital organ of the administration. It is also called "soul" and is a significant key to planning.

During the First World War, the US army adopted a rating system for evaluating military personnel for the first time. The performance appraisal roots in the early 20th century and traces to Taylor's pioneering "Time and Motion" studies. From 1920 to 1930, industrial units adopted relational wage structures for hourly-paid workers, which continued up to mid-fifties. It is a performance appraisal, merit rating, behavioral assessment, employee evaluation, personnel review, progress report, staff assessment, service rating, etc. However, widely used terms are performance appraisal or evaluation.

It is the process of deciding how employees do their job. Performance refers to the degree of accomplishment of the tasks that make up an individual's job and indicates how well nursing personnel is fulfilling the job requirements.

PERFORMANCE APPRAISAL

Definitions

According to the Oxford English Dictionary, "Appraise" means "estimate the value or quality". Yoder Dale defined it as a comparatively formal, systematic program of individual employee evaluation. Cleveland et al. viewed performance appraisal as the method of evaluating the behavior of employees in the workplace, including both quantitative and qualitative aspects of job performance

Performance is the individual ability to carry out a specified task. Individual ability focuses on the total behavior of the individual: the individual knowledge, skill to perform the activities, and the attitudes and interaction with other people. Hence performance appraisal in the context of administration is judging the ability of the individual employee. It is a procedure, way, or method to decide the skills. It also acts as a yardstick to control. It is the process of evaluating the relative worth or ability of an individual employee against predetermined job-related performance standards per job descriptions.

Characteristics

The following list shows the characteristics of performance appraisal:
- Performance appraisal is a formal systematic procedure usually involving three steps: setting work standards, assessing employee's actual performance against set standards, and providing feedback to the employees to improve deficiencies.
- It is to find out how well the employee is performing the job.
- The employee must know about their evaluation.
- It measures the actual performance of employees and guides them for future improvement.
- Performance appraisal is not job evaluation; it is a future-oriented activity as it aims at employee development.
- It is both formal or informal, but formal is more objective as well as systematic.

Purposes

I: Employees based

1. *To act as a yardstick for promotion:* As already has been mentioned that it is one of the measures that can be used as a controlling method because the performance reports are considered at the time of promotion, especially when the development is through seniority basis.
2. *To measure job performance:* The foremost objective of performance appraisal to measure what an employee does or to review the performance of the employees over a given period. So the employees will come to know their strengths and weaknesses and where they stand. And thereby helps to judge the gap between the actual and the desired performance.
3. *To improve shortcomings:* When the employees come to know their weaknesses and merits, and the management asks them to improve on those points, hence it is through performance appraisal they get the opportunity to improve upon weak points.
4. *To identify training needs:* Helps to identify training needs and planning for training programs.
5. *To decide salary and wages:* Helpful in determining the salary and payments based on the employees' performance.
6. *To act as a motivational force:* It acts as a motivational force for the employees to become more efficient and develop competition attitude among team members.
7. *To have a base for counseling:* Performance appraisal provides support for advice if required performance improvement.
8. *To have organizational control:* It helps the management in exercising organizational control and strengthens the relationship and communication between superior-subordinate and management employees.
9. *To provide feedback to employees:* It is through performance appraisal that gives feedback to the employees regarding their past performance.
10. *To have a periodic review of progress:* It helps to have a periodical review of progress by identifying individual employee's potentials.
11. To allow the employee to evaluate themselves.

II: Institutional based

1. To assess organizational objectives
2. To measure work standards
3. To remove grievances of the employee
4. To assist in planning and evaluating human resources.

III: Specific

1. *To decide on promotion:* It serves as a useful basis to decide on transfers, promotion, and demotion or job change.
2. *To take compensation-related decisions:* It serves as a basis for wage and salary adjustment. Under the merit system, the employee receives the raises based on performance.
3. *To plan training and development programs:* It can serve as a guide for formulating suitable training and development programs.
4. *To measure performance supervisors and managers in developing team leaders:* It provides a measure of the effectiveness of the supervisors and managers in developing the team members who work under their direction.
5. *To provide performance feedback:* It enables the employee to know how well he or she is doing on the job.
6. *To have a base for personal development:* The supervisors help the subordinates by guiding and counseling to do better and thus help them to improve.

Principles

The following lists the principles of performance appraisal:
- Performance appraisal must be objective and behaviorally oriented.
- The objectives should be in behavioral terms.

- The criteria should be well defined and should be known to staff.
- The methods used for appraisal based on the goals, standards, and criteria framed for appraisal.
- It requires documentation and discussions with the employee.

Consideration for Planning Performance Appraisal

1. **Determine what is to appraise**
   Determine the content matter based on the job analysis. The job analysis consists of a set of tasks and responsibilities and conditions of a specific job. It may be quantity wise or quality wise. Quality of performance consists of quality of work; mental quality—ability to learn, adaptability, and reasoning power; supervisory attributes—leadership, organizing capabilities, and cooperation; and personal traits in terms of personal characteristics observable in employee's job activities—honesty, self-control, initiation, appearance, attitude toward work, and fellow employees, and capability for further development.
2. **Determine who is going to be appraised and by whom?**
   Their immediate supervisors and superiors evaluate their subordinates at different levels. The appraiser should have thorough knowledge about the job content and criteria for appraising while performing the job. The appraiser should also know what is more important and what is relatively less important and need to prepare the reports and make a judgment without bias.
3. **Determine why to appraise?**
   The appraiser should be aware of the purposes of the appraisal. In the governmental sector, it is usually done annually termed as annual confidential report and considered at the time of promotion. It may be for other purposes, as mentioned under the purpose section of this chapter.
4. **Determine when to appraise?**
   The superior usually conducts informal appraisals. Otherwise, they plan to do an annual appraisal regularly.
5. **Determine how to appraise?**
   Decide the methods and tools for evaluation. The tools should be valid and reliable.

APPROACHES TO PERFORMANCE APPRAISAL

Traditional Approach

The traditional method is concerning past performance. The primary purpose of the traditional approach is to make a decision and justify the salary and perks of the employees only and not relating to the development of employees. It judges the organizational performance as a whole by the past achievements of its employees.

Modern Approach

The purpose of the performance appraisal under the contemporary approach is the development of employees and taking corrective actions timely to achieve organizational goals within the time frame and to re-plan. It is formal and structured. Its purpose is to identify training needs and to plan training programs for employees. Hence the modern approach is future oriented.

PERFORMANCE APPRAISAL PROCESS

Performance appraisal is an ongoing process of assessing the performance of an employee within a given period by a supervisor. It measures the actual performance of the employee, the strengths and weaknesses, and the scope for improvements. It includes the following steps, as shown in **Figure 31.1**:

1. **Set standard and develop criteria**
   Setting up the standards serves as the benchmark against the performance to measure. It is used as the base to compare the actual performance of the employees. It should focus on the desired results of each job. Frame the criteria to judge the performance of the employees as successful or unsuccessful and the degrees of their contribution to achieving objectives of the organization. The standards must be clear, in measurable terms, and must be understood by all concerned.
2. **Communicate the standards**
   The performance appraisal process involves appraiser and appraisee to evaluate performance. An appraiser should be thorough with the job description that will help the appraiser to set the goals and targets and objectively analyze the results. The person should know the standards. Communicate standards to evaluators.
3. **Measure actual performance**
   After the standards are framed, accepted, communicated, the actual performance is measured. It requires the use of selected methods and ratings to evaluate the performance. It is the most challenging task in the performance appraisal process.

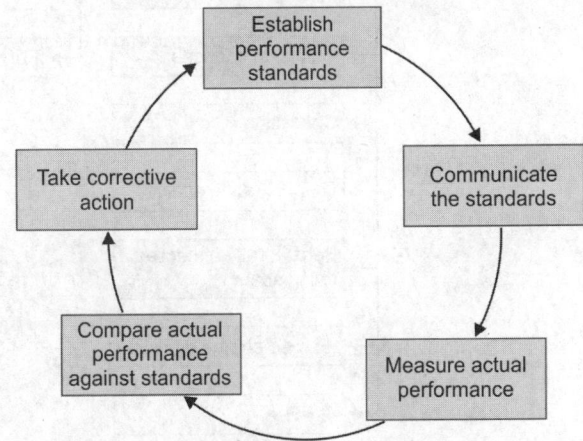

Fig. 31.1: Performance appraisal process.

4. **Compare actual performance against standards and discuss the results**
   During this stage, compare the actual performance with the set of standard performance. Whatever be the results they should be communicated and presented with the appraisee.
5. **Taking corrective action, if required**
   The last step of this process takes corrective action, if necessary. Immediate effects are to set the things right back on track. The remedial measures seek to find out how and why performance deviates.

METHODS OF PERFORMANCE APPRAISAL

Individual Methods

Individual methods of performance appraisal (**Fig. 31.2**) are as follows:

1. **Confidential reports:** The government organization usually relies on this method. This method is one of the old and traditional ways of evaluating employees. A confidential report is a detailed report about the employee and generally prepared at the end of every year by the immediate superior. It has information about the employee's strengths, weaknesses, and performance. It also contains information about the employee's personality traits (qualities) and his or her behavior
2. **Essay appraisal method:** This is the simplest method of rating an employee. Under this method, the rater expresses, in detail, the employee's strong and weak points. The assessor also gives suggestions for improvement. This method is highly subjective and not free from bias.
3. **Critical incidence technique:** Under this method, the appraisee rates the employees based on essential events or takes a snapshot of the incidence and writes a brief report about the incidence. It includes both negative and positive points. There is a scope for discussion on performance in this method. However, some supervisors may be biased while recording the incidents.
4. **Checklists:** A checklist is a set of descriptive statements about the employees and their behavior. The rater has to tick mark "Yes" or "No" for each statement. This method is simple, convenient, less time consuming, and more economical. However, it requires time to prepare structured statements.
5. **Graphics rating scales:** It is one of the conventional techniques of performance appraisal. The appraisee indicates along with a continuum quality and quantity of performance of the employee. It indicates different degrees of a particular trait. The continuum has anchors as "outstanding," "good," "fair," and "unacceptable" to help in the rating process. It includes both personal and job-related performance factors of the employees. This method is not free from bias.
6. **Behaviorally anchored rating scales:** Behaviorally anchored rating scale (BARS) is relatively a new method. BARS is systematically developed checklists using critical incidents in combination with graphic rating scales. There are behavioral statements that describe important job performance qualities as good

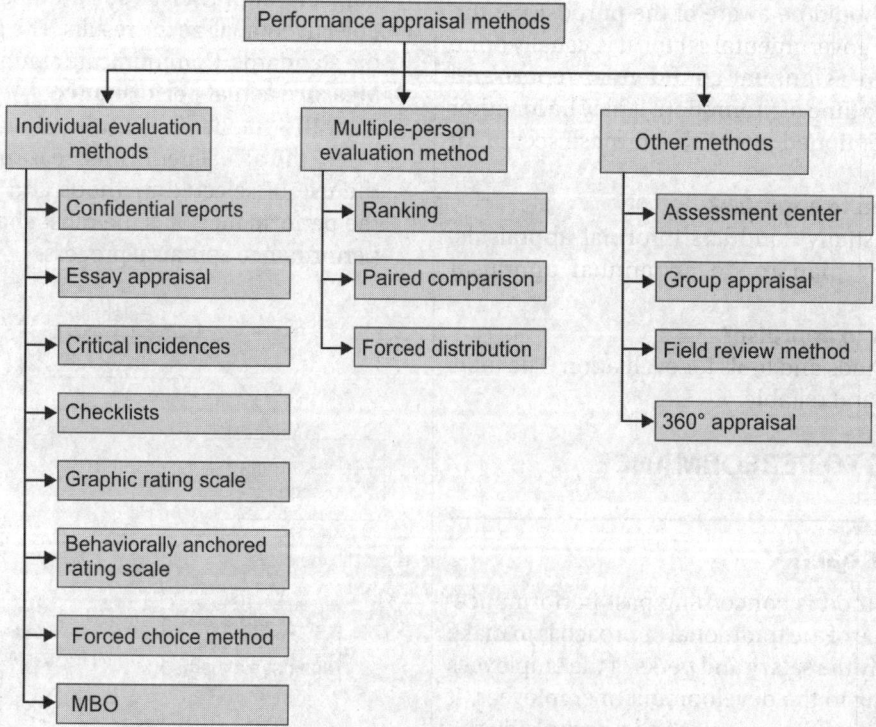

Fig. 31.2: Performance appraisal methods.

or bad. These statements derive from significant events. They are time consuming and costly to construct. The scales need validation to be updated.

7. **Forced choice method:** This method is useful to reduce bias. There are several sets of pair phrases, two of which may be positive and two may be negative, and appraisee is asked to indicate which of the four sentences is the most and least descriptive of a particular employee and thereby increasing the objectivity in the evaluation of the employees' performance.

8. **Management by the objective method:** As already discussed in one of the previous chapters, management by objective (MBO) is participative goal setting, choosing a course of actions and decision-making process **(Fig. 31.3)**. The employees and the superiors sit together, identify common organizational goals, and set their goals, the standards of their performance, and decide the line of action. Observe employee for the actual performance and compare with the standards set, and feedback is provided to rectify the mistakes and plans are modified. The appraisee should record directly and immediately observe job-related behaviors.

Multiple-person Evaluation Methods

The list below shows the multiple-person evaluation methods:

1. **Ranking method:** Ranking scale is a simple, quick, and the most convenient means of an appraisal. Rank an employee against others based on their relative levels of performance. The evaluator is asked to evaluate the employees from highest to lowest on a specific overall criterion. This method allows expressing the relative position of each employee in terms of numerical rank. The employee scoring the highest is first and then selects the next highest and so on. This method has limited value for performance as it is not readily determinable, and differences in ranks do not indicate absolute or equal differences among the employees.

2. **Paired comparison:** In this method, one employee is compared with all other employees in the group for only one trait at a time. The evaluator puts a tick mark against an employee who will be better of two and assign the final ranking by the number of times the employee is better than others by using a formula $N(N-1)/2$, where N is the total number of compared employees.

3. **Forced distribution method:** The appraiser forcibly evaluates the staff according to the standardized distribution scale. He or she considers at least two criteria for rating on five points scale and places employees between two extremes. This method is objective but challenging to construct a set of statements.

Other Methods

There are also some other methods for performance appraisal:

1. **Assessment centers:** This is a system or organization where several employees assessed by various experts using various techniques such as roleplaying, simulation exercises, and transactional analysis. The appraiser ranks the performance of each employee in order of merit. The purpose of the appraisal is for promotion, training, and development.

2. **Group appraisal method:** In this method, several appraisers do the rating, including the immediate supervisor. The group uses multiple techniques to evaluate the employee. The actual performance is compared with the standard, finds the gap, discusses, and suggests the improvement. This method eliminates personal bias, but it is time consuming.

3. **Field review method:** Under this method, the employee is evaluated by another person, not by his or her immediate supervisor. The appraiser prepares a report based on records of output and information that he or she gets from his or her immediate supervisor. He or she also interviews the employee to assign rating using standardized forms.

4. **360° feedback appraisal:** This system is also known as multirater feedback. It is the most comprehensive method of assessment. The input comes from multiple sources about the employees' performance. The management takes evaluation feedback from the superior, subordinates, peer groups, or team members, clients, and also from the appraisee. Self-appraisal is the cornerstone of this method. It gives a chance to the employee to look at her strengths and weaknesses. Superiors rate the actual performance; subordinates can evaluate specific abilities such as communication, delegating, motivating, and leadership qualities. A team will evaluate cooperation and other attitudes of the employee. A 360° appraisal is more appropriate to

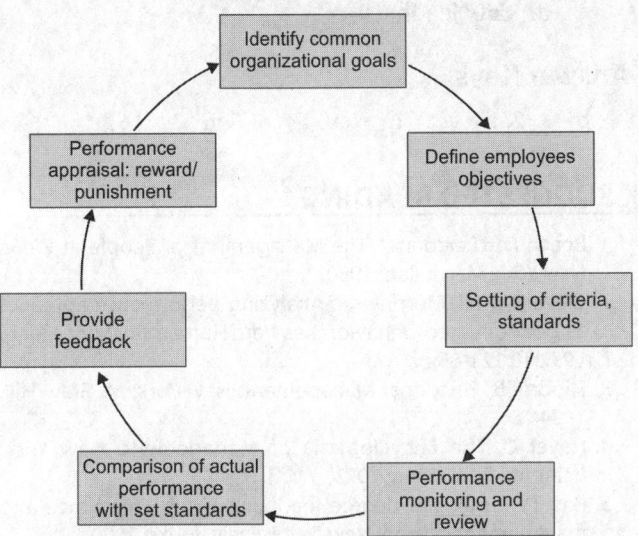

Fig. 31.3: Management by objective process.

assess the leadership and management abilities of the managers.

GUIDELINES FOR EFFECTIVE PERFORMANCE APPRAISAL

Following is the list of guidelines for effective performance appraisal:
- It should provide consistent, reliable, and valid information.
- The appraisal techniques should rely on a job analysis and job descriptions.
- The appraisal forms, procedures, techniques, and tools should be standardized.
- The means should be practicable.
- The appraisers should be thorough and undergo training on evaluation procedure and should be a friendly and good listener.
- He or she should begin with positive comments and always reinforce the positive points.
- The employees must know the evaluation parameters, the purpose, time, and getting feedback on their evaluation beforehand.
- The appraiser must document the expected standards for nursing practice and job responsibilities, past performance, performance to be developed, and recommendations for future improvement.

CHAPTER HIGHLIGHTS

- Performance appraisal is the process of evaluating the ability of an individual employee against predetermined job-related performance standards.
- It has both employees-based and institutional-based purposes and acts as a development and control measure.
- Performance appraisal must be objective, behaviorally oriented, and criterion based.
- There are various methods of conducting performance appraisal, including individual, multiple-person evaluation, and other methods such as filed review and 360° approaches.
- The organization must have specific guidelines for developing a performance appraisal system.

REVIEW QUESTIONS

I. Essay Type Questions
1. Define performance appraisal. Discuss its purposes.
2. Performance appraisal is a formal and structured process. Discuss.
3. Enumerate different methods of performance appraisal. Describe in detail the individual methods of performance appraisal.
4. What do you mean by multiple-person evaluation? Describe the ranking and paired comparative method of evaluation in detail.
5. Discuss various guidelines for an effective performance appraisal system.

II. Short Notes
1. MBO as a method of evaluation
2. Confidential reports
3. Approaches to performance evaluation
4. Principles of performance appraisal
5. Characteristics of performance appraisal

III. Multiple Choice Questions
1. The quality of performance when a person can learn, adapt, and reasoning power is:
   a. Quality of work   b. Mental ability
   c. Supervisory ability d. Personal traits
2. Which of the following approach is concerning with the past performance of employees?
   a. Traditional approach
   b. Modern approach
   c. Informal approach
   d. Formal approach
3. What is the main purpose of annual confidential report especially in government organizations?
   a. Measuring performance
   b. Periodically reviewing progress
   c. Providing feedback
   d. Considering at the time of promotion
4. Which method of performance appraisal used to rate the behavior of employees through a set of statements?
   a. Confidential report
   b. Graphic rating scale
   c. Checklist
   d. Behaviorally anchored rating scale
5. Which method of performance appraisal various experts use through various methods to evaluate several employees?
   a. Assessment centers
   b. Group appraisal
   c. Field review
   d. 360° feedback

Answer Keys

1. b   2. a   3. d   4. a   5. a

SUGGESTED READING

1. Beach DS. Personnel: The Management of People at Work. New York: Macmillan; 1980.
2. Cleveland JN, Murphy KR. Analyzing performance appraisal as goal-directed behavior. Res Pers Human Resour Manag. 1992;10:121-85.
3. Flippo EB. Personnel Management. New York: McGraw-Hill; 1984.
4. Heyel C. The Encyclopedia of Management. New York: Reinhold Publishing; 1973.
5. Rao TV, et al. 360-degree feedback and performance and management system. New Delhi: Excel Books; 2000.
6. Walker H, Jones H. A guide to peer appraisal. Nurs Manag. 2004;11(1):22-4.

32 CHAPTER

Discipline and Grievance Procedure

CHAPTER OUTLINE

- ⊃ Discipline
  - ✦ Definitions of Discipline
  - ✦ Purposes of Discipline
  - ✦ Prerequisite for Discipline
  - ✦ Types of Discipline
  - ✦ Characteristics of Disciplinary System
  - ✦ Discipline Rules
  - ✦ Principles of Discipline
- ⊃ Indiscipline
  - ✦ Causes of Indiscipline
  - ✦ Consequences of Indiscipline
- ⊃ Steps of Progressive Discipline
  - ✦ Penalties for Misconduct/Indiscipline
  - ✦ Role of Nurse Administrator in Maintaining Discipline
- ⊃ Employee Grievance
  - ✦ Meaning and Definitions
  - ✦ Features
  - ✦ Reasons for Grievances
  - ✦ Forms of Grievances
  - ✦ Consequences of Grievances
  - ✦ Grievance Handling Procedure

LEARNING OUTCOMES

After completion of this chapter, the learner will be able to:
- Define and understand the concept of discipline
- Describe the aims and objectives of the discipline
- Discuss the characteristics of a discipline system
- Describe different types and approaches to the discipline
- Explain the principles of disciplinary action
- Explain various components of discipline
- Discuss the disciplinary procedure
- Define employees' grievance
- Discuss practical ways of handling employees' grievance

KEY TERMS

Discipline, indiscipline, penalty, discipline system employee grievance, Grievance handling procedure

INTRODUCTION

Every organization needs well-defined discipline rules and regulations. Effective disciplinary rules and regulations are essential to maintain order in the nursing organization. A discipline is required to have a productive and positive work environment.

DISCIPLINE

Definitions

The word "discipline" comes from the Latin word "disciplina," which means teaching, learning, and growing. Discipline can be training or molding of the mind and character to bring about desired behaviors. The constructive discipline uses discipline as a means of helping the employees to grow, not as a punitive measure.

- Discipline is the force that prompts individuals or groups to observe rules, regulations, standards, and procedures deemed necessary for an organization.
  —*Richard D Calhoon*
- Discipline indicates the spirit and confidence with which the members of the organization perform their task.
  —*SK Datta*
- Discipline means an orderly and systematic behavior which is opposite to confusion. It is a derivative of word "disciple," which means learner or follower one who takes another as teacher or leader. —*RC Goyal*
- International Labor Organization (ILO) refers "discipline" as a control mechanism to ensure

compliance with organizational objectives. It is used to control those who deviate from performance and behavioral standards. Discipline means voluntary and willing compliance of rules and regulations and instructions and also the development of the right habits of conduct in work with others at the workplace. Discipline refers to a set of actions imposed by the organization on its employees for failure to follow the organizational rules, standards, and policies.

Purposes

The aim of discipline is as follows:
- To take appropriate action against the misconduct of employees
- To develop and protect other employees
- To improve organizational efficiency
- To improve the functioning of the organization
- To create a positive work culture
- To implement a code of conduct for guiding employees
- To teach a discipline work culture
- To develop human capacity and stimulate efficiency
- To create a spirit of tolerance and good interpersonal relationship
- To impart an element of certainty to give and seek direction and responsibility.

Prerequisite

Three essential requisites can help in maintaining discipline: self-discipline, orderly behavior, and punishment.
1. **Self-discipline:** This is the discipline that an employee has from oneself, has her or his principles of life, and adopts a particular pattern of behavior. The employee needs to have self-knowledge, courage, and committed and have internal consciousness.
2. **Orderly behavior:** To be in discipline, the employee should have orderly conduct.
3. **Punishment:** It is a preventive measure to take action against indiscipline.

Types

There are two types of discipline: positive and negative disciplines:
1. **Positive discipline**
   It is a type of discipline whereby the employee maintains discipline willingly by following established rules and regulations of the organization. The environment the employee feels is creative in the organization. Each employee feels accountable for her or his work, motivated to accomplish group and organizational goals. The superior tries to make the subordinates educate the value of discipline. It is a willful discipline. It is a type of developmental approach to shaping the behavior of nurse employees by providing favorable consequences for the right behavior and avoiding physical punishments.

2. **Negative discipline**
   It is a type of control whereby the employee is forced to obey rules and regulations that may be fear of getting the punishment, warnings, and penalties. It is a form of punitive discipline. In this type of control, the employees have low morale, more destructive, and give low work output. They are frustrated due to an unhealthy work environment. It is a negative approach to maintain discipline. It is usually a traditional approach to managing the regulation in the organization, where managers used to be autocratic. But at times, this approach may be used in maintaining discipline.

Characteristics of Disciplinary System

The following lists the characteristics of disciplinary system:
- The employees should be aware of the code of conduct or conduct rules.
- There should be a timely inquiry in case of break of conduct rules.
- The disciplinary officer should impersonal and consistent.
- There should be a system of warning to the employee not following a code of conduct.

Discipline Rules

To maintain discipline and behavior among the employees and to prevent them misusing the powers given to them as per position and for their end, the government has formulated and enforced a code of conduct or conduct rules.

The primary purposes of discipline rules are to maintain the correct behavior toward superiors, to protect the integrity of the officials, and to regulate the activities.

Principles of Discipline

The list below shows principles of discipline:
- There should be a sound standard of conduct, codes, and norms in the organization.
- Employees should be aware of the rule of conduct, codes, and norms.
- Conscious efforts should be made to create conditions for easy acceptance of the laid down norms.
- Implement standard of behavior, codes, and norms promptly and review time to time.
- Take disciplinary action, if required, quickly, privately, thoughtfully, and consistently.
- Take disciplinary action in a systematic way.
- Use progressive and development approach in dealing with disciplinary action.

INDISCIPLINE

The word "indiscipline" means the absence of discipline among employees. Indiscipline depicts in the form of confusion, chaos, abuse, etc.

Causes

The following results in indiscipline:
- Lack of awareness of organizational rules and regulations
- Incorrect philosophy of discipline
- Lack of well-defined code of conduct
- Absence of any procedure to handle grievances
- Improper attitude toward employees' problem
- False promises made by superiors
- Favoritism
- Poorly defined employees' expectations
- Misuse through dividing people and exploitation of subordinates
- "Divide and Rule" policy in the organization
- Inappropriate supervision
- Communication barriers
- Low morale and motivation among staff
- Poor employees' selection and orientation
- Poorly selected and trained supervisors
- Unfair management practices such as wage discrimination, discrimination in job assignment, distribution of workload, too strict, noncompliance of promotional, and transfer policies
- Personal frustrations and misunderstandings.

Consequences

Indiscipline can lead to inefficiency on the part of employees; unhealthy and unsafe work environment; change in behavior or misbehavior: inconsistent behavior and risky behavior; disturb the peace; and negligent toward her duties.

Progressive Disciplinary Process

Progressive discipline is a process that deals with job-related behavior of the employees when they do not meet expected and communicated performance standards. The purpose of this program is to correcting and improving the misbehavior of employees. There are two ways to improve the performance behavior of the problematic employees, oral reprimand, and written reprimand.
1. **Oral reprimand:** The supervisor may have verbal interaction with the employee to discuss the problem behaviors and the expectations to change the practices which are a form of oral reprimands.
2. **Written reprimand:** The other way is a written form; the supervisor documents if the behavior continues or if an employee commits a serious offense.

Steps of Progressive Discipline

There are five steps in dealing with progressive discipline. These are informal feedback—verbal warning, letter of counsel—written notice, letter of reprimand, suspension—final warning, and termination.
1. **Informal feedback—verbal notification:** Take informal feedback and give a verbal warning to an employee on receiving a complaint from superior for the misconduct. Before even verbal warning, initial inquiry and counseling are done to confirm that the employee is aware of the problem. If the problem continues, the employee gets a verbal warning.
2. **Letter of counsel—written warning:** It is a written warning of unacceptable behavior or unsatisfactory work performance and kept in the official personnel file.
3. **Letter of reprimand:** It includes a written description of warning and consists of a review of any prior related corrective action, a thorough statement of the circumstances causing current corrective action, and a clear picture of future expectations.
4. **Suspension—final warning:** It is the final warning. During the suspension, the employee may either get a salary or may be without pay, depending on the severity of the offense. The notification has the reasons for the action. The employee may be removed from the work immediately before conducting an investigation where there is suspected theft, a disorderly conduct, or a threat to other employees or clients.
5. **Termination:** If all the above steps are against an employee, the employee may get a termination order.

Penalties for Misconduct/Indiscipline

There are significant and minor penalties awarded for employees for their misconduct.

A. Major penalties: Demotion, dismissal, transfer, discharge, withholding increments, etc. are the significant penalties awarded for the employees for their serious misconduct. The procedure for significant penalties/punishment is as follows (**Fig. 32.1**):
1. **Written complaint:** The first in progressive discipline is to take a report of misconduct.
2. **Preliminary inquiry:** This is a fact-finding inquiry conducted informally to find out the nature and extent of delinquent's fault.
3. **The decision to start formal departmental inquiry:** The appointing authority decides for the preliminary investigations.
4. **Suspension:** The appointing authority decides for suspension of the employee depending on the report of departmental inquiry.
5. **Charge sheet:** Allegations against the delinquent if proved in the form of specific charges, the charge sheet issued personally, or through registered post.
6. **Appointment of inquiry officer:** The disciplinary officer will simultaneously nominate an officer to conduct a further inquiry after suspension.
7. **A written statement of defence:** The charged officer submits a written comment of the defence report to the inquiry officer according to the direction mentioned in the charge sheet.
8. **Recording of evidence by inquiry officer:** The inquiry officer records the evidence given by the charged officer. The accused officer has the right to cross-examine

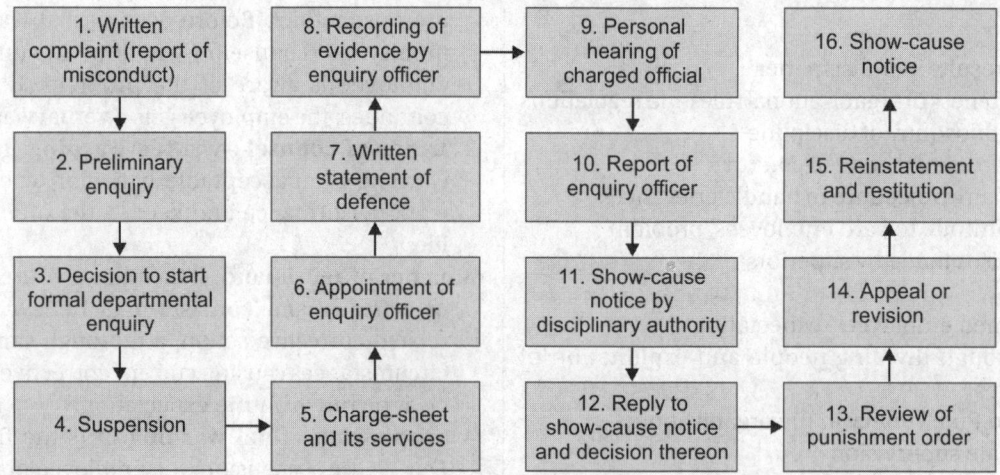

Fig. 32.1: Showing the disciplinary process.

the witnesses brought in by the department and her witnesses in defence.
9. **Personal hearing of charged official:** The accused official can make an oral submission.
10. **Report of inquiry officer:** The inquiry officer makes the report, submits in duplicate to the disciplinary officer, and also gives his or her opinion.
11. **Show-cause notice by disciplinary authority:** The disciplinary officer decides to award punishment and is issue a show-cause notice to charged officer.
12. **Reply to show-cause notice and decision thereon:** Upon objective consideration of reply, the disciplinary authority can reduce his conclusion to a concise, reason out the order, and communicate to the charged person.
13. **Review of punishment orders:** In some instances, the penalized official can request the disciplinary officer to reconsider the order.
14. **Appeal or revision:** The charged official can appeal for a reconsideration of order to the next higher authority.
15. **Reinstatement and restitution:** In case a suspended official exonerates the charges by the disciplinary authority, he or she is reinstated as a matter of course and restores his or her original position. However, if the appellate reinstates a dismissed, he or she is allowed to regain his or her job if his or her acquittal is honorable.
16. **Show-cause notice:** In case the disciplinary officer proposes withholding of emoluments of a reinstated official for suspension period, he must first issue a show-cause notice to her before taking final action.

B. Minor penalties: The minor penalties are in the form of oral warning, written warning, fines, loss of privileges, etc. No formal charge sheet issued for the minor indiscipline and no need to appoint a regular inquiry officer. The most common action is taking an explanation for misconduct.

Role of Nurse Administrator in Maintaining Discipline

Nurse administrator should follow the below criteria to maintain discipline:

- Make your expectations clear to subordinates
- Develop a positive attitude toward employees
- Appreciate if assistants take the initiative and self-disciplined
- Treat them as mature persons
- Have trust in your staff and accept their potentialities
- Spend time with them and have meetings with them
- Generate positive work culture in the department
- Make rules and policies available to all the employees
- Encourage open communication with subordinates
- Formulate friendly implementations of policies
- Carefully keep a record of employees' behavior that prompt disciplinary action
- Investigate carefully and be prompt if the staff has any grievances
- Be empathetic to the complaints
- Avoid severe disciplinary procedures that may backfire
- Take corrective and constructive action
- Allow employees feedback in the disciplinary process.

EMPLOYEE GRIEVANCE

Meaning and Definitions

Employee grievance is a formal procedure whereby the employee expresses any dissatisfaction or feeling of injustice regarding the work situation. It is a feeling of discontent or injustice expressed by an employee about the job and its nature and about the management policies and procedures.
- According to Jucius, "a grievance is an expressed dissatisfaction, whether valid or not, arising out of anything connected with the organization that an employee thinks, believes, or even feels to be unfair or inequitable."
- According to ILO, "Grievances are defined as breaches of the collective agreement, custom, and practice, the statute law, common law, natural justice or as any problem of a sufficient nature to cause a disturbance of the workplace equilibrium." It refers to a complaint

of one or more employees concerning wages and allowances, working conditions, interpretations of service conditions covering such areas as overtime, job assignment, and termination of service. It is in the form of complaint.

Features

The features of employee grievance are as follows:
- It is a form of discontent or dissatisfaction related to employment.
- It arises due to any genuine or imaginary feelings or reasons.
- It may or may not express.
- Initially, the employee may complain of verbally or in writing. Without taking any action, it can grow into a grievance.
- There is no fulfillment of expectation of the employee.
- It relates to a problem of interpretation or perceived non-fulfillment of one's expectation from the organization.
- It may affect the performance or work.

Reasons for Grievances

Every employee has certain expectations that he/she thinks must be fulfilled by the organization. When the expectations are not performed by the organization, its consequences might result in grievance. It may occur due to the following reasons in the hospital:
1. **Salary and compensation:** When employees feel that their salary, bonus, and benefits are not appropriate or less as compared to other employees in the organization.
2. **Work environment:** Improper working conditions, poor physical conditions, and unsafe workplace.
3. **Supervision:** Attitude of supervisors toward employees such as the perceived notion of bias and favoritism.
4. **Feeling of harassment:** Employees suffer from feelings of victimization, neglect, and unable to adjust with their colleagues.
5. **Management politics:** Irrational management policies with respect to promotions, transfers, assignments, workloads, granting leaves, fines, and disciplinary rules.
6. **Lack of appropriate codes and processes:** The weak management system and work culture may also take a form of grievances.

Forms of Grievances

Grievances can be of the following types:
1. **Factual:** When the grievance is with a valid reason or when the legitimate needs of the employees remain unfulfilled.
2. **Imaginary:** It means that the employee's dissatisfaction is without any valid reason. In this case, management is not at fault.
3. **Disguised:** When the employee is dissatisfied with the reasons that are unknown to her. It may be due to under pressure or a heavy heart.

Consequences of Grievances

If the grievances are not identified and redressed correctly and timely, they may adversely affect employees, managers, and organization as a whole. The complaints affect the individual performance and poor quality of services in spite of high investment in the highly qualified nursing workforce and sophisticated technology. These can:
- Take the form of collective disputes
- Lower the morale and efficiency of the nurse employees
- Increase the rate of absenteeism and turnover among nurses
- Reduce the level of commitment and sincerity by the nurses
- Result in frustration and dissatisfaction among nurse employees
- Lower work output
- Result in loss of working hours
- Increase wastage and costs
- Deteriorate teaching and research programs
- Strain superior-subordinate relation
- Increase indiscipline cases
- Unrest
- Strike, etc.

Grievance Handling Procedure

Every organization should have a valid grievance handling procedure to redress the grievance effectively. It should provide a formal framework, setting limits on the arbitrary management authority and power.

The grievance procedure should be sound, simple, clear, short, and unambiguous based on legislation. The trained staff must handle promptly and should take action immediately. One must formulate a grievance committee in the organization that can keep track of the functioning of the grievance handling procedure and makes necessary changes to improve it.

Steps in Grievance Handling Procedure

Following are the steps in grievance handling procedure:
1. **Identify/acknowledge the complaint:** Management must identify the charge by direct observation, grievance procedure, gripe boxes, open door policy, and exit interview, etc., if not expressed by the employee. The management immediately acknowledges the complaint put forward by the employee.
2. **Define the grievance correctly:** After identifying complaints, acknowledge and define it precisely.
3. **Gather the facts:** The managers should gather relevant and sufficient facts explaining the grievance's nature. It may be facts, opinions, and data.

4. **Analyze the data and finding the cause of grievance:** The information gathered should be analyzed and identifies the actual cause of complaint to take remedial action.
5. **Decision-making:** Identify the alternative course of action and its consequences based on grievances; then decide the best alternative considering the policy of the organization.
6. **Immediate redressal:** Redress grievance immediately by implementing the decision.
7. **Implementation and follow-up:** Follow the application at every stage.

Guidelines in Grievance Handling Procedure

The list shows the guidelines in grievance handling procedure:
1. Treat each complaint as important
2. Spend adequate time with the complainant and be relaxed during the process
3. Get all facts and figure and avoid preconceived notions about the involved parties
4. Practice attentive listening skills and control your emotions
5. Ensure privacy
6. Settle down the grievance at the lower level
7. Maintain proper records
8. Be proactive and always make the process win–win.

CHAPTER HIGHLIGHTS

- Discipline is voluntary and willing compliance with rules and regulations and instructions.
- It is a set of actions imposed by the organization if employees fail to follow the organizational rules, standards, and policies.
- Self-discipline, orderly behavior, and punishment are essential to maintain discipline.
- The employees may maintain discipline either willingly or forcefully. Lack of control may create confusion, chaos, and inefficiency.
- Progressive discipline is a process to correct and improve the misbehavior and misconduct of employees. It starts with a verbal warning, written warning, reprimand, suspension as a final warning, and termination.
- For misconduct, either major or minor penalties awarded for employees depending on their seriousness of the fault.
- Employee grievance is employee expressions for any feeling of injustice related to employment conditions. These may be factual, imaginary, or due to under pressure.
- A grievance committee in the organization handles grievances in a systematic way.

REVIEW QUESTIONS

I. Essay Type Questions
1. Define discipline. Why is it essential to maintain discipline in the organization?
2. What are the various types of discipline? Discuss it in detail.
3. Describe various stages of progressive disciplines in detail.
4. Explain the procedure for awarding significant penalties.
5. Define grievance. What are the common reasons for grievances among nurses?

II. Short Notes
1. Principles of discipline
2. Features of grievance
3. Causes of indiscipline
4. Grievance handling the procedure
5. Role of nurse administrator in the handling grievance procedure

III. Multiple Choice Questions
1. A type of discipline whereby the employees follow the rules and regulations willingly is:
   a. Positive discipline
   b. Negative discipline
   c. Progressive discipline
   d. Self-discipline
2. Which type of warning is applicable for an employee on receiving a complaint from superior for her misconduct?
   a. Written   b. Oral
   c. Reprimand   d. Suspension
3. Which of the following is considering a major penalty?
   a. Oral warning   b. Written warning
   c. Fine   d. Charge sheet
4. A form of complaint expressed by employees toward injustice regarding work situation?
   a. Injustice   b. Indiscipline
   c. Grievance   d. Misconduct
5. A type of grievance where employees' dissatisfaction is without any valid reason is:
   a. Imaginary   b. Factual
   c. Disguised   d. Dispute

Answer Keys
1. a   2. b   3. d   4. c   5. a

SUGGESTED READING

1. Available from http://ezinearticles.com/?Discipline-And-Disciplinary-Actions-In-Organisations&id=2004328. (Accessed Jan 2018).

2. Available from http://www.ilocarib.org.tt/Promalco_tool/productivity-tools/manual10/m10_8.htm. (Accessed Jan 2018).
3. Clara J. Grievance handling do nurses need this skill? Nurs J India. 1997;88(11):245-6.
4. Employee grievance. [Online] Available from http://hr.powergridindia.com/HRWebSite/RTIInfo/DisciplinaryProceduresGuidelines.pdf. (Accessed Jan 2018).
5. Ganong WL. Grievance handling. J Nurs Admin. 1974;4(1):11.
6. ILO: Examination of grievances and communication within undertakings. Geneva: ILO; 1965.
7. Jucius MJ. Personnel Management. Homewood: Richard D Irwin; 1997.
8. Katharina SK. Approaches to employees' grievance handling in hospitals. J Acad Hosp Admin India. 1992;4(1):43-6.
9. Mark IL. The eight essential steps In grievance processing. Disp Resol J. 1999;54:81-6.
10. Metzger N. Handling grievances: guidelines for RNs. Hosp Prog. 1979;60(9):69-71, 94.
11. Potgieter S, Muller M. A model for handling grievances in nursing services. Curationis. 1997;20(3):33-40. Abstract (Pub Med).
12. Trish Sa, Sinha RP, Kumar A. Approaches to higher productivity in the health care system. J Acad Hosp Admin. 1991;3:1-8.
13. Yesudian CAK. Impact of hospital administration training-A study, IIMB. Manag Rev. 1987;2:193-209.

33 Stress Management

CHAPTER OUTLINE

- Work Stress
  - Definitions of Stress
  - Defining Work Stress
  - Nature of Stress
  - Types/Levels of Stress
  - Stages of Stress
- Sources of Stress
- Consequences of Workplace Stress
- Approaches to Stress Management
  - Individual Coping Strategies
  - Cognitive Restructuring Strategies
  - Stress Inoculation Training
  - Employee Assistance Programs
  - Organizational Coping Strategies
- Nurse Managers' Role in Stress Management
- Tips for Reducing Stress at the Workplace

LEARNING OUTCOMES

After completion of this chapter, the learner will be able to:
- Recall and understand the concept of work stress
- Discuss the nature and types of stress
- Enlist multiple sources of stress
- Evaluate and apply various approaches to stress management
- Highlight the role of nurse managers in reducing nurses' work stress
- Discuss tips for reducing stress at the workplace

KEY TERMS

Stress, work stress, stages of stress, eustress, distress, burnout, stress management

INTRODUCTION

Stress at the workplace becomes a concern to organization administrators. Among the health-care professionals, especially nurses have generally considered a high-risk group regarding work stress and burnout. Nurses' environment includes an enclosed atmosphere, time pressures, excessive noise or extremely quiet, sudden swings of from intense to mundane tasks, no second chance, unpleasant sights and sounds, and prolonged standing hours. The hospital nurses do experience an increased level of stress and are the highest in particular nursing units due to multifactors.

WORK STRESS

Definitions of Stress

The stress is a physical science word that refers to external pressure or a load of an object. Canadian endocrinologist Hans Selye introduced the term "stress" in medicine in 1949. According to him, stress is the response and adjustment of body functioning with the various internal and external environmental stimuli/factors. It is a form of regulation and maintains body homeostasis.

According to Looker and Gregson, it is a disparity of imbalance between requirement and ability to cope with demand. George Engel defined it to all processes, whether originating in the external environment or within the person, which imposes a need or requirement upon the organism, the resolution, or handling of which necessitates or activity of the mental apparatus before any system is involved or activated.

Stress refers to mind and body's response or reaction to a real or imagined threat, event or change. The risk, development, or modification is commonly called stressors. Stressors can be internal (thoughts, beliefs, attitudes) or external (loss, tragedy, change).

Defining Work Stress

The Occupational Safety and Health Administration at the National level The National Institute for Occupational

Safety and Health (NIOSH) defines it as the mismatch between job demand and capabilities, resources, and needs of employees. The resources are physical, emotional, economic, social, or spiritual. Thus, workplace stress occurs when the challenges and demands of work become excessive, the pressures of the workplace exceed the worker's ability to handle them, and job satisfaction turns to frustration and exhaustion.

Nature of Stress

Stress helps a person to prepare mentally and physically to cope with the responsibility. The person adapts oneself to the burden, either external or internal and tackles it consequently through several defense mechanisms. In normal circumstances, there are three phases of stress, i.e. the first phase is alarm phase that prepares individuals to take action; the second phase is a resistant phase that helps an individual to adopt stress; and the third phase is the exhaustion phase that develops if the individual continues to have stress. Stress is positive or negative depending on individual emotional, behavioral, and psychological responses to stress-related factors.

Types/Levels of Stress

Figure 33.1 depicts the types/levels of stress.
1. **Eustress:** Eustress is a positive or friendly stress that stimulates a person to function better. It acts as a physical and mental ability trigger. The individual's abilities to control stress exceed its requirements; therefore he or she is in a positive state of preparation and is in balance or within tolerable limits. The low-to-moderate amount of stress can act constructively. As a positive influence, stress can compel us to act. The moderate level of stress can increase effort, stimulate creativity, and encourage enthusiasm at work.
2. **Distress:** Distress is a negative stress or burn out that may cause illness. It is harmful to both individuals and the organization. In this case, job demand exceeds the employee's abilities. It may break down employees' physical and mental systems resulting in low performance and brought on by very intense stress and reacted through absenteeism, turnover, errors, accidents, dissatisfaction, and reduces performance. As a negative influence, it can result in feelings of disruption, rejection, anger, and depression, which in turn can lead to health problems such as headache, upset stomach, rashes, insomnia, ulcers, high blood pressure, heart disease, and stroke.
3. **Burnout:** The burnout is a form of exhaustion resulting from repeated emotional pressure. Our body tries to keep in mental and physical balance (homeostasis), but continued negative stress may disturb that balance.

Stages of Stress

Hans Selye explained stress through general adaptation syndrome (GAS), a way that the body tries to keep in balance. There are mainly three stages of stress: alarm, resistance, and exhaustion stage.
1. **The alarm stage:** The alarm stage is the initial mobilization by which the body meets the challenges posed by the stressor. Upon identifying the stressor, the brain sends biochemical messages to all the body systems. Respiration increases, blood pressure rises, pupils dilate, and so forth.
2. **Resistance stage:** If the stressors continue, the GAS proceeds to the resistance stage. The person is now fighting with stressors and gives rise to tension, anxiety, and fatigue. The resistance may be high or low to a specific stressor. The person is more prone to illness during this stage.
3. **Exhaustion stage:** If the stressors continue, the body of a person exhausts its ability to adapt. The symptoms are similar to the alarm stage. The person will fight or flight.

SOURCES OF STRESS

Work stress or occupational stress among nurses is due to a variety of organizational and personal-related factors. The empirical evidence indicated that in addition to nursing itself, organizational and managerial characteristics create stress among nurses. The primary cause of job stress is employees' characteristics and working conditions, which can lead to the risk of injury and illness **(Fig. 33.2)**. The following are the significant sources of stress:
1. **Organizational factors:** Studies indicate that organizational and management characteristics are the cause of stress among nurses. Shift pattern, the behavior of doctors, and the behavior of nurse managers are significant stressors among organizational factors, in addition to nursing itself. The origin of stress can be due to physical, psychological, or social factors. The significant predictors of stress are as follows:
    - *Workload:* The excessive workload in terms of actual workload, due to a shortage of staff or time pressure, increasing responsibilities, nonnursing work, can lead to emotional exhaustion among the nurses.

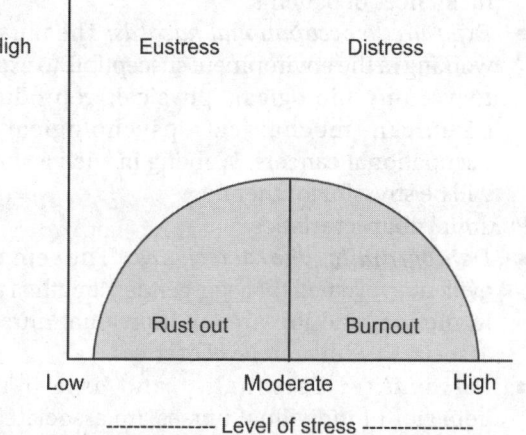

Fig. 33.1: Types/levels of stress.

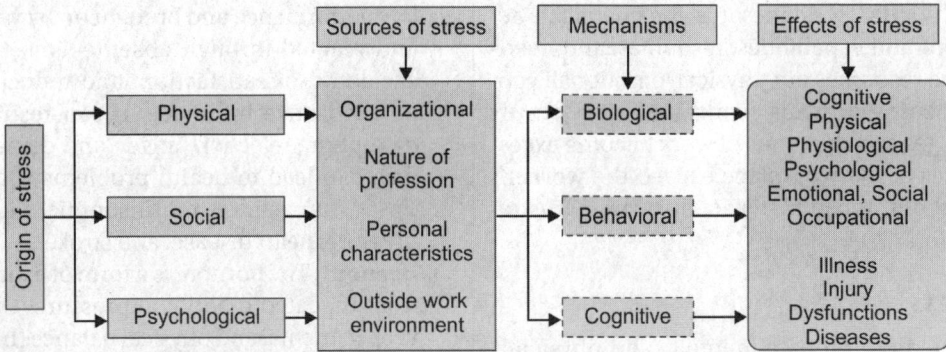

Fig. 33.2: Origin, sources, and effects of stress.

- *Understaffing:* The shortage of staff during the morning, evening, and night duties can lead to extra work or burden among the nurses, and there will be time pressure to complete the task, which can be the cause of stress and burn out among nurses.
- *Job content:* If there is hectic, monotonous, or routine work, unpleasant tasks and work of low social value can lead to frustration among the staff. The nurses working in a hazardous environment have a fear of getting infections.
- *Working hours:* Long, unsocial, strict, and inflexible duty hours. The nurses who work for more than 35 hours or more per week are likely to report high risk than the nurses working for fewer hours and in the regular shift.
- *Shift duty pattern:* Frequent shift duty pattern of odd hours, especially the night duties, changes the lifestyle and behavior of the nurses.
- *Undefined job:* One of the predictor of stress as reported by nurses is unclear job descriptions, unit, and organization **Lack of task autonomy, accountability, and feedback:** Accountability without independence at times becomes the source of stress between nurse administrators and supervisors.
- *Lack of career development:* Job insecurity, lack of promotional avenues, lack of opportunity for growth, and advancement can cause stress among nurses.
- *Physical facilities/environment:* Inadequate, unpleasant, or dangerous physical facilities, e.g. poor ventilation, lighting, temperature, crowding, noise, air pollution, or ergonomic problems, are the stressors at the workplace. Lack of adequate equipment and articles to provide the care and lack of facilities for rest during the long hours of duty can also be the predictors of low productivity and can lead to frustrations among nurses.
- *Social environment:* Lack of support from the nurse administrators; lack of family-friendly policies; poor interpersonal relationships with coworkers, doctors, nurse administrators, and other team members; and lack of staff support, autocratic behavior of the supervisors, and conflict with doctors are the predictors of psychological stress among nurses. The problematic relationship among team members also increases stress among them, and they can develop anxiety and feelings of fear.
- *Communication barriers:* Ineffective communication can lead to stress among staff; for example, the team or its individual member, if not informed ahead of time for the change of duty, may feel frustrated while reporting.

2. **Professional service-related factors:** The nature of nursing is not free from stress. It is considered as one of the stressful occupations. Following are some of the critical contributory factors of stress among nurses:
    - *Caring for suffering and death and dying patients:* The patients suffering from pain, disability, long term and acutely ill, death, and dying can be the source of stress for nurses. Having daily contact with suffering patients and nurses can get psychological trauma associated with witnessing death and dying.
    - *Severe patients and their family members:* At times, the nurses are experiencing critical and demanding patients, and their family members can be the sources of stress among nurses.
    - *Working with psychiatry patients:* Nurses may face emotional exhaustion in working with aggressive patients, especially with suicidal and violent incidences of patients.
    - *Exposure to occupational hazards:* The nurses are working in the environment susceptible to exposure to various biological, physical, reproductive, chemical, mechanical, psychological, and occupational cancers. Working in such a situation will be stressful for them.

3. **Personal characteristics**
    - *Demographic characteristics:* The empirical evidence revealed that age, gender, length of tenure in the job, and job area of individual nurses are associated with their level of stress.
    - *Personality:* Personality and interpersonal behavior of individual nurses are associated with various dimensions of stress. The nurses with state

anxiety of personality "A" and have a problematic relationship; and with uncooperative behavior with coworkers, doctors, and head nurses usually have psychological stress.
- *External locus of control:* The nurses who believe that outside forces are controlling their fate in the job environment are more stressful than other nurses who think that they can control potentially adverse effects in their job.
- *Competency:* The nurses, if not competent, may be scared and not confident to handle the situations that will be under stress.
- *Lack of preparation:* Nurses who are not emotionally mature can have a high level of stress to deal with the patients.

4. **Other factors**
   - Death or sickness in the family
   - A temporary setback or other personal problem
   - A poor support structure
   - Instability between work and family or own life
   - Lack of self-esteem
   - Financial issues.

CONSEQUENCES OF WORKPLACE STRESS

I: General consequences
Effects of stress can vary among individuals; however, the stress can be classified into cognitive, biological or physiological, emotional, behavioral, and occupational.

1. **Cognitive:** Cognitive symptoms relate to the understanding and knowledge functioning of the body. The common symptoms are related to memory, decision-making, indecisiveness, concentrate, judgment, negative thinking, thoughts, worrying, etc.
2. **Biological or physiological:** Due to stress, the individual suffers from physiological symptoms that are psychosomatic. The physiological symptoms are headache, body ache, constipation, nausea, vomiting, loss of appetite or excessive eating, sleep disturbance, tachycardia, chest pain, skin allergy, heartburn, etc.
3. **Emotional and psychological:** The individual can develop specific emotional and psychological symptoms due to increased stress; the symptoms vary from individual to individual. These symptoms are a feeling of loneliness, agitation, irritability, loss of patience, anxiety, feeling tense, and depression.
4. **Behavioral:** Due to stress, the individual can develop many behavioral symptoms such as remain isolated, silent, not taking responsibilities, consuming alcohol, cigarette smoking, or other substance to relax, nail biting, teeth grinding, excessive exercising or shopping, and unnecessary reacting to unexpected problems. Rule out a medical or psychological condition if anyone is experiencing stress.
5. **Occupational:** Absenteeism; poor interpersonal relations with coworkers, doctors, head nurse, and patients; poor performance; nursing errors; job dissatisfaction; negativities for the job; and decreased motivation are some reasons of occupational stress. The findings of the studies revealed a strong negative association of nurses' occupational stress and job satisfaction.

II: Consequences of long-term stress
1. **Physical and physiological**
   - *Cardiovascular disease:* The persistent stress resulted in many cardiovascular diseases such as hypertension, chest pain, and angina.
   - *Musculoskeletal disorders:* The literature also documented that stress is the main contributory factor for many musculoskeletal disorders such as backache and body ache.
   - *Gastrointestinal and metabolic disorders:* The studies indicated stress is one of the risk factors for many gastrointestinal diseases such as peptic ulcer, intestinal ulcers, diabetes, and even cancer.
2. **Psychological:** The literature also documented that many psychological problems among health workers are due to occupational stress and has reported that almost 75% of patients seek psychiatric consultation. There is an increase in mental problems such as anxiety, depression, and feeling of insecurity among nurses. They also indulge in substance use such as drugs, alcohol, and suicides, which are more common among those who have burned out.

APPROACHES TO STRESS MANAGEMENT

Individual Coping Strategies
It includes programs in which the employees learn about the causes and consequences of occupational stress, cognitive coping skills, and time management, which are intended to change how they can organize their working situation. It also includes relaxation and meditation techniques, which can reduce stress.

1. **Time management:** The inability to manage time could be one of the stressful situations in a job. If the nurses know how to manage their time and have a plan for doing it along with the necessary room to deal with unexpected crises or emergencies, they will feel more positive and will have fewer tensions. Nurses who feel less stress are better able to take care of themselves and their patients.
2. **Relaxation/meditation:** Relaxation/meditation techniques are complementary methods. Meditation is a way of focusing on something in a relaxed state in a quiet environment.
   - *Physiologically oriented methods:* The aim is to achieve deep muscle relaxation through contracting and relaxing major muscle groups. In muscle relaxation technique, a trained instructor teaches the participants about deep breathing and deep relaxation exercises and advices them to practice daily for 15 minutes by using tape recorder.

- *Meditation-relaxation technique:* In this technique, instruct the participants to sit quietly and meditate for 15–20 minutes once or twice a day. The participants begin each meditation session by calming and relaxing the body, and then they spend the remaining time working with a mantra (meditation sound).
- *Cognitive-oriented method:* Imagery and meditation have relaxation effects. It includes three cognitive processes: focusing, passivity, and receptivity with an outcome of a calm mind and relaxed body functions.
- *Biofeedback:* It is another popular relaxation technique. It is a separate intervention evaluated by Murphy but usually employed in combination with relaxation. During the practice of relaxation exercises, observe and record some of the internal processes of the participant by the use of sophisticated equipment. The equipment measures temperature, muscular tension, heartbeat, and blood pressure. Once you are aware that your internal body responses are in a state of stress, you can begin to make adjustments by changing the environment and adopting other stress releasing methods.

3. **Other individual coping strategies:** Keeping pet; saying prayers; singing aloud; laughter therapy; having a good sleep; aerobatics; spending time with children; taking a walk; making friends; and cultivating interests in gardening, reading, writing, and cooking, are also helpful in forgetting the worries and controlling stress.

Cognitive Restructuring Strategies

These strategies aim at the reduction of stress and the coping skill strategies directed toward the development of personal strategies aimed at improving skills and competencies to meet the job demand. It involves training in positive coping self-statements (e.g. I can do this work, or I can handle the situation) that encourage the person to assess conditions, prepare to face stressors, and to cope with stress.

Stress Inoculation Training

The program focuses on activities such as time management, communication skills, conflict resolution, and problem-solving skills. Most of the studies use a method of education and discussion.

Employee Assistance Programs

In this program, a form of psychotherapy is given to highly stressed individuals either outside or in a psychological clinic. A brief therapeutic model is comprising two weekly sessions of therapy, followed by a third session 3 months later. Two modes of prescriptive treatment are a short cognitive-behavioral and exploratory treatment and a brief relationship oriented.

Organizational Coping Strategies

1. **Organizational change:** The regulatory change approach is useful to apply to reduce stress in case of excessive workload. It is in two forms:
   a. *Organizational-wide program:* According to Jones, take the following steps to organize an organizational-wide schedule to reduce stress among employees:
   - Assess stress levels of employees
   - Review and modify causative organizational factors of stress
   - Work out a series of policies and procedures concerning interdepartmental communication, organization, and personnel policies to reduce stress
   - Inform employees about work out modifications in policy and procedures in small conference sessions
   - Provide a series of video-cassette training modules to all employees to make them understand personal and occupational stress and methods of reducing stress and improving coping skills
   - Set up a comprehensive employee assistance program for employees to discuss their problems, both work-related and personal issues.

   b. *Organizational developmental program:* The program is aiming to create a corporate culture and provisions to meet individual needs and eliminate the causes of stress. This approach involves the participation of all employees of an organization to diagnose and solve the problems by taking the following steps:
   - Ask all employees to list down three things they consider best in their department and the three things they think worst and urgently need modification
   - Discuss their responses in a general meeting and report to the head
   - Form a group of volunteers among employees to gather additional information and make recommendations for improvement.

2. **Stress management training program:** The program should include the general building awareness about job stress, securing top management commitment and support for the program, and nurses' input and involvement in all phases of the program and to conduct the program.
   - *Identifying the problem:* Obtain information about nurses' perceptions regarding their job conditions and perceived levels of stress by holding group discussions and conducting the survey.
   - *Analyze data:* Analyze the information gathered to identify stressful job conditions, levels of stress, health status, and job satisfaction level.

- *Planning intervention:* After gathering information and level of stress among employees, plan intervention, and implement the intervention.
- *Evaluation:* Evaluate the impact of the intervention and accordingly make modifications.

NURSE MANAGERS' ROLE IN STRESS MANAGEMENT

The nurse managers can play an essential role in stress management of nurses by adopting the following approaches:
1. Design jobs to provide stimulation and opportunities for nurses to use their skills
2. Clearly define nurses' roles and responsibilities
3. Plan orientation programs for the newly joined staff
4. Give nurses opportunities to participate in decisions and actions in inpatient care
5. Improve communications and provide a supportive environment
6. Provide performance counseling to staff to identify the ways to improve the skills and performance and to understand the work environment as well as his or her strengths and weaknesses
7. Provide an empathic climate where he or she can discuss his or her tensions, conflicts, concerns, and problems
8. Organize group meetings to solve the problems.

TIPS FOR REDUCING STRESS AT WORKPLACE

The following lists the tips for reducing stress at workplace:
1. **Recognize the sign and symptoms of excessive stress:** Do not ignore the signs of stress.
2. **Take care of yourself:** Pay attention to your physical and emotional health. Use physical stress-relieving strategies. Do exercises; break up the activity into two or three shorter segments. Get sound sleep.
3. **Prioritize and organize your responsibilities:** Manage your time by creating a balanced schedule, do not commit yourself, try to leave earlier in the morning, and plan regular breaks and relax. Also, manage the task by prioritizing tasks, delegating responsibilities, and be willing to compromise.
4. **Improve emotional intelligence:** Manage your emotions in positive and constructive ways. Communicate with others in ways that overcome differences, repair wounded feelings, and defuse tension and stress.
5. **Improve upon bad habits:** Eliminate self-defeating behaviors. Flip your negative thinking.
6. **Improve communication:** Share information with employees and define employees' roles and responsibilities. Make interface friendly and efficient.
7. **Be role models:** Act as positive role models, especially in times of high stress.
8. **Consult your employees:** Give them opportunities to participate in decisions, value their feelings, praise excellent work performance, both verbally and officially. Provide opportunities for career development.
9. **Cultivate a friendly and social climate:** Provide opportunities for social interaction among employees. Establish a zero-tolerance policy for harassment.
10. **Keep yourself physically and mentally fit:** Follow a healthy lifestyle. Be positive.

CHAPTER HIGHLIGHTS

- According to Hans Selye, stress is the response and adjustment of body functioning with the various internal and external environmental stimuli/factors.
- Work stress is a mismatch between job demand and capabilities, resources, and needs of employees.
- There are three levels of stress: eustress, distress, and burnout. The eustress is a physical and mental ability trigger; moderate stress requires to act. The burnout is the extreme level of stress; the individual can go in a crisis.
- There are mainly three stages of stress: alarm, resistance, and exhaustion stage.
- The primary sources of stress at the workplace are organizational, professional, personal, and other external factors.
- The individuals can have general and long-term consequences due to stress that can affect their health and work efficiency.
- There are many coping strategies at the individual and organizational level to cope with stress.
- Nurse managers can play a vital role in reducing the stress level among nurses through implementing various strategies.

REVIEW QUESTIONS

I. Essay Type Questions
1. Define work stress. Discuss various types of stress.
2. What are the sources of stress? Discuss it in detail.
3. Describe the general consequences of workplace stress affecting the health and work performance of nurses.
4. Enumerate different types of approaches to stress management. Explain individual coping strategies in detail.
5. Discuss the role of the nurse manager in the stress management of nurses.

II. Short Notes
1. Stages of stress
2. Consequences of stress
3. Organizational coping strategies
4. Sources of stress
5. Eustress versus distress

III. Multiple Choice Questions

1. Who introduced the term "stress" in Medicine?
   a. Looker and Greyson
   b. Hans Selye
   c. George Engel
   d. Schmidt
2. Which type of stress is harmful to both individual and organization?
   a. Rust out
   b. Burnout
   c. Distress
   d. Eustress
3. At what stage of stress, an individual continues fighting with a stressor that develops anxiety, tension, and fatigue?
   a. Alarm stage
   b. Resistance stage
   c. Exhaustion stage
   d. Crisis stage
4. Which of the following is the professional service-related stressor?
   a. Lack of career development
   b. Financial issues
   c. Lack of self-esteem
   d. Caring death and dying patients
5. The stress prone symptoms that relate to understanding and knowledge functioning of the body is:
   a. Biological
   b. Behavioral
   c. Cognitive
   d. Emotional

Answer Keys

1. b   2. c   3. b   4. d   5. c

SUGGESTED READING

1. Blair A, Littlewood M. Sources of stress. J Commun Nurs. 1995;40:38-9.
2. Clegg A. Occupational stress in nursing: A review of the literature. J Nurs Manag. 2001;9:101-6.
3. Deckard GJ, Rountree BH, Hicks LL. Nursing productivity: A qualitative view of performance. Nurs Econ. 1988;6:184-8.
4. Lee J, Graham AV. Students' perception of medical school stress and their evaluation of a wellness elective. Med Edu. 2001;35:652-9.
5. McVicar. Workplace stress in nursing: A literature review. J Adv Nurs. 2003;44:633-42.
6. Michie S, Williams S. Reducing psychological ill health and associated sickness absence: A systematic literature review. Occup Environ Med. 2003;60:3-9.
7. Michie S. Causes and management of stress at work. Occup Environ Med. 2002;59:67-72. Available from http://www.cdc.gov/niosh/docs/99-101/.
8. Russler MF. Multidimensional stress management in nursing education. J Nurs Educ. 1991;30:341-6.
9. Selye H. The Stress of Life. New York: McGraw-Hill; 1976.
10. Sky Hudgins. The Importance of Stress Management for Nurses. International Council of nurses. 2008. Available from www.statswsheet.com. [Accessed October 2008].

34 CHAPTER

Occupational Health and Safety

CHAPTER OUTLINE

- Occupational Health and Safety
  - Occupational Health
  - Occupational Safety
  - Importance of Occupational Health and Safety
- Occupational Hazards
  - Meaning
  - Why Hospitals Have a Risk of Occupational Hazards?
  - Common Occupational Hazards in Hospitals
  - Common Occupational Diseases
- Prevention of Occupational Hazards
  - The Constitutional Employees' Right to Health
  - Occupational Health Laws
  - National Policy on Safety, Health, and Environment
  - Indian and the International Labour Organization
  - Health and Safety Program at the Local Level
- Nurses' Role in the Prevention of Occupational Hazards/Diseases

LEARNING OUTCOMES

After completion of this chapter, the learner will be able to:
- Define and understand the concept of occupational health and safety
- Identify the burden of occupation diseases
- Appreciate the importance of occupational health and safety
- Explain common occupational hazards
- Discuss general methods of prevention of occupational hazards/diseases
- Elaborate on various occupational health and safety acts
- Describe nurses' role in the prevention of occupational hazards/diseases

KEY TERMS

Occupation health and safety, occupational hazards, occupational health and safety acts, occupational health laws

INTRODUCTION

The health and safety of employees are an essential aspect of an organization's smooth and effective functioning. Nurses as care providers are the key persons in the healthcare system in the delivery of health in every setting. The health of care providers, in whose hands the health of others rest, is equally important to keep them healthy, and ensure safety.

Safety brings organizational effectiveness. Good health and safety performance ensure an accident-free environment. It helps in improving employee morale, reducing absenteeism and enhancing productivity, minimizing occupational injuries and illnesses, and increasing the quality of services. There is a need to identify hazards, their evaluation, and control of risks.

OCCUPATIONAL HEALTH AND SAFETY

Occupational Health

World Health Organization defines occupational health as a multidisciplinary activity. It concerns the health and safety of employees. It focuses on preventing and controlling occupational work-related disorders, injury, impairment, or disease affecting an employee during employment. It also aims at eliminating the risk factors and workplace conditions for the health and safety of people at work. International Labour Organization (ILO) and World Health Organization (WHO) emphasize the promotion of the highest degree of physical, mental, and social well-being of employees, the prevention health problems, the protection of workers from risks of diseases, and providing an environment that should be free from occupation hazards.

Occupational Safety

Safety is the "absence of danger," and occupational safety means "the absence of danger at work." It relates to exposure to a hazard accident. It is the protection of employees from occupational hazards. It is the health and well-being of people employed in a work environment.

Occupation health and safety are concerning physical, social, and mental well-being of workers as a whole. The United States Congress Occupational Safety and Health Act passed to prevent employees from workplace illnesses and promoting the safety of employees. India has also had legislation on occupational safety and health for 50 years.

Importance of Occupational Health and Safety

The nature of work plays a central role in employee's health since most nurses spend at least 8 hours a day in the workplace and with patients suffering variety of problems, both infectious and noninfectious, admitted in the hospital.

Aims and objectives of occupation health and safety

The following list shows the aims and objectives of occupation health and safety:

- To promote and maintain the highest degree of physical, social, and mental well-being of employees
- To prevent the adverse effects on the health of employees caused by their working conditions
- To reduce injuries, accidents, infections, and absenteeism
- To protect the employees in their employment from risks of occupational health hazards
- To improve the organizational effectiveness by improving the quality of nursing care
- To place and maintain the professional environment for the employees to adapt their physical and mental needs with the adaptation of their work.

OCCUPATIONAL HAZARDS

Meaning

According to the Dictionary, occupation hazards are the dangers to health associated with occupation or work environment. It includes the risk of accident and of contracting occupational diseases or can lead to the death of an individual at the workplace.

Why Hospitals Have a Risk of Occupational Hazards?

There are many reasons to have a risk of occupational hazards in the hospital. Hospital is not like other factories where occupational safety can be measured by industrial accident rates instead in such a setting; occupational safety is more concerned about illnesses and diseases that are arising from the workplace. The hazard risks in the hospitals are mainly due to the hospital environment, physical layout and working conditions, and nature of the profession.

1. **Hospital environment**
   Nurses come in direct contact with patients having infections, suffering from infectious diseases, chest infections, and bacterial and viral infections. The person handling such patients has a higher risk of getting infections. These are hospital cross-infections, e.g. tuberculosis, typhoid, hepatitis, rabies, scabies, cough, cold, fever, and bronchitis. The staffs working in radiotherapy or chemotherapy unit are susceptible to infertility, chromosomal defects, etc.
2. **Physical layout and working conditions**
   Overcrowding, poor sanitation, poor air ventilation, inadequate lighting arrangement, lack of safe drinking water facility, lack of retiring place, facilities for tea, food, unsafe working conditions, such as unguarded machinery, slippery floors, or inadequate fire precautions, can lead to specific physical hazards and gastrointestinal and respiratory diseases.
3. **Profession itself**
   - *Nature of work:* Due to the nature of work such as long-standing duties, all types of physically strenuous tasks, e.g. shifting patients from trolley to bed, and other nursing procedures, etc. This nature of work can lead to problems of the musculoskeletal system such as backache, cervical spondylosis, leg cramps, and body ache.
   - *Night duties and regular shift duties:* Night and shift duties can also lead to problems of the musculoskeletal system and of gastrointestinal, e.g. nausea, vomiting, and indigestion. Changes in lifestyle patterns can even give rise to psychosomatic and psychosocial issues like family adjustment problems, unhappily married life, divorce, etc.
   - *Stressful workplace:* Nursing staff is also working in very stressful conditions where they are caring for acutely ill and dying patients. Their stressful and painful situations can affect their psychological well-being and can create psychosomatic problems such as emotional upset, depression, mania, and cardiovascular diseases such as hypertension, anxiety, and heart palpitation angina.
   - *Lack of promotional avenue:* Stagnation, low-social prestige although noble profession can lead to rejection, frustration, and little job satisfaction that can affect their personality and mental health.

Common Occupational Hazards in Hospitals

There are several categories of insidious risks, i.e. those hazards that are dangerous but which may not be visible), including as shown in **Table 34.1**.

1. **Biological hazards**
   Biological hazards are commonly known as occupational infections that arise due to infectious agents such as bacteria, viruses, fungi, infectious waste, and parasitic infestations. Biological hazards exist throughout all health-care settings. The examples are

TABLE 34.1: Common health hazards about location and occupation in hospitals.

	Types of hazards	Location	Personnel at risk
Biological	AIDS, hepatitis B, and cytomegalovirus	All the wards including emergency, Operation theatre, renal, dental, labs	Doctors, nurses, dental staff, lab staff
	Rubella, Tuberculosis	Obstetrics, pediatrics, child care wards, labs	Pregnant staff. Nurses, lab staff, physicians, student
Physical	Noise	Workshop, laundry, kitchen, ICU, cardiac coronary unit, OT	Persons working in workshop, kitchen, nurses, doctors, and technicians
	Vibration	Vibrating machines, monitors, vehicles	Nurses, servants, cleaners, drivers
	Thermal	Central Sterile Services Department (CSSD), OT, kitchen, laundry	CSSD workers, nurses, OT staff including nurses, kitchen workers, laundry workers, and nurses
	Illumination	All areas	All staff
	Radiation	X-ray, wards, OT, physiotherapy and dental unit	Radiologist, radiographers, nurses, doctors
Chemical	Cleansing, compounds, disinfectants	All areas	Cleaning staff, nurses, servants
	Cytotoxic	Pharmacy, wards, waste disposal	Pharmacists, nurses, doctors, garbage collector
	Ethylene oxide Glutaraldehyde	CSSD	Nurses, ward servants, assistants
	Methyl methacrylate	Dental, OT	Dental staff, surgeons, nurses
	Solvents	Lab, all areas	Technicians, scientists, cleaners
	Waste anesthetic gases	Dental, OT, recovery	Dentists, dental staff, nurses, surgeons, anesthetist
Ergonomics	Manual handling	Patient areas, stores	Those who handle patients and loads
	Postural, constraints	All areas	All staff
	Occupational, overuse syndrome	All areas	Keyboard, clerical, cleaners, physicians, drivers
Psychosocial	Patient relative, contact, lack of control, shift work, overwork, threats to physical security	All areas	All staff

occupational pulmonary tuberculosis, viral hepatitis B and C, HIV infection/AIDS, Severe Acute Respiratory Syndrome (SARS), occupation dermatosis, and other infectious diseases due to hospital-acquired infections.

2. **Physical hazards**

Physical hazards arise from the extreme level of noise, vibration, lighting, temperatures, ionizing, and nonionizing radiation. Excessive noise can cause annoyance and stress, increased accident rates, hearing impairment, and hearing loss. The extreme vibrations cause congestion of pelvic and abdominal organs. The physical hazards due to thermal include thermal stress, both cold (hypothermia, frostbite, etc.) and heat exhaustion (headache, dizziness, fainting, lack of concentration, anorexia). Poor and defective illumination causes eye strain, fatigue, accidents, etc. Nonionizing radiation leads to cataracts, skin erythema, burn, etc. The exposure to high ionizing radiation such as X-rays and gamma rays affects various organs of the body such as skin, bone, lungs, and blood. The radiation also has an effect on reproductive function such as sterility, abortions, stillbirths, and congenital genetic disabilities.

3. **Chemical hazards**

Chemical hazards arise from liquids, solids, dust, fumes, vapors, and gases. Toxic chemicals in use in hospitals include cleaners used by contracted cleaning staff. The staff may develop skin allergy, contact dermatitis, irritation to eyes, throat, and lungs.

Exposure to mercury in liquid form occurs from accidental spills that occur during sterilization and centrifugation of thermometers in central supply areas or through inhalation, or skin contact causes stomatitis, gastrointestinal disturbances affect the kidney, and organic mercury can affect the central nervous system. The exposure to organic solvents, metals, acid mists, and sterilizing agents (ethylene oxide) can affect the various systems of the body including the skin, nervous system, kidney, gastrointestinal system, and blood-forming organs and increases reproductive functions and breast cancer risk among women in occupational settings. Exposure to ethylene gas has an association with the occurrence of disease on reproductive organs and results in mutagenic changes, neurotoxicity, and sensitization.

Health hazards from e-waste recycling due to a chemical such as beryllium, found in computer motherboards, cadmium in a chip is poisonous and can lead to cancer, bleeding from throat and breathlessness, lung ailments including asthma, bronchitis, and chronic lung infections.

4. **Ergonomic hazards**

Ergonomic hazards occur due to heavy lifting, loading of application of high vibration, pushing, walking, repetitive motions, poorly designed types of machinery, broken instruments, and chipped articles. The most common hazards are musculoskeletal disorders. The most important locations are shoulders, arms, knees,

lower backache, injuries of muscles and tendons, ligaments, and bones. Nurses used to suffer from low backache pain, cuts, burns, needle stick injuries, etc.
5. **Psychosocial hazards**
Psychosocial hazards occur due to psychological risk factors such as inadequate personal support system, workplace stress, safety hazards, environmental exposures, severe patients and relatives, lack of control over work situation, shift work, overwork, threats to physical security, and low wage. The environmental; physical factors such as noise, thermal, radiation, poor lighting, and chemical factors; and individual social factors such as personality, interpersonal relationship, and age. These factors can cause psychological problems such as anxiety, dissatisfaction, depression, burnout, headache, backache, hypertension, diabetes, peptic ulcer, leg cramps, sleep disturbances, and some behavioral issues such as absenteeism, poor interpersonal relation, social isolation, nonparticipation, and substance use.

Common Occupational Diseases

Following are some of the common occupational diseases:
- Hypertension, coronary heart diseases
- Behavioral and psychosomatic disorders such as headache, backache, diabetes, peptic ulcer, leg cramps, sleep disturbances, gastrointestinal problems, etc.
- Gastrointestinal diseases such as peptic ulcer
- Respiratory nonspecific chronic illness and asthma
- Musculoskeletal disorders such as low backache, shoulder and neck pain, muscle cramps.

PREVENTION OF OCCUPATIONAL HAZARDS

The Constitutional Employees' Right to Health

Article 21 of the Indian Constitution has the provision of protection of life and personal liberty of a person. A worker has the fundamental right to health; medical aid, while in service or after retirement, is a fundamental right. The Directive Principles of State Policy secure the health and strength of workers, men and women, and the tender age of children. There is also a provision of just and humane conditions of work and maternity relief.

Occupational Health Laws

Some occupational health laws are listed below:
1. **Health Provisions Under the Factories Act, 1948**
   The Factories Act, 1948, based on the British Factories Act, is amended from time to time in India. The Factories (Amendment) Act was implemented on 1 December 1987. But this Act does not cover hospitals. The Factories Act 1948 protects workers from long hours of manual labor. Under this act, employees should work in healthy and sanitary conditions. They should precaution for their safety and prevention of accidents.
   - *Section 10* of the Act states that a State Government may appoint qualified medical practitioners as "certifying surgeons" to discharge the following duties: The young person's engaged in hazardous works must undergo an examination. The persons who are working in the substance used or new manufacturing processes or the place that may cause injuries must work under medical supervision.
2. **Chapter IX of the Act**
   This act has the provision of health, safety, and welfare measures for the workers in factories and prohibits women and children from working in certain occupations.
3. **The Employees' State Insurance Act, 1948**
   Under the ESI Act, the insured workers have benefits of cash in the case of sickness, maternity, and employment injury; the ESI Act also provides pension to the dependants in case of the death of the insured worker who died of employment injury and medical benefit to workers.
4. **Occupational health protection (safety)**
   Occupational health safety by ILO/WHO committee in June 1977 recommends that each member should adopt laws and regulations on occupational and security to the individual nature of nursing work and of the environment in which it is carried out. They should also have access to occupational health service recommendations and where occupational health services are not set up. Following recommendations must be followed and ensured by the employers, each member, and organizations:
   a. *Medical measures*
      - Pre-placement examination: Nursing personnel must undergo a medical exam on taking up and terminating an appointment (47-1).
      - Regularly assign the wok, keeping in mind the specific risk to their health. If suspected, advice to undergo regular medical tests.
      - Assure objectively and confidentially in the examination provided.
      - Notify industrial accidents or diseases, if recognized to the competent authority.
      - Carry out periodical inspection of the working environment and conduct studies to find out the particular risk of exposure for health.
      - Maintain and analyze health records regularly.
   b. *Environment sanitation and engineering measure (1981 recommendations)*
      - Appropriate structural features, maintenance, and repairs of working place
      - Provision of sufficient lighting, ventilation, odor, temperature, humidity, and cleanliness
      - Prevention of harmful physical and mental stress due to the condition of work
      - Radiation protection
      - Working facilities for changing and storing clothes

- Supply of safe drinking water and other welfare facilities.
c. *Working time and rest periods (VIII, 1977)*
  - The working hours should not exceed more than 40 hours per week.
  - The working day, including overtime, should not exceed 12 hours.
  - There should be meal break, rest break, and week rest.
  - There should be a provision for leaves and security.
d. *Measures for pregnant women and children*
  The regular assignment of pregnant women and parents of young children should not be prejudicial to their health.
e. *Mental health*
  There should be counseling sessions for nursing personnel, especially those who are working intensive care and emergency units as they might at risk of rejection, low job satisfaction, emotional instability, and other psychological problems.
5. **Occupational Safety and Health Act, 1989**
  The Act addresses the occupational safety concerns of health-care workers but could not be worked out. In July 2001, Bio-Medical Waste (Management & Handling) Rules, 1998, had a provision of "Accident Reporting" concerned with waste management and handling.
6. **Occupational safety and health institutions**
  There are two leading institutions devoted to occupational health and safety: Central Labour Institute, Mumbai and Regional Labour Institutes in Kolkata, Kanpur, and Chennai under Ministry of Labour and National Institute of Occupational Health (NIOH), Ahmedabad and Regional Institutes in Kolkata and Bengaluru under the Indian Council of Medical Research (ICMR) Ministry of Health. The National Institute of Occupational Health (NIOH) is quite active as a research institute, providing enough training of staff to get aware of health-care facilities of the dangers surrounding them and take adequate precautions to avoid hazards and appropriate measures in case of accidents.
7. **IS 18001:2000 Occupational Health and Safety Management Systems**
  The standard prescribes requirements for the system that is concerning the health and safety of employees and providing information regarding its specification.

National Policy on Safety, Health, and Environment

The main objective of policy on safety and health at the national level is to reduce occupational risks and health-related problems. It also aims to provide a database for better monitoring and improving performance. Its focus is to make the public aware of safety and health at the workplace.

Indian and the International Labour Organization (ILO)

India is a founder member of ILO. ILO sets up the "International Labour Standards" in the form of Conventions and Recommendations. ILO concerns with worker's fundamental rights, protection, social security, labor welfare, occupational safety and health, women and child labor, migrant labor, indigenous and tribal population, etc.

Health and Safety Program at the Local Level

1. **Nosocomial infection control**
  The hospital's Infection Control Nurse and Infection Control Committee are concerning with the prevention, surveillance, and control of nosocomial infections. The hospitals must have an Infection Control Program in the hospital's Infection Control Manual. The manual must outline the principles, strategies, policies, and procedures for infection control in the hospital. All staff should be familiar with the manual. There should be regular feedback on the surveillance of nosocomial infection. The hospital must adhere to standard safety measures for infection control.
2. **Patient safety**
  The hospital must have standard operative protocols for patient safety. For example, keeping bed rails up particularly for those patients with an altered conscious state from medication or illness, maintenance of equipments, bathroom/toilet aids particularly for the elderly or disabled, walking aids for the disabled, and during recovery, prevention of pressure ulcers, carefully applying hot water bottle if required to the unconscious patients, and prevention of chemical burns, etc.
3. **Food safety**
  Hospital kitchens prepare meals for inpatients, and in many cases, prepare meals for the staff canteen. The food storage, handling, and preparation should be done to the highest standards to avoid any risk to already sick or compromised patients.
4. **Disaster management**
  There should be disaster management protocols in all the hospitals at different levels.
5. **Biomedical waste management issues**
  The major components of such a waste management system include the following:
  - *Waste segregation at the source:* There should be sharp containers, biohazard bins, general waste bins, and cytotoxic bins; all standardized and color coded.
  - *Waste streams:* These should be general, contaminated, cytotoxic/pharmaceutical, body parts.
  - *Storage and transport:* There should be the provision of cold storage for contaminated waste and body parts; transport in safe, leak-proof containers.

- *Waste treatment:* The hospital must have the provision of sterilization of contaminated waste (steam autoclave); incineration of cytotoxic, pharmaceuticals, and body parts in an incinerator meeting all relevant standards and statutes.
- *Waste disposal:* There should be clear-cut guidelines for Local Council approved engineered sanitary landfill.

6. **At the community level**

Hospitals should take a proactive role in the community to:
- Promote health worker through safe workplaces and facilitating fitness programs, weight reduction, smoking cessation, and stress relief for their workers.
- Promote public health in the community by being a lead agency for injury prevention through a collaborative safe community project.
- Increase commitment to quality assurance activities to maximize patient protection against adverse outcomes.
- Promote environmental health by support for waste reduction, reuse, and recycling; use of energy-efficient, environmentally friendly buildings; and greener, organic gardens.
- Provide a written "Routine Practices" document that is easily accessible.

NURSES' ROLE IN THE PREVENTION OF OCCUPATIONAL HAZARDS/DISEASES

Nurses can play a vital role in the prevention and promotion of occupational health and safety. She should be aware of the extent of problems that occur due to occupational hazards.

A. At operational level
1. The nurse may identify the need, assess, and plan interventions to reduce the risk of hazardous exposure.
2. Advocates necessary research ultimately leading to risk reduction and prevention strategies in the workplace.
3. Engage in routine health surveillance procedures, periodic health assessment, and in evaluating the results from such screening processes and maintain a high degree of alertness to any abnormal findings.
4. Follow universal standard precaution and standard safety measures. Use personal protective devices where required.
5. Use appropriate techniques and body posture for lifting and poisoning of patients.
6. Take proper sleep, especially after night duties.
7. Follow policies and intervention guidelines.
8. Report incidents to appropriate authority.

B. At administrative level
- Ensure the availability of protective equipment and cleansing agents
- Establish a sharp program
- Establish an immunization program for all nurses
- Provide personal protective equipment (PPE) such as shield aprons and safety glasses
- Establish procedures for the use of diagnostic equipment and PPE
- Minimize exposure time to radiation
- Ensure the post of warning signs appropriately
- Promote rest breaks
- A well-planned rotation plan with rest breaks during night shift and the day off after night duty
- Maintain the right work environment and culture.

CHAPTER HIGHLIGHTS

- Occupation health and safety are about the physical, social, and mental well-being of workers as a whole.
- Occupation hazards are the dangers to health associated with occupation or work environment.
- The typical occupational hazards in the hospital are biological, physical, chemical, ergonomic, and psychosocial hazards.
- There is safety legislation at constitutional, national, and the local level to prevent and control health hazards of the workplace.
- Nurses at the operational and administrative levels play a vital role in maintaining occupational health and safety.

REVIEW QUESTIONS

I. Essay Type Questions
1. Define the term "Occupation Health and Safety"? Discuss its aims and objectives.
2. Define occupational hazards. Explain why hospitals have risk occupation hazards.
3. Describe common occupational hazards in hospital.
4. Discuss various ways of preventing and controlling occupational hazards in the hospital.

II. Short Notes
1. Occupational Safety & Health Act, 1989
2. Health and safety programs
3. Nurses' role in preventing occupational health hazards
4. Chemical hazards in hospital
5. Occupational health laws

III. Multiple Choice Questions
1. Which of the following chemical from e-recycling causes health hazards?
   a. Organic solvent   b. Ethylene oxide
   c. Mercury   d. Beryllium
2. Which type of hazard occurs due to exposure to radiation?
   a. Physical   b. Chemical
   c. Biological   d. Ergonomic

3. Which of the following are the risk factors of ergonomic hazards?
   a. Liquids, solids, dust, fumes, and gases
   b. Noise, vibration, lighting, and temperature
   c. Heavy lifting, pushing, and repetitive motions
   d. Stress, shift duties, and overwork
4. Which occupational disease has possible symptoms of headache, backache, diabetes, peptic ulcer, or sleep disturbances?
   a. Gastrointestinal   b. Psychosomatic
   c. Cardiovascular   d. Musculoskeletal
5. According to ILO, how many maximum working hours should be in a week?
   a. 48 hours   b. 42 hours
   c. 40 hours   d. 36 hours

Answer Keys

1. d   2. a   3. c   4. b   5. c

SUGGESTED READING

1. Alli BO. Fundamental principles of occupational health and safety. Geneva: International Labour Office; 2001.
2. Ando S, Ono Y, Shimaoka M, et al. Associations of self-estimated workloads with musculoskeletal symptoms among hospital nurses. Occup Environ Med. 2000;57:211-6.
3. Available from http://www.kznhealth.gov.za/occhealth/policyocc.pdf. [Accessed April 2018].
4. Available from https://www.who.int/occupational_health/regions/en/oehemhealthcareworkers.pdf. [Accessed April 2018].
5. Bongers PM, Kremer AM, Laak J. Are psychosocial factors, risk factors for symptoms and signs of the shoulder, elbow, or hand/wrist?: A review of the epidemiological literature. Am J Ind Med. 2002;41:315-42.
6. ILO. Beyond deaths and injuries: The ILO's role in promoting safe and healthy jobs', the International Labour Organisation, 2008.
7. Jin K, Sorock GS, Courtney T, et al. Risk factors for work-related low back pain in the People's Republic of China. Int J Occup Environ Health. 2000;6:26-33.
8. John Tingle, Alan Cribb (Ed). Nursing law and ethics. Oxford: Blackwell Science; 1995.
9. Josephson M, Lagerström M, Hagberg M, et al. Musculoskeletal symptoms and job strain among nursing personnel: A study over three years. Occup Environ Med. 1997;54:681-5.
10. Kaushal V, Kumar S, Singh S, Shyama NS, Sharma DK. Hospital risk management-strategy to enhance safety. Int J Med Toxicol Legal Med. 2007;10(1):1.
11. Larese F, Fiorito A. Musculoskeletal disorders in hospital nurses: a comparison between two hospitals. Ergonomics. 1994;37:1205-11.
12. Lugah V, Ganesh B, Darus A, Retneswari M, Rosnawati M R, Sujatha D. Training of occupational safety and health: Knowledge among healthcare professionals in Malaysia Singapore Med J. 2010;51(7):586-91.
13. National Institute of Occupational Safety and Health. Safety and Health Topic: Health Care Workers. State of the Sector Healthcare and Social Assistance. Available from http://www.cdc.gov/niosh/docs/2009-138/. [Accessed April 2018].
14. Preventing Needlestick Injuries Among Healthcare Workers. (n.d.). Available from https://www.who.int/occupational_health/activities/5prevent.pdf. [Accessed April 2018].
15. Sepkowitz KA, Eisenberg L. Occupational deaths among healthcare workers. Emerg Infect Dis. 2005;11:1003-8. Available from www.cdc.gov/ncidod/EID/vol11no07/04-1038.htm. [Accessed September 2018].
16. Smedley J, Egger P, Cooper C, et al. Manual handling activities and risk of low back pain in nurses. Occup Environ Med. 1995;52:160-3.
17. Trinkoff AM, Lipscomb JA, Geiger-Brown J, et al. Musculoskeletal problems of the neck, shoulder, and back and functional consequences in nurses. Am J Ind Med. 2002;41:170-8.

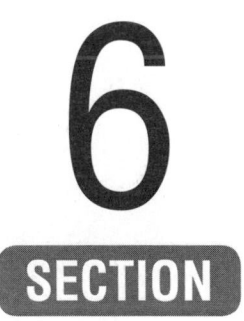

SECTION 6

Directing and Leading

35. Directing and Motivation
36. Communication
37. Effective Supervision
38. Nursing Leadership
39. Conflict Management
40. Collective Bargaining, Unions, and Professional Associations

CHAPTER 35

Directing and Motivation

CHAPTER OUTLINE

- Directing
  - Meaning of Directing
  - Features of Directing
  - Roles and Functions of Directing
  - Principles of Directing
  - Directing Process Activities
  - Techniques of Directing Process
- Motivation
  - Defining Motivation
  - Motivation Process
  - Types of Motivation
- Motivation and Performance
  - Influencing Factors of Motivation
  - Factors Causing Demotivation
- Models of Motivation
- Motivational Theories
- How to Create a Motivating Climate?
- Role of Nurse Managers to Motivate Staff

LEARNING OUTCOMES

After completion of this chapter, the learner will be able to:
- Recall and understand the concept of directing
- Analyze the importance of directing
- Explain the principles of directing
- Recall the concept of motivation
- Explain types of motivation
- Understand the ways of affecting behavior and performance
- Explain various models and theories of motivation
- Discuss the role of nurse managers in motivating staff

KEY TERMS

Directing, motivation, extrinsic, intrinsic, behavior, performance

INTRODUCTION

Directing/leading is the heart of the management process and is its third function to achieve the organizational goal. It helps the nursing managers to supervise and control the activities of nursing staff working under them. Proper directions play a vital role in maintaining a healthy working environment. How the managers are communicating, guiding, motivating, and supervising is reciprocal to the accomplishment of organizational objectives. It is the central point around which other functions of management revolve. It is also called the spark of life of control.

DIRECTING

Meaning of Directing

- Directing or direction means issuing of instructions to the subordinates, supervising them, motivating them, and providing leadership to contribute to the best of their ability for the achievement of nursing organizational goals. It is also known as "actuation."
- Direction is a complex function that includes all those activities which are designed to encourage subordinates to work effectively and efficiently.

  —*Koontz and O'Donnell*
- Directing is what to do and in what manner through dictating the procedures and policies for accomplishing performance standards.

  —*Earnest Dale*
- Directing consists of a process or technique of issuing instructions and carrying out operations as originally planned.

  —*Human*
- According to Dictionary meaning, direction is something that provides direction or advice as to a decision or course of action.
- Activating deals with the steps a manager takes to get subordinates and others to carry out plans.

  —*Newman & Warren*

In nursing management, from top to operational, direction takes place wherever a superior-subordinate relationship exists. It includes all the activities issuing orders, instructing, inspiring, guiding, motivating, leading, and supervising that take place at the workplace to achieve the goal of the nursing organization. In other words, directing involves communication, leadership, supervision, and motivation. It also consists of making provision for the necessary facilities and creating a work environment whereby nursing personnel may perform to the best of their abilities.

Features of Directing

1. The direction is a function required at all levels of nursing management. Every nurse manager provides guidance and inspires her subordinates to do the best nursing care.
2. The direction is the function to initiate the action and helps in converting plans into performance.
3. The directing is the continuous activity of communicating, leading, and motivation throughout the organization.
4. The directing is concerned with the human element.
5. Direction has dual functions: getting the things done through subordinates and providing the opportunity to superiors to do more meaningful work.

Roles and Functions of Directing

1. Direction initiates actions to achieve desired outcomes in an organization.
2. Direction attempts to integrate employees' effort by identifying their capabilities.
3. Direction facilitates changes in the organization and keeps the elements such as supervision, motivation, leadership, and communication effective.
4. Direction ensures that every employee works for organizational goals.
5. Direction tries to get the best from the employees. It provides a way to channelize the efforts and utilize their capabilities.
6. It increases efficiency and effectiveness in the organizational functioning.

Principles of Directing

The purpose of direction is to achieve the organizational goal. The managers must follow principles of directing to fulfill those objectives (Fig. 35.1):

1. **Harmony of objectives:** Harmony of objectives means that employees' goals should go side by side with the organizational goals. There should be harmony between these goals and their objectives; then, only the organization will progress. And it is possible through effective and appropriate directions given by the superiors.
2. **Principle of scalar chain:** Principle of scalar chain states that chain of superiors and subordinates raging from top to bottom level. It establishes a superior-subordinate relationship and also defines the authority of superiors. Communications in the hierarchy flow from top to bottom and from lower to top level. A clear-cut line of authority must follow for giving instructions, orders, commands, and guidance.
3. **Unity of command:** Unity of command exists when subordinate gets orders and instructions from one superior only. Otherwise, there will be confusion, conflict, disorder, and indiscipline in the organization. Therefore, the subordinate should report to one supervisor alone.
4. **Appropriate techniques:** The nurse managers should use correct direction techniques to ensure the efficiency of direction. The methods must be suitable to the superior, the subordinate, and the situation. These are authoritarian, consultative, and free rein.
5. **Direct supervision:** Effective supervisor makes direct personal contact with his or her subordinates for giving any direction. Such direct contact improves the morale and commitment of employees. Therefore, wherever possible, make use of direct supervision.
6. **Effective leadership:** This principle states that supervisors should be effective leaders instead of doing the same things as subordinates are doing to secure maximum output from them.
7. **Understanding and comprehension:** The supervisor must convey the directions to their subordinates. Instructions must be clear and comprehensive for the subordinates to understand.
8. **Effective communication:** The success of directions depends on the effective communication between superiors and subordinates. The downward communication should be apparent.
9. **Use of informal communication:** Organizations should have informal groups because the information passes very quickly, and management can take appropriate steps in time.
10. **Utilization of the maximum individual efforts:** The supervisors should use effective directional techniques to maximize the personal attempt to accomplish organizational goals.
11. **Clear orders:** The instructions or the rules given by the superiors should be unambiguous, concise, logical, and acceptable by the subordinates.

Principles of directing process
- Principle of harmony of objectives
- Principle of scalar chain
- Principle of unity of command
- Principle of appropriate techniques
- Principle of direct supervision
- Principle of effective leadership
- Principle of understanding
- Principle of maximum individual contribution
- Principle of effective communication
- Principle of clarity
- Principle of efficiency
- Principle of follow through

Fig. 35.1: Principles of directing process.

12. **Follow-up:** Directing is a continuous process. It should have the means of evaluating the performance of employees and provide feedback to them. After giving the directions, they should follow them.

Directing Process Activities

Directing is a process of giving instruction, guidance, and oversee the performance of the workers by the managers to achieve predetermined goals. There are five elements of the effective directing process: supervision, motivation, leadership, communication, coordination and cooperation, and commanding **(Fig. 35.2)**:

1. **Supervision:** Supervision involves guiding the efforts of others to achieve stated work output. Direct control is the day-to-day relationship between nurse manager/supervisor and operational level nurses that cover training, motivation, mentoring, coordination, and maintenance of discipline to achieve the nursing organizational goals. Adequate supervision is the key to a possible direction. There should be the closeness of control, group cohesiveness, proper delegation, and good human relation for effective monitoring.
2. **Motivation:** Motivation is the core of a compelling direction. It is one of the factors affecting human behavior and performance. It implies to engage the nurses in action by ensuring that a channel to satisfy the motive becomes available to them. The nurse manager can activate the hidden capabilities of their subordinates by motivating them to do the work. There are many ways to motive employees by giving financial increase such as the increase in salary and increments or nonfinancial incentives such as providing better working conditions, job security, flexible timings, and recognitions. Motivational strategies should be competitive, productive, comprehensive, and flexible. These strategies must consider diverse needs such as physiological, safety, security, psychological, ego, and economic needs of employees.
3. **Leadership:** Leadership is an essential factor for a successful direction and for the organization to accomplish its goals. It is a continuous process of influencing and supporting subordinates to work enthusiastically toward achieving goals. A good leader brings life into the group and motivates them for actions.
4. **Communication:** Communication is essential in the process of directing. It is a form of sharing and exchanging information between superior to subordinates. It is the element of understanding between them. Effective communication is required for command and instructions by the superiors and facilitates work, increases motivation, brings change, optimizes patient care, increases nurses' satisfaction, and facilitates coordination.
5. **Coordination and cooperation:** Coordination and collaboration are another important activity in the directing process. Coordination is a result of deliberate action of collective effort and is must. Coordination is essential to coordinate and channelize various activities of subordinates and to create team spirit among them. It is easy to achieve predetermined objectives of organization through collective efforts. Coordination allows orderly arrangement of group efforts to provide unity of actions to achieve common goals. It has a much broader concept than cooperation in management. Cooperation, in contrast, refers to the willingness of individuals to help each other. It reflects attitudes of employees in helping each other and is a result of voluntary action. Coordination is only possible if employees cooperate. However, both are important in management and required to issue orders, instruction, motivate, guide, and supervise employees.
6. **Order giving:** Order giving is the most critical element of direction. The nurse managers give instructions and orders to their subordinates as to how to do the work. He or she assigns the work per the job descriptions. Order giving needs a high degree of efficiency to motivate the subordinate to do the job; otherwise, it leads to dissatisfaction among assistants. Orders can be specific or general, oral or written, formal or informal, and immediate or planned and requires following up before and after execution.

Techniques of Directing Process

There are mainly three techniques used by managers in directing immediate subordinates, as discussed below:

1. **Delegation of authority:** Delegation of authority is conferring power by managers to others to accomplish a particular assignment. It is an essential means of directing function. Managers have to rely on others to achieve a task. Delegation of authority is a means of direction through sharing power with subordinates and providing them the opportunity to learn. It helps in the following ways:

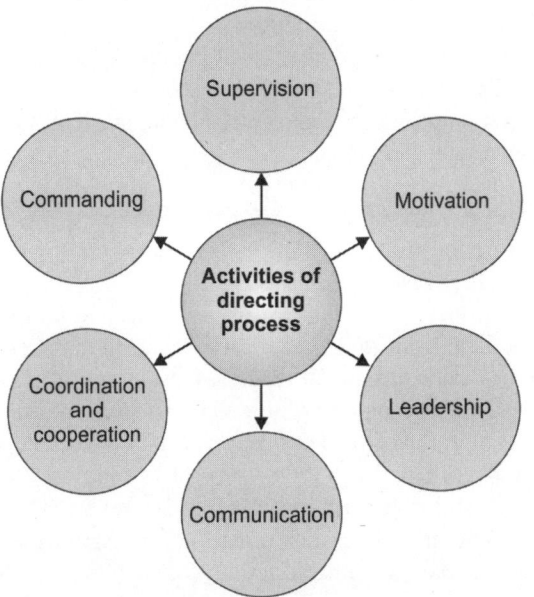

Fig. 35.2: Activities of the directing process.

- Delegations of authority can bring trust among employees and offer the chance to be responsible.
- It motivates subordinates and develops them to be future managers.
- It reduces the workload of superiors.

Delegation of authority also has many disadvantages. Give it with caution. There are many reasons or barriers to effective delegation. We will discuss this part in detail in the chapter on the delegation of authority.

2. **Issuing orders and instruction:** It is essential to mangers to issue orders and guidance to their subordinates from time to time to accomplish a task. Ordering is a device and force of authority used by managers to direct their subordinates and to get the work done. Orders should be prepared in advance and known to their immediate subordinates so that they can obey their instructions. Managers should not personalize while giving orders, and all should be treated equally, keeping their capability and experience. Give orders according to the situation and discuss it with subordinates. According to Koontz and O'Donnell, a good order should have the following essentials:
   - The order must be reasonable and give per overall objectives of the organization.
   - The orders must be short, concise, and complete to make employees understand what you expect from them.
   - The order must be time bound. Specify time limit and provide guidelines.
   - Try to give orders in written form that helps in fixing the responsibility.
   - Orders must follow a chain of command, i.e. subordinates must get orders only from one superior. Otherwise, it will create confusion.
   - The superior must consider the orders feasible to implement.
   - The subordinates must follow orders issued by superiors. Make sure that orders are implemented per plan.

3. **Supervision:** Supervision is an essential technique in the directing process. It is a means of direction, guidance, and controlling workforce to accomplish the assigned task. Managers should directly supervise the work of subordinates. It provides link between superiors and subordinates to understand them as well as their problems. Managers can provide direct assistance and guidance if required time to time.

Supervisors can follow strict supervision where all powers are concentrated with the supervisors or can use democratic oversight, where subordinates are involved in the decision-making process, or they can use free-rein leadership style where subordinates are independent of work. All these techniques can use in any situation and types of subordinates, their capabilities, and amount of supervision required. The main aim of supervision is to subordinate toward the achievement of objectives effectively and efficiently on time.

MOTIVATION

Motivation is the heart of management. The motive is an inner state that activates and directs action toward some goals. It is a challenging task for managers to keep the staff motivated to perform well in the workplace. The manager has to know the act of each employee and what might drive each one individually. By understanding employees' needs, managers can understand what rewards to use to drive them.

Defining Motivation

Motivation derives from "motive," which means to move, to act to satisfy a need or want. Any consideration, idea, or object is prompting the individual to act or move to accomplish motivational needs. It also means impulse or urges in an individual to do work.

- According to Scott, motivation is the process of stimulating people to action to accomplish desired goals.
- McFarlands defines motivation as a way to direct and control urges, drives, desires, aspirations, or the behavior of human beings.
- Motivation is a type of force that motivates people to act. It assists in explaining the cause and way of human behavior.
- Motivation is an internal condition that activates one's behavior, giving its direction. Motivation has also defined as a desire or need, which directs and energizes behavior toward a goal.

Motivation Process

Motivation is a process and has three elements: driving state, the behavior activation by the state, and the goal. The cycle begins when an individual feels something is lacking or feels a need. A need is a physiological or psychological state of deprivation that compels a person for some action for its satisfaction. It ranges from basic survival need to achieve a need for power and self-actualization. It differs from want, which refers to what a person would like to have, irrespective of what he or she needs it.

The need causes a driving state within an individual. A drive is an aroused condition that directs the behavior of an individual to avoid discomfort or to fulfill that urge and compel to act. A motive is an internal force that determines the action of a person. It directs, explains, and predicts the behavior of a person along a channel and defines the choices to make. There are many types of motives, such as innate and acquired motives, physiological, social, personal, stimulus, and unconscious motives. When the motive is at work, it creates tension. The tension, in turn, arouses a person to do some activity to relieve stress. Motive includes needs, basic drives, likes, and dislikes, interests,

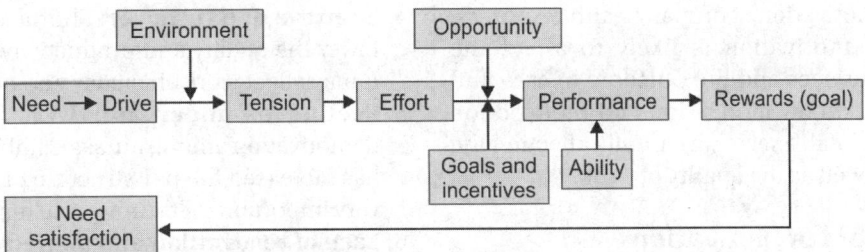

Fig. 35.3: Motivation process.

desires, and attitudes, since all these direct us to do some action or to behave in a manner called the instrumental behavior.

The instrumental behavior helps a person to reach the goal, which is the satisfaction of some state of need. The person feels relief. The goals can be positive or negative. The cognition factor, which includes memory, perception, thinking, and feeling, is essential for motivation. The cycle is completed but will start again when some need is felt and persistently put an action (effort) to achieve the goal (reward) and satisfy its need **(Fig. 35.3)**. In contrast, without requirement, the drive state will continue.

There are mainly three characteristics of motivation: activation, persistence, and intensity of effort. Activation or initiation of behavior deals with the direction of efforts and choose the best out of alternative practices or actions. Persistence means putting the efforts to continue despite obstacles. It deals with how one can sustain and stop reactions. Intensity means how much a person tries in a given task or action to achieve a goal.

Types of Motivation

A. **Intrinsic motivation:** Intrinsic motivation refers to motivation that originates within the person and willingly. It is the actual self-motivation. It is the personal gratification and feeling of fulfillment, rather than just achieving a goal.
B. **Extrinsic motivation:** Extrinsic motivation comes from the external environment, such as rewards, money, incentives, popularity, competition, and punishment, to achieve something. It is of the following types **(Fig. 35.4)**:
 1. *Affiliation motivation:* Affiliation motivation is a drive that relates to people on a social basis. There is an intense desire of an individual to associate with different people in social matters. The individuals must have favorable attitudes toward others, and they need to cooperate with them.
 2. *Competence motivation:* Competence motivation allows the person to perform high-quality work. The person is motivated to solve the problems and strive to be skillful and creative. They learn from their experiences.
 3. *Achievement motivation:* In this type of motivation, the person has a concern for more and more

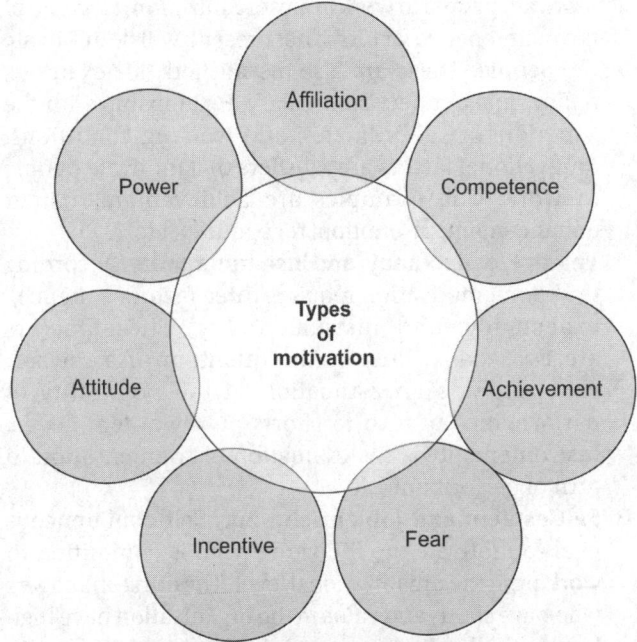

Fig. 35.4: Types of motivation.

 achievements and accomplishments. He or she wishes to achieve objectives and climb up on the ladder of success.
 4. *Fear motivation:* The person gets motivated by known or unknown fear and acts contrary to his or her original intention. It is good to accomplish the work quickly but for a short time, not always.
 5. *Incentive motivation:* Incentive motivation arises due to incentives and rewards for doing a task. In some instances, the employees put an extra effort to get a prize. It is a form of extrinsic motivation.
 6. *Attitude motivation:* It signifies the way the employees perceive their future and react accordingly. It must reveal self-confidence among employees. Employees, if having a positive attitude toward the work, will be motivated to work.
 7. *Power motivation:* Power motivation is a powerful drive to influence people. It helps in bringing desired changes in the organization.

MOTIVATION AND PERFORMANCE

Work performance depends on the level of motivation. The performance and quality of the health system rely on the variety and motivation of human health resources. Therefore, nurses' motivation is likely to affect the delivery of health services and the outcome of care and performance of work. Low motivation and reduced job satisfaction hurt the health sector, harmfully affecting the job performance as well as the quality of work.

Influencing Factors of Motivation

1. **Hygiene and motivational factors:** According to Herzberg (1959), hygiene and motivational factors motivate people to work in any organization. Hygiene or the maintenance factors, if not present, will de-motivate the people. These are also dissatisfiers, for example, policy, rules, supervision, salary, relationship with the superiors or subordinates, and working conditions. Motivational factors are satisfiers that motivate people to work. The examples are achievement, career enhancement, promotion, recognition, etc.
2. **Valence, expectancy, and instrumentality:** According to Vroom, motivation requires three factors "valence," expectancy, and instrumentality. These factors are essential to denote the quantum of a reward; expectancy is an estimation of the possibility of performance in turn to efforts put by an employee. Instrumentality is the estimation of compensation in turn of performance.
3. **Self-esteem and job enrichment:** Self-confidence is vital to motivate the individual who is committed to working at the organizational level. The nurse managers who have status and value in the organization have high levels of self-esteem.
4. **Attribution:** Attribution is either internal or external characteristics of a person that describes their behavior. The personality traits and motivation ability are the internal factors, and work environment and facilities available are the external factors that determine the behavior of an individual.

Factors Causing Demotivation

1. **Workplace hazards:** There are many risks in health care that have the potential to cause serious injury. One of the most common risks health-care professionals, including nurses, may encounter sharp injuries. Some of these injuries can expose nurses to blood-borne infections that are potentially life-threatening, e.g. Hepatitis B and C.
2. **Shift duty pattern and long working hours:** Working hours and shift duty patterns can affect the social life of nurses. At times it may affect their social relationships and may have a risk of isolation and loneliness. They may have less time to take care of their children and also less time to spend with their family members.
3. **Night duty:** Due to the night shift, sleep, waking, digestion, and other physiological functions of nurses may affect them. They may have disorientation and feelings of fatigue.
4. **Shortage and turnover:** Shortage and turnover may lower the quality and productivity of nursing the care. It may affect work efficiency and performance.
5. **Feeling of underpaid:** It is another factor for demotivation among nurses. Although the government has increased the pay structure of the nurses, which is very important for the nurses to remain in the hospitals.
6. **Lack of recognition and appreciation:** Many people think that a nursing degree is not as respected as a medical profession, although they take care of the patients and do a relatively large amount of work. So lack of appreciation can harm the stress and job satisfaction of the nurses and could adversely influence staff turnover.

General demotivating factors are unfair and detrimental criticism, public humiliation, rewarding the nonperformers, failure or fear of failure, the success that leads to compliance, lack of measurable objectives, low self-esteem, lack of priorities, negative self-talk, office politics, unfair treatment, mediocre standards, frequent change, and responsibility without authority.

MODELS OF MOTIVATION

The goal of most organizations is to benefit from positive employee behavior in the workplace by promoting a win–win situation for both the organization and workers. The following models and theories can be applied:

1. **MARS model of individual behavior:** The MARS model of individual behavior is an excellent medium for creating a win–win relationship between the employer and employees. The MARS model depicts the behavior of an individual. Individual behavior is the outcome of internal and external factors (**Fig. 35.5**). MARS is an acronym of the four primary elements, i.e. motivation, abilities, role perception, and situational factors. The values, personality, opinions, attitudes, and stress form a basis for shaping individual behavior and performance.
2. **Four-drive model of employee's motivation:** Lawrence and Nohria "four-drive model" is based on four drives drive to "Acquire and Achieve"; drive to "Belong and Bond"; drive to "Challenge and Comprehend"; and drive to "Define and Defend." This

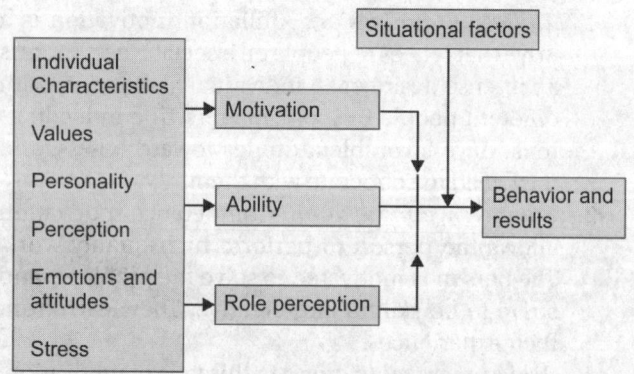

Fig. 35.5: MARS model of individual behavior.

model is efficient and useful to motivate the employees at the individual as well as the organizational level. At the individual level, understanding what the motivational drivers are on any given day or about work can help clarify and define what the motivators are for success. At the manager level, utilizing the four-drive model is an excellent tool for communicating with the employees. At the organizational level, a four-drive model is a tool that can be used across the organization to drive specific organizational goals. These drives are as follows:

- *Acquire and achieve:* This drive is the most important to motivate the employees. Typically these are extrinsic rewards such as pay, office, and bonus and intrinsic rewards such as a sense of achievement.
- *Belong and bond:* This drive is to create positive personal relationships with others at the workplace, which can lead to a feeling of love and belongingness.
- *Challenge and comprehend:* This drive is to understand how to fit in, what things mean, how to solve and overcome challenges, and make meaningful contributions.
- *Define and defend:* The derive activates when a belief, team, or an organization threatens.

MOTIVATIONAL THEORIES

The industrial psychologists and behavioral scientists had a significant contribution to developing motivational theories. Work motivation research is part of individual psychology. The doctrines of work motivation traditionally have both personal and situational characteristics.

Need-based Theories

Hierarchy of Needs Theory

Abraham Maslow proposed a hierarchy of needs theory. According to Maslow, each has a hierarchy of needs. There are five types of requirements. An individual has to satisfy each level of need before to think for the next one. These needs are physiological, safety, social, esteem, and self-actualization needs.

1. **Physiological needs:** These needs are necessary and essential needs for survival. It includes the need for food, water, air, and sleep. According to Maslow's theory, all other requirements will not be felt or be a source of motivation without meeting physiological needs.
2. **Safety needs:** Each need for protection from physical and emotional harm. These are medical insurance, job security, and financial reserves.
3. **Social needs:** The individuals also have social needs. They need to have social interactions with others in society. They should have a feeling of a sense of belonging, affection, acceptance, and friendship.
4. **Esteem needs:** Each has self-esteem needs. These are either internal or external. The sense of belongingness, respect, and achievement account for internal esteem needs and social status; recognition is the external form of esteem needs.
5. **The self-actualization needs:** It is the highest level of need and followed by fulfilling the other lower needs. This particular need is concerning with the contemplation and achieving full potential and dreams. The truth, justice, and wisdom are examples of self-actualization needs.

These needs provide the scope for the constant growth of the individual. The individual must try to achieve all these needs by putting the best effort and try to do better than before.

Existence, Relatedness, and Growth Theory

Clayton Alderfer is the originator of existence, relatedness, and growth (ERG) theory. It has its basis on Maslow's hierarchy of needs theory. Existence relates to motivators for existence. It includes the need for survival, such as physiological and safety needs. Relatedness is the motivation for seeking a good interpersonal relationship. It includes social and external esteem needs. Growth means a desire for personal growth and development. It consists of a higher level of needs such as internal esteem and self-actualization needs

Fredrick Herzberg Two-factor Theory

Herzberg's theory of motivation includes hygiene factors and motivators. The theory explains the factors that motivate individuals by identifying and satisfying their individual needs (**Fig. 35.6**).

The hygienic factors are dissatisfiers, such as policies, rules, supervision, working conditions, safety, and security on the job. Motivator factors are intrinsic to the situation, such as achievement, recognition, new responsibilities, and advancement and growth opportunities. The management must identify dissatisfiers' factors and try to use various measures to enrich or restructure employees' jobs to satisfy and motivate them.

Acquired-needs Theory

David McClelland proposed the acquired-needs theory. It is a three-need theory. According to acquired-needs theory, individuals acquire three types of needs as a result of their life experiences. These are the need for achievement, affiliation, and power (**Fig. 35.7**).

1. **Need for achievement (nAch):** Achievers seek to appreciate frequent recognition of how well they are doing. They prefer to work alone and take a risk in doing different works, but avoid high risks where there is a

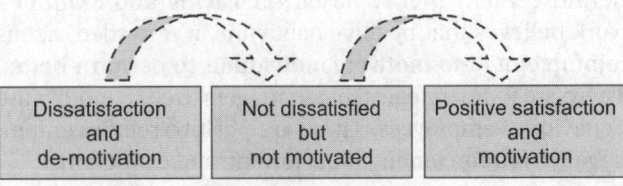

Fig. 35.6: Two-factor theory.

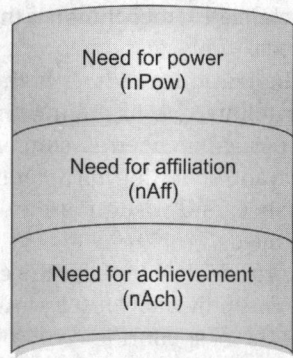

Fig. 35.7: McClelland's acquired-needs theory.

significant chance of failure. They hardly go for money, provided it gives feedback and recognition. They set moderate, realistic, and achievable goals.

2. **Need for affiliation (nAff):** The need for affiliation look for harmonious relationships with other people. They seek approval rather than recognition and try to project a favorable image of themselves. They prefer working with others and enjoy lots of social activities. They ask to belong, join groups, and organization.
3. **Need for power (nPow):** Power seekers want to power to control other people or achieve higher goals. They try to make more suggestions in meetings and help others. They enjoy the competition and winning and do not like to lose.

Process-based Theories of Motivation

It describes the ways and means of motivating employees according to their behavior. It aims to fulfill and satisfy their required needs by awarding for their performance. The motivation varies from situation to situation and individual to individual. **Figure 35.8** depicts the concept of a process theory of motivation. There are various process-based theories, such as equity theory, reinforcement, and expectancy theory.

Equity Theory

Adams proposed the equity theory. According to this theory, the individuals feel motivated when they perceive that superior treats them equally in terms of their input and output ratio with the input–output ratio of comparison person or a referent.

$$\frac{\text{Person Output}}{\text{Input}} = \frac{\text{Referent Output}}{\text{Input}}$$

Reinforcement Theory

Reinforcement theory based on Pavlov and Skinner's work believes that positive behaviors, if rewarded, act as reinforcement to motivate individuals to perform better. There are four strategies that managers used to modify the behavior of employees. These are positive reinforcement, negative reinforcement, punishment, and extinction.

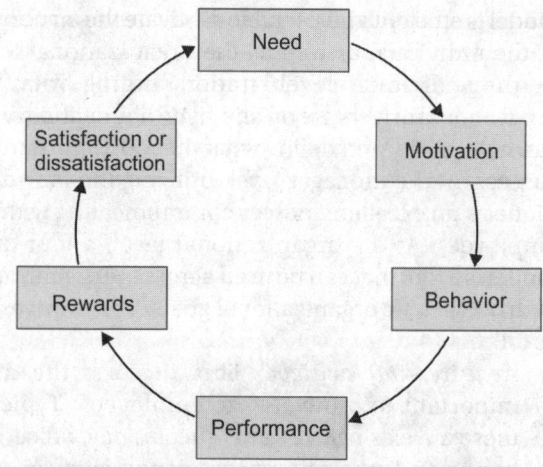

Fig. 35.8: Process theory of motivation.

Positive and negative reinforcement methods increase the desired behaviors, and the other two ways decrease the frequency of negative expression. Positive reinforcement brings positive response followed by favorable consequences; negative reinforcement brings positive reaction followed by removing adverse effects. Whereas managers use punishment strategy to reduce undesirable behaviors by presenting adverse effects, and extinction is the method of decreasing the frequency of unwanted behavior by removing awards/incentives following an undesirable behavior.

The Expectancy Theory

The expectancy theory proposed by Porter and Lawler believes that individuals motivate by perceiving a high level of effort that leads to performance (expectancy); excellent performance leads to a better outcome (instrumentality), and the better result leads to value or reward (valence). The individuals get motivated by simple calculation of expectancy, instrumentality, and valence in which they evaluate their situations.

Motivation = Expectancy × Instrumentality × Valence

The managers try to influence the expectancy by hiring knowledgeable and skilled employees or organizing training programs to have trained and experienced employees, adequate facilities, and encouragement by the employer. They connect the award system, bonuses, and merit pay with performance to influence instrumentality. They also try to find out the awards that the employees' value and make awards more attractive to motivate them.

HOW TO CREATE A MOTIVATING CLIMATE?

The employees can be more productive if the workplace of an organization is comfortable and pleasant. The nurse administrator can play an important role to create a motivating climate to encourage staff to put in their best by observing the following tips:

1. **Motivate yourself before you motivate your subordinates:** Explore yourself and consider what motivates the subordinates. Understand their feelings and support them so that they will be prompted to do the work.
2. **Keep organizational goals with individual goals:** Managers and supervisors should know what they want from their subordinates. They should be clear to organizational goals. To motivate them, keep their goals with organizational goals.
3. **Know the motivators of your subordinates:** Motivate each employee in different ways. Asking them, listen to them, and observe them.
4. **Recognize that supporting employee motivation is a process, not a task:** Sustain an environment where each staff can strongly motivate themselves as supporting employee motivation is an ongoing process.
5. **Appreciation:** Show verbal praise immediately after any staff completes his or her work/project successfully. It should be specific and honest.
6. **Transparency:** Create an atmosphere of openness. All the staff should be treated equally and informed about the decision to avoid any ill-feeling among the team.
7. **Rewards:** Encourage an atmosphere of healthy competition among the staff, so that they should be motivated to put their best in the department.
8. **Management loyalty:** Be loyal to your staff, and then only they will be faithful to you. Try to understand your feelings.
9. **Management concern:** Treat your staff as individuals and help them with their problems. It will help to create a healthy and safe environment.
10. **Excellent infrastructure:** Try to provide a unique work environment where the staff can work, relax, and have fun that enhances the quality of work and employee satisfaction. Provide them a little privacy, canteen, etc.
11. **Have one-on-one meetings with each staff:** Staff is motivated more if you show concern toward them and give attention. Get to know their families, their hobbies, etc. Have individual meetings with them.
12. **Delegation:** Delegate appropriate responsibilities and authority to your subordinates so that they can carry out specific tasks. It allows them to take a stronger role in their jobs, which usually means more fulfillment and motivation in their work, as well.
13. **Participative:** Encourage each staff to participate in all the activities that can give them a sense of affiliation, acceptance, and recognition.
14. **Warmth supports the team:** Respect the individual potential of each group. Correct; guide them, if doing something wrong positively and appropriately. There should not be any panic or fear in them.
15. **Provide feedback:** Convey the staff about the outcome of their activities and contributions toward organization and improvement in the nursing services. Acknowledge their work and efforts and celebrate their successes. It will help them to motivate them to work at their best.

ROLE OF NURSE MANAGERS TO MOTIVATE STAFF

Nurse managers play an essential part in motivating their staff. Staff need to be motivated to have quality patient care, to develop their efficiency, and to reduce absenteeism.

- Focus on needs and wants of individual staff
- Recognize each team as a unique individual and use accordingly appropriate strategy to each group
- Act as a role model, active listener, supporter, and encourager for demotivated team
- Recognize differences among staff and treat them well
- Give them respect and dignity—a feeling of belonging
- Set realistic goals and make work interesting
- Throw a challenge
- Have effective communication
- Practice nonfinancial rewards for right action
- Provide positive reinforcement
- Create a climate for the independent and motivating working environment; help them
- Make them responsible and give them a feeling of belonging and ownership
- Create a competitive and healthy environment
- Use problem-solving approach
- Motivate staff through individual guidance and counseling.

CHAPTER HIGHLIGHTS

- Directing is the continuous activity of communicating, leading, and motivation throughout the organization.
- Directing is a continuous process that follows various principles.
- The main elements of directing are supervision, motivation, leadership, communication, and order given.
- Motivation is the process of motivating people to act to accomplish the desired goals.
- It has three elements: driving state, the behavior activation by the state, and the goal, and three characteristics: activation, persistence, and intensity of effort.
- Both intrinsic and extrinsic motivation are essential for performance.
- Many organizational and personal factors motivate and demotivate the employees that may affect their performance.
- MARS and four-drive models of motivation describe factors affecting the motivation of employees at the individual and organizational levels.
- Most of the motivational theories are hierarchy need based.
- Nurse managers must try to create a work climate to motivate staff.

REVIEW QUESTIONS

I. Essay Type Questions
1. What do you mean by "Directing"? Discuss its features.
2. Enumerate principles of directing. Describe the essential elements of directing.
3. "Motivation is the core of compelling direction." Discuss.
4. Define the term "motivation"? Describe the motivation process.
5. Discuss in detail the factors influencing motivation and demotivation among employees.
6. As a nurse manager, how would you create a motivational climate in a nursing unit?

II. Short Notes
1. Roles and functions of directing
2. Herzberg two-factor theory
3. Role of the nurse manager to motivate staff
4. Types of motivation.

III. Multiple Choice Questions
1. Which principle of directing states that subordinates should get orders and instructions from one superior only?
   a. Unity of command
   b. Harmony of objectives
   c. Direct supervision
   d. Effective leadership
2. The process of influencing and supporting subordinates to work enthusiastically to achieve the goal is:
   a. Motivation   b. Supervision
   c. Direction   d. Leadership
3. Effective monitoring is one of the essential elements in directing; it includes:
   a. Activation of hidden capabilities of subordinates by motivating them to work
   b. Commanding and giving instructions to subordinates to facilitate work
   c. The closeness of control, group cohesiveness, and good human relation
   d. Ordering to motivate subordinates to do the job
4. An aroused condition that directs the behavior of an individual to act is:
   a. Drive   b. Need
   c. Motive   d. Tension
5. Which type of motivation relates to people on a social basis?
   a. Extrinsic   b. Intrinsic
   c. Affiliation   d. Attitude
6. The need concerning with contemplation and achieving full potential in Maslow's hierarchy need is:
   a. Social need   b. Safety need
   c. Esteem need   d. Self-actualization
7. Which theory of motivation explains the factors that motivate individuals by identifying and satisfying their individual needs?
   a. Hierarchy need theory
   b. Herzberg two-factor theory
   c. Acquired-needs theory
   d. Process theory
8. Who proposed acquired-needs theory?
   a. McClelland D   b. Fredrick H
   c. Clayton Alderfer d. Maslow A

Answer Keys
1. a 2. d 3. c 4. a 5. c 6. d 7. b
8. a

SUGGESTED READING

1. Available from https://ebrary.net/2814/management/models_organiational_behaviour.
2. Bobbins SP. Organisational Behaviour. New Delhi: Prentice Hall; 1997.
3. Cunningham JB, Eberle T. A guide to Job Enrichment and Redesign. Personnel. 1990; 57.
4. Davis K. Evolving models of organizational behavior. Acad Manag J. 1968;11(1):27-38.
5. Davis K. Human Behaviour at Work. New York: McGraw Hill Book Co.; 1991.
6. Dimock ME. Administrative Vitality. New York: Harper Brothers; 1975.
7. Hackman JR, Oldham GR. Development of the diagnostic job survey. J Appl Psychol. 1975;60:159-70.
8. Luthans F. Organisational Behaviour. New York: McGraw Hill Book Co.; 1995.
9. Newstrom J, Davis K. Organization Behavior: Human Behavior at Work. New York: McGraw-Hill; 1993.
10. Newman WH, Warren EK. The Process of Management. New Delhi: Prentice-Hall a; 1985.
11. Terry GR, Franklin SG. Principles of Management. Delhi: ABS; 2000.

36 CHAPTER

Communication

CHAPTER OUTLINE

- Communication
  - Meaning and Concept
  - Features of Communication
  - Purposes of Communication
  - Importance of Communication
- Communication Process
- Types of Communication
- Channels of Communication
- Effective Communication
  - Barriers and Problems in Communication
  - Elements of Effective Communication
  - Features of Effective Written Communication
- Communication Pattern in Nursing

LEARNING OUTCOMES

After completion of this chapter, the learner will be able to:
- Recall and understand the concept of communication
- Describe the process and mechanism of communication
- Explain the different types of communication
- Explain the concept of interpersonal communication
- Describe various communication channels used in the hierarchy of nursing services
- Understand multiple barriers and problems encountered for effective communication
- Discuss the features of effective communication
- Describe measures to develop effective communication

KEY TERMS

Communication, communication process, channels, barriers, effective communication, communication pattern

INTRODUCTION

Communication is the life source for any organization. Effective communication is essential to accomplish all managerial functions. It is vital for directing and controlling in the organization. In the formal organization, the employees perform various activities to achieve their common objectives. It is through communication, which provides an exchange of information and sharing of ideas.

COMMUNICATION

Meaning and Concept

The term "communication" is a derivative of the Latin word "communis" means common. In other words, it means if a person communicates with another, it establishes a collective group of understanding. According to the dictionary, it is imparting thoughts, opinions, or information by speech, writing or signs.

According to Newman et al., communication is an exchange of facts, ideas, opinions, or emotions by two or more persons. Hoben referred it to a verbal interchange of thought or idea. In the words of Hudson, the means of conveying information from one person to another are communication.

Leagens defined it as a process by which two or more people exchange ideas, facts, and feelings and have a common understanding of its meaning and use of message. It is the process of passing information and knowledge from one person to another (Keith Davis). The communication is not only concerned with sending or receiving a message but involves understanding as well. It is a bridge of understanding between two or more people. Hence it is a two-way process.

Features

The salient features of communication are as follows:
- Communication involves at least two people who send the message and the second who receives the message.
- It is a two-way process, and the process does not complete until the receiver has understood the message.
- It is to create an understanding in the mind of the receiver of information.
- It will be in various forms: orders, instructions, reports, suggestions, observations, and so on.
- The message may convey through words spoken or written or gestures.

Purposes

Communication helps in the following ways:
- It provides a channel to establish and disseminate the goals.
- It facilitates the development of plans for the achievement of goals.
- It aids in the management and utilization of workforce.
- It helps manage, lead, direct and motivate employees to contribute right things.

Importance

Effective communication is an essential requirement of sound management to perform its basic functions, i.e. planning, organizing, leading, and controlling.

1. **Foundation of planning:** Communication serves as a foundation of planning. A nurse manager can receive suggestions and comments from subordinates at the time of the formulation of a rotation plan, assignment, etc. who, in turn, communicate to them for implementation.
2. **Facilitation:** Communication facilitates in achieving goals. Nurse managers must communicate effectively with their subordinates to achieve team goals.
3. **Decision-making:** Communication facilitates decision-making by providing the right type of information at the right time to the decision-makers.
4. **Unity of direction:** Communication provides integration, of course, to various activities of the department.
5. **Basis of motivation, cooperation, and improving nurses' morale:** Communication promotes motivation among the staff by clarifying and informing about the work by the nurse managers and gets the collaboration. It is an essential tool for motivation, which can improve the morale of nurses.
6. **Effective coordination:** Communication helps to achieve effective coordination in the organization. Top-level nursing managers can communicate its policies, objectives, and programs to their subordinates and can receive his or her suggestions in turn. It will help the management to keep in touch with the performance of various nursing units in the health institutions.
7. **Congenial nurse manager-nurse relation:** Communication develops understanding between the nurse managers, supervisors, and nurses of operational levels. The nurse manager cannot get the work done from the nurse unless they are communicated effectively of what he or she wants to do. It leads to harmonious human relations and socialization of nurses in the nursing organization, thereby improving their work performance and work output.
8. **Device for handling employees' grievances:** Communication is a useful device for achieving the participation of nurses. Nurse manager receives the complaints, claims, and suggestions from the nurses and takes appropriate corrective actions.
9. **Modification of the behavior of staff:** Communication facilitates change among nurses. A well-informed nurse will have a better attitude than a less-informed nurse.
10. **Effective control:** Communication helps in control by transmitting information about the performance of nurses through supervision working in various nursing units—a different method of communication, e.g. rounds, reports, meetings.

COMMUNICATION PROCESS

Communication is a dynamic and circular process that involves a series of actions and reactions and takes various steps. It is a process involving the exchange of facts, viewpoints, and ideas between staff placed in different positions in the organization to achieve a goal. The communication process starts with the communicator or the sender who encodes or formulates an idea or message to communicate to another person known as a receiver, a person who decodes the message. The message may be expressed verbally or nonverbally through a channel (media), and the communication process also has feedback in the form of a response, which is essential at each step. In between, there may be many barriers, such as noise **(Fig. 36.1)**. The communication process has the following elements:

1. **Communicator:** The communicator is the sender or a source that initiates or encodes the communication process and takes the initiative to start a dialogue.

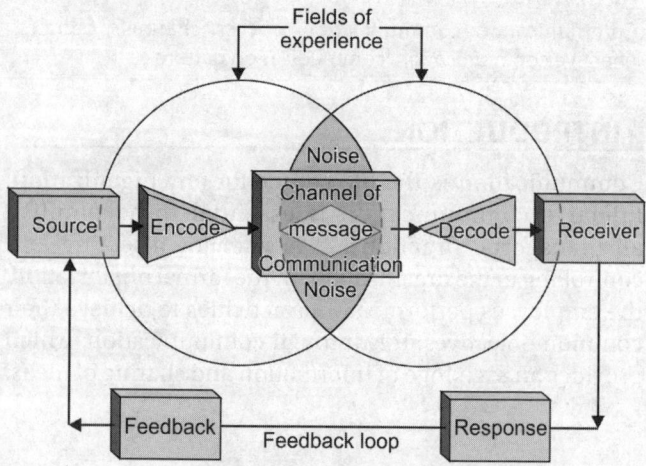

Fig. 36.1: Communication process.

2. **Encoding:** It is organizing the idea of messages by the communicator, who decides the method of communication, either verbal or nonverbal, and means of sending correspondence.
3. **Message:** It may be facts, opinions or information. The sender organizes the word. It is in the form of either verbal or nonverbal. The message must be in the form that the receiver must understand it.
4. **Channel:** A channel of communication is the way of carrying a message from the sender to the receiver. There are many ways of communicating a message such as written, spoken, verbal, nonverbal, and mass media. The sender must select the most appropriate channel to convey the message keeping in mind the time and urgency of the message.
5. **Receiver:** A receiver or a decoder is a person who receives and interprets or decodes the message. A receiver is responsible for responding and giving feedback on the news.
6. **Decoding:** Decoding is the process of understanding the message.
7. **Feedback:** A receiver that reads and interprets the message is responsible for providing feedback to the sender immediately. The handset also decides the way and means of sending back the response. It is the backbone of effective communication. It helps to stimulate and reinforces an idea to communicate.

Noise: Noise is an interruption that affects the communication process adversely. The sources of sounds can be both internal and external.

TYPES OF COMMUNICATION

Communication can be formal and informal, downward, upward, lateral, diagonal, external, verbal, and nonverbal (**Fig. 36.2**).

According to the Relationship

Formal Communication

Formal communication is a form of communication that follows a chain of command through a line of authority in a hierarchy of an organization. It is an official communication.

Advantages
- It ensures the orderly flow of information.
- It follows the official chain of command.
- It facilitates control of subordinates by superiors.

Disadvantages
- It is generally very slow as it follows the formal chain of command.
- It delays decision-making especially when the number of positions is in the hierarchy.

Informal Communication

A type of communication that does not follow a chain of command and occurs outside the official network. It is personal communication. It usually exists along with the formal notification. It is unplanned, neither written and nor recorded. It is also known as grapevine, as the conversation spread like grapevine in the organization. But it helps in making teams and also helpful in developing an interpersonal relationship.

Advantages
- It develops better human relations in the organization.
- The people feel social satisfaction.
- It is very fast as it is free from all the barriers.
- It serves to fill the gaps in informal communication.
- It allows the management to know the attitude employees about management.
- It facilitates the administration to share information on matters with the nurses.
- It is a supplement in those cases where formal communication does not work.

Disadvantages
- It carries some degree of error in it.
- It can spread imaginary rumors within the organization.
- It can bring misunderstanding among employees.
- It can bring inefficiency in the organization.
- It leads to making hostility against nurse administrators.

Table 36.1 depicts a comparison between formal and informal communication.

According to the Direction

1. **Downward communication:** As the name indicates, it flows from a higher level to the lower level in the

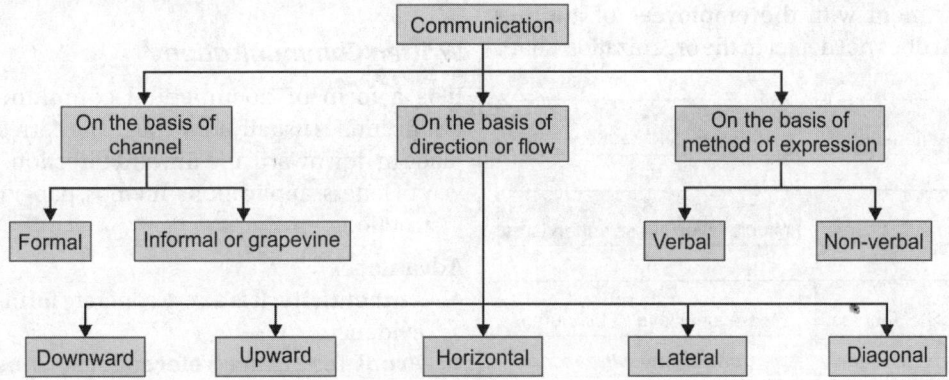

Fig. 36.2: Classification of communication.

TABLE 36.1: Comparison of formal and informal communication.

Formal communication	Informal communication
Follows the official chain of command	Based on a personal relationship
It originates as per the need of the organization	The psychological need is the base for informal communication
Generally accurate, based on facts	May not be authentic
It is slow and follows the hierarchy and expensive method of information transmission	It is nonexpensive, oral, and carries information rapidly
It is rigid as it follows official path	It is flexible as it moves freely
Chances of distortion of the message are minimal	Chances of misuse of the word are very high
The position is significant	Has no relevance of the position
Only official message	Public opinion in the organization

organization. It is a formal communication. The conversation takes place between superior and subordinates. It flows from chief nursing officer to staff nurses **(Fig. 36.3)**.

2. **Upward communication:** It is a type of formal notification, flows from a lower level to a higher level in the organization. The conversation takes place between subordinates to superior. It flows from staff nurses to chief nursing officer in the nursing organization **(Fig. 36.3)**. It takes place to report the functioning of the organization, sharing views and ideas, and participating in decision-making. It can be in oral or written forms.

3. **Lateral communication:** It is a type of formal communication and takes place at the same levels or with different departments in the organization.
   Advantages
   - It facilitates the coordination of work.
   - It economizes time and helps in improving understanding.
   - It helps to check on the power of the top managers.
   - It promotes cooperation among team members.
   - It provides emotional support to staff.
   - It is a means of sharing information.
   - It helps to resolve intra and interdepartmental conflicts.

4. **Diagonal communication:** It is a type of formal communication that takes place between the managers of one department with the employees of another department. It does not depict in the organization chart.

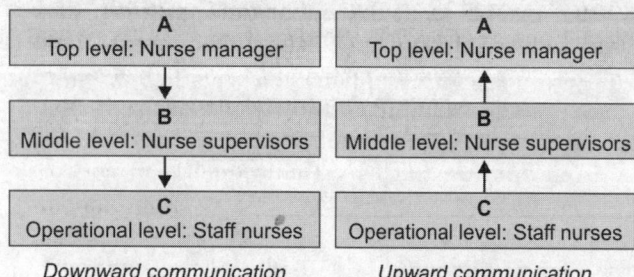

Fig. 36.3: Downward and upward communication.

5. **External interface:** A type of communication takes place between the manager of the department with the outer group or outside the organization for an official purpose is an external communication.

Communication According to Expression

Verbal Communication

Verbal communication is oral communication that uses spoken or written form. It may be face to face, telephonic, or using other media. Speeches and discussion are examples of oral communication. Verbal communication is a secure communication that helps in building trust and rapport.

Advantages
- **Understanding and transparency:** As oral communication serves as interpersonal, it provides more understanding and openness among managers, supervisors, and operational level staff.
- **Scope for flexibility:** Oral communication has no element of rigidity and allows changes in the decision-making.
- **Instant feedback:** The decision can be made quickly without delay, as the feedback is an integral part of the communication process.
- **More effective:** Oral communication is more effective because it is easy to resolve the problems face to face or direct contact between the staff.
- **A cost-effective way of communication:** Oral communication saves not only time but also the money and effort.
- **Encourage morale:** Oral communication promotes receptive and encouraging morale among nurses and essential for team building and synergy.
- **More specific:** It helps in conveying the message with the desired pitch and tone.

Disadvantages/limitations
- It is less authentic unless the conversation is audio or video recorder.
- Possibility of misunderstanding if words are not clear and not understood.
- At times there can be arising conflict situation when there is a slip of the tongue by a person.
- It may create confusion or delay the action if not used authentic.

Written Communication

It is a form of documented communication. Formal notification is usually in writing. The correspondence takes place in downward and upward direction. These are in the way of letters, applications, memos, papers, reports, orders, instructions, etc.

Advantages
- **Authenticity:** It is a very concrete form of documentary evidence.
- **Proof for future reference:** It is useful for future reference purposes.

- **Bulk communication:** It can be easily distributed to many employees, thus making it a bulk communication method.
- **Cheaper means of communication:** It is a more affordable means of communication when used or sending and receiving messages to distance places.
- **More transparent and specific:** Written notes are written carefully, and hence drafted more precise and accurate.

Disadvantages
- Written communication has a lack of feedback, the absence of modulations to convey the message effectively, etc.
- Very expensive for transmitting short messages.
- It is generally formal.
- If poorly drafted, it can create misunderstanding and confusion.
- There is a lack of secrecy in written communication.

Nonverbal Communication

Other than oral and written communication, nonverbal communications are essential to express emotions, attitudes, and reactions. The person, if not able to express message verbally or in writing, can communicate in this form. Eye contact, gestures, movement, and postures are types of nonverbal communication. Eye contact is most useful in gaining someone's trust. Gesture allows to interest the person by showing the bigger picture of saying. Movements used to attract people to have more interest in speech. Good posture reflects confidence, trust, and power.

CHANNELS OF COMMUNICATION

A network is a structured fabric of the organization, made up of channels that are interconnected.

Formal Communication Channels

These are "Through Proper Channel," which means that the path of communication flows through the line of authority linking a position to its line superior, i.e. the range of superior-subordinate authority relationships. There are five types of a communication networks in an organization: chain, circle, wheel, inverted V and free flow **(Fig. 36.4)**.

1. **Chain communication:** The message flows in the direction of the vertical line along the scalar chain of command is chain communication. It flows from top to bottom or from bottom to top. Thus the flow of communication takes place through a scalar chain of command, and there is no horizontal communication.
2. **Circular network:** In this type of channel, the communication flows in a circle. Each staff can communicate with his or her adjoining colleagues. It is a prolonged form of the communication channel.
3. **Wheel communication:** In this type of communication channel, the subordinates communicate with and through nurse managers. All the contacts pass through a nurse manager who acts as the hub of a wheel.
4. **Free flow communication:** Under such a communication channel, there is no restriction on the flow of conversation. This network is informal and highly flexible.

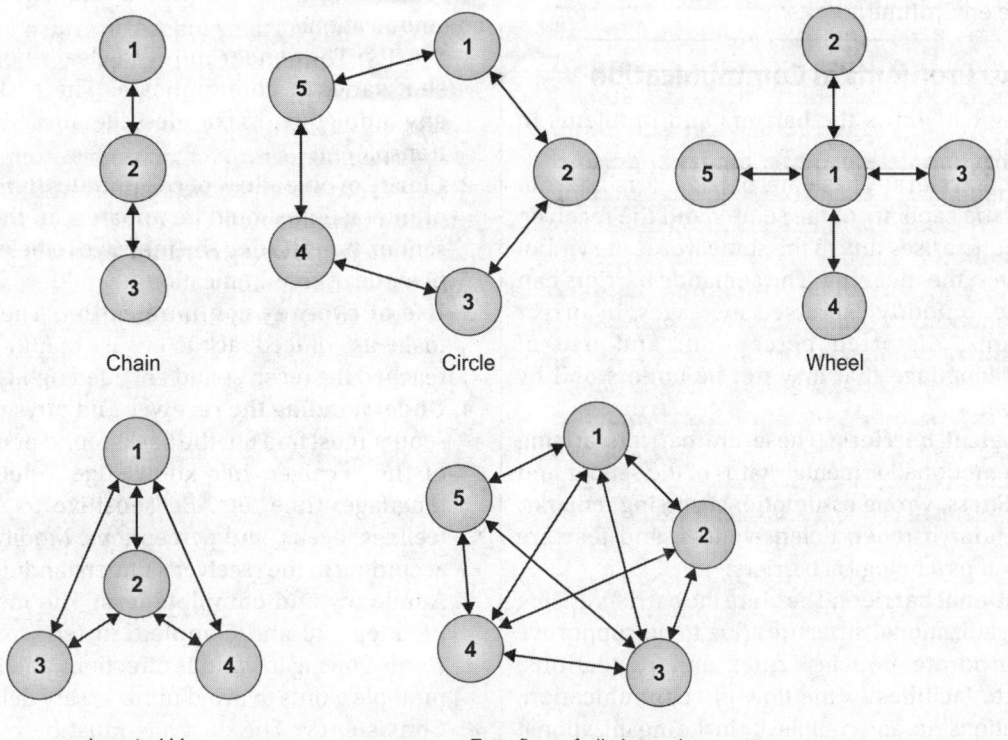

Fig. 36.4: Networks of communication.

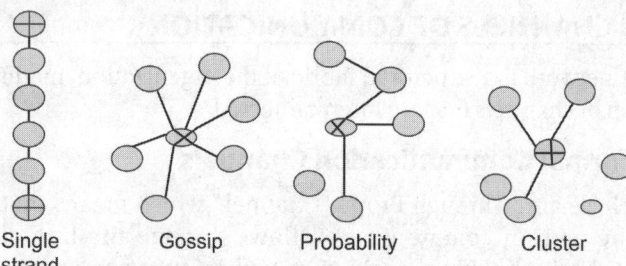

Fig. 36.5: Informal communication channel.

5. **Inverted V:** In this communication network, the staff communicates with immediate superior as well as superior's superior. The communication flows faster.

Informal Communication Channels

These are various forms (Fig. 36.5):
- **Single strand:** The staff communicates with other staff through the intervening team.
- **Gossip:** The staff communicates nonselectively.
- **Probability:** The staff communicates randomly with other staff according to the law of probability.
- **Cluster:** The staff communicates with only those staff that he or she trusts.

EFFECTIVE COMMUNICATION

For the success of any organization, there is a need for effective communication. It is the heart of the organization. It might be the result of the accurate transmission of information by the sender and the receiver and encoding, decoding by them, the media used, and the environment.

Barriers and Problems in Communication

The following list shows the barriers and problems in communication:
1. **Semantic barriers:** These are barriers arising from the linguistic capacity of the sender and the receiver. The difficulty arises due to the same words or symbol means the same meaning. The semantic barriers can occur due to poorly expressed messages, incorrect translations, distorted perception, and use of technical language that may not be understood by the receiver.
2. **Psychological barriers:** These are barriers arising from the emotional or mental status of the sender and receiver. Stress, wrong assumptions, passing remarks, attitude, poor listener, defensiveness, and fear are examples of psychological barriers.
3. **Organizational barriers:** These are the barriers arising within organizational structures due to no supportive or no corporate policies, rules and regulations, inadequate facilities to the flow of communication, status relationship, and complexity in the organizational structures.
4. **Personal barriers:** Unfavorable attitude of managers/supervisors toward subordinates, fear of challenge to authority, lack of confidence in subordinates, lack of subject knowledge, skills, perceptual variations, disorders of sense organs, ignoring a communication, lack of awareness, lack of time are examples of personal barriers causing inefficient communication process.
5. **Environmental barriers:** One of the significant hurdles of communication in a workplace is the ecological and physical barrier. High intensity of light for visual communication, high temperature, humidity, bad ventilation contribute distortion in sending and receiving a message are examples of the physical obstacles. Other environmental restrictions include competing for stimulus where it becomes challenging to pass on the message orally if confirmation giving information simultaneously within hearing distance, sometimes-loud music or traffic noise creates a barrier in the communication process.
6. **Mechanical barriers:** Mechanical barriers include any disturbances, which interfere with the fidelity of the physical transmission of the message. A telephone in poor working condition creates a mechanical barrier. In mass communication, automatic barriers also include smeared ink in the printed matter, a rolling screen on TV, a type too small to be read in the newspaper.

Elements of Effective Communication

The following elements play a major role in effective communication:
1. **Clarity:** The sender must be clear about what he or she wants to communicate. There should not be any ambiguity. Make message attractive, brief, and transparent.
2. **Clarity of objectives of communication:** The purpose of interaction should be apparent in the mind of the sender, transmitting the message to help in the choice of mode of communication.
3. **Use of two-way communication:** The sender must make use of feedback to ensure that the message has reached the receiver and encoded rightly.
4. **Understanding the receiver and physical setup:** The sender must find out the background or understanding of the receiver, her knowledge, education status, language, time, etc. Be sensitive to the receiver's feelings, needs, and perceptions. Modify the message according to the receiver's understanding.
5. **Adequacy and completeness:** The message should be adequate and complete in terms of the type of words flowing in various directions and the number of multiple words to avoid unnecessary delay.
6. **Consistency:** The message must be consistent with plans, policies, programs, and goals.

7. **Timing:** The messages should be reached in time with the receiver to get the desired response in time.
8. **Appropriate language and symbols:** Use proper grammar and words that should be decoded by the receiver.
9. **Credibility:** Have credibility in communication. The sender must maintain trust and credibility while communicating.
10. **Excellent listener:** Be a good listener. Maintain good eye contact, ask appropriate questions, do not interrupt in between and change subject, express emotions with control, and listen responsively, be patient. Do not lose your temper.
11. **Use of simple language:** Emphasize the use of simple and clear words in the messages.
12. **Noise reduction:** Identify the source of noise and then eliminate that source. Interact with the communicator in a noise-free place.
13. **Control over emotions:** Make effective use of body language while communicating and do not show emotions. Be aware of the tone and pitch used for communication.
14. **Avoid overloading of messages:** Prioritize the work and should not overload with the work. Spend quality time with the subordinates and should listen to their problems and feedbacks actively.
15. **Constructive feedback:** Avoid giving negative feedback if to be given delivered constructively.
16. **Select the appropriate channel:** The managers should adequately select the channel of communication. Simple messages should be conveyed orally; use written means for delivering multiple messages.
17. **Flexibility in meeting the targets:** Have flexibility in achieving the goal and should not put much pressure on employees to reach their objectives.
18. **Use of multiple channels of communication:** Reinforce messages to have effective communication.
19. **Use an informal channel of communication:** Make effective use of grapevine type of connection to deliver formal messages. The nurse manager will come to know the problems faced by them while rendering the care to the patients.
20. **Maintain transparency with team members and subordinates:** Maintain openness in communication and have easy access with assistance. Also, avoid discussing essential matters during lunchtime as the employee is altogether in a different mood.
21. **Be confident:** Confidence in communication is essential and adopts a positive approach.

Features of a Effective Written Communication

Following are the features of effective written communication:
1. **The clear message:** The message must be clear and use of the appropriate medium. Handwriting must be legible and clear and deal with each aspect separately and clearly.
2. **Completeness:** The message must be complete. Organize the news appropriately. Verify the contents of the message for any omission, and organize the word in a logical sequence. Unify the individual sentences and paragraphs.
3. **Coherence:** The ideas expressed in the paragraph should be in sequence and clear. Follow the smooth flow and transparency in the message.
4. **Conciseness:** Omit unnecessary words and sentences from the message. The message must be short and specific. It must convey meaning and must be attractive. Use precise words and avoid vague judgmental descriptions.
5. **Credibility:** Write correct and complete sentences in the message. The message must be clear, which brings credibility.
6. **Correctness:** The message should be free from technical and grammatical errors—express the tone and style of communicating clearly. The statement and content must be technically accurate and specific.
7. **Continuity:** The message should be in continuity. Avoid jargon and use few words.

COMMUNICATION PATTERN IN NURSING

Communication pattern in nursing varies from hospital to hospital in India as well as abroad. Evidence from elsewhere revealed that at Sweet Dell (pseudo-acronym), direct communication, a vertical chain of command acts as a filter that resulted in inefficient and disrupted information flow between medical and direct care staff, limiting the flow and quality of information available for clinical decisions and also reduced cognitive diversity.

In India, the study in district hospitals of North India in the 1990s reveals that there is no direct communication per the chain of command between nursing administrators of the district hospital and state nursing administrator at the directorate level. There is a vertical chain of command; communication flows through medical administrator/chief medical officer/medical superintendent to the medical administrator of health directorate to nursing administrator/assistant nursing director. In the nursing unit, communication flows upward, downward, horizontal, and outward of all level nurses **(Fig. 36.6)**.

1. **Communication of nurse administrator with medical administrators:** The nurse administrators communicated with medical administrators for providing the information regarding the census of the hospital, health conditions of the critically ill patients, medicolegal cases, and admitted hospital staff every day. Also, communicate verbally during the rounds and inform about the problem arising in maintaining sanitation. They write the requirements of material supply every month and of condemnation of articles every 3 months.
2. **Communication of nurse administrator with subordinates:** Nurse administrators receive verbal

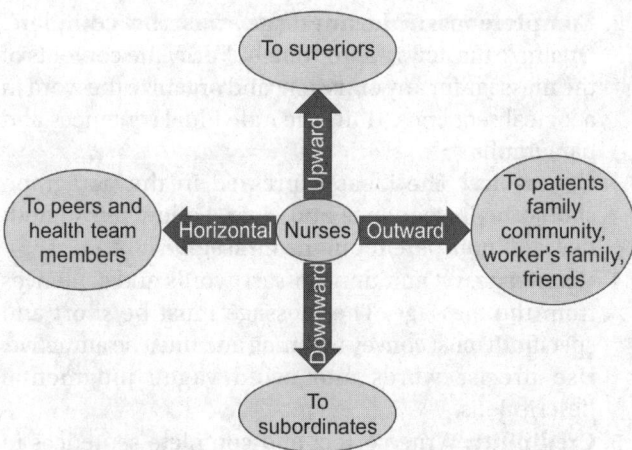

Fig. 36.6: Communication direction in a clinical setting.

and written information from night sisters and communicate to the evening sister about the census, health condition of the critically ill patients, medicolegal cases, and admitted hospital staff every day and during the rounds.

3. **Communication pattern of nurse supervisors:** The nurse supervisors usually report about sanitation with the nurse administrators and patients with bedside nurses, and for personal problems, they approach the nurse administrators.
4. **Communication pattern of bedside nurses:** Communications of bedside nurses occur with doctors related to patients, and for sanitation, they report to the nurse supervisor. They attend social events almost with medical and nursing personnel.

CHAPTER HIGHLIGHTS

- Communication is a dynamic and circular two-way process of exchange of facts, ideas, opinions, or emotions by two or more persons.
- The communication process includes a series of elements such as communicator, encoding, message, channel, receiver, decoding, and feedback.
- Communication is the center of management functions. It is formal and informal, downward, upward, lateral, diagonal, external, verbal, and nonverbal.
- In an organization, communication follows both formal and informal channels to convey and receive messages.
- Communication barriers can arise due to sematic, psychological, environmental, personal, and organizational problems.

REVIEW QUESTIONS

I. Essay Type Questions
1. What do you mean by "communication"? Describe its salient features.
2. Describe in detail the process of communication.
3. "Effective communication is an essential requirement of sound management." Discuss with suitable illustrations.
4. Describe various types of communications exist in an organization.
5. What are the different channels of communication observed in an organization?

II. Short Notes
1. Formal versus informal communication
2. Elements of effective communication
3. Barriers in communication
4. Communication pattern in nursing

III. Multiple Choice Questions
1. Encoding in the communication process means:
   a. A source that initiates the communication process
   b. Organization of idea of messages by the communicator
   c. The way of carrying a message from the sender to the receiver
   d. The interpretation of the message by the receiver
2. Which type of communication follows a chain of command through a line of authority in a hierarchy of an organization?
   a. Verbal
   b. Nonverbal
   c. Formal
   d. Informal
3. Which one of the following types of communication flows from a higher level to the lower level in an organization?
   a. Downward   b. Upward
   c. Lateral   d. Horizontal
4. The communication barriers that arise due to linguistic problems of sender and receiver is:
   a. Semantic
   b. Personal
   c. Environmental
   d. Psychological
5. Which one of the following communication channels where the subordinates communicate with and through manager?
   a. Chain   b. Circular
   c. Wheel   d. Cluster

Answer Keys
1. b   2. c   3. b   4. a   5. c

SUGGESTED READING

1. Albrecht, Halsey J. Supporting the staff nurse under stress. Nurs Manag. 1991;22(7):60-61, 64.
2. Davis K. Grapevine communication among lower and middle managers. Pers J. 1969:272.

3. Elements of the Communication Process—All About Business (n.d.). Available from https://www.mbaknol.com/business-communication/elements-of-the-communication-pro. [Accessed Jan 2018].
4. Explaining the Stages of Communication Process Information (n.d.). Available from https://www.ukessays.com/essays/information-technology/explaining-the-stages-of-. [Accessed Jan 2018].
5. Gibb JR. Defensive communication. J Commun. 1961;11(3):141-8.
6. Hersey P, Blanchard K. Management of Organizational Behavior: Utilizing Human Resources, 4th edition. Englewood Cliffs, NJ: Prentice-Hall; 1982.
7. Oral Communication—Meaning, Advantages, and Limitations. (n.d.). Available from https://www.managementstudyguide.com/oral. [Accessed Jan 2018].
8. Patz JM, Biordi DL, Holm K. Middle nurse manager effectiveness. J Nurs Admin. 1991;21(1):15-24.
9. Peterson LW, Halsey J, Albrecht TL, McGough K. Communicating with staff nurses: Support or hostility? Nurs Manag. 1995;26(6):36-8.
10. Pincus JD. Communication: Key contributor to effectiveness—the research. J Nurs Admin. 1986;16(9):19-25.

37 CHAPTER

Effective Supervision

CHAPTER OUTLINE

- Supervision
  - Meaning and Concept
  - Definitions
  - Purposes of Supervision
  - Importance of Supervision
  - Principles of Supervision
- Supervision Styles
- Forms of Supervision
- Responsibilities of a Nurse Supervisor
- Role of a Nurse Supervisor
- Essential Qualities of a Nurse Supervisor
- Steps of Supervision
- Techniques and Tools Used for Supervision
- Tips for Effective Supervision

LEARNING OUTCOMES

After completion of this chapter, the learner will be able to:
- Recall and understand the concept of supervision in nursing
- Describe the importance of proper supervision in nursing
- Apply the principles of supervision at the workplace
- Enumerate styles and forms of supervision
- Discuss various tools and techniques used for supervision
- Describe the qualities of a good nursing supervisor

KEY TERMS

Supervision, styles of supervision, normative, formative, restorative, tools and techniques

INTRODUCTION

Supervision is one of the essential components of staffing. It involves the management, direction, and leadership of employees. Supervision operates in all functions of administration, i.e. planning, organizing, leading, evaluating, and staffing. Monitoring is generally about overseeing the efforts of people. Often, in an organization structure, these people (even though usually part of management) report to a manager who sets guidelines and overall goals for their organization that they use to create goals and directions for the people reporting to them. It influences the course of the organization, has an impact on employees' job satisfaction and retention, and is critical to quality service delivery. Supervision can only be adequate if the supervisors are competent technical experts and trainers.

SUPERVISION

Meaning and Concept

The word supervision is a derivative of two Latin words, "super" means "above" and "'video" means "see," involving overseeing or superintending the work of others. Supervision means "overseeing" as a higher vision. It refers to guiding and controlling subordinates for their tasks. It conveys different ideas to different people. To some, it may be "inspection and checking" of work performance. To others, it means direction accompanied by authority. It also means safeguarding the personnel from making mistakes. Hence, supervision can be viewed as a work-control method and also considered to be a supportive and guiding process. Thus, supervision means directing, investigating, guiding, helping, and advising subordinates in their performance to achieve the established objectives of the organization.

It is a teaching–learning process that provides constant observation, monitoring, and evaluation. The concept of supervision has changed from the past. Now the emphasis is on participative, democratic/person-oriented leadership in supervision than autocratic. In nursing, it consists of all activities that express leadership in the improvement of learning and teaching of nursing care in nursing service. The aim of nursing supervision is to improve human, individual, and scientific nursing care of patients and nurses.

Definitions

- Supervision is described as the watching, overseeing, and critical intense directing of a course of action or particular activities. It is the act, process, or function of supervising.
  —*Department of Health, 1993*
- Supervision employs to designate the fundamental duties at the very bottom or first level of management hierarchy, the job that bears the formally assigned authority and responsibility for planning and controlling the activities of subordinate, nonsupervisory employees usually on a direct, face to face basis.
  —*Sartain and Baker*
- Supervision is observing the subordinates at work to ensure that they are working according to plans and policies of the organization and to help them in solving the problems.
  —*Terry*
- Supervision is a process by which the subordinates are guided according to their needs by the immediate superiors so that they can make the best use of their knowledge and skill and improve their abilities to do their job efficiently and effectively to fulfill the objectives of the organization.
  —*Williamson*
- Nursing supervision is a service devised to enhance patient care by promoting, stimulating, and fostering personal growth and welfare. It is primarily concerned with the personnel. It is also concerned with the physical facilities and equipment and ease and difficulty of the quality of staff.
  —*Perrodin CM*
- Supervision is a form of teaching that involves advising, helping, inspiring, leading, and liberating.
  —*Jean Barrette*

Thus, supervision is direction, guidance, and control of the working force to ensure that they are working according to plan, policy, program, and instructions. It is a two-way dynamic and social process to fulfill organizational goals. It is an ongoing process interwoven with motivation, performance appraisal, staff development, and leadership. Supervision is assisting staff to perform in the best way possible to yield the best results in the realization of organizational goals.

Objectives

Main Objectives

- To see the completion of the task on time
- To promote continuous improvement in the performance.

Specific Objectives

- To meet the predetermined goals of the department
- To ensure the working of employees according to their job description
- To evaluate the quality of care rendered by the staff
- To motivate staff to use talents and potentialities
- To guide individual staff to achieve their personal goals
- To help staff to adjust with the environment
- To promote teamwork.

Purposes

The following list shows the purposes of supervision:

1. **To accomplish work:** Good supervision always ensures the completion of work within the expected framework. Superiors at various levels supervise their subordinates. The nurse managers in their area ensure appropriate availability of resources and conducts ward rounds to make sure that nurses are performing their duties per plan.
2. **To evaluate performance and provide feedback:** During supervision, nurse manager observes each staff for his or her performance, assesses their weak areas and strengths that will help his or her to correct weaknesses, and encourages and appreciates his or her strong points.
3. **To improve staff efforts individually and collectively:** The purpose of supervision is to not directly finding fault and punishing defaulters. Instead, it aims at enhancing staff efforts separately and together. Intelligent supervision will enable nurse managers to look ahead for shortcomings that may interfere in the progress of the organization and accordingly can take remedial actions at the appropriate time.
4. **To make subordinates self-directed:** Supervision helps and motivates subordinates to become self-directive and ethical decision makers.
5. **To bring a sense of security:** Good supervision provides a sense of security and develops confidence among them to make decisions.
6. **To bring personal and professional growth:** Good supervision helps subordinates to grow personally and professionally to achieve quality care.
7. **To help in solving clinical, managerial, and personal problems:** Superiors help subordinates to use various evidence-based alternatives to solve client, administrative, and personal problems through supportive guidance and teaching.
8. **To encourage teamwork:** Nurse manager as a supervisor plays a vital role in establishing a work culture to work together as a team, share their views, and discuss their ideas to bring improvement in practice.
9. **To bridge the gap between personal and organizational goals:** Supervisor guides and motivates subordinates to give their best to bridge the gap between individual and organizational goals.
10. **To improve the quality of nursing care:** Good supervision always aims to improve the quality of nursing care based on standards.

Importance

Supervision helps subordinates as follows:
- To promote optimum functioning of each staff and unit
- To improve knowledge and skills of subordinates according to their needs
- To develop the right attitude toward work, coworkers, and clients and their families
- To perform the best to achieve the goal of nursing organization
- To coordinate services within the department and organization to achieve the goal
- To develop and improve the nursing standard
- To formulate new policies
- To interpret the policies and objectives of the organization and suggest ways and means improve them
- To protect the public by reducing negligence and errors by the staff
- To establish a good interpersonal relationship between superiors and subordinates, between subordinates, and between organization and society
- To set personal goals according to organizational goals
- To create a physical, psychological, and social environment to work.

Principles

The principles of supervision are as follows:
1. It is an ongoing and continuous teaching–learning process.
2. It is employee centered rather than task centered.
3. It is cooperatively planned and focused on the attainment of the goal.
4. It should have objectives, methods, and criteria for judging.
5. It has a basis on the job description and individual needs of staff.
6. It stimulates subordinates for their self-development.
7. Supervisor must be technically and academically competent.
8. Proper supervision respects the individuality of subordinates.

SUPERVISION STYLES

Autocratic Supervision

Autocratic supervision is a type of supervision in which the supervisor considers himself or herself in an authority position and expects subordinates to work according to his or her direction. There is no scope of involving subordinates in decision-making. The supervisor commands and has full control over their subordinates.

Democratic Supervision

Democratic supervision is participative and consultative. The supervisors follow democratic principles while dealing with subordinates. They involve them mentally and emotionally in the decision-making process, consult them, and welcome their suggestions in all matters such as preparing duty plan and time schedules. They have confidence and trust in their subordinates. They involve them in issues of the departmental and give them based on their recognition. The supervisor gets cooperation from subordinates, motivates, boosts their morale, recognizes their skills and potentials, and helps them to increase their efficiency.

Laissez-faire/free-rein Supervision

Laissez-faire is independent supervision. The supervisor determines and interprets policy, programs, protocols, and work per job assignment. The supervisor only guides subordinates and leaves them free to work on their own within the framework of instructions.

FORMS OF SUPERVISION

Clinical Supervision

Clinical supervision is a facilitated process to reflect on practice. It focuses on analyzing issues and problems, clarifying goals, identifying strategies for goal attainment, and establishing an appropriate plan of action. The success of clinical supervision depends on creating a value-based work culture for the personal development of staff.

Managerial Supervision

The managerial supervision focuses on balancing managerial work such as weekly workload, administrative procedures, meetings, planning and strategy, data collection, audit activity, recruitment and retention issues, and communication. It is more of managerial work and supervising these parameters by using various methods. The supervisor needs managerial skills to manage and supervise subordinates.

Personnel Supervision

Personnel supervision deals with issues related to interpersonal, job pressure, and the motivation of subordinates. Supervision should allow staff space to express negative or positive feeling related to their work. Supervisors try to create a work culture, so that every staff feels free to work as a team. The supervisors act as mentors and exhibit participative and democratic styles to deal with subordinates. They encourage staff to give their best output.

Professional Supervision

Professional supervision reflects the supervisor's role as an expert within the multiprofessional team to identify specific training or development needs. The supervisor encourages subordinates to explore areas that required improvement.

RESPONSIBILITIES OF A NURSE SUPERVISOR

The responsibilities of a nurse supervisor are as follows:
1. **In general**
   Administrative: Assigning duties, preparing duty roster, provide material, etc.
   Teaching: Providing technical guidance
   Helping: Helping by solving problems
   Linking: Acting as a communicator, the link between superiors and subordinates
   Evaluating: Carrying out performance appraisal.
2. **Toward superiors**
   - Identify and carry out activities of superiors
   - Suggest measures for improving the efficiency of the staff
   - Act as a liaison between higher authority and subordinates
   - Refer matters to the next supervisors for proper intervention.
3. **Toward subordinates**
   - Assist in selecting, orienting, and inducting new staff
   - Teach and help subordinates, assign duties, make duty roaster, and appraise their performance
   - Involve subordinates in planning patient care
   - Conduct meetings, conferences, rounds, and guide subordinates
   - Develop a spirit of dedication, teamwork, cooperation, and harmony among the staff
   - Deal subordinates as individuals to maintain a high standard of performance always.
4. **Coordination and cooperation**
   - Involve in effective planning of nursing unit
   - Allocate just and fair workload
   - Anticipate difficulties and problems
   - Maintain coordination with other team members
   - Look for newer methods of improvement.

ROLE OF A NURSE SUPERVISOR

The three main roles of a supervisor are normative, formative, and restorative **(Fig. 37.1)**.
1. **Normative**
   The supervisor focuses on setting standards, objectives, implementing policies, procedures, standards of care or quality desired in care output, ensuring efficient and effective delivery of care, management, and quality control of professional practice, performance appraisal, and maintaining discipline. The supervisor helps subordinates to know their expectations, how much, how well, and how soon by giving work direction, protocols, schedules, etc. Functions of a supervisor include the following:
   - Setting standards, objectives

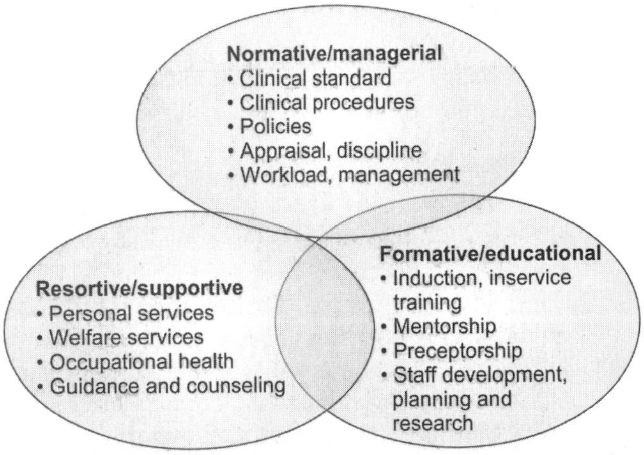

Fig. 37.1: Role of the nursing supervisor.

   - Assessing staff workload
   - Preparing the duty roster
   - Assigning duties/clients
   - Estimating the requirement of equipment and supplies
   - Managing material and other resources
   - Identifying problems and helping nurses to solve problems
   - Doing performance appraisal and giving feedback
   - Maintaining discipline.
2. **Formative**
   Supervisors also play a formative role. It is an educative role aiming for the development of subordinates. The supervisor helps subordinates to know what they can do to improve their performance in the future. They perform various educative activities, such as:
   - Organizing orientation program for newly joined/posted staff. Informing them about their job responsibilities by providing job descriptions, the methods they should use, personnel with whom and how they will work, and or community wherein they will work by interpreting policy and procedure manuals
   - Planning and conducting in-service education programs according to the needs of the staff and organization
   - Conducting skill training programs and demonstration to improve their skills
   - Encouraging them to attend continuing education programs, workshops, seminars, and conferences, and library searches to update their knowledge and skills
   - Teaching subordinates by sharing knowledge and providing technical guidance
   - Conducting planned and unplanned clinical rounds, conferences, and meetings
   - Making an effort to have informal staff development programs
   - Participating in planning research, guidance and counseling, and individual and group conferences.

3. **Restorative**
   The restorative or supportive role of a supervisor is essential to create a therapeutic relationship. This aspect of supervision addresses the needs for staff support through management to minimize occupational stress.
4. **Other major roles**
   - *As a communicator:* The supervisors act as communicators between the operational and other members of the team. They facilitate the flow of communication. A free flow of communication among staff members is necessary for teamwork.
   - *Performance evaluator:* Performance appraisal is a vital role of a supervisor. Supervisor creates awareness among subordinates regarding their performance and sends confidential reports to superior to consider at the time of promotion. Each supervisor is to do a performance appraisal of their subordinates and gives them feedback. It provides an opportunity for them to improve.
   - *Rewarding and punishing role:* Supervisors reward subordinates on their excellent performance through recognition, appreciation, promotion, etc. and punish them for poor performance by informing superiors, taking disciplinary action, transferring to another unit, or dismissal.

ESSENTIAL QUALITIES OF A NURSE SUPERVISOR

The 10 essential qualities of a nurse supervisor are listed below:

1. **Conceptual and personal qualities**
   The supervisor must have conceptual and personal attributes. The supervisor should be honest, have a sense of humor, and have a balanced personality. He or she should be capable of discharging the responsibilities assigned to him or her. The supervisor should be innovative, creative, and inspiring; able to take the initiative; be enthusiastic, intelligent; and have self-awareness, decisiveness, persistence, adaptability, thoroughness, and sociability. He or she should be reliable, objective, cooperative, and responsible and have good physical and mental health. He or she should have a vast horizon of life, be farsighted, and be a person of character, integrity, and commitment.
2. **Sharing and caring qualities**
   Supervisors must know all staff, their work, conduct, skill, training, knowledge, success, failure, habit, temperament, liking, disliking, and all that they can know. They should understand the spirit of their staff and adjust their behaviors accordingly. They should also let them know about themselves. It will develop a friendly attitude and create oneness and mutual trust on both sides.
3. **Tactful**
   A supervisor should be tactful enough to handle all managerial situations and should have a logical attitude to convince staff. He or she should take care of all resources and recognize the qualities and potentials of subordinates.
4. **Emotional stability**
   A supervisor must be mentally mature and should not lose her patience and temper quickly. A successful supervisor has a sound temperament and plans things in such a way that things happen as he or she wants.
5. **Unbiased and fair**
   The supervisor must treat all staff working under his or her supervision impartially. He or she should be fair to all. He or she should not prejudice against any of his or her staff; otherwise, it will create tension, bitterness, and, later, trouble.
6. **Leadership qualities**
   Supervisor must possess all qualities of a leader and must have the capability to appreciate; respect human dignity and individual worth of staff; recognize individual differences; understand the potentialities of each staff and delegate function; and authority where and when required; should be resourceful, foundational, and critical thinker; and should have personal discipline; and should accept and bring changes. The supervisor must lead a group of staff who look at him or her for guidance and direction. He or she should boost their morale to lead them effectively.
7. **Communication and relationship qualities**
   Supervisors must have excellent communication and relationship-building skills. They should have the ability to work with different types of staff. They should have shared decision-making skills, interdepartment and team-building spirit, academic relationships, and influencing behavior. They need to exhibit supportive behaviors in working with staff and so on. They should use language that is easily understood by the team. The nurse supervisor must be a good listener to make communication effective.
8. **Professional qualities**
   Supervisors must be professionally trained and should have professional and personal accountability in career planning. They should adhere to a code of ethics and believe in evidence-based clinical and management practices. They should try to focus on advocacy for clinical practice. They need to be members of professional organizations and work for professional uplift.
9. **Technical and teaching qualities**
   A supervisor should have knowledge of work that he or she is supervising. She must have experience in clinical practice, patient care delivery model, staffing, work schedule, ability to evaluate, ability to encourage personal and professional growth, teaching abilities, and positive attitude. She can be successful if she knows the technical aspects of the concerned job.
10. **Organizing and managerial qualities**
    A supervisor is a part of management. The nurse supervisors must, therefore, possess the knowledge

of management functions. They must have self-confidence, problem-solving and decision-making abilities, and delegating skills. The supervisor must be resourceful, democratic, dynamic, and passionate and must maintain group cohesiveness. He or she should be a source of inspiration and have the ability to design the workplace system. He or she must be able to manage and develop human, material, and other resources. The supervisor must involve in quality improvement and risk management. He or she should know about patients' safety, hospital, unit, and health policy and must be able to organize training programs. She must command respect and should be able to maintain discipline in the department and inculcate a spirit of cooperation among subordinates. Supervisor means:

S—supervise—human, material, and other resources
U—utilize—men, money, equipment, and methods
P—plan—work, staffing, techniques, and objectives
E—enforce—rules–regulations, policies, protocols, standards, and practice guidelines
R—relate to human resource—communication and interpersonal relationship
V—validate—performance, transfer, and promotion
I—instruct—methods, procedures, protocols, and safety
S—show—role model, democratic, and leadership behavior
O—organize—work, unit, and department
R—regulate—control, coordination, and work.

STEPS OF SUPERVISION

The three major phases of supervision are as follows:
1. **Preparatory phase**
   During this phase, the supervisors carry out the following activities:
   - Identify the expected relevant problem
   - Assess the performance of individual staff
   - Study hospital policy, routine, rules, regulations, guidelines, procedure manuals, job specification, standard norms, and targets
   - Prioritize areas, activities, and tasks related to nursing care
   - Prepare a checklist for observation and prepare a plan, schedule, and content for supervision.
2. **Supervision phase**
   During the supervision phase, the supervisor does the following activities by using job description, task description, weekly time table, and other tools for supervision:
   - Establish contact with subordinates, clients, and their relatives and also with other team members
   - Review objectives with subordinates
   - Review job description
   - Observe nursing staff's motivation and interest in work
   - Observe the performance of all tasks of the staff concerning skill, attitude, organization of resources, and its utilization
   - Identify gaps and needs for follow-up action.
3. **Reporting, feedback, and follow-up phase**
   The supervisors perform the following activities during this phase:
   - Prepare a report of observations made during supervision
   - Provide feedback to staff
   - Submit a report to superior
   - Plan for follow-up actions such as:
     - Organization of in-service training programs
     - Reorganization of time table/work plan/duty roster
     - Guidance and counseling of staff members
     - Individual and group conferences
     - Initiating staff welfare activities.

TECHNIQUES AND TOOLS USED FOR SUPERVISION

Tools are means, and procedures are the ways of doing something. Tools and techniques used for supervision are viewed as a control method. The selection of tools and technology for supervision depends on the type of organization, the aim of supervision, personality, and ability of the supervisor, activities performed by subordinates, and immediate circumstances. The sound, democratic principles must be kept in mind while using these tools and techniques. The techniques and tools used in supervision are as follows:

1. **Direct observation**
   Use both participatory and non-participatory methods to observe nurses directly at the time of performing duty. During observation, evaluate them for their performance, competency, and style of functioning. Evaluate whether they are applying scientific principles, theories; and understand their weak areas that need to be corrected through guidance, counseling, and organizing training programs. The supervisor can also use various tools such as observation checklist, rating scale, and observation guide.
   a. *Observation checklist:* The observation checklist is a record of relevant information to be observed. It is also a convenient recording device. It provides a way to record a "Yes" or "No" answer to denote the presence or absence of characteristics or qualities helpful in the evaluation of the performance of staff. It comprises a list of all expected skills and behaviors in the form of statements, and space is provided for a supervisor to tick mark whether a particular behavior/activity is carried out. Being the observer, the supervisor is required to check operations performed by the staff within a given period. Score these statements subsequently and the total score on the observation checklist will be

equal to the sum of scores for items checked for him or her.

b. *Rating scale:* The rating scale is a widely used technique by supervisors to evaluate the performance of subordinates. It is a tool to assess both the work and qualities of subordinates. It indicates varying degrees of a particular trait. The continuum has anchors as "outstanding," "good," "fair," and "unacceptable" to help in the rating process.

c. *Behaviorally Anchored Rating Scale:* Behaviorally Anchored Rating Scale (BARS) is a relatively new method. These checklists are systematically developed using critical incidents in combination with graphic rating scales. These can be used by the supervisor to assess predetermined critical areas of job performance. The scale comprises sets of behavioral statements that are developed from critical incidents and describe the performance of an individual.

2. **Verbal and written reports**

Oral and written reports such as anecdotal reports, critical incidence reports, and confidential reports can be used as tools to evaluate and guide subordinates.

a. *Anecdotal reports:* The anecdotal records are written documents used to record ongoing specific observation on the knowledge, skill, and attitude of an individual subordinate. It provides cumulative information the individual's performance. It should be brief, objective, and focused on specific performance and recorded during or immediately after an activity. These types of reports can be analyzed, shared, and used for further improvement by the supervisor.

b. *Critical incidence reports:* These reports are used to document any unusual occurrence or incidence, such as falls or medication errors in the delivery of client care. A supervisor can use this report to rate subordinates based on critical events or a snapshot of incidence and write a brief report about the incidence. The report can include both negative and positive remarks. This method helps to improve the management and treatment of patients by identifying high-risk patterns and initiating in-service programs to prevent future problems.

c. *Confidential reports:* The confidential report is one of the old and traditional methods of evaluating employees by supervisors. A confidential report is a detailed report about employee and generally prepared at the end of every year by the immediate superior. It contains information about the way the subordinate has carried out his or her duties; about his or her strengths, weaknesses, major failure, and achievements; and also about his or her personality, character, ability, and relation with colleagues. It should also mention the opinion on promotion, guidance, and assistance required to correct deficiencies. The supervisor must assess subordinates periodically for his or her work.

3. **Nursing rounds**

Nursing rounds are bedside visits made by nursing professionals to evaluate treatment, assess the current course, and document the patient's progress or recuperation. It is a useful method to supervise, evaluate, and guide nurses working at different levels in hospitals and the community. Practices regarding the purpose of rounds and the frequency of nursing rounds vary from hospital to hospital and depend on the level and extent of supervision coverage. Data of the district hospital of North India revealed that nursing administrators/supervisors supervise the work of nursing/other personnel by making nursing rounds. The types of nursing rounds are as follows:

a. *Patients'/clinical rounds:* Both nursing administrators and supervisors conduct clinical rounds. Nursing administrators usually perform the clinical rounds randomly during the morning and night hours. Nursing supervisors also do clinical rounds at the time of handing and taking over, along with staff nurses on duty or during morning hours independently of their respective units. These rounds are useful to assess the quality of care and the condition of patients and to identify the problems of patients and the significant ones. It is also helpful to get feedback from patients and to share patients' experiences regarding nursing and treatment. It aids in supervising the functioning of units.

b. *Hospital administrative rounds:* Daily the nurse administrators conduct these types of rounds independently or with medical administrators to ensure and monitor sanitation of hospitals/units and the functioning of units. Nursing supervisors during evening duty conduct rounds in various units of the hospital, including emergency. These types of rounds are useful to ensure the functioning of units, to provide administrative satisfaction to the hospital by ensuring proper provision and maintenance of adequate equipment and supplies, and by eliciting ideas and suggestions for improved working conditions.

c. *Ward sanitation rounds:* Nursing supervisors usually conduct rounds to check sanitation periodically in their respective units and provide feedback and suggestions to improve accordingly.

d. *Teaching nursing rounds:* The teaching rounds are mainly for education and skill development purposes. Nursing supervisors conduct teaching rounds with staff nurses and students at the bedside with caution.

e. *Medical rounds:* Practices of accompanying the unit medical head in medical rounds vary from hospital to hospital. In a few hospitals, the unit medical head conducts round with his or her medical team;

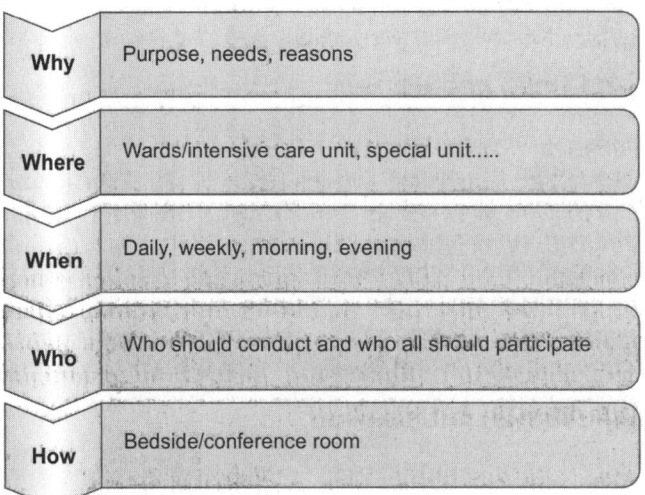

Fig. 37.2: Planning for organizing nursing rounds.

and in many hospitals nursing supervisors and staff nurses may attend medical rounds in their respective units/assigned patients where most decisions concerning patient care, prognosis, or continuity of care are made. During medical ward rounds, nurses can contribute by supplementing clinical information and providing extra details about patient assessment.

The supervisor must organize nursing rounds systematically by keeping in mind its purpose and need. The supervisor can decide where to conduct, when to perform, and who should do and how to lead (**Fig. 37.2**).

4. **Conferences**

   Both individual and group clinical conferences are essential methods in supervision used for teaching-learning and evaluation purposes. Conferences are usually conducted in a conference room adjoining the nursing unit/ward.

   a. *Individual conferences:* Individual conference is a one-on-one strategy on an individual basis that takes place between staff nurse and supervisor depending on the focus of discussion. These are generally short, lasting about 2–5 minutes to discuss various issues such as examining an ethical dilemma, the cultural aspect of care, and issues related to patients, families, and communities.

   b. *Group conferences:* In group conference, a group of staff nurses (usually 3–12) interacts, and the supervisor as a mentor exchanges ideas and expressions with them. Staff nurses are mainly involved in discussions, and solutions are derived from their own experiences or opinions, which are applied to patient problems. These are organized to set objectives and criteria for nursing care and to plan methods for improving care. To solve problems that may interfere in rendering care and in evaluating the results of efforts.

   c. *Nursing care conferences:* Two or three staff nurses in a group report on various aspects of patient care. Supervisor leads the discussion and the staff nurses in a group freely participate by asking questions or giving suggestions.

5. **Manuals and protocols**

   Manual is a document containing a set of information on a particular subject. It is a guide or a ready reference for nurse managers. Different types of manuals are available in the hospital, such as hospital policy manual, nursing policy manual, nursing service manual, ward policy manual, nursing law manual, and nursing procedure manual. Nursing policy manual usually reflects the philosophy, goal, aims, and objectives of nursing services approved by the administrator and indicates a course of action/procedures or standards, guidelines, and protocols to be utilized by nursing staff in various situations. The nursing service manual reflects the organization and administration of the nursing department, its functions, qualifications, interdepartmental relations of nursing personnel, etc. The administrative protocol is a system of rules and acceptable behaviors used by managers. Nursing clinical protocols are clearly defined detailed plan/outlining of nursing care/actions or standing orders regarding treatment in emergencies or in the absence of a doctor. It describes why, where, when, and by whom but does not represent the method of a procedure. Both manuals and protocols can be used to control, supervise, and guide staff.

6. **Performance evaluation**

   Performance evaluation is an essential controlling method in staff management used by supervisors. Nursing supervisors assess subordinates to measure and improve their performance, plan training programs based on their needs, and give them feedback. They also review their progress periodically, guide and counsel them to do better, and provide an opportunity for self-evaluation. Essay appraisal method, forced-choice method, critical incidence technique, checklist, rating scales, ranking method, management by objective, multiple-person evaluation methods, group appraisal method, and 360° feedback appraisal method are the examples of performance evaluation tools and techniques.

7. **In-service and continuing education programme**

   Nurse managers and supervisors organize in-service and continuing education programs for its nursing staff to improve and update their knowledge, skills, competencies, and overall performance. They provide opportunities for staff to develop personally and professionally.

TIPS FOR EFFECTIVE SUPERVISION

The following tips should be adhered for effective supervision:

- Don't overburden staff and exert undue pressure
- Give autonomy to staff depending upon personality, expertise, capabilities, knowledge, competence, and experience
- Be professionally and technically competent
- Encourage staff in decision-making
- Communicate freely with subordinates
- Provide good leadership
- Be flexible and be a good planner, organizer, and coordinator
- Create a suitable climate for productive work
- Encourage innovation, allowing free flow of ideas
- Share positive experiences
- Understand the situation and the problem
- Adopt a positive and supportive attitude for supervision
- Focus on continued and sustained staff growth
- Communicate and maintain a free flow of information, which creates a feeling of uncertainty in the minds of subordinates
- Keep in mind the rule of confidence/classified information
- Motivate subordinates; give personal notes of appreciation and small gestures of kindness
- Be fair and believe in justice and say no to favoritism
- Decide on facts; as far as possible, try to keep feelings out of the decision-making process
- Be acceptable: respect is earned, not demanded. You have to make yourself fair as a leader.

CHAPTER HIGHLIGHTS

- Supervision means directing, guiding, and advising subordinates in their performance to achieve the established objectives of the organization.
- It is of three types, namely, autocratic, democratic, and laissez-faire.
- The various forms of supervision are clinical, managerial, personnel, and professional supervision.
- The supervisor performs various general functions, with superiors, subordinates, and coordinating services.
- The leading roles of a supervisor are normative, formative, and restorative. He or she also performs the role of a communicator, performance evaluator, and rewarding and punishing part.
- Supervision is a process and has preparatory, supervision, reporting, feedback, and follow-up.
- A supervisor can use various methods and tools to supervise subordinates.

REVIEW QUESTIONS

I. Essay Type Questions
1. Define the term "supervision". Discuss its objectives and purposes.
2. What is the importance of supervision in nursing? Describe the essential qualities of a nurse supervisor.
3. Discuss the various styles of supervision used by a supervisor.
4. Describe the various steps undertaken by a nurse supervisor to supervise staff nurses.
5. Explain in detail various tools and techniques used by a supervisor.

II. Short Notes
1. Forms of supervision
2. Nursing rounds
3. Conferences as a tool of supervision
4. Role of a supervisor

III. Multiple Choice Questions
1. A type of supervisory style in which the supervisor expects subordinates to work according to his or her directions:
   a. Autocratic
   b. Democratic
   c. Participative
   d. Laissez-faire
2. Which form of supervision focuses on issues related to interpersonal, job pressure, and motivation of subordinates?
   a. Clinical
   b. Managerial
   c. Personnel
   d. Professional
3. Which one of the following roles of a supervisor aim for the development of subordinates?
   a. Evaluative
   b. Formative
   c. Normative
   d. Restorative
4. Which of the following attributes depict the conceptual and personal quality of a supervisor?
   a. A supervisor must understand the spirit of the staff and adjust his or her behavior accordingly
   b. A supervisor should be cautious to handle all the managerial situations
   c. A supervisor must treat all staff impartially
   d. A supervisor should be honest and have a sense of humor
5. A systematically developed checklist that uses critical incidents in combination with graphics rating scale is:
   a. Behaviorally Anchored Rating Scale
   b. Rating scale
   c. Observation checklist
   d. Semantic rating scale

Answer Keys
1. a   2. c   3. b   4. d   5. a

SUGGESTED READING

1. Agarwal DV. Management: Principles, Practices, and Techniques. New Delhi: Deep & Deep Publications; 1984.
2. Bernard JM, Goodyear RK. Fundamentals of Clinical Supervision, 2nd edition. Boston, MA: Allyn & Bacon; 1998.

3. Bones K. The basis of proper supervision and getting the most from your clinical supervisor. Nurs Times. 2000;96(4):45-8.
4. Busby A, Gilchrist B. The role of the nurse in the medical ward round. J Adv Nurs. 1992;17(3):339-46.
5. Chagon J, Russell RK. Assessment of supervisee developmental level and supervision environment across supervisor experience. J Counsel Develop. 1995;73:553-8.
6. Gallon S. Clinical supervision training manual. Portland, OR: Northwest Frontier ATTC; 2002.
7. Glover D. Reflections on supervision. Nurs Times. 2000;96(5):47-50.
8. Hill K. The sound of silence-nurses' non-verbal interaction within the ward round. Nurs Crit Care. 2003;8(6):231-9.
9. Jones A. Expanding the skills needed in clinical supervision. Nurs Times. 1997;93(50).
10. Manias E, Street A. The interplay of knowledge and decision making between nurses and doctors in critical care. Int J Nurs Stud. 2001;38(2):129-40.
11. Manias E, Street A. Nurse-doctor interactions during critical care ward rounds. J Clin Nurs. 2001;10(4):442-50.
12. Nicklin P. A practice-centered model of clinical supervision. Nurs Times. 1997;93(46):2.
13. O'Hare JA. Anatomy of the ward round. Eur J Intern Med. 2008;19(5):309-13.
14. Perrodin CM. Supervision of nursing service personnel, 8th edition. New York: The Mac Milan Co; 1964.

38 Nursing Leadership

CHAPTER OUTLINE

- Significance of Leadership
- Leadership
  - Meaning
  - Definitions and Concepts
  - Features of Leadership
- Leadership and Management
- Theoretical Approaches to Leadership
- Leadership Styles
  - Nurses' Leadership Styles
- Effective Leadership
  - Need for Effective Leadership in Nursing
  - Importance of Effective Leadership
  - Outcomes of Effective Leadership
  - Qualities of Effective Leader
  - Leadership Competencies and Skills
- Leader and Leadership Development

LEARNING OUTCOMES

After completion of this chapter, the learner will be able to:
- Understand the concept and significance of leadership
- Familiarize with the changing trends of defining nursing leadership
- Define nursing leadership
- Discuss the features of nursing leadership
- Differentiate between leadership and management
- Familiarize with classical studies and theoretical approaches to leadership
- Describe leadership styles concerning nursing leaders
- Discuss the concept of effective leadership
- Enlist the qualities of an effective leader
- Explain the essentials of competencies required for nurses
- Describe leader development and leadership development
- Explain various methods adopted for the development of leaders and their leadership behaviors

KEY TERMS

Leadership, management, attributes, followers, theoretical approaches, leadership development, competencies, leadership behaviors

INTRODUCTION

Effective leadership is key to a successful organization. Good leadership helps, solves these tasks, and provides a cushion for absorbing the impact of difficulties that crop up in any administrative activity. Complexity and size of an organization tend to develop a bureaucratic form of administration. An organization thus needs capable leaders who can lead the members to accomplish organizational goals. The leaders need to exercise authority in a better way to make organization decisions. The coordination and cooperation among team members are the key to the success of an organization.

In the health-care sector, leadership equally holds an essential place among health administrators and managers. Nursing is an important section of the health-care force. Nurses in nearly all countries give direct care and manage the work of others. Professional nurses in leadership positions are responsible for many of the health services provided in the communities, hospitals, and long-term care settings. Because of the amount of their responsibility and given their high number, sound and effective leadership and management by nurses is an essential prerequisite for the achievement of the global strategy of health.

SIGNIFICANCE OF LEADERSHIP

Listed below are the two major significances of leadership:
1. The importance of leadership arises from the openness of the organization as a system and from the fact that it operates in a changing environment, because effective change over requires leadership to build stabilizing

devices of the organization for coping with altered requirements.

2. It arises from the nature of individual membership in organizational settings. The employees who form an organization are the members of society. The extra organizational activities influence the behavior of the individual. Other factors, e.g. the turnover and replacement, introduce unique experience and personality in the organization. All these changes demand adaptation on the part of an organization, which can be possible with the aid of people in leadership roles.

LEADERSHIP

Meaning

Leadership is the art of getting others to do something. Leadership originated from the word "lead" means "to go." In the action verb, it is "to guide," "to be the first," "to go ahead." The leaders typically are the ones who go first. According to Harper Collins Dictionary, it is the ability to lead, and as a modifier, it is leadership qualities. Thus, leadership means to guide, to hold command, and to get the work done through subordinates.

Definitions and Concepts

The definitions and concepts of leadership are as follows:
- Keith Davis viewed leadership as the ability to make others follow and meet the set objectives. It helps people to work together and motivate them to achieve their desired goals.
- Hersey and Blanchard defined leadership as a process to achieve a set goal by influencing the activities of people in a given situation. It is the outcome of leader, follower, and selected environmental variables.
- Leadership, according to Northouse (2004), is a process whereby an individual influences a group of individuals to achieve a common goal.
- Sullivan and Garland (2010) viewed leadership as an activity or a process that requires interpersonal skills to influence people to achieve a particular goal.
- Leadership is defined as "the relationship in which one person influences others to work together willingly on related tasks to obtain the leader's desires."
- Porte-O'Grady (2003) considered leadership a process to motivate people to identify a goal, to take action, support, and motivate them to achieve that goal.

Leadership requires influencing attitude, beliefs, and feelings of people to achieve set goals. The person who guides or directs becomes the leader, and the people whom they lead are the followers. There is always an interaction between leader and followers. This interaction is also purposeful. The leaders try to influence the followers or groups to fulfill purpose or objective. Thus, this activity of changing people to strive willingly for group objectives is called leadership.

Leadership is the interaction between the leaders and followers, and the goal being task accomplishment or overall organizational objectives. The flow of influence is from leader to follower and vice versa within the context of a particular situation. The situation may change. Hence, in every case, where one is trying to influence the behavior of another individual, leadership is operating.

The four factors of leadership are leader, followers, situation, and communication. Thus, the process of leadership is a function of a leader, followers, and a situation. According to McGregor:

$$L = f(e, f, s)$$

L stands for leadership; f for followers; and e, f, and s are the situational characteristics.

The situational characteristics are the leaders' characteristics, followers' personalities, attitudes, needs, organizational characteristics, nature of task performed, and other factors. Interaction or communication is also significant in the process of leadership (**Fig. 38.1**).

Features of Leadership

The features of leadership are as follows:
- It is a continuous process and does not end at all. A leader guides his or her followers, whenever necessary.
- There is a relationship between the leader and the followers, which arises from their functioning.
- The followers work willingly and enthusiastically to achieve those goals.
- It provides an experience of help to follower to attain common goals. Leaders give recognition and importance to individuals.
- It exercises in a particular situation at a given point of time and under a specific set of circumstances. Thus, there is no style of leadership that applies to all the conditions.

LEADERSHIP AND MANAGEMENT

Lead means to guide on the way, especially by going in advance; to direct on a course or in a direction. The term "manage" is to address, which requires a skill to lead subordinates and manage the work of subordinates.

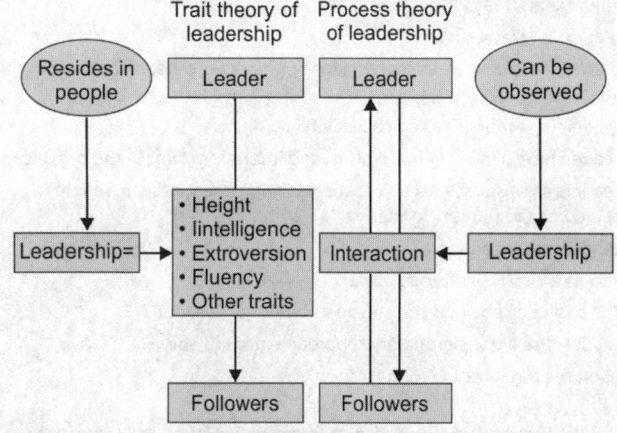

Fig. 38.1: Model of leadership.
Source: Northouse PG. Leadership: Theory and practice (5th ed). London: Thousand Oaks, CA, Sage, 2010.

Leadership and management are the two concepts having a symbiotic and synergistic relationship. To achieve organizational goals successfully, management and leadership skills need to integrate.

Difference Between Leadership and Management

It is essential to understand that leadership and management differ in many ways, which are listed below:

1. Leadership is a synthesis, and management is analysis. Analysis is breaking down the whole into parts. Synthesis/integration is to combine separate components to form a whole. A leader synthesizes solutions; management subdivide the solutions after analyzing the problems.
2. Leadership has a long-term impact, but management has short-term goals. Leaders' decisions impact the future of an organization; they bring vision and motivate the organization to achieve the goals. Manager's role is more of managing the day-to-day activities, supervising the subordinates, getting the work done, measuring performance, etc.
3. Leadership is a part of management. Management is a broader term.
4. Leadership is concerned with influencing subordinates to climb up to the next level. Management is the process of getting the work done or executing the plan.
5. Management operates in a formal structure of the organization; leadership operates in both organized and informal groups.
6. Leaders exercise informal authority, and managers use formal power.

Table 38.1 represents the difference between leadership and management.

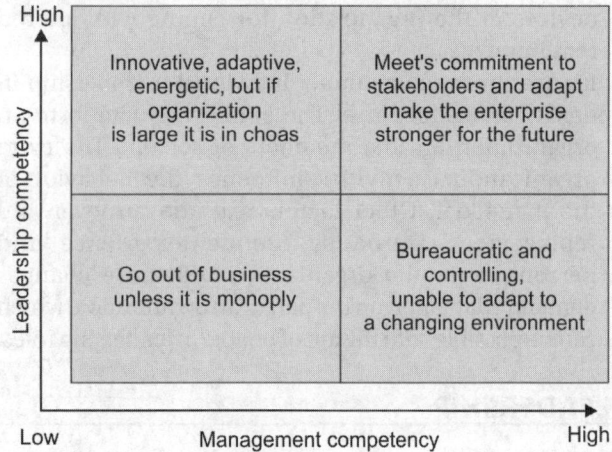

Fig. 38.2: Leadership vs management competency quadrant.

Nurse managers need to have both leadership and managerial skills because of the dramatic and rapid changes in nursing. They must strive for the integration of leadership characteristics throughout every phase of the management process. When management exists without leadership, the organization is often unable to change; and when guidance is without supervision, the organization is as active as its charismatic leader. Integrating leadership skills with management skills is necessary for an individual to become an effective leader-manager since leadership and managerial skills are a mix of transactional and transformational leadership styles **(Fig. 38.2)**.

THEORETICAL APPROACHES TO LEADERSHIP

The two major theoretical approaches to leadership are as follows:

TABLE 38.1: Difference between leadership and management	
Leadership	**Management**
Leadership is a part of the management	Management is a broader term
The focus is on vision and purpose	Managers do things efficiently to get the results
Leadership creates systems that managers manage and changes them in fundamental ways	Management makes systems to work through the years
Leaders empower followers	Manager's control subordinates
Leadership is concerned with influencing to contribute toward organizational goals	A manager plans, organizes (leads), and controls the various organizational activities
Leadership emphasizes on collectivity	Management emphasizes on individualism
Leadership operates in both formal and informal groups in the organization	The management works in the legal structure of the organization
Leaders are inspirational and charismatic and energizes the people to overcome the barriers to change	Managers are productive and effective
Leaders are proactive	Managers are reactive as far as futurity is concerned
People are led by informal power	Leaders direct subordinates by using formal authority
The source of power is the personal abilities of a leader	The source of power is the authority delegated by position
Leaders use a transformational approach in leadership	Management uses a transactional approach
Align the organization to the vision	Organize the team, subordinates, execute the plans, supervise, evaluate
Use the bottom-up approach; synthesize all the issues and solve them holistically	Use the top-down approach, analyze the problems into specific problems, and then address each of them

Classical Studies on Leadership

Several studies and a considerable body of knowledge are available on leadership. A review of classical studies has set the stage for established and emerging theories of leadership.

1. **The Iowa leadership studies:** The series of studies have been conducted in the late 1930s by Ronald Lippitt and Ralph K White under the direction of Kurt Lewis at the University of Iowa. The study analysis showed different styles of leadership that produced different complex reactions from the same or similar groups. Although study generalization was dangerous, it had crucial historical significance.
2. **The Ohio State leadership studies:** A team of researchers from psychology, sociology, and economics conducted studies at Ohio State University studies in 1945. They developed the Leader Behavior Description Questionnaire (LBDQ) to analyze leadership styles in numerous groups and situations. They found two types of leadership behaviors, i.e. consideration and initiative.
3. **The early Michigan leadership studies:** At the same time, a survey on leadership was conducted at the Research Center of the University of Michigan, USA. Twelve high–low productivity pairs were selected for examination. Nondirective interviews were conducted on 24 section supervisors and 419 clerical workers. Results showed high-producing employee-centered section supervisors.

Theoretical Approaches

As early as 1830, Hegel reportedly wrote the first book about leadership. By the mid-20th century, the researchers became interested in finding out the factors that resulted in high and low productivity. Chapter 8 covers leadership theories.

The primary leadership theories, such as Bass and Avolio's transformational and transactional leadership, are used to frame the research design and tools to find out the leadership styles.

Leadership Styles

Meaning

Leadership is practiced by leadership style, which is the total pattern of leaders' actions toward followers. It represents the philosophy, skills, and attitudes in practice of a leader. Leadership style means how a person plays a role; the way he or she reacts, how he or she decides, how he or she interacts, and treats other people. Leader behavior is the mixture of all styles over some time, but one style tends to be dominant at one time.

Types

I. **According to dimensions**
   1. *Goal attainment style:* It is a type of behavior a leader exhibits to attain a goal.
   2. *Adaptation style:* A type of behavior a leader adapts at a time to decide to direct the group.
   3. *Balanced style:* A type of behavior a leader exhibits to attain a balance of goal attainment and adapting practices with subordinates.

II. **According to the leader's approach to influence**
   1. *Transactional leadership:* A type of leadership wherein a leader has relationship with the follower to exchange information and ideas. The leader gives rewards to the followers for his or her excellent performance and punishment for not performing and complying with the instructions.
   2. *Transformational leadership:* A type of leadership wherein a leader is inspirational and ideal for the followers. They are clear about their goals and vision and allow followers to participate in decision-making.

III. **According to a leader's approach in decision-making**
   1. *Autocratic or directive:* In this type of leadership behavior, the leader considers a position of authority and expects subordinates to follow. The subordinates are made aware of what to do, but not why. The leader sets the goals and expects them to be accepted, along with methods of achieving them. The leader defines the problem, diagnoses the problem, generates, evaluates, and chooses among alternative solutions.
   2. *Autocratic with the involvement of subordinates*
      - A leader may define the problems but ask subordinates to gather information regarding the issues.
      - A leader may work on identifying problems and its solutions but takes subordinates' opinions to understand and review and for getting feedback from them.
      - A leader may also define the problem but discusses either with an individual member (individual consultative style) or with a group (group consultative style) to get alternative solutions.
      - A leader may present the problem and ask the group to identify the cause of the issues and solutions and to select the best alternative (group decision style).
   3. *Participative:* Leaders present their analysis of problems and proposals for action to members. The members as a group define the problem, identify the cause, and alternative solutions, and select the best one. A leader acts as a facilitator of a work group and invites criticism and comments.

IV. **According to a leader's influence and maintenance functions**
   1. *Socioemotional style:* A leader emotionally influences subordinates to get the work done. They have interpersonal and emotional intelligence skills, are more supportive and accept subordinates, and are concerned about their welfare.
   2. *Task style:* Leaders are concerned about a particular task. He or she frames the deadline, method, and

standard of the responsibility and expects the subordinates to perform accordingly. They are usually directive leaders. They want to achieve the outcome.
3. *Combination of task and socioemotional style:* Leaders have both task and socioemotional qualities to get the work done from subordinates.

V. **According to authority used by a leader**
1. *Autocratic:* Autocratic leaders allow minimal team participation in the decision-making process and sometimes even ignore the opinions of their subordinates. They are not concerned about the abilities and welfare of subordinates.
2. *Democratic:* The democratic leaders delegate authority to their subordinates. Leaders inform subordinates about the overall purpose and goal of the organization and allow them to participate in decision-making and problem solving. Leaders value the individual characteristics and abilities of each subordinate. Democratic leaders use personal and positional power to draw out ideas from employees and motivate them to set their own goals, develop their plans, and control their practice. Thus, democratic leaders seek advice from their subordinates and try to reach a consensus within their teams.

Nurses' Leadership Styles

The leadership styles among nurses are as follows:
1. **Relationally focused leadership styles**
   - *Transformational style:* Leaders motivate subordinates to work beyond their capacities and expectations.
   - *Individualized consideration:* Leaders are concerned with satisfying the individual needs of subordinates.
   - *Resonant style:* This style is based on the emotional intelligence of the leaders, which inspires, coaches, develops, and includes others even in the face of adversity.
2. **Task-focused styles**
   The task-focused leaders articulate clear role expectations, create well-defined communication channels, and focus on tasks and attaining goals. They exhibit the following leadership styles:
   - *Active management-by-exception style:* A leader focuses on monitoring task execution for any problems to maintain current performance levels.
   - *Laissez-faire styles:* These are similar in that they conceptualize as passive avoidance of issues, decision-making, and accountability.
   - *Passive-avoidant leadership style:* The leader either takes action after the problem becomes serious (passive) or avoids making any decision at all.
   - *Transactional leadership style:* It emphasizes the transaction or exchange that takes place among leaders, colleagues, and followers to accomplish the work.
   - *Dissonant leadership style:* This is characterized by pacesetting and commanding forms that undermine the emotional foundations required to support and promote staff success.
   - *Instrumental leadership style:* It focuses on the strategic and task-oriented developmental functions of leaders.

EFFECTIVE LEADERSHIP

Need for Effective Leadership in Nursing

Effective leadership is vital to guide for solving complex problems related to nursing care delivery. It is critical in delivering high-quality care, ensuring patient safety, and facilitating positive staff development. It is not confined to the executive level of nursing organizations but equally necessary at supervisory and operational levels.

Leadership in nursing is required to make decisions, for delegation, for resolving conflict, and for acting intelligently. They should also nurture and care and be socioemotional with team members.

Importance of Effective Leadership

Effective leadership is considered crucial in the following ways:
- Enables nurse leaders to handle situations effectively
- Improves work output and quality of work
- Improves employees job satisfaction and morale
- Reduces absenteeism, turnover, and shortage
- Maintains healthy work environments
- Provides positive outcomes for organizations, patients, and healthcare providers
- Enables effective change management
- Improves the standard of patient care.

Outcomes of Effective Leadership

1. *Staff satisfaction*
   Job satisfaction: The highest job satisfaction is associated with a variety of relational focused leadership styles such as socioemotional, consideration, inspirational, resonant, and transformational leadership but significantly lowers with more task-focused forms of leadership such as instrumental, management by exception, and laissez-faire leadership.
   - *Satisfaction with their leader:* Data revealed a significantly higher satisfaction with their leader having charismatic, resonant, and transformational leadership and reduced satisfaction with their leaders having management by exception, transactional and laissez-faire, and dissonant leadership styles.
   - *Satisfaction with job mobility options, job security, financial rewards, and time to spend with patients:* These are significantly higher in association with

resonant, empowering, initiating structure and consideration styles of leadership in association with dissonant (pacesetting and commanding) styles of leadership.

2. **Staff relationships**
   - *Organizational commitment:* Significantly increased organizational commitment with transformational leadership, supportive leadership, consideration, and charismatic leadership, whereas lower organizational commitment with management by exception and instrumental leadership styles, with the leadership practice of inspiring a shared vision.
   - *Nurses' intent to stay:* Data revealed significantly higher consideration for leadership by the nurses to remain in the organization compared to leaders having decision decentralization.
   - *Nurses' intent to leave:* Significantly higher with management by exception leadership and lower with charismatic leadership.
   - *Actual retention:* Significantly more upper with consideration and significantly lower following decision decentralization.
   - *A decrease in turnover:* Leader–member exchange and transformational leadership practices.
   Staff health and well-being: Staff health is better, while anxiety, emotional exhaustion, and stress were reported lower with transformational leadership, empowering leadership, supportive leadership, resonant leadership, and nurse-assessed nurse manager ability, leadership, and support of nurses. Nurse emotional exhaustion and poorer psychological health are associated with dissonant leadership and management by exception.
   - *Job tension:* Decreased when nurses had a positive perception of nursing leadership.

3. **Healthy work environment**
   - *Nurse empowerment:* Greater nurse empowerment with transformational leadership, connective leadership, leadership empowering behaviors, and motivational leadership.
   - *Culture and climate:* Better in association with leadership support for improvement, structural leadership, initiative structure, and change-oriented leadership.
   - *Role clarity:* Greater and conflict and ambiguity reduce in association with transformational leadership and initiating structure activities.
   - *Teamwork:* Teamwork between physicians and nurses was reported to be better in association with resonant leadership, more exceptional nurse manager ability, guidance, and support of nurses, and leader-empowering behaviors.
   - *Other characteristics:* Innovation, group cohesion, nursing work group collaboration, conflict management, and nursing models of care—significantly higher in association with consideration leadership, resonant leadership, socioemotional leadership, change-oriented leadership, leader-empowering behaviors, nurse manager ability, guidance and support of nurses, transformational leadership, and peer leadership.

4. **Organizational productivity and effectiveness**
   Factors reflecting individual, team, and organizational productivity and efficiency were reported to be higher in association with charismatic, transformational, and change-oriented leadership. Significantly reduced efficiency and productivity are associated with management by exception, transactional, laissez-faire, and peer leadership.

Qualities of Effective Leader

Leadership has three P's—person (a leader), people (followers), and purpose (goal). A person (leader) influences a group of people to work to achieve a goal and has a deep-rooted commitment to accomplish the goal (**Fig. 38.3**). An effective leader is a catalyst in facilitating effective interaction among workforce, materials, and time. He or she is a synergist who unifies the efforts of followers with his or her diverse skills.

The nursing administrator, supervisor, head nurse, and nursing staff in team nursing are all leaders. They should have the following qualities:
1. Knowledge of self
2. Integrity and sincerity
3. Clarity of vision and goals
4. Commitment and willpower
5. Innovative and ambitious
6. Persistent and self-confident
7. Good communication skills
8. Tactful and thoughtful
9. Flexible and reliable
10. Objective and cooperative
11. Progressive and enthusiastic
12. Organizational skill
13. Emotionally intelligent
14. Managerial competencies
15. Conflict managerial skills
16. Problem-solving abilities
17. Technically competent
18. Teaching skills

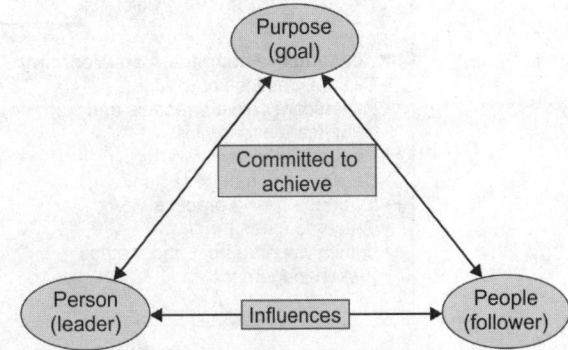

Fig. 38.3: Prerequisite for leadership.

19. Role model
20. Source of motivation.

Leadership Competencies and Skills

Competency has become an issue of vital importance in nursing administration. Advancement, globalization, and unexpected situations challenge the responsibilities of nurse managers. Nurse managers need to be competent to provide a cushion for absorbing the impact of difficulties that crop up in any managerial activity and also to cope with the hospital's competitive and high-tech environment apart from his or her job assignments **Figure 38.4** depicts the competencies and skill required for nurse executives/administrators.

In Indian scenario, the overall leadership competencies (LCs) of nurse managers working in critical care on parameters of knowledge, technical and teaching, organizational and management skills, conceptual and personal attributes, human resource management are found to be approximately 75% as compared to the desired >86% (Vati et al.; **Fig. 38.5**).

LEADER AND LEADERSHIP DEVELOPMENT

Definitions

Definitions of leader and leadership development are as follows:

- Leader development typically focuses on individual-based knowledge and the skills and abilities associated with formal leadership roles
- McCauley et al. (1998) defined leadership development as a process to expand the potentials of employees by effectively engaging in leadership roles and methods
- Leadership development focused on building and using interpersonal competence.

Difference Between Leader Development and Leadership Development

Leadership development is different from leader development. These differ in approach, concepts, competence base, and the skills required for the development. **Table 38.2** shows the distinction between leader development and leadership development.

Methods to Improve Leadership Effectiveness

A study conducted in the Indian scenario revealed various factors that can help in the development of LCs among nurse managers working in a specialty area **(Fig. 38.6)**. To develop leadership talents and induce positive attitude toward certain leadership qualities among nurse managers, and also keeping in mind the other factors, the following methods can be adopted to improve the leadership effectiveness among the nurse leaders.

Leadership Training Programs

These are most effective in bringing short-term as well as long-term change. The success of training depends on the need for behavioral change, the commitment of trainees to change, and the support they get from the organization. The training must focus on teaching relationship and communication skills and inculcating other characteristics such as openness, extroversion, and motivation, ability to integrate and manage emotions. They must emphasize teamwork, collaboration, and empowerment. These programs are as follows:

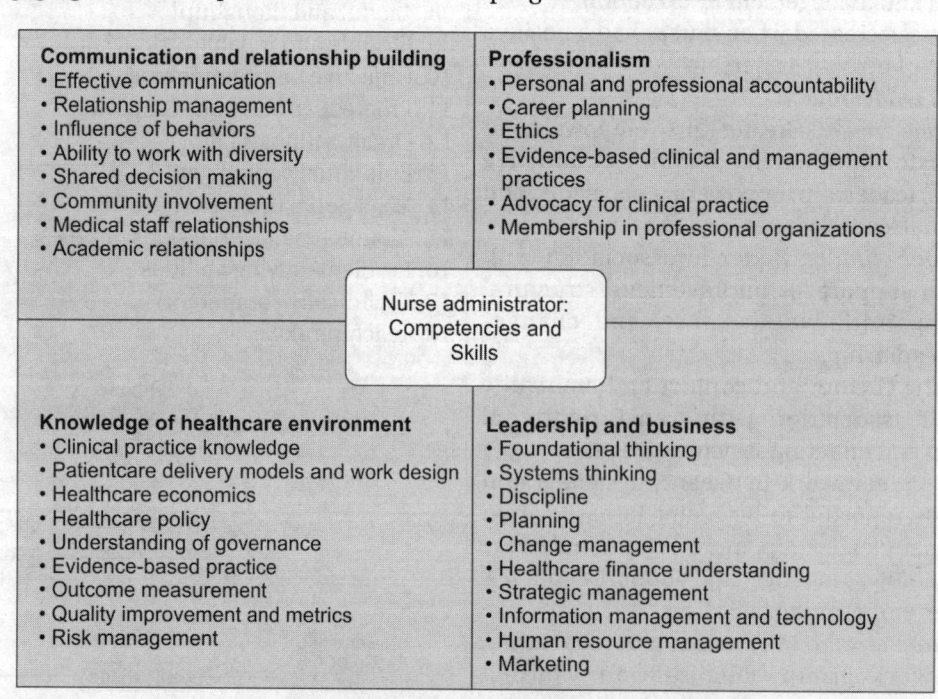

Fig. 38.4: Competencies and skills of nurse executives.
Source: AONE nurse executive competencies. Nurse Leader 2005. pp. 50-6.

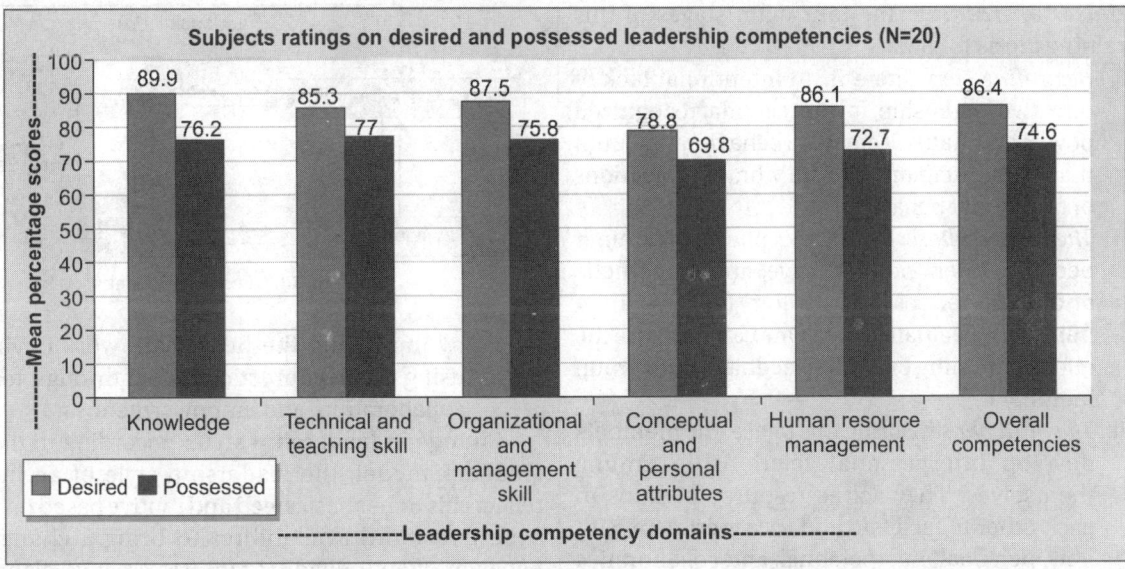

Fig. 38.5: Desired and possessed leadership competencies among nurse managers.

TABLE 38.2: Difference between leader development and leadership development.

	Leader development	Leadership development
Approach	Human	Social
Concepts	Individual: Personal power, knowledge, trustworthiness	Relational: Commitment, mutual respect, and trust
Competence base	Intrapersonal	Interpersonal
Skills required	Self-awareness: Emotional awareness, self-confidence, accurate self-image Self-regulation: Self-control, trustworthiness, personal responsibility, adaptability Self-motivation: Initiative, commitment, and openness	Social awareness: Empathy, service orientation, political awareness Social relationship

1. **Classroom-based training:** Classroom teaching is quite popular and effective. But there are chances that the trainees may not apply the change in behavior in an actual situation. Traditional classroom-based training has limited effectiveness in developing leaders. Once the course is over, participants adopt the previous practice.

2. **Sensitivity training or T group:** T group training is a small-group interaction process. It is highly unstructured and requires people to become sensitive to others' feelings through group activity. The number of participants varies from 10 to 12.

   Objectives
   - To make participants sensitive to emotional reactions and in expression in themselves and others
   - To motivate the participants to develop personal values and goals to solve their personal and social problems democratically and scientifically
   - To inculcate a sense of achievement of behavioral effectiveness among the participants.

   Types of groups: The different types of groups in training are as follows:
   i. *Stranger lab group:* All the participants are from various organizations, and they are strangers to each other.
   ii. *Cousin lab group:* All the participants are from the same organization but different units. They know each other but not very well.
   iii. *Family lab group:* All participants are from the same units and know each other quite well.

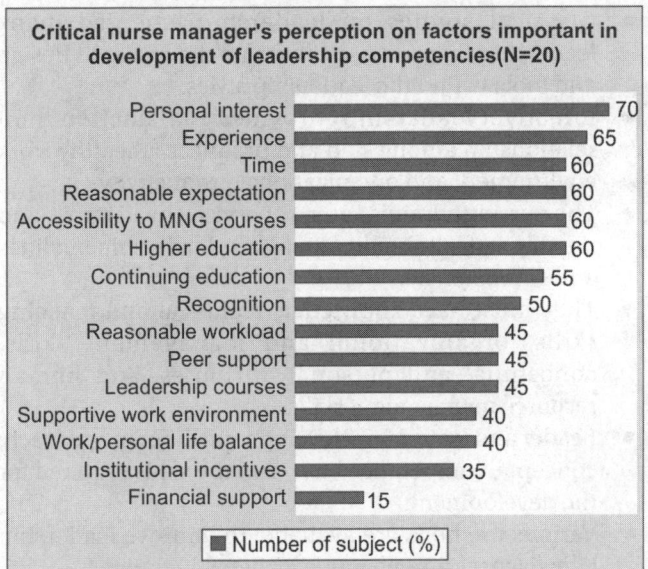

Fig. 38.6: Influencing factors of leadership development.

Phases of training: The four main stages of this training are as follows:
  i. *Beginning step:* There is an intentional lack of directive leadership, formal agenda, recognized power, and status. It creates a behavioral vacuum that the participants fill with vibrant projections of traditional behavior.
  ii. *The second phase:* During this phase, the trainer becomes open, nondefensive, and empathetic and experiences his or her feelings in a minimally evaluative way. One can measure the effect of training by getting feedback from group members.
  iii. *The third phase:* During this phase, the members develop interpersonal relationship among themselves. They act as resource persons to each other to facilitate and try experiment with new, personal, interpersonal, and collaborative behaviors.
  iv. *Last phase:* During this phase, the relevance of the experience in terms of "back home" situation and problems are explored.

  All four events are applicable in a strange lab. Another lab group requires some adjustment and attention to have intergroup linkage through interviews and confrontation sessions to solve problems and interpersonal issues.
3. ***The 360° feedback:*** The 360° feedback is a method to gather perceptions of an individual's performance from peers, direct reports, supervisors, and, occasionally, other stakeholders.
4. ***Coaching:*** It is for improving individual performance and enhancing organizational effectiveness and is an ongoing process. Little empirical evidence are available on the impact of coaching on leadership development.
5. ***Mentoring:*** It is useful for individual personal development. Open organizational programs tend to involve the pairing of a junior manager with a more senior manager or an executive outside the direct chain of command. It is helpful to provide learning opportunities, and, at the same time, one can supervise and evaluate subordinates.
6. ***On-site programs:***
    - *Contact with caregivers:* It is one of the ways to improve leadership among nurses. The nurse managers and nurses must have direct contact with their caregivers. It will help them to practice and observe leadership skills in the form of self-efficacy.
    - *Empowerment:* The efforts by the organization to "empower" nurses promote positive work behaviors and attitudes, including leadership behavior.
    - *Transformational/relational leadership practices:* Up to 12 months after the program, participants can practice this type of leadership skills.
    - *Improvement of healthcare work environments:* The dynamic clinical leaders can bring a change by improving the healthcare work environment using the best practice model through teamwork, collaboration, and empowerment.

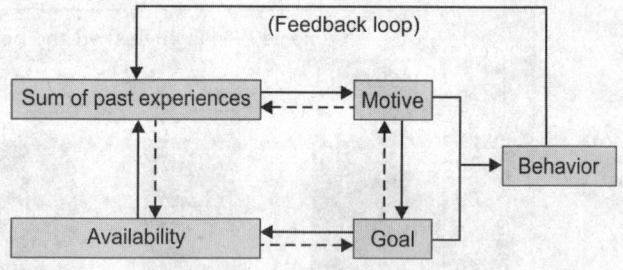

Fig. 38.7: Feedback model.

Change in leadership style: According to the Fiedler feedback model, the leadership style of an individual reflects his or her basic need and motive based on previous experience and availability. To bring a change in the behavior of an individual requires creative planning and patience. A need for the training of leaders is required to change their behaviors and modify the work environment, evaluation, and feedback **(Fig. 38.7)**.

The training and development programs, such as T group training and team-building approach, can encourage the leaders to adopt specific normative behavior. Recognize the conditions under which one can perform best and try to modify the situations that do not suit. It is easy to change the environment instead of changing ones' behavior.

CHAPTER HIGHLIGHTS

- Leadership is a continuous process to achieve a defined goal by influencing the activities of people in a given situation.
- Leadership is the interaction between the leaders and followers to accomplish the goal.
- Leadership and management are the two concepts having a symbiotic and synergistic relationship; both need to integrate.
- Classical studies on leadership emerged many leadership theories used to frame the research design and tools to find the leadership styles.
- Effective leadership provides satisfaction and relationship among staff and produces a healthy work environment and organizational productivity.
- The nursing administrator, supervisor, head nurse, and nursing staff all should possess the leadership qualities and competencies.
- They must have knowledge, technical and teaching skills, organizational and management skills, conceptual and personal attributes, and human resource management skills.
- Leader and leadership development differ in approach, concepts, competence base, and the skills required for the development.
- Various methods are available to improve leadership effectiveness among nurse leaders.

REVIEW QUESTIONS

I. Essay Type Questions
1. Define the term "leadership." Discuss its significance and characteristics.
2. Describe classical studies of leadership.
3. What do you mean by leadership style? Describe the various leadership styles.
4. Differentiate between leader development and leadership development.
5. What is the importance of effective leadership in nursing? Describe its outcomes.

II. Short Notes
1. Management versus leadership
2. Qualities of an effective leader
3. Leadership competencies
4. Methods of developing leadership

III. Multiple Choice Questions
1. What is the most important factor in the leadership process?
    a. Leader
    b. Follower
    c. Task
    d. Communication
2. Which of the following is concerned with leadership?
    a. That focuses on vision and purpose
    b. That emphasizes individualism
    c. That is result oriented
    d. That uses the transactional approach
3. Which one of the following competencies relate to professionalism?
    a. Ability to work with diversity
    b. Advocacy for clinical practices
    c. Understanding of governance
    d. Human resource management
4. Who was the pioneer of the path–goal theory?
    a. Lewin
    b. Fiedler
    c. Robert House
    d. Likert
5. In which type of leadership, a leader develops a relationship with followers to exchange ideas?
    a. Transactional
    b. Transformational
    c. Directive
    d. Participative

Answer Keys
1. d   2. a   3. b   4. c   5. a

SUGGESTED READING

1. Akerjordet K, Severinsson E. The state of the science of emotional intelligence related to nursing leadership: An integrative review. J Nurs Manag. 2010;18(4):363-82.
2. Antrobus S, Kitson A. Nursing leadership: Influencing and shaping health policy and nursing practice. J Adv Nurs. 1999;29(3):746-53.
3. Davis K. Human Behaviour at Work. New Delhi :Tata McGraw-Hill Company Ltd., 1975.
4. Dunham J, Fisher E. Nurse executive profile of excellent nursing leadership. Nurs Adm Q. 1990;15(1):1-8.
5. Hersey P, and Blanchard KH. Management of Organisational Behaviour. New Jersey: Engle wood Cliffs, Prentice Hall, 1977.
6. Huque H. Nursing leadership development strategies. NJI. 1988; 39(1):324.
7. Jooste K. Leadership: A new perspective. J Nurs Manag. 2004;12(3):217-23.
8. Koklavani NZ. The way for effectiveness leadership. NJI. 2008; 99(4):85-7.
9. Leadership Vs. Management—Practical Management. (n.d.). [online] Available from http://practical-management.com/Leadership-Development/Leadership-Vs-Management. [Accessed on May 2019].
10. McCauley C, Moxley R, and Van Velsor E. (eds.). Handbook of Leadership Development. San Francisco: Jossey- Bass Publication, 1998.
11. Northouse PG. Leadership : Theory and practice (5th ed.). London: Thousand Oaks, CA, Sage, 2010.
12. Northouse PG.Leadership: Theory and Practice, (3rd Edition), London: Sage Publications, 2004. available at www.sagepub.co.uk/upm-data/9546_017487ch02.pdf. [Accessed Jan 2020].
13. Porter-O' Grady T, and Malloch K. Quantum Leadership: A Textbook of New Leadership. Boston: John & Bartlett, 2003. (Cross reference) Available from (online) Leadership Roles and Management Functions in Nursing: Theory ... https://books.google.co.in › books
14. Roussel L, Swansburg RC, Swansburg RJ. Management and Leadership for Nurse Administrators, 5th edition. Boston, MA: Jones and Bartlett Publishers; 2009.
15. Sullivan EJ, and Garland G. Practical Leadership and Management in Nursing. Harlow: Pearson Education Limited, 2010.
16. Sullivan EJ, Decker PJ. Effective leadership and management in nursing, 7th edition. London: Prentice-Hall; 2009.
17. Tofino J. Transformational leadership in health care. Nurs Manag. 1995;26(8):42-7.
18. Venkatesan L. The importance of critical thinking for nursing leadership. Ind J Nurs Midwifery. 1999; 12(3):23-6.

39 Conflict Management

CHAPTER OUTLINE

- Organizational Conflict
  - Meaning and Definitions
  - Conflict Process
  - Factors Influencing Conflict
  - Elements of Conflict
  - Types of Organizational Conflict
  - Dimensions of Conflict
  - Impact of Conflict
- Conflict Management
  - Different Managerial Styles in Handling Conflicts
  - Steps in Conflict Management
  - Conflict Management/Resolution Strategies

LEARNING OUTCOMES
After completion of this chapter, the learner will be able to:
- Understand the concept of organizational conflict
- Describe organizational conflict process
- Enlist the influencing factors and elements of conflict
- Discuss different types of organizational conflict
- Explain the dimensions and impact of conflict
- Describe the different managerial styles of handling conflicts
- Explain the steps of managing organizational conflict
- Describe conflict-resolution strategies

KEY TERMS
Organizational conflict, conflict process, models, conflict management, managerial styles, resolution strategies

INTRODUCTION

Organizational conflict often results in differences between two or more individuals in an organization. Organizational conflict can be positive or negative. Positive conflict allows an organization to improve its operations to overcome a lack of resources and has the scope to increase productivity and improve performance. Negative conflict can result in a disruption of organizational operations and profit loss. Constant conflict in an organization can create a challenging work environment and low productivity. The conflict originates from a disagreement between two individuals or groups and their attitudes, values, and expectation clashes. Poor communication is also the cause of organizational conflicts. Conflicts need to resolve by cooperation and common consensus of the affected parties.

ORGANIZATIONAL CONFLICT

Meaning and Definitions

Early definitions of conflict had focused on a wide variety of different phenomena (Mack and Snyder, 1957; Fink, 1968). Pondy (1967) had sorted these definitions into several categories: antecedent conditions, emotions, perceptions, and behaviors.

- Conflict refers to a struggle or contest between people with opposing needs, ideas, beliefs, values, or goals. Conflict may escalate and lead to nonproductive results, or disputes can be beneficially resolved and lead to final quality products.
- Conflict is a social situation where two parties have differences in their attitudes, values, and opinions that may affect the achievement of their goals. Conflicts are inevitable and need to manage to avoid negative impacts on the individual or organization.

Conflict Process

Organizational conflict is a process where a series of events and reactions takes place. Different models describe the conflict development process in their own ways **(Fig. 39.1)**.

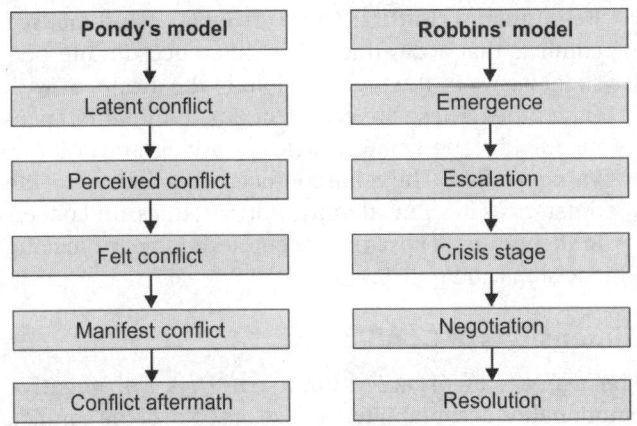

Fig. 39.1: Conflict development process.

Pondy's Model (1967)

Pondy's model of conflict development describes five main stages of conflict process:

Stage 1: Latent conflict: During this stage, no conflict is present, but many factors may influence the possibility of conflict. Organization conflicts arise due to task interdependence of departments in complex organizations, differences in their goals and setting priorities, line and staff functions, incompatible performance criteria and standards, inequality in allocating resources.

Stage 2: Perceived conflict: One or more parties become aware of the conflict and begin to analyze it. When a party or subunit perceives its goals obstructed, conflict enters the second stage. Each group seeks the source of the conflict and finds reasons for problems.

Stage 3: Felt conflict: Both parties respond emotionally to each other and their attitudes polarize into "us-versus-them." Anger, frustration, and hostility prevail with each other. In this stage, cooperation between units decreases, and small problem escalates into colossal conflict. Thus, organizational effectiveness declines.

Stage 4: Manifest conflict: Both parties try to get back at each other. There is fighting and open aggression as well as passive aggression. Adversarial behavior (jealousy, hatred, anger and frustration, apathy, rigid rules adherence, and violence) is exhibited, leading to stress and threat, which in turn increases emotional responses and negative arousal.

Stage 5: Conflict aftermath: It is the last stage in the conflict. It results if conflicts remain unsolved by the manifest stage, and it may affect the organization adversely. The conflicts solved before this stage will prove decisive.

Stephen P Robbins' Model

The Robbins' model describes five stages in the conflict process:

1. **Emergence stage:** It is the first stage in development conflicts. Conflict arises due to favorable conditions for disputes. It starts with a possible difference or incompatibility (latent phase) between the parties in their values, attitudes, and goals. Due to personal and communication problems, the conflict may enter into a stage of cognition and personalization stage. A dispute at this stage arises at an individual level.
2. **Escalation stage:** During this stage, *conflict*, if not solved, is at the institutional *level*. Both parties use noncooperative attitude and avoidance tactics.
3. **Crisis stage:** During *the crisis stage*, the conflict is severe. None of the parties wants to resolve the dispute and negotiate with each other. It is an emergency stage when there is a need to solve the conflict.
4. **Negotiation stage:** During this stage, both parties discuss, negotiate, and reach a consensus to resolve the conflict. They realize the emotional intensity and attachment and agree to negotiate. This stage is the de-escalation stage; both parties compromise and bargain for any kind of settlement.
5. **Outcome or resolution stage:** During this stage, if parties negotiate and arrive at a settlement, it may result in positive (functional) or negative (dysfunctional) conflict.

Factors Influencing Conflict

Factors affecting conflict are as follows:
- Rules and procedures or constraints upon the interaction process, such as decision rules and negotiating procedures
- Complex adaptive system (CAS) of the health-care system, and conflict usually occurs at different levels simultaneously
- Differences in knowledge, power, and control experienced by the various disciplines. While most conflicts involve some difference between disciplines
- Work stress that affect employee commitment and the higher level of stress may cause conflict and job dissatisfaction
- The religion and languages differences between clients and health-care providers
- Healthcare involves people interacting with other people and thereby issues about personal or religious values crops up
- Behavioral predispositions viewed as habits
- Social pressures or normative forces on the conflict parties
- Issues concerning workplace safety can also be the factors of conflict between health care workers and the organization
- Individual factors such as emotional intelligence, personality, incompetency, attention deficit affect conflict, conflict management, and commitment to an organization.

Elements of Conflict

Cadotte and Stern (1979) described the following aspects of conflict:
- **Conflict potential:** Conflict potential is the extent that the actions of one party are likely to (or perceived to) hinder the goal attainment of the other.

- **Dependence (or power):** The party determines the level of dependence of one party on another by the value of the inputs invested in the relationship. The level of control is inversely related to the level of dependency between the parties.
- **Conflict perception:** Conflict perception is one party's judgment of whether the other party is interfering with the attainment of its goals. Conflict exists in case of an actual disagreement or dispute.
- **Resultant force:** Resultant force is the pressure that one party uses to persuade the other to change its goals, objectives, and perceptions of reality to meet its desires. It may be either coercive or noncoercive. Coercive pressure frequently causes more disruption in the relationship than does noncoercive force.
- **Conflict aftermath:** It is the outcome of the conflict resolution and directs future interactions between the organizations. This model also incorporates a feedback mechanism by which future conflict episodes are favored or influenced by previous conflict resolution results.

Types of Organizational Conflict

The five types of organizational conflict are as follows:
1. **Intrapersonal conflicts:** These conflicts occur within the individual due to frustration, role conflict, and competing goals. The frustrated individuals behave indifferently and may be antisocial, aggressive, and uncooperative. These may affect the performance of the individual in the workplace.
2. **Interpersonal conflicts:** Interpersonal conflict is the conflict between individuals of the organization. Disputes may arise due to personal differences in education, experiences, cultural background, personality style, or the communication gap in the organization. It may also be due to incompatible roles and work stress caused by competition, workload, lack of resources, etc. in the organization.
3. **Intragroup conflicts:** Intragroup conflict occurs within the group, team, or department. These conflicts involve more than one person in a group due to the inability to conform to group dynamics.
4. **Intergroup conflicts:** Intergroup conflict occurs between different groups, teams, and departments. These disputes arise due to competition for resources, work independence, and status struggle.
5. **Interorganizational conflict:** Interorganizational conflict arises in different organizations to compete against one another.

The primary sources of organizational conflicts are a task, relationship or process.
- **Task conflict:** Task conflicts are commonly occurring in the workplace. These are due to disputes/differences in opinion regarding work assignment, human resources, procedures and policies, organizational goals, functions, and process of working.
- **Relationship conflict:** These are relationship-focused conflicts that occur due to the differences in interpersonal issues in the organization, in the group, or with each other. These are common due to the differences in individual personality, style of working, and attitude.
- **Value conflict:** The value conflicts occur because of the differences in value identity, norms, ethics, and beliefs in the groups. These may occur at the time of making decisions and policies.

Dimensions of Conflict

The aspects of organizational conflicts are negative emotionality, acceptability, the size or scope of the conflict, importance, group communication norms, and resolution potential. Each of these dimensions applies to all types of conflict.
- **Negative emotionality:** The dimension of emotionality refers to the amount of negative affect exhibited and felt during the conflict. It is associated with poor group performance and low member satisfaction. Emotion includes anger, which provides for violence, frustration, uneasiness, discomfort, tenseness, resentment, annoyance, irritation, fury, and rage.
- **Acceptability:** The acceptability dimension refers to group norms about conflict and communication. Group norms are standards that guide group members' behavior. Acceptability norms increased both the positive effect of constructive conflict and the negative impact of destructive conflict on group performance and member satisfaction.
- **The size or scope of conflict:** The nature of conflicts depends on the size or scope of a dispute and its duration. Conflicts are perceived as more dangerous when they involve more significant number of people, more events, or more considerable influence over future interactions.
- **Importance:** Other predictors of group performance, beyond the frequency or number of times conflict episodes occur within groups, are its importance. If the issue is of great importance and vital to the life and success of the group, then it is more dangerous.
- **Group communication norms:** These may also influence the effect of conflict. Groups with open and direct expressions of conflict would be less likely to experience explosive conflict, but at times, can increase the amount of negative and positive conflict within groups.
- **Resolution potential:** Resolution potential refers to the degree to which the conflict appears possible to resolve. It positively influences the constructive effects of conflict on performance and satisfaction and decreases the adverse effect. The main determinants of whether a member perceives conflict as resolvable include characteristics of the members (e.g. experience, personalities), group structure (e.g. interdependence, leader involvement), and dimensions of conflict (importance, emotionality, acceptability).

Impact of Conflict

The Positive Effect of Task-focused Conflict

Task-focused conflicts affect the group and organizational outcomes:
- Improve decision-making outcomes
- Increase group productivity
- Make use of potentials and capabilities of groups
- Encourage discussion that helps groups to perform better.

The Negative Effect of Relationship-focused Conflicts

There is a negative association between relationship conflict, productivity, and satisfaction in groups:
- Relationship conflicts interfere with performance because it may reduce threats, increase power, and attempt to build a relationship rather than working on the task.
- It decreases goodwill and mutual understanding, which hinders in accomplishing organizational tasks.
- Time is often spent on interpersonal aspects of the group rather than on technical and decision-making tasks.
- It may create negative, irritable, suspicious, and resentful members.
- Chronic relationship conflicts may also affect group functioning.
- It led members to lose sight of the mission; and they become more defensive and blame each other.

CONFLICT MANAGEMENT

Different Managerial Styles in Handling Conflicts

Kilmann and Thomas (1974) described five styles to handle conflicts based on two dimensions: assertiveness and cooperativeness **(Fig. 39.2)**.

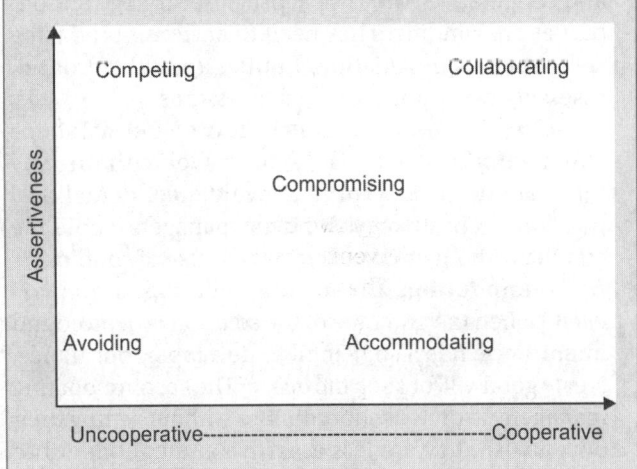

Fig. 39.2: Two-dimensional taxonomy of five conflict-handling modes.

TABLE 39.1: Conflict styles and prospective behaviors.

Conflict styles	Dimensions	Behaviors
Competing: forcing	Assertive and uncooperative	Pursues own concerns at others expense
Collaborating: problem solving	Highly assertive and cooperative	Identify concerns of others, active listener, and have a nonthreatening confrontation
Compromising: sharing	Moderately assertive and cooperative	Partially satisfies both parties
Avoiding: withdrawal	Less assertive and uncooperative	Neither pursues his or her concerns nor those of others
Accommodating: smoothing	Less assertive and highly cooperative	Favors subordinate without setting their own goals

Assertiveness is concerned with satisfying one's concerns, and cooperativeness is when the individual tries to meet others' interests. The emerging styles are competing, accommodating, avoiding, collaborating, and compromising **(Table 39.1)**, which the managers can use according to the situation.

- **Competing:** The competing way is helpful in situations where there is a need to make a quick decision and handle vital issues. The competing managers are highly assertive but uncooperative with subordinates. They make their own decisions without listening to other views. They use arguments, position power, assert feelings, and opinions of subordinates, and have a rationale for their actions. Although it is helpful to increase creativity and enthusiasm, it can lead to violence.
- **Collaborating:** Collaborative mode is useful in a situation involves constructing an integrative solution through compromise, improving the relationship, and having commitment. The collaborative managers are highly assertive and cooperative. They try to use a win–win strategy to solve conflicts. They try to give chance for everyone to participate in emerging into some concrete solution through collaboration actively. The manager needs to have collaboration skills such as active listening, nonthreatening confrontation, identifying concerns, and analyzing inputs. They need to initiate the problem-solving process and should have a high level of commitment. They are highly qualified and knowledgeable to accept responsibility to solve the problem. This type of mode is truly worthy but very difficult to follow. Many of the managers need the training to do it very well.
- **Compromising:** The compromising mode is appropriate in situations while dealing with issues of moderate importance, and both parties have equal power status. It is also suitable to resolve conflicts temporarily due to time constraints or if there is a strong commitment to resolve the dispute. The compromising managers are both moderately assertive

and cooperative. They use a lose–lose strategy or both parties are winning. They need to have compromising skills such as negotiation, finding a middle ground, assessing value, and making concessions.
- **Avoiding:** The avoiding strategy is useful in situations when conflicts are likely to solve without any intervention. It is a form of avoidance, denial and postponement strategy. Avoiding managers ignore the conflict without intervening in the cause of conflict.
- **Accommodating:** The accommodating strategy is useful when the outcome of the solution is of profound importance. It is also helpful to develop performance, create goodwill, or keep the peace. The accommodating managers favor their subordinates without setting their own goals. They are less assertive and confident but highly cooperative. It is useful to resolve the problem immediately; but in the long run, it may create a problem. They need to have accommodating skills such as forgetting desires, selflessness, and ability to obey orders.

Steps in Conflict Management

According to *Borisoff* and Victor, **one needs to take five steps to manage conflict, which they called the "five A's."**
1. **Assessment:** This step involves the identification of the problem. In this stage, the manager gathers the information about the problem from the parties. It will help them to decide the conflict-handling mode.
2. **Acknowledgment:** The next step is acknowledgment. During this step, both parties listen to each other, understand, and acknowledge each other's viewpoints.
3. **Attitude:** During this stage, the parties do realize that fundamental differences are observed between people based on culture, intelligence levels, gender, and other factors.
4. **Action:** The parties begin to find a way to correct the problem by discussing the options/alternatives.
5. **Analysis:** During this stage, the parties agree on the solution they choose. They summarize all the information and decide on a solution.

Conflict Management/Resolution Strategies

Conflict management is essential to resolve conflicts, though all disputes cannot necessarily be determined. Conflict management techniques depend on the problem source. Following are the management strategies:
1. **By modifying task relationships:**
    - *Organizational restructuring:* Try to analyze the problem, and if it is found that the issues are related to organizational structure such as in communication, hierarchical relationship, or in reporting, try to modify the structural variables to reduce the communication and measurability problems.
    - *Increasing integration:* To overcome disputes related to resources and subunit orientations, integrate processes such as task forces, teams, and individual roles.
    - *Change in hierarchy and decentralizing authority:* Use democratic leadership and top-bottom approach to involve employees in decision-making and make them accountable. Conflict reduces because employees know their superiors.
2. **Organize in-service training on conflict and conflict management:** All health-care institutions must organize in-service training programs on conflict and conflict management for health-care providers. It should be a part of their training. Training must include basic conflict principles and approaches and practical skill practice on conflict resolution skills such as in negotiation, mediation, and facilitation.
3. **Improve communication skills:** Communication is at the heart of conflict and conflict resolution. The health-care providers must use active listening by hearing, understanding, repeating, or reframing what the other person is saying. Ensure that another person must understand the message clearly.
4. **Understand different communication styles and responses to conflict:** It is crucial to understand different methods of communication, especially during the conflict resolution stage. During that stage, every individual may respond differently, particularly, in response to stressful situations.
5. **Modify the behavior and attitude of individuals:** Each differs in their perception, attitude, and values; they react differently in different situations. The employees working in various divisions and functions have different ideas about accomplishing organizational goals. Managers can use the following ways to modify their behaviors:
    - Be proactive instead of reactive
    - Control anger especially over unimportant issues
    - Try to make people realize their mistakes indirectly
    - Admit mistakes and poor decisions if taken
    - Develop a conducive environment to allow parties to share their grievances
    - Develop a system to resolve the conflict between management and unions
    - Use a third-party negotiator
    - Make a policy to exchange/rotate/terminate individuals.
6. **"Four R's" of conflict resolution:** According to Engleberg and Wynn, "four R's" used to manage conflict are as follows:
    i. *Reason out:* Find out the reason or the cause of the conflict. Try to focus on conflict, don't get involved emotionally and gather detailed information about the problem.
    ii. *Observe reactions:* After gathering information, observe the response of the parties involved in the conflict. Try to analyze the attitudes, either destructive or positive, to conflict. If devastating, try to work with them to convert into positive responses to conflict.

iii. *Results*: Try to find out the consequences of the conflict that remain unresolved and pro and cons of managing conflict.
iv. *Work on resolution:* Decide alternatives strategies to resolve the conflict based on the cause. Select the best strategy/conflict management behavior to resolve the dispute, so that both parties do not lose. Consider relationship building, the importance of conflict, consequences, readiness of the parties, and outcomes of disengagement. The resolution must be specific, mutually acceptable, appropriate, realistic, and time based.

CHAPTER HIGHLIGHTS

- Conflict is a social situation where two parties have differences in their attitudes, values, and opinions that may affect the achievement of their goals.
- The five main stages of conflict process are latent, perceived, felt, manifest, and aftermath conflict stage.
- Many personal and organizational factors contribute to initiating conflicts that have either positive or negative effects on organizational performance.
- Conflicts may be intrapersonal, interpersonal, intergroup, intragroup, or interorganizational.
- Depending on the nature of disputes, managers use different managerial styles, procedures, and strategies in handling conflicts.

REVIEW QUESTIONS

I. Essay Type Questions
1. Define organizational conflict. Describe in detail conflict process.
2. Discuss the different types of organizational conflicts.
3. Explain various dimensions of conflicts.
4. What are the different styles that managers can use to handle organizational conflicts?
5. Describe in detail various strategies managers can use to resolve conflicts.

II. Short Notes
1. Factors contributing to conflicts
2. Elements of conflicts
3. Positive and negative effects of conflicts
4. Four R's of conflict resolution

III. Multiple Choice Questions
1. The stage at which many factors influence the possibility of conflict is:
   a. Latent   b. Perceived
   c. Felt   d. Manifest
2. The stage at which none of the party wants to resolve the dispute is:
   a. Emergence   b. Escalation
   c. Crisis   d. Negotiation
3. Which one of the following is the feature of the "aftermath stage" of conflict?
   a. Both parties try to find out the source and reason for conflict
   b. Both parties do not reach to conclusion and conflict remains unsolved
   c. Both parties respond emotionally to each other
   d. Both parties try to get back at each other
4. Which of the following style do managers use when they are highly assertive and cooperative?
   a. Competing
   b. Compromising
   c. Collaborating
   d. Accommodating
5. At what stage in conflict management, both parties listen and try to understand each other's viewpoints?
   a. Assessment   b. Analysis
   c. Attitude   d. Acknowledgment

Answer Keys
1. a   2. c   3. b   4. c   5. d

SUGGESTED READING

1. Managing and Resolving Conflict in a Team - UK Essays. Available from (online) https://www.ukessays.com/essays/management/managing-and-resolving-conflict-in-a-team-management-essay.php. [Accessed Jan 2020].
2. Baker KM. Improving staff nurse conflict resolution skills. Nurs Econ. 1995;13:295-317.
3. Blake RR, Mouton JS. Solving Costly Organization Conflict. San Francisco, CA: Jossey-Bass; 1964.
4. Borisoff D, and Victor DA. Conflict Management: A Communication Skills Approach. 2nd ed. Boston: Allyn and Bacon, 1998.
5. Cadotte ER, and Stem LW. A Process Model of Interorganizational Relations in Marketing Channels 1979. (Cross reference) in Research in Marketing, Vol. II, Jagdish Sheth, ed., Greenwich, Conn.: JAI Press, 1979.127-158. Available (online) https://journals.sagepub.com › doi › pdf.
6. Dalton DR, William DT, Michael JS, et al. Organization structure and performance: A critical review. Acad Manag Rev. 1980;5:49-64.
7. Dotun O, Fong S, Elmore G, Korwin D, and Azziz R. The associations between residents' behavior and the Thomas-Kilmann Conflict MODE Instrument. Journal of Graduate Medical Education March 2010; 2(1):118-25.[online] Available from https://www.jgme.org/doi/full/10.4300/JGME-D-09-00048.1. [Accessed Jan 2020].
8. Fink CF. Some conceptual difficulties in the theory of social conflict. Journal of Conflict Resolution 1968; 12(4), 412–60. Available from (online) https://doi.org/10.1177/002200276801200402. [Accessed Jan 2020].
9. Fontaine D, Gerardi D. Healthier hospitals? Nurs Manag. 2005;36(10):34-44.
10. Lewicki RJ, Stephen EW, David L. Models of conflict, negotiation, and third-party intervention: A review and synthesis. J Organ Behav. 1992;113:209-52.

11. Mack RW, and Snyder RC. The analysis of social conflict—toward an overview and synthesis. Available from (online) https://doi.org/10.1177/002200275700100208. [Accessed Jan 2020].
12. Pinkley RL. Dimensions of conflict frame: Disputant interpretations of the conflict. J Appl Psychol. 1990;75:117-26.
13. Pondy LR. Organizational conflict: Concepts and models. Adm Sci Q. 1967;12:296-320.
14. Spector PE. Introduction: Conflict in organizations. J Organ Behav. 2008;29:3-4.
15. Steven L, King JA. Managing conflict constructively in program evaluation. Evaluation. 2005;11(4):415.
16. The five stages of conflict | eHow.com. [online] Available from http://www.ehow.com/info_8070222_five-stages-conflict.html#ixzz1JZLnBfV0 by Sage Kalmus, eHow. [Accessed March 2011].
17. The Thomas-Kilmann Model-Conflict Resolution. Available from (online) http://www.managetrainlearn.com/page/conflict-resolution-model. [Accessed Jan 2020].
18. Thomas KW. Conflict and conflict management. In: Dunnette MD (Ed). Handbook of Industrial and Organizational Psychology. Chicago, IL: Rand-McNally; 1976. pp. 889-935.
19. Wall JA, Ronda RC. Conflict and its management. J Manag. 1995;3:515-58.

40 CHAPTER

Collective Bargaining, Unions, and Professional Associations

CHAPTER OUTLINE

- Collective Bargaining
  - Defining Collective Bargaining
  - Objectives of Collective Bargaining
  - Focus of Collective Bargaining in Nursing
  - Characteristics of Collective Bargaining
  - Process of Collective Bargaining
  - Merits and Demerits of Collective Bargaining
  - Types of Collective Bargaining
- Role of Trained Nurses Association of India in Bargaining and Policies for Strike
- Health-care Laws
- Employee Unions
- Professional Associations

LEARNING OUTCOMES

After completion of this chapter, the learner will be able to:
- Recall and understand the concept and process of collective bargaining
- Discuss the objectives and characteristics of collective bargaining
- Enlist merits and demerits of collective bargaining
- Explain various types of collective bargaining
- Discuss TNAI role in negotiation and policies
- Describe different health-care labor laws
- Define employees' unions and professional associations
- Enumerate features and objectives of unions and associations
- Discuss the legal status and growth of associations in India

KEY TERMS

Collective bargaining, health-care labor laws, employees' unions, professional associations, legal status

INTRODUCTION

In India, the concept of collective bargaining as trade unions was conceived in the 20th century and attained its significance after 1962. The term "collective" in the collective negotiations applies to employers and employees as they come together and put a joint effort to establish mutually agreeable terms and conditions for employment. The phrase "collective bargaining" was coined by Sydney, Beatrice, and Webb, while Great Britain is known as the "home of collective bargaining." Negotiation is the process of cajoling, debating, discussing, and even threatening to reach to a concrete agreement among the representing parties.

Due to rapid social change and dissatisfaction with values and norms, the nurses are also striving toward collective bargaining to meet their professional and personal needs. Although a professional association has represented the nursing profession, say the Trained Nurses Association of India since 1908, interest in labor unions is increasing due to administrative practices that support investment in labor unions.

COLLECTIVE BARGAINING

Defining Collective Bargaining

- Collective bargaining is a process of negotiation that involves a set of procedures by which employee representatives and employer representatives negotiate to obtain a signed agreement that describes conditions of employment, especially wages, hours, and benefits.
- The National Association of Manufacturers (USA) defined collective bargaining as a process by which management and labor may explore each other's problems and viewpoints to develop a framework of employment relations for their mutual benefit.

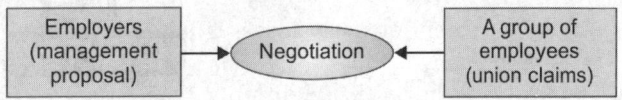

Fig. 40.1: Process of collective bargaining.

- Collective bargaining is a process of a cooperative agreement between the representative of both employers and employees to regulate working conditions and employment-related issues **(Fig. 40.1)**.
- Collective bargaining is a technique or a procedure adopted by unions and management for compromising their conflicting interests.
- Collective bargaining in nursing is the procedure opted by nurses to reach a cooperative agreement regarding employment terms and rights, and the duties are known as collective bargaining. Collective bargaining aims to resolve issues about wages, working conditions, health and safety, and working hours of nurses. These may be a useful tool to gain control over nursing practice and to attain professional, personal, and economic goals (Breda, 1997).

Objectives of Collective Bargaining

- To reach an agreement on issues related to employment, status, administrative matters such as working conditions and safety, wages, salary, autonomy, staffing, benefits, cadre, promotions, etc.
- To maintain employee–employer relation bilaterally
- To protect the interests of employees through a joint effort
- To negotiate voluntarily to gain mutual benefits and loss by both sides
- To resolve the differences between employees and management through negotiation.

Focus of Collective Bargaining in Nursing

There are many reasons that nurses start bargaining collectively at the organizational, local, state, and national levels. In India, nurses have associations at the national, state, and local level in the service side as well as in teaching team. The committees formulated to discuss issues such as cadre, staffing, and working conditions. Salary, benefits, and working conditions were the primary focus of collective bargaining. But in recent times, negotiation extended to almost all aspects of employee–employer relations, thereby covering a large area. The focus of collective bargaining in nursing is as follows:
- Union recognition and scope of the agreement
- Management rights
- Union security
- Strikes and lockouts
- Activities and responsibilities
- Career, wages, salary structure
- Working conditions
- Job rights and seniority

- Discipline
- Promotions
- Grievances handling
- Health and safety.

Characteristics of Collective Bargaining

1. **Bipartite process:** It is a two-way process where the employees' and employers' representatives negotiate directly.
2. **Equality:** Both the parties in the collective negotiations should maintain balance.
3. **Voluntarily negotiation:** Both parties negotiate freely to go bargaining. They have discussions, mutual trust, and understanding.
4. **Formal process:** It is a legal process to regulate specific employment-related issues at the national and organizational levels.
5. **Flexible:** It is an ongoing and flexible activity.
6. **Improvement:** It aims to improve the employer–employee relationship in the organization to resolve specific conflicts.
7. **Representation:** It takes place between the representatives of employees and employers.
8. **Dynamic:** Collective bargaining is progressive and continues to change over a period and grows and expands the way of agreement.
9. **Continuous:** Collective bargaining is an ongoing process, which begins with the agreement and goes on negotiating.

Process of Collective Bargaining

Collective bargaining is a process of several activities and comprises seven main steps, including enforcement of agreement **(Fig. 40.2)**:
1. **Preparatory phase:** During the preliminary period, identify negotiation teams. The negotiation teams

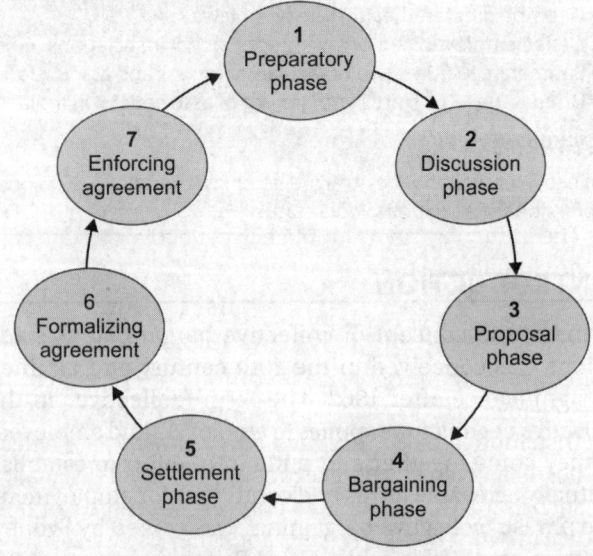

Fig. 40.2: Collective bargaining process.

must be representatives of both the parties. The parties should have the knowledge and skills to discuss and negotiate. The team must identify the exact problem, gather relevant information related to the topic, and examine the situation and issues for negotiation before the discussion.
2. **Discussion phase:** Set an appropriate time and make a conducive environment for negotiation. Have discussions. Maintain mutual trust and understanding. Both parties must have good listening skills, ask questions, observe, and summarize.
3. **Proposal phase:** The proposal phase starts with the initial opening of statements. Both parties discuss and brainstorm to decide possible options to resolve issues.
4. **Bargaining phase:** During the bargaining phase, both parties try to solve problems.
5. **Settlement phase:** During the settlement phase, both parties have a consensus to agree on a joint decision and negotiated change.
6. **Formalizing the agreement:** After agreeing upon, draft a formal document of agreement. It should be simple, clear, and concise. Both parties sign the final deal and abide by its terms and conditions.
7. **Enforcing the agreement:** To have the deal valid and meaning, enforce or implement it immediately.

Merits and Demerits of Collective Bargaining

Merits

- It provides an opportunity to negotiate regarding professional and employment issues.
- It promotes employees' democracy and their participation with management.
- It helps in maintaining a harmonious relationship between the employee and the employer.
- It emphasizes on the interests and benefits of employees and management.
- It eliminates unnecessary expenditure and avoids bitterness among employees and management.

Demerits

- The collective bargaining process may not be always fair.
- Power and politics often influence the decision.
- The immediate consequence of collective bargaining if not fulfilled is strike or lockout.

Types of Collective Bargaining

Collective bargaining consists of four types, which are listed below:
1. **Distributive or conjunctive bargaining:** It is a type of negotiation that takes up economic issues for discussion, such as wages, salaries, and bonuses. It is more competitive in which one party gains and other party loses.
2. **Integrative or cooperative bargaining:** In an integrative type of negotiation, both parties may gain, or at least neither party loses. It tends to be more cooperative.
3. **Productive bargaining:** In this type of talk, the management has control over the employee–employer relationship. Substantial benefits are measured based on productivity standards.
4. **Composite bargaining:** A kind of negotiation wherein both parties agree on wages with equity.

Role of Trained Nurses Association of India in Bargaining and Policies for Strike

According to the Trained Nurses Association of India (TNAI), it cannot legally act as a negotiating body because its members include nurses working in government, private, and voluntary organizations. To settle issues, nurses working in different organizations joined the associations of paramedical and followed their terms and conditions. But with the time, nurses had their associations. The TNAI formulated the following bargaining guidelines and policies:

- **Formulation of grievances committee:** The TNAI members must formulate a grievances committee comprising nurses of various cadres after consulting the government, either union/state or employing agencies. The primary purpose of expressing this type of committee is to solve local, personal, or professional issues.
- **Formulation of the committee at the state level:** At the state level, there should be a committee that must comprise of state-level representative nurses and a representative from TNAI. The purpose of this committee is to act as an arbitrator to deal with the cases referred by the local grievances committee.
- **Recognizing organizations and nurses association as negotiating bodies:** The TNAI members help the organization and nurses' association to fight for their rights through collective bargaining and create opportunities through their executive committees at the state level. In collaboration with the nurses associations at the state level and TNAI, the state branch may allow nurses to go on strike under specific terms and conditions.

HEALTH-CARE LAWS

Introduction

According to dictionary, law is a rule of conduct established by an authority able to enforce its will. It is a controlling regulation to which an agent or power acts. The health-care laws are rules applied to patients, health-care providers, payers, and vendors of health-care organizations. These laws are concerning with the health of the individuals and population at large. Health-care laws are in the form of statutory requirements, contract laws, medical malpractice, medical laws, administrative laws, regulatory laws, public health laws, and consent. These are related to practice, client, and health-care providers.

These laws form the legal framework for health that governs the rights and responsibilities of the government, health-care providers, society, and the population at large. Based on these health-care laws, health organizations and institutions make strategies, policies, and mandates. These guide them to commit to achieving health-care goals and create a drive for their actions. These act as the boundaries as to what an organization and individuals should do and what should not be done.

Purposes

Health-care laws help to achieve the following:
1. Establish and meet the health policy and its goals
2. Safeguard health issues of the public at large
3. Provide occupation safety and health at work
4. Protect people from infectious diseases
5. Create and establish a health system structure
6. Establish a health institution, its mandate, duties, and responsibilities
7. Enforce and maintain health-care practice standards
8. Regulate health services and health institutions
9. Set and maintain the standards of health training institutions
10. Protect the rights of consumers
11. Monitor the safety and efficacy of pharmaceuticals and devices
12. Gather and preserve the health information data.

Health-care Laws in India

In India, there are various health-care laws that relate to the following **(Table 40.1)**:
1. Commissioning of the hospitals, e.g. Society Registration Act (1960)
2. Qualification, practice, and conduct of health professionals, e.g. Medical Council Act (1956), the Indian Nursing Council Act (1947)
3. Storage and sale of drugs and safety and efficacy of medications, e.g. Drug and Cosmetic Act, 1945 (Amendment, 1982)
4. Biomedical Research, e.g. Breeding of and Experiments on Animals (Amendment) Rules (2005)
5. Management of Patients, e.g. Pre-Natal Diagnostic Techniques (PNDT) Act (1994), Medical Termination of Pregnancy (MTP) Act (1997)
6. Medicolegal aspect, e.g. Consumer Protection Act (1986)
7. Safety of patients, public, and staff, e.g. Biomedical Waste Management Handling Rules (1998 and 2000), Environment Protection Act (1986)
8. Employment of manpower, e.g. ESI Act (1948), Maternity Benefit (Amendment) Act (2008), Indian Trade Union Act (1926)
9. Professional training and research, e.g. Indian Nursing Council Rules for starting colleges and schools
10. Business aspects of hospital, e.g. Charitable and Religious Trust Act (1920), Contract Act (1967).

TABLE 40.1: Health-care laws in India.

S.No.	Health-care laws
1.	Andhra Pradesh Medical Practitioners registration (Amendments) Act, 1968
2.	Andhra Pradesh Allopathic Private Medical Care Establishments (Registration and Regulation) Rules, 2007
3.	Andhra Pradesh Medical Practitioners (Amendments) Registration Act, 1986
4.	Arbitration and Conciliation Act, 1996
5.	Consumers Protection Act, 1986
6.	Constitution of India (Article 19, 32, 226, etc.)
7.	Companies Act, 1956
8.	Consumers Protection (Amendment) Act, 2002
9.	Contract Labour (Regulation and Abolition) Act, 1970
10.	Factories Act, 1948
11.	Industrial Dispute Act, 1947
12.	Indian Medical Council Act and Amendment Acts
13.	Indian Medical Central Council (Amendment) Act, 2002
14.	IMC (Professional conduct, Etiquette and Ethics) Regulation, 2002
15.	Indian Contract Act
16.	Indian Partnership Act
17.	Indian Panel Code, 1860 (Chapter XIV—offenses affecting the public health, safety, convenience, decency, and morals)
19.	Medical Termination of Pregnancy (Amendment) Act, 2002
20.	Transplantation of Human Organ Act, 1994 (Bare Act) and Transplantation of Human Organ (Amendment) Rule, 2002
21.	Payment of Gratuity Act, 1972
22.	Payment of Wages (Amendment) Act, 2005
23.	Narcotic Drugs and Psychotropic Substances Act, 1985
24.	Narcotic Drugs and Psychotropic Substances (Amendment) Act, 2005
25.	Registration of Births and Deaths Act, 1969
26.	Workmen Compensation Act, 1923
27.	Workmen Compensation (Amendment) Act, 2000

EMPLOYEE UNIONS

Employee associations and unions are part of human resource administration. Unions and associations are nothing but the organizations of employees formed to promote and protect their interests through collective action.

Trade union is the employee's association formulated to achieve specific purposes to advance and protect the interests of its members. Webb, Sidney, and Beatrice viewed it as a wage earners' association formed to maintain and improve the working conditions of its employees. Trade union is a formal association to protect the interests of its members through collective actions.

Features of Unions

The five main features of unions are as follows.
1. It is an association of employees.
2. It is relatively permanent.
3. It secures certain economic and social benefits to members.

4. Its focus is on joint, coordinated action and collective bargaining.
5. It regulates the relationship between employees and management.

Objectives of Unions

- To bargain for wages and salaries
- To insist on the compensation for the work per the nature of the job
- To see the minimum payments paid to the employees
- To ensure that deserving employees get due promotions
- To ensure adequate retirement benefit provisions to meet employee's financial needs for the rest of the life
- To fight for the provision of proper working place, weekend holidays, sick leaves, free medical aid, etc.
- To negotiate to improve the social conditions within the services and to improve the human relations within the organization
- To fight against improper implementation of personnel policies in respect of recruitment, selection, promotions, transfers, training, etc.
- To work as a guide, consulting authority, and negotiating machinery in overcoming the personal problems of members
- To safeguard the organizational health through various methods evolved for grievance redressing and techniques adopted to reduce absenteeism, turnover, and improve employee relations.

Purposes

- To solve the problems of the employees
- To secure better wages and working conditions
- To enhancement of self-respect and dignity
- To fulfill social needs and stability of employment and other issues during service.

Legal Status and Growth of Employees' Associations/Unions in India

- Articles 19 and 309 of the Indian Constitution are concerned with the legal status of public employees' associations. The employees' organizations in government are usually active from the postindependent period. The Amalgamated Society of Railway Servants of India and Burma (1897) formed by the Anglo-Indians and domiciled Europeans employed in railways who established the association of public employees to seek the redress of grievances.
- The Indian Civil Service Association came into being in 1918.
- In 1922, the All India Railway Men's Federation was formed and soon after Postal and Telegraphs Employees Union formed.
- After the First World War, Mahatma Gandhi and his followers aspired the civil servants to establish the associations.
- International Labour Organization (1919) gave the impetus of the establishment of more unions and associations.
- Employees' organizations were formed after the formation of the All India Trade Union Congress and the enhancement of Trade Union Act, 1926.
- In 1937, many conditions were prescribed for an association of civil servants.

PROFESSIONAL ASSOCIATIONS

Introduction

A professional association is a body of persons that brings together members of the same profession to exchange information and experiences professionally to keep the members updated and to advance their profession. It is a professional organization where a group of persons of the same profession comes together to facilitate the achievement of specific purposes.

Nursing Welfare Association, Nursing Teachers Association, Trained Nurses Association of India, Student Nurses Association are examples of a professional association in nursing.

Features of a Professional Association

1. Members engage in the same profession.
2. It facilitates to achieve specific purposes especially providing services.
3. It controls the entry in the profession and maintains its standard.
4. It represents the profession in discussion with other association/bodies.
5. It expresses the interest of professional members and the public.
6. It concerns the career advancement of its members and profession.
7. It has a legal identity and is recognized by the government.
8. It can enter into agreements and is responsible for its actions.
9. It grants designation and certification.
10. It should provide structure and governance to the profession.

Objectives of Professional Associations

1. To provide a shared vision and purpose to the profession.
2. To promote a sense of commitment and motivation to its members.
3. To develop a sense of ownership for their actions.
4. To provide a platform for discussions and to exchange the ideas and experiences about the profession.
5. To establish a common viewpoint regarding practice and standards of the profession.
6. To give a voice to the profession by organizing workshops, conferences, and meetings.

7. To ensure professional credibility and power.
8. To emphasize professional development by organizing continuing education and development programs.
9. To develop and implement professional regulation and standards to protect the public at large.
10. To produce skilled and competent professionals who can provide a high standard of care by reviewing the curriculum.
11. To have a link with the consumers, policy makers, the government, and health professionals.
12. To increase its membership by adopting various leadership strategies.

According to LD White, the objectives of professional associations are as follows:
- To promote personal acquaintance among individuals with shared interests and problems
- To give suggestions for improvement and advancement
- To encourage research in the profession by organizing a periodical conference for the exchange of ideas and experience, so that the best intentions may be selected and applied to improve the efficiency of the administration
- To issue literature for the spread of the latest information relating to their field
- To bring the employees nearer to those to whom they can confide for their failure and successes
- To disseminate professional knowledge among many people and stimulate joint and individual research and help in solving problems about the profession
- To bring efficiency and boost the morale of its members
- To promote and protect the interests of members
- To develop and train staff and members
- To obtain data on wages and conditions of work
- To deal with safety and health at the workplace and working environment
- To initiate steps to improve public image and public relations.

Types of Professional Associations

According to Balthazard, the four types of professional associations are as follows:
1. **Member-benefit professional associations:** These associations exist to serve the benefits and interests of its members. The focus is to create value for the members and abide by a code of ethics. It is the platform to discuss, exchange information, and advocate on behalf of members. But it lacks legitimacy status.
2. **Designation-granting professional associations:** These associations exist to serve the interest of its members and grant one or more designation per their qualification. The certification is not the purpose of the association; instead, members have the right to use the name.
3. **Certifying bodies:** These associations provide certification to those having established qualifications and serving the interest of the members. These may or may not protect the investment of the public.
4. **Professional regulatory bodies:** Professional regulatory bodies are the professional association that serves the interest of both the profession and the public at large. These have legal status and authority delegated by law. It develops and establishes the standards of qualification, practice standards, and conduct. It has a professional code of ethics and regulation for the members. These are also certified bodies and grant certification for the requirement to practice. Indian Nursing Council and the State Nursing Council are the examples of such professional regulatory bodies.

Professional Association Versus Employee Unions

Both professional association and employee unions are working to achieve the same goal, i.e. to raise the professional status and welfare but with differences in its nature, priorities, approaches, etc. A professional association and an employee union/association differ in many ways **(Table 40.2)**.

When they work together, both professional associations and employee unions may help in achieving the goal of the nursing profession. They seem to be the two sides of the same coin, comprising interest in job, working for the welfare of nurses; to raise the profession status, more work autonomy, cadre, service conditions, anomalies of pay scales, career opportunity, shortage of nursing personnel, lack of equipment and supplies, working conditions, and allied matters pertaining to nursing profession.

CHAPTER HIGHLIGHTS

- Collective bargaining is a negotiating process between the representatives of employers and employees to regulate working conditions and other issues.
- It is bipartite, flexible, and a formal ongoing process where both parties negotiate freely to resolve specific conflicts.
- The process is to undergo various phases before reaching the agreement and enforcement of arbitration.
- It may be of distributive, integrative, productive, or composite type based on its outcome.
- Trained Nurses Association of India formulated the bargaining guidelines and policies.
- The health-care laws are rules applied to patients, health-care providers, payers, and vendors of health-care organizations. Based on these health-care laws, health organizations and institutions make strategies, policies, and mandates.
- Employee unions are the associations or organizations of employees formed to promote and protect their interests by collective action.

Chapter 40: Collective Bargaining, Unions, and Professional Associations

TABLE 40.2: Differences between a professional association and employee unions/association.

Employee unions/association	Professional association
Regulates relation between its member employees and their employers/management	Represents the Interest of its members to the profession and the public, to government, employers, or other agencies
Deals with work-related rights or issues of employees at institutional-specific levels	Advocates interest of the profession, deals with issues of broader scale, and also takes up an institutional-specific level
Takes an active role in working life ➤ Negotiates for better pay, benefits, promotion, institutional-related working problems ➤ Handle and bargain grievances with management/employer ➤ Helps members with issues arising at the workplace ➤ Represents all employees' members under its authority	Preserves professional standards ➤ Supports the development of social support ➤ Promotes research and studies ➤ Disseminates information through journals, newsletters, conferences, workshops, seminars, etc. ➤ Has a good network with other agencies, associations and through journal subscriptions ➤ Establishes a standard code of conduct, policies for the improvement of the profession
Uses more aggressive methods	Uses dynamic methods of negotiations and bargaining
Openly negotiates the interest of employees' rights, demands, grievances, needs, privileges, salary, hours of work, working conditions, etc.	Indirectly confers the benefit of employees' rights, claims, complaints, obligations, and opportunities to raise professional status and welfare

- A professional association is an organization where a group of persons of the same profession comes together to facilitate the achievement of specific purposes.

REVIEW QUESTIONS

I. Essay Type Questions
1. Define collective bargaining. Discuss its characteristics.
2. Describe the process of collective bargaining.
3. Define health-care laws. Describe its purposes.
4. What are the characteristics of professional association?
5. Discuss the role of TNAI in collective bargaining.

II. Short Notes
1. Merits and demerits of collective bargaining
2. Types of collective bargaining
3. Employee union
4. Types of professional association

III. Multiple Choice Questions
1. Which phase of collective bargaining starts with the initial opening of a statement to decide possible options?
   a. Preparatory   b. Proposal
   c. Bargaining   d. Settlement
2. Name the type of negotiation in which both the parties may gain.
   a. Integrative   b. Distributive
   c. Productive   d. Composite
3. The Consumer Protection Act (1986) relates to which one of the following health-care law?
   a. Commission of hospitals
   b. Management of patients
   c. Business aspects of hospital
   d. Medicolegal aspect
4. Which type of professional associations exists to serve the interest of its members and has the right to its name?
   a. Member benefit
   b. Certifying bodies
   c. Designation granting
   d. Regulatory bodies
5. In which year the Indian Civil Service Association came into being?
   a. 1918   b. 1919
   c. 1922   d. 1926

Answer Keys

1. b   2. a   3. d   4. c   5. a

SUGGESTED READING

1. Aiken LH, Havens DS, Sloane DM. The magnet nursing services recognition program. AJN. 2000;100(3):26-35.
2. Balthazard C. The four types of professional organizations. Human Resources Professional Association, 2017. Available (online) https://www.hrpa.ca/Documents/Regulation/LinkedIn-Articles/01-The-four-types-of-professional-organizations.pdf. [Accessed July 2019].
3. Bloom JR, Parlette GN, O'Reilly CA. Collective bargaining by nurses: a comparative analysis of management and employee perceptions. Health Care Manage Rev. 1980;5(1):25-33.
4. Breda KL. Professional nurses in unions: Working together pays off. Journal of Professional Nursing March-April 1997; 13(2): 99-102. Available from (online) https://doi.org/10.1016/S8755-7223(97)80010-5. [Accessed June 2019].
5. Budd K, Warren L, Patton M. Traditional, and Non-traditional Collective Bargaining strategies to improve the patient care environment. OJIN 2004; 9(1): Manuscript 5. Available from (online) http://ojin.nursingworld.org/MainMenuCategories/ANAMarketplace/ANAPeriodicals/OJIN/TableofContents/Volume92004/No1Jan04/CollectiveBargainingStrategies.aspx. [Accessed Jan 2020].
6. Buerhaus PI. Economic pressures building in the hospital employed RN labor market. Nurs Econ. 1995;13(3):137-41.
7. Buerhaus PI. Shortages of hospital registered nurses: causes and perspectives on public and private sector actions. Nurs Outlook. 2002;50(1):4-6.
8. Bureau of Labor Statistics—Wikipedia. (n.d.). [online] Available from https://en.wikipedia.org/wiki/Bureau_of_Labor_Statistics. [Accessed Jan 2020].

9. Friedlander R. Stress, self-esteem, and well-being among female health professionals: a randomized clinical trial on the impact of a self-care intervention mediated by the senses. PLoS One. 2017;12(2):e0172455.
10. Functions of a Professional Association. Available from (online) www.strongprofassoc.org › uploads › 2016/05 › PAS-Module-4-May2016. [Accessed July 2019].
11. Legislation & Common Law: Indian Legal System. (n.d.). [online] Available from http://www.legalservicesindia.com/article/587/Legislation-&-Common-Law-:-Ind.
12. Our Legal World—All About Law: Indian Bare Acts—Central … (n.d.). [online] Available from https://www.ourlegalworld.com/2019/03/indian-bare-acts-central-and-states-laws.h.
13. Ramaswamy EA, Ramaswamy U. Industrial and labour. New Delhi, India: Oxford; 1981.
14. Reproductive - Center for Reproductive Rights. Available from (online)https://reproductiverights.org/sites/default/files/documents/RRareHR_final.pdf. [Accessed Jan 2020].
15. Useche S, Ruiz J, Vanegas C, Sanmartin J, Alfaro E. Workplace burnout and health issues among Colombian correctional officers. PLoS One. 2019;14(2):e0211447.
16. WHO | Health laws Available from (online) https://www.who.int/health-laws/legal-systems/health-laws/en/. [Accessed July 2019].
17. Yoder D. Personnel management and industrial relations. Prentice-Hall; 1972.

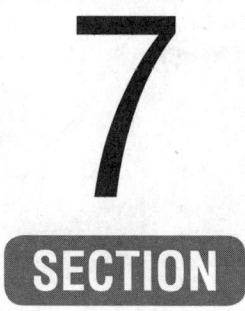

Organizational Behavior and Human Relations

41. Fundamentals of Organizational Behavior, Human Relations, Public Relations, Publicity, and Public Education
42. Group, Group Formation, and Group Dynamics
43. Power, Organizational Politics, Lobbying, and Advocacy
44. Team Management and Time Management

41 CHAPTER

Fundamentals of Organizational Behavior, Human Relations, Public Relations, Publicity, and Public Education

CHAPTER OUTLINE

- Organizational Behavior
  - Concept and Meaning
  - Importance and Scope
  - Organizational Behavior Models
- Human Relations
  - Defining Human Relations
  - Areas of Human Relations
  - Elements of Human Relations
  - Prerequisites for Good Human Relations
  - Principles of Human Relations Approach
  - Advantages of Good Human Relations
  - Role of the Nurse Manager to Develop Human Relations
- Public Relations
  - Concept of Public Relations
  - Nature of Public Relations
  - General Consideration
  - Aims of Public Relations
  - Functions of Public Relations
  - Advantages of Public Relations
  - Elements of Public Relations
  - Factors affecting Hospital Public Image
  - Organizing Public Relations Program
- Publicity and Public Education
  - Definitions
  - Characteristics of Publicity
  - Purposes of Publicity and Public Education
  - Means of Publicity and Public Education
  - Nurses, Role in Improving Hospital Public Relations

LEARNING OUTCOMES

After completion of this chapter, the learner will be able to:
- Understand the concept of organizational behavior
- Appreciate the significance and scope of organizational behavior
- Describe various models of organizational behavior
- Recall and understand the idea of human relations and public relations
- Discuss the elements of human relations and public relations
- Describe the principles of human relations
- Enlist the advantages of human relations and public relations
- Discuss the role of the nurse manager to develop a human relationship
- Discuss the aims and functions of public relations
- Enumerate factors affecting hospital public image
- Organize a public relations program
- Describe the characteristics and means of publicity
- Discuss the role of nurses in improving hospital public relations

KEY TERMS
Organizational behavior, human relations, self-disclosure, public relations, publicity, public education, public image

INTRODUCTION

Organizational behavior (OB), human relations, and public relations are vital aspects to any organization, especially in the present scenario of technical and modern advancement. Organizational behavior of an organization depends on its philosophy, values, vision, goals, and corporate culture, and its processes such as leadership, communication, group dynamics, quality of work life, and the motivation level of employees.

Human relations skills are essential for the nurse managers working in the hospitals to effectively work as group members and build cooperative effort within the team he or she leads. Moreover, the human element works miracles in increasing efficiency and production as a result of the right relationship with the employees. It helps to bring about productivity, a work culture, the essence of responsibility, and accountability.

Public relations refers to building, bridging, and establishing rapport with general public. Public relations professionals in both private and public sectors serve as advocates for service and profit motive by maintaining a positive relationship with the public and recognizing the growing importance of good public relations to the success of their organization.

ORGANIZATIONAL BEHAVIOR

Organization behavior (OB) has its evolution since 1800 by Robert Owen, the father of personnel management, who first emphasized the importance of the human needs of the employees in the organization. In 1835, Andrew Ure added the value of the human factor by providing welfare facilities and other compensations to workers. Later, in 1990s William Gilbreth, Taylor, Fayol, Elton Mayo, Maslow, Henry Mintzberg, and Peter Drucker developed theories related to OB. Peter Drucker, who was the father of modern management, emphasized the importance of change and innovation and improvised the methods to get the best from the people in the organization.

Concept and Meaning

Organization behavior is the study of human behavior at work. According to Luthar, it concerns with understanding, predicting, and controlling the behavior of people at work in the organization. It studies how the individuals behave with each other, with a group in the organization during their working schedule. It tries to understand the impact of the behavior of individuals, groups, and the structure of an organization on its performance.

Organization behavior has an interdisciplinary approach and is an applied science since the principles of multiple disciplines involved in this field. Psychology studies how the individuals respond to a stimulus; sociology contributed to finding out the relationship of individuals with each other and with the group. Social psychology studies the behavior of individual and organization, conflict, threats, and stress; anthropology contributed to study the customs, traditions, social norms, and group dynamics. Political science has its contribution to understanding power and organization politics and economics studies to find out the effect of monetary and nonmonetary incentives on improving the performance of employees in the organization.

It is normative and value centered since it studies the group norms and values of individuals to improve their performances. It is humanistic and optimistic as it deals with directing and controlling the behavior of individuals to get the maximum output. Its focus is to accomplish organizational objectives, personal satisfaction, and personal and group goals. Therefore, OB requires a whole-system approach to improve the effectiveness of the organization, keeping in mind the aspiration and achievement of individuals. OB system comprises formal organization system, individual system, and social system **(Fig. 41.1)**.

The formal organization system has a structure, which is the interface between technology and human resources, represented by hierarchy and functional specialization. The

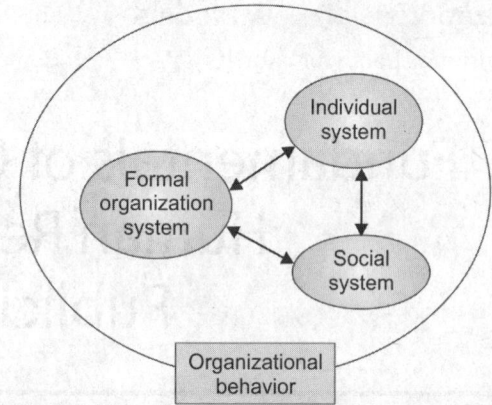

Fig. 41.1: Concept of organizational behavior in an organization setting.

hierarchy depicts a superior and subordinate relationship. It influences the individual system and social system. In the individual system, individuals interact with each other. Each varies in personality, attitude, perception, and motivation. Groups form the social system in the organization. The formal organization has formal groups, but human resources tend to form informal groups. These informal groups are essential to influence the individual system to bring changes in the organization and facilitate integration in the social group. Thus, the formal organization system tries to make use of the individual system to integrate a social system to achieve its objectives.

Importance and Scope

The scope and importance of OB are as follows:
- OB helps to understand the behavior of individuals in a better and scientific way in a situation in an organizational setting.
- It aids to manage, control, and direct human resources in a better way and try to maintain cordial social relation in the organization.
- It seeks to solve the organizational problems at the individual and group levels.
- It uses power and sanction in a better way and is able to apply the best leadership behavior, communication, organization climate, and organization adaptation strategies.
- It studies the relationship of individuals with their social environment.
- At the individual level, it examines the personality, perception, attitudes, values, job satisfaction, learning, and motivation of individuals as each one is unique.
- At the group level, it studies group dynamics, communication, leadership behavior, power, and politics.
- At the organizational level, it studies different organization structures, culture, change management, innovation strategies, and development to improve its function and performance and behavior of individuals.
- It tries to find out the best organization as a social system where the individuals and groups interact with each other and have a mutual interest in the pursuit of accomplishing organizational goals.

Organizational Behavior Models

Organizational behavior models operate on cognitive, behavioristic, and social learning framework. The different models of OB are autocratic model, custodial model, supportive model, collegial model, system model, and S-O-B-C model.

1. **Autocratic model:** The autocratic model was the most prominent one during the 1800 and 1900s. It explains that employers and managers have decision-making power, whereas the employees are to follow the instructions of managers. The managerial orientation is toward authority, and managers are the dictators. They have the right to give command to the employees. The employees are expected to follow orders. The management decides what is the best. It involves very close and strict supervision to get the expected performance from employees. The performance result is minimal. The employees depend on their bosses and, they get fewer wages, are less skilled. This model is comparable with McGregor "X" theory and Likert system of using punishment, fear, and threat means to get the work done. The drawback of this model is its high human cost, primarily caused by micromanagement. This model is useful in organizational crisis and to guide managerial behavior when there are no popular alternatives.

2. **Custodial model:** The managerial orientation issue is the use of incentive and reward schemes. The basis of this model is to satisfy organizational human resources. According to this model, the organization provides economic security to its employees. They are offering high salaries and other benefits such as health benefits, financial incentives to increase the satisfaction level of employees, to reduce absenteeism, and turnover. The employee's security needs to be met in this type of model. The employees now show the loyalty and dependency towards the organization, but their level of performance is not very high. The organizational climate psychologically contends, and employees are happy, may not be productive.

3. **Supportive model:** The basis of this model is leadership rather than on the use of power or money. The aim is to support employees in their achievement of results and participation. The emphasis is to fulfill the status and recognition needs of the employees. According to a supportive model, organizational climate helps the employees to achieve their higher order of needs. The employees may say "we" instead of "they." They are highly self-motivated and have a feeling to participate in various activities of the organization. The organizational climate is positive, where the employees are encouraged to give their ideas to improve performance. The employees work under supportive supervision. The organization under participative leadership provides space and a favorable climate for employees to make their own decisions and responsibility to improve their performance. This model is less successful in developing nations where employees have priority for physiological needs.

4. **Collegial model:** The collegial model is partnership based on the team concept. Employees develop a high degree of understanding with each other and share common goals. They are responsible and self-disciplined as they set the standards. The self-actualization need of the employees is the prime concern. The manager's role is to guide the team, creating a motivating environment. The team members work together, solve the problems, and look for better methods for better performance to accomplish organizational goals. The employees as a team feel needed, useful, and some degree of fulfillment with a worthwhile contribution.

5. **System model:** The system model reflects the values underlying positive OB. The managers focus their attention on helping employees develop feelings of hope, optimism, self-confidence, empathy, trustworthiness, esteem, courage, and resiliency. The managers at all levels show compassion, project self-worth in one's bearing, and can read the social situation and respond appropriately. They use language effectively to explain and persuade and are more authentic. They support employees' commitment to short- and long-term goals, give timely and acceptable feedback, and encourage employees to feel comfortable with change and uncertainty. They create a positive work culture where employees feel more ease and family atmosphere is provided so that they give their best performance. Employees go beyond self-discipline and reach a state of self-motivation. This type of work culture allows employees to meet their needs of a higher order, such as social status, esteem, autonomy, and self-actualization needs. The employees are more dedicated, emotionally attached, and loyal to the organization. They are concerned with the success of the organization and do what is suitable for the organization.

The above five models are closely related to human needs. Each model is built upon the accomplishment of others. The managers need to identify each model and also use and measure its effectiveness **(Table 41.1)**.

6. **S-O-B-C model:** S-O-B-C is another modern model of OB proposed by Fred Lutheran. It describes the mechanism of human behavior, how the individuals respond to the situation that results in their actions. S-O-B-C stands for S—situation, which is more than a stimulus. It includes all types of environmental stimuli such as physical, psychological, and sociocultural, O—organism that provides for physical and physiological aspects of individuals, B—behavior that consists of both overt and covert behaviors of the individual, and C—consequences that also consists of both overt and covert. The consequences may further modify the stimulating situation or create a new location to lead in the right direction **(Fig. 41.2)**.

TABLE 41.1: Comparison of different models.

Variable	Autocratic model	Custodial model	Supportive model	Collegial model	System model
Basis of model	Power	Economic resources	Leadership	Partnership	Trust, the community, meaning
Managerial orientation	Authority	Money	Support	Team concept	Caring, compassion
Employee's orientation	Obedience	Security	Job	Responsibility	Psychological ownership
Employee's dependency	Boss	Organization	Participation	Self-discipline	Self-motivation
Employee's need met	Subsistence	Security	Recognition	Self-actualization	Wide range
Performance	Minimal	Passive cooperation	Awakened drive	Moderate enthusiasm	Passion and commitment

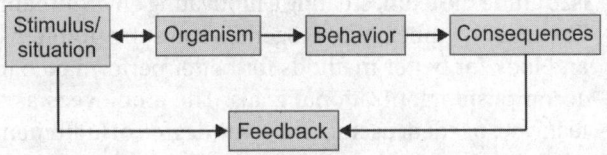

Fig. 41.2: S-O-B-C model of organizational behavior.

According to this model, it is essential to understand and evaluate the cause of the behavior of individuals who react to a given situation. It is also necessary to analyze the circumstance under which an individual behaves in a way and modify accordingly.

HUMAN RELATIONS

As a member of the health-care team, the nurse must know the science of human relations to understand human behavior and to develop a positive attitude toward the profession. The nurse manager should have full regard for the values of the right human relations and need to think that the nurses are working under him or her to an end if an organization is to succeed, monitor, and maintain the relationships among the people in that organization.

Defining Human Relations

Human relations is the ability to work effectively through and with other people. It is a phenomenon of organized human activity directed toward the promotion of cooperative and happy work relationships. It is getting the work done by people with their hearts in the job. It is motivating people to work to the best of their capacity. It includes a desire to understand others, their needs and weaknesses, and their talents and skills.

In a workplace setting, human relations involve an understanding of how people work together in groups, satisfying both individual needs and group objectives. In the broadest sense, the study of human relations has two goals—personal development and growth and achievement of an organization's objectives.

Areas of Human Relations

1. **Self-esteem:** Self-esteem is at the core of most issues in human relations. Self-confidence is the highest level of need. High self-esteem is the key to performance and high-quality work, primarily when the work directly affects other people.
2. **Mutual respect:** Mutual respect is the favorable consideration or regard that two people have for each other, can exist only when self-esteem is stable. Without trust, mutual respect is meaningless. There is a need for maintaining trust and mutual respect by all the members to perform at their best.
3. **Self-awareness and self-disclosure:** Self-awareness is the knowledge about yourself as perceived by others. Self-disclosure is a form of the communication process of telling about yourself to others.

Elements of Human Relations

Elements of human relations are as follows:
1. **Human need satisfaction:** According to Maslow's theory, the hierarchy of needs are physiological, safety, social, esteem, and self-actualization needs. These needs are prepotent for motivating behavior.
2. **Motivation:** Motivation is the act of stimulating an individual or oneself to contribute the utmost to achieve the desired objectives. At the workplace, the managers inculcate motivation through various means such as monetary, positive reinforcement, allowing participation, and job enrichment.
3. **Status and defined roles:** Give appropriate status and set each one's role in the organization. Encourage them to participate in staff and professional development.
4. **Informal social groups:** It is essential to have social gatherings to exchange views and to share their feelings.
5. **The spontaneity of group formation:** These are a form of association through which they can work together and can make decisions for the betterment of employees.

Prerequisites for Good Human Relations

For a good human relations, it is essential to have the following features:
- Respect the human dignity of employees
- Understand the personality of each individual and give recognition
- Encourage personality development
- Be fair, honest, and cooperative
- Be punctual and observe punctuality
- Understand the past and future behavior of subordinates
- Direct, change, and control the behavior of subordinates
- Stimulate, encourage, and motivate them for advancement
- Have provision for right incentives for excellent accomplishments
- Listen and avoid arguments

- Keep an open mind and act on "what's right"–not on who's right.

Principles of Human Relations Approach

The eight principles of human relations approach are listed below:

1. **Principle of recognition and appreciation:** It means that human beings, along with financial gains, need attention and admiration.
2. **Principle of fair treatment:** The principle of appropriate treatment means that in the human relations approach treat the staff like human beings and not as machines. Understand their feelings and emotions.
3. **Principle of informal relations:** It means that informal relationship is essential in the right human relations in the organization along with formal ties.
4. **Principle of job security and job satisfaction:** This principle means that staff needs job security and job satisfaction to work enthusiastically.
5. **Principle of effective communication:** The principle of effective communication means no conflicts and misunderstandings among the members.
6. **Principle of decentralization:** It means that the provision of greater autonomy and decision-making power to individual staff, and different departments aid in maintaining human relations. Emphasize informal communication channels also.
7. **Principle of participatory decision-making:** It means that participation provides greater autonomy to individual employees to improve human relationships.
8. **Principle of self-motivation:** The employees who can set their own task-related goals and monitor their performance should be self-motivated. The purpose of managers in such an organization is to design and implement organizational structures that reward such self-motivation and autonomy and to negotiate working relationships with subordinates that foster effective communication in both directions.

Advantages of Good Human Relations

Listed below are the advantages of a good human relations:
- Excellent human relations has a significant impact on the efficiency, productivity, and profitability of an organization.
- It reduces the incidences of absenteeism, strike, and acts of indiscipline.
- It is more preventive than curative.
- It can provide a nurse manager information about each staff and group needs.

Role of the Nurse Manager to Develop Human Relations

In the subsequent list, the nurse manager plays a role in developing human relations:
- Recognize the importance of the individual and deal with in a human manner.
- There must be a mutual understanding of their position.
- The employees and administrators should have a common interest, i.e. the accomplishment of organizational goals.
- Focus on joint discussion, exchange of views, and excellent communication.
- Set a good example for your employees.
- Help them to feel that they are essential members of the team.
- Try to understand your employees.
- Be fair and impartial in all the matters.
- Develop your employees for promotion.
- Plan your work carefully and keep your perspectives. Give clear, concise, and complete instructions. Tell them "what" and "why."
- Get result, develop safe, efficient employees; give them the right tools for the job.
- Know the details of all the principles, policies, and laws.
- Know your duties, responsibilities, and authorities.
- Evaluate your effectiveness.

PUBLIC RELATIONS

The term "public relations" is ubiquitous and often misused and misapplied, vague, and misunderstood. But in a hospital context, this aspect is inherent in each activity of the hospital and administrative decision behind it. It is a bonus benefit from the hospital activities. It built up the exact image of an organization.

Public relations is in existence from time immemorial. Any goodwill gesture between at least two individuals naturally culminates in enhancing the quality of the relationship. In Ramayana, Hanuman sets an example of public relations par excellence. Krishna created a paradigm of excellent public relations while conducting dialogues and consultation, even at the war theater of the great epic Mahabharata. In history and culture, various examples of public relations personalities are Ashoka, Kautilya, and Akbar, and even during the freedom movements.

Meaning and Definitions

The term public, though frequently in use, is not easy to define. The general public is vague. In the case of hospitals, the term "public" includes all the staff working in the hospital, management, clients, relatives, and family members. It implied to the community in general.

Institute of Public Relations, USA, defines public relations as a deliberate, planned, and sustained activity to have a mutual relationship between the organization and the public at large. Baus Herbert M referred to public relations as the application of various behavioral sciences such as philosophy, psychology, sociology, and communication to understand human behavior.

According to Harlow, public relations is a distinctive management function. It deals with management issues and keeps management informed about public opinion. It maintains mutual understanding, acceptance, and cooperation between the organization and the public. It uses research and sound and ethical communication as its principal tools.

Nature of Public Relations

Public relations is concerned with identifying and evaluating public attitudes, and a process of planning and executing programs of public interest to carry general understanding and acceptance (Scott, 1965). Public relations is merely finding out what people like to do and what they do not want to do and doing less about it. Public relations is an essential effort in understanding and letting others understand.

Public relations is both art and science. It is an art in the sense that one has to conceive and use creative ideas in building the bridges of understanding, and it is science as it designs technologies that help people to continue to understand each other.

Public relations involves a two-way communication process between an organization and its public and also include communication to change the mindsets of the people in a particular direction. Public relations as a form of communication is used to persuade or influence people using ethical means. The following three ways are involved in a conversation:
- Awareness: The message should reach the public.
- Acceptance: The public should agree with the message.
- Action: The public should act or interact accordingly.

General Consideration

Following are the general considerations for public relations:
- Mostly the hospital administrator acts as the public relations in charge. He or she may employ some assistant who should be a skilled person in the public relations process.
- Some hospitals appoint public relations officer (PRO)/welfare officer to manage the public relations department.
- Public relations refers to building, bridging, and establishing understanding and rapport with the general public.
- The person responsible for public relations must plan, organize, and evaluate the function of public relations programs.
- It is a two-way process between hospital and public that needs effective communication and understanding.
- Formal and informal contacts should be established between employees and the public.
- The public needs proper information and facts regarding hospital services through publicity, propaganda, advertising, and education.

Aims of Public Relations

The four main aims of public relations are the following:
1. To enhance the image of excellence, quality, reliability, and respectability of an organization
2. To eliminate misunderstandings and misgivings
3. To promote a healthy relationship between the public and administration
4. To have public support.

Functions of Public Relations

The following are the functions of public relations:
- To establish the relationship between organization and society
- To develop reciprocal understanding and goodwill
- To analyze the public perception and attitude toward the organization
- To identify the organization policy with the public interest
- To execute the programs for communication with the public.

Advantages of Public Relations

The main advantages of public relations are as follows:
1. Public relations helps the hospitals to secure and maintain the goodwill of the community to accomplish the purpose up to their satisfaction.
2. The public can fully utilize the services rendered by the hospital.
3. It also helps to orient the staff working in the hospital about the public programs.
4. It reflects the reputation of the hospital as it depends upon the type of public image.
5. It will help them to visualize the extent and type of services rendered by the hospital and the attitude of staff members toward ordinary people.
6. The staff learns adjustment, patience, and understanding of the sick and their families to meet the patient's need, in spite of technical perfection.

Elements of Public Relations

According to Raymond, the following are the elements of public relations:
- A planned effort or management function
- The relationship between an organization and its public
- Evaluation of public attitudes and opinions
- An organization's policies, procedures, and actions
- Steps were taken to ensure that said policies, procedures, and activities are in the public interest and socially responsible
- Execution of action and/or communication program
- Rapport, understanding, and acceptance.

Factors Affecting Hospital Public Image

The three factors that influence public image are services rendered by the hospital, health providers, and the means of publicity/public education:
1. **Services:** The hospital provides various types of services to the patient once admitted, e.g. medical, nursing, laboratory, dietetics, and rehabilitation. Emergency and outpatient departments are the most sensitive areas.

2. **Health providers:** The staff working in hospitals, their knowledge, skills, and attitudes toward the clients is critical. How they provide the services, how they react and interact, what their view, are they motivated to do the work, affect the public image.
3. **Means of publicity and public education:** The types of modes and methods used for the promotion should reach the public, and the public should understand the information.

Organizing Public Relations Program

The following are the steps to organize a successful program under public relations:
1. **Identification of need:** Identify the need of the public to organize any program. It should be need based.
2. **Careful planning:** Determine what community wants and plan various methods, the time, and who all will be involved. Get cooperation from all concerned, department, administration, public, and other agencies. Observe ethical standards.
3. **Implementation:** Implement the program per plan.
4. **Evaluation:** Evaluate the outcome of the program. Observe public reaction and take feedback and suggestions from them.
5. **Replanning:** Revamp if required.

PUBLICITY AND PUBLIC EDUCATION

People are ignorant of the fact concerning hospitals. Hospital staff have also made little effort to explain the hospital's functions and services to the public and use of their goodwill toward the hospital. It is through favorable publicity, the community can take advantage of the services provided, and the hospital may be able to extend its usefulness. Hence, the propaganda must be directed toward the best interest of the community. The main aim of publicity is to sell the ideas and means of its accomplishments.

Definitions

Publicity is a cooperative plan of utilizing every possible legitimate and ethical means of informing the public of the benefits it can expect to derive from its hospitals. It is an act or device designed to attract public interest. According to Collins English Dictionary, publicity is a process of drawing the attention of the public, about the organization, products, and services using mass media.

Publicity provides evidence-based facts, engaging and newsworthy to media such as radio, television, magazines, newspapers, and journals (Yale, 1991). Advertising is a method of publicizing information from an outside source used by the media because the information has news value (Broom et al., 2000). Publicity refers to information designed to appear in any medium of communication to keep the name of a person or company before the public or of creating public interest in their activities (Risberg, 1988).

Characteristics of Publicity

The characteristics of publicity are as follows:
1. Publicity material should appeal to emotions and intellect.
2. Publicity must have continuity.
3. Publicity must proceed from general to specific.
4. Quality of promotion should be maintained.
5. The advertisement should be positive, not negative.

Purposes of Publicity and Public Education

The following are the purposes of publicity and public education:
- To develop public understanding and appreciation of hospital including nursing services
- To foster an attitude of genuine goodwill on the part of the public toward the hospital
- To stimulate a greater desire for personnel to understand the work of the hospital and to have close contact with staff and public
- To have cooperation with other agencies in the community
- To encourage to utilize facilities provided by the hospital
- To clarify the public about the position of the hospital as the principal source of skilled and continuous nursing
- To improve the health and welfare condition of the community by encouraging the use of hospital facilities and getting feedback from them
- To promote the use of hospital by the majority of people.

Means of Publicity and Public Education

Publicity and public education are achieved by adopting the following methods:
1. **Written mode:** Use accurate and up-to-date facts, since errors are more dangerous to reputation. Coordinate all written publicity to accomplish one purpose. The information should be presented interestingly, in short, and designed to read by the public. It should be a focus on knowledge what the public desires. Various ways to publicize through written words are as follows:
    - *News items:* The news item in the media is the most commonly used field. Organize conferences with the city editors of newspapers. Maintain friendly relations with them. The information may come in the form of straight news stories, editorials, feature elements, historical columns, and society columns or news pictures.
    - *Contests and school papers:* Hospitals can invite school groups for games and paper readings on the subjects dealing with the hospital services.
    - *Magazines:* Magazine in the form of newsletters where the day-to-day events can be published.
    - *Hospital bulletins:* These are also suitable publicity mode.

- *Information booklets to patients:* To render the information regarding the hospital, rules, and regulations, timings for the visitors, etc.
- *Discharge cards:* This gives the information regarding the treatment follow-up.
- *Annual reports:* Annual report is vital to acquaint the people with the services of the hospital.

2. **Spoken words:** Effective verbal communication is necessary to convey the message to the public, which are as follows:
   - *Satisfied patients:* The patients will appreciate if it renders quality care.
   - *Medical and nursing staff:* Words and acts are essential for all patients and their relatives.
   - *Hospital personnel:* When talking with the patients, give a clear picture of the hospital. Hence, their attitudes are essential. Teach all the staff about basic facts concerning the hospital.
   - *During meetings:* The best position to discuss details concerning the institute is in the meetings, primarily administrative and governing body meetings by the public officer or the concerned person.
   - *Radio and television:* These are good media for publicity to inform people and to educate them. Radio and television telecasts must occur at regular intervals. There should be fix time or day in a week. The program should be in series. Particular attention must give to make it interesting, better entertaining.
   - *Teleconferencing:* This is advance technology where the patients and people can take advice and discuss their health problems.

3. **Visual means:** The impression received through the eyes is beneficial and lasting. One can use television, tours, exhibits, motion pictures, LCD projection media, and Internet by having websites for this purpose.

4. **Multiple means:** Using combinations of methods for health education forum, meetings sponsored by hospitals, community health meetings, and community programs for publicity are quite useful in disseminating educational information to the masses.

Nurses' Role in Improving Hospital Public Relations

The role of nurses in improving hospital public relations is as follows:
- Delivering and ensuring high-quality patient care
- Attending the clients on admission
- Providing orientations to clients and relatives
- Informing about rules and regulation
- Educating and guiding them about the care and other health matters
- Maintaining privacy
- Ensuring the client is getting all hospital services in the proper way, e.g. dietary services
- Ensuring environmental sanitation and cleanliness
- Attending complaints and suggestions from them.

CHAPTER HIGHLIGHTS

- Organization behavior is the study of human behavior in an organizational setting.
- Organization behavior has a normative and interdisciplinary approach and is an applied science.
- Organization behavior system comprises formal organization system, individual system, and social system.
- The different models of OB are autocratic model, custodial model, supportive model, collegial model, system model, and S-O-B-C model.
- Human relations is the ability to work effectively through and with other people.
- Self-esteem, mutual respect, self-disclosure, and self-awareness are the main areas of human relations.
- The managers need to follow the principles of the human relations to understand the past and future behavior of individuals and direct, change, and control their behavior.
- Public relations is a deliberate, planned, and sustained activity to have a mutual relationship between an organization and the public at large.
- Three main factors influence public image, services, health providers, and the means of publicity and public education. It needs careful planning to organize in the hospital.
- Publicity is a process of drawing the attention of the public, about the organization, products, and services using mass media. The various ways to publicize are through written words, spoken words, visuals, and other means.

REVIEW QUESTIONS

I. Essay Type Questions
1. Define organization behavior. Describe its importance and scope.
2. Enlist various models of organizational behavior. Describe any one in detail.
3. Define the term "human relations." Discuss its main areas.
4. Explain the principles of human relations why it is vital to have good human relations in the organization.
5. What do you understand by public relations and publicity? Describe its purposes and advantages.

II. Short Notes
1. Collegial model of organizational behavior
2. Role of the nurse manager in maintaining human relations
3. Elements of human relationships
4. Means of publicity and public education
5. Organizing public relations program

III. Multiple Choice Questions

1. Organizational behavior is normative because it:
   a. Deals with directing and controlling the behavior of individuals
   b. Studies the relationship of individuals with each other
   c. Understands power, organization politics, and economics
   d. Studies the group values of individuals to improve their performance.
2. Which discipline contributes to study the customs, traditions, social norms, and group dynamics?
   a. Sociology
   b. Anthropology
   c. Psychology
   d. Social psychology
3. Which one of the following organizational behavior models emphasizes team concept and self-discipline employees?
   a. System
   b. Custodial
   c. Collegial
   d. Supportive
4. Which one of the following organizational behavior models explains the employers' role to make the decision?
   a. Autocratic
   b. S-O-B-C
   c. Custodial
   d. Supportive
5. Which principle of human relations emphasizes the provision of greater autonomy and decision-making power to subordinates?
   a. The principle of participatory decision-making
   b. The principle of informal relation
   c. The principle of effective communication
   d. The principle of decentralization
6. The public relations is an art because:
   a. It designs technologies that help people to continue to understand each other
   b. One has to conceive and use creative ideas in building understanding
   c. It deals with identifying and evaluating public attitudes
   d. It influences people using ethical means
7. A deliberate, planned, and sustained activity to have a mutual relationship between organization and public is:
   a. Organizational behavior
   b. Human relations
   c. Public relations
   d. Publicity
8. Who created a paradigm of excellent public relations through dialogues and consultation in history?
   a. Krishna
   b. Ashoka
   c. Kautilya
   d. Akbar

Answer Keys
1. d 2. b 3. c 4. a 5. d 6. b 7. c
8. a

SUGGESTED READING

1. Available from http://www.citehr.com/69683-understanding-organizational-behavior-ob.html. [Accessed July 2019].
2. Available from https://ebrary.net/2814/management/models_organiational_behaviour. [Accessed July 2019].
3. Bobbins SP. Organizational Behaviour. New Delhi: Prentice-Hall; 1997.
4. Cunningham JB, Eberle T. A Guide to Job Enrichment and Redesign. Personnel. 1990; 67(2): 56-7.
5. Davis K. Evolving models of organizational behavior. Acad Manag J. 1968;11(1):27-38.
6. Davis K. Human Behaviour at Work. New York: McGraw Hill Book Co.; 1991.
7. Dimock ME. Administrative Vitality. New York: Harper Brothers; 1975.
8. Evolution of Management Thoughts (managerial Function). (n.d.). [online] Available from https://www.civilserviceindia.com/subject/Management/notes/evolution-of-manageme. [Accessed July 2019].
9. Felgen J. A Caring and Healing Environment. Nurs Adm Q. 2004;28(4):288-301.
10. Hackman JR, Oldham GR. Development of the diagnostic job survey. J Appl Psychol. 1975;60:159-70.
11. Jones J, Schilling K, Pesut D. Barriers and benefits associated with nurses information seeking related to patient education needs on clinical nursing units. Open Nurs J. 2011;5:24-30. Epub 2011 Feb 24. (Pub Med).
12. Kapoor B. Importance of human relations in nursing. Nurs J India. 1998;89(11):252-3.
13. Kyle B. Henry S. Dennison, Elton Mayo. Human relations historiography. Manag Org History. 2006;1:177-99.
14. Luthans F. Organisational Behaviour. New York: McGraw Hill Book Co.; 1995.
15. Melnechenko KL. To make a difference: Nursing presence. Nurs Forum. 2003;38(2):18-24. (Pub Med).
16. Newman WH, Warren EK. The Process of Management. New Delhi: Prentice-Hall; 1985.
17. Newstrom J, Davis K. Organization Behavior: Human Behavior at Work. New York: McGraw-Hill; 1993.
18. Nisberg JN. The Random House Handbook of Business Terms. New York: Random House, 1988.
19. No author listed. Communicating with patients and carers. Nurs Times. 2000;96(24):43-6. (Pub Med).
20. Scott WR. Special issue on professionals in organizations. Administrative Science Quarterly 1965; 10(1):65-81. Available from (online) https://www.jstor.org/stable/2391650?seq=1. [Accessed Jan 2020].
21. Stuenkel DL, Nguyen S, Cohen J. Nurses' perceptions of their work environment. J Nurs Care Qual. 2007;22(4):337-42. (Pub Med).
22. Subbiah N, Workshop report. Nursing Journal of India. FindArticles.com. [Online] Available from http://findarticles.com/p/articles/mi_qa4036/is_200305/ai_n9298232/. [Accessed September 2011].
23. Terry GR, Franklin SG. Principles of Management. Delhi: AITBS; 2000.
24. The Human Relations Approach—Docshare01.docshare.tips. (n.d.). [online] Available from http://docshare01.docshare.tips/files/10637/106373587.pdf. [Accessed July 2019].
25. Turkel MC, Ray MA. Creating a caring practice environment through self-renewal. Nurs Adm Q. 2004;28(4):249-54.
26. Weber J. Creating a holistic environment for practicing nurses. Nurs Clin North Am. 2007;42(2):295-307, vii. (Pub Med).

42 CHAPTER

Group, Group Formation, and Group Dynamics

CHAPTER OUTLINE

- Group and Group Formation
  - Defining a Group
  - Importance of a Group
  - Characteristics of a Group
  - Types of Groups
- Purposes of Groups
- Group Formation and Development
- Group Dynamics
  - Concept of Group Dynamics
  - Elements of Group Dynamics
  - Group Dynamics in Nursing Management

LEARNING OUTCOMES

After completion of this chapter, the learner will be able to:
- Understand the concept of group and group dynamics
- Discuss the importance and characteristics of a group
- Describe the types of groups and the focus areas of group dynamics
- Familiarize with the process of forming groups
- Describe various theories of group development
- Define multiple elements of group dynamics
- Appreciate the application of group dynamics in the nursing management

KEY TERMS

Group dynamics, group, group norms, group cohesiveness, leadership, group formation, group development

INTRODUCTION

A group is an entry point for growth, and the dynamics of a group are fundamental to find out the success of the group. The importance of a group on productivity was appreciated in 1930 by Elton Mayo and his associates. The concept of groups was studied scientifically in the last decade of the 19th century onward. The idea of group processes and group dynamics developed and accelerated since the 1980s.

Groups affect the functioning of the organization and are essential to achieve goals. These form the foundation of human resources in the organization. Due to the complexity of health organizational activities, it becomes virtually difficult for healthcare providers to cope at a satisfactory level. Hence, it is crucial to have a group of people working together as well as a team for them to combine their knowledge and abilities to solve complex problems.

The nurse manager must know both group behavior and individual behavior. In the group the nurse manager influences personal work, job satisfaction, and effective performance. Apart from this, a nurse is to work with groups of people in the clinical area; therefore, a basic knowledge of group dynamics and cultural diversity is essential to deal with them and to lead a focus group, quality improvement team, and so on.

GROUP AND GROUP FORMATION

Defining a Group

A group consists of individuals working together for a common objective. According to Collins dictionary, a group comprises persons bound together by common social standards, interests, etc. The team consists of a group of people organized to work together. Brown (1988) opines that a group must have two or more members. According to Erofeev, Glazer, and Ivanitskaya (2009), a group has two or more members interacting with each other and sharing a common purpose. The organization is also a "group" having a group of people who interact and work together to achieve a common goal of that organization.

Importance of a Group

A group is formed with certain objectives and importance, and some of them are listed below:
- Groups help members to participate in making it more effective.
- Groups cooperate to complete work effectively in the organization.
- A group uses creative and innovative ideas compared to a single individual.
- Group efforts motivate individuals, their attitude, and behavior to accomplish work.
- A group can satisfy the needs of its members.

Characteristic of a Group

From the sociological point of view, a group must have two or more freely interacting individuals, collective norms, collective goals, and shared identity. According to Jarlath F Benson, a group should have a set of people engaging in frequent interactions; individuals must identify with one another and define themselves and by others as a group. They share their beliefs, values, and norms about the areas of common interest. The members of group come together to work on everyday tasks and for agreed purposes. A group must have a democratic atmosphere and involve interested group members. A group should have constructive criticism and consensus in decision-making. There should be clarity in the task, roles, and assignments. All members must have emotional stability. There should be regular assessment of performance, purpose, and process. A group should possess the following characteristics:

1. **Goal-oriented activities:** The members of a group should have goal-oriented activities and share some common goals.
2. **Well organized:** Social groups tend to have different roles, rules, regulation, and a set of norms that give them a unique identity.
3. **Interdependency:** The members in a group are interdependent on each other, influencing their actions and bringing changes in their personalities.
4. **Power structure:** The group members may exercise autocratic or democratic power, depending on the type of group. Group can be hierarchical where power is vested in the highest authority of the group or it can be vertical, where the power is vested in every member of the group.
5. **Group structure:** Group structure revealed a pattern of relationships among members who hold the group together to achieve specific goals. The group structure is framed based on its size, functions, norms, and cohesiveness.
   a. *Group size:* Group size varies from two people to a considerable number of people. A group may be large or small. In a large group, the member's participation and satisfaction are less when compared to a small group. In a small group, the members have intimacy, and each one has the opportunity to participate and share views.
   b. *Group functions:* A group has three main functions, i.e., task functions, maintenance functions, and self-interests. These functions make the group effective and productive.
      i. **Task functions:** A group performs the following primary duties:
         ○ Initiating: A group takes the initiative to define a problem, propose tasks, and give suggestions to solve a problem.
         ○ Information giving and seeking: A group must state its beliefs, offer and find facts, and provide suggestions.
         ○ Clarifying ideas: A group clarifies doubts of members by interpreting and suggesting alternatives with examples.
         ○ Bringing closure: A group must discuss every matter with its members by summarizing, restating, and offering solutions.
         ○ Consensus testing: A group must take consensus to make any decision.
      ii. *Maintenance functions:* Each group needs social–emotional support to be effective. The group members play the following maintenance roles:
         ○ Encouraging: The members appreciate the contribution made by other members and help them in the future.
         ○ Improving: The work environment can be improved by expressing group feelings, by sensing moods and relationships, and by sharing feelings.
         ○ Harmonizing: In a group, the members try to reconcile their differences and reduce group tension.
         ○ Compromising: The group members compromise with each other's actions by admitting errors, solving problems, and looking for alternatives.
         ○ Communication: The members in a group attempt to have excellent conversation, facilitate the participation of others, and suggest ways through discussion and sharing.
         ○ Standard setting: The members of a group try to set standards, group norms, rules, and roles.
      iii. *Self-interest functions:* Group members may also have self-interests instead of getting attracted to group performance. They may dominate, put pressure on group, manipulate the things, or may divert the mind of members for their self motive.
6. **Interaction among members:**
   a. *Unorganize social interaction:* Groups may have disorganized communication which is just for

recreation and casual enlightenment. However, these are useful for successful adjustment, personality development, and coincidental education.
b. *Collaborative group interaction:* Collaborative group interaction is to pool out the characteristic findings for reference readings, experiments, and experience. These are useful for augmenting, rounding out, and clarification of unfamiliar knowledge.
c. *Logical group interaction:* A consistent group interaction is mainly for discussing to reach a conclusion. These are useful to solve a common problem, achieve a cooperative decision with consensus, and formulate or refine group policies.

Types of Groups

1. **Formal groups:** Formal groups are functional groups established by an organization to achieve the organizational goals and the overall corporate mission. These are permanent groups designed and planned by top management to achieve organizational goals.
2. **Task groups:** Tasks groups are temporarily formed to achieve a specific task at a particular time. These groups have informal temporary committees and the task force to solve the problem.
3. **Informal groups:** Informal groups are operating in all organizations. These are in the form of associations, unions, etc. and formed by themselves. These are very effective and powerful. They have an informal communication network forming a part of the grapevine to the organizations. These are formed as an interest group, membership group, friendship group, or reference group.

Purposes of Groups

1. **Organizational functions:**
   - To assist in accomplishing complex, independent tasks
   - To help in generating new ideas and solutions
   - To coordinate interdependent efforts
   - To provide problem-solving mechanisms for various problems
   - To aid in implementing complex decisions
   - To encourage a feeling of cohesiveness among group members, enhancing the capabilities of group members
   - To provide opportunities for individual members to grow
   - To socialize and train new entrants
   - To develop leadership qualities
   - To help members become self-reliant
   - To increase participation of members at all levels
   - To organize, utilize, and exploit the ideas of group members.

2. **Individual functions**
   - To satisfy the personal need for affiliation
   - To enhance an individual's self-esteem and sense of identity
   - To provide an opportunity for individuals to test and share their perceptions of social reality
   - To reduce an individual's anxiety and feeling of insecurity.

Group Formation and Development

There are general tendencies among individuals to form a group. It may be a similarity attraction effect, exposure, that is, the people to whom the individuals are exposed repeatedly, and reciprocity. The various other reasons to join, form, and develop groups are as follows:

- **Organizational motives:** Organizations form groups to plan and group various activities of the organization efficiently and logically.
- **Personal motives**: Groups are formed by for their interest in their workplace. These are informal or interest groups, and the members join this group voluntarily.
- **Individual attraction:** Individual attraction is based on similar attitudes and personality, and economic standing is one of the reasons to form a group.
- **Similar interests**: Individuals may be motivated to join an informal or interest group because the activities of the group appeal to them.
- **Goal achievement:** Individuals may also be motivated to join a group because of its goals.
- **Need for affiliation:** People also form groups to satisfy their need for attachment.
- **Instrumental benefits:** Sometimes people also form groups to provide help so that others are benefited.

Theories on Group Development

1. **Classic approach:** George Homans developed the traditional method. According to this theory, groups are formed due to sentiments, interactions, and activities. Having everyday events, individuals communicate and promote positive or negative attitudes with each other. Communication of the individuals is the primary element in this theory.
2. **Social exchange theory:** As the name indicates, according to this theory, a group is formed due to social exchange among individuals. They meet to expect a mutual benefit from each other based on trust and obligation. There should be a positive relationship to attract and affiliate to a group.
3. **Social identity theory:** According to this theory, the group members have recognition and fulfill the need for self-esteem. A group may exist based on its demographic characteristics, cultural background, or organizational values. Individuals feel a sense of belongingness and are motivated to contribute to

similar groups. An individual is self-satisfied being a member of the group.

4. **Schutz's three-stage model (1958, 1966):** The three-stage model by Schutz suggests that each group, irrespective of its nature undergoes three interpersonal phases in the same sequence, namely inclusion, control, and affection.
   a. *Inclusion:* It is the initial stage of the forming a group. During this phase, individuals are primarily concerned about their acceptance in the group. They try to know each other and focus on belongingness issues, such as attention, acknowledgment, recognition, and identity.
   b. *Control:* During this stage, the team members focus on leadership and structure issues. Each member tries to establish a comfortable interchange and degree of initiation concerning power, influence, and responsibility.
   c. *Affection:* In this stage, the members become emotionally close. They develop positive behavior, such as intimacy and personal confidence.

5. **Tuckman's four-stage model:** In the 1960s, Bruce Tuckman established the most common framework for examining the "how" of group formation. Bruce Tuckman's model for group development is basically for the team to grow, to face challenges, to tackle the problems, to find the solution, to plan, and to deliver results. The model describes the following four linear stages of group development to take a decision (Fig. 42.1).
   1. *Forming:* The forming stage is an orientation phase. During this stage, the team members meet and get to know each other. They start building rapport and friendship with each other. The team learns the purpose of the group, the opportunities, and challenges as well as the rules to follow. In this stage, group members are formal in fear of exposing information to each other. Members exchange some personal data, are enthusiastic about knowing how the group works, and make new friends. Initially, they do not know the issues and objectives of the team. They see the goal and start work without knowing their exact roles. Mature team members behave appropriately. The supervisor behaves as a group leader and tries to evaluate how each member of the team can work as an individual and how the member responds to work pressure.
   2. *Storming:* During this stage, the group is likely to observe the highest level of disagreement and conflict. Members come to know each other's position and level, open up to each other, and confront each other's ideas and perspectives. They also address issues related to problem, resolution, individuals as well as group roles. They show and share personal anger, frustration, and dissatisfaction, and there is internal competition for leadership or to influence the group. Members need to develop tolerance and patience. Usually, the supervisor observes as the group as a nonparticipant and does not interfere in decision-making. The team is motivated to resolve their differences amicably.
   3. *Norming:* The norming stage is a consolidation phase of group development. The members recognize individual differences and expectations from each other. They start developing a sense of belongingness and cohesion. At this stage, they are clear about their roles, responsibilities, and positions.
   4. *Performing:* Performing phase is a stage of maturity. The group attained a feeling of cohesiveness. They become well organized, work independently and also in a group. The acceptance level toward each other is maximum, and they try to resolve conflict through group discussion. The group members know their roles and are flexible in their work schedule to achieve the maximum output. The members are self-reliant and independent in making decisions through a rational process.
   5. *Adjourning:* Adjourning is the last stage of the group development process in temporary groups. Wrapping up becomes the priority at this stage. Few members feel satisfied due to task accomplishment but some feel depressed. They often experience sadness and closure and they prepared to leave.
6. *McGrath's time, interaction, and performance theory:*
   According to McGrath's (1991) time, interaction, and performance (TIP) theory, different teams have various ways of achieving the same goal. He suggested four modes of group activity, i.e., inception, technical problem solving, conflict resolution, and execution.
   a. **Inception:** Inception mode is an acceptance stage in which a group develops goal-oriented tasks.
   b. **Technical problem-solving:** After developing goal-oriented tasks, the group starts solving technical problems. Each one of them tries to find alternative solutions to the problem from a technical point of view.

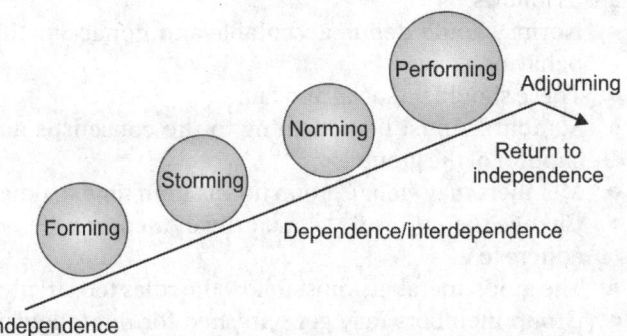

Fig. 42.1: Stages of group development.

c. **Conflict resolution:** In this phase, the group members focus on selecting the best policy to resolve conflicts.
d. **Execution:** In the execution mode, the members implement the best solution to achieve the goal.

GROUP DYNAMICS

Concept of Group Dynamics

The two words, group and dynamics, coin group dynamics. A group is a social unit of two or more individuals who have a set of beliefs and values in common and follow the same norms and work to achieve specific tasks or goals. The word "dynamics" means the flow of activities that lead the group toward the establishment of its set goals. The word dynamics is a Greek word, meaning the study of "force." Thus, the term group dynamics refers to the forces operating wide in groups for social interaction and interest.

Group dynamics mean the interactions between people who discuss in a group setting. It also refers to the structures and processes with which groups form and function. It reveals a group's characteristics, formation, and functioning. It is a social process by which people interact face to face in small groups. It is the study of groups and group processes and the interrelationships among members of a group.

In 1896, Gustave Le Bon, a French social psychologist, developed the concept of group psychology. Later on, William McDougall (1920), Sigmund Freud (1922), Wilfred (1961), William (1958, 1966), Ernest Johns, and other scholars contributed to the field of group dynamics. Tuckman is renowned for the four stages of a group formation. Kurt Lewin (1947, 1948, and 1951) was the founder of group dynamics and coined this term and studied that individuals and groups act and react differently in different situations.

Elements of Group Dynamics

Group dynamics are concerned with why and how groups develop. The focus areas of group dynamics are group communication, group conflicts, group decision-making, group morale, group problem-solving, group leadership, group norms and values, and group process. Group norms and cohesiveness are the prime concerns of group dynamics and discussed below:

Group Norms

Group norms are acceptable standards of behavior within a group that are shared by the group members. These reflect the rules that the group members follow. These are stated explicitly and implicitly and describe acceptable and unacceptable behavior. Norms specify beliefs, attitudes, and expectations common for group members. Michael Argyle explains group norms as the guidelines or rules regarding acceptable behavior framed by a group. These are criteria to monitor the functioning of the group members.

Purposes of group norms: The purposes of group norms are as follows:
- To facilitate group survival
- To maximize their chances of task success and minimize chances of task failure
- To make the group more organized
- To achieve the objectives of the group
- To define and predict acceptable and unacceptable behavior
- To monitor the conduct of its members
- To avoid embarrassing situations
- To express the values of the group
- To make the members identify themselves with the group
- To reflect the level of commitment, motivation, and performance of the group
- To discipline the members of a group to make them work regularly and adequately
- To reduce absenteeism and turnover among employees
- To regulate each action of the group members
- To help groups meet the aims of performing successfully and keeping the morale high.

Types of norms
1. **Performance norms:** This criterion defines and monitors the performance of the members. This also determines the effort put by everyone to achieve a goal.
2. **Reward-allocation norms:** This determines rewards to allocate according to the performance of group members.
3. **The norm of equality:** The rule of justice means equal treatment of all members of the group.
4. **Equity norms:** The equity norm suggests that every member must share the same reward for the same performance. The member who puts maximum effort and has skill receives the highest compensation.
5. **Social responsibility norms:** It states that the members who fulfill the needs of social responsibility will receive the largest share of the reward.
6. **Behavior norms:** These norms define the behavior standard of individuals while working on a day-to-day basis.

Characteristics of norms: The characteristics of norms are as follows:
- Norms should define acceptable and nonacceptable behavior.
- These should be social and fair.
- Standards must be according to the consensus and support of the group.
- Members may violate group norms from time to time.
- Change the norms if the majority of members do not adhere to it.
- The group members must follow the rules too strictly.
- Group members may get punished for not following standards.

Group Cohesiveness

Defining group cohesiveness: According to Likert, cohesiveness is the attractiveness of the members toward the group or resistance of leaving it. According to Aswathappa, it is the extent to which each member like others and how far each one wants to remain as a member of a group. According to Festinger, it is the entire field of forces that acts on the members to stay in the group. It is the bonding of group members and their desire to remain part of the group. It includes all forces that make an individual to be in the group and stay in the group. These forces are strong liking, belongingness, similar choices, attitudes, goals, and needs. The group members have a sense of group feeling to perform to achieve the stated goals.

Loyalty and commitment of the members to each other are the ingredients of group cohesiveness. The group members work together in a group, support, and have trust in each other and are generally produced to achieve their goals.

Advantages of group cohesiveness: The advantages of group cohesiveness are as follows:
- It can teach high morale among group members.
- The group members become loyal and committed to work.
- It helps members to have a feeling of belongingness and security.
- The members actively participate and regular at their work.
- The members put their maximum effort to achieve the organizational goals.
- The members have a maximum satisfaction level.
- It increases work productivity and satisfaction of employees.
- There are fewer chances of conflicts and differences among members.
- The members show less anxiety to their work.

Factors influencing group cohesiveness: The factors affecting group cohesiveness are as follows:
- Smaller groups, special norms, and practices
- Interpersonal attraction among the members
- Social structure and leadership style of the group
- The ability of group members to achieve goals
- Type of interdependence among the group members
- Mutual understanding, support, and self-esteem among members
- Time spent together and frequent interaction
- Excellent quality and amount of communication
- Loyalty, commitment, and satisfaction of the group members
- The attractiveness of the group's goals and activities
- Maintaining group culture and group norms
- Group's relationship to its outside environment
- Intense competition with other groups
- A severe external threat to survival.

Effects of group cohesiveness
a. **Positive results:** The employees feel greater satisfaction with their work. Employee turnover and absenteeism will be low. The members will have high empowerment and show greater productivity. All members participate in decision-making and problem-solving related activities.
b. **Adverse effects:** Top cohesive groups can be detrimental to organizational performance if their goals misaligned with organizational goals. They can also be more vulnerable to the group. They will not be serious about solving the problems, working on various alternative solutions, and implementing the best alternative. They used to be very slow in making decisions and go on making excuses for not accomplishing the goals on time. They may fail to examine risks and may get biased in processing the available information to solve the problem.

Methods to Develop Leadership in a Group

The following methods should be adhered to develop leadership in a group:
- Start a discussion with open-ended questions
- Encourage all members to participate in discussion openly
- Appreciate participation and contribution of members
- Pay equal attention to all members
- Do not be partial and consider everyone's opinion
- Have patience and listen to the ideas of all members
- Focus on the goal of the group
- Observe every one's perceptions
- Make all the members understand the meaning of a team
- Make all the members clear about the statements
- Repeat and conclude the main ideas and feelings
- Do not ask questions frequently
- Take consensus, summarize the ideas, emphasize the facts, and encourage to discuss again.

Group Dynamics in Nursing Management

The nurse managers must know group dynamics, various types of group, group formation, group norms, and group cohesiveness. Following are the ways that they can apply at their workplace to achieve the organizational goals:
- The nurse manager can promote healthy informal groups to improve morale among nurses since the accomplishment of the organizational goals and high productivity depend on how much is the morale of the employees influenced by informal groups.
- Nurse managers need to function in a group to promote problem-solving and acceptance of responsibility.
- The nurse manager needs to know how groups function to facilitate effectiveness. Since each member of the group plays an essential role in achieving the work of

the group and each member is different in his or her personality, it has a different way of doing the work.
- The nurse manager can improve the work environment by maintaining the therapeutic interpersonal relationship with the team group. In the performance of these roles, the group members share the power of the organization and its management.
- Nurse managers with the working knowledge of group dynamics can use their experience to assemble groups. Such knowledge is vital in the selection of the chair of committees, task forces, and other groups of clinical nurses. It is essential for selecting nurses for organizational committees
- Group training creates awareness of the roles the members play and the opportunity to manage them, so that they become productive. Group training can contribute to the theory of nursing practice and management.
- The concepts of group dynamics a nurse manager can apply while conducting continuing education and in-service education program for professional nurses through role-plays and case studies.
- Knowledge of group dynamics is essential for nurse managers to improve leadership competencies and to facilitate group discussions and communication. Groups are a common feature of most of the experiences of all nurses in such roles as outcome management; team coordination; and teaching of students, patients, and family.

CHAPTER HIGHLIGHTS

- Group dynamics are the interactions between people who discuss together in a group setting and concerned with why and how groups develop.
- The size, functions, norms, and cohesiveness of a group form the group structure. A group should have constructive criticism and consensus in decision-making.
- The two types of the work group are formal groups and informal, and groups are formed due to multiple reasons.
- Many approaches/theories are involved in developing different types of groups, such as traditional theory, social exchange, social identity, Schutz's three-stage model, and Tuckman's four-stage model.
- Group norms and cohesiveness are the primary focus areas of group dynamics. Group norms are acceptable standards of behavior within a group and are the attractiveness of the members toward the group or resistance to leave it.

REVIEW QUESTIONS

I. Essay Type Questions
1. Define group dynamics. Describe the functions of a group.
2. Enumerate the reasons to form groups. Discuss the different types of groups.
3. Define group cohesiveness. Explain factors influencing group cohesiveness.
4. Enlist theories and models of group development. Discuss any one theory or model in detail.

II. Short Notes
1. Purposes of a group
2. Tuckman's theory
3. Group norms
4. Group cohesiveness

III. Multiple Choice Questions
1. A pattern of relationship among members holding a group together to achieve a goal is:
    a. Group size
    b. Power structure
    c. Group function
    d. Group structure
2. Under which type of functions in group dynamics encouraging and harmonizing roles of a group are categorized?
    a. Maintenance   b. Task
    c. Self-interest   d. Interdependency
3. Which type of interaction is mainly for discussion to solve an issue in a group?
    a. Collaborative   b. Organized social
    c. Logical   d. Unorganized social
4. At which stage in Schutz's model, the team members focus on leadership and structural issues?
    a. Inclusion   b. Control
    c. Affection   d. Adjourning
5. At which stage in Tuckman's model, the group observes the highest level of disagreement and conflict?
    a. Forming   b. Norming
    c. Storming   d. Performing

Answer Keys

1. d   2. a   3. c   4. b   5. c

SUGGESTED READING

1. Arrow H. Stability, bistability, and instability in small group influence patterns. J Pers Soc Psychol. 1997;72:75-85.
2. Aswathappa K. Human Resource Management- Text and Cases. (7th ed.), New Delhi: McGraw Hill Education (India) Private Limited, 2013.
3. Available from http://journals.plos.org/plosone/article?id=10.1371/journal.pone.0161281. [Accessed Jan 2018].
4. Available from http://www. hrdq.com/products/gda.htm. [Accessed Jan 2018].
5. Bion WR. Experiences in Groups and Other Papers, New York, Basic Books, 1961.
6. Brown R. Group Processes: Dynamics within and between Groups. UK: Wiley, 1988.
7. Earnest J. The Elements of Figure Skating (rev. ed.). London: Allen and Unwin, 1952.

8. Festinger L, Schacter S, Back K (Eds). Social pressures in informal groups: A study of human factors in housing. New York: Harper and Brothers, 1950.
9. Ivanitskaya LV, Glazer S, Erofeev DA. (2009). Group dynamics. Available in Johnson JA. (Ed), Health Organizations: Theory, Behavior, and Development (pp. 109"C136). Boston: Jones & Bartlett. Jex, SM, & Beehr, TA, 1991.
10. Judith TR, Mary ST. Clinical Leadership in Nursing, 1st edition. Philadelphia, PA: Saunders; 1998.
11. Katz D, Kahn R. The Social Psychology of Organizations, 2nd edition. New York: John Wiley & Sons; 1978.
12. Lewin K, Dorwin Cartwright (Ed). Field theory in social science. New York: Harper, 1951.
13. Lewin K, Lewin GW (Ed). Resolving social conflicts: selected papers on group dynamics [1935-1946]. New York: Harper and Brothers, 1948.
14. Lewin K. Frontiers in group dynamics: Concept, method and reality in social science; social equilibria and social change. Human Relations 1947; 1(1): 5-41.
15. Likert R. New Patterns of Management. New York: McGraw-Hill Book Company, 1961.
16. Luthans F. Organizational Behavior, 10th edition. Boston, MA: McGraw-Hill; 2005.
17. McDougall W. The Group Mind: A Sketch of the Principles of Collective Psychology. New York: Putnam's, 1920.
18. McGrath JE. Groups: Interaction and Performance. Englewood Cliffs, NJ: Prentice-Hall; 1984.
19. Morgan BB, Salas E, Glickman AS. An analysis of team evolution and maturation. J Gen Psychol. 1994;120(3):277-91.
20. Poole MS, Holmes ME. Decision development in computer-assisted group decision making. Hum Commun Res. 1995;22(1):90-127.
21. Schutz W. FIRO: A Three-Dimensional Theory of Interpersonal Behavior. New York: Holt, Rinehart & Winston, 1958
22. Schutz W. The Interpersonal Underworld. (Updated version based on 1958 work). Palo Alto, CA: Science and Behavior Books, 1966.
23. Sigmund F. Group Psychology and the Analysis of the Ego. London: The International Psycho-Analytical Press, 1922.
24. The Role of The Group Leader—Angelfire. (n.d.). [online] Available from http://www.angelfire.com/ns/southeasternnurse/GroupDynamicsCulturalDiversity.htm. [Accessed Jan 2018].
25. Tubbs S. A Systems Approach to Small Group Interaction. New York: McGraw-Hill; 1995.
26. Tuckman BW, Jensen MA. Stages of small-group development revisited. Group Org. Studies 1977;2(4):419-27.
27. Tuckman BW. Developmental sequence in small groups. Psychol Bull. 1965;63:384-99.
28. Tuckman BW. Developmental sequence in small groups. Psychol Bull. 1965;63:384-99.
29. What is a group? | Infed.org. (n.d.). [online] Available from http://infed.org/mobi/what-is-a-group/. [Accessed July 2019].

43
CHAPTER

Power, Organizational Politics, Lobbying, and Advocacy

CHAPTER OUTLINE

- Power
  - Meaning and Definitions
  - Types of Power
  - Sources and Result of Power
- Organizational Politics
  - Historical Perspective
  - Definitions
  - Characteristics of Organizational Politics
  - Factors Influencing Political Behavior
  - Managing Organizational Politics
- Lobbying and Advocacy
  - Meaning
  - Importance of Lobbying
  - Advocacy Skill for Lobbying
  - Opportunities for Lobbying and Advocacy
  - Role of Nurses in Lobbying and Advocacy

LEARNING OUTCOMES

After completion of this chapter, the learner will be able to:
- Understand the concept of power and organizational politics
- Describe the bases of power in the organization
- Explain how the information relates to power in the organization
- Discuss the consequences and contingencies of power
- Explain the perspectives of organizational power and politics
- Discuss the main characteristics of organizational politics
- Describe the types of political activity found in the organization
- Describe factors and conditions that encourage organizational politics
- Identify ways to control dysfunctional organizational politics

KEY TERMS

Power, organizational politics, lobbying, advocacy, political activity

INTRODUCTION

Organizational power and politics are regarded as critical factors affecting various organizational practices. Power and politics inextricably interwove with the fabric of an organization's life. Power is one of the attributes of a successful organization. Power is the ability of a person, group, or organization to influence others and requires the perception of the dependence of one individual over another.

Power is an essential organizational behavior theme as it determines its culture and, ultimately, its success.

Power and politics are ever present and necessary features of organizational life. Without them, the organization is unable to accomplish its objective. However, one can abuse power for their personal or political goals. Power is necessary to influence an individual or group. Nurses are to use position and power to influence patients, physicians, other health-care professionals, and coworkers.

POWER

Meaning and Definitions

The concept of power is often confused with authority, and no universal description of the term exists. Power means "to be able to." We, as a nurse leader, can use power in a very constructive way. Styles and Hall viewed power as central to the development of nursing as a profession. Bierstadt defined power as the ability to employ force. Roger considered power as the potential to influence others. It is the ability and willingness to change the behavior of others to produce specific intended effects.

The ability to use power requires particular strengths, energy, and concrete actions. French defined power as a force that person A has over person B, which is "equal to a maximum force which A induces on B—the maximum force which mobilizes B in the opposite direction."

Chandler (1992) defined power as a means to control, influence, or dominate, whereas Kanter (1993) referred it as the ability to get things done, to mobilize resources, and to understand and use to achieve the goal. It includes caring and empowering patients (Benner, 2001). It is a tool for professional excellence in nursing to enhance the quality of care and for professional promotion (Sepasi et al., 2016).

Types

Power can be classified in various ways. It may be formal and informal. A person has the official authority by position in the hierarchical structure of an organization. It is legitimate or legally bestows by post. The informal or intimate power is personal and created by the person through social interaction and its influence, rather than authority. The person may influence others through persuasion, dialogue, debate, charisma, or personality style. The following are the types of power:

Legitimate Power

Legitimate authority is also a position of strength. It is legal and formal. This power is bestowed on a person holding a job in an organization. All the employees have position power according to organizational rules and regulations. For example, the managers have the power to direct and command their subordinates to achieve preset goals. Legitimate power is like a formal authority that one can create, grant, change, or withdraw by management. The structure in an organization identifies legal authority by position and location in the hierarchy, level of responsibility, and social placement. Usually, higher level positions exercise more power than lower level positions in a classical hierarchical organizational structure.

According to Hardy and Clegg (1996), legitimate power has two perspectives, namely, the functionalist and critical perspectives. The power exercised during decision-making as a part of a deliberate strategy to achieve the intended outcome is the functional perspective of power. But when the dominant group in an organization attempts to exercise the ability to manipulate things is a critical perspective of power.

Reward Power

Reward power involves positive sanctions. It is directly proportioned to rewards valued by others. Higher the perceived values of such rewards, greater the power. The manager who praises and recognizes sends a memorandum of thanks but holds the influence. Organizational rewards are in the form of promotion, better assignments, salary increase, bonus, and other monetary benefits. Power is derived from the ability of an individual.

Coercive Power

Coercive power involves negative sanctions. A subordinate perceives the failure to comply with the wishes of the superior may lead to punishment or some negative outcome. In coercive power, usually, managers use some form of punishment such as the threat of dismissal, suspension, demotion, or strictly enforcing rules, and assigning unfavorable tasks. The subordinate may get psychological harm. The coercive power is directly proportioned to the number and severity of the sanctions over which the manager has control. Since the coercive power can create resentment and hostility among employees, its use is often successful in the short run.

Expert Power

Expert power is exercised as a result of one's knowledge, experience, and skill of an individual. It is a personal power originating from the expertise of a person. The people will acknowledge and follow the individuals having knowledge and skill in that field. Nurses can exercise this power, whatever the position they hold.

Referent Power

Leaders possess referent power due to their traits, personality, and identity. This power can influence others having those characteristics. Others often imitate people with referent power due to their actions, attitudes, and dress. A person who is respected by others for whatever reason has referent power over those people. The referent power comes from within the person. The persons who get emotionally involved with the persons having referent power are likely to give respect and willing to follow them.

Information Power

The information power is a type of power that persons exert by having information as perceived by others. The data is powered when there is control over the flow and interpretation of data and coping with uncertainty. It comes from legitimate or expert sources. The control over data is shared in highly bureaucratic organizations.

Connection Power

Connection power is a type of power that comes from a connection of a person with a very influential or highly renowned person. People use this type of force to achieve their own goals.

Sources and Results

Both organizational and individual factors are the primary sources of power. Influence power is primarily based on organizational factors. Coercive, reward, and legitimate power are obtained from their position in the organization. Whereas the cause of other forces such as expert and

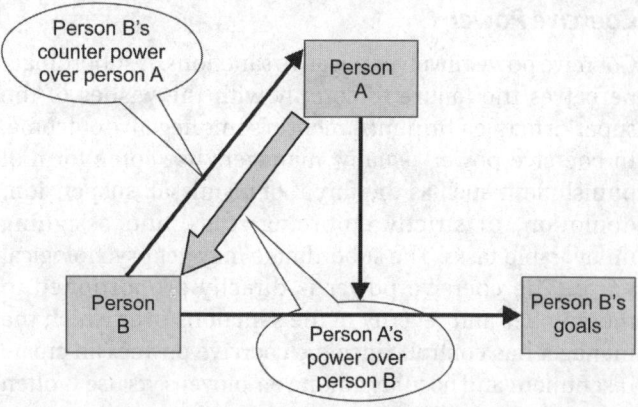

Fig. 43.1: Concept of power.

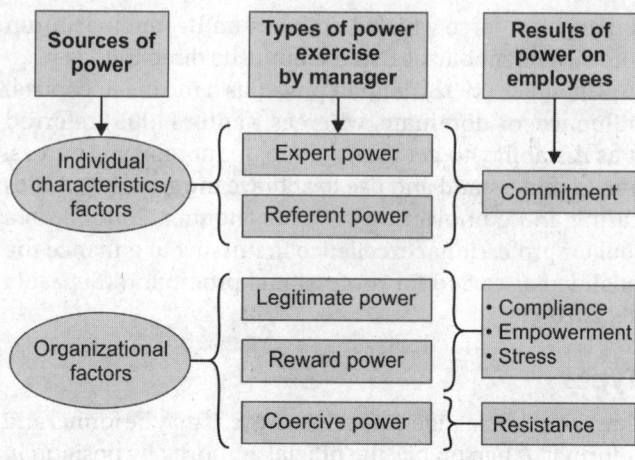

Fig. 43.2: Powers, its sources, and results.

reference power is primarily characteristics of an individual **(Fig. 43.1)**. Some managers possess managerial and other competencies and hence can exercise all types of controls.

The manager who exercises different powers from different sources has an impact on his or her employees. It resulted in commitment, compliance, and resistance among employees. The managers with expert and referent power have highly committed employees. The managers with legitimate and reward power will give room to or tend to produce compliance, empowerment, and stress among employees. The managers using coercive power will find to be resistant to the subordinates working under them **(Fig. 43.2)**.

Legitimate Power Outcome

The subordinates hardly challenge the use of legitimate power by their superiors. However, the excellent way of making the request and following it up is significant for ensuring the subordinate's future compliance and the growth of the superior's referent power. Command managers overuse this power and ignore participatory leadership approaches. Hence, the managers must be sensitive to employees' needs.

Reward Power Outcome

Reward power is the ability of a person to control the allocation of reward. The manager must be sure that the employee has done the job before awarding compensation. This type of power, if exercised by the managers, can bring compliance among employees; they will feel empowered and the work stress may reduce. Empowerment is power sharing, the delegation of power or authority to subordinates in the organization. If not used or in case of bias in using this power by the manager, it can lead to ill feeling among the employees, and they will work under stress.

Coercive Power Outcome

Usually, coercive power is a negative sanction. Using coercive control is a natural response when something goes wrong. But the consequence of using power is often resistance from employees' side, and they resent it. It is a challenging form of punishment to use successfully in an organization. This type of power should be used very carefully and within the legal and rules framework.

Expert Power Outcome

Managers can use expert power most effectively to address employee concerns. They can win the confidence and trust of employees; they respect their abilities, knowledge, and competencies. By use of this type of power by the managers, the employees will be very committed to their work.

Referent Power Outcome

By using this type of power, the employees will be committed to work. A manager who wants her employees to be punctual, considerate, and creative should use a kind of power.

ORGANIZATIONAL POLITICS

Each organization comprises people with varied personal interests and goals. Politics refers to means of recognizing and, ultimately, reconciling competing interests within the organization. In any organization, at any given moment, several people are seeking to gain and use power to achieve their needs. This pursuit of power is political behavior.

Historical Perspective

The concept of organizational politics began in the 1970s, with a focus on the aspects of power and bureaucracy in the workplace, specifically focused on management and leadership. There was fragmented exposure in the literature before the 1980s. In 1983, organizational politics found its way into the research and textbooks on organizational behavior in publications by Robins, Hellriegel, Slocum, and Woodman. In 1980, Mintzberg coupled politics with influence and considered to constitute one among several systems of impact in the organization.

Definitions

Organizational politics is an attempt to influence others using discretionary behavior and linked to dysfunction in organizations to gain personal objectives.

Mintzberg (1983) referred to organizational politics as an informal, illegitimate, and uncertified individual or group behavior that results both in games and positive change. Decisions are not made rationally or formally but rather through compromising accommodation and bargaining.

Pfeffer (1981) described organizational politics as those behaviors used for their preferred personal outcomes at the time of uncertainty or disagreement. It is an intentional social influence process in which action is strategically designed to maximize short-term or long-term self-interests (Parker et al., 1995).

The politics may be in the form of attacking and blaming others, controlling information, not disclosing to any others, cultivating networks, creating obligations, forming coalitions, and trying to impress others to achieve their gains.

Characteristics of Organizational Politics

Vigoda (2006) describes organizational politics as the unique domain of interpersonal relations in the workplace. Its main features are as follows:
- The readiness of people to use power in their efforts to influence others
- To secure personal or collective interests
- To avoid adverse outcomes within the organization.

Factors Influencing Political Behavior

Politics is an essential skill in managers who wish to get things done. The art of how to get them on your side is crucial at any rank and it involves human resource implications. However, even today, most of the studies dealing with organizational politics suggest that it is a predominantly negative phenomenon. The following six main factors influence political behavior (**Fig. 43.3**):

Vague Objectives

Due to vague objectives, there is more room available for playing politics by the employees. Some people may use ambiguity to manipulate the situation for their benefit.

Scarce Resources

When resources are limited, people tend to use politics to make sure that they get the maximum benefit.

Changes in Technology and Environment

Organizational effectiveness is a function of the organization's ability to appropriately respond to an unpredictable environment and adapting to complex technological developments. Thus, political behavior is liable to improve when the internal technology is sophisticated and the external environment is highly volatile.

Nonprogrammed Decisions

Sometimes the organizations make a lot of nonprogrammed decisions on specific issues without any set standards due

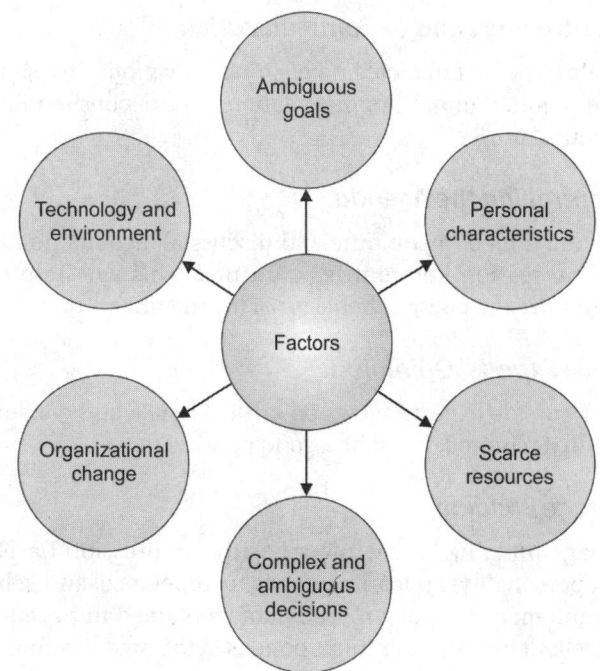

Fig. 43.3: Factors influencing organizational politics.

to complexity. Managers make decisions on intuition guesses and affected by their politics.

Change Management

During change management and changes in the organizational structure and policies, the people in powerful positions can play politics. They may restructure, develop a new division, and introduce new strategies per their political behavior.

Personal Characteristics

Some people, due to their personalities, have a strong need to seek power for themselves and use political tactics to acquire more power.

Managing Organizational Politics

The extreme politics in any organization is dangerous; it can demoralize other people, destroy loyalty, and make them uncooperative. Most of the time, people may use their time and energy in attacking and counterattacking. The employees who work in such an environment have low job satisfaction and commitment toward their work. They hardly pay attention to quality work and remain absent. They make excuses for making decisions. Though it is impossible to eliminate political behavior in organizations, it is possible to reduce it. The managers need to understand the cause of politics and try to take action accordingly. Managers can apply the following techniques:

Controlling the Information

Try not to disseminate critical information to others. The people who will not disclose the information, get the political power.

Controlling Lines of Communication

Follow the hierarchical line of communication. Give only the required minimum information to have considerable political power.

Controlling the Agenda

Conduct meeting on time and discuss all agenda points in the session before it is adjourned. This will help to minimize the political behavior of the members.

Seek Experts' Opinion

Get outside experts' views on critical issues and consult them if required. It can be a good political move.

Image Building

Image building is creating a positive impression based on personality, appearance, style, competence, and self-confidence of a person. The managers need to have an excellent image to minimize politics in the organization.

Building Alliance

To build an agreement is another technique of gaining political power. It is necessary to have a coalition with the right people.

Eliminate the Factors Causing Organizational Politics

Try to assess the organizational factors causing politics among employees and try to solve by:
- Providing enough resources
- Setting clear goals
- Developing performance standards
- Introducing rules and regulation
- Letting the employees verbalize their grievances
- Taking quick actions if somebody indulges in too much politics
- Managing change effectively, having meetings with them periodically, and seeking suggestions
- Removing political norms if any
- Recruiting employees who are least involved in politics
- Give employees more control over their work.

LOBBYING AND ADVOCACY

Meaning

According to business dictionary, lobbying is defined as "the act of attempting to influence leaders to create an activity that will help a particular organization." Originally it was used to influence and buy the president by the political advocates at the hotel's lobby to access grant.

Lobbying is a form of advocacy of influencing decisions made by the government by individuals or lobby groups. Advocacy is a process or act of supporting a cause or proposal. The professional lobby group or lobbyists are the people who try to influence legislation, regulation, or other government decisions or actions on behalf of a professional group. They are the elected officials of professional organizations and work for professional interest.

Importance of Lobbying

Lobbying is considered crucial due to the following reasons:
- To raise awareness of a concern
- To promote a solution to the concerned issue
- To influence others to take action or lead a change in regulation, legislation, and other decisions.

Advocacy Skills for Lobbying

To promote safe practice environment, quality of care, and nurses' status and uplift the nursing profession, nurses at different levels have the responsibility to work through appropriate channels to address concerned issues. The code of ethics in nursing also identified a range of advocacy skills and activities. Nurses involving in advocacy must have the following advocacy skills:

Problem-solving Skills

Lobbyists must have problem-solving skills. They need to identify the problem to address and develop goals and strategies and need to work out various activities for each recognized event. They should be masters to prepare memorandum/agenda specifying the issue. They should know the appropriate time to put a request before the decision maker as well as how to approach them. They need to have patience, to negotiate and compromise skills, and have collaboration with other agencies.

Communication Skills

Lobbyists are advocates for professional nurses. They voice on behalf of the group, and they bring nurses together to address concerned issues and possible solutions. Therefore, they must have both verbal and written communication skills. They should discuss the mass in brief and to the point. Communication should be evidence based and with supporting documents. At the end of the address, provide a leaflet depicting critical aspects of issues and strategies.

Influencing and Leadership Skills

The lobbyists must have competence, must build trust and credibility, and must have leadership qualities to influence decision makers to agree with proposed solutions of the identified issues. They can make use of persuasion skills, which is an important key to exert influence.

Collaborating Skills

Collaboration with coworkers, departments, and other agencies is essential to achieve a goal. Lobbyists must have a positive collaborative relationship to gain support from them to address common issue, goals, strategies, and actions; they need to build trust, credibility, and mutual respect and work with them closely, making them understand about the concerned issue, seeking appropriate support, and informing them about the progress.

Opportunities for Lobbying and Advocacy

Nurses have great opportunities while working in the following capacities as:
- Members of various committees in the department (hospital, educational institute) or organization
- Member of councils (International Nursing Council, Indian Nursing Council, State Nursing Council, and other boards)
- Member of professional association, e.g. Trained Nurses Association of India (TNAI)
- Associating with organization-wide activities for nurses and the nursing profession
- Conducting various surveys on employees, client satisfaction, and submitting reports to decision makers to focus their attention toward concerned issues and possible solutions
- Attending meetings to raise awareness about relevant issues
- Teaching students and nurses at the bedside
- Educating the public about the role of nurses and the nursing profession to assess, plan, intervene to address healthcare issues.

Role of Nurses in Lobbying and Advocacy

Professional nurses have multitasks related to advocacy in nursing practice. They can support through teaching, mentoring, peer review, involving in professional associations, community service, and updating knowledge and skill in advocacy.

1. **Role of TNAI in lobbying**
   - To promote legislation and to speak on behalf of nurses regarding legislative action
   - To promote and protect the economic welfare of the nurses
   - To represent nurses and to serve as their spokesman with allied national and international agencies
   - To serve as the official representative of TNAI and as a member of International Council of Nurses (ICN)
   - To promote high standards of healthcare to nursing practice
   - To advance professional, educational, economic, and general welfare of nurses
   - To have affiliation with the ICN; Commonwealth Nurses Federation, government committees and councils, and other organizations.
2. **Role of Indian Nursing Council in lobbying**
   - Promotion of health and healthcare proposals and commenting on planned legislation as well as proactively advising, altering, and offering suggestions to the government on matters affecting the nursing profession, including service conditions
   - With the Government of India
     - Sanctioning of budget and grant in aid
     - Sanctioning of the scales of pay and allowances for the offices and staff of the council
     - Collection of information from the State Nursing Services and the School of Nursing having special projects
     - Declaration under Section 10,14,15, of INC Act
   - Involved in the operational management and regulation of services in the interest of society.
3. **Nurse administrator/manager role in lobbying**
   Nurse managers can play an important advocacy role in the following issues:
   a. *Adequate resources*
      - Staffing requirement, scheduling
      - Involving in the budgeting process for staffing and advocating on equipment and supplies
      - Improving staff knowledge and skill on advocacy
      - Collaboration between nurse managers and staff nurses
      - Being a member of the purchase committee.
   b. *Advocacy for a healthy work environment*
      - Development of conflict-resolution skills
      - Delegating ownership
      - Recruitment, development, and retaining staff
      - Induction program
      - Change management.
4. **Nurse educator role in lobbying**
   Nurse educators can play an important role in developing nurse advocates by organizing staff development programs for in-service nurses and mentoring nurses in practice.
5. **Nurse practitioner role in advocacy**
   Nurses working with patients are advocates for patients. They should have open and genuine dialogues with them, establish a real therapeutic relationship, exercise power, and find the appropriate situation to advocate. They need to use coping strategies to face barriers to patient advocacy by finding opportunities and by persistence. And they should search for an expansion of knowledge and skill through in-service training and advance professional qualifications for support.

CHAPTER HIGHLIGHTS

- Power is the ability and willingness to change the behavior of others to produce specific intended effects.
- There are many types of power, such as legitimate, reward, coercive, expert, referent, information, and connection power.
- Both organizational and individual factors are the primary sources of power. The managers empowering power from different sources influence their employees accordingly.
- Organizational politics is an intentional social influence process in which action is strategically designed to maximize short-term or long-term self-interest. The

managers need to understand the cause of politics and try to take actions accordingly.
- Lobbying is a form of advocacy of influencing decisions made by the government by individuals or lobby groups.
- Advocacy is a process or act of supporting a cause or proposal. Professional nurses have multitasks related to advocacy in nursing practice.

REVIEW QUESTIONS

I. Essay Type Questions
1. Define "power." Explain the different types of powers.
2. Describe sources and outcome of powers.
3. Explain the concept of organizational politics. Describe the factors influencing political behavior.
4. Describe various methods of managing organizational politics.

II. Short Notes
1. Legitimate and reward power
2. Lobbying and advocacy
3. Advocacy skills for lobbying
4. Role of nurses in advocacy

III. Multiple Choice Questions
1. The ability and willingness to change the behavior to provide specific intended results are:
   a. Politics   b. Power
   c. Lobbying   d. Advocacy
2. Which type of power leaders possess due to their traits, personality, and identity?
   a. Legitimate   b. Expert
   c. Referent   d. Reward
3. The outcome of power exercised on employees by managers possessing expert and referent powers is?
   a. Empowerment   b. Stress
   c. Resistance   d. Commitment
4. The lobbyists having competence, build trust, and creditability use which type of skills?
   a. Influencing   b. Communication
   c. Problem solving   d. Collaborating

Answer Keys
1. b 2. c 3. d 4. a

SUGGESTED READING

1. Baum HS. Organizational politics against organizational culture: A psychoanalytic perspective. Hum Res Manag. 1989;28(2):191-206.
2. Bellinger G. Bureaucracy and organizational politics. [online] Available from http://www.systems-thinking.org/bop/bop.htm. [Accessed Feb 2018].
3. Benner P. From Novice to expert: Excellence and Power in Clinical Nursing Practice (Commemorative Edition). Upper Saddle River, NJ: Prentice-Hall Health; 2001.
4. Bierstadt R. An analysis of social power. American Sociological Review 1950; 6: 7-30.
5. Chandler GE. The source and process of empowerment. Nurs Adm Q. 1992;16(3):65-71.
6. Clegg SR, Hardy C, Nord WR (ed). Handbook of Organization Studies. New Delhi: SAGE Publications India Pvt. Ltd., 1996.
7. Drory A, Romm T. The definition of organizational politics: A review. Hum Relat. 1990;43(11):1133-54.
8. Ferris GR, Frink DD, Galang MC, Zhou J, Kacmar M, Howard JL. Perceptions of organizational politics: Prediction, stress-related implications, and outcomes. Hum Relat. 1989;49(2):233-66.
9. French JRP, Jr, and Raven BH. The basis of social power. In Catwright (ed) Studies in Social Power. Ann Arbor MI: Institute for Social Research, University of Michigan; 1959. pp. 150-67.
10. Gibson CH. A concept analysis of empowerment. J Adv Nurs. 1991;16(3):354-61.
11. Hall RH. The professions, employed professionals, and the professional association. Professionalism and the empowerment of nursing: Papers presented at the 53rd convention, 1982, pp. 1-15. Washington DC: American Nurses' Association. (Cross ref.)
12. Manojlovich M. Power and empowerment in nursing: Looking backward to inform the future. OJIN: The Online Journal of Issues in Nursing Jan 31, 2007; 12 (1), Manuscript 1. DOI: 10.3912/OJIN.Vol12No01Man01.
13. Hellriegel D, Slocum JW, and Woodman RW. Organizational Behavior. South-Western College Pub., 2001.
14. Laschinger HKS, Sabiston JA, Kutszcher L. Empowerment and staff nurse decision involvement in nursing work environments: Testing Kanter's theory of structural power in organizations. Res Nurs Health. 1997;20:341-52.
15. Madison DL. Organizational politics: An exploration of managers' perceptions. Hum Relat. 1980;33(2):79-100.
16. Manojlovich M. Predictors of professional nursing practice behaviors in hospital settings. Nurs Res. 2005a;54(1):41-7.
17. Miller BK, Rutherford MA, Kolodinsky RW. Perceptions of organizational politics: A meta-analysis of outcomes. J Bus Psychol. 2008;22(3):209-22.
18. Mintzberg H. The Nature of Managerial Work: Theory of management policy series, California: Prentice-Hall, 01-Jan-1980.
19. Parker PS, Ogilvie DT. Gender, Culture, and Leadership: Towards a culturally distinct model of African-American womwn executives' leadership strategies. Leadership Quarterly, 1996; 7 (2): 187-214.
20. Pfeffer J. Managing with Power: Politics and Influence in Organizations, Boston: Harvard Business School Press; 1992.
21. Pfeffer J. Power in organizations. The University of Michigan: Pitman Pub., 1981.
22. Rafael AR. Power and caring: A debate in nursing. Adv Nurs Sci. 1996;19(1):3-17.
23. Robins SP. Organizational behavior Pennsylvania: Prentice Hall, 2001.

24. Rogers CR. A theory of therapy, personality, and interpersonal relationships, as developed in the client-centered framework. In: S Koch (Ed), Psychology: A study of a science. (Vol. III). New York: McGraw-Hill, 1959.
25. Ronald L. The value of health and the power of prevention. Int J Workplace Health Manag. 2008;(2):95-108.
26. Sepasi RR, Abbaszadeh A, Borhani F, Rafiei H. Nurses' perceptions of the concept of power in nursing: a qualitative research. J Clin Diagn Res. 2016;10(12):LC10-15.
27. Styles MM. Society and nursing: The new professionalism. Professionalism and the empowerment of nursing: Papers presented at the 53rd convention; 1982. pp. 16-26. Washington DC: American Nurses' Association. (Cross ref.).
28. Thompson JD. Organizations in Action. New York: Mc-Graw-Hill; 1967.
29. Vigoda-Gadot F, Drory A. Handbook of Organizational Politics. Northanpton Massachusetts: Edward Elgar Publishing Inc., 2006.

44 CHAPTER

Team Management and Time Management

CHAPTER OUTLINE

- Team Management
  - Concept and Meaning of Team
  - Team versus Working Group
  - Importance of Team Approach
  - Composition and Types of Teams
  - Significance of Teamwork
  - Characteristics of a Successful Team
  - Essential Ingredients of a Successful Team
  - Designing a Team-based Organization
  - Stages to Develop Teams
  - Factors Affecting the Development of Teams
  - Strategies for Team Management
- Time Management
  - Meaning and Definitions
  - Time Management Process
  - Principles of Time Management
  - Importance of Time Management in Nursing
  - Advantages of Time Management
  - Common Time Wasters and Possible Solutions
  - Effective Time Savers
- Effective Time Management
  - Barriers to Effective Time Management in Nursing
  - Strategies for Effective Time Management
  - Tools of Task Prioritization
  - Criteria for Good Time Management System
  - Approaches to Effective Time Management
  - Common Time Management Tips

LEARNING OUTCOMES

After completion of this chapter, the learner will be able to:
- Recall and understand the concept of team
- Describe the characteristics of a successful team
- Design a team-based organization
- Appreciate various stages to develop teams
- Identify factors hindering the development of teams
- Propose and apply multiple strategies for team management
- Recall and understand the concept of time management
- Describe basic time management principles and its outcomes
- Appreciate the importance of time management in nursing
- Enlist the typical time wasters and its remedies
- Identify barriers to utilizing effective time management by nurses
- Describe strategies to plan effective time management

KEY TERMS

Team, team management, working group, time management, time wasters, time management strategies

INTRODUCTION

Nursing organizations today must survive and grow in this electronic, advanced era and rapidly changing environment of the health sector. The nurse administrators and supervisors need to bring relevant changes in the work setup for continuous improvement in nursing, quality management, and delivery of nursing services in time. To fulfill this aim, they need to work in various types of work groups in which the nurses can work with synergy. Such groups can take the form of a team.

Teams are mandatory and especially within the healthcare organization. Each member of the team has to play a vital role in meeting the needs of clients to their satisfaction. Cooperation and collaboration among health professionals as a team will help in providing high-quality clinical care and increase job satisfaction among staff (Begley, 2009).

Time management is one of the tools to improve the effectiveness and efficiency of any organization. It is an essential key to success and means to improve work performance and nursing practice. The idea of time management is in existence for more than 100 years. It is an art by itself. It is one of the causative factors to stress, but those who follow, create an action plan, act, grab opportunities and have passion for time and work can do wonders and succeed personally and professionally.

TEAM MANAGEMENT

Together empowering to achieve more.
—*Anonymous*

Concept and Meaning of Team

To function well, a human being body requires all the organs to work together in perfect coordination, and even if a single organ gets damaged or inactive, the entire system does not work efficiently. This is valid for organizations also, where everybody must work together to achieve the organizational goal. It carries the perception of togetherness, collaboration, interdependence, sharing of success and failures, and a sense of community.

Meaning of Team

According to Katzenbach and Smith (1993), a team comprises a small skilled group who commits to accomplishing a common purpose and goal and be accountable to each other for their performance. It works in an organized manner independently and cooperatively to achieve its organizational goals. The members have short-term and long-term interactions. The teams may be of executive, departmental, operational, and planning working group levels. Short-term teams might include a team to develop an employee onboarding process, an organization to plan the annual company party, or a team to respond to a specific customer problem or complaint.

A team is a group of people working together toward a common goal. A nursing team is a group of professional and nonprofessional nursing personnel working together in planning, giving, and evaluating patient-centered care to a group of patients.

Team Versus Working Group

In an organization, employees work in groups, but we cannot call all groups as teams. Because there are specific attributes attached to sides that make them different. Katzenbach and Smith had made an effort to state the fundamental difference between a team and a working group **(Table 44.1)**. It indicates that an organization is more than just a group of individuals working together.

Importance of Team Approach

- Teams are the best way for an organization:
  - to improve productivity or effectiveness of the care rendered to the clients
  - to make work more meaningful
  - to give nurse employees a sense of unity and belongingness.
- Teamwork prompts nursing staff to perform any task without taking any credit.
- Team has the potential to create positive synergy. Team members interact with each other and create a learning environment.
- Units are the building blocks of the organization. They satisfy employees' need for social interaction, status, recognition, and respect. It carries the perception of togetherness, collaboration, interdependence, sharing of success and failures, and a sense of community.

Composition and Types of Teams

A team is composed of a group of people working together to have a common goal. Irrespective of the number of people, be it 2 or 200, it is one entity. In organizations, teams usually fall into one of two primary groups: permanent teams and temporary teams. The most common types of teams in an organization are as follows:

1. **Task force or cross-functional team:** This team consists of employees of the same hierarchical level but from different departments to accomplish a particular task.
2. **Problem-solving team:** It is a type of temporary team assembled to share a problem. It is composed of 5 to 12 employees from the same department who meet regularly to discuss the possible alternatives to improve quality, efficiency, and the work environment.
3. **Self-managed work team or self-directed work team:** An ongoing group of employees who share a joint mission and collectively manage their affairs within the predetermined boundaries is referred to as a self-managed work team. Usually, this team comprises of 10–15 employees who take responsibility for their former supervisors. This team practices collective control and decision-making to decide work assignments.
4. **Committees:** A committee is a temporary or permanent group of people assembled to act upon some matter.
5. **Work group:** A work group is a permanent group of workers who receive direction from a designated leader.

TABLE 44.1: Working group versus team.

Working group	Team
Working group has a strong and focused leader	Team has shared leadership roles
Each member has individual accountability	Members have mutual accountability of their performance
Purpose of the working group is similar to the organizational mission	The team itself delivers specific team purposes
Individual work product	Collaborative work product
Conducts efficient meetings	Encourages open-ended discussions and active problem-solving meetings
In working groups, the focus is to measure the effectiveness	The focus is to measure work performance directly by assessing collective work products
They discuss, decide, and delegate work	The team discusses, decides, and does the real job together
Skills are random and varied	Skills are complementary
Work groups have neutral or negative synergy	Teams have a positive synergy

6. **Quality circle:** It consists of employees who belong to the same area. They should meet regularly to discuss and solve work-related problems to improve work opportunities.

Significance of Teamwork

- Performance can be enhanced through improved productivity, quality, and better patient care.
- A team approach can be made cost-effective by reducing errors, absenteeism, and turnover, since the clients get a feel that the staffs are valued and are contributing toward achieving the goal.
- Team-based culture enhances innovation, creativity, and flexibility.
- Team provides a sense of self-control, self-worth, human dignity, identification with the work, and self-fulfillment to its team members.
- Groups also provide an opportunity for the employees to gain respect and dignity for managing themselves, resulting in employees having a better quality of work-life and reduced the work stress.

Characteristics of a Successful Team

As the very word identifies, TEAM stands for:
T: Together
E: Everyone
A: Achieves
M: More
Following are the characteristics of a great team:

- The team members must be aware of a common goal and outcome.
- The team has to be diverse. The team comprises employees who think differently, too intuitive thinkers as well as logical thinkers.
  The team members take responsibility to carry on their assignments.
- The team members should have mutual respect and shared vision about where the team is heading.
- Team members speak respectfully to one another and about one another and listen without interrupting.
- They express opinions, feelings openly, and honestly.
- Team members make commitments seriously and keep them.
- They support the team and each other.
- Focus on problems and solutions, not blame and shame.

Figure 44.1 depicts a team-effectiveness model by Lloyd.

Essential Ingredients of a Successful Team

Based on various research studies, the following are the critical ingredients for a capable team (**Fig. 44.2**):

1. **Apparent team goal:** Team goals should be evident, so that one can specify to achieve objectives. The goal should motivate the team members and make them

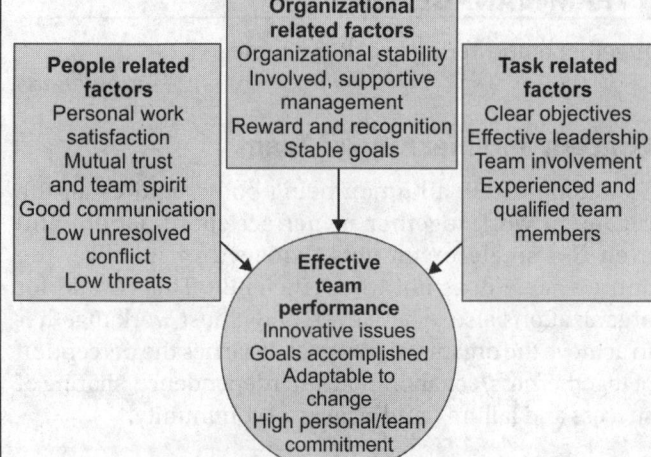

Fig. 44.1: Team effectiveness model.

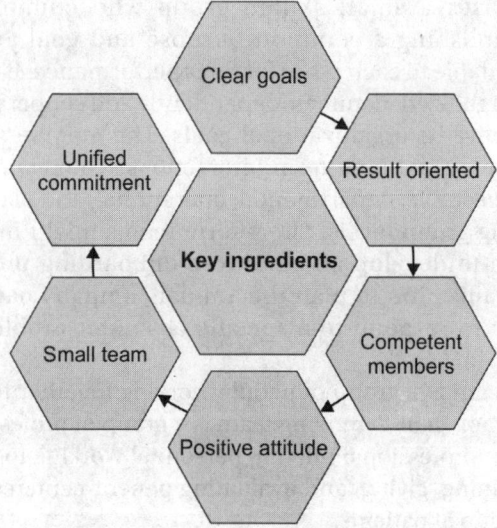

Fig. 44.2: Key ingredients of a successful team.

feel worthwhile and vital. The team leader clears the purposes of the members.

2. **Result-driven structure:** The specific teams need to have clear roles for the group members, a sound communication system, a method to diagnose individual performance, and an emphasis on facts-based judgments. The group with appropriate structures can meet the needs of the group as well as accomplish team goals.

3. **Competent team members:** A group should be composed of the right number and mix of members to accomplish all the tasks assigned to the groups. They should give training and enough information to remain competitive. They should be competent in interpersonal skills and teamwork. They need to have the ability to do the job as well as solve problems. They should be open, supportive, action oriented, and having a definite personal style. They should work in a collaborative way.

4. **Positive attitude:** All team members should be positive thinkers. They should have enough self-confidence, self-respect, and respect for other team members.

5. **Team size:** The team size should be as small as possible. The members should start functioning as a committee.
6. **Unified commitment:** Excellent teams develop a sense of unity or identification. Generate such a team spirit by involving the members in all aspects of the process.
7. **Collaborative climate:** Team members need to have trust toward each other, be open, and be honest, should there be a cooperative environment. Effective team leader ensures a collaborative environment by making effective communication, by demanding and rewarding collective behavior and guiding the members through the team's problem-solving efforts.
8. **Standards of excellence:** Teams must have standards of excellence to derive members to perform at their optimum level. The rules have to be very clear, concrete, to enable all team members to perform up to standards. The team leader makes expectations clear, reviews results, and encourages members to perform at the highest level.
9. **Organizational support and recognition:** Teams that are supported by resources or facilities, recognized for team accomplishments and rewarded collectively for better performance, can achieve excellence.
10. **Effective leader:** Leadership is the central driver of a team's effectiveness, influencing the team through cognitive, motivational, affective, and coordination. An effective team leader must:
    - Always be on the lookout for distraction, tangents, and unproductive or ancillary issues. It is the team leader's responsibility to get it back on track if the leader spots the project going astray
    - Keep the team focused on the goal
    - Maintain a collaborative climate
    - Build confidence among the members
    - Demonstrate technical competence
    - Set priorities
    - Manage performance
    - Change leadership style to suit the changing situation
    - Allow the team members to participate in the decision-making process
    - React positively
    - Keep frequent checks on team spirit and individual morale levels.

Designing a Team-based Organization

The following are the few tips to design or build a capable team:
1. **Consensus building:** Team should be limited to no more than 12 members. Conduct meetings as it is an excellent way of fostering team spirit and team working habits.
2. **Trust:** Promote trust through delegation, openness of conduct, and communication.
3. **Communication:** Team must spend plenty of time together. It enhances bonding. Inform the team members about all facts and figures, agenda, and minutes relevant to their overall responsibilities. Intend communication can be through informal direct conversation, telephonic, e-mail, fax, video, etc. or open communication.
4. **Achieving potential:** The team power, individual brains, and personalities involved must be encouraged to collaborate in generating results.
5. **Skills and role clarity:** One of the secrets of a successful team is observing the skills of team members to the type of task they are required to perform. They should also be clear about their roles and even the functions of all other members with whom they have to interact. This understanding enables the members to act immediately as a team according to the needs and requirements of a particular situation, without waiting for someone to issue an order.
6. **Diversity:** Managing diversity is a balancing act in a team approach. There can be conflicts among the members while working in a group. The disputes can be emotional, textual, constructive, destructive, argumentative, open, or suppressed, which are to be resolved among team members.
7. **Rewarding performance:** The team performance must be rewarded financial or nonfinancial means, so that the members can be motivated to work better and best.
8. **Adapting to change:** This is an essential function of nurse managers. Ensure that teams adjust to external changes. The team should recognize the need for change and be flexible enough to accept it. Listen carefully to the team's reaction toward any change. Members can be involved in the decision-making process.
9. **Training a team:** Arrange training sessions for team members that can help them to improve their technical skills and develop managerial and personal relations among the group.
10. **Make team members emotionally intelligent:** The members must learn to collaborate and cooperate and bring synergy in the team. Use the 360° feedback to make aware of their strengths and weaknesses and then efforts are made to change their behavior.
11. **Empower team:** Team members must be empowered to make the required decisions. Delegate authority to team members, so that they can function effectively.
12. **Positive reinforcement:** Provide positive feedback and recognize and give rewards to team members. It will improve their motivational level and thereby performance.

Stages to Develop Teams

The four developmental stages in team building are as follows:
1. **Forming:** Forming is the first stage in the development of teams. During this stage, the team members gain self-awareness and seek acceptance from other members. They need to adapt to the group or fit in that

environment. They focus on role definition and form bonding and raise questions about the purpose of a team, available resources, time constraints, their roles, strengths, and weaknesses of other members.

2. **Storming:** It is characterized by turbulence and stress as members become more task oriented. Members face several problems related to personality, trust building, and goal orientation. So resolution is one of the tools to make this stage successful, which is possible by effective leadership. The team leader needs to provide clear direction and encourage the members to adopt specific roles and focus on the group.
3. **Norming:** In this stage, the members feel less threatened and become goal oriented. Their conflict level reduces, and they focus on purposes and goals. Work efficiency increases, morale improves, and the group becomes more confident.
4. **Performing:** This stage is about productivity, quality decision-making, progression toward the stated goals, and personal growth of team members. The team performance is optimal.

Factors Affecting the Development of Team

- Resistance to change by team members
- The team members have problems such as aggression, competition, shaming, and blaming, which are not tackled properly
- Blurred purposes, goals, and roles of members
- An incompetent and ineffective leader.

Strategies for Team Management

- Involve both management and staff in the team-building process, so that all team members understand the importance of their involvement
- Designate qualified staff to provide coaching and to mentor the opposing team
- Make the team members aware of their roles, the purpose of a team, and team goals
- Approach the team members in an assertive manner
- Allow each member to provide feedback on problematic situations
- The leader must communicate one-to-one basis
- Listen carefully and actively, use all senses to assess verbal and nonverbal messages
- Avoid blaming and shaming; provide feedback to all team members
- Discuss short-term goals and develop an action plan
- Arrive at a consensus regarding mission and goals
- Define member's roles and responsibilities
- A leader must clarify boundaries
- Determine the resources required to accomplish goals
- Periodically review team development, progress, and goal attainment
- Develop a collaborative relationship to create effective teams and use them to improve the delivery of nursing services, treatment outcomes, and patient satisfaction.

TIME MANAGEMENT

Successful people are those who act. The world is full of dreamers, but dreams remain just dreams if they do not realize by an action plan.
—*Sir Thomas*

Meaning and Definitions

Time management is a set of skills used to utilize time effectively. Time management is a process of arranging, organizing, scheduling, and budgeting one's time to achieve more productive work and productivity. Lakein referred to it as a process of determining needs, setting goals, prioritizing, and planning activities to achieve those goals. It is concerning planning and allocating time.

Time management is a product of organizing skills; however, some processes may not apply to everyone in the same way. It is the use of procedures that are designed to help the individual to achieve his or her desired goals. It involves clusters of behavior that are deemed to facilitate productivity and alleviate stress.

Time planning is one of the elements or skills of time management, which includes making optimal use of plan, organizing, directing, and controlling. It refers to skills, techniques, systems, and a set of principles required to manage time effectively.

From the above definitions, time management is behaviors aiming to use time effectively while performing certain goal-directed activities such as time assessment behaviors, planning practices, and monitoring behaviors. Time assessment behaviors make aware of the past, present, and future and self-awareness of one's time use. It includes attitudes, cognitions, which help to accept tasks and responsibilities that fit within the limit of one's capabilities. Planning behaviors involve setting goals, scheduling tasks, prioritizing, making to-do lists, grouping tasks that aim at effective use of time. Monitoring behavior aims at observing one's use of time while performing activities, generating a feedback loop that allows a limit to the influence of interruptions by others.

Time Management Process

Time management is a cyclic process and follows various steps such as goal setting, review time utilization, matching time utilization patterns with goals, planning and prioritizing, self-monitoring, and time shifting and adjustment **(Fig. 44.3)**.

Step 1: Goal setting

It is the first step in time management. During this stage, identify professional and personal goals with realistic short-term and long-term time frames for attainment. Assign each target with a priority number or letter in the order of importance.

Step 2: Reviewing time utilization

During this stage, review your way of spending time and list down the productive and time-waster activities.

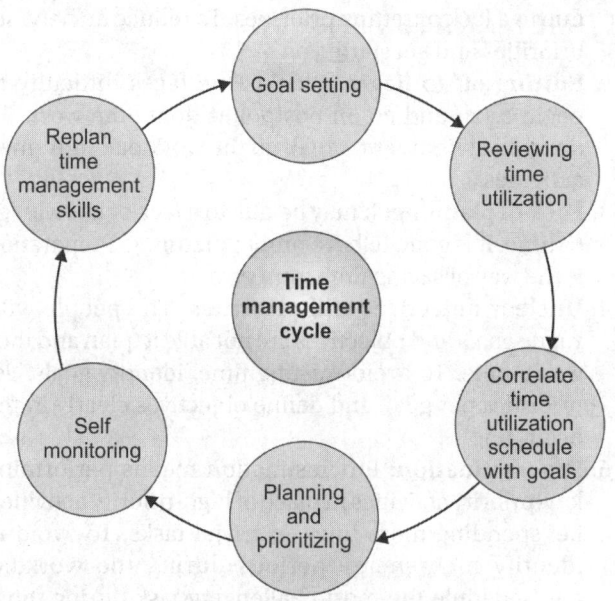

Fig. 44.3: Time management cycle.

Step 3: Correlate time utilization schedule with goals
During this stage, try to correlate the identified personal and professional goals with the calendar. Identify hurdles and time wasters in goal attainment. Apply the Pareto principle of 80/20 (spent 80% time in top 20% of the most important work).

Step 4: Planning and prioritizing
Plan and prioritize for better time management. Use a priority time management matrix. Try to identify time wasters. Identify and prioritize needs. Keep schedule in blocks.

Step 5: Self-monitoring
Identify major time wasters. Monitor all the activities and plan accordingly.

Step 6: Replan time management skills
During this stage, try to avoid time wasters and plan time management behaviors. Be cool for uncontrollable time wasters but get back to the track. Correct time-waster behaviors and modify the time plan.

Principles of Time Management

Time needs to be managed forcefully. Measure the success of time management by the quality of both work and personal life. Time management needs setting priorities and taking charge of the situation and time utilization. It is changing those practices or activities that may cause a waste of time by using different methods to maximize the use of time. The principles of time management are as follows:

1. **Value time:** Set your time ahead. Winners are always on time. They never wait for tomorrow. For them, tomorrow only adds to stress and disorganization. Prepare yourself in advance and plan appropriately.
2. **Positive attitude:** Look at the positive side of situations and avail opportunities. Act according to the case.
3. **Goal oriented:** Identify the goals both long term and short term. Plan activities according to plans.
4. **Scheduling:** Make a list of activities and schedule a regular time to each planned activity.
5. **Prioritize tasks:** Prioritize tasks according to its importance and urgency, such as how critical or essential, how important, can be put off, can delegate, and can ignore? Cross tasks on completion and reprioritize as the need arises.
6. **Divide large tasks:** Break an enormous task into a series of small jobs to accomplish the task on time.
7. **Be organized:** Plan a schedule for each activity. Put things or files away on completion. Put items/archives that are often used in a more accessible location. Throw things away if they are no longer needed.
8. **Manage workload efficiently:** Do not say "yes" for too many things. Try to live to the priorities of your own, rather than the preferences of others. Learn how to say "NO."
9. **Follow a routine:** Make a daily, weekly, monthly, quarterly, and annual routine and follow it. Methods help to ensure not to forget to do things. Be proactive and make checklists of often-repeated tasks.
10. **Delegate work effectively:** Learn to delegate is one of the most challenging tasks. Delegate work to trusted subordinates. Initially delegate small tasks to test them.
11. **Document work:** Record each activity immediately after completion. Do not forget to enter critical points. Do not leave it to begin at the end of the shift.
12. **Manage meetings:** Meetings are a fact of everyday business. To get the most out of a meeting, be productive and informative in the least amount of time. Poorly managed meetings can waste time. Therefore, be well organized, consistent, and assertive that can help managers to manage sessions efficiently.
13. **Control interruptions:** To conduct meetings, plan venue having fewer interruptions. Set an appropriate time limit to control breaks and then quickly go back to work.
14. **Manage your health:** It is essential to maintain your health. Moderation is the key, allow time to relax and for reflection. Give yourself extra time to take care of your health.
15. **Balance work and home life:** Schedule specific times to spend with family or friends regularly and keep the appointment at your convenience. Family time should not disturb your work life.
16. **Self-evaluation:** Keep a record of time spent. Evaluate yourself to make sure that the way you are prioritizing tasks is in line with your goals. There is often a gap between what you think that you are doing and what you are not doing. Things ought to run smoothly per plan.

Importance of Time Management in Nursing

1. Time management helps nurses to ensure that they complete all their work before the end of their each

shift. They also need to regularly check on patients while handling any contingencies or emergencies that arise, so the ability to prioritize is vital.
2. Time management is vital for nurses to make quick and wise decisions regarding patient care.
3. It allows them to prioritize needs, decide on interventions and outcomes, and implement the most critical interventions first.
4. Time management reduces the cost of services, saves time, and eliminates time wasters. It will help them to allocate their time to establish and maintain therapeutic nurse–patient relationships, implement the nursing process to maximize patient outcomes and to complete work assignment efficiently.
5. Planning and implementing adequate time management reduces stress among nurses, as they know what is to be done in each time, and keeping the necessary room to deal with unexpected crisis in their schedule.
6. Proper time planning and management can produce better results at a low cost. It contributes to high-quality care.

Advantages of Time Management

1. **Manages workload efficiently:** Time management helps in managing workload easily by planning and estimating outcome-based time and proper utilization of time on high-priority tasks.
2. **Improve the quality of work:** Quality of work can improve time management. It shows positive results in job performance and academic performance.
3. **Positive attitudinal and stress-related outcomes:** There is a positive relationship between attitudinal and stress-related issues. With proper time management, the persons have job satisfaction, less work–family interference. It helps to reduce frustration, irritability, anger, and stress.
4. **Impact of time management on accomplishing work:** There is a positive outcome in the completion of tasks in managing time. People can meet deadlines on time and feel a sense of accomplishment.
5. **Self-awareness about the work:** People come to know about the workload, the time required for each activity, and the way to complete work on time with time management.
6. **Improves the quality of life:** Time management helps you to organize personal life and work life systematically.

Common Time Wasters and Possible Solutions

Table 44.2 lists both external and internal time wasters. One should avoid time wasters to achieve the goals. Some of the time wasters are discussed below, with possible solutions.

1. **Anxiety and less motivation:** This may be due to the heavy workload that allows putting things off and also due to a lack of setting priorities. To reduce anxiety, set priorities and get started
2. **Putting off to begin a task:** One faces difficulty to begin a job and go on postpones doing the work. To open an assignment, break up the workload into small activities.
3. **Lack of planning:** It may be due to a lack of knowledge or time. It is good to have proper planning. Preparation is the way of saving time from errors.
4. **Unclear objectives and priorities:** The people with vague goals and objectives are not able to plan and they waste time. To avoid wasting time, identify goals. Set priorities per goal, and define objectives clearly in the beginning.
5. **Procrastination:** Procrastination means performing low-priority activities in place of high-priority activities, i.e. spending more time on trivial tasks. To avoid it, identify high-energy periods during the workday and schedule the most challenging task during those periods. Prioritize work. Divide complex tasks into smaller tasks. Define deadlines to develop a time frame and fit the job into the schedule. Deal with unpleasant tasks first. Prepare an action plan and prioritize all activities and functions every week.
6. **Perfectionism or slow skilled:** Perfectionism means to be very efficient and slow competent. It is one of the time wasters. To overcome it, develop reasonable standards of practice. Strive for excellence by doing a job well and using the resources provided by the organization. Seek guidance and suggestions from other experienced nurses.
7. **Daydreaming**: Dreaming without any purpose hinders in achieving the goal. To avoid daydreaming, check energy level and concentration and accordingly plan.
8. **Interruptions:** There can be many interruptions at work, e.g. telephone calls, noise, etc., which can disturb your work. Identify those interruptions and try to avoid them.
9. **Socializing idle conversation:** It is a time waster. Follow useful discussion per the situation demands.

TABLE 44.2: Common external and internal time wasters.

External	Internal
1. Too many interruptions	1. Anxiety and low motivation
2. Unrealistic time estimate	2. Putting off starting a task
3. Lack of planning	3. Indecisiveness
4. Unclear goals, objectives, and priorities	4. Inefficiency
5. Idle socializing at the workplace	5. Procrastination
6. Doing urgent rather than meaningful work	6. Perfectionism or slow skills
7. Too many and ineffective meetings	7. Stress
8. Unscheduled visitors	8. Daydreaming
9. Poor organization	9. Not being able to say "no"
10. Poor work environment	10. Leaving task unfinished
11. Poor delegation	
12. Trying to get other's cooperation	
13. Bureaucratic "red tape"	

10. **Stress:** Extreme stress and burnout affect work. One has to find some suitable methods and should reduce the stress.
11. **Inability to say "no":** Saying "yes" to works of others. It is one of the significant obstacles in achieving the goal. Introspect yourself and ask what you can do and say no to the rest.
12. **Incomplete tasks:** Habit of not completing work fully. It is one of the time wasters. The solution to this is to complete the first task and then move on to the next.

Effective Time Savers

- Follow proper decision-making process
- Do only one task at a time
- Establish daily, short-term, midterm, and long-term goals
- Correspond using quick methods and media without wasting time
- Throw away unwanted things
- Set deadlines at the personal level and also for the organization
- Do not spend time on time wasters
- Get rid of busywork
- Maintain schedule per plan
- Use management tools to remind and follow the activities
- Delegate the work to trusted subordinates and educate them
- Try to have a simple way of doing things
- Keep enough time to accomplish high-priority work
- Adjust priorities as a result of a new task.

EFFECTIVE TIME MANAGEMENT

Barriers to Effective Time Management in Nursing

Success in the nursing profession requires fine-tuned time management skills. Utilization of time in an effective way is the key to success rendering quality care. Identify barriers in the workplace. The common obstacles to time management for nurses are disorganization, distraction, perfectionism, procrastination, and rigidity.

1. **Disorganization:** It is the inability to organize work accurately. Keep things in place to avoid confusion. So it is crucial to keep the necessary stuff in defined areas. Follow the schedule and keep all materials and information ready in hand.
2. **Distraction:** There are many reasons for getting distracted in the workplace. It may be due to telephone calls, patients, rounds, visitors, and so on. Try to avoid distractions. Be mentally stable and be polite with others even in the busiest time.
3. **Procrastination:** It is a negative behavior that delays important work for unnecessary reasons. It involves performing low-priority activities in place of high-priority activities. So it is vital to be positive. Identify high-energy periods, set priorities, and visualize the result. Define deadlines to develop a time frame
4. **Perfectionism:** Although perfection in work is paramount, but at times, it can lead to procrastination. The pressure to complete work causes chaos and confusion among people. Develop reasonable standards of practice to avoid too much perfectionism. Do the job well by using resources effectively.
5. **Rigidity:** Rigidity is essential in performing specific tasks, e.g. to keep a schedule. But to bring change in processes, it is necessary to be flexible in carrying out activities.
6. **Poor planning or unrealistic planning:** To manage time is to control time by proper planning. Planning takes time. List down all activities for a day and review time frames to determine whether the time assigned to each event is realistic. Analyze the use of time.

Strategies for Effective Time Management

A day has 24 hours, which equals to 1,440 minutes or 86,400 seconds. Everybody gets the same number of hours, minutes, and seconds each day. Different individuals follow different ways to manage their time well. Following strategies can help to manage time effectively:

1. **Four generations of time management:** Four generations of time management approach given by Stephen R Covey is a broad categorization of numerous methods to time management. According to this approach, each generation builds on another and each one moves to achieve greater control over previous one.
    a. **First generation:** During this stage, prepare notes and checklists, which act as reminders. Make a list of tasks and arrange them on a priority basis. Use notes to remind you to complete the scheduled tasks during the day. It helps them to keep on track to complete the job on time.
    b. **Second generation:** Schedule the activities by using calendars, appointment books, time planners, and even computers. Write down timings and venues of meetings and important events. Time managers of the second generation are in favor of effective planning, try to attempt to look ahead, and prepare well in advance by scheduling tasks.
    c. **Third generation:** The third generation is also called "schedule and prioritize" generation. It reflects the current time management field and focuses on setting specific, long-term, intermediate, and short-term goals and targets. Individuals, who believe in this generation, identify and prioritize tasks, clarify values, and compare the worth of activities based on their relationship. It focuses on the concept of daily planning. Such managers may maintain their task list on the computer, by using organizer/appointment book and make a

significant contribution, efficient scheduling, and control on time.

d. **Fourth generation:** The fourth generation of time management is "being efficient and proactive." People who fall in this generation, understand and appreciate the difference between urgent and important tasks. Attempt to accomplish critical tasks; usually, they forget to do essential activities. It will cost them in their life and need time, simply because they were not urgent. The central theme of this generation is to get started, persist, and persevere.

2. **The Pickle Jar Theory:** The Pickle Jar Theory for time management is one of the strategies to have adequate time management. This theory has a basis for making time for things that matter. Following are the main criteria of this theory:
   a. **Prioritization:** Prioritization means doing essential tasks first. It will help to complete more jobs in a given time. Identify "most important tasks" and "just filler tasks" that don't need to be done or are not that important.
   b. **Focus on important things first:** Other criteria for effective time management are to focus on the important stuff first and minimize distractions. For example, if you first put stones, then pebbles, and then the sand will fit more into the pickle jar than doing it another way around.
   c. **Room for rest and recreation:** To manage time effectively, make room for rest and recreation, i.e. allow room for sand. Relaxation will help in completing tasks on time and with as little stress as possible.

3. **Time management matrix approach:** Time management matrix approach is a management model by Stephen Covey in his book *The 7 Habits of Highly Effective People*. This approach provides a way to prioritize tasks, determine goals, and commitments **(Table 44.3).**

TABLE 44.3: Time management matrix

	Urgent	Not urgent
Important	1. Necessity—Reduce tasks that need immediate attention. Reactive "firefighting" Crises Pressing problems Medical emergencies Deadline-driven tasks	2. Quality—improve your habits, proactive actions that reduce quadrant 1 Preparation Preventive Values clarification Planning Relationship building True recreation Personal growth
Not important	3. Deception—Try to manage things such as Interruptions Phone calls, e-mails Meetings Many pressing issues	4. Waste—Avoid time-wasting activities Busywork Some phone calls, e-mails Time wasters Escape activities Excessive TV

All workplace tasks are divided into important/unimportant tasks in the vertical axis and urgent/not urgent tasks in the horizontal axis of a table. As a result of these two criteria, the model creates four squares "quadrants" that are keys to time management performance. One can significantly change the size of four quadrants within the time matrix.

a. **Quadrant 1—urgent and important:** This quadrant is known as *quadrant of necessities*. It includes tasks that are both urgent and important, compelling and require immediate attention, and essential and need more initiative to make things happen and contribute to achieving mission, values, and goals. Personal, medical, professional true emergencies, crises, and essential deadline-driven projects or problems are examples of these types of activities. These activities are firefighting as one cannot avoid time spent on these activities but can reduce if prepared to tackle. The managers who fall under this quadrant are crisis managers, problem-minded people, and deadline-driven producers.

b. **Quadrant 2—important but not urgent:** This quadrant is known as *quadrant of quality*. It is a quadrant of personal, proactive, power, and heart of effective personnel management. Mangers of this quadrant deal with tasks that are not urgent but important; they think of building a relation, focus on mission, statement, long-term planning, preventive, maintenance, preparation, etc. They are opportunity minded, feed excuses, and starve problems. The critical activities of mangers that fall in this quadrant are (1) identifying their roles, (2) setting goals for the next 7 days, (3) scheduling time, and (4) reviewing the schedule daily. They focus on organizing work every week, rather than on a daily basis, and plan time on productive tasks such as office work, business, recreation, relaxation, education, etc. that results in vision, perspective, balance, discipline, control, and quality life with few crises.

c. **Quadrant 3—urgent but not important:** This quadrant is known as *quadrant of deception*. This quadrant includes tasks that are urgent but not important. They spend most of the time reacting to critical things. They assume an important one, but they are not really. They believe in daily planning. These are activities that are short-term focused but allow interrupting our working lives, such as answering every phone call. They feel victimized and have a shallow or broken relationship. Productive time managerial people live out of this quadrant and spending more time in quadrant 2.

d. **Quadrant 4—neither urgent nor important:** This quadrant is known as *quadrant of waste*. It includes things that are neither urgent nor important. Sometimes people mistake this quadrant for recreation. People who fall under this quadrant are irresponsible, fired from a job, and dependent on others. They are time wasters and lead careless lives. Productive time managerial people live out of this quadrant and spending more time in quadrant 2.

Tools of Task Prioritization

Task prioritization can be achieved using the following list of tools:

1. **Paired comparison:** Paired comparison is a sort of analysis to evaluate the criteria that are vague, subjective, or inconsistent. It helps to prioritize options by comparing each item on a list with all other details based on its importance in priority list.
2. **Grid analysis:** It is a type of analysis performed by considering many factors to prioritize the items as the most important.
3. **Action priority matrix:** It is a quick and straightforward diagramming technique involving an intelligent approach for making highly efficient prioritization decisions. The evaluator plots the value of each task against the effort it will consume. By doing this, the most significant rewards in the shortest possible time will quickly spot "quick wins," which soaks up time for little eventual reward, avoiding "hard slogs."
4. **Pareto analysis:** The main aim of this analysis is to identify the most significant changes to be mad according to the problems identified. It is focused on different types of problem in a group and prioritizes the most common problem and method of resolving those problems.
5. **Nominal group technique:** It is a method to prioritize various issues by the group. To have a consensus of the group, each member has to participate in the discussion. It will help to make a consensus to arrive at the priority list.

Criteria for Good Time Management System

- Setting goals and deadlines daily, weekly, monthly, quarterly, half-yearly, and yearly
- Make a daily schedule and a list of tasks with priorities
- Schedule time for specific activities
- Have planned communication and other meetings
- Delegate activities with a deadline and checkpoints
- Identify and prepare time management techniques for handling specific time management problems such as crises, interruptions, etc.
- Organize and manage materials, files, projects, etc.
- Clarify job assigned to each member of the team
- Keep all management tools ready, such as monthly, weekly calendars, etc.
- Spend at least 20% of the time for planning.

Approaches to Effective Time Management

Following are a few approaches that can help nurses to manage time effectively:

1. **L-E-A-P-S Approach:** This acronym stands for:
   a. **List down all the activities/tasks:** Prepare a list of all events, both productive and time wasters.
   b. **Estimate time:** Estimate the time required to carry out each activity/task.
   c. **Allow time for unexpected things:** Keep time allowance for unexpected work, errors, and interruptions.
   d. **Prioritize activities/tasks:** Use either ABC's approach or the time management matrix to prioritize the activities/tasks. In the ABC's approach, A stands for "the most important" job, B "the important but not so urgent one," and C stands for jobs that will not require attention immediately. Review all activities at the end of the day and replan accordingly for the next day.
2. **"Plan, pick, and play" approach:** Prioritize and learn to be assertive in dealing with nurse managers, patients, and colleagues.
   a. **Plan:** Planning saves time. Have a clear idea before starting work. Prepare a schedule for each shift.
   b. **Pick:** Prepare a list of the assigned job. Prepare a priority list of each activity according to urgency. Document each event after completion. Again make a list according to priority for the next period. Time management for nurses concerns the second and most crucial part of the job, i.e. patient care. Replan, after fulfilling the first need of the patient.
   c. **Play or relax:** Plan time for relaxation and a healthy work–life balance.
3. **Scheduling tasks and activities approach:** The tasks and activities scheduling approaches are concerned with self-discipline. Management tools such as time planner, calendar, etc. help in being self-disciplined These are useful in managing time effectively. Write down all activities in a time planner and this will help to stay on task. Keep in mind the following points to schedule tasks:
   - Review job descriptions. Compare job descriptions with real job activities.
   - Discuss role expectations with the head nurse. Conduct a time study and analyze the time spent by a nurse manager to carry out all activities. Prepare a chart of fixed commitment.
   - Spend time for planning. Prepare a list of activities, both productive and nonproductive. Develop daily goals.
   - Prepare a weekly schedule and daily checklist.
   - Identify time wasters. Try to avoid or reduce distractions and utilize time for productive activities.
   - Think positive and reduce stress.

Common Time Management Tips

- Set realistic goals for tasks and activities
- Analyze workload in personal and professional lives
- Break longer tasks into smaller ones

- Identify and prioritize tasks according to their importance and urgency
- Prepare an action plan to organize tasks and activities
- Group similar jobs together
- Priority-wise allocate time to each activity
- Set personal and work-related goals according to priority
- Do weekly planning; begin with challenging tasks, and allocate sufficient time to complete the most critical tasks
- Be assertive with team members and seniors; learn to accept tasks that you can do
- Make accurate decisions and know commitments and limitations
- Set start and finishing time for each activity
- Conduct meetings in an organized way; deal carefully with employees and avoid wasteful communication
- Avoid other time wasters while at the workplace
- Delegate work as much as possible to lessen your workload and save time
- Handle paperwork efficiently as it is a time-consuming affair
- Organize the work area systematically
- Be familiar with standoff procedures.

CHAPTER HIGHLIGHTS

- A team is a group of people working together toward a common goal. A working group has a strong and focused leader, and each member is accountable for one's work.
- The organizations have both permanent and temporary teams. Four developmental stages in team building are forming, storming, norming, and performing.
- Time management is a process of arranging, organizing, scheduling, and budgeting one's time, more productive work, and productivity.
- Time management is a cyclic process and follows various steps. It reduces the cost of services, saves time, and eliminates time wasters.
- The common obstacles of time management for nurses are disorganization, distraction, perfectionism, procrastination, and rigidity.
- Different individuals follow different ways to manage their time well.

REVIEW QUESTIONS

I. Essay Type Questions
1. Define the term "team management." Explain different stages of developing a team.
2. Describe strategies of team management.
3. Enlist time wasters. Discuss the time management process.
4. Explain approaches to effective time management.
5. Describe various strategies of time management.

II. Short Notes
1. Time management system
2. Principles of time management
3. Team-based organization
4. Barriers to team development

III. Multiple Choice Questions
1. A group of skilled persons commits to accomplishing a common purpose for their performance is:
   a. Team b. Organization
   c. Working group d. Committee
2. The purpose of a successful team is:
   a. To conduct meetings and have discussions
   b. To measure work efficiency and effectiveness
   c. To discuss, decide, and delegate work
   d. To measure the work performance by assessing collective work
3. Which type of team shares a joint mission and collectively manage their affairs?
   a. Problem-solving team
   b. Self-managed team
   c. Cross-functional team
   d. Quality circle team
4. Which one of the following terms is used for performing low-priority activities in place of high-priority activities?
   a. Perfectionism b. Distraction
   c. Procrastination d. Disorganization
5. In the time management matrix, which one of the following terms is used to depict a quadrant of personal, proactive, power, and heart of effective personnel management?
   a. Quadrant of necessities
   b. Quadrant of qualities
   c. Quadrant of deception
   d. Quadrant of waste

Answer Keys
1. a 2. d 3. b 4. c 5. b

SUGGESTED READINGS

1. Adams GA, Jex SM. Relationships between time management, control, work-family conflict, and strain. J Occup Health Psychol. 1999;1:72-7.
2. Arnold E, Pulich M. Improving productivity through more effective time management. Health Care Manag. 2004;23:65-70.
3. Barling J, Kelloway EK, Cheung D. Time management, and achievement striving interact to predict car sale performance. J Appl Psychol. 1996;81:821-6.
4. Claessens BJC, Eerde WV, Rutte CG, et al. A review of the time management literature. Pers Rev. 2007;36:255-76.
5. Conte JM, Mathieu JE, Landy FJ. The nomological and predictive validity of time urgency. J Organ Behav. 1998;19:1-13.
6. Covey SR. The 7 Habits of Highly Effective People. New York: Simon & Schuster; 1989.

7. Denne B St. John. Teamwork across boundaries. Health Prog. 1999;80(5):58-62.
8. Fisher K. Leading Self-directed Work Teams: A Guide to Developing New Team Leadership Skills. New York: McGraw-Hill; 1993.
9. Fox ML, Dwyer DJ. Stressful job demands and worker health: An investigation of the effects of self-monitoring. J Appl Soc Psychol. 1996;25:1973-95.
10. Green P, Skinner D. Does time management training work: An evaluation. Int J Train Dev. 2005;9:124-39.
11. Hall BL, Hirsch DE. An evaluation of the effects of a time management training program on work efficacy. J Organ Behav Manag. 1982;3:73-98.
12. Katzenbach JR, Smith DK. The discipline of teams. Harv Bus Rev. 1993;71(2):111-20.
13. Lakein A. How to Get Control of Your Time and Your Life. New York, NY: P.H. Wyden, 1973.
14. Malhotra M. Managing teams effectively in the organizations of today. Paper read in a seminar on "Human Relations in Organizations" organized by the Department of Psychology, Panjab University, on February 8, 2002.
15. Mitchell TR, James LR. Building better theory: Time and the specification of when things happen. Acad Manage Rev. 2001;26:530-47.
16. Robbins SP. Organizational Behaviour. New Delhi: Prentice-Hall; 2004.
17. Sarp N, Yarpuzlu AA, Mostame F. Assessment of time management attitudes among health managers. Health Care Manag. 2005;24:228-32.
18. Stewart GL, Manz CC, Sims HP. Team Work and Group Dynamics. New York: Wiley; 1999.
19. Waterworth S. Time management strategies in nursing practice. J Adv Nurs. 2003;43(5):432-40.

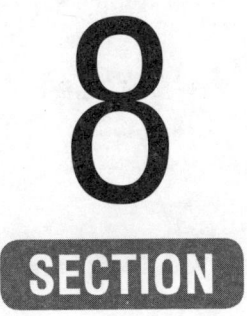

SECTION 8

Material Management

45. Material Management: Concept, Principles, and Procedures
46. Equipment Management, Planning Equipment and Supplies, and Condemnation
47. Procurement and Purchasing
48. Inventory Control and Inventory Accounting System

45 CHAPTER

Material Management: Concept, Principles, and Procedures

CHAPTER OUTLINE

- Material Management
  - Concept
  - Definitions
  - Classification of Materials
  - Aim and Objectives
  - Purposes of Material Management
  - Importance of Material Management
  - Advantages of Material Management
  - Functions of Material Management
  - Principles of Material Management
  - Elements of Material Management
- Procedure of Material Management System

LEARNING OUTCOMES

After completion of this chapter, the learner will be able to:
- Understand the concept of material and material management
- Discuss aims, objectives, and principles of material management
- Describe functions, needs, purposes, and importance of material management
- Enlist the management techniques used in material management
- Explain the procedural steps of material management

KEY TERMS

Material, equipment and supplies, equipment-related consumable items, material management, stock, condemnation, stock value

INTRODUCTION

Materials are the major cost factor in an organization. In health organizations, about 40% of budgetary allocation is on procurement and management of stores. Every organization, big or small, needs proper feeding for good results. It requires planned and progressive provisioning and purchase to keep the machinery running. It can be achieved only through effective material management.

MATERIAL MANAGEMENT

Concept

Materials are things required to carry out work or making something. These are things needed for the smooth functioning of the organization. According to Webster, the word material "relates to the production and distribution of economics, goods, and social relationships of owners and laborers." Materials referred to equipment, apparatus, and supplies procured, stocked, and utilized by an organization. Management means bringing together the available resources to achieve a specific objective. Integrated material management is a close coordination of all departments that are concerned with the utilization of materials. It is an integrated approach or set up for which the material manager is responsible for interrelated functions and in position to exercise control and coordination to ensure the proper balance of conflicting objectives of individual features.

Definitions

- Material management includes all the activities from forecasting requirements to utilizing and up to the disposal of the material. The materials vary from simple housekeeping to sophisticated equipment, depending on the type of hospital.
- Material management deals with managing materials such as drugs, supplies, and equipment to deliver health-care services. It concerns with planning, organizing, and controlling the flow of materials from their initial purchase, internal operations, and to the distribution at service point.
- Integrated material management includes material planning, indenting, purchase systems, reducing

uncertainties in demand and supply, handling and transportation, storage, issuing materials, inventory management, and disposal of obsolete, surplus and scrap materials.
- According to Judith, material management is managing and controlling medical, surgical, clerical, interdepartmental services, and equipment from acquisition on the floor to disposition. Housley referred to it as management and control of materials, including goods, services, and equipment, from procurement to disposal. It is a technique or a method concerning material management from purchasing to destination.

Classification of Materials

The hospital uses a large variety of materials for patient care. Material ranges from consumables, stationery to even equipment besides the pharmaceuticals and optical goods. The department undertakes standardization of products, i.e. grouping items of similar specifications to facilitate the department to forecast and plan its material requirements.

1. **General classifications:** Materials are generally classified into the following:
   a. The material used in the hospital is of seven categories: capital assets, consumables, hospital wear, printing and stationery, linen, instruments, and consignment.
   b. Materials can be under four heads: drugs, equipment, materials, and supplies. In the government setup, the focus is almost wholly on the fourth class, i.e. supplies.
   c. The material categorized as drugs, supplies including linen, equipment, and instruments, monitors, etc., facilities related.
   d. Another classification is as below:
      - Medical items include pharmaceutical, surgical, consumable, and protective materials.
      - Capital equipment and accessories
      - Catering equipment
      - Electrical, mechanical, civil materials used for maintenance work
      - Housekeeping materials
      - Linen.
2. **Classification based on the cost criteria:** The material categorized on cost is commonly known as the "ABC" group. ABC stands "Always Better Control." "A" category of material is under strict control and supervision and requires a right estimate. "B" category of equipment is under reasonable control. The middle-level manager manages this category of material based on a rigid requirement. "C" category of items is under common control of storekeepers and purchases these materials on usage estimates.
3. **Classification based on time toleration of non-availability criteria:** The material classified on time toleration of nonavailability is commonly known as the "VED" group. VED/VEN stands for "vital essential desirable/not so essential," "V" category of items cannot tolerate its nonavailability. These items are required to be all the time available. "E" group items cannot tolerate its nonavailability for 2–3 days due to the availability of alternative items. "D" category items may wait for a longer time for its availability.

Materials are one of the essential resources to accomplish the goals of the health-care organization. The health administrators need to plan a material management system to ensure an adequate supply of material to improve expected demand pattern with a minimum amount of money blocked in procuring nonproductive manner, and it is paramount importance to supply that material of the right quality to its destination at the right time to consumers.

Aims and Objectives

The material management aims to have the right quality of material, the right quantity of supplies of materials, at the right time, at the right place, and for the right cost. Its objectives are as follows:
- To ensure the supply of availability of material right quality, quantity, at the right place, and at the right time
- To obtain the correct quality of materials at the lowest possible price
- To maintain a high inventory turnover
- To maintain continuity of supply, preventing interruptions of flow of materials
- To avoid a surplus of material
- To develop reliable sources of supply
- To ensure proper distribution at every level
- To ensure efficient utilization of available materials.

Purposes of Material Management

The following list shows the purposes of material management:
1. To gain an economy in purchasing
2. To have a reserve stock during an emergency or out of stock
3. To maintain consumption fluctuations
4. To provide satisfactory services to customers
5. To satisfy clients at the time of replenishment.

Importance of Material Management

Material management is a matter of prime importance. The efficiency with which it is performed often determines the success of an organization. In the health sector, it is concerning with distributing drugs, supplies, and equipment required by the staff to deliver health services. It concerns the flow, conservation, and utilization of the materials as well as the quality and cost of the materials.

Material management is a managerial tool to deliver the supply at the right quality, the right quantity at the right time. It needs reasonable inventory control, sound methods of condemnation, and disposal to improve the efficiency of the organization.

Advantages of Material Management

1. **Material management**
   - Control of inventories is made more accessible and simple
   - Eliminates losses caused by the deterioration of surplus materials
   - Reduces clerical work
   - Reduces cost and improves profitability and rate of return on investment
   - Minimizes assorted problems of delivery schedules, emergency orders, and storage
   - Reduces emergency or rush orders
   - Brings better regulation inflow of materials
   - Ensures better storage and facilitate the better-coordinated movement of materials into the production line.
2. **Integrated material management**
   - Ensures better accountability by having centralization of authority and responsibility for all aspects of material functions
   - Facilitates better coordination of various features of material management
   - Encourages effective communication and thus enhances better performance
   - Promotes adaptability to electronic data processing for collection, collation, and analysis of data
   - Improves team spirit and therefore provides an opportunity for growth and development.

Functions of Material Management

1. **Material management**
   1. Material planning and programing
   2. Purchasing and outsourcing
   3. Inventory control
   4. Storekeeping and warehousing
   5. Codification
   6. Standardization and evaluation of all products
   7. Transportation and material handling
   8. Inspection and quality control
   9. Cost reduction through value analysis
   10. Disposal of surplus/obsolete material
   11. Distribution.
2. **Material management department**
   1. Optimum material acquisition
   2. The optimum size of the inventory
   3. Optimum inventory turnover rate
   4. Good vendor relationship
   5. Material cost control
   6. Effective issuing and distribution
   7. Elimination of losses and pilferage.

Principles of Material Management

The list below shows the principles of material management:
1. **Principle of effective management and supervision:** It means that material management must follow principles of planning, organizing, staffing, directing, controlling, reporting and budgeting for its effective management and monitoring.
2. **Principle of sound purchasing:** Material management must ensure the sound purchasing process through sound purchasing methods. There should be an effective purchase system.
3. **Principle of negotiations:** It means that one must arrive at a common understanding through bargaining on contract for purchasing, specification, price, and payments, etc. There should be skillful and hard poised negotiations in material management.
4. **Principle of simplicity:** Material management system should be simple in operation, and everybody associated with it should understand its functioning.
5. **Principle of productivity:** Material management system must reduce cost and improve profitability and rate of return on investment through inventory management.
6. **Principle of controlling:** There should be a simple inventory control program in the material management system.
7. **Principle of codification:** In material management, a coding system must follow. Assign codes to all categories of material.
8. **Principle of standardization and specification:** It means that standardization and specification must follow for the acquisition of material.
9. **Principle of prioritizations:** Principle of prioritization means to procure material on a priority basis.

Elements of Material Management

The following are the elements of material management (Fig. 45.1):
1. **Demand estimation:** Estimating and calculating the requirement of supplies and equipment are the most crucial element in material management. Prepare a list

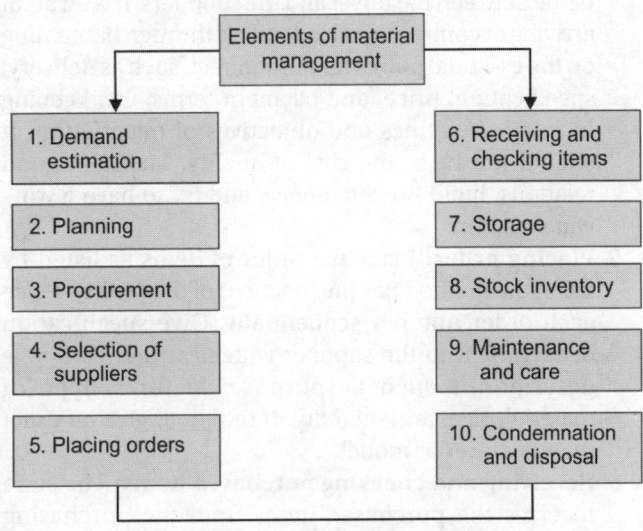

Fig. 45.1: Elements of material management.

of items, quality, and quantity required, the delivery time, and frequency of delivery. One should make a particular, careful, and technical study of material needs to formulate a procurement program. Provide supporting data for appropriations and expansion of grants.

2. **Planning:** Planning is vital to have the right quality, the quantity of material at the right time, and the correct cost. The plan requires at all stages and levels of management. Planning is a listing of necessary equipment and their cost estimation. Keep in mind the previous levels of performance and anticipated activity and consumptions of required items at the time of planning. Other factors, such as lead time and frequency of orders and stock level, are also considered at the time estimating and planning the number of materials. Estimate the costs of ordered materials within budget.

3. **Procurement:** Procurement is an essential element in material management. It is a process of obtaining material from the preparation and processing through to receipt and approval of the invoice for payment. One has to take many steps from need assessment to delivery stage. It is concerning with gain, buy, purchase, and acquires the material. Check items for quality and quantity per order. Procurement of material depends on various factors such as prioritizations of purchase of equipment based on need and budget, fixing price, calling for at least three tenders/quotations, opening and finalizing tender, and placement of orders, receiving the material and making payment.

4. **Selection of suppliers:** Select a supplier keeping in mind the price, quality, delivery time, guarantees and warranties, reputation, and reliability of suppliers. Compare the costs of different suppliers. Whenever possible, obtain quotations from at least three suppliers to compare the prices. Negotiate with the supplier for value, quality, and delivery time, etc. Negotiation is a battle between the buyer and the suppliers. It is an art of arriving at common understanding through bargaining on the essential points for the contract, such as delivery, specification, price, and payment terms, etc. keeping in mind the ethics and objectives of negotiation. It should not be at the cost of quality. Maintain good relations, build up confidence, and try to have a win-win situation.

5. **Placing order:** Place the order of items as listed by using the method per the practices of the facility. Place each order number sequentially. Give specification of each item to the supplier with clear and complete descriptions such as purpose, features, type of material, size, and quantity. If required, give an exact manufacturer or model.

6. **Receiving and checking purchased items:** The store receives the purchased items from the purchasing department. There are different types of stores, such as drug stores, linen stores, medical stores, and surgical stores. Inspection of those items is an essential element in material management. Check each piece for its quality per specification ordered. Get receipts of all purchased items and forward them for payment.

7. **Storage:** After receiving the requested material, it ensures that the issue of material for usage is adequately preserved to prevent loss or damage. The store must have enough space to store the materials. These should be protected from fire, pest, and seepage and should be kept at the temperature as prescribed. All materials received must be entered in the ledger and should be in safe custody.

8. **Stock inventory:** Inventory is a list of nonexpendable supplies and equipment kept in the organization. It includes the number of goods or materials in hand. It is an essential tool in the inventory management system. The in-charge of stock should have a copy of it and should check inventory at regular intervals to check its condition and location of supplies and equipment. It helps to identify the purchasing requirement. There should be an annual stock verification of all stores, wards, departments, units, etc.

9. **Maintenance and care:** Proper maintenance of equipment is essential to preserve capital investment. Take care of all the material and instruments. These should be in working order and periodically calibrated for effectiveness and accuracy. These should be cleaned, checked for any damage, and report if any defect or out of order regularly. There should be clear instructions for staff using equipment regarding the care and maintenance of equipment.

10. **Condemnation:** Condemnation is another vital element in material management. Each facility has a condemnation committee to review used materials, especially nonfunctioning and obsolete items. The committee plans to have condemnation periodically to condemn nonfunctioning and outdated items after proper checking of records, physical inspection, and unserviceable report, etc. All departments must make a record of all condemned items and do entries in stock registers. Dispose of these items per guidelines.

There are the following management techniques used for different purposes in material management:

1. Value analysis, standardization: for right item
2. Inventory control: for right quantity
3. Cost–benefit analysis and value analysis: for right price
4. Vendor research: for right source
5. ABC, VED, etc. analysis: for the right method
6. Operation research: for right delivery.

PROCEDURE OF MATERIAL MANAGEMENT SYSTEM

The material management system has the following steps (Fig. 45.2):

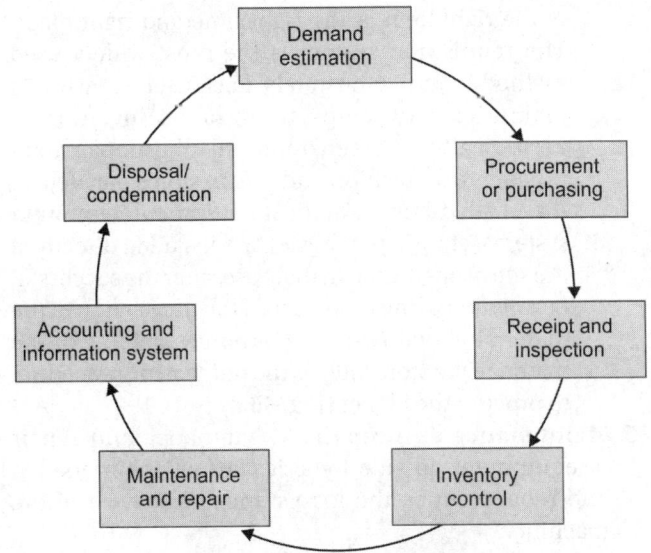

Fig. 45.2: Procedure for material management.

1. **Demand estimation/planning and budgeting:** The first step in handling the problem of supply is determining requirement needs. To estimate demand, one needs to consider three factors, i.e. the kind of articles required, the quantity of each requested item, and the time and frequency of delivery. Formulate a procurement program based on the material requirement. Provide supporting data for its appropriations. Demand estimation is concerning with cost balance, material specification, and value analysis.
   a. *Cost balance:* Material management is involving balancing the cost of the material. The price of the item includes both its actual cost and carrying (inventory) cost. The carrying cost is the cost of storing for distributing. The carrying value has 20–30% of the price. It includes interest on capital (15%), storage cost (racks, almirah, building), workforce cost, deterioration cost, pilferage cost, obsolescence, ordering costs, insurance cost, and stock out the cost. If stock increases, carrying costs will increase. Similarly, if the ordering cost rises, the carrying cost will increase.
      - The economic order supply includes both carrying and order costs. Using the following formula, one can get the economic order quantity.
      - Economic order quantity = $\sqrt{2AS/I}$, whereas A = annual consumption, S = ordering cost, and I = inventory cost (carrying cost)
      - Optimum review period is related to the number of orders and calculated by using the following formula:
        Optimum review period = $\sqrt{288 \times \text{cost/order/inventory cost} \times \text{carrying cost}}$
   b. *Material specification:* Material specification is the character of the material required. The material specification classifies material. It classifies the material in a precise and defined way. It gives the exact character of the articles required, quality or grade, the nature of their construction, and all other required special attributes. It facilitates and smoothens the work of service and reduces the purchasing process.

   The preparation and use of proper specifications depend on the system of supply. According to Thomas, it enhances the reputation of the purchaser for exact knowledge of his needs. It informs the dealers that swiftness during a purchase agreement is not a part of the purchaser's policy—a certainty that encourages competition among the most desirable vendors (quotation) and secures the lowest prices. It saves the time of dealers, while incomplete descriptions, in contrast, require a significant amount of time. It also keeps the time of purchasing officers in answering questions of possible bidders and avoids the danger of cooperation between the dealers and those who are to receive and use the articles purchased.
   c. *Value analysis:* Value analysis is the management technique in material management to identify incurred nonessential costs and to reduce the cost. It examines the quality (right item) and price of the item.
2. **Procurement:** After determining the supply requirement, the next step in material management is procuring the required material. Each institute has its rules and regulation regarding acquisitions of materials. Many institutes have centralized medical stores for the procurement of drugs and supplies. State governments also use a system of fixed-rate contracts or running rate contracts. The objective of purchase is to secure the articles specified when and where needed and at the lowest obtainable prices. It has various operations like selecting the vendors, arranging the purchase price, time and place of delivery, verification of shipments, and settlement and payment of vendors' remuneration claim.
3. **Receiving and inspecting the material:** After receiving the supply in the store, control is necessary to ensure the quality of materials. The store-incharge, which is representative of the supplier and representative from the purchase committee of the hospital, verifies the delivered items against the invoice. Verification ensures the things per the order placed. **Figure 45.3** depicts the procedure followed by receiving the supply.
4. **Inventory control:** Inventory control includes storing, issuing, and delivery. It is one of the vital functions of material management.
   a. *Storing:* The stores must be easily accessible to both suppliers and consumers. It must have adequate space to accommodate all drugs and supplies. Plan the layout of stores according to the type of

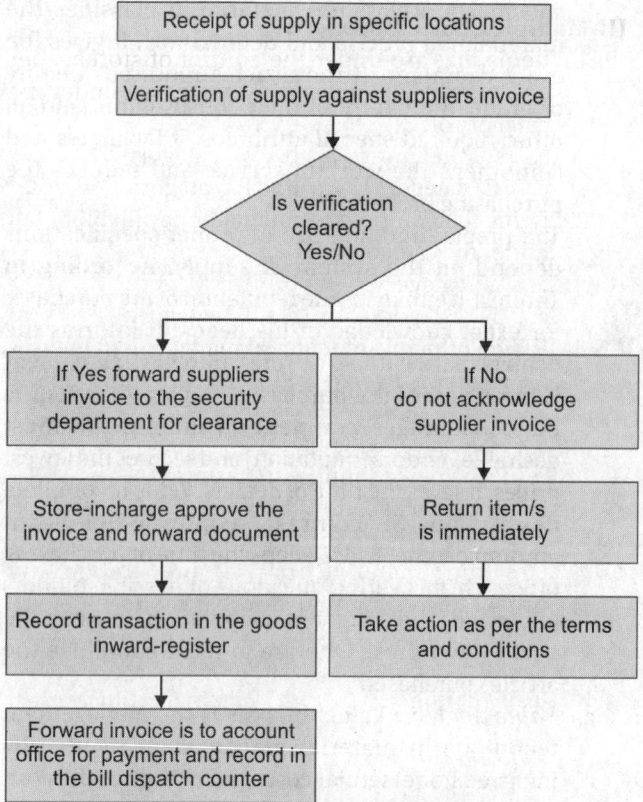

Fig. 45.3: Receiving and verifying the procedure.

material. Alphabetical arrangements help in the identification and retrieval of amounts. Medical supplies required controlled temperature and humidity and protection from lights. There should be a provision of refrigeration to store all sera and vaccines. Stock the minimum and maximum level of each item and consider the level of reordering, buffer stock policies, analysis of the movement pattern of each item, and minimum pilferage.

The central stores undertake centralized storing of all items. In some hospitals, the convenient stores take this responsibility except pharmaceutical products, food items, and bulk equipment installed at the site of operation.

b. *Issuing and distribution:* The stores ensure an uninterrupted supply of materials to the various departments to ensure the smooth and efficient functioning of the hospital. The hospital must have a systematic procedure of issuing and distribution. Sound store system keeps a continuous issue, accurate stock status reports, timely detection of discrepancies, and prompt clearance of goods inward note to expedite bill payment, reduction in losses, etc.

Distribution usually involves transportation to various units or health-care delivery system. It is an intricate process focusing on the distribution of the right item at the right time and right place. The requisition system is the most widely used method in Indian hospitals. Each user department maintains and keeps track of its inventories. Periodically or when required, the department prepares a requisition and sent to stores that deliver the needed items. Medical equipment, computer systems, etc. are purchased and installed directly at the site of operation. In that case, after the successful installation of the item, record the transaction in the material issued register. On nonavailability of the material, the store follows the purchasing procedure to procure the object **(Fig. 45.4)**.

5. **Maintenance and repair:** Maintenance and repair of equipment go side by side. Proper maintenance and repair reduce the losses and breakdown of the machine.
6. **Accounting and information system:** The accounting and information system aids in controlling the material management system. Accounting handles the financial matters associated with procurement.
7. **Disposal and condemnation:** Dispose of surplus products and nonfunctional equipment that are either functional but obsolete or nonfunctional and obsolete or beyond economic repair, operational but hazardous, useful but no longer. It is essential to decrease in holding costs and in storage capacity. All the hospitals have a condemnation committee. Dispose of the used material either by selling to other hospitals or scrap dealers.

The hospital also undertakes periodic write off of the items that are not fit to use. The store maintains complete details about each item in the hospital, including their expiry dates. The store immediately disposes of any expired items.

The user department informs the store in writing to dispose of any equipment. The store immediately arranges for removal of the same from the user department. Before removing the material, cannibalize parts so that one can use the usable parts of the

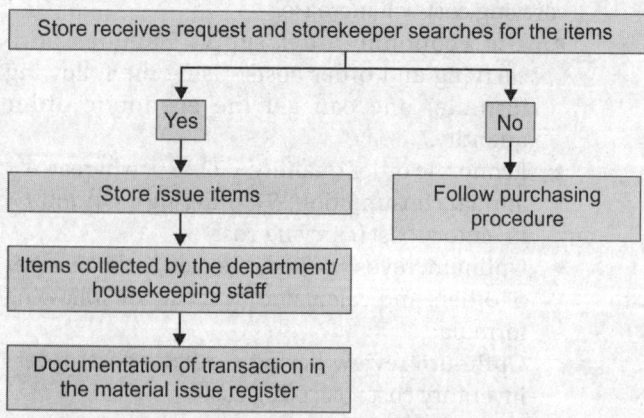

Fig. 45.4: Issuing and distribution system of material.

Chapter 45: Material Management: Concept, Principles, and Procedures

discarded machine in the future for another device of the same type.

CHAPTER HIGHLIGHTS

- Materials include equipment, apparatus, and supplies procured, stocked, and utilized by an organization.
- Material management includes all the activities of the store from the stage of forecasting of requirements to utilization to the final disposal.
- Material ranges from consumables, stationery to even equipment besides the pharmaceuticals and optical goods, and classified in many ways.
- It concerns with provision of drugs, supplies, and equipment needed by the staff to deliver health services.
- Material management is based on principles and involved in carrying out many equipment and supplies-related functions.
- Significant elements of material management constitute demand estimation; planning; procurement; selection of supplies; placing orders; receiving and checking items; storage; maintaining stock inventory; maintenance; and care, condemnation, and disposals of equipment. Every facility follows its procedures for material management.

REVIEW QUESTIONS

I. Essay Type Questions
1. Define material management. Discuss its importance and purposes.
2. Enumerate principles of material management.
3. Describe elements of material management in detail.
4. Discuss procedure of material management system.
5. Describe functions of material management.

II. Short Notes
1. Classification of material
2. Objectives and advantages of material management
3. Procurement
4. Condemnation

III. Multiple Choice Questions
1. Items that are under the control of storekeeper and purchased on usage estimates fall under the category of:
   a. "A" category
   b. "V" category
   c. "C" category
   d. "E" category
2. Items that cannot tolerate its nonavailability fall under the category of:
   a. "V" category
   b. "E" category
   c. "N" category
   d. "B" category
3. Which principle of material management focuses on minimizing cost and improving profitability and rate of return on investment?
   a. Principle of negotiation
   b. Principle of sound purchasing
   c. Principle of controlling
   d. Principle of productivity
4. Obtaining material from the preparation and processing of a requisition from receipt and approval of invoice is:
   a. Procurement
   b. Storage
   c. Ordering
   d. Demand estimation

Answer Keys
1. c   2. b   3. d   4. a

SUGGESTED READING

1. Available from http://apps.who.int/medicinedocs/documents/s17710en/s17710en.pdf. [Accessed July 2019].
2. Housley CE. Hospital Material Management. Rockville, Md: Aspen Publishers; Inc.; 1978.
3. Kowalski JC. Material management is crucial to overall efficiency. Healthcare Financial Management. [Online] Available from Find Articles.com. [Accessed Dec 2011].
4. Kulkarni GR. Management Accounting for Hospitals. Mumbai: Ridhirai Enterprise; 2003.
5. Kumar R, Goel SL. Hospital Administration and Management, Vol I. New Delhi: Deep & Deep Publication.
6. McGibnoy. Principles of Hospital Administration. New York: Putnam's Sons; 1969.
7. Schulz R, Johnson AC. Management of Hospitals and Health Services: Strategic Issues and Performance, 3rd edition. St Louis: CV Mosby; 1990.

46 Equipment Management, Planning Equipment and Supplies, and Condemnation

CHAPTER OUTLINE

- Equipment and Supplies
  - Meaning
  - Types of Equipment
  - Equipment Management
  - Equipment Management Cycle
- Stock Verification
  - Nurses' Role in Equipment and Supply Management
  - Role of Nurse Managers in Maintaining Equipment and Supply
- Planning of Equipment and Supplies
  - Goals of Planning
  - Objectives
  - Equipment Planning Process: Prerequisites
  - Steps in the Planning Process
  - Planning Tools
- Condemnation of Equipment
  - Criteria for Condemnation
  - Condemnation Committee
  - Procedure for Condemnation
  - Disposal of Equipment

LEARNING OUTCOMES

After completion of this chapter, the learner will be able to:

- Understand the concept of equipment and supplies
- Enlist types of equipment and supplies
- Describe equipment management and its cycle
- Acquaint with different department of equipment and supply
- Explain the process of annual physical stock verification
- Describe the nurses' role in equipment and supply management
- Discuss the role of nurse managers in maintaining equipment and supply
- Explain condemnation of equipment procedure
- Develop goals and objectives for planning equipment and supplies
- Elaborate the planning process of equipment and supplies
- Enumerate essential tools used in planning equipment and supplies

KEY TERMS

Equipment, supplies, equipment management cycle, planning tools, condemnation

INTRODUCTION

Equipment and supplies are some of the critical parts of overall material management. Functional, accurate, and safe clinical equipment and supplies are the requirement in the provision of health services. Well-maintained equipment will give nurses greater confidence in the reliability of its performance and contribute to a high standard of client care. Equipment management is an essential issue for safety and cost in modern hospital operations.

EQUIPMENT AND SUPPLIES

Meaning

Equipment

The term "equipment" means all items necessary for the functioning of all services of the hospital including accounting and records, maintenance of buildings, laundry, nursing units, etc. The hospital requires both movable and fixed equipment. These are devices, tools, and instruments used in the hospital.

Supplies

Supplies are those items that are used up or consumed; hence, the term "consumable" is for supplies. The supply in the hospital includes drugs, surgical goods (disposables, glassware), chemicals, antiseptics, food materials, stationeries, the linen supply, etc.

Types of Equipment

There are verities of equipment and supplies to carry out the function of hospitals.

Various equipment and technologies (health technology) used in the health facility are as follows:

A: Categorization I:
1. Medical equipment: These include equipment, such as (1) pharmaceutical, (2) surgical, (3) protective, and (4) consumable items. These are those items that are used up during the operation of equipment (e.g., film, reagents, gel)
2. Capital equipment and accessories
3. Catering items
4. Electrical/mechanical, civil material for maintenance work
5. Housekeeping
6. Laundry equipment
7. Office equipment
8. Printing and stationary

B. Categorization II:
1. Diagnostic equipment
2. Treatment equipment
3. Life support
4. Medical monitors
5. Medical lab equipment
6. Medical devices, such as apparatus, appliances, and other articles including software
7. Surgical instruments
8. Fundamental clinical specialists
9. Sterilization related

C. According to World Health Organization (WHO), equipment and health technologies are classified into various categories as given in **Table 46.1**:

TABLE 46.1: Various types of equipment and health technologies.

S. No.	Category	Description
1.	Medical equipment	Equipment used for medical diagnosis, monitoring, and treatment of patients
2.	Communication equipment	Equipment used for communicating information, such as telephones and paging systems
3.	Office furniture	Office furniture, such as desks, chairs, or filing cabinets
4.	Service supply equipment	These include supply installations, such as electrical installations, water, sewage pipelines, and gas supplies
5.	Laundry and kitchen equipment	Equipment required for kitchen, such as cookers, or equipment required for laundry activities, such as cold rooms and washing machines
6.	Workshop equipment	Workshop equipment, such as hand tools, bench tools, or test instruments
7.	Walking aids	Items, such as wheelchairs and crutches
8.	Training equipment	Equipment required during training courses, such as overhead and slide projectors, video, and tape recorders
9.	Equipment-specific supplies	Items, such as consumables, accessories, spare parts, and maintenance materials used with the equipment
10.	Biomedical waste treatment plant	It includes incinerators, septic tanks, or biogas units
11.	Health facility furniture	Furniture, such as beds, cots, trolleys, and infusion stand
12.	Office equipment	Office equipment, such as computers, photocopiers, calculators, and record systems
13.	Plant for cooling, heating	Machinery, e.g. air conditioners, compressors, and lift
14.	Vehicles	Any conveyance, such as ambulances, cold-chain motorbikes, mobile workshops, and buses
15.	Fire fighting equipment	Such as fire blankets, buckets, and extinguishers
16.	Energy sources	A source of energy, such as generating sets, solar panels, or transformers
17.	The fabric of the building	Items that are part of integral structure or framework of a building, such as doors, windows, or roofs
18.	Accessories	Items that connect the machine to the patient (e.g., leads, probes), assist with the use of the device (e.g., trays, footswitches), or adapt its performance
19.	Fixtures built into the building	Items installed into the fabric of the building, such as ceiling-mounted operating theater lights, scrub-up sinks, and fume cupboards

Equipment Management

Equipment management includes all activities from the selection and acquisition through incoming inspection, acceptance, maintenance, and eventual condemnation and disposal.

Medical equipment management recognized within the medical logistics domain. The purpose of equipment management is to ensure that equipment used in inpatient care is functional, safe, and meet the mission and objective of the medical facility. Quality equipment management must focus on the preservation of material, regular planned replacement, and improved performance through internal processes.

Many departments, such as equipment users, purchase, procurement, maintenance, finance, administrative, and support are involved in equipment management. It also includes representatives from planning, financial, clinical, technical, and logistic areas depending on size, autonomy, and decentralization of authority.

Equipment Management Cycle

Various activities undertaken in equipment management cycle shown in **Figure 46.1**:

1. **Planning and budgeting:** Planning is the first phase of equipment management. Careful planning of equipment is essential to maintain quality care. It is vital to plan equipment requirements according to the budget. Information, such as actual clinical requirement, available qualified users, approved and reassured source of the recurrent operating budget, confirmed maintenance services and support, and adequate environment support is essential to consider at the planning phase. There should be a clear-cut policy on the acquisition, utilization, and maintenance of equipment.

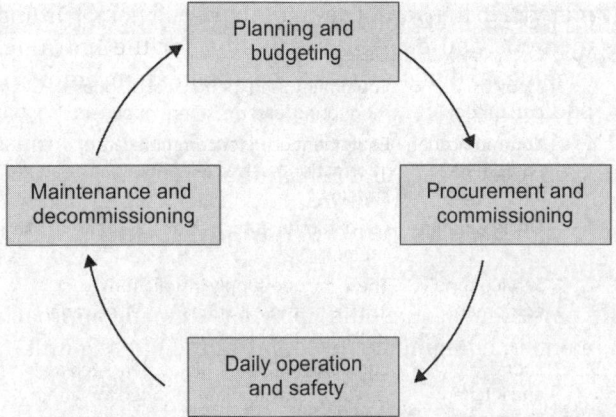

Fig. 46.1: Equipment management cycle.

2. **Procurement and commissioning:** Procurement and commissioning are concerning with the acquisition of equipment management. Procurement is the process of obtaining equipment and supplies through purchasing or other means. It is important to procure the right equipment, of the right quality, in the right quantities, on time, in the right place, and at the right cost. It ensures delivery, installments, and testing functioning (commissioning) procedures to get the equipment ready for use. It includes various activities, such as selection, supply, delivery, storage, installation, testing, training, etc.

Commissioning is a process of checking and ensuring functioning and safety of newly installed equipment before being used. It is done through testing and making adjustments in newly installed equipment. Both supplier and expert hospital technical staff do commissioning. If suppliers require to do commissioning, the hospital technical staff must monitor the process to record any technical fault. A link should be maintained between user and supplier and observe any supplier's technical services.

Hospital has separate stores and purchase sections under material management that also the take care of equipment. The purchase officer directly supervises the material, and in the stores, the store officer supervises. The storekeepers and other staff function under the store section. The purchase section is responsible for compilation of all demands, finalization of specification, floating of tender inquiry, placement of supply orders, monitoring of liabilities, record keeping, etc., whereas the store department is responsible for initiation and compilation and demands, receipt of goods, testing, and quality control, record keeping in stock ledgers, issue of equipment, bill verification, maintaining supply.

3. **Daily operation and safety:** Daily operation and safety are another important areas in equipment management. It focuses on the management of the effective utilization of equipment. Various committees, such as infection control committee, purchase committee, training committee, equipment users, section heads, technical staff, maintenance, support service staff, procurement, finance staff, and others can coordinate in managing daily operation and safety of the equipment. Ensuring the effective and safe operation of equipment includes the following:

- Planning and organizing in-service training programs for equipment operators and managers
- Planning and allocating recurrent budgets to cover equipment-related requirement, such as references, manuals, guides, etc.
- Monitoring for the effective utilization of equipment
- Inclusion of staff-related activities:
    ♦ Making staff accountable for their use and handling of equipment by assigning them, proper handing, and taking over
    ♦ Encourage and train them on how to use and handle a particular equipment
    ♦ Provide them guidelines and reference material
    ♦ Checking equipment daily and in every shift for its functioning their performance
    ♦ Inventory check by the head of the department
    ♦ Regular maintenance of equipment, etc. by the maintenance department
    ♦ Purchasing of correct consumable and cleaning materials by procurement and purchase department
    ♦ Checking stocks of different department stores by the main store department
    ♦ Developing a suitable environment and discipline among staff.

4. **Maintenance and decommissioning:** Proper maintenance of equipment is essential to obtain sustained benefits and to preserve capital investment. Equipment must be in working order and periodically calibrated for effectiveness and accuracy. There should be a maintenance department, adequate supply of maintenance material, and spare parts availability, stationery, office space, technical reference material, and adequate access to transport by maintenance staff. Each hospital has a separate department/workshop for maintaining and repairing equipment. A biomedical engineer is usually appointed to supervise this critical activity. Each department maintains a history sheet of all the high-tech equipment. The sister in charge of the unit is responsible for getting the equipment repaired and also for maintenance.

Areas that need priority for maintenance are sterilization, electricity supply, water supply, laundry, kitchen, refrigeration, sewage, and sanitation air conditioning among medical equipment are the equipment related to operation theaters, syringes, anesthetics, basic lab, X-rays, delivery, and basic diagnostics require to priorities. VED/VEN (vital, essential, desired/not so essential) system can be opted to prioritize equipment maintenance and repair work. It is essential for repairing existing old equipment; dismantle old units if required, decommissioned material must be deleted to keep the inventory current.

Good management practice should include guidelines for equipment users regarding its care and cleaning, safety procedures, checking for functional and performance, and maintenance-related activities with time frames monthly and quarterly. Nearly all significant hospitals have hospital clinical engineering departments/workshops which takes up this management responsibility.

Stock Verification

The organizations usually have annual physical stock verification. The deputed officers do annual physical stock verification of all wards, stores, departments, and units within the hospital. They check entries and ground balance with the stock ledger. They also note down the significant losses and substantial surplus and inform to the head of the institution.

Nurses' Role in Equipment and Supply Management

Managing supplies and equipment involves much more than keeping the storage area neat. Managing a hospital's nursing department includes managing the supplies and equipment needed for patient care and treatment. Determining quantities that are cost efficient and best for the patients and ordering stock are one way the nursing manager helps keep the department running smoothly. The head nurse/nurse manager is responsible for the proper management of equipment and supplies required for patient care. The critical roles of nurse managers are as follows:

1. **Procuring:** The procurement process involves several steps. The practical nurse manager must be aware of the requirement of supplies and equipment for daily operations. They send requisition per the condition through the proper channels. The nurse manager must know the basics of the procuring system of the hospital. Some hospitals adopt a unique code system for procuring various items. In many hospitals, ward-aide assists nurse managers and places the indents.
2. **Receiving and inspecting:** The ward sisters must investigate and count the material carefully on receiving the indent from stores. They must check for the expiry dates, match with the requisition, and must label all the items received. They make entries in the appropriate registers.
3. **Storing:** Each ward has a store with wardrobes. Store the supplies and equipment received from the respective store inappropriate places. Protect the materials from any damage and loss. It should be in safe custody. There should be adequate space for storing materials. Storing items group wise and alphabetically will help in identifying the object.
4. **Issuing, distributing, and maintaining inventory:** Nursing managers must ensure an adequate supply of material in the ward. They must have policies regarding methods and days of distribution for the morning, evening, and night staff and maintain an inventory of equipment.
5. **Maintenance of records:** The nurse managers must keep records of equipment and supply.

Role of Nurse Managers in Maintaining Equipment and Supply

The nurse manager should apply a systematic approach to maintain equipment and supply in the nursing unit. It includes input, process, and output and feedback steps.

Input: The main objective of the input component is to ensure an adequate supply of equipment and supplies of a nursing unit. The nurse managers need to:
- Participate in estimating the demand for equipment and supplies
- Know about hospital policy for procuring, indenting, stocking, etc.
- Know about nursing norms for equipment and supply per nursing council
- Develop ward policy per requirement
- Communicate higher authority about the gap between demand and supply
- Conduct meetings with superiors and subordinates to estimate requirements of materials
- Prepare guidelines for handing and taking over for the staff.

Process: The objective of the process phase is to maximize the proper utilization of available equipment and supply by the team and adequate maintenance of equipment and supplies. The nurse managers need to:
- Maintain an up-to-date inventory of equipment and supplies
- Send requisition monthly, weekly, and daily per the policy
- Have inventory control and maintain buffer stock for emergency
- Distribute material adequately for the evening and night shift
- Conduct supervisory rounds; check daily and periodically emergency, general, and life-saving equipment regularly
- Assign and delegate the work to junior staff; make them accountable for any loss and misuse of materials and supplies
- Make sure the proper utilization of articles and supplies by the nurses
- Communicate all the team members about the "out of stock" and nonfunctioning equipment and materials
- Develop an orientation plan for the patients and their relatives about the availability and nonavailability of particular article, equipment, and supplies
- Maintain record and report of equipment and supplies
- Condemn the nonfunctioning and outdated equipment per policy.

Output: The main objective of this phase is the maximum utilization of available equipment and supplies to render quality patient care.
- All the staff must know hospital and ward policies related to equipment and supplies.
- There should be an adequate and regular supply of equipment and other supplies without any interruption.
- All materials and articles should be in working order.

PLANNING OF EQUIPMENT AND SUPPLIES

Equipment and supplies are an essential part of health care. These are necessary means in diagnosis, monitoring, and treatment of patients suffering from disease conditions. These are also the means to control the environment by supplying heat and light and to provide necessities, e.g., water, electricity, feed patients, transport patients, and staff. Therefore it is imperative to focus on planning equipment and supplies to maintain quality health services.

Goals of Planning

Following are the goals of planning:
1. To plan and budget for equipment and supplies per directives/policies
2. To develop planning tools
3. To estimate realistic equipment-related allocation
4. To prepare long-term plans and budget
5. To review annual plans and budget
6. To monitor progress to improve planning and budgeting.

Objectives

The list below shows the objectives:
- To get the current equipment situation
- To develop a plan for equipment
- To calculate expenditure required
- To extend the short-term and long-term plans
- To make the budget calculation
- To devise methods to review progress and for monitoring.

Equipment Planning Process: Prerequisite

According to guidelines given by government, organization, and professional bodies are the following prerequisite:
1. Have policies for purchasing and donations/disposable/condemnation of equipment and supplies
2. Get the model equipment list containing standardized/minimum equipment and supplies required for the facility, e.g., for 50-bedded hospital
3. Use a bottom-up approach; involve all concerned at a suitable decentralized level for need assessment, bulk bye equipment, and supplies.

Steps in Planning Process

Following are the steps in equipment planning process (Fig. 46.2):

1. **Need identification and setting goals:** Identify the annual requirement for equipment and supplies. Set objectives of supplies and equipment planning. Based on developing a yearly action plan, goals and procedures must be clearly defined to set activities priority wise. Prepare an annual action plan that should indicate goals and activities for submitting estimates of equipment and supplies.

   These activities are as follows:
   - Annual inventory update
   - Reviewing of the equipment development plan (EDP)
   - Reviewing of the equipment training plan (ETP)
   - Costing annual needs (EDP and ETP)
   - Reviewing core equipment expenditure plan and planning annual purchase, rehabilitation, corrective and training activities, yearly equipment budget, and feedback plans
   - Updating long-term plan and equipment and supplies expenditure plan.

2. **Gather current stock and supply data:** To estimate equipment and supplies requirements, one should have a clear picture of the present situation of stock and supplies. The current stock information can easily be available from equipment inventory.

   Equipment inventory is a compilation of record sheets containing lists of equipment found in all departments. It may be a list, catalog, or may be in a computer program. It covers a wide range of items with possible types of equipment along with their expected product lifetimes. Items in the inventory are arranged per facility policy, may be alphabetically, location wise, manufacturer wise, by usage/function, age wise, or by inventory code wise. Design equipment inventory system and code-numbering system.

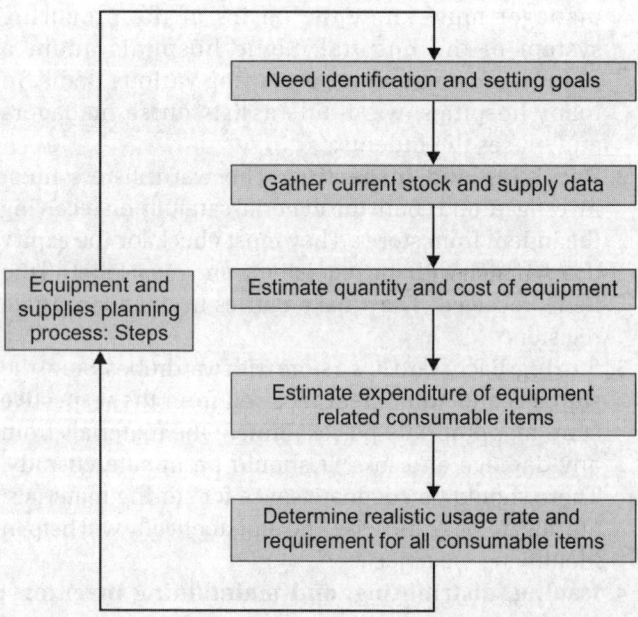

Fig. 46.2: Steps in equipment and supplies planning process.

It should be updated regularly on receiving new equipment, sending equipment for repairing, the material found nonfunctional, every month, quarterly, and annually. Equipment inventory is useful (1) to identify any deficiency in stock and supplies, (2) to help in planning replacement and disposing of policies, (3) to implement purchasing and donation policies, and (4) to calculate equipment and costs.

3. **Estimate the quantity and cost of equipment:** The stock value is the estimation of the quantity and cost of the material. Consider the following steps to calculate the stock value of equipment:
   a. Gather information about current and up-to-date prices of required equipment from various sources, such as from suppliers, manufacturers' websites, and other sources. Allow depreciation over time and link replacement and maintenance estimates in current prices.
   b. Compile a reference equipment price list for each department by listing specific prices for the type of equipment. A reference equipment price list provides with approximate costs for any material.
   c. Estimate new stock value by using any one of the following methods:
      - A rough estimate based on multiplying the approximate number of equipment by reference prices
      - Exact estimate based on the precise amount of material (determined from equipment inventory) and then increasing the number of equipment using reference prices
      - Forecast for the future requirement based on the amount of equipment required (determined from model equipment list-standard list) using reference prices.
   d. Use only the correct stock value for planning and budgeting.
   e. Keep on revising prices and stock value periodically to have up-to-date current reference equipment price list.
   f. Apart from the cost of equipment, identify and allocate spending costs. Spending/purchase cost must include operating cost, maintenance cost, transport and installation cost, cost of recoding and evaluating, staff cost, training cost, administrative and other costs depending on the type of equipment.

4. **Estimate expenditure of equipment-related consumable items:**
   a. Estimate equipment-related consumable items required in different departments. Prepare a detailed list of all types of consumable items. Equipment-related consumable items are as follows:
      - Equipment consumable, e.g., paper, battery, etc.
      - Replacement accessories, e.g., probes, lamp, etc.
      - Spare parts
      - Maintenance material
      - Equipment cleaning material
      - Safety material, e.g., protective clothing
      - Energy supplies
   b. Find out the different types of expenditure currently spent on equipment from "equipment expenditure record." There are usually two types of funds for purchasing equipment: 1. Capital funds, and 2. recurrent funds.
      - *Capital funds:* Capital funds are allocated and utilized for purchase of new equipment, replacing existing equipment, buying additional new material for preinstallation work, support services, or repairing equipment. In capital funding, a large amount of money spent on purchasing stuff.
      - *Recurrent funds:* Recurrent funds cover small regular expenses weekly or monthly basis. It is also known as actual lifetime cost, i.e., on daily operational, maintenance, and administrative requirement. It is allocated and utilized on (1) maintenance of equipment, (2) buying equipment-related consumable items, (3) purchase spare parts of materials, (4) for administrative expenses, such as buying stationery, maintenance services, and energy cost, and (5) for ongoing training expenses.
   c. Estimate running costs that should include capital expenditure and recurrent expenditure for maintenance, consumable items, and training expenses.
   d. Calculate usage rate for equipment-related consumable items.

5. **Determine realistic usage rate and requirements for all equipment-related consumable items:**
   a. Investigate and finalize the type of equipment-related consumable items requirement
   b. Find out the rate of use, i.e., quantity needed per day, per week, or per month to deliver service to patients by consulting departments/already prepared list, maintenance departments, referring departmental and store records, and getting information from suppliers
   c. Calculate the annual recurrent funding requirement
   d. Calculate correct reordering quantities and timing. After getting feedback from the health management team, the storekeeper calculates the right reordering quantity, and also enters these items in the stock register. After entering these items in the stock register, become "stockable" items
   e. Confirm equipment and technical data specification before final selection of model during the procurement
   f. Update information and review annually usage rate.

Planning Tools

1. **Reference materials:** Reference material is the literature on equipment and its details. These reference materials can refer to planning and budgeting. There

are different types of materials available in a variety of forms from various sources. Sources of getting reference materials are as follows:
a. *Manufacturers and their representatives:* Get brochures of various equipment from manufacturers and their representatives in free of cost
b. *Bulk suppliers:* Bulk suppliers can also provide procurement catalogs free of charge
c. *Ministry of health:* Obtain the list of registered manufacturers from the ministry of health
d. *Other organizations:* Obtain reference materials, such as model equipment list, equipment specification, list of manufacturers' operators, and service manual, list of registered manufacturers by request or copies on payment
e. *Internationally on payment or on subscription:* Get other reference material, such as books on various equipment-related subjects, service manuals, equipment evaluation, and hazard reports, technology assessment, journals, and internationally advice regarding equipment issues from internally on payment or subscription
f. Explore more sources from suppliers, manufacturers, international agencies, and other international agencies
g. CD-ROM, video, DVD on equipment-related subjects
h. Internet websites
i. Storing in computers system as electronic copies after scanning.

2. **Vision:** The vision of an organization used as a planning tool. View in terms of intervention, and procedures can direct planners to determine the type of equipment that is required based on the kind of services provided by a particular health facility.

3. **Model list of equipment:** Model list of equipment is a standardized list of equipment specifying a minimum requirement for each health-care intervention in a particular type of health facility/organization. These are prepared by professional bodies, accreditation bodies, government, and the World Health Organization to meet minimum requirements. Mostly these are made based on the type of hospitals/facility, beds, type of services provided, budget, standard, etc. and by doing equipment analysis by using clinical, technical, and economic data through computer software programer. World Health Organization has recommended the "Essential Health Care Technology Package" for determining the equipment list.

4. **Purchasing and donation policies:** Policies can guide in the acquisition process to decide which type of equipment for procurement when to procure, why to procure, and how to procure with priority. These policies are at the government and organizational levels. The plans must indicate the valid reason and order of preferences in purchasing equipment.

Following *criteria* help in deciding quantity and type of equipment required and included in the standard list:
a. *Need:* Estimate equipment and supplies based on depreciation, the missing item from the minimum requirement, requirement for additional equipment, or per directives of government or professional bodies. Estimate per the capacity of the facility, necessity of running services without unique material, and for safety point of view.
b. *Appropriateness:* Equipment selected should be (1) suitable for the organization, for operating staff, for local maintenance service availability, and local conditions; (2) acceptable to the team and patients, and (3) compatible with existing equipment and consumable supplies and existing utility and energy sources.
c. *Quality and safety:* Equipment and supply must meet performance and safety standards, such as International Standard Organization (ISO), pharmacopeia specification, international electrotechnical commission (IEC) standard mark. These should be durable, easy to clean, disinfect, and sterilize. Pack and label all equipment and procure from registered manufacturers and suppliers.
d. *Affordable and cost-effective:* Selection of items must be based on price and quality. These should be affordable and must check the budget for operational running costs including maintenance, consumables and accessories, spare parts, electricity, safe disposal, and training costs.
e. *Source:* Source of supplies and equipment is another essential criterion. Manufacturers and suppliers, imported supplies, donations, and used supplies are the primary sources for the procurement of supplies and equipment. Procure items from registered manufacturers and suppliers, ensure performance and safety standards and its brand for imported supplies, and budget other costs during planning and budgeting process. Buy carefully used supplies if it is in the right conditions, tested, with service and repair manuals, and other terms and conditions.
f. *Usability and maintenance:* Equipment and supplies must be easy to operate, clean, and maintain. Each item procured must have warranty/guarantee card, manual and guidelines, after-sale technical and maintenance support, easy availability of spare parts, and equipment-related consumable items.
g. *Material:* Material make is an essential criterion under the equipment and supplies planning process. The material of these items should be of suitable quality materials, such as tungsten carbide or stainless steel, which last long.

Metal items rust easily and need to clean and sterilize regularly. Glass items are fragile and break easily, and most of the glass items are made up of plastic to overcome the drawbacks of glassware items. Plasticware materials are of different types based on the required temperature resistance, chemical resistance, flexibility, and transparency of the things.

  h. *Disposable or reusable:* This is another criterion in planning the type of items to be procured. It depends on policy, affordability, facilities for sterilization of reusable, periodicity, and reliability in supply. Some supply, such as syringes and gloves can be disposable designed for the single use.

5. **Replacement and disposable policies:** There should be criteria/procedures for replacement and disposable or condemn articles. Develop utility and disposal criteria to study equipment for technical skills. The materials beyond repair get damaged, unsafe, unreliable, technically obsolete, no longer economically to repair, or whose spare parts are not available need to be disposed of and replaced by new articles. There should be guidelines for each facility for safe disposal of equipment, instruments, and materials and supplies per National Waste Management Guidelines and should be a part of the planning process.

6. **Generic equipment specification and technical data:** Generic equipment specification and technical data provide a base for planning equipment and supplies. Each purchase planning list must-have item details and order information. Item details should include its specification, quantities, technical and environmental data, such as interrupted power supply, location, temperature, humidity, etc. It should also include the details of terms and conditions, i.e., quality, delivery, and payment terms for items to be ordered.

CONDEMNATION OF EQUIPMENT

Condemnation is an act of judging material including equipment; articles, linen, etc. are unfit/unsafe for use, nonfunctional, scrapped, and surplus, need to dispose of, and technically obsolete.

Criteria for Condemnation

Following are the criteria for condemnation:
- Nonfunctional and beyond economical repair (unserviceable): These are items having a high cost of repairing than its current value after depreciation and life of the equipment.
- Nonfunctional and technically obsolete: These are nonfunctioning, and its parts and service are no longer available equipment.
- Functional but clinically obsolete: These equipment are in working order but cannot be put into use being outdated and require replacement due to rapid improvement/change in technology/design.
- Surplus items: These are functional items but are not required for use and lying in the stores for more than 5 years.
- Scrap items: These are process waste, broken, and any other materials not covered above but have got resale value.
- Functional but hazardous: Equipment that has been damaged by contamination.
- Empty items: These include empty containers, crates, bottles, and drums.

Condemnation Committee

The hospital formulates its condemnation committee/board to condemn the nonconsumable items having at least five members. The numbers vary from hospital to hospital. It comprises the following members:
- Medical superintendent/chief medical officer
- Joint medical superintendent
- Nursing superintendent/senior most nursing staff
- Biomedical engineer/head of department/supplier/service agency, etc.
- Administrative officer.

The committee meets annually once and completes the condemnation of all unused items.

Procedure for Condemnation

The following list shows the procedure for condemnation:
- Send all store items found nonfunctional in the nursing units, theaters, and departments to main stores.
- The office in-charge of main stores follows the procedure for condemnation.
- List down all torn linen items in the wards, theaters, and other departments and send it to the nursing superintendent for consolidation that places before the condemnation committee for approval.
- The committee inspects/examines items according to laid down criteria for condemnation and certify after proper scrutiny of records, physical inspection, unserviceable records, purchase value, etc. Estimate the life of equipment per the manufacturer's description. The service agency certifies the condition of material, which is beyond economical repair and proposes the disposable value of items that are for condemnation. The committee is empowered to condemn things up to the fixed amount for each item.
- Each ward/department maintains proper records of all the items condemned and do appropriate entries in their ledger book.

Disposal of Equipment

The following list shows the disposal of equipment:
- The condemned articles are stored and disposed of or thrown away or kept in an allocated area for scrapped equipment.
- Keep functional but clinically obsolete items for research or training purposes.
- Dispose of the equipment safely per biomedical waste management hospital policy/guidelines.

- Either tender system or public auction may be conducted depending on the earning revenue value of disposing items fixed by the competent authority.
- Immediately after the approval of competent jurisdiction to declare the materials surplus/obsolete/unserviceable must delete from stock ledgers with suitable entries in the general disposal register. These entries should tally with the items condemned and removed from the main stock register of instruments, accessories, furniture, etc.
- The store officer physically hands over the items sold with its details to the party and issue gate pass to facilitate security check, etc.
- Store officer records disposal or removal of items in the disposal register to keep a permanent record.

CHAPTER HIGHLIGHTS

- Equipment and supplies are one of the essential parts of overall material management.
- Four activities, i.e., planning and budgeting, procurement and commissioning, daily operations and safety, maintenance and decommission equipment under the equipment management cycle.
- Planning equipment and supplies are essential to maintain quality health services.
- There are many equipment planning tools used in planning equipment and supplies.
- Five significant steps of planning equipment are to estimate equipment requirements, need identification, and setting a goal, gathering current stock data, determine stock value, assess the expenditure of material-related consumable items, calculating usage rate, and requirement of consumable items.
- Condemnation is an act of judging material including equipment and linen, are unfit/unsafe for use, nonfunctional, scrapped, and surplus, need to dispose of, and technically obsolete.
- Each hospital formulates its condemnation committee and has a set condemnation procedure.

REVIEW QUESTIONS

I. Essay Type Questions
1. What is meant by equipment and supplies? Describe the steps of the equipment management cycle.
2. Enlist prerequisites in the equipment planning process. Describe its steps in detail.
3. Describe planning tools used in estimating equipment requirements.
4. Describe the process of condemnation.

II. Short Notes
1. Criteria for selecting supplies and equipment
2. Model list of equipment
3. Equipment inventory
4. Condemnation committee

III. Multiple Choice Questions
1. Which one of the following item is consumable?
   a. Equipment   b. Materials
   c. Supplies   d. Accessories
2. A process of checking and ensuring new equipment for its functioning and safety is known as:
   a. Inspection   b. Commissioning
   c. Maintenance   d. Decommissioning
3. Compilation of record sheets containing lists of equipment is:
   a. Inventory control
   b. Model list of equipment
   c. Reference equipment price list
   d. Equipment inventory
4. The stock value of equipment means:
   a. Depreciation in value overtime
   b. Quantity and cost of equipment
   c. Approximate price of equipment
   d. Running cost of equipment
5. "Appropriateness" criteria in selecting supply and equipment means:
   a. Equipment must meet performance and safety requirements
   b. Equipment should be easy to operate, clean, and maintain
   c. Equipment must be within the budgetary lineup
   d. Equipment should be suitable and compatible with existing equipment
6. In purchase planning, the order information must include:
   a. Specification and quantity of equipment
   b. Quality, delivery, and payment
   c. Specification and payment
   d. Quality and quantity of equipment

Answer Keys
1. c   2. b   3. d   4. b   5. d   6. b

SUGGESTED READING

1. Available from http://apps.who.int/medicinedocs/documents/s17710en/s17710en.pdf. [Accessed July 2019].
2. Housley CE. Hospital Material Management. Rockville, Md: Aspen Publishers, Inc; 1978.
3. Kowalski JC. Material management is crucial to overall efficiency. Healthcare Financial Management. [Online] Available from Find Articles.com. [Accessed Dec 2011].
4. Kulkarni GR. Management Accounting for Hospitals. Mumbai: Ridhirai Enterprise; 2003.
5. Kumar R, Goel SL. Hospital Administration and Management, Vol I. New Delhi: Deep & Deep Publication.
6. McGibnoy. Principles of Hospital Administration. New York: Putnam's Sons; 1969.
7. Schulz R, Johnson AC. Management of Hospitals and Health Services: Strategic Issues and Performance, 3rd edition. St Louis: CV Mosby; 1990.

CHAPTER 47

Procurement and Purchasing

CHAPTER OUTLINE

- Procurement
  - Definitions
  - Objectives
  - Procurement Process
  - Budgetary Process in Procurement
  - Procurement Process for Consumable Items
- Purchasing
  - Meaning
  - Key Steps of Purchasing
  - Principles of Purchasing
  - Points to Remember While Purchasing

LEARNING OUTCOMES

After completion of this chapter, the learner will be able to:
- Understand the concept of procurement and purchasing
- Enlist the objectives of the procurement system
- Describe in detail the procurement process
- Explain the method of the budgetary process
- Describe steps in the purchasing process
- Describe principles of purchasing
- Elaborate the points to keep in mind while purchasing materials including equipment

KEY TERMS

Procurement, purchasing, procurement process, consumable items, procurement system, the purchasing process

INTRODUCTION

The provision of adequate material in departments is of prime importance for carrying out various activities to render patient care as well as for meeting its needs. Procurement is a significant step in material management. Usually, the hospital has a central store and procurement/store officer under the control of the medical superintendent is recruited, who manages the materials.

PROCUREMENT

Definitions

Procurement means the acquisition of material and services to carry out various activities in any organization. It is sourcing and purchasing of goods or commodities by an organization, institution, or a person. It simply means the purchase of products from suppliers at the lowest possible cost.

It is a process of obtaining material from preparation and processing. Defense Acquisition University referred to it as an act of buying equipment and services for the government. The organization purchases the items and external suppliers. It is a process that involves a series of activities such as giving an order, receiving, reviewing, and approving items from suppliers. It specifies the method of maintaining relationships with the supplier to have a high level of service.

Objectives

The following list shows the objectives of procurement:
- To acquire needed supplies as inexpensively as possible
- To obtain high-quality supplies
- To ensure prompt and dependable delivery
- To distribute the procurement workload by avoiding the period of idleness and overwork
- To optimize inventory management through appropriate procurement procedures.

Procurement Process

Following is a proven step-by-step technique of procurement process that will help control successfully to achieve its goals (Fig. 47.1):

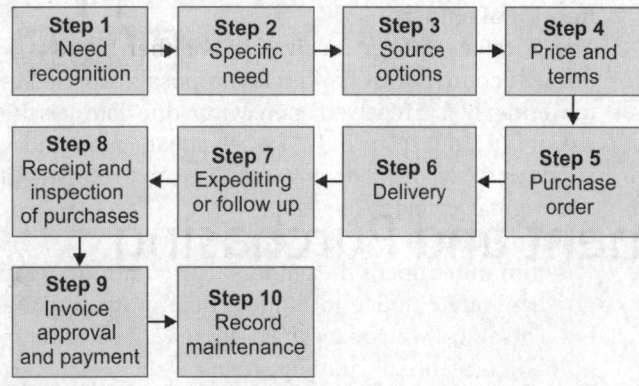

Fig. 47.1: Procurement process.

Step 1: Need recognition
Recognize the need for procuring the materials for the department either from internal or external sources. The items may include reordered or new things for the unit.

Step 2: Specific need
Decide the specifications of items for purchasing. Take the help of suppliers to visit the department or from the engineering department.

Step 3: Source options
Determine the source to obtain the product. The hospital might have an approved vendor list. Identify suppliers using purchase orders or research a variety of other sources such as magazines, the Internet, or sales representatives.

Step 4: Price and terms
Do survey from all sources or at least three suppliers to get the best price of the required product before finalizing the cost and terms.

Step 5: Purchase order
After finalizing the product place order to buy. The purchase order must mention the name of the product with specifications and conditions, cost, service, and any additional requirements.

Step 6: Delivery of item
The supplier delivers the purchase order either personally or per requirement and get acknowledged from the receiver.

Step 7: Follow-up or expedition
The expedition is following up on purchase order within the time of the service or materials delivered.

Step 8: Receipt and inspection of purchases
On delivery of the product by the supplier, check the material for quantity and quality per the order placed.

Step 9: Approval of invoice and payment
At the time of payment, the finance department checks the invoice, receipt, and original purchase order that should match. In case of any discrepancies, resolve before the payment by the finance department. The department makes payment in any mode per requirement.

Step 10: Record maintenance
The department does proper documentation and keeps a record of the purchase order, and items received receipts, tax paid, etc. Each item has its code. The purchase records require for tax purpose and purchase orders to confirm warranty information. These records are a reference for future purchases as well.

Budgetary Process in Procurement

The following list shows the budgetary process in procurement (**Fig. 47.2**):

1. **Need assessment**
   Assess the need for having the equipment/item in the department.
2. **Finding the budget**
   Each department has a budget to purchase materials. But sometimes the department indents even without a specific budget with the approval of head of institution.
3. **Priority selection of material**
   Assess the requirement of equipment/material for procurement and infrastructure requirement. Formulate a committee. Depending on the policy, the department either directly purchases or forwards a request to the central store for purchasing.
4. **Standards and specification**
   Get a detailed specification and standard of product per the requirement before placing indent.
5. **Placing indent**
   The head of the department indents the item with proper specification and quantity and estimates the cost, its utility, and the operational period. The head of the department then sends it to the store department to verify its stock and render a no-stock certificate wherever applicable. After ascertaining from the store department, it directly communicates to the purchasing department to check for details. The purchase officer places it before the relevant standing purchase committee. After getting the approval by the purchase committee, consider the indent item for purchasing.
6. **Select the appropriate method for procuring**
   a. *The open tender:* Use the open-tender method for all high-cost items. The notice inviting tender should be short, clearly worded. Provide a brief description of the material for procurement, the qualification of suppliers, the date of receipt of bid,

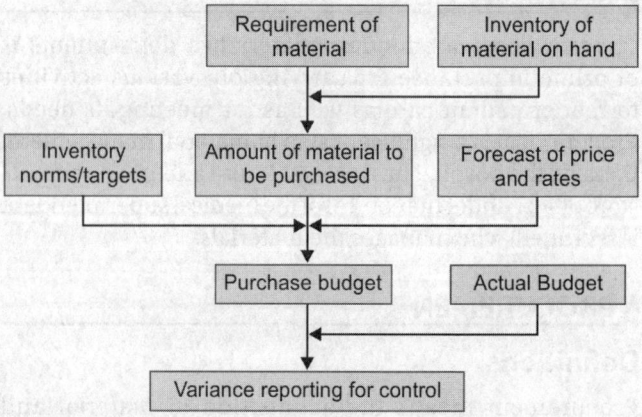

Fig. 47.2: Budgeting process in procuring items.

the date, time, and venue of opening the tenders. It is public bidding, resulting in low prices, published in newspapers. The term is usually 1 month. Send the quotations on time mention date and time in the tender form. Typically, the organization follows two packets or two bin systems. Two separate packets are technical bid and financial bid. The validity of tenders is generally 3 months (90 days). The tender amount as earnest money is 2% or, as decided, is payable along with all quotations. One fifth is withheld, in case of default.

b. *Limited tender:* In the limited tender, invite the bids from limited suppliers (about 8–10). Reduce the lead time for these tenders.

c. *Procurement by negotiation:* It is a conversation and battle between the buyer and the suppliers. It is an art of arriving at common understanding through bargaining on the essential points for the contract, such as delivery, specification, price, and payment terms, keeping in mind ethics and objectives of negotiation **(Fig. 47.3)**. Maintain good relations and try to have a win–win situation. The principles of negotiation are as follows:
- Put yourself in supplier shoes
- Consultation is essentially an artful communication
- Be a good listener, and let the supplier speak
- Satisfy the supplier needs
- Talk to a proper person
- Build up confidence
- Always ask for a discount
- Take one point at a time
- Negotiate bulk price.

d. *Direct procurement:* The direct acquisition is applicable for the purchase of proprietary, low priced, small quantity materials from a single supplier at his quoted price. Usually, the departments do direct procurement of items in case of emergency purchases.

e. *Rate contract:* It specifies the rate asked by a firm to store supply during the period covered by the agreement.

f. *Spot purchase:* It is purchasing items on the spot through a committee, which comprises officers from stores, accounts, and purchasing departments.

g. *Risk purchase:* It is the cost difference recovered from the first supplier in case that fails to deliver the ordered item and purchased from another supplier.

7. **Receipt of tenders**
The purchase officer receives bids either by post or through courier or by hand. The proposals dropped in the tender box. If received open within due date, it is the risk of the bidder. The bids, if received late, mark those as late or delayed and do not open. Return to bidders in the original envelope as sealed.

8. **Opening tenders**
The committee opens the tenders. The committee may give a separate notice to bidders before opening the bid. The officer who opens the bidding will read out the particulars of the solicitation.

9. **Evaluating tenders**
Evaluate tenders logically and scientifically. Make a comparative statement of all the bids. The tender must contain details such as rate, delivery schedule, make, and taxes of items. The conditional tenders should not be accepted. Negotiate with the lowest bidder only wherever necessary. Make a separate evaluation for technical and financial bids. Invite tenders for discussion to arrive at a threshold level of acceptability. The bidders who technically acceptable shall be allowed to withdraw their price bids and send a revised request again in a sealed envelope or to adhere to the original price bid sent. Open the price bids, evaluate each one, and award the contract the lowest evaluated bidder.

10. **Placement of orders**
Once the purchase proposal is approved, the purchase officer prepares the purchase orders and arranges to send it to the vendor. The purchase order shall contains the make and model of the item with description, rate, and quantity-ordered amount and terms and conditions.

11. **Follow-up of orders**
Be in touch with the supplier after placing the order. Keep following the supplier until the delivery of items.

12. **Receipt and inspection of material**
The material received at the entry point is checked thoroughly for quantity and quality by the indenter. The documents obtained are also verified against the supplier's packing slip and purchase order. Record in the receiving report all the discrepancies between the materials, incomplete supply, etc. Document the received items with signature and date. Enter the serial number of the item in the receiving report.

13. **Invoice approval and payment**
After the approval of the invoice, the payment is made to the supplier by the finance department of the institute.

Procurement Process for Consumable Items

The list below shows the procurement process for consumable items:
- Place an order with a description of the consumable or nonstock materials.
- Enter the consumable materials with a short text description as the main identifiable characteristic without assigning a number.

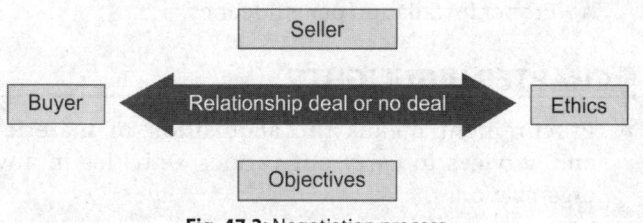

Fig. 47.3: Negotiation process.

- The purchase requisition is subject to approval, based on the predefined parameters, before being converted to a purchase order and issue to a vendor.
- There is no inventory in the system.

PURCHASING

Meaning

Purchasing is a method of buying required materials through payment in various modes from suppliers/vendors. It is a process that involves a series of activities. As a system, each step has input (information), throughput and output, and feedback **(Fig. 47.4)**.

The purchasing process varies from organization to organization, but the fundamental procedure remains the same. The purchasing process begins with buying and acquiring particular material with a specification. It is one of the functions in the supply cycle. The main principle of purchasing to buy the right equipment in the right quantity, of the right quality, at the correct cost, from right source and place, from right supplier/vendor, at the right time. It involves a process of selecting the right sources of supply, finalizing terms and conditions of purchasing, placing a purchase order, follow-up, maintaining a cordial relationship with suppliers, approving the final cost, evaluating, and rating suppliers.

Key Steps of Purchasing

Figure 47.5 depicts the key steps of purchasing:
1. **Purchase/requisition**
   Identify the need, what to buy, and how much of it and when it is needed to deliver.
2. **Supplier selection**
   Identify supplier, price, and lead time.
3. **Purchase order**
   Place an order for purchase. The purchase officer identifies the items to procure according to the quantity required.
4. **Fulfillment**
   Supplier procures the items and sends to the buyer.
5. **Order receipt**
   Check the details for quality and quantity per the order placed.
6. **Supplier invoice/payment**
   The supplier sends the invoice, which is processed by the finance department before the supplier payment.

Principles of Purchasing

The following are the principles of purchasing:
1. **Principle of need assessment:** Identify the need for items with the specifications for purchasing.
2. **Principle of the aim of purchasing:** The ultimate objective for purchasing is the right quality, right quantity, correct prices, right source, right time and place, with the right mode of transportation and the right attitude.
3. **Principle of appropriate methodology:** Consider the proper technique such as value analysis, material intelligence, purchase research, SWOT analysis, purchase budget, and lead time analysis.
4. **Principle of the centralizing system:** Centralize the purchase system and have back up of proper systems management.

Points to Remember While Purchasing

1. **In General**
   - There should be the proper specification of all items.
   - Invite quotations from reputed suppliers.
   - Compare item for the basic price, freight and insurance, taxes, and levies.
   - Ensure quantity and payment discounts.
   - Discuss payment terms.
   - Have the delivery period and guarantee.
   - Check vendor reputation (reliability, technical capabilities, convenience, availability, after-sales service, sales assistance).
   - Shortlist for better negotiation terms.
   - Seek order acknowledgment.
2. **Purchase of an equipment**
   Check for:
   - Latest technology
   - Availability of maintenance and repair facility, with minimum downtime
   - Postwarranty repair at reasonable cost
   - Upgradeability
   - Reputed manufacturer
   - Availability of consumables
   - Low operating costs
   - Installation
   - Proper installation per guidelines.

CHAPTER HIGHLIGHTS

- Procurement means the acquisition of material and services to carry out various activities in any organization.

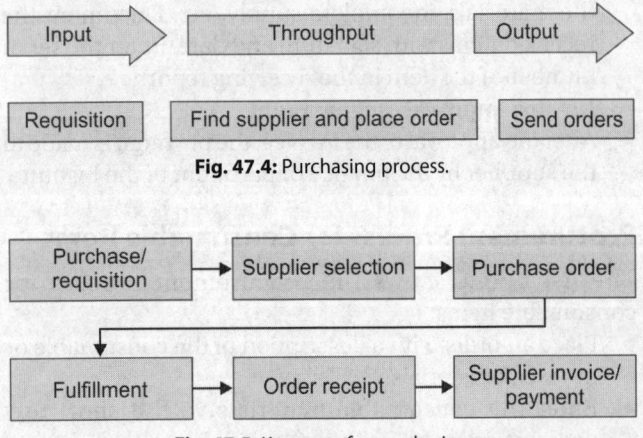

Fig. 47.4: Purchasing process.

Fig. 47.5: Key steps for purchasing.

- The step-by-step technique of procurement and budgetary process helps control successfully to achieve its goals.
- Purchasing is a method of buying required materials through payment in various modes from suppliers/vendors. There are multiple steps in the purchasing process.

REVIEW QUESTIONS

I. Essay Type Questions
1. Define the term "procurement." Describe in detail the procurement process.
2. Explain in detail the budgetary process in procurement.
3. What do you mean by purchasing? Discuss its procedure in detail.

II. Short Notes
1. Principles of purchasing
2. Open tender method of procuring
3. Methods of procuring materials

III. Multiple Choice Questions
1. Under which process the acquisition of materials and services falls to carry out activities?
   a. Purchasing   b. Procurement
   c. Budgeting   d. Commissioning
2. Minimum how many suppliers required getting the best price of the required product before finalizing the cost?
   a. Three   b. Four
   c. Five   d. Six
3. What is the duration of the validity of tenders in general?
   a. 6 months   b. 4 months
   c. 3 months   d. 1 month
4. Which one of the following terms used for the cost recovered from the first supplier in case that fails to deliver the ordered item and purchase from another supplier?
   a. Spot purchase   b. Rate purchase
   c. Direct purchase   d. Risk purchase
5. Which principle of purchasing specifies value analysis, SWOT analysis, material intelligence, etc.?
   a. Principle of appropriate methodology
   b. Principle of centralized system
   c. Principle of purchasing
   d. Principle of need assessment

Answer Keys

1. b   2. a   3. c   4. d   5. a

SUGGESTED READING

1. Chandorkar AG. Hospital Administration and Planning. Hyderabad: Paras Medical Publishers; 2004.
2. Gupta S, Kant S (Eds). Hospital Stores Management: An Integrated Approach, 1st edition. New Delhi: Jaypee Brothers Medical Publishers Pvt Ltd; 2000.
3. Kant S, Pandaw CS, Nath LM. A management technique for effective management of the medical store in hospitals. J Acad Hosp Adm. 1997;89:41-7.
4. Kent C, Hunter D. Management material. Nurs Times. 1997;29(5):36-7.
5. Mac Eacharan, Malcolm M.T. Hospital Organization, and Management. Illinois: Physician Record Company; 1962.
6. McGibons JR. Principles of Hospital Administration, 2nd edition. New York: GP Putnam and Sons; 1969.
7. McAllister JC. Challenges in purchasing and inventory control. Am J Hosp Pharm. 1985;42(6):1370-3. (Pub Med).
8. Procurement and Supply Cycle. [Online] Available from https://www.cips.org/en-SG/knowledge/procurement-cycle/. [Accessed June 2019].
9. Procurement Management Process—The 2019 Guide. [Online] Available from https://kissflow.com/procurement-process/. [Accessed June 2019].
10. Satyanarayana P. Material management. J Acad Hosp Adm. 1994;31:21-6.

48 Inventory Control and Inventory Accounting System

CHAPTER OUTLINE

- Inventory Control
  - Concept of Inventory and Inventory Control
  - Objectives of Inventory Control
  - Importance of Inventory Control
  - Basic Principles of Inventory Control
  - Maintaining Inventory Control
  - Inventory Stock Levels
  - Inventory Control Techniques
  - Inventory Ordering Techniques
- Inventory Control System

LEARNING OUTCOMES

After completion of this chapter, the learner will be able to:
- Understand the concept of inventory, inventory control, and inventory system
- Appreciate the importance of inventory control
- Enumerate the objectives of inventory control
- Describe various types of inventory costs
- Discuss how to achieve control
- List down the significant activities of inventory control
- Define setting up of different stock levels
- Apply basic principles of inventory control
- Explain techniques of inventory control
- Classify and describe in detail types of inventories
- Explain inventory model for quantity and inventory replenishment
- Describe inventory accounting system

KEY TERMS

Inventory, inventory control, inventory system, inventory cost, accounting system, inventory techniques

INTRODUCTION

The proper inventory controls and processes can save millions in health-care costs by enabling a hospital to efficiently order and store only the right amount of supplies needed for patient cases while tracking fees, tier pricing, and patient charges associated with supplies.

INVENTORY CONTROL

Concept of Inventory and Inventory Control

Inventory

Inventory is the blocked working capital of an organization in the form of materials, which is usually zero. Yet, there is a need to maintain an inventory. The inventory is a stock to ensure uninterrupted supplies and to have future economic value. It provides a cushion between the estimated and the actual demand for materials. It is anything that is bought and held before use. It includes all the materials, parts, supplies, expenses, and in-process or finished products recorded on registers or books by an organization and kept in its stocks for some period.

Inventory Control

Inventory control is the process of measuring and regulating inventory according to the predetermined criteria such as size for order, safety stock (SS), minimum level, maximum level, order level, etc. Inventory control means stocking an adequate number and kind of stores so that the materials are available whenever required and wherever required. Inventory control keeps the optimal balance of material. It is a system that indicates type and quantity of material for order, the time for ordering equipment, and the amount to keep in stock.

Chapter 48: Inventory Control and Inventory Accounting System

Inventory control minimizes the total cost of inventory. It includes physical control of materials, preserving materials, minimizing obsolescence and damaged through timely disposal and efficient handling, and maintaining store records and stocking. The store officer is responsible for the physical verification of stocks and reconciliation them with book figures, the inventory ordering quantities, setting stock level, lead time (LT) analysis, and reporting.

According to Dave Kaczmarek, inventory control refers to controlling product availability and balancing the costs of ownership with the costs of procuring, which includes purchasing, receiving, and paying. It is the technique of maintaining the size of the inventory at some desired level, keeping in view the best economic interest of an organization. It is concerning with minimizing the total cost of the stock.

Objectives of Inventory Control

- To supply the materials on time
- To give maximum clients' service by meeting their requirement timely, effectively, efficiently, smoothly, and satisfactorily
- To reduce or minimize investment in inventories
- To minimize idle time by avoiding stock out and shortages
- To prevent the lack of stock
- To reduce the losses due to deterioration, obsolescence, damage of stock
- To meet unforeseen future demand
- To average out demand fluctuations
- To balance various inventory costs such as carrying cost, order cost, etc.

Importance of Inventory Control

- It provides and maintains excellent customer service.
- It enables a smooth flow of materials through the production process.
- It removes the uncertainty of requirement and procurement of items.
- It ensures a reasonable utilization of equipment.
- There is a possibility of a discount on purchasing in bulk.
- It defines inventory control and inventory system.
- It provides maximum supply service with maximum efficiency.
- It fills a gap between forecast and actual requirement for a material.
- It ensures an adequate level of inventory in the store.
- It eliminates duplication in ordering.
- It keeps in mind the requirements fluctuations and lead time and price in bulk buying.
- It minimizes transportation cost, inventory costs, and waiting time.
- It monitors the loss of material and utilization of stocks.
- It facilitates cost accounting activities and disposes of obsolete and nonfunctioning store items.

Basic Principles of Inventory Control

1. **Principle of SS:** The principle of SS means to keep stock usage at an average rate during the extension of LT. The SS is the difference between the worst-case scenario (WCS) and the average weekly usage (forecast) (AWU) during the LT period.

$$SS = (WCS - AWU) LT$$

In contrast, LT is the time spend in deciding stock replenishment and actual availability of the goods. It should be logic; it should have all steps, including order (Purchase Order (PO)/Manufacturing Order (MO)) processing time, Quality Control (QC) check/quarantine, etc. It should be "effective"; it stands that all steps must be as short as possible. It should be "attainable," which means it should remain reasonable and not too optimistic. It should be "dependable," which means that it should have the reliability of LT and supplier quality assessment program.

2. **Principle of average inventory ('INV' stands for Inventory and 'AVG' stands for Average):** The average inventory is the sum of the SS and half the reorder quantity (ROQ).

$$INVAVG = SS + 1/2 ROQ$$

3. **Principle of reorder point:** The reorder point (ROP) is the sum of the SS and the quantity used during the LT.

$$ROP = SS + (AWU \times LT)$$

According to this principle, items for which annual consumption is high, place the orders frequently to keep inventory level as low as possible. Items for which annual consumption is not high, maintain enough stock and place orders less frequently.

Maintaining Inventory Control

The primary activities in inventory control are planning, procuring, receiving, and inspecting, recording, storing and issuing, and physical verification of product items. Follow-up, material standardization, and substitution of material are also the activities of inventory control. Maintain inventory control by undertaking the following measures:

- Purchase items at economical price at a proper time and in enough quantity
- Provision of suitable and secured location with enough space
- Follow inventory identification system.

Inventory Stock Levels

Stock levels are liable to revise according to the fluctuations in the cost of holding the stock, the cost of placing an order, and the cost of shortage.

1. **Minimum level:** The minimum level is the level maintaining the minimum stock for smooth production. Calculate the minimum standard by subtracting the

reorder level from average usage per period multiplied by average time to obtain delivery.

Minimum level = Reorder level − Average usage per period × Average time to obtain delivery

2. **Maximum level:** The maximum level is the level of stock beyond which the stock is difficult to maintain. Calculate the maximum level by subtracting the re-order level from expected minimum consumption in units during the least time to obtain delivery plus ROQ.

Maximum level = Reordering level − Expected minimum consumption in units during the least time to obtain delivery + ROQ

3. **Average stock level:** The average stock level is half of the maximum and minimum stock level.

Average stock level
$$= \frac{\text{Maximum level} + \text{Minimum level}}{2}$$

4. **Reserve stock:** Reserve stock is the excess usage requirement during standard LT.
5. **Reorder level:** Re-order level is the stock level at which to place another order. Re-order level is the stock level in which there is maximum usage of stock in the maximum reorder period.

Re-order level = Maximum reorder period × maximum usage.

Inventory Control Techniques

There are many techniques based on the analysis to apply for inventory control. These are always better control (ABC) analysis; vital, essential, and desirable (VED) analysis; fast moving, slow moving, and nonmoving (FSN) analysis; scarce, difficult, and easy (SDE) analysis; high, medium, and low (HML) analysis; *XYZ* analysis; government, ordinary, local, and foreign (GOLF) analysis; and seasonal off-seasonal (SOS) analysis.

There are thousands of items required in hospitals. The administrator is to identify these vital few from trivial many and exercise tight control on them to achieve the primary objective of reduction in the cost of inventory. Analyze items in the hospitals by using various classifications, but the most widely used rating is ABC and VED analysis. These types of reports are in practice in medical stores since 1981 on the recommendations of the Administrative Reform Committee.

ABC Analysis

ABC analysis is an essential supply chain technique in inventory control. It is a ubiquitous tool in all the stores having stock of large inventory items. ABC classification is a system of categorization of objects/inventory in three classes, with each type having a different management control associated and based on the cost factor or their annual consumption value.

ABC analysis popularly known as "always better control" or alphabetical approach is a beneficial approach to material management based on Pareto's principle of "vital few and trivial many" based on the capital investment of the item and cost criteria or in simple term based on annual consumption value of the said item (annual consumption value=quantity consumed × cost of the article). It is selective inventory control (SIM) since this method is a means of categorizing inventory items according to the potential amount to be controlled.

According to Pareto's theory, 10% of items consume about 70% of the budget, which are Group A items. The next 20% consume 20% of the budget, which are Group B items, and the remaining 70% items account for just 10% of the budget, which are Group C items.

"A" items: These are small in number but consume a large number of resources and are managed by top management. These items must have tight control, a rigid estimate of requirements, strict and closer watch and require low SSs. These items consume significant portions of funds.

"B" items: These have reasonable control. These items are purchased based on rigid requirements and reasonably have strict watch and control. Safety stocks are maintained moderately. Middle-level managers manage these items.

"C" items: These items are more abundant in number but consume a lesser amount of resources and must have ordinary control measures. The purchase is based on the usage estimates but requires high SSs. **Table 48.1** depicts the comparison of items based on ABC analysis.

TABLE 48.1: Comparison of items based on ABC analysis.

S. No	Items A	Items B	Items C
1	High consumption value	Has moderate value	Has low consumption value
2.	Very strict control	Moderate control	Loose control
3.	No or meager safety stock	Low safety stocks	High safety stocks
4.	Frequent ordering	Once in 3 months	Bulk ordering once in 6 months
5.	Maximum follow-up and expediting	Periodic follow-up	Follow-up and facilitating in exceptional cases
6.	Weekly control statement	Monthly control reports	Quarterly control reports
7.	Maximum value analysis	Moderate value analysis	Minimum value analysis
8.	Accurate forecasting in material management	Estimation based on record	Rough estimation
9.	Many sources for each item	Two or more reliable sources	Two reliable sources
10.	Minimization of waste, obsolete, and surplus	Quarterly control over the surplus and obsolete items	Annual review over the surplus and obsolete items
11.	Central purchasing	Combination purchasing	Decentralized purchasing
12.	Maximum effort to reduce lead time	Moderate attempt to reduce lead time	Minimum clerical efforts
13.	Handled by top management	Middle management can control	Can be fully delegated

Chapter 48: Inventory Control and Inventory Accounting System

TABLE 48.2: ABC analysis.

Item no.	Annual consumption units	Unit cost (₹)	Annual consumption value (₹)	Annual consumption value (₹) in descending order	Item no.	Cumulative annual consumption value (₹)	Cumulative %	Category and cost %	
11	20,000	0.25	5,000	24,000	17	24,000	46.28	A	70%
12	30,000	0.20	6,000	10,000	15	34,000	65.57	A	
13	10,000	0.10	1,000	6,000	12	40,000	77.14	B	20%
14	500	0.30	150	5,000	11	45,000	86.78	B	
15	5,000	2.00	10,000	4,500	19	49,500	95.47	C	
16	8,000	0.05	400	1,000	13	50,500	97.39	C	
17	6,000	4.00	24,000	700	18	51,200	98.14	C	10%
18	700	1.00	700	400	16	51,600	99.51	C	
19	9,000	0.50	4,500	150	14	51,750	99.81	C	
20	50	2.00	100	100	20	51,850	100.00	C	

Principles of ABC Analysis
- The analysis depends on its annual consumption values rather than the unit cost.
- The limits for ABC categorization are not uniform but depends on the size of the organization, its inventory as well as the number of items controlled.
- The analysis does not rely on the importance of things instead based on the material price, material credibility, and availability status of material, material physical characteristics, and frequency of material usage.
- It also depends on the degree and characteristics of controls exercised by the management: The necessity of control, the need of which material placed under control, and the particular features of the material.

Method of ABC Analysis
Based on the annual usage, tabulate the consumption value of all the items in the store. List down each item and its consumption value separately and then rearrange the list in descending order beginning with the item of the highest value and ending with the item of the lowest value. Follow the below steps for calculation:

1. Gather all the inventory data and make a list of all the store items with the unit price/item and yearly consumption.
2. Calculate annual usage (in ₹).
   (Annual consumption in units × unit costs = annual consumption value)
   For stores, it will be quantity issued × unit rate/item.
3. Arrange items in the descending order according to the total value of consumption (annually) per piece in rupees.
4. Assign item numbers against their annual usage.
5. Find out cumulative annual usage/consumption cost and in percentage.
6. Classify items according to their percentage consumption value (price).

Those items that together form 70% of the total yearly usage value or select the top 10% of all the details have the highest rupee percentage may be categorized as "A" items. These are item numbers 17 and 15.

Items that fall under 20% of the total annual usage value or select the next 20% of all the things with the next highest rupee percentage categorized as "B" items. These are 11 and 12.

The items fall under 10% of the total annual usage value, or the next 70% of all the items with the lowest rupee percentage categorized as "C" items **(Table 48.2)**. ABC analysis does not stress on items that are less costly but may be vital. Place the orders based on classification, but this analysis does not provide a direct solution.

Advantages of ABC Analysis
The list shows the advantages of ABC analysis:
- It maintains investment in inventory.
- It is easy to manage stock and control the wastage of costly items.
- It aids in maintaining safety to the total cost.
- It helps in exercising selective control with a large number of items.
- It rationalizes the number of orders and thus reduces the inventory.
- It depicts visible results in a short period.
- ABC analysis helps the managers to control the inventories, primarily "A" items.
- It helps in pinpointing the obsolete stocks and reducing administrative costs.

Disadvantages of ABC Analysis
The list shows the disadvantages of ABC analysis:
- It needs proper standard and coding of inventory items.
- It concerns with a cost value of material and not it's functioning.
- It is challenging to have periodic reviews on ABC analysis.

Applicability
ABC analysis finds its applications in the following:
- It has universal application for fields requiring selective control.
- It extends almost all aspects of material management, such as purchasing, receiving, and inspection.
- It can be used in any setting to control the cost.

VED Analysis

VED analysis means vital, essential, and desirable analysis. The materials are classified based on criticality that on a functional basis. The degree of criticality is whether equipment vital to the process, essential, or desirable for the procedure.

"V" stands for "vital" items. These items are necessary for the hospital functioning, and shortage can cause havoc, e.g. oxygen supply. These items need to stock in large quantity to ensure smooth operation.

"E" stands for "essential" items. These items are necessary to maintain the quality of the services. Without these items, the functions may not interrupt but may affect efficiency and expenses. These items need to stock in a sufficient amount to ensure a regular flow of work, e.g. antibiotics, intravenous fluids, etc.

"D" stands for "desirable" items. These items one easy to procure when required. The unavailability of these items will not interfere with the treatment, e.g. tonics, cough syrups, B. complex, etc.

The basis of the VED classification is on the shortage and cost of materials. However, it is a subjective analysis. For "vital" items, one cannot tolerate the lack; for "essential" items, one can tolerate the deficit for a short period, whereas for "desirable" items, the deficiency does not matter.

Advantages of VED Analysis
The advantages of VED analysis are as follows:
- It is useful for monitoring and controlling stores and spares inventory.
- It determines the criticality of an item and its effect on production and other services.
- It classifies spare parts or objects based on the necessity of things. Maintain a large stock of inventory of "V" items and keep the minimum stock of "D" items.
- It helps to control and maintain the stock of various types.

Combination of ABC and VED Analysis
By combining ABC and VED analysis, based on the consumption value and the criticality, it will give fruitful results **(Table 48.3)**.

Advantages
- It aids management in materializing the policy and the service standard.
- It controls the stock levels by visualizing the inventory carrying cost.

Fast-moving, Slow-moving, and Nonmoving Analysis

Meaning
FSN is "fast-moving, slow-moving, and non-moving" classification based on the consumption pattern of the items or design of issues of items from stores.

TABLE 48.3: Combination of ABC and VED analysis bases.

	V	E	D	Category	Item	Cost
A	AV Constant control regular follow-up	AE Moderate stocks	AD No stock	Category 1	10	70%
B	BV Moderate stocks	BE Moderate stocks	BD Low stocks	Category 2	20	20%
C	CV High stocks	CE Moderate stocks	CD Meager stocks	Category 3	70	10%

Category 1: Needs close monitoring and control
Category 2: Moderate control, *Category 3:* No need for control.

Method
Consider the date of receipt or last date of issue, whichever is later to determine the number of months that have elapsed since the previous transaction. Group the items in 12 months. Review nonmoving articles periodically to prevent expiry date.

Analysis
For analysis, consider the issuing of things/items of the past 2 or 3 years. If there is no issuing of the item during that period, it falls under "N" item. Up to 10–15 issuing of the items in that period falls under "S" item, whereas the things exceeding such limits during that period fall under "F" item. The period of consideration and the limited number of issues vary from organization to organization.

The demand for fast-moving (F) items is very high. Thus special care should be taken in respect of these items; otherwise, the work may suffer due to a shortage of such things. All obsolete inventories contribute to nonmoving (N) items. It may be due to a change in technology or specification or may not be in use for a longer time.

Advantages
The advantages of FSN analysis are as follows:
- It avoids investing nonmoving or slow items.
- It facilitates timely control.
- It is useful in controlling obsolescence.

SDE Analysis

Meaning
SDE stands for scarce, difficult, and easy to procure items. "S" stands for "scarce" items, which are difficult to acquire and generally require source development. These items need to either import or in short supply. The top-level management manages these types of things. There is a need to maintain a big SS of such items. "D" stands for "difficult" items. These items are available indigenously but difficult to procure. These items need to purchase from distant places and trying to get reliable suppliers. It is necessary to maintain a SS for these types of things. "E" stands for "easy" items. These items are accessible to purchase in the local markets. Only minimum SS needs to maintain such things.

Criteria
SDE analysis has the basis of problems encountered in the procuring and the accessibility of items.

Advantages
The following list shows the advantages of SDE analysis:
- It takes into account the LT.
- It is useful when there is a scarcity of items.
- It helps in determining the method of buying.
- It aids in fixing up the responsibilities of buyers.

HML Analysis
Criteria
The primary criterion of HML classification is the unit value of the item. Based on the unit value, the materials are of high-value materials, medium value materials, and low-value materials.

Analysis
List out all the items in the descending order of unit value, and the management may fix the limits for determining three categories.

Advantages
Following are the advantages of HML analysis:
- It aids in controlling over-consumption at departmental level.
- It helps in deciding the frequency of physical verification.

XYZ Analysis
Criteria
XYZ classification is on the value of the inventory stored.

The X items are those whose inventory values are high, while Z items are those whose inventory values are low. And Y items are those who have moderate inventory stocks. Usually, XYZ analysis is in conjunction with ABC or HML analysis. **Table 48.4** depicts XYZ analysis in conjunction with ABC.

Advantages
Following are the advantages of XYZ analysis:
- Identifies few items accounting for a large amount of money locked up in the stock
- Helps to take steps for liquidation /reduction.

GOLF Analysis
GOLF stands for government, ordinary, local, foreign.

Criteria
GOLF analysis is carried out based on the source of the material.

Method
A particular procedure needs to follow for procuring imported items. The usual process may not work in respect of these items. For another type of material, a separate method requires to follow.

TABLE 48.4: *XYZ* analysis in conjunction with ABC.

Class of item	A	B	C
X	Minimize the stock with those items having low inventory value (Z category)	Convert the stock to those items having low inventory value (Z category)	Dispose of the surplus stocks
Y	Convert the stock to those items having low inventory value (Z category)	–	Have tight control
Z	–	Reviewing stocks levels twice a year	–

SOS Analysis
SOS stands for seasonal and off seasonal items. "S" stands for seasonal items, and OS stands for off-seasonal. The analysis identifies items into:
- Seasonal available only for a limited period
- Seasonal available throughout the year
- Off-seasonal items quantity ned to determine on different consideration.

Strategy for procurement
- **For seasonal items, but available only for a limited period:** Procure and stock the material requiring for 1 year.
- **For seasonal items, but available throughout the year:** Calculate the requirement to purchase during the season after comparing the saving cost on account of lower prices.
- For off-seasonal items, estimate the requirement based on different parameters **(Table 48.5)**.

Inventory Ordering Techniques
Economic Order Quantity
Economic order quantity (EOQ) or fixed ordered quantity system is the technique of ordering materials whenever stock reaches the reorder point. It deals when the cost of procurement and handling of inventory are at the optimum level with and minimum total cost. In this technique, the order quantity is more significant than a single period requirement, so that ordering cost and holding cost balanced out.

Steps for calculation of EOQ
- A = Demand for the year of an item in terms of rupees
- S = Ordering costs in rupees
- I = Carrying cost per rupee per year expressed as a decimal
- Q = Quantity per order in rupees
- EOQ = Number of order × S + Average inventory × I = $\sqrt{2AS/I}$

Assumptions of EOQ
- Demand for the product is constant.
- LT is constant.
- Price per unit is constant.

TABLE 48.5: Item classification, their bases, and uses.

Technique	Basis	Main use
ABC (always better control)	Value of consumption	To control inventories
VED (vital, essential, desirable)	Criticality of item	To determine the stocking levels
FSN (fast moving, slow moving, not moving)	Consumption pattern of items	To control obsolescence
SDE (scarce, difficult, easy to obtain)	Problem faced in procurement	Lead time analysis and purchasing strategies
HML (high, medium, low)	The unit price of material	To control purchasing
XYZ	Value of items in storage	To review the inventory and their uses at scheduled intervals
GOLF (government, ordinary, local, foreign sources)	Source of materials	Procurement strategies
SOS (seasonal off-seasonal items)	Nature of supplies	Procurement/holding strategies for seasonal items

- Inventory carrying cost has a basis on average inventory.
- Ordering cost is constant per order.
- All the demands of the product will be satisfied.

Then the EOQ model
- EOQ = $\sqrt{2AS/IU}$
- A = Demand for the year of an item in terms of rupees
- S = Ordering costs in rupees
- I = Carrying cost per rupee per year expressed as a decimal
- U = Unit cost of procuring an item

Weaknesses of EOQ Formula
- Erratic usage
- Faulty basic information
- Costly calculations

Advantages
- It is an easy technique to estimate inventory to order.
- It is useful for avoiding some expenditure that is not generally required.
- The ordering cost consists of stationary, stock quantity, storage, and receiving.

Reorder Limit Method

It is the method of ordering a fixed quantity, usually the EOQ, either as and when the stocks reach the reorder limit (ROL) or at the end of a predetermined review period if the stocks have fallen below the ROL.

1. There is a fixed ordering quantity (the EOQ) and checked for reaching the ROL
   The ROL determined by adding the LT requirements to SS.
   ROL = Safety stock + LT requirements
2. There is a fixed ordering quantity (the EOQ) and reviewed periodically, either the stocks have fallen below a ROL. If the stock is lower than the ROL, place the order for EOQ. Otherwise, if it is above the ROL, no action needs to be taken till the next review point.
   The reorder point, R, is calculated as follows:
   $R = B + SD(L+P/2)$
   R = Reorder point (in units)
   B = Safety stock (in units)
   SD = Average daily sales (units/day),
   L = Average LT (in days)
   P = Review time (in days)
   The average stock works out to SS + ½ of EOQ

Periodic Ordering Method

The stocks receive at fixed intervals of time (known as review period and orders placed for a variable quality). There is no fixed ordering quantity. Determine the ordering amount as the difference between the actual stocks held at the time of periodic review and the maximum inventory level (M).

Maximum inventory level = SS + consumption rate (LT + review period)

Depending upon whether the LT is greater or lesser than the review period, apply one of the following two rules in fixing the ROQ.

If LT < review period, ordering quantity = M – actual stock held at the time of review

If LT > review period, ordering quantity = M – (actual stock held at the time of review + quantity on order)

Optimum Review Period

The optimum review period can calculate using the following formula:

Optimum review period (in months) =
$$\frac{288 \times \text{Cost per order (in Rs)}}{\text{Annual usage (in units)} \times \text{unit cost (in Rs)} \times \text{annual inventory carrying a cost}}$$

Safety Stocks

The SSs become necessary to avoid "stockouts" if the rate of consumption increased and or the LT gets extended from the values considered for the replenishing systems. Calculate SS by finding out the above two variations occur over a period to maintain n additional quantity of capital.
- When consumption variation is very high, Safety stock = (Maximum rate of consumption – normal rate of consumption) × LT.
- If there is a high variation in LT, Safety stock = Normal consumption rate × (maximum LT – normal LT)

INVENTORY CONTROL SYSTEM

The inventory system is a set of policies and controls that monitors levels of inventory and determines what standards should be maintained when stocks replenish and how large orders should be. The inventory control system includes all aspects of managing lists of the organization.

The inventory management or accounting system is a process of managing the flow of materials efficiently, utilizing workforce and equipment effectively, coordinating internal activities. Inventory management provides information to managers who make accurate and timely decisions to manage their services. These days the organizations rely on the computerized inventory management system.

Factors in Inventory Control Management

There are mainly four factors in inventory control management viz the cost of holding the stock, the cost of placing an order, and the cost of shortage, i.e., what is lost if the stock is insufficient to meet the demand, and up to date and accurate record keeping.

1. **Ordering cost:** It is the cost of ordering the item and securing its supply. It includes the expenses for raising the indents, purchase requisition by the user department till the execution of the order, and receipt and inspection of the item, the salaries and wages of store personnel employed, the rent of store, stationery, and other consumables used by the store, etc.
2. **Inventory carrying (holding) cost:** It is the cost incurred for holding the volume of inventory and measured as a percentage of the unit cost of an item. It includes capital cost, obsolescence cost, deterioration cost, tax on stock, insurance cost, storage and handling cost, the salaries and wages of store personnel employed, the rent of store, stationery and other consumables used by the store, etc.
3. **Out of stock/shortage cost:** It is a loss that occurs or which may occur due to the non-availability of materials. It includes break down or delay carrying out the work, backorders, loss of goodwill, etc.
   Other costs include capacity cost—overtime payments, layoffs, and idle time; set up price and overstocking prices.
4. **Inventory record systems:** The organization may use either the perpetual system or the periodic system to record the transaction involving inventory or account for inventory. So inventory records are kept using either one of these systems
   - *Perpetual inventory system:* Perpetual means continuous. Perpetual inventory system implies constant maintenance of stock records, and in its broad sense, it covers both regular stock-taking as well as up to date recording of store books. It is a method of recording store-balances after every receipt and issue to facilitate regular checking and to obviate closing down for stocktaking. It is a system where an organization keeps continuous, moment-to-moment records of the number, value, and type of inventories that it has.

Features

The features of perpetual inventory system are as follows:
- This system comprises three parts: Bin card, store ledger, and continues stock taking. Bin card is a record of receipts, issues, and closing balances of items of stores.
- Store ledgers are inventory control system records in the form of leaf cards for easy removal and insertion. These are for all costly items.
- Continues stock taking is a method of verification required for restricted items based on their utility.
- Every day selected numbers of items to need to match with the ledger book and bin card.
- Inventory accounts need to update after each purchase.
- The inventory subsidiary ledger needs updating after each transaction. Inventory quantities need to update continuously.
  - *Periodic inventory system:* Periodic means at specific points in time. In a conventional/regular inventory system, the quantity of inventory on hand requires to is determine regularly once a month, quarterly, or at the beginning and end of each year. There is no mention of in-between records. This system does not keep continuous, moment-to-moment records of inventories.

Features

The features of periodic inventory system are as follows:
- It has a record of all acquisitions of inventory of the accounting period by debits to a purchases account.
- The total in the purchases account at the end of the accounting period added to the cost of the inventory on hand at the beginning of the period.
- No updating after each purchase of stock in inventory subsidiary ledger.
- No continuously updating of inventory quantities instead of an updated periodic basis.

CHAPTER HIGHLIGHTS

- The inventory a stock to ensure uninterrupted supplies and to have future economic value.
- Inventory control means stocking an adequate number and kind of stores so that the materials are available whenever required and wherever required.
- There are mainly three principles of inventory control: the principle of SS, the principle of average inventory, and the principle of ROP.
- The principle of SS means to keep stock usage at an average rate during the extension of LT.
- The average inventory is the sum of the SS and half the ROQ.
- The ROP is the sum of the SS and the quantity used during the LT.
- There are many techniques base on analysis to apply for inventory control such as ABC analysis, VED analysis, FSN analysis, etc.

- There are mainly three types of inventory ordering techniques: EOQ, ROL, and periodic ordering method.
- The inventory system is a set of policies and controls that monitors levels of inventory and determines what standards.
- There are four factors in inventory control management, namely the cost of holding the stock, the cost of placing an order, the cost of shortage, and accurate record keeping.
- The organizations use either the perpetual system or the periodic system of inventory control.

REVIEW QUESTIONS

I. Essay Type Questions
1. Define inventory control. Discuss the basic principles of inventory control in detail.
2. Enlist inventory control techniques. Describe ABC analysis in detail.
3. Describe inventory ordering methods.
4. What do you mean by the "Inventory system." Describe factors affecting the inventory management system.

II. Short Notes
1. Principle of safety stock
2. Inventory stock levels
3. VED analysis
4. Reorder limit method

III. Multiple Choice Questions
1. Which method deals with measuring and regulating inventory?
   a. Inventory system
   b. Procurement
   c. Inventory control
   d. Purchasing
2. Safety stock means:
   a. To keep stock usage at an average rate during extension of lead time
   b. To maintain enough stock and place orders less frequently
   c. To purchase items at economical price at a proper time in enough quantity
   d. To place the orders frequently to keep the inventory level as low as possible
3. Which of the following is the basis of the ABC analysis technique?
   a. Unit cost value
   b. Consumption pattern of the items
   c. Degree of criticality
   d. Annual consumption value
4. Which type of items requires minimum safety stock?
   a. Scarce items   b. Easy to obtain
   c. Moving items   d. Difficult items
5. Which of the following method used for ordering material when the stock reaches to reorder point?
   a. Control purchasing method
   b. Periodic ordering method
   c. Economic order quantity method
   d. Reorder limit method

Answer Keys

1. c   2. a   3. d   4. b   5. c

SUGGESTED READING

1. Available from http://www.iimm.org/knowledge_bank/6_purpose-of-inventory-management.htm. [Accessed July 2019].
2. Curt Werner "Simple things count in inventory control - Cover Story." Healthcare Purchasing News. [Online] Available from FindArticles.com. [Accessed December 2011].
3. Devanani M, Gupta AK. ABC, and VED analysis of the pharmacy store of a tertiary care teaching, referral health care institute of India. Pharmaceut Manag. 2010;2:105-7.
4. Gopalakrishnan P, Sundaresan M (Eds). Material Management: An Integrated Approach, 1st edition. New Delhi: Prentice-Hall of India, Pvt Ltd; 1985.
5. Gupta S, Kant S (Eds). Hospital Stores Management: An Integrated Approach, 1st edition. New Delhi: Jaypee Brothers Medical Publishers Pvt Ltd; 2000.
6. Inventory control. [Online] Available from https://www.accountingtools.com/articles/what-is-inventory-control.html. [Accessed July 2019].
7. Inventory Control Systems. [Online] Available from https://www.inc.com/encyclopedia/inventory-control-systems.html. [Accessed July 2019].
8. Kant S, Pandaw CS, Nath LM. A management technique for effective management of the medical store in hospitals. J Acad Hosp Adm. 1997;89:41-7.
9. McAllister JC. Challenges in purchasing and inventory control. Am J Hosp Pharm. 1985 Jun;42(6):1370-3. (Pub Med).
10. Ray DB. Hospital inventory management. J Acad Hosp Adm. 1994;6(1):9-12.
11. Sikder SK, Aggarwal AK, Das Jaya Krishnan N. Inventory control by ABC and VED analysis in medical stores depot of CGHS Delhi. Health Population: PerspectIssues. 1996;19:165-72.
12. Thawani VR, Turankar AV, Sonatakke SD, et al. Economic analysis of drug expenditure in Government medical college hospital Nagpur. Indian J Pharma. 2004;36:15-9.

SECTION 9

Controlling

49. Fundamentals of Controlling
50. Quality Assurance and Quality Management
51. Nursing Service Standards
52. Nursing Audit
53. Accreditation

49 — Fundamentals of Controlling

CHAPTER OUTLINE

- Controlling
  - Meaning and Definitions
  - Objectives
  - Features of Controlling
  - Importance of Controlling
- Principles of Effective Control
- Steps in the Controlling Process
- Limitation of Control

LEARNING OUTCOMES

After completion of this chapter, the learner will be able to:
- Understand the concept of controlling
- Discuss the features and importance of controlling
- Enumerate principles of controlling
- Describe steps of controlling and its limitation

KEY TERMS

Controlling, controlling process, effective control

INTRODUCTION

Controlling is a fundamental and essential function of management. It runs at all levels of the organization. Planning is the beginning of the managerial role, and control may be said to be a final stage. Managers' effectiveness depends on ability in exercise of control. It is a never-ending activity and is essential for accomplishing objectives. Planning is concerned with setting goals and objectives and developing plans. Control is a process that enables managers to get their programs and policies implemented and takes appropriate actions to achieve objectives of the organization. In controlling, managers make sure that performance or things are going by plans. They also confirm that the standards, principles, and procedures are laid down.

CONTROLLING

Meaning and Definitions

Control means comparing actual happening with predetermined standards or objectives. Controlling is measuring and correcting the performance of activities per plans of subordinates to achieve predetermined goals and objectives. Control is also a tool to detect and correct significant variations in the results of the planned activities.

George Terry defined controlling as to determine what to accomplish, i.e. evaluating the performance, if necessary, applying corrective measures so that the performance takes place according to plans. According to Singh, controlling is concerned with examining, observing, reviewing, measuring, and evaluating the performance of the people according to the operational plan for the achievement of their predetermined goals.

Koontz and O'Donnell refer control like planning is ideally forward looking, and the best kind of managerial control corrects deviations from plans before they occur. Management control is the process of assuring that resources are obtained and used effectively and efficiently by the managers to accomplish an organization's objectives (Anthony).

The control consists of verifying whether everything occurs in conformity with the plans adopted, the instructions issued, and principles established. It has for its object to point out weaknesses and errors to rectify them and prevent a recurrence. It operates on everything, things, people, and actions.

Objectives

The following list shows the objectives:
1. To measure performance or progress
2. To compare actual performance with standards

3. To find out any deviations or gap in performance
4. To devise and take corrective actions immediately.

Features of Controlling

Box 49.1 depicts the essential characteristics of control.

1. **Controlling is a continuous process:** Controlling is an ongoing, never-ending process. It is in exercise at all times and has defined patterns and time. Managers need to ensure that everything is on the right course per the plan.
2. **Controlling is forward looking:** Controlling is always focused on the outcome or future and not on the past. However, it is concerned with measuring the performance of history to suggest appropriate corrective measures for future action. It is exercised with the view to guard against the future to avoid repeated mistakes. Return of the past is the base for determining the control for future.
3. **Controlling is a dynamic process:** Controlling is not only a continuous process but also a dynamic process. To carry out planned action plans effectively and to maintain managerial control operation, there should be some elements of flexibility in the control system to adjust with shortcomings in the program.
4. **Controlling is exercised at all levels:** The head of an organization exercises overall control, and it is required to monitor at all levels. All departmental heads are assigned the job and responsibility to control their department, although the nature, scope, and limit of control vary. They need to ensure that all activities are carried out by the laid down objectives and action plan on time.
5. **Controlling is a coordinating activity:** Controlling is a process in which numerous work-related activities are required to be integrated to verify and ensure whether everything occurs in accordance to the plan adopted. Under the control system, the managers observe subordinates for their performance and check records for their appropriateness. Coordination is essential to carry out such types of activities to achieve goals, and necessary measures can be taken to correct shortcomings if any.
6. **Control is related to planning:** Planning is the first step in management, as mentioned earlier, whereas controlling is the final step. The managers adopt all controlling measures/methods and incorporate them into the operational plan because of organizational objectives. Control is exercise by measuring the performance of individuals and the functioning of an organization. After implementing plan, they make efforts to see the completion of the objectives. Accordingly they plan corrective measures and take appropriate actions in case of any discrepancies. Hence planning provides a base for controlling for evaluating performances. Without planning, it is difficult to compare the actual performance with standard.
7. **Control is an essence for action:** In the control system, immediate steps are required to correct things if it goes wrong. The primary purpose of the controlling system is to detect the defaults in any operation, including performance of subordinates, and to take appropriate actions immediately to correct those errors. Thus the immediate response is the essence of control.
8. **Controlling is a preventive process:** Controlling is preventive, too, as immediate actions are taken to prevent and avoid future losses and shortcomings. It is an act of guiding and verifying, based on evidence and results.
9. **Controlling is concerning with individuals:** Controlling is concerning with performance of individuals who are involved in various activities of management. It includes the execution of plans, material management, financial management, and so on. The managers check shortcomings and financial lapses. Hence they also control individuals to measure their performance involving in these activities.
10. **Controlling is an end function:** Controlling judges the performance of all the operations carried out as well as compare the actual performance of the system with the standards/criteria laid down to find out any gap. It is also concerning correcting or fulfilling those gaps by taking immediate action. Hence controlling is also looking back (process or implementation plan) to devise appropriate measures to accomplish desired and predetermined objectives.

Importance of Controlling

Control is an integrated and coordinating function of management, which helps to achieve stated targets and ensure performance per plan. The importance of control in management is as follows:

- **Ensuring performance:** Controlling provides performance per predetermined standards and objectives. It devises, takes, and follow-up timely corrective measures if found any deviation from the plan.
- **Forward looking:** It draws lessons for taking proper measures for the present and the future and makes long-term planning possible through follow-up.
- **Maintains coordination:** All activities are regulated and coordinated by controlling. It keeps a continuous check on all events and guides them to achieve predetermined goals through coordinated guidelines.
- **Improves efficiency and effectiveness:** The main focus of the controlling system is to achieve the organizational objectives. It ensures that the actual

---

Box 49.1: Features of controlling.

- A continuous process
- Forward looking
- A dynamic process
- Exercised at all levels
- A coordinating activity
- Related to planning
- An essence for action
- A preventive process
- Concerning with individuals
- An end function

performance conforms per standards laid down. It necessarily improves organizational efficiency and effectiveness.
- **The basis for future action:** Control provides the base for the next operation. Based on actual performance analysis, if the performance is not by the plan, it helps in taking corrective actions in the future. It also helps management to avoid repetition of past mistakes in future.
- **Facilitate decision-making:** The controlling system facilitates decision-making. Whenever there is a shortcoming in actual performance, the control helps in deciding the follow-up and future course of action.
- **Maximizes contribution:** Performance evaluation is one of the tools of control. Everybody knows that they will be evaluated for their performance regularly. They try to put their best effort into being the best in their performance and try to improve upon previous work. In this way, control maximizes employees' contribution to achieving organizational goals.
- **Source of motivation:** Control also acts as a source of motivation. With the help of control, employees are evaluated as efficient or inefficient according to their performance through predetermined standards. They try their best to achieve the criteria laid down to them. They also keep in mind that their performance is under check. This pressure acts as motivation for them to compete with each other in delivering the best performance.

PRINCIPLES OF EFFECTIVE CONTROL

Effective control over the organization is vital to make sure that all the activities conform to plans. During planning, standards are laid down, and these standards form a key to control. It is the basis for evaluation and measured in quantitative form. To make control system practical, basic requirements or the principles need to follow. These basic principles traced out by Koontz O'Donnell are described in **Box 49.2**.

1. **Principle of appropriateness:** Principle of relevance states that restrictions should be appropriate and adequate and should reflect the nature and needs of activities. There are different departments in the organization, and each department has various actions to perform. Hence controls must be designed according to the type of services and needs of the department concerned to serve the interests of the organization effectively.

2. **Principle of readiness:** The principle of preparedness means that an active control system detects projected deviations before they occur. It prompts timely reporting to take corrective measures immediately. The time factor is significant in reporting as well as for deciding course of action. If controls are to remain valid, both reporting of deviations and follow-up course of action should be done immediately without any delay. The control must lead to corrective measures.

3. **Principle of forward looking:** Principle of prospective states that an active control system suggests corrective actions of future conform to the standards laid down. Control is to detect shortcomings from standards and to prescribe practical corrective actions.

4. **Principle of exceptions:** Principle of limitations or exception means that focusing priority on deviations that have more considerable significance in achieving laid down objectives than to that deviations/defective, which have importance. Adequate controls must reveal exceptions at strategic points of relevance.

5. **Principle of clarity:** Effective control system must have clear, specific control measures. The employees must be clear about the standards of performance. The controls must be well defined and should not leave any room for arguments for employees.

6. **Principle of flexibility:** The principle of flexibility in the control system means that the control plan must be so flexible that it can work during unforeseen circumstances and quickly adjust in any change in the environment.

7. **Principle of profitability:** The principle of profitability states that designing control techniques and methods in such a way that should maximize output with minimum use of workforce, money, and material and time.

8. **Principle of recognition:** According to the principle of gratitude, the employees must accept control standards. They should be aware of the criteria of evaluating performance; otherwise it will be difficult at the time of implementation.

9. **Principle of motivation:** Principle of motivation states that controls should motivate both employees and managers. It should be a motivating act rather than a hindering factor in achieving organizational goals. It should be used in a positive sense to improve performance rather than giving punishment. Employees must be clear about the standards of performance and method of evaluation.

10. **Principle of understandability:** Principle of understandability applies to both managers and employees. The managers must understand various techniques of controlling and control tools. They should know how to operate and analyze the information gathered. Explain the control tools adequately to everyone in the organization. They should understand the importance of performance evaluation and devising and implementation of

> **Box 49.2: Principles of effective control.**
> - Appropriateness
> - Readiness
> - Forward looking
> - Exceptions
> - Clarity
> - Flexibility
> - Cost effectiveness
> - Recognition
> - Motivation
> - Understandability
> - Objectivity
> - Communication

various control measures. It will help in the application of control techniques.

11. **Principle of objectivity:** An active control system must have operationally defined standards. Control tools should be valid and consistent, reliable, and easy to operate. There should be objectivity in assessing and analyzing the performance of managers.
12. **Principle of communication:** The controlling system must have proper and prompt flow of information. The seniors must communicate standards to the subordinates; they should be aware of performance criteria. There should be appropriate feedback. The performance must reach the managers at the earliest and take prompt action. The level of performance and steps suggested for improvement should be communicated to subordinates so that they can start working per suggestions. Effective control is possible if the flow of information takes place in both upward and downward directions.

STEPS IN THE CONTROLLING PROCESS

Controlling is the process of assessing current performance against predetermined standards as per plan to ensure adequate progress and satisfactory performance to achieve organizational goals within a given period. There are following steps in the controlling process **(Fig. 49.1):**

1. **Setting control criteria/standards:** The setting up criteria or standards is the first step in control, which serves as a benchmark against the performance measurement. Standards are the established criteria that are used to measure the results. Develop a list of key result areas for control. Define each key area as possible in quantitative terms. It includes in terms of services provided, working hours, physical quantity, or in monetary terms such as costs, revenues, and other criteria of performance.

   The standards should be flexible, transparent, easily understandable, and measurable terms. After setting the standard, decide the level of performance, as satisfactory, average, unsatisfactory, and the degrees of individual contribution to the achievement of organizational goals and objectives. Thus standards are the criteria to measure against actual results.
2. **Communicate standards:** Communicate criteria for control to measure performance to everyone in the organization. The subordinates must be involved to set the goals and targets and standards. Give a clear explanation about rules before implementing them.
3. **Measure actual performance:** The next step in the controlling process is the measurement of actual performance. Various controlling methods are employed to measure actual performance against set criteria/standards. It will help management to find out either the work is being done according to plans or not. It is the most critical and challenging task in the control

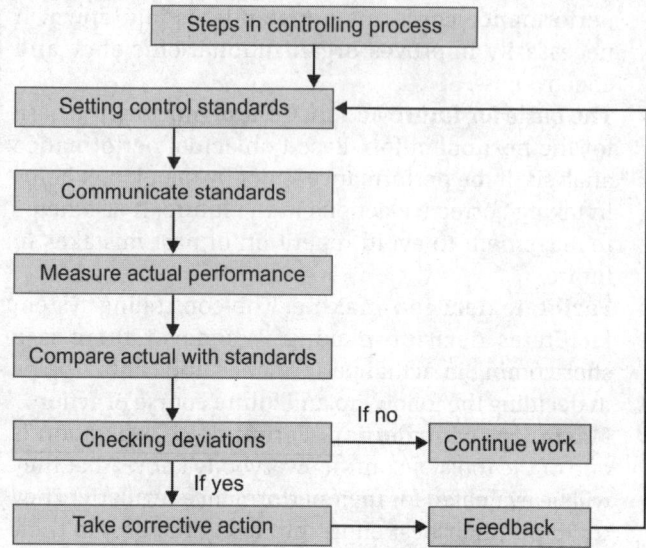

Fig. 49.1: Steps in the controlling process.

process. Project in time the action to correct for the deficiencies, if detected.
4. **Compare actual with standards:** After measuring actual performance, the next step in the controlling process is to compare actual performance with the standards set. The primary purpose of comparing actual with criteria is to find out whether things are going per plan or not.
5. **Checking deviations:** After comparing actual with standards, the next step that should be taken by the management is to find out (1) deviations, if any, (2) the level of variation, and (3) the cause of change. Decide some permissible limits at the time of setting standards to take action. Monitor for any deficiencies to take corrective actions immediately per plan. Communicate and discuss the findings with the concerned employees.
6. **Taking corrective action:** After finding out shortcomings, take appropriate corrective action immediately. Immediate steps are to set the things right back on track. Corrective measures may include revision of the plan, reframing goals and objectives, or modifying plan of action through reassigning duties, or appointing additional staffing or even through better directing.
7. **Feedback:** Taking feedback is essential after each step to know the impact of each action. After receiving corrective measures, make sure that whether things are going now per plans, whether the action taken has brought the desired results, or not.

LIMITATION OF CONTROL

The limitations of the controlling system are as enumerated below.
1. **The controlling system is expensive and time consuming:** Controlling system involves many persons

in assessing performance, finding out deviations, and taking corrective actions. All these activities require a lot of time and money to execute controls.

2. **Difficulty in setting the standard:** Criteria must be in measuring terms to assess the performance. There is specific qualitative attribute such as motivation and coordination that may not be possible to express in quantitative words, are difficult to control.

3. **Uncontrollable external factors:** There are certain external factors such as government health-care policies; changes in technology may affect the functioning of the organization. These factors are difficult to control and can make internal control ineffective.

4. **Noncooperation from subordinates:** Communicate goals, objectives, standards, and action plans to everyone in the organization. Since the effectiveness of the control process depends upon its acceptability by the subordinates. If they are not involved and not aware of action plans, they may oppose and show noncooperation toward work. It may increase pressure among them being regularly monitored and evaluated for their performance.

CHAPTER HIGHLIGHTS

- Controlling is a continuous, integrated and coordinating, forward looking, and dynamic process. It is exercised at all levels to improve organizational efficiency.
- Control is a process that enables managers to get their plans and policies implemented and take appropriate actions to achieve the objectives of the organization.
- Controlling is concerned with examining, observing, reviewing, measuring, and evaluating the performance of the people according to the operational plan for the achievement of their predetermined goals.

REVIEW QUESTIONS

I. Essay Type Questions
1. What do you mean by control? Describe its characteristics.
2. Describe various steps required in controlling process.

II. Short Notes
1. Importance of controlling
2. Principles of effective control

III. Multiple Choice Questions
1. Controlling is closely related to:
   a. Fixing of authority
   b. Setting objectives
   c. Fixing of responsibility
   d. Assigning tasks
2. The reason to exercise control is:
   a. Whenever something is wrong
   b. When efficiency is to be improved
   c. When errors are to be rectified
   d. Regularly, at all the times
3. Controls are:
   a. Static   b. Forward looking
   c. Rigid   d. Fixed
4. Which principle of control explains that priority must be focused deviation that has greater significance in achieving laid down objectives than just have importance?
   a. Principle of exception
   b. Principle of promptness
   c. Principle of flexibility
   d. Principle of appropriateness

Answer Keys

1. b   2. d   3. b   4. a

SUGGESTED READING

1. Bobbins SP. Organisational Behaviour. New Delhi: Prentice Hall; 1997.
2. Cunningham JB, Eberle T. A Guide to Job Enrichment and Redesign. Personnel. 1990; 67(2): 56-7.
3. Davis K. Evolving Models of Organizational Behavior. Acad Manag J. 1968;11(1):27-38.
4. Davis K. Human Behaviour at Work. New York: McGraw Hill Book Co.; 1991.
5. Dimock ME. Administrative Vitality. New York: Harper Brothers; 1975.
6. Hackman JR, Oldham GR. Development of the Diagnostic Job Survey. J Appl Psychol. 1975;60:159-70.
7. Luthans F. Organisational Behaviour. New York: McGraw Hill Book Co.; 1995.
8. Newstrom J, Davis K. Organization Behavior: Human Behavior at Work. New York: McGraw-Hill; 1993.
9. Newman WH, Warren EK. The Process of Management. New Delhi: Prentice-Hall; 1985.
10. Terry GR, Franklin SG. Principles of Management. Delhi: ABS; 2000.

CHAPTER 50

Quality Assurance and Quality Management

CHAPTER OUTLINE

- Historical Perspectives of Quality Assurance
- Quality Assurance and Quality Management
  - Concept of Quality
  - Approach to Quality
  - Purposes of Quality
  - Quality Assurance to Quality Management
- Total Quality Management
- Quality Circle
- Models of Quality Assurance and Quality Management
- Quality Evaluation Systems in Healthcare
- Six Sigma in Healthcare

LEARNING OUTCOMES

After completion of this chapter, the learner will be able to:
- Familiarize with historical perspectives of quality assurance
- Understand the concept of quality and related terms
- Enlist the purposes of quality
- Explain total quality management (TQM)
- Describe various models of quality assurance and quality management
- Discuss quality circle, its principles, importance, and elements
- Explain quality evaluation systems in healthcare
- Describe Six Sigma and its models

KEY TERMS

Quality, quality assurance, quality improvement, quality circle, continuous quality management, total quality management, quality evaluation system, Six Sigma

INTRODUCTION

Nurses are accountable to society for the quality of nursing care. Moreover, ensuring quality has become necessary in the healthcare system due to modern healthcare technology, increased competition, privatization, and awareness among the clients. Nurses have accountability toward patient care, keeping in mind the patient's rights; the cost of health services demands quality assurance in nursing.

As a result of advancement in healthcare technology, increased competition, privatization, and awareness among the clients, the healthcare system has become well aware of the need to ensure quality. The evolution of nursing as a scientific discipline has accountability toward patient care, keeping in mind the patient's rights; the cost of health services demands quality assurance in nursing. Quality is a multifaceted and an all-encompassing word and needs to be perceived in totality to avoid misinterpretations.

HISTORICAL PERSPECTIVES OF QUALITY ASSURANCE

- The quality notion in healthcare dates back to the mid-nineteenth century in England. In 1842, Dr Edwin Chadwick, a public health activist and a pioneer from Britain, recommended sanitary police to monitor the hygienic condition.
- In 1854, Florence nightingale, a leading nurse during the European Crimean War, written several quality criteria in nursing care considered to be the first nursing care standards in history.
- In 1918, the American College of Surgeon provided the criteria and standards for accreditation for Hospital Standardization Programme, adopted by the Joint Commission on Accreditation of Hospitals (JCAHO) in 1952.
- In 1966, Dr Avedes Donabedian first introduced three measures of quality: Structure, process, and outcome for monitoring and assessing the quality of care. "Structure" includes as the input both human

and physical resources for delivery of healthcare to the patients; "processes" included all procedures and activities required to deliver care by providers and support system; and "outcomes" included results and outputs of the care process, e.g., morbidity and mortality rate and patient satisfaction.
- In India, a Consumers Protection Act enforced for quality care implemented in 1986. The quality Assurance Project in the United States in 1990 and the World Health Organization is also working on this issue.

QUALITY ASSURANCE AND QUALITY MANAGEMENT

Concept of Quality

Quality is not something that happens by chance. It is the result of grit and determination to change the mindset and overcome the odds.

The ideas of quality in healthcare grounded in the works of industrial experts. In industries, the importance of quality first appreciated in the 1940s and 1950s and defined in various ways:

John D McClellan defines quality as the degree to which a product conforms to specification and quality standards. According to the National Association of Quality Assurance Professionals, it is a degree of excellence, being provided and documented, based on the best knowledge available and achievable at a particular facility.

The quality is a level to which the patient care improves the probability of desired results and reduces the chance of undesired effects. Donabedian proposes three definitions of quality:
1. **The absolutist description:** The possibility of benefit and harm to health valued as quality, with no attention to cost.
2. **The individualized definition:** Quality focuses on the patient's expectations of benefit and harm and other undesired consequences.
3. **The universal definition** includes the cost of care, the benefit/harm continuum, and the distribution of healthcare.

American Medical Association, 1991, defines quality as the degree to which care services influence the probability of optimal patient outcomes. Quality of nursing practice is possible to achieve when the organization's processes and activities are designed and implemented to meet the needs and expectations of the receiver on a competent, consistent, and continuous basis (INC, 2006).

Approach to Quality

Juran developed a trilogy approach to quality, i.e., quality planning, quality control, and quality improvement **(Fig. 50.1)**. *Quality planning* determines the customers and their needs to develop products and design processes to produce those products; *quality control* is the evaluation

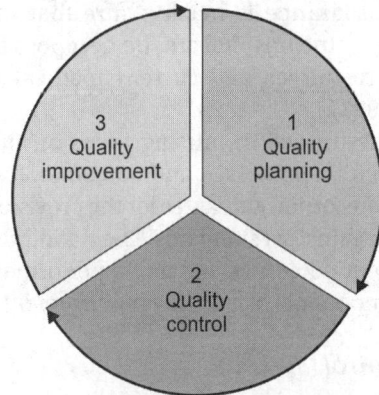

Fig. 50.1: Juran's concepts of quality.

of performance to identify discrepancies between actual performance and goals, and *quality improvement* establishes an infrastructure and the project teams to carry out process improvement.

Purposes of Quality

Following are the purposes of quality:
1. To meet the external and internal needs and expectation of the customers
2. To meet the demand of the population for the care
3. To establish standards and variance control
4. To reduce the deficiencies and negligence
5. To achieve excellence of care
6. To bring improvement in care and services
7. To utilize healthcare resources efficiently
8. To deliver quality care and services
9. To fulfill the desire for recognition and strive for excellence
10. To set a benchmark.

Quality Assurance to Quality Management

Quality Assurance

Different scholars defined the term "quality assurance" differently. Significant definitions are as follows:

Donabedian, 1982, defines quality assurance as a degree of judging care that contributes to valued outcomes. Marker 1998 considered quality assurance of nursing practice is the nursing standards used in evaluating the improvement of client care.

QA is the process for objectively and systematically monitoring and evaluating the quality and appropriateness of patient care and for resolving identified problems. "Appropriateness" referred to the extent to which a particular procedure or treatment is efficient is neither excessive nor deficient and provided in a setting best suited to the patient's needs (Joint Commission).
1. QA is designing a product or service and controlling its production, so well that quality is inevitable." "In healthcare, the activities and programs intended to guarantee or ensure the quality of patient care" (The Joint Commission).

2. Quality assurance is making sure that the services provided by the hospital are the best possible in given existing resources and current medical knowledge (WHO, 1992).

Quality assurance in nursing focus on nursing care delivery structure, processes, and outcomes. It viewed as a program for the formal guarantee for the provision of quality nursing care against set standards. The standards of nursing care for patient outcomes and nurse performance are the essential components of a quality management approach.

Quality Control

Quality control is the process of measuring actual performance and comparing it with goals to act upon accordingly. There are various methods to measure quality control. According to Shubin, quality control means the recognition and removal of identifiable causes of defects and variation from the set standard. Henry Fayol considered it as a control consists of verifying whether everything occurs in conformity with the plan adopted, the instruction issued, and principles established. Its object is to point out weaknesses or errors to rectify and prevent occurrence. It operates in everything—things, people, and actions.

Quality Improvement

The quality improvement is the process or processes of reducing variance. It is a process to achieve a new level of performance or quality that is superior to the previous one. According to JCAHO, there are the following characteristics/tenets of quality improvement:
- The commitment of the organization to set quality priorities reorient the organization to a customer focus and function as a role model
- Defining quality and incorporating into mission and planning documents
- Exploring the needs and expectations of customers, both internal and external and make changes to meet those needs
- Involving employees with quality improvement and focusing on quality-driven daily activities
- Targeting improved quality toward work processes instead of individuals
- Emphasizing quality improvement by design rather than quality by inspection
- Using formal problem-solving methods and statistical tools to make decisions.

According to the USAID QA project, the following steps must be in place before the intervention processes for improvement can begin:
1. Plan for quality, setting, and communicating a standard
2. Identify, prioritize, and define key improvement opportunities (IOs)
3. Organize a quality team
4. Analyze and study the IOs for root causes
5. Develop alternative solutions and actions for improvement
6. Implement, monitor (against thresholds), and evaluate efforts and restart the cycle.

Tools of quality improvement
The important tools of quality improvement are as follows:
- **Flowcharts:** A flowchart is a pictorial representation of the steps or tasks in a process depicted by using standard and special symbols **(Fig. 50.2)**. It clarifies the process and identifies inefficiencies.
- **Fishbone diagram:** Fishbone is a cause-and-effect diagram. It identifies factors or causes contributing to a specific problem. Diagonal lines drawn off the mainline depict major associated categories of causes **(Fig. 50.3)**. Generally, these categories are people, policies, equipment, and procedures in the organization and identified through brainstorming.
- **Histogram:** A histogram is a frequency distribution data graph. It is useful in data analyzing quality improvement. It provided a visual summary of the data and constructed by graphing frequency values on the vertical axis and categories evenly spaced on the horizontal axis in a logical order.
- **Pareto chart:** The Pareto chart is a histogram displaying the most significant factors contributing to a problem. It is similar to a histogram with frequency values on the vertical axis and categories on the horizontal axis. With the Pareto, however, the most frequent causes of the problem plotted on the graph in the descending order. Therefore, it separates the significant reasons for the insignificant ones.

Continuous Quality Improvement

In the 1980s, QA is replaced by constant quality improvement. It is a coordinated and integrated approach to improve processes that affect the outcome. Later on, performance management replaced continuous quality improvement (CQI). There are three critical programs

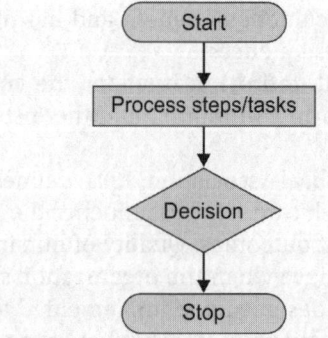

Fig. 50.2: Steps delineating the flowchart process.

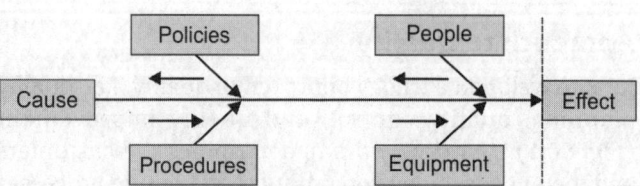

Fig. 50.3: Components of a fishbone diagram.

Chapter 50: Quality Assurance and Quality Management

TABLE 50.1: Quality assurance to quality improvement.

Quality assurance	Value added	Quality improvement
Externally required QA coordinator-driven parallel management	Commitment, leadership, and strategic quality planning	Internally motivated management driven is the function of management
Delegated to a few organization-oriented problem/people focused	Involvement/education customer-driven and product/service design improvement	Involved all customer oriented and process focused
Follows organizational structure	Systems orientation to delivery of care	Monitors the flow of care
Pretends to assure (quality endpoints) 10-step process exclusively	Continuous improvement Planned, systematic approach to development	Pushes to improve Routine improvement processes

under CQI, namely awareness, measurement, and improvement. JCAHO added the CQI philosophy in the accreditation policy and focused on the quality paradigm shift from quality assurance to quality improvement **(Table 50.1)**.

Quality Management

Quality management encompasses various activities, such as program design, involving personnel from different disciplines, goal setting, and administrative support. Education of staff, recruitment, and retention of qualified staff and similar issues become defined targets in control of quality. In quality management, changes in any aspect of service design must consider from the whole.

International Organization for Standardization (ISO) developed coordination and unification of industrial standards. ISO 9000 family of standards deals with quality management. Standard ISO 9001:2000 applies to hospitals. Many organizations already implemented and certified quality management.

Definitions

- Quality management is a process by which people are mobilized to achieve quality goals. It becomes the umbrella under which all operations and activities related to quality fall.
- Quality management is a three-part (trilogy) approach, i.e., quality planning, quality control, and quality improvement. *Quality planning* involves determining who the customers are and what their needs are, then developing products based on those needs and designing processes to produce those products, *quality control* is the evaluation of performance to identify discrepancies between actual performance and goals, and *quality improvement* establishes an infrastructure and the project teams to carry out process improvement.
    —*Dr Joseph M Juran*
- Quality management in healthcare is a continuous process and not a result. It is an ongoing pursuit of excellence through constant process control at every step, with the total commitment of the top management, involvement of all staff and is aimed at providing to the consumers, services at acceptable quality.
    —*Joshi SK (2009)*
- Total quality management is an approach that seeks to integrate all resources and functions with the aim of a unified thrust focused on meeting the customers' needs and the organization's objectives.

Purposes of quality management
Quality requires at all levels of healthcare services to:
- Meet the needs and expectation of the customers
- Standardize services and control variance
- Minimize errors and thus attain excellence in care
- Bring effectiveness in delivering services
- Bring improvement in care and services
- Meet increased demand for quality care
- Bring efficiency in resources utilization and thus reduces costs
- Fit into the pressure of competition and to enhance marketing
- Fulfill the desire for recognition and certification and to strive for excellence
- Fulfill ethical code to provide the best and most appropriate care accessible to the patient
- Attract attention in the field and will encourage other individual, organizations, or systems to emulate and follow (benchmarking).

Objectives of quality management
The primary aim of quality management is to improve quality and to reduce waste by focusing on the needs of employees and patients (McLanghlin and Kaluzncy, 1994). Specific objectives highlighted by Slee and Slee (1991) and Gillem (1988) are as follows:
- To establish particular quality goals
- To have a shared responsibility in improving quality
- To educate and train the employees
- To formally recognize efforts to improve quality
- To identify specific projects/areas that promise to improve quality
- To provide necessary resources, both real and financial
- To regard employees as not only a provider but also a user of the services
- To focus continually on methods of improving the quality of care.

Characteristics of quality management
The principal features of quality management are as follows:
- The quality management system must give equal emphasis on three aspects, i.e., structure, process, and outcome. It should be output oriented and process driven.

- It should be patient focused with essential criteria, such as availability, accessibility, appropriateness, effectiveness, efficiency, affordability, and timeliness and must be need based.
- There should be a system of continuous monitoring/checking of various processes of healthcare delivery at every step to find out any deviation and to rectify immediately.
- Staff must be trained and should be aware of protocols and must have the highest level of motivation and commitment to defect prevention.

Principles of quality management

The principles of quality management are as follows:
1. Quality is as conformance to requirement.
2. The system of quality is prevention.
3. The performance standards are zero defect.
4. The measurement of quality is the price of non-conformance.
5. Quality management is management accountability.
6. Quality management should be teamwork.
7. It should focus on continuous improvements in services.

Process (steps) of quality management

Phillip B Crosby views quality management as for quality improvement and emphasizes 14 steps to undertake for quality management. These steps can be applied to implement quality management programs in healthcare organizations **(Fig. 50.4)**:

1. **Management commitment:** This is one of the essential steps in the implementation of quality management in the organization. Management defines boundaries, creates and exhibits full understanding, and supports for quality improvement. Management plays a vital role as a leader.
2. **Formation of quality management team:** The next step in quality management is to form a quality management team. It should comprise a team leader who should be a senior person with leadership qualities and should be authoritative and knowledgeable as well.
3. **Training of management and staff:** Under the quality management program, educate and train all staff including management, about the quality management. Teach the scope of work, resources required, time frame, and impact of the program. Impart training in a group of different levels, such as senior management staff, and lower-level staff separately.
4. **Development of quality culture:** In quality management, it is crucial to create a quality culture. It includes the creation of a new system of values, beliefs, and behaviors of all staff where everybody must think and talk about quality and participate in a quality program. Create quality awareness among everyone in the organization.
5. **Development of quality policy and procedures manual:** Quality policy and Quality procedure manual are the apex documents in the organization. It should provide detailed information about the quality system, its scope, various processes, operations, and methods of implementing quality management system (QMS).
6. **Defining key areas and objectives for improvement:** It is essential to identify a critical area that requires improvement as well the purposes of those vital areas. Define critical areas, such as improvement in patient safety, patient care, medication, documentation, etc. and development objectives of each key area. These objectives should be in measurable terms, time bound, and specific, e.g. reduction of medication error to 1%.
7. **Mapping of processes of organization**: Process mapping means identification of all practices being carried out in the organization and details of each process to find out the best evidence-based practices for developing the working protocols or standardized operative procedures.
8. **Development of hospital information system:** Develop a hospital information system to gather and process-related information and further to generate the data required for feedback on the quality of care.
9. **Formulation of standards and measurement criteria:** Standards serve as a benchmark against to measure the quality. Criteria are attributes, such as Health care-associated infection (HCAI), neonatal mortality, staffing in the medical ward, and standards are quantitative values against each set criteria for measurement or comparison. For example, the nurse–patient ratio in medical ward 1:3 round the clock or HCAI not >5%, etc.
10. **Implementation of the quality management system:** Per the plan, after carrying out above-mentioned steps, implement quality management system.
11. **Management review of the quality management system:** After the implementation of QMS to improve

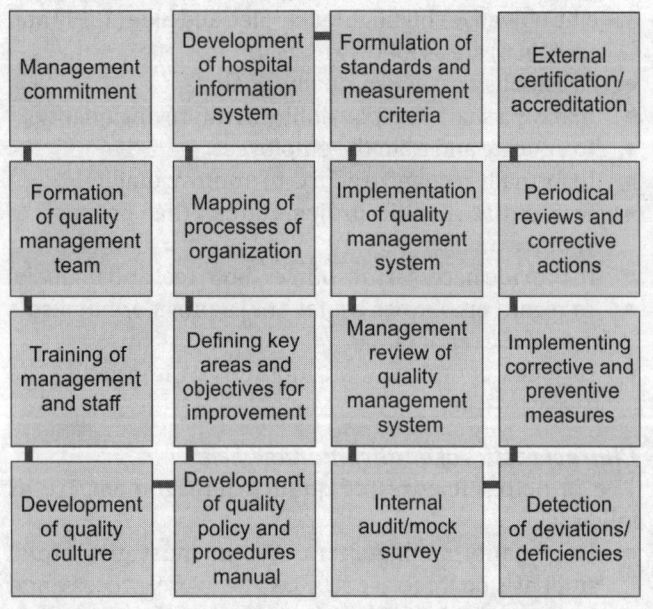

Fig. 50.4: Quality management process.

the quality, its effectiveness in terms of its suitability to the organization and any change is required. If QMS docs show the expected results, management review may lead to change the policies/procedures, allocation of resources, and even change in quality system. During management review, it must ensure whether QMS implemented is going in the right direction or not and whether it requires any significant change.

12. **Internal audit:** Internal audit for quality management is also known as a mock survey. It is carried out after 3 months of implementation of the QMS program. It should be done by trained internal auditors to assess whether the organization is ready for external audits by certified accreditation body—National Accreditation Board for Hospitals and Health Care Providers (NABH) in Indian setting.
13. **Detection of deviations/deficiencies:** During an internal audit or mock survey, if there is any defect or deviation further analyzed to assess causes to take appropriate remedial measures on time.
14. **Implementing corrective and preventive measures:** In case deficiencies are detected, communicate and discuss with staff about the error and its causes and the obstacles they are facing in attaining goals. Recognize the team who participated and take corrective measures.
15. **Periodical reviews and corrective actions:** Monitor performance continuously. Conduct periodic management reviews until the results are found satisfactory. The quality team must communicate with employees regularly. Do it all over again to emphasize that quality improvement never ends.
16. **External certification/accreditation:** As mentioned above, that internal audit or mock survey is aimed to assess the readiness of the organization for the final accreditation audit. If any deficiency found during the interior inspection, take corrective measures to ready for the last accreditation by the accrediting agency.

TOTAL QUALITY MANAGEMENT

Quality management is considered an organized, coordinated, and integrated approach to manage/improve processes that affect patient outcomes. It is an integrated system of CQI aimed at meeting customers' expectations. *Quality management* is the process by which people are mobilized to achieve quality goals. Quality management becomes the umbrella under which all operations and activities related to quality fall.

Contributors to TQM

Total quality management was the work of Deming, Juran, and Crosby. Their contributions to TQM has three paths and one journey **(Table 50.2)**. Hospitals in developing countries had integrated the TQM philosophy and dramatically changed their management approach.

Objectives of TQM

The objectives of TQM are as follows:
1. To establish specific quality goals
2. To improve quality as a responsibility shared by all employees
3. To educate and train the employees
4. To formally recognize efforts to improve quality
5. To identify particular projects that promise to improve quality
6. To provide necessary resources, both real and financial

TABLE 50.2: Contributors to "total quality management" and their contributions.		
W Edward Deming	*Joseph M Juran*	*Phillip B Crosby*
Quality is continuous improvement through reduced variation	Quality is fitness for use.	Quality is conformance to requirements
The 14 points	**The quality trilogy**	**The four absolutes of quality management**
➤ Create consistency of purpose toward improvement of product and service	Quality planning	➤ The definition of quality is conformance to specification
➤ Adopt the new philosophy	Quality improvement	➤ The system of quality is prevention
➤ Cease dependence on mass inspection	Quality control	➤ The performance standards are zero defect
➤ End awarding business on price tag alone	**The 10 steps of the quality improvement process**	➤ It is the price of nonconformance
➤ Improve consistently and forever the system of production and service	➤ Build awareness of the need and opportunity for improvement	**The 14 steps of quality improvement**
➤ Institute training on the job	➤ Set goals for improvements	➤ Define, create, and exhibit management commitment
➤ Institute leadership	➤ Organize to reach the goals	➤ Form quality improvement team
➤ Drive out fear	➤ Provide training throughout the organization	➤ Measurement to determine areas for improvement
➤ Breakdown barrier between staff areas	➤ Carry out projects to solve the problems	➤ Develop cost of quality measures
➤ Remove slogans, exhortations, and targets for the workforce	➤ Report progress	➤ Create quality awareness in everyone
➤ Eliminate numerical quotas for the workforce and also for people in the management	➤ Give recognition	➤ Take corrective action on problems previously identified
➤ Remove barriers to pride of the quality	➤ Communicate results	➤ Zero-defect planning
➤ Encourage education and self-improvement for everyone	➤ Keep score	➤ Employee education of all employees in the company
➤ Take action to accomplish the transformation	➤ Maintain annual improvement part of the conventional systems and processes of the company	➤ Zero-defect day is held to let all employees know there has been a change
		➤ Goal setting for individual and groups
		➤ Error causes removal by employees sharing with management the obstacles they face in attaining goals
		➤ Recognition for those who participate
		➤ Quality councils to communicate regularly
		➤ Do again and again to emphasize that quality improvement never ends

7. To regard employees as not only a provider but also a user of the services or results produced by antecedent events in the process of rendering on episode or regimen of care
8. To focus continually on methods of improving the quality of care.

Principles of TQM

The principles of TQM are as follows:
1. It is a multidisciplinary and interdisciplinary approach to examine organizational processes.
2. It is an overall approach to management to identify problems and follow a process similar to that used in the nursing process: Fixing an existing problem, preventing problems, changing systems to address the root causes of issues, and managing innovation.
3. It focuses on work processes, customer orientation, and statistical data analysis.
4. The emphasis is on management accountability, teamwork, and continuous improvements.
5. It needs systems, tools, and techniques that can convert this approach into realities.
6. It creates client focus, long-range plan, continuous improvement, daily process management, and employees' involvement.

QUALITY CIRCLE

Quality circle is a system to identify and recognize employees and allow them to participate and integrate with a system. It will help to satisfy their "ego" needs and to motivate them to work efficiently. The concepts of Maslow's theory are the base of the philosophy of quality circle. It has its origin in Japan in 1962 by Dr Deming, and Dr Juran created an International Association of Quality Circles in the United States in 1977. It focuses on the participative management style by using evidence, basic statistics, group dynamics, and job satisfaction.

Principles of Quality Circle

The principles of quality circle are as follows:
- To understand employees to improve work life
- To develop active cooperation and mutual trust among employees
- To involve all including lower-level employees
- Human development

Elements of Quality Circle Program

Ricker described the following features:
a. **People building philosophy:** Quality circle program will work if there is a sincere desire on the part of management to help their employees to grow and develop through the quality circle.
b. **It is voluntary:** It is visible proof to all the employees that it is for their benefit. They are entirely free to take or not take advantage of it.
c. **Employees help others to develop:** Since all the employees will not understand and use the techniques very quickly, so they must help each other. It is the way to grow and develop their capabilities.
d. **Everyone's participation:** Quality circles are participative; therefore, the manager must see that each employee will contribute to solving the problem.
e. **The emphasis for training:** In-service education programs initiated to make the employee more and more productive and to make them aware of the latest technology. Management must also receive management skills by undergoing various management-training programs.
f. **Encouragement for creativity:** There is a non-threatening environment for ideas. The organization gets suggestions from employees seriously and gives a chance to experiment with them.
g. **Supportive management:** The management must give emphasis on quality circles, devote some time with the employees, and give some advice and some commitment in the beginning.

MODELS OF QUALITY ASSURANCE AND QUALITY MANAGEMENT

American Nurses' Association Model

American nurses' association (ANA) model developed by Long and Black in 1975, is the first proposed and accepted model of quality assurance. It is a cyclic model. It helps in the self-determination of the patient and family, nursing health orientation, patients' rights to quality care, and nursing contributions. **Figure 50.5** depicts the essential components of the ANA model:
1. **Identify value:** These are rights and benefits patient/client from economic, social, psychological, and spiritual perspectives, organization philosophy, and the providers of nursing services.

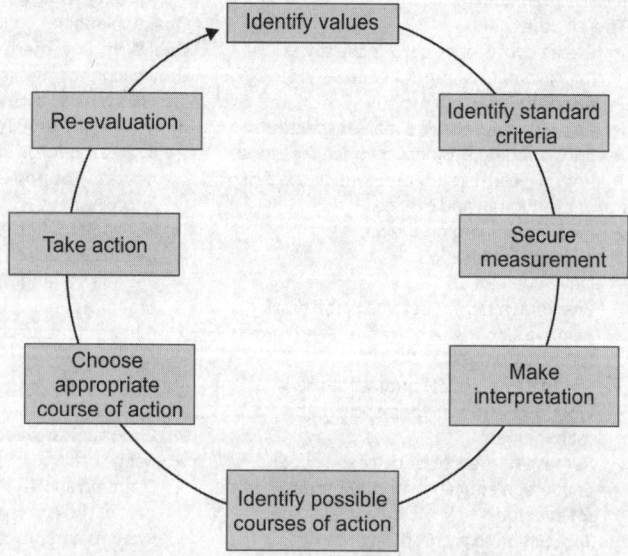

Fig. 50.5: ANA model of quality assurance.

2. **Identify standards and criteria:** Identify standards and criteria for quality assurance. These can be derived from the philosophy and objectives of the organization. These are of three types:
   a. *Structure standards:* Standards of the structure are defined by licensing or accrediting agencies. Another standard of structure includes an organizational chart which shows supervisory methods, communication patterns, staff patterns, and sometimes staff assignments.
   b. *Process standards:* These are the standards related to the quality of patient care. An agency can choose to use standards of care set forth by professional organizations.
   c. *Outcome standards:* Outcome standards reveal the results of nursing care.
3. **Secure measurement:** Measurements needed to determine degree of attainment of criteria and standards are as follows: Nursing audit, utilization's reviews, and review of agency documents, self-studies, and evaluation of physicals facilities are used to measure structural standards; peer review, client satisfaction surveys, direct observations, questionnaires, interviews, audits, and videotapes are used to measure process standards; and research studies, client satisfaction surveys, client classification, admission, readmission, discharge data, and morbidity data are used to measure outcome standards.
4. **Make interpretations:** The base for interpolation is to meet the degree of predetermined criteria about the strengths and weaknesses of the program. The rate of compliance compared with the expected level of criteria accomplishment.
5. **Identify a course of action:** Identify the course of action according to the compliance level. Convey positive feedback and reinforce the team if the compliance is above the normal or the expected standard. Improve conditions if the efforts are below the expected level. Try to find out the cause of the problem and the possible solution to solve the issues.
6. **Choose an action:** Select the best alternative from various alternative courses of action. It is essential to analyze the pros and cons of each choice in terms of environmental conditions and the availability of resources.
7. **Take action:** It is essential to establish each one's accountability to take appropriate action. Assign each one's responsibility and prepare a time frame to implement the proposed courses of action.
8. **Re-evaluation:** It is the last step in quality assurance. Reevaluate the process according to preset criteria to interpret whether the course of action has improved the deficiency or remedied. If there is an improvement, offer positive reinforcement. In case of the defect, if any, repeat the problem-solving process.

Thus according to this model, all the quality assurance systems involve appraisal of quality standards followed by an action for quality improvement at each stage of the cycle. The cycle is an open system as it allows ideas of continued quality improvements.

Donabedian Model

Donabedian quality framework is a method of measuring quality as structure, process, and outcome in the mid of the 1960s. A structure may directly influence the outcome (**Fig. 50.6**).

According to the model, "structures" include the adequacy of healthcare facilities, the qualifications of practitioners, and the financial aspects of care. The "processes" were the aspects of care. And "outcomes" are the precise and concrete measurements of the effectiveness of care.

FOCUS–PDCA Model: Quality Management Model

FOCUS-PDCA is an acronym used for an approach to problem-solving, and it stands for find, organize, clarify, understand, select (FOCUS)-plan, do, check, act (PDCA). This model is an improvement methodology, devised in 1930, to create a culture of continuous improvement resulting in a higher level of excellence.

The main concepts of FOCUS are to (1) find a process to improve, (2) organize a team that knows the process, (3) clarify current knowledge of the process, and (4) understand causes of variation. After understanding the problem and selecting solutions, use PDCA model, plan the improvement effort; do they plan, follow all steps of an action plan, check the difference in results, act on these results, i.e., write policy, train the staff, and continue to monitor (**Fig. 50.7**).

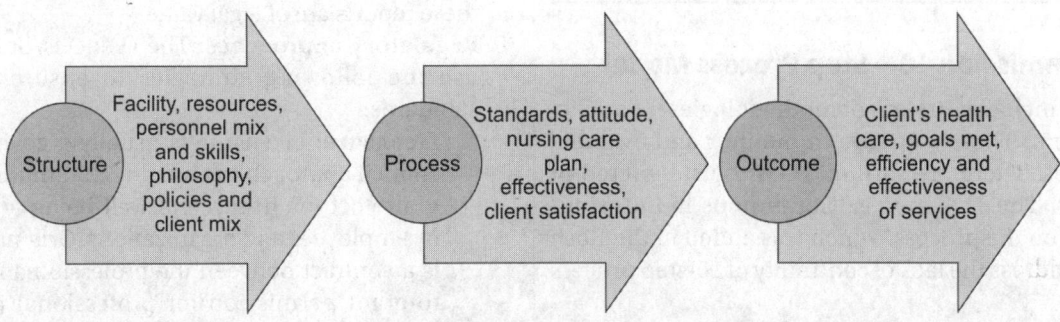

Fig. 50.6: Donabedian model of quality assurance.

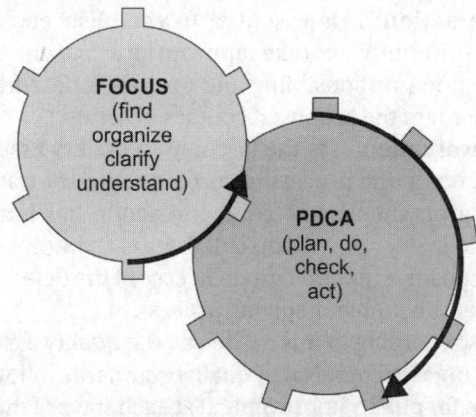

Fig. 50.7: FOCUS–PDCA model.

QUALITY EVALUATION SYSTEMS IN HEALTH CARE

1. **Audit systems:** There should be a proper audit system in the organization. Audits are a retrospective review of documentation and records against a set of predetermined criteria.
2. **Quality awards:** The organization receives various awards to maintain quality in many countries, such as the European Foundation for Quality Management (EFQM) and the Baldrige Award in the United States.
3. **Peer assessment:** It is a process whereby one healthcare practitioner usually a physician will evaluate the care of a peer and assist change toward a better outcome. These are designed to monitor client-specific aspects of care appropriate for certain levels of care. The audit has been the primary tool used by the peer review committee to ascertain quality of care.
4. **Utilization review:** The utilization review activities are to assure the care needed and the cost appropriate for the level of care. There is a prospective assessment of the necessity of care before implementation, concurrent, a review of the necessity of implementing nursing care, and retrospective analysis of the need for services received by the client after implementing care.
5. **Evaluation studies:** Evaluation studies can be conducted using various quality assurance models. The main models are Donabedian, structure-process-outcome model, the tracer model, and the sentinel model. The tracer model is a measure of both the process and outcome of care. It revealed differences in the outcome as a result of nursing care standards. The sentinel method is an outcome measure for examining specific instances of client care.
6. **Clients' satisfaction:** There are various ways to evaluate the satisfaction of customers; it can be done by using telephone interviews and mailed questionnaires to measure structure, process, and outcome.
7. **Incident reviewing:** It is a process of reviewing incidents that occurred in the hospital during the stay of patients. The critical incidents by a physician/nurse wrong administration medication and negligence in carrying out procedures. The report must specify the name, age, exact time and place, description of the occurrence, precautionary measures, and conditions of the patient before and after the incident, etc. since these reports are of legal value.
8. **Regulatory approaches:** The agencies/organizations use the following strategies to ensure minimum standards:
   a. **Licensure:** Licensure is usually a governmental/council approach to ensuring minimum standards to protect the health and well-being of the public by employees and organizations. Original licensure is a contract between the profession and the state to grant permission for professional practice. It

TABLE 50.3: Joint commission 10—step process model and rush model with suggested TQM tools.

Joint Commission 10-step process	Suggested TQM tools
1. Assign responsibilities	–
2. Delineate scope of care/service	Brainstorming affinity diagram
3. Prioritize aspects of care/service. Categorize as high volume, high risk, problem prone, or high cost of poor quality Identify at least two projects to address Flowchart the process	Pareto chart Talley/check sheet Prioritization matrix Brainstorming Matrix diagram, flowchart
4. Establish indicators for identified projects	Affinity diagram, flowchart analysis
5. Establish thresholds for evaluation based on customer expectations	Run or control chart
6. Collect and analyze data	Talley sheet
7. Evaluate the effectiveness of care and document the level of improvement	Pareto or scatter diagram, histogram Run or control chart, fishbone diagram
8. Determine and implement appropriate actions	–
9. Evaluate the effectiveness of action and document the level of improvement	Talley/check sheet Pareto, run or control chart Histogram
10. Communicate results	Pareto, run or control chart or flowchart, histogram, the display matrix
11. Continuous monitoring/improving on the process	Run chart, control chart

Joint Commission 10—Step Process Model

The model includes 10 steps or methodologies for quality management. These steps are to monitor and evaluate the services. There are various TQM tools depicted in **Table 50.3**. The 11th step is 'Continuous monitoring/improving on the process,' which was added in the Rush Model to address the lack of continuity of 10-step process model.

requires written regulations to define the scope and limits of the professional's practice.
b. **Accreditation:** It is a process of validation in which colleges, universities, and other institutions of higher learning are evaluated and certify its competency, authority, and credibility. It is usually a voluntary, nongovernmental approach to grant recognition to those organizations that meet agreed-upon quality standards. In India, the Indian nursing council, State nursing councils, and affiliated universities have established the minimum criteria for each education program and guidelines for inspecting nursing education programs. In the part of the accreditation process, these bodies, per norms, regularly appoint inspectors to check approved/newly establishing education institutes physically and get feedback through duly filled Performa, supporting documents, and with their comments. Based on reports, if any deficiency found, they send compliance reports to the institution to correct within stipulated time.
c. **Certification:** Certification is the confirmation of or certifying specific characteristics of an object, person, or organization through documentary proof. It is also a voluntary, governmental, or nongovernmental approach to grant recognition to individuals and organizations that have met high standards in specialized areas.
d. **Credentialing:** It is the formal recognition of professional or technical competence and attainment of minimum standards. It has four main objectives: To produce a quality product, to confer a unique identity, to protect the care provider and public, and to control quality.
e. **Registrations and renewal of registrations:**
    - *Registration for "Nurse" and "Midwife":* The professional nurse registered as "nurse" (RN) and "midwife" (RM) under the State Nursing Council, where she will apply. Licensure is allowed at a time only in one state. He or she should have recognized qualification either Diploma in Nursing (General Nursing and Midwifery) or BSc Nursing from Indian Nursing Council recognized institution. They registered under the State Nursing Council Act.
    - *Registration for Auxiliary Nurse and Midwife:* Auxiliary Nurse and Midwife registered as RANM under the State Nursing Council, where she will apply. Licensure is allowed at a time only in one state. He or she should have recognized the qualification of auxiliary nurse and midwife (ANM) from an institution recognized by the Indian Nursing Council. They registered under the State Nursing Council Act.
    - *Renewal of registration:* It is necessary to maintain the quality of nursing practice. In India, most of State Nursing Councils renew the registration of nurses after every 5 years without any criteria (in some states) and before renewing the certification to practice he/she should have 150 hours of attendance in Continuing Nursing Education (CNE) in the form of workshop, or CNE (in some states). He/she needs to submit proof of employment, attested copies of 10th, 12th, nursing degree or diploma, original previous nursing, and midwifery registration certificate.
    - *Registration of additional qualification:* In some states of India, nursing councils have provision to register extra/higher qualification or renew the registration of candidates who had already registered as RNRM with their basic requirements.
    - *Secondary registration:* This is the registering qualified candidate with concern State Nursing Council from where he/she is trained and then registering the same qualification once again to other State Nursing Council where he/she wants to practice.

SIX SIGMA IN HEALTHCARE

Meaning and Definitions

Bill Smith at Motorola in 1986 developed three quality improvement methodologies, i.e., quality control, TQM, and zero defects. A defect is the nonconformity of a product or service to its specifications. Six Sigma developed at Motorola to systematically improve processes by eliminating defects. Six Sigma stands for six standard deviations (SDs) from mean. Sigma (σ), a Greek letter used to describe variability or an SD in mathematical or statistics terms. SD is a measure of dispersion (spread) indicates how far away a measured result is from the average (the center of data).

According to Craig Tonner, Six Sigma is a rigorous and systematic methodology that utilizes facts and statistical analysis to measure and improve organizational, operational performance, practices, and systems by identifying and preventing "defects" in service-related processes to accomplish effectiveness.

Six Sigma aims at improving customer–client satisfaction and thereby profitability by reducing and eliminating defects. It may relate to customer satisfaction, service quality, and cost minimization. It also aims at reducing cost and continuous improvement in service/care.

Concepts of Six Sigma

Six Sigma as a Metric

The term "Sigma" is often used as a scale for levels of "goodness" or quality and offers a way of measuring the performance capability of existing systems or processes.

TABLE 50.4: Measuring performance capability.

Sigma	Defects per millions
3.0	66,807
4.0	6,210
5.0	233
6.0	3.4

It is a statistical unit of measure that reflects the likelihood that an error will occur. Using this scale, "Six Sigma" equates to 3.4 defects per one million opportunities (DPMOs). DPMO allows taking the complexity of the product/process into account.

Historically, it is easy to strive for three-sigma processes (where all the data points fall within 83 SDs). Three-sigma processes, on the other hand, still allow 66,807 defects (errors) per million opportunities. But by achieving Six Sigma, the failure rate is minimized to 3.4 defects (errors) per million opportunities or a 99.9996% success rate **(Table 50.4)**.

Rule of thumb is to consider at least three opportunities for a physical part/component—one for form, one for fit, and one for function in the absence of better considerations. Therefore, Six Sigma started as a defect reduction effort in manufacturing and applied to other business processes for the same purpose.

Six Sigma as a Methodology

Six Sigma is a method of improving quality by removing defects and their causes in various operations and activities. It concentrates on those outputs which are essential to customers. It relies on a statistical analysis of data and robust problem-solving techniques. It focuses on an organization to understand and managing clients' requirements, aligning key service processes to achieve those requirements, utilizing data analysis to minimize variation in those processes, and drive rapid, and sustainable improvement to service processes.

Six Sigma as a Management System

It is a management system since used as a strategy in the organization to establish a high-performance system by:
- Setting client-focused high objectives and prioritizing resources for projects
- Mobilizing teams to attack top impact projects and results directing efforts to ensure improvements
- Gathering and analyzing data to make decisions to improve service.

Six Sigma is a mix of three and is a powerful combination of tools, concepts, techniques, and principles designed to improve process performance. It is a quality barometer that provides a systematic approach that eliminates defects. It is essentially client centric in its path.

Six Sigma Methodologies

It has two critical methodologies: DMAIC and DMADV, and other methods are CDOC(conceptualize, design, optimize, and control), DCCDI(define, customer concept, design and implement), and DCDOV(define, concept, design, optimize, and verify), etc.

1. **DMAIC:** "**D**efine opportunities, **M**easure performance, **A**nalyze opportunity, **I**mprove performance, **C**ontrol performance" is a rigorous, data-driven problem-solving process. It is an improvement system to improve existing services of the below standard and try for incremental improvement. It consists of the following five steps:
    a. *Define* relates to defining the process improvement goals that should be consistent with customer demands and organizational strategy or describe the problem.
    b. *Measure* the current services/processes and collect relevant data for future comparison or measure current practices and results.
    c. *Analyze* to verify results. Determine what the relationship, and attempt to ensure that all factors consider and analyze all data for critical connections.
    d. *Improve* or optimize the services (process) based on the analysis using techniques like improving by implementing changes to the service (process).
    e. *Control* is to ensure that any variances corrected before they result in defects/negligence.
2. **DMADV:** The DMADV process (define, measure, analyze, design, verify) is an improvement system used to develop new processes or services/products at Six Sigma quality levels. It can also be employed if current services (process) require more than just incremental improvement. It consists of the following five steps:
    a. *Define* the goals. Design activity that is consistent with customer demands and enterprise strategy or defines the problem.
    b. *Measure* and identify critical to qualities (CTQs), service capabilities, and assess risk.
    c. *Analyze* the service capabilities to develop and design alternatives and to evaluate design criteria to select the best design.
    d. *Design* every detail, optimize the design, and plan to verify a design. This phase may require simulations.
    e. *Verify* the design, implement the process, and handover to process owners.

Green belt and black belt execute both six sigma processes, and six sigma master black belt oversees it.

Six Sigma Quality Team

1. **Six sigma green belt:** They are six sigma practitioners or the organizational employees who apply six sigma to their jobs. They are trained in the methodology and tools to need to work effectively on a process improvement team. They may act as team members under the direction of a Black Belt or may lead their own less complicated, high impact projects that are directly related to their daily work.

2. **Six sigma black belt:** Black Belt team is on-site six sigma experts. They are highly skilled in applying statistical tools and methodologies. They develop and lead cross-functional teams and advise management on prioritizing, planning, and launching six sigma projects. They execute projects in the organization.
3. **Six sigma yellow belt:** Six sigma yellow belt experts are usually the individual process owners and operators who act as team members on six sigma projects. They have a basic knowledge of six sigma and are often responsible for the development of the process. They are also for running smaller process improvement projects using the PDCA and enables yellow belts to identify processes. They feed information to Green belts and black belts working on larger system projects.

External six sigma experts address the most complicated process improvement projects and provide training to black belts, green belts, and yellow belts. They make them understand about the functioning of computers and statistical software in-depth, which are essential components for exploring data in the department and data simulation, screening data for errors, manipulating data and performing transformations.

Principles of Six Sigma

The principles of six sigma are as follows:
1. Six sigma is customer oriented in terms of quality, cost, delivery, safety, etc. A customer/client is anyone who receives a product, service, or information.
2. It is chance oriented. It tries to grab opportunities—an opportunity represents by every chance to get something right or get it wrong.
3. It believes in zero tolerance for defects—3.4 DPMOs, i.e., defect free, hence plan systematically to eliminate defects/negligence or errors as near to perfection as possible.
4. It defines success and develops indicators to measure success or failure of the process, referred to as defects per million opportunities.
5. It serves as a mechanism for cultural transformation in the organization and based on professional ethics and governance.

6. It is data oriented and needs to use sound techniques in decision-making.

Six Sigma Model

Beth Lanham and Pamela Maxson-Cooper developed the six sigma model in 2003 based on the steps of DMAIC Six Sigma (**Fig. 50.8**). The model has excellent practicability in healthcare settings because of its feasibility to standardize processes by using statistical methods. It tries to reduce the chance of occurring 3.4 errors per million. It is specially tested to answer nursing to reduce medical errors and enhance patient safety.

Tools of Six Sigma System

The tools of six sigma system are as follows:
1. **A question-asking method:** The *5 Whys* is used to find out the cause–effect relationships underlying a particular problem. It is to know the leading cause of the problem.
2. **Analysis of variance:** Analysis of variance (ANOVA) is the test of the statistical significance test applied in determining the variations.
3. **Control chart:** It is also known as the "Shewhart chart" or "process-behavior chart." The chart is critical to control and improve the process. It determines either method is in a state of statistical control or not by differentiating significant change from the natural variability of the process. It also helps to eliminate errors by determining the source of variation. It predicts the future performance of the process is in control.
4. **A critical-to-quality tree:** It is a quick tool generally used at the beginning of a project to translate general customer requirements into specific quantified requirements.
5. **Fishbone diagram:** It is a cause-and-effect diagram showing the causes of a specific event arranged in categories, such as the six Ms, eight Ps, or four Ss and also shows cause-and-effect relationships among various variables. The diagram gives a shape of a fishbone or a skeletal of a fish labeled as a fishbone diagram.

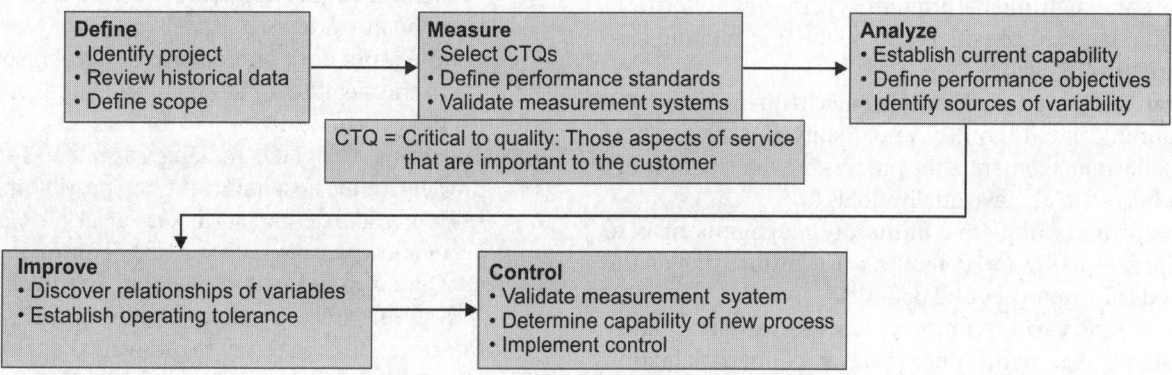

Fig. 50.8: Six sigma model based on DMAIC methodology.

The six Ms are machine (equipment), method (process), materials, measurement (management), man (people), and mother nature (environment). The eight Ps include price, promotion, people, processes, place/plant, policies, procedures and product (or service). The four Ss are surroundings, suppliers, systems, and skills.

6. **Process capability:** A process is a series of steps taken in combination with input like tools, materials, methods, and people engaged in producing a measurable output. Process capability is the capability of a process to meet its purpose as managed by an organization. It measures the variability of a process and compares variability with a proposed specification.

7. **Pareto chart:** It is a particular type of bar chart where the values arranged and plotted in descending order. The graph accompanies a line graph showing the cumulative frequency of each category from left to right. The vertical axis on the left side depicts the frequency of occurrence, and the vertical axis on the right side is the cumulative percentage of the total number of events/total cost/or total of the particular unit of measure. It represents the most common sources of defects, the highest occurring type of error, or reasons for customer complaints, etc. It uses 80–20 rule, i.e., 80% of the problems stem from 20% of the causes.

8. **Run chart:** It is a graph that depicts observed data in a time sequence. The data usually is the output or performance of a process. The horizontal (x) axis represents the time and the output under observation on the vertical (y) axis. A horizontal reference line indicates the average mean or median of the data.

9. **Thought process map:** It presents thoughts, ideas, and questions at the beginning of the project. It helps to identify the objectives and actions of the project. All the information gathered is recorded in a set format.

10. **Cost–benefit analysis:** It is the process to analyze the total expected costs against the total expected benefits of one or more actions to choose the best or the most profitable and suitable alternative.

CHAPTER HIGHLIGHTS

- Quality assessment and quality control in healthcare date back to the midnineteenth century in England; Florence nightingale brought several quality criteria in nursing care considered to be the first nursing care standards in history.
- Juran developed a trilogy approach to quality as quality planning, quality control, and quality improvement.
- Quality management is the process by which people are mobilized to achieve quality goals.
- The primary objective of quality management is to improve quality and to reduce waste by focusing on the needs of employees and patients.
- There are various approaches to evaluate quality systems, e.g., audit, peer reviews, client satisfaction surveys, regulatory strategy, etc.
- Six sigma is a rigorous and systematic methodology that utilizes facts and statistical analysis to measure and improve organizational and operational performance.

REVIEW QUESTIONS

I. Essay Type Questions
1. Define quality and enlist purposes of quality.
2. Enumerate objectives of total quality management and discuss its principles.
3. Describe the American nurses' association model of quality.
4. How the Donabedian model of quality differs from quality management model?

II. Short Notes
1. Total quality management
2. Historical development of quality
3. Donabedian model
4. Quality evaluation systems in healthcare

III. Multiple Choice Questions
1. Who first noticed a positive correlation between adequate nursing care to wounded soldiers and a decrease in mortality rate among a group?
   a. Edwin Chadwick   b. Florence nightingale
   c. Emery Grove   d. Abraham Flexor
2. In which year, the American College of Surgeon created criteria and standards for accreditation under Hospital Standardization Programme that were later adopted by Joint Commission on Accreditation of Hospitals:
   a. 1854   b. 1910
   c. 1918   d. 1952
3. Who developed the trilogy approach to quality?
   a. McClellan   b. Crosby
   c. Donabedian   d. Juran
4. Which one is Donabedian individualized definition of quality?
   a. Quality focuses on the patient's expectations of benefit or harm and other undesired consequences
   b. The profit and damage to health are quality, with no attention to the cost
   c. The population values the cost of care, the benefit/harm continuum, and the distribution of healthcare
   d. The input both human and physical resources to the healthcare system associated with the delivery of healthcare to the patients
5. According to WHO, making sure that services provided by the hospital are the best possible in given existing resources and current medical knowledge:
   a. Quality planning   b. Quality control
   c. Quality assurance d. Quality improvement
6. A system where participation of employees is integrated with a system to motivate them to work effectively is:

a. Quality control
b. Quality improvement
c. Quality management
d. Quality circle

Answer Keys

1. b   2. c   3. d   4. a   5. c   6. d

SUGGESTED READING

1. Brindha V. Quality assurance in nursing. Nightingale Nurs Times. 2006;2(2):9-11.
2. Brook N. Nurse-led discharge planning improves the quality of care. Nurs Times. 2001;97(19):40.
3. Casanova JE. Status of quality assurance program in American hospitals. Med Care. 1990;28(11):1104-09.
4. Cohen T. Human resources and quality assurance. Hosp Top. 1990;68(2):35-8.
5. Coyne C, Killien M. A system for unit-based monitors of quality of nursing care. J Nurs Admin. 1983;17(1):26-32.
6. Crosby PB. Quality is Free. The Art of Making Quality Certain. New York: New American Library; 1979.
7. Das B. Quality nursing care. Nurs J India. 1994;80(10):242.
8. Darr K. Risk management and quality improvement: Together at last—Part 2. Hosp Top. 1999, Spring; 77(2):29-35. [Online] Available from http://www.ncbi.nlm.nih.gov/pubmed/10847926.
9. Donabedian A. Criteria and standards for quality assessment and monitoring. QRB Qual Rev Bull. 1986, Mar;12(3):99-108. [Online] Available from http://www.ncbi.nlm.nih.gov/pubmed/3085044.
10. Donabedian A. Some issues in evaluating the quality of care. Am J Public Health. 1988;71:409-12.
11. Duffy JR, Hoskins LM. The quality caring model. ANS Adv Nurs Sci. 2003;26(1):77-88. [Online] Available from http://www.ncbi.nlm.nih.gov/pubmed/12611432.
12. Fromburg R (Ed). Monitoring and Evaluation in Nursing Services. Joint Commission on Accreditation of Hospitals; 1996.
13. Gupta SK, Kant S. Quality dimensions in hospital infection control. J Acad Hosp Admin. 2002;14(1):51-5.
14. Juran JM, and Gryna FM. Juran's Quality Control Handbook, 4th ed. New York: McGraw-Hill, 1988.
15. Katz JM, Green E. Managing Quality—A Guide to System-Wide Performance Management in Health Care, 2nd edition. St. Louis: Mosby; 1997.
16. Keill P, Johnson T. Optimizing the performance through process improvement. J Nurs Care Quality. 1994;9(1):1-9.
17. Khan Y. Factors affecting quality assurance in nursing care. Nurs J India. 1999;90(8):173-4.
18. Lundquist MJ, Axelsson A. Nurses' participation of quality assurance. J Nurs Manag. 2007;15(1):51-8.
19. Melum MM, Siniores M. The next generation of health care quality. Hospitals. 1989;63(3):80.
20. Nagpal N. Analysis of current nursing situation-existing standards of nursing. Paper presented at the workshop on "Planning process of nursing services at the State level for HFA 2000 AD" at the NIHFW New Delhi; 1987 Oct.
21. Patterson CH. Standards of patient care: The Joint Commission's focus on nursing quality assurance. Nurs Clin North Am. 1988;23(3):625-37.
22. Paul V. Quality measurement across borders: Needs and options. World Hosp Health Services. 2006;42(1):19-22.
23. Reddy BK, Arundhathy M, Acharyulu GVRK. A strategy for successful TQM in a corporate hospital—A study using six sigma. J Acad Hosp Adm. 2002;14(2):7-14.
24. Sherman JJ, Malkmus MA. Integrating quality assurance and total quality management/quality management. J Nurs Adm. 1994;24(3):37-41. [Online] Available from http://www.ncbi.nlm.nih.gov/pubmed/8133323.
25. Singa SB, Anneli S. Evaluation of patient-focused health care from a systems perspective. Syst Res Behav Sci. 2000;17(6):513.
26. Tabish SA. Continuous quality improvement in health care organisations. J Acad Hosp Adm. 1995;8(2-1):11-8.

51 Nursing Service Standards

CHAPTER OUTLINE

- Nursing Standards
  - Concept of Nursing Standards
  - Characteristics of Standards
  - Advantages of Adopting Standards
  - Importance of Nursing Standards
  - Types of Standards
- Taxonomy of Standards
- Setting and Measuring Quality Standards
- Role of Nurse Administrators in Developing Standards
- Barriers and Constraints in Developing Nursing Standards
- Developed Nursing Practice Standards
- Role of Regulatory Bodies in Regulating Nursing Standards

LEARNING OUTCOMES

After completion of this chapter, the learner will be able to:
- Understand the concept of nursing standards
- Enlist characteristics of nursing standards
- Identify the advantages and importance of standards
- Explain in detail the taxonomy of nursing standards
- Describe how to develop quality standards
- Appreciate standards designed by regulatory bodies
- Discuss the methods of evaluation used in maintaining standards
- Describe the role of nurse administrators in developing standards for nursing practice
- Discuss barriers and constraints encountered in developing standards for nursing service
- Exemplify a sample for standards and norms in nursing services

KEY TERMS
Standard, nursing standards, norms, taxonomy, quality, setting standards

INTRODUCTION

Standards are an essential part of health care. Due to the shifting paradigm of healthcare and demographics, increasing the cost of healthcare with scared resources, it is vital to think for cost-effectiveness. Nurses among all healthcare professionals can contribute toward the profitability of healthcare by providing competent and ethical quality care and allow an organization to measure its level of quality. A professional characteristics framework forms a foundation for the standards. It is the standards through which the organization translates quality into professional terms and allows the organization to measure its level of quality. A professional characteristics framework forms the foundation for the standards.

Nurses have been leaders in the field of standards development. Since nursing is the most significant health professionals providing care to individuals, families, groups, communities, and populations in a multiplicity of settings, standards have an essential role in guiding nursing practice. Standards enable nurses to promote safe, competent, and ethical practice. Today nurses are developing standards at a variety of levels and in a range of settings.

A workshop was held in Calcutta on August 1992 by the Nurses' Research Society of India (NRSI), in partnership with the Royal College of Nursing of the United Kingdom, Dynamic Quality Improvement Programme (DQIP), introduced an approach to quality improvement to nurses in India interested in evaluating and improving the care they provide. Since then, three sites have implemented the system for standard setting and audit (dynamic standard setting system), which is the method for evaluating care used within that approach.

Indian Nursing Council has made efforts to develop and testing of standards for maintaining uniformity in nursing education and nursing practice. There is still a need to establish, monitor, and enforce standards of professional practice and conduct in India.

NURSING STANDARDS

Concept of Nursing Standards

Standard

Standards are the benchmark of achievement based on a desired level of excellence. As such, standards become model to be initiated and may serve, in turn, as the basis of comparisons (The Oxford Dictionary, 1964). Donabedian defines standards as professionally developed expressions of a range of acceptable variations from a norm or criterion. Whereas a *criterion* refers to a predetermined element to compare aspects of quality of medical service, and *norms* are "measures" of usually observed performance. A standard is a descriptive statement of the desired level of performance to judge the quality of structure, process, or outcomes.

Nursing Standards

The nursing care standard is "a descriptive statement of desired quality to evaluate nursing care given to a patient." A nursing standard is used as a target or gauze to measure the performance. A standard can be a planning tool if used as a *target* and a control device when used as *gauze* to measure and evaluate actual performance. Nursing practice standards are statements that describe the expected desirable and achievable level of performance to measure actual performance.

Characteristics of Standards

- A standard must be in writing form.
- Standards should define a set of rules, actions, or outcomes.
- Standards are in writing for customers, staff members, and systems.
- Authority must approve standards.
- Standards must be specific, measurable, appropriate, reliable, and timely carried out.

Advantages of Adopting Nursing Standards

- To define quality levels and provide the basis for quality control of services
- To promote professional nursing practice by regulating, directing, and evaluating nursing practice
- To enable patient/client to judge the adequacy of nursing care
- To provide guidelines to nurse researchers in identifying and exploring relationships between nursing practice and patient care outcomes
- To give instructions for nurse administrators to support and facilitate safe, competent, and ethical nursing practice within their agencies
- To provide guidelines for nurse educators in setting objectives of educational programs
- To provide a framework for developing specialty nursing standards
- To facilitate articulation of the role of nursing within the health-care center.

Importance of Nursing Standards

Standards are necessary to demonstrate professional dedication to the public, government, and other stakeholders in maintaining public trust and upholding the criteria of its professional practice. Standards are important because:

- Standards are vehicles in the organization that translates quality into operational terms and hold everyone (patient, care providers, support personnel, management) in the system accountable for their part.
- These also allow the organization to measure its level of quality.
- Standards, indicators, and thresholds are the elements that make a quality assurance system work in a measurable, objective, and qualitative manner.
- It helps to bring the health workers' knowledge and control over the variation in the healthcare system (Berwick, 1991).
- It is crucial to keep variation within limits of control (Deming, 1986).
- It helps to reduce variations in healthcare by defining what an organization expects for the day-to-day inputs, processes, and outcomes of healthcare and services.
- Standards maintain public trust and uphold criteria of its professional practice.
- Standards guide nursing practice.
- Standards enable nurses to promote safe, competent, and ethical practice.

Types of Standards

Standards range from broad, profession-specific standards to detailed care standards established by a specific agency **(Fig. 51.1)** that illustrates the relationship among the various types of nursing standards for practice. The base depicts the standards for practice of the regulatory body, which describes expectations regarding nursing practice across the profession. In contrast, the specific client-care standards drawn at the apex of the figure are client focused and explain specific nursing actions and interventions required to achieve desired client outcomes in a particular setting. This range of standards represents mutual and congruent expectations concerning the standards for the nurse in practice (Smith, 1991).

TAXONOMY OF STANDARDS

1. *According to domain*
   a. *Structure standards:* Structural standards establish guidelines for organizational patterns and support

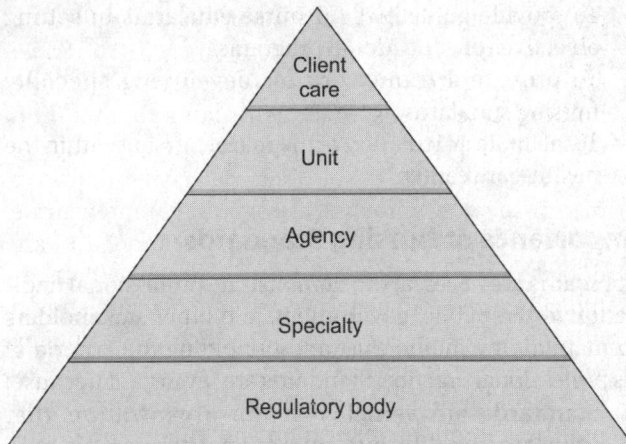

Fig. 51.1: Pyramid of nursing standards.

structures for providing healthcare. It defines rules to deliver services and outline legal parameters that govern performance expectations. These are nonnegotiable and cannot be modified. These define the scope of authority within which individual or group representing organization may function.

Structure standards include mission, philosophy, goals, policies, and job descriptions of the organization/department, physical setting, physical facilities, equipment, staffing, educational backgrounds, and job assignments. For example, structure standards for an intensive care unit may specify the number of square feet per patient, equipment available at the bedside, and availability of specially trained nurses at a ratio of 1:1.

b. *Process standards:* Process or performance standards define how the service is to be carried out. It defines operational norms and translates organizational values into actions and those processes in writing for which the organization will be held accountable. It is negotiable, flexible, and based on the analysis of situations and individual's decisions. Procedures, protocols, practice guidelines, plans, and documentations are examples of process standards. A process standard might specify an initial nursing care plan established within 24 hours of admission.

c. *Outcome standards:* These are part and parcel of every process. These define both desirable results to achieve and avoid undesirable consequences. These evaluate the effects of actions and processes. Outcomes are attached to all process standards and are in writing form for every procedure, practice, guidelines, and plan. The Institute of Medicine (IOM) has identified that process and outcome must go hand in hand. Effective methods increase the likelihood of relevant results. Processes need to change if results are not met (IOM, 1999).

2. *According to context*

According to context, the standards in terms of structure, process, and the outcome are standards of service, standards of practice, and standards of governance **(Table 51.1)**.

TABLE 51.1: Sample table of taxonomy of standards according to context.

Domain	Context		
	Standards of service	Standards of practice	Standards of governance/performance
Structure			
Process			
Outcome			

a. *Standard of service:* A standard of care focuses on the patient. Joint Commission has defined "standard of care" as those activities or outcomes of nursing activities focuses on patients' status or expectations.

These are a specific detailed plan of care for individuals having a health problem. The standards of care become the basis for determining the level of care delivered and for the quality improvement within the organization as well as for cost analysis. Each nursing department should have standards and norms. The above table depicts a sample proforma for standards and criteria for nursing services.

b. *Standards of nursing practice:* "Standards of nursing practice" focusses on the structure and process domain/elements used by the nurse and nursing service to provide patient care (Patterson). It describes what the nurse does or how he or she provides nursing care to the patient to achieve the expected outcome. These are authoritative statements that describe an acceptable level of professional nursing performance. The standards of practice, therefore, define professional practice.

c. *Standards of performance:* Standards of performance used by the Joint Commission relate to how well nurses must perform against identified standards of performance specified in the job description for evaluation purposes. The Joint Commission on Accreditation of Healthcare Organizations (JCAHO) standards of performance include assessment of competency of nurses, establishing standards of patient care, and practice of nurses.

Table 51.2 depicts a sample proforma for standards and norms for nursing services.

Nursing Service Standards from the Accreditation Manual for Hospitals

The Joint Commission publishes consensus standards for use in the accreditation of hospitals and other healthcare organizations. Standards address the structure, process, and outcomes of the patient care activity across a health-care organization's scope of service. The standards focus on the provision, management, and monitoring of hospital-based nursing care:

1. There should be an organized nursing department/service.
2. A qualified nurse administrator should head the nursing department/service and integrate it appropriately with the medical staff and with other hospital staff that provides and contribute to patient care.
3. The nursing department/service should meet the nursing care needs of patients and to maintain established standards of nursing practice.
4. The nursing department/service assignments in the provision of nursing care should commensurate with the qualifications of nursing personnel and are designed to meet the nursing care needs of patients.
5. Individualized and goal-directed nursing care should provide to the patients through the use of the nursing process.
6. The nursing department/service personnel should prepare appropriate education and training programs for their responsibilities in the provision of nursing care.
7. Written policies and operative procedures guide the standards of nursing care.
8. As part of the hospital's quality assurance program, the quality and appropriateness of the patient care provided by the nursing department/service should monitor and evaluate and resolve the identified problems.

TABLE 51.2: Sample proforma for standards and norms for nursing services.

Standard	Criteria	Indicators
Structure	Professional qualification	➤ Registered nurse with General Nursing/BSc Nursing/MSc Nursing ➤ The well-adjusted personality of the nurse ➤ Flexible in dealing
	Qualities and competence	➤ Maintaining ethical standards ➤ Possess knowledge and skill
	Physical facilities	➤ Nursing station ➤ Rooms/wards provide easy mobility of the machine ➤ Space between the beds ➤ Adequate lighting ➤ Telephone facilities ➤ Provision of O_2 and suction ➤ Adequate water supply, etc.
	Nurse–patient ratio	1:3 or 1:5
	Physical environmental	➤ Therapeutic climate ➤ Client's physical safety ➤ Reception room ➤ Treatment room ➤ Conference room ➤ Store room
Process	➤ Assessment ➤ Identification data ➤ Recognition of symptoms ➤ Recording	➤ Collect pertinent data ➤ Perceptual disorders ➤ Cognitive disorders ➤ Physical ailments ➤ Affective disorders ➤ Physical examination ➤ Any untoward behavior ➤ Establishes a therapeutic relationship with the client
	Nursing diagnosis	Develop nursing diagnosis
	Expected outcomes and planning	➤ Assist client to set realistic goals ➤ Develop a nursing care plan
	Implementation	Provide skilled nursing care per plan
	Evaluation	➤ Assess the client's progress ➤ Modified care plan and makes an alternative course of action
Outcome	Short-term care	➤ The client's participation in the therapy ➤ Client's kept up regular appointments ➤ Develop trusts in nurse ➤ Recognizes his needs, abilities, strengths, and limitations. ➤ Self-dependent
	Long-term care	➤ The client's participation in the therapy ➤ Client's kept up regular appointments ➤ Develop trusts in nurse ➤ Recognizes his needs, abilities, strengths, ➤ Limitations. ➤ Self-dependent

SETTING AND MEASURING QUALITY STANDARDS

Setting standards is an important activity; it should plan, implement, and review continuously. As the mentioned standard is a statement of expectations that defines the structure, process, and outcomes, it should be an ongoing dynamic process that continually incorporates the experience and perspective of healthcare professionals and staff members throughout its development.

Methods of Setting Nursing Standards

Professional standard techniques, comprehensive review systems, and process appraisal techniques are used in nursing to set/prepare standards in the nursing profession.

a. **Professional standards:** The professional standard category contains the various guidelines and standard documents that healthcare professionals have published as a basis for quality assurance. These based on structure, process, and outcome quality assurance model are given by the American Nurses' Association as discussed in quality assurance.

b. **Comprehensive review:** Many professional bodies specify standards and guidelines for practice applied in all settings. These standards are at a high level of generality and use as a framework for exercising in specific standards settings. The nursing profession has adopted the opposite strategy. It provides guidelines for a process for local standard-setting on the assumption that later on, it can develop the local and specific general standards. For example, the Royal College of Nursing's Dynamic Standard Setting System (DySSSy) established in 1965 (UK) to implement at the ward level.

It facilitated local standard setting as well as quality appraisal and improvement.

c. **Process appraisal:** The process appraisal techniques focus primarily on an assessment of the quality of processes of care. It includes procedures and activities of the health professionals. It consists of all technical, interpersonal, and moral issues and provides access, diagnosis, treatment, discharge, aftercare, and health education and promotion. Process standards developed in nursing than in any other professional area and almost all instruments for measuring process quality designed for use in nursing

Steps to Set Nursing Standards

Following steps are considered while setting standards (Fig. 51.2):

1. *Identify the basis for setting standards*
   - The standard should be desirable and useful.
   - There should be positive aptitude and attitude to develop a standard.
   - There should be sufficient resources for developing, implementing, and maintaining standards.
   - There should be an ability to promote established standards.
   - One has to take responsibility to develop standards.
2. *Develop a checklist*
   - Do proposed standards effectively address the identified?
   - Are new standards need to develop, to revise, or modify?
   - Are proposed standards likely to improve the quality care?
   - How will implementations of the proposed standards affect the cost of providing care?
   - Will an anticipated increase in cost be justified by any expected improvement in quality care?
   - What significant barriers to the implementation of the proposed standards exist?
   - Does the standard-setting organization have appreciated resources and services available to help healthcare organizations to interpret and implement the proposed standards?
3. ***Develop nursing standards:*** Follow seven-step methodology to develop nursing standards (Fig. 51.3)
   a. *Identify the system that requires standards*: Identify high volume, high-risk, and problem-prone function per the priority and also use standard criteria for selection among possibilities as based on importance, feasibility, impact, and cost.
   b. *Identify a panel of experts to address standard*: The team should include the right persons to address issues necessary to complete a task (Barassard, 1989). Usually, five to eight members will be the most effective team. It should include qualified under their experiences, training, and role in the organization. Include technical experts and someone from the authority within the organization.
   c. *Identify inputs, processes, and outcomes of the system*: The team must identify elements for each of the components, i.e. input, processes, and result of the system.
      - List down the desired outcome for an activity
      - Lists the processes of outcomes to occur and inputs that the processes require.
      - Prepare tools that are useful for identifying inputs, processes, and outcomes.
   d. *Define quality characteristics*: The team then decides on the quality characteristics of each essential element and then define a standard for that.
   e. *Develop a draft of standards*: Steps are as follows:
      i. Choose a format: Mostly format is in the form of the statement. Algorithms are usually applied for process standards; case management plans, nursing care plans, and critical paths are especially used for practice standards; and clinical care protocols for used as practice guidelines to render nursing care.
      ii. Gather background information: Information gathered through reviewing literature related to nursing theories, philosophies, existing nursing practices, and nursing processes; consulting experts; benchmarking; and reviewing past experiences.
      iii. Draft standards: Delphi method or flowchart methods can be selected to draft standards or to begin with "seed" standards.

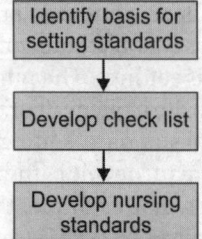

Fig. 51.2: Steps for setting standards.

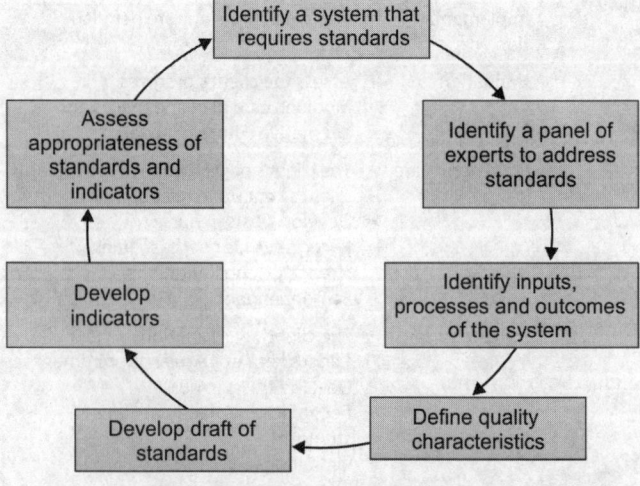

Fig. 51.3: Steps of developing standard.

TABLE 51.3: Checklist to determine the suitability of standards and indicators.

S. No.	Criterion	Yes	No
1.	Are standards appropriate to the organization		
2.	Are the standards valid		
3.	Are the standards reliable		
4.	Do the standards have clarity		
5.	Are standards applicable		
6.	Are the indicators measurable		
7.	Are various methods (staff meetings, questionnaires, etc.) used to finalize standards		
8.	Is feedback of client/staff taken and incorporated		
9.	Is the team reviewed standards		
10.	Is a revision of developed standards carried out before implementation		

f. *Develop indicators for standards*: Indicator is a well-defined objective and measurable variable used to monitor the quality and appropriateness of a vital aspect of care. It is compliance to standard and measures variance from the desired level of standard. An indicator can be a structure, a process, or an outcome, about which data collected during monitoring activities (Donabedian A). An index can include structure, process, and outcome elements used in the measurement of one aspect of nursing care and should be in measurable terms.

g. *Assess the appropriateness of standards and indicators*: Appropriateness is a ratio or degree of congruence between what the patient needed and the care given by a nurse. It is the extent of nursing care provided in the inappropriate setting, best suited to patient's needs. Use a checklist to assess the appropriateness of standards **(Table 51.3).**

Measuring Nursing Standards

Nursing Research Society of India (NRSI), in partnership with the Royal College of Nursing of the UK, discussed an approach to quality improvement in nursing care and developed "Standard setting and audit system (dynamic standard setting system)" to evaluate care that was implemented in three hospitals in one of the workshops on "Dynamic Quality Improvement Programme (DQIP)", held at Calcutta in August 1992.

Indian Nursing Council has made efforts to develop and evaluate standards for maintaining uniformity in nursing education and nursing practice. The nursing standards are evaluated through inspection, accreditation, and self-assessment.

Inspection: Inspection can be made more effective and purposeful by the use of standards. A government agency/professional body/financial institution can conduct the investigation, a sort of official examination. Ideally, setting standards should be a joint process and assess performance against the criteria.

Accreditation: Accreditation is a process of setting standards and measuring compliance. The standards set through a consultative process with consumers. After judging, standards are subjected to periodical and ongoing reviews to ensure their continual appropriateness.

Currently, accreditation generally rests with autonomous organizations, as applied to Government or individual professional bodies or associations. Independent accreditation bodies conduct certification in the United States, Canada, Australia, and England.

Self-assessment: Self-assessment being one's performance can be useful to analyze one's strengths and weaknesses in the performance. It is done by the following:
a. An individual nursing department can do a self-assessment to establish its standards and measure its performance periodically
b. Departments can do a self-assessment for particular program-specific standards.
c. Standards can also be set to measure against other similar institutions or professional groups for sharing experiences to achieve an optimum level of nursing care.

ROLE OF NURSE ADMINISTRATORS IN DEVELOPING STANDARDS

The purpose of nurse administrator has been identified by "Development of guidelines for standards for nursing practice (1999)" committee, which is as follows:
1. *Initiator*: As an initiator, he or she creates awareness/sensitizes nurses at first- and second-level leadership positions on nursing standards.
2. *Facilitator*: As a facilitator, he or she develops implements, monitors, and evaluates standards for nursing practice at all times.
3. *Procurement*: He or she procures and keeps a record of necessary infrastructure required for developing, implementing, maintenance, and monitoring standards for nursing practice.
4. *Formulation of the committee*: He or she forms a core group or a committee for developing, implementing, monitoring, and maintaining standards for nursing practice.
5. *Staff development*: He or she assures on-the-job orientation and in-service education to enhance the implementation and monitoring of standards for nursing practice.
6. *Auditing and reviewing of standards*: He or she ensures verification and reviewing of standards for nursing practice.
7. *Change agent*: As an educator, he or she gives orientation to nursing personnel regarding the need for standards of nursing practice; stimulates, and motivates the nurses to implement and maintain standards of

nursing practice and also trains core group to develop, implement, monitor, manage, and evaluate the criteria for nursing practice.
8. *Evaluator*: As an evaluator, he or she monitors the implementation of standards for nursing practice and also evaluates the auditing and reviewing process for updating standards of nursing practice.

BARRIERS AND CONSTRAINTS IN DEVELOPING NURSING STANDARDS

The obstacles and constraints in the development of standards for nursing services are related to policies, nursing human resources, equipment, and other materials, physical facilities, budget, and monitoring systems (Fig. 51.4).

1. *Nonavailability of written policies*
   - Absence of laid down rules
   - Lack of appropriate written policies for nursing practice
   - Lack of specific job descriptions of various categories of nursing personnel in different health care settings
   - Absence of system regarding renewal of registration of practice nurses
   - Lack of political and professional support for improving standards for nursing care
   - Inadequate autonomy and accountability of nursing practice.
2. *Nursing human resources issues*
   - There is an insufficient nurse–patient ratio in totality and different shifts in hospitals and other healthcare settings.
   - There is a lack of awareness regarding concepts of standards, sensitivity to need of standards and knowledge as regard for developing, implementing, and monitoring of standards for nursing practice.
   - Lack of strategies for regular updating of knowledge and skills in various clinical areas of nursing practice.
   - Inadequate and inappropriate supervision and control of nursing services provided by nursing personnel at all levels.
   - Lack of adequately prepared nurse administrators for planning and organizing nursing services.
   - Lack of promotional avenues for nurses at all levels due to limited cadre in nursing.
   - Absence of recognition, appreciation, and motivation for nursing personnel in planning, organizing, and providing nursing care.
   - Absenteeism and increased turnover rate among nurses.
   - Lack of proper utilization of nurses.
3. *Lack of equipment and supply*
   - Inadequate quantity of equipment and supplies to provide the nursing care
   - Low quality and substandard equipment
   - Lack of training in handling various equipment, machines, and monitors in advanced clinical practice
   - Lack of stationery items.
4. *Inadequate physical facilities*
   - Inappropriate and insufficient physical setup of the hospital
   - Poor sanitation
   - Shortage of water and electricity supplies
   - Improper drainage and waste disposal facilities.
5. *Budget constraints*: Uncertainty for the commitment of adequate financial support for development and implementation of standards for nursing care.
6. *Inadequate monitoring system*: No auditing system is in practice to evaluate nursing care given. Inspection or accreditation of the hospitals is not the concern.

DEVELOPED NURSING PRACTICE STANDARDS

Nursing practice standards are a set of activities expected from a professional group of nurses, classified according to practice areas, consistent with areas for code of ethics and professional conduct. Each area has specific standards, the rationale for each standard, and the performance criteria, i.e. selected behaviors to achieve standard or indicators. Various associations and regulatory bodies have developed standards for their nurses.

The American Nurses' Association Nursing Practice Standards

The American Nurses' Association (ANA) nursing standards articulate who, what, where, why, when, and

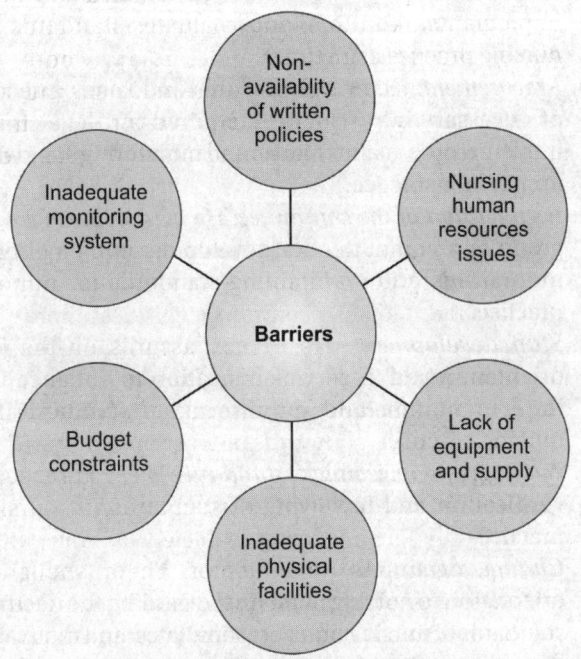

Fig. 51.4: Barriers in developing standards.

how of practice. There are 16 ANA standards of practice, 6 standards of practice, and 9 standards of professional performance (Annexure 1).

The Canadian Nurses' Association Practice Standards

There are 25 Canadian Nurses' Association (CNA) standards of practice: eight standards of professional responsibility, eight standards of knowledge-based practice, five standards of ethical practice, and four standards of provision of service to the public (Annexure 2).

Practice Standards in India

There are 21 standards of practice: five standards of professional responsibility and accountability, three standards of nursing practice, two standards of communication and interpersonal relationships, three standards of valuing human beings, six standards of management, and two standards of professional development (Annexure 3).

ROLE OF REGULATORY BODIES IN REGULATING NURSING STANDARDS

The nursing councils and professional organizations play a vital role in maintaining the nursing practice and education standards in India **(Fig. 51.5)**.

The councils regulate and control the registration of nurses, auxiliary nurse midwives, multipurpose health workers, and health visitors practicing in states to give recognition to training institutions, to grant affiliation and withdraw recognition, to conduct examinations, and certification, etc.

1. **Maintaining nursing standards:** It involves the nursing activities for the care of clients. The main activities are as follows:
   a. *Regulation and control of registration of nurses:* Any person who fulfills academic qualifications and training as prescribed rules shall register, on payment; any person shall renew his or her enrollment in the manner prescribed by regulations and on payment of renewal fees; make entries in the register, from time to time, to revise the same and issuing certificates of registration in accordance with the provisions of the Act by the state councils to maintain live register.
   b. *Approval for registration of Indian and foreign nurses:* According to the Indian Nursing Council Act, 1947, the Indian and international nurses having foreign qualifications can get consent for registration under section 11(2) (a). Indian citizens possessing international nursing qualifications after examining individually and after equivalency in regard to syllabi with the recommendation of equivalence committee and conformation from concerned foreign authorities, of which eligible nurses, get approval for registration in India.
   c. *Approval for a job to foreign nationals:* The international or national nurses possessing foreign qualification can work in charitable institutions for a limited period with the support of President, Indian Nursing Council (INC), and grants temporary permission for employment in these institutions if their requirement found at par by the equivalence committee.
   d. *Licensing and supervision:* Every licensing authority exercise general supervision and control on the nurses, auxiliary nurse midwives, female health workers, and female health assistants/health supervisors practicing within the area under its jurisdiction.
      ♦ Only registered nurses and midwives can practice in hospitals and institutions. Persons who are not registered or not in the list should not practice; if they do so, there is a penalty for fraudulent use of a certificate.
      ♦ No registered hospital, nursing home, or diagnostic center shall employ nursing personnel who do not possess the minimum required qualification laid down in the Indian Nursing Act, 1947.
   e. *Developing nursing practice standards:* The practice of standards for nurses in India can be used as a parameter for evaluating performance and as a measure of quality control. Licensing authority and various nursing associations and organizations develop nursing standards.

The trained nurses' associations had described the national standards to member nurses. The specialty nursing organizations, e.g. Society of Midwives-India (SOMI), Association of Psychiatric Nursing, Nursing Research Society of India (NRSI), are working on these issues. The councils and nursing associations prescribe the minimum staffing pattern, recruitment policies, pay remunerations, etc. infrastructure to the recognized establishments, code of ethics, and professional conduct.

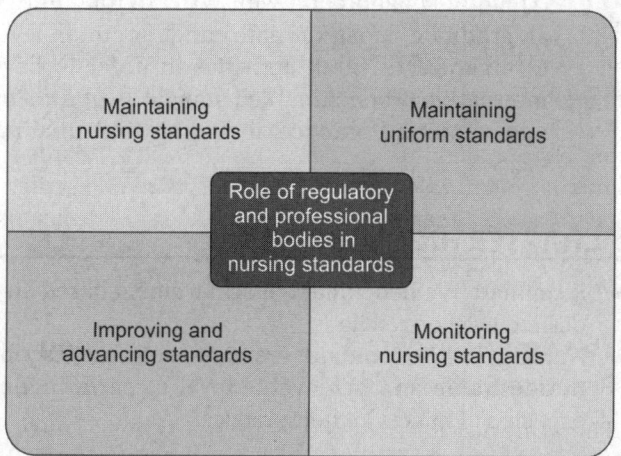

Fig. 51.5: Role of regulatory and professional bodies in nursing standards.

2. **Maintaining uniform standards:** Regulatory bodies maintain uniform standards of nursing education by the following:
   a. *Recognition of training institutions:* No nursing educational institute can start without prior approval of the Indian Nursing Council, State Council, and the Government. The council may prescribe by the regulations and after inspections and such inquiry as it deems fit, recognize, or sanction approval to any institution for the training of nurses.

   The council may withdraw recognition from any such institution after it's an inspection by representatives of the council. The order of such withdrawal shall be in writing and shall be served in the manner as laid down by regulations.

   b. *Affiliation:* The council may request accordance with rules, and after inspection, training institute, if found fit, affiliates to any institution or hospital for preventive, promotion, curative, and rehabilitative nursing care of patients.
   c. *Development and implementation of curriculum:* Nursing councils have the power to make regulations, develop, and prescribe the standard curricula for the training of nurses, midwives, and health visitors, for training courses for teachers of nurses and training in nursing administration and revise time to time. Prescribe the conditions for admission to courses of instruction as aforesaid.
   d. *Certification:* The council prescribes minimum standards of examination and other requirements to be satisfied to secure qualifications recognition under this Act. The state councils conduct an exam of the diploma course and prepare a schedule for written and practical examination to issue certificates after successful completion of the study.
   e. *Meetings:* To maintain quality of nursing education in the country and to understand the problem/issues of each State Nursing Registration Council (SNRC) and evolve consensus between INC and SNRC conduct meetings with the state registrars.
3. **Monitoring nursing standards:** The councils follow uniform standards of education by:
   a. *Inspections and accreditation:* First inspection conducted on receipt of the proposal received from the institute to start any nursing program by the Indian Nursing Council as well by the State Nursing Council. Re-inspect those institutions, which are found unsuitable. Nursing Council conducts periodical (after 3 years) inspection of the recognized institution to monitor the standards of nursing education and the adherence of the norms prescribed by the Nursing Council. Thus recognizes institutions/organizations/universities imparting Master's degree/Bachelor's degree/PG diploma/diploma/certificate courses in the field of nursing.
   b. *Withdrawal of recognition:* Indian nursing council has the power to withdraw the recognition of qualification in case the institution fails to maintain its standards, and that an institution recognized by a State Council for the training of nurses, midwives, auxiliary nurse midwives, or health visitors does not satisfy the requirements of the council.
   c. *Regulation of policies and rules of conduct:* The council regulates the training policies and programs in the field of nursing and prescribes rules of conduct and disciplinary action against nursing schools/colleges in the state.
   d. *Continuing education:* The nursing organizations and councils implement quality of nursing education by organizing and inviting nurses to participate in various refresher courses, workshops, seminars, and conferences for nurses of all levels.
   e. *Approval of degrees awarded by foreign universities:* INC recognizes Degree/Diploma/Certificate awarded by foreign universities/institutions on a reciprocal basis, thus maintaining the standard in nursing education.
4. **Improving and advancing standards:** To improve the standards of nursing education and nursing practice and to have international standards, the councils and nursing organizations have taken various steps:
   a. *Promotion of research activities:* Indian nursing council constituted National consortium for PhD in Nursing through six study centers connected by videoconferencing facilities since 2005–2006. Nursing Research Society of India also supports the development of nursing research activities in universities and healthcare institutions to set the nursing care standards.
   b. *Training of nurses:* For advancing the standards of nursing education and practices in India, a Memorandum of Understanding (MOU) was signed at New Delhi on 11th April 2006 between Indian Nursing Council and Sir Edward Dunlop Hospitals (I) Ltd in collaboration with WHO to train nurses at graduate, postgraduate, and doctoral level to organize research activities in order to have international benchmarked standards of nursing education and practice, including credentialing, etc.

CHAPTER HIGHLIGHTS

- A standard is a benchmark of achievement based on a desired level of excellence.
- Nursing practice standards are statements that describe the desirable and achievable level of performance expected of nurses in their practice.

- According to the domain, standards are structure, process, and outcome. *Structure standards* are nonnegotiable, define rules for delivering services, and establish guidelines for organizational patterns, support structures for providing health care; *process standards* are negotiable; identify ways to carry out services and operational norms that translate corporate values into actions, and *outcome standards* define both desirable results achieved and undesirable results that to be avoided.
- According to context, standards are of service, practice, and governance. *Standards of care/service* are activities or outcomes of nursing activities, focus on patients' status or expectations; *standards of nursing practice* focus on the structure and process domain/elements used by the nurse and nursing service to provide patient care; and *standards of performance* relate how well nurse must perform against identified standards of performance specified in job description for evaluation purposes.
- There are three steps to set standards—identifying the basis for setting standards; preparing checklist; and developing standards. A seven-step methodology to develop nursing standards.
- Nursing councils, associations, and organizations develop practice standards in nursing and classify according to practice areas include code of ethics and professional conduct.
- The nursing standards measure through inspection, accreditation, and self-assessment. Nurse administrators play an essential role in developing standards in nursing.
- The barriers and constraints in the development of standards for nursing services are related to policies, nursing human resources, equipment, and other materials, physical facilities, budget, and monitoring systems.
- The nursing councils and professional organizations play a vital role in maintaining the nursing practice and education standards.

REVIEW QUESTIONS

I. Essay Type Questions
1. Define nursing standards and enlist purposes and the advantages of having standards in nursing.
2. Discuss the taxonomy of standards.
3. Describe seven-step methodology to develop nursing standards.
4. Write barriers and constraints in the development of standards for nursing service.
5. Discuss the role of nursing councils and professional organizations in maintaining nursing standards.

II. Short Notes
1. Standards of service
2. Role of nurse administrators in developing standards
3. Evaluation of standards
4. Monitoring nursing education standards

III. Multiple Choice Questions
1. A predetermined element to compare aspects of the quality of medical service is:
   a. Norm   b. Standard
   c. Criterion   d. Quality
2. The nursing standard, when used as a planning tool, is:
   a. Target   b. Gauze
   c. Rule   d. Authority
3. To demonstrate a profession dedicated to the public, government, and other stakeholders in maintaining public trust and upholding the criteria of its professional practice are necessary to have:
   a. Guidelines   b. Standards
   c. Control   d. Quality care
4. A type of standard that define operational norms and translates organizational values into actions and those processes in writing for which the organization will be holding accountable is:
   a. Structure   b. Outcome
   c. Process   d. Service
5. An indicator which is well-defined objective and the measurable variable used to monitor quality and appropriateness of an important aspect of care can include:
   a. Structure, process, and outcome
   b. Structure and outcome
   c. Process and outcome
   d. Structure and process
6. A process of setting standards and measuring compliance through a consultative process that is subjected to periodical and ongoing review to ensure their continued appropriateness is:
   a. Inspection   b. Accreditation
   c. Self-assessment d. Audit

Answer Keys

1. c 2. a 3. b 4. c 5. a 6. b

SUGGESTED READING

1. American Nurses Association. Standards of Clinical Nursing Practice, 2nd edition. Washington, DC: Author; 1998.
2. American Nurses Association (ANA). Scope and Standards for Nurse Administration, 2nd edition. Washington, DC: Author; 2004.; 2000.
3. American Nurses Association (ANA). Nursing: Scope and Standards of Practice. Washington, DC: Author; 2004.

4. Bensen DS, Van Osdol W. Quality Audit Systems For Primary Care Centers. Methodist Hospitals of Indiana, Inc; 1990.
5. Canadian Nurses Association. Framework for the Practice of Registered Nurses. Ottawa: Author; 2007.
6. Canadian Association of Nephrology Nurses and Technologists. Standards for Nursing Practice; 2001. [Online] Available from http://www.cannt.ca/standards/nursing.
7. Claflin N. Nursing standards of patient care and standards of nursing practice- a practical approach. J Health Qual. 1993;15(3):25-7, 30-3.
8. Joint Commission on Accreditation of Healthcare Organizations Standards: HR.3.10, (EP7); HR.3.20; HR.3.10 (EP1, EP4) NR 1, NR 2, NR 3. 2004 Comprehensive Accreditation Manual for Hospitals: The Official Handbook (CAMH).
9. Ministry of Health and Family Welfare: Report of Development of standards for nursing practice. New Delhi: WHO Project: IND-HRH-031/98; 1999.
10. Nurse in Scope Advancement. [Online] Available from http://www.csgna.com/scope.htm.
11. Nursing Association Standards of Practice, Standards of Practice Survey. [Online] Available from http://www.cgna.net/standards.htm.
12. Standards nsg\Canadian Nurses Association—Standards and Best Practices.htm.

ANNEXURE 1

American Nurses Association (ANA) Standards

ANA STANDARDS OF NURSING SERVICE

1. The nursing department has the responsibility and authority for the practice of nursing in the health-care facility.
2. Allocate the finance to the nursing department necessary to carry out the departmental program.
3. The nursing department promotes safe and therapeutically effective nursing care through the implementation of established standards of nursing care.
4. It has delineated responsibilities in the health facility's disaster plan.
5. It has written personnel policies, which can be expected to attract, qualified nursing programs, and opportunities for staff development.
6. It develops a written agreement with the educational institution for the use of the clinical facilities by nursing students, which ensures the safety and welfare of the patients.
7. It initiates and promotes studies of and where feasible, research on administrative, supervisory, and nursing care practices.
8. It ensures and provides the physical facilities, supplies, and equipment needed to carry out the objectives and standards of the nursing department.
9. It continuously evaluates its administrative, supervisory, and nursing care practices.

ANA STANDARDS OF CARE/PRACTICE

Standard 1: Assessment: *Measurement Criteria*

- The systematic and ongoing data collection process
- Holistic data collection involves clients, family, and others, as appropriate
- A priority of data collection activities determined by the client's immediate condition and anticipated needs of the client or situation
- Uses proper evidence-based assessment techniques and instruments
- Uses analytical models and problem-solving tools
- Analyzes available relevant data, information, and knowledge to identify patterns and variances
- Relevant data documented in a retrievable format.

Standard 2: Diagnosis: *Measurement Criteria*

- Diagnoses or issues from assessment data
- Validate diagnoses with clients, family, and others, as appropriate
- Diagnoses or problems documented to facilitate the determination of expected outcomes and plan of care.

Standard 3: Outcome Identification: *Measurement Criteria*

- Formulate outcomes with clients, family, and others, as appropriate
- Culturally appropriate anticipated results derived from diagnoses
- Considers associated risks, benefits, and costs, and current scientific evidence, and clinical expertise
- Defines expected consequences considering associated risks, benefits, and fees, and current scientific evidence, in terms of clients, family, ethical consideration, environment, and situation
- Outcomes include a time estimate for attainment
- Findings provide direction for continuity for care
- Modifies results based on changes in the status of the client and evaluation of the situation
- Documents expected outcomes as measurable goals.

Standard 4: Planning: *Measurement Criteria*

- Develops an individualized plan considering client characteristics or the case, including age, culturally appropriate, and environmentally sensitive
- Develop a plan with clients, family, and others, as relevant
- The plan includes strategies that address each of identified diagnoses or issues, promotion, and prevention of disease
- Provides continuity within the plan
- Incorporates a timeline within the plan
- Establishes the plan priorities with clients, family, and others, as appropriate
- Utilizes the plan to give direction to the health-care team
- The plan reflects current statutes, rules and regulations, and standards.
- Integrates current trends and research affecting the care
- Considers the economic impact of the plan
- The plan uses standardized language/recognized terminology.

Standard 5: Implementation: *Measurement Criteria*

- Implements plan
- Documents implementation
- Uses evidence-based interventions particular to the diagnosis or problem
- Utilizes community resources and systems to implement a plan
- Collaborates with nursing colleagues and others.

Standard 5a: The Nurse Must Coordinate Care Delivery: *Measurement Criteria*

- Coordinates implementation of care
- Employs strategies to improve health and a safe environment
- Documents the coordination of care.

Standard 5b: Health Teaching: *Measurement Criteria*

- Provides health teaching that addresses healthy lifestyles, risk-reducing behavior, developmental needs, activities of daily living, and preventive self-care
- Seeks opportunities for feedback/evaluation of the effectiveness of strategies.

Standard 6: Evaluation: *Measurement Criteria*

- Evaluation of outcomes is systematic, ongoing, criteria based, and related to structures and processes in the plan and timeline
- Involving client and other care providers in the process, as appropriate
- Effectiveness of planned strategies evaluated by client responses and attainment of expected outcomes
- Documents the results of the evaluation
- Revise plan using ongoing assessment data (as needed)
- Disseminates results (as appropriate, by state and federal laws and regulations) to clients and others involved in care or situation
- ANA Standards of Professional Performance.

Standard 7: Quality of Care: *Measurement Criteria*

- Documents nursing process
- Initiates changes in nursing practice by using the results of quality improvement activities
- Uses innovation in nursing practice
- Participates in quality improvement activities to quality and effectiveness of nursing practice.

Standard 8: Training and Education: *Measurement Criteria*

- Participates in continuous educational activities
- Commits to lifelong learning
- Gets experiences that reflect current practice
- Maintains records
- Develops clinical and professional skills.

Standard 9: Evaluating Professional Practice: *Measurement Criteria*

- Provides age-appropriate care in a culturally and ethnically sensitive manner
- Engages in self-evaluation regularly by identifying an area of strength and areas for further professional development
- Obtains informal feedback regarding own practice from clients, peers, colleagues, and others.
- Participates in systematic peer review, as appropriate
- Provides rationales for practice beliefs, decisions, and acts as a part of the informal and formal evaluation processes.

Standard 10: Collegiality: *Measurement Criteria*

- Discusses with peers and colleagues about client care
- Provides peers with feedback regarding their practice or role performance
- Interacts with colleagues and team
- Maintains therapeutic and caring relationships with peers and colleagues
- Contributes to an environment conducive to the education of healthcare providers.

Standard 11: Collaboration: *Measurement Criteria*

- Communicates patient, family, and healthcare providers regarding care and the nurse's role in the provision of that care
- Collaborates with appropriate individuals in creating a documented plan focused on outcomes with decisions related to care and delivery of services that indicate the communication.

Standard 12: Ethics: *Measurement Criteria*

- Uses the current Code of Ethics for Nurses with Interpretive Statements (ANA) to guide practice
- Provides care to preserve and protect client autonomy, dignity, and rights
- Maintains client confidentiality within regulatory parameters
- Act as a client advocate and fosters skills for self-advocacy
- Maintains a therapeutic/professional client–nurse relationship
- Demonstrates commitment to practicing self-care, managing stress, and connecting with self and others
- Contributes to resolving ethical issues of clients, colleagues, or systems (i.e. ethics committees)
- Reports illegal, incompetent, or impaired practices.

Standard 13: Research: *Measurement Criteria*

- Utilizes the best available evidence to make decisions
- Participates in research activities.

Standard 14: Resource Utilization: *Measurement Criteria*

- Evaluates factors and impact on practice when choosing practice options that would result in the same expected outcome

- Assists the client and family to identify and secure appropriate/available services to address health-related needs
- Assigns or delegates task, based on the needs and condition of the client, potential for harm, stability of the client's situation, the complexity of the job, and predictability of the outcome
- Assists client and family to become informed consumers about options, costs, risks, and benefits of treatment and care.

Standard 15: Leadership: *Measurement Criteria*

- Engages in teamwork
- Creates and maintains healthy work environments
- Defines a clear vision, goals, and prepare a plan
- Commits to continuous, lifelong learning
- Provides health teachings
- Demonstrates creativity and flexibility
- Have a passion for quality work
- Promotes the advancement of the profession.

ANNEXURE 2

Canadian Nurses Association (CNA) Standards

1. **Professional Responsibility: Indicators**
    1.1. The registered nurse is accountable at all times for his or her actions.
    1.2. The registered nurse follows current legislation, standards, and policies relevant to the profession or practice setting.
    1.3. The certified nurse questions policies and procedures are inconsistent with therapeutic patient/client outcomes, best practices, and safety standards.
    1.4. The registered nurse engages in and supports others in the continuing competence process.
    1.5. The registered nurse participates in quality improvement activities.
    1.6. The certified nurse practices competently.
    1.7. The registered nurse regularly assesses his or her practice and takes the necessary steps to improve personal competence.
    1.8. The registered nurse ensures his or her fitness to practice.

2. **Knowledge-based Method: Indicators**
    2.1. The registered nurse supports decisions with evidence-based rationale.
    2.2. The registered nurse uses appropriate information and resources that enhance patient care and achievement of desired patient outcomes.
    2.3. The registered nurse demonstrates critical thinking in collecting and interpreting data, planning, implementing, and evaluating all aspects of nursing care.
    2.4. The registered nurse exercises reasonable judgment and sets justifiable priorities in practice.
    2.5. The certified nurse practices within his or her level of competence.
    2.6. The registered nurse documents timely, accurate reports of data collection, interpretation, planning, implementing, and evaluating nursing practice.
    2.7. The registered nurse supports, facilitates, or participates in research relevant to nursing.
    2.8. The registered nurse applies nursing knowledge and skill in providing safe, competent, ethical care. Regulated members perform restricted activities authorized under the HPA regulations that they are qualified to act if they are appropriate to the area of practice.

3. **Ethical Practice: Indicators**
    3.1. The certified nurse practices with honesty, integrity, and respect and complies with the CNA Code of Ethics (2002).
    3.2. The registered nurse reports unskilled practice or professional misconduct to the appropriate person, agency, or professional body.
    3.3. The certified nurse advocates protecting and promoting a client's right to autonomy, respect, privacy, dignity, and access to information.
    3.4. The registered nurse assumes responsibility for ensuring that their relationships with clients are therapeutic and professional.
    3.5. The certified nurse advocates for practice environments that have the organizational and human support systems and the resource allocations necessary for safe, competent, and ethical nursing care.

4. **Provision of Service to the Public: Indicators**
    4.1. The certified nurse collaborates with the client/family and other members of the health-care team regarding activities of care planning, implementation, and evaluation.
    4.2. The accredited nurse uses communication and team-building skills to enhance client care.
    4.3. The registered nurse is accountable for the supervision of other healthcare team members, and nursing students.
    4.4. The registered nurse explains nursing care to clients and others.

ANNEXURE 3

Nursing Practice Standards in India

PROFESSIONAL RESPONSIBILITY AND ACCOUNTABILITY

Standard 1: Nursing care based on the quality assurance model: The performance criteria are as follows:
- Demonstrate an understanding of the concept of quality assurance model
- Analyze and identify needs and problems
- Use relevant tools and processes to evaluate care
- Take appropriate action to improve quality.

Standard 2: Nursing care is professionally managed and ethically justified: The performance criteria are as follows:
- Demonstrate knowledge of current ethical issues in healthcare
- Maintain professional conduct and follow the code of ethics
- Participate effectively in ethical decision-making
- Demonstrate managerial skills
- Demonstrate a humanistic approach to management.

Standard 3: Nursing care provided within the legal framework: The performance criteria are as follows:
- The nurses should be aware of legal boundaries for their practice.
- They should perform activities that fall within those boundaries.
- They should recognize a breach of law related to practice and report to the appropriate authority.

Standard 4: Document nursing care: The performance criteria are as follows:
- Demonstrates an understanding of the value and implications of maintaining records.
- Maintains legible, complete, and accurate records
- Keeps records systematically and safely
- Maintains confidentiality of records.

Standard 5: Nurse accepts responsibility and accountability for their actions: The performance criteria are as follows:
- The nurse assumes and delegates responsibility within the scope of nursing practice and competence
- She consults other members of the nursing team when requisite nursing care is beyond her competence
- Consults other healthcare professionals as and when required.

NURSING PRACTICE

Standard 1: Nursing care reflects practice standards to adhere: Nurses are to:
- Demonstrate an understanding of standards for nursing practice
- Demonstrate adherence to the satisfactory level of practice standards
- Maintain records of the care that are congruent with practice standards.

Standard 2: Delivery of nursing care reflects the nursing process approach: The performance criteria are as follows:
- Conduct a systematic, complete, and accurate nursing assessment of their clients and groups
- Formulate a plan of actions based on priority needs
- Collaborates with individuals and groups in formulating the plan of care
- Implement the care per the policy
- Evaluate the outcomes of actions taken and revise the plan of care.

Standard 3: Nursing care should provide in a safe environment: The performance criteria are as follows:
- Ensure a safe and therapeutic environment in care settings
- Adhere to standard safety measures and universal precautions to prevent infections
- Follow guidelines for biomedical waste management
- Sensitize coworkers, individuals, and groups about the importance of a safe environment.

COMMUNICATION AND INTERPERSONAL RELATIONSHIPS

Standard 1: Nurse fosters a productive interpersonal relationship with the clients and families: The performance criteria are as follows:
- Maintain rapport with clients and their families
- Demonstrate effective communication skills
- Demonstrate the ability to listen attentively and patiently
- Respond empathetically and constructively to a concern expressed by them
- Foster environment that is conducive for communication
- Maintain interpersonal relationship within professional boundaries.

Standard 2: Nurse initiates strategies to promote the learning of clients and groups: Nurse needs to:
- Identify learning needs of client and groups
- Optimize learning opportunities for them
- Conduct planned and incidental teaching
- Evaluate the outcome of the teaching-learning process.

VALUING HUMAN BEINGS

Standard 1: Nursing care enhances the dignity, individuality, and self-esteem of individuals and groups: Nurses are expected to:
- Convey respects to individuals in all dealings

- Promote and support self-awareness, self-esteem, and self-determination among individuals.

Standard 2: Nursing care reflects active pursuit for the rights of all individuals, and in particular the vulnerable groups: The performance criteria are as follows:
- Describe the constitutional and legal rights of individuals
- Inform and educate an individual about their rights
- Seek consent of individuals after adequate and factual information
- Respect the rights individuals and families to refuse care after ensuring that they understand the consequences of refusal per policy
- Mobilize support of health team members, families, and communities for the protection of the rights of vulnerable groups.

Standard 3: Nursing care reflects gender sensitivity toward the needs of women related to their health: The performance criteria are as follows:
- Describe the cultural, social, economic, and political context in which women live
- Promote and support self-awareness, self-esteem, and self-determination among women
- Enhance the dignity of them as reflected in dealing with them
- Promote health-seeking behavior in women.

MANAGEMENT

Standard 1: Management of nursing services reveals effective management techniques: The performance criteria are as follows:
- Demonstrate understanding of different management techniques
- Applies appropriate management techniques based on situational analysis
- Initiate activities for the enhancement of own managerial skills.

Standard 2: Management of nursing services reflects the use of quality assurance model: The performance criteria are as follows:
- Appreciate the significance of the Quality Assurance Programme for quality nursing care
- Demonstrate an understanding of Quality Assurance Programme and own role in the implementation
- Involve team members in the development and implementation of Quality Assurance Programme.

Standard 3: Management of nursing services organizes and utilizes resources efficiently: The performance criteria are as follows:
- Assess the essential requirement of funds for the delivery of quality nursing care
- Demonstrate an understanding of the system for procuring, using and monitoring of resources
- Delegate responsibilities to appropriate team members for inventory control
- Ensure preventive maintenance of equipment.

Standard 4: Management of nursing services contributes to the development and implementation of institutional policies in conformity with statutory regulations: The performance criteria are as follows:
- Demonstrate an understanding of institutional policy and statutory regulations
- Provides to framing and reviewing the institutional policy as per statutory regulations
- Communicate the policies, rules, and regulations to concerned persons and ensure compliance.

Standard 5: Management of nursing services develops and implements staff development and welfare programmes: The performance criteria are as follows:
- Prepare a plan for the staff development
- Facilitate implementation of staff development-related services
- Participate in continuing educational programs
- Motivate the nurses for participation.

Standard 6: Management of nursing services ensures disaster preparedness: The performance criteria are as follows:
- Participate in an institutional plan for disaster preparedness
- Organize training and drill for the members of the disaster management.

PROFESSIONAL DEVELOPMENT

Standard 1: Nursing care reflects the commitment to ongoing education and professional growth of self and others: The performance criteria are as follows:
- Participate in continuing education program
- Review current literature
- Participate in professional meetings to professional journals
- Identify learning needs.

Standard 2: Nursing care includes activities, which focus on the advancement of a profession: The performance criteria are as follows:
- Identify the requirements for change in scope of nursing practice
- Participate in research activities
- Conducts nursing research
- Interpret and utilize research findings in nursing practice
- Contribute to advancement in nursing.

52 CHAPTER

Nursing Audit

CHAPTER OUTLINE

- Nursing Audit
  - Audit
  - Clinical Audit
  - Definition of Nursing Audit
  - Objectives of Nursing Audit
  - Importance of Nursing Audit
  - Advantages and Disadvantages of Nursing Audit
  - Bases of Nursing Audit
  - Types of Nursing Audit
- Nursing Audit Process
- Role of Nurse Managers in Nursing Audit

LEARNING OUTCOMES

After completion of this chapter, the learner will be able to:
- Discuss the historical background of nursing audit
- Define audit, nursing audit, and clinical audit
- Enlist objectives of nursing audit
- Discuss the importance of nursing audit
- Enumerate advantages and disadvantages of nursing audit
- Describe bases for nursing audit in the hospital setting
- Explain different types of nursing audit
- Discuss the process of nursing audit
- Define the role of nurse managers in nursing audit

KEY TERMS

Audit, nursing audit, clinical audit, audit process, debit, standard

INTRODUCTION

An audit has become a mechanism for assessing and improving the quality of work and identifying ways of improving the efficiency of care. Due to an increase in the complexity of healthcare and awareness among people for their rights necessitate that nurses to become accountable for their practice.

The concept of audit rooted as early as during the Crimean war of 1853–1855 undertaken by Florence Nightingale. It was first advocated by Ernest Codman (renamed as a valid medical auditor) in 1912 on monitoring surgical outcomes. The first report of the nursing audit of the hospital was published in 1955.

In the United States, since 1974, a medical audit has become a legal requirement for patients to ensure standards of care. In 1990, the American Institute of Certified Public Accountants issued a revised guide entitled Audits of Providers of Health Care Services to replace its 1972—Hospital Audit Guide.

In India, health survey and planning committee appointed by Government of India (Mudaliar Committee Report, 1961) reported that medical audit is a new concept and till 1992; it remains as a maiden concept, but now professional review is becoming increasingly aware of rights, cost, and minimal standards of healthcare, and in the near future, hospital including nursing services will be audited or accredited. Accredited agencies are already on the move toward this motto.

NURSING AUDIT

Audit

The term "audit" means "an official examination of a business or financial records to see that they are true and correct." It is also an official examination of the quality or standard of something. According to the Medical Dictionary, an audit is a systematic reviewing of documentation to find out the level of the quality of the services rendered in a given situation.

An audit is a process by which someone looks at the result of an activity and makes a judgment about whether done to the level expected, as set out by preset rules, guidelines or standards.

Clinical Audit

1. The clinical audit is the systematic and critical analysis of the procedure used for diagnosis, care, and treatment, associated use of resources, and the effect care has on the outcome and quality of life for the patient (Department of Health, London, 1993).
2. Clinical audit is multiprofessional, patient-focused check, leading to cost-effective, high-quality care delivery in the clinical teams (Batstone and Edwards).
3. Clinical audit is a clinically led initiative to improve the outcome of patient care via structured review—clinicians examine their practice and results against agreed standards and modify their practice where indicated (Mann, 1996).

Definition of Nursing Audit

1. According to the Medical Dictionary, a *nursing audit* is a review of the performance record of patients specifying nursing care through established criteria. *A nursing audit* is a formal, detailed systematic review of records or observation of nursing actions to assess the quality of nursing care by comparing the documented evidence with accepted standards and criteria (RANF, 1985).
2. *The nursing audit* is the examination of a patient record to determine the degree to which nursing care was satisfactory according to prescribed standards and to collect data as a base for corrective action (Donovan).
3. *A nursing audit* is a form of quality assurance. It is a systematic and critical analysis of nursing care carried out by nursing personnel by using available resources and the outcomes for patients/clients to make appropriate improvements according to the report.

The nursing audit is an umbrella term used for nursing in totality, whereas clinical examination is a part of the nursing audit. The nursing audit is the evaluation of nursing services by nursing personnel, including nurse administrators, through observation, questioning, and records. It is a method by which nurses compare actual practice against preset standards and identify areas for improving their care. It is also a method of examining the quality of nursing care systematically.

Objectives of Nursing Audit

The following list shows the objectives of nursing audit:
- To evaluate and try to improve the expected quality of nursing
- To measure the level of quality of patient care against standards
- To minimize the cost of rendering nursing care
- To have a basis for detecting nursing negligence
- To take remedial measures towards cost-effectiveness
- To provide education to all nursing personnel through self-education
- To prevent shortcomings from reoccurring
- To provide a database for planning resources by getting information on what resources are being used redeployment for productive use
- To improve knowledge and skill by learning from past mistakes
- To avoid external auditing.

Importance of Nursing Audit

The list below shows the importance of nursing audit:
- It serves as a valuable indicator to measure quality care.
- It focuses on care provided and not on the care provider.
- It helps in improving the quality of nursing.
- It facilitates to attain more efficient use of health-care resources.
- It assists in maintaining the quality and accuracy of nursing records.

Advantages and Disadvantages of Nursing Audit

Advantages
- Its utilization as a method of measurement is in all areas of nursing.
- It may be a useful tool as a part of the quality assurance program in documentation.
- It is a process to understand its outcomes.

Disadvantages
- Since many of the components overlap that makes analysis difficulty.
- It is time consuming.
- It requires a team of trained auditors.
- It deals with information.

Bases of Nursing Audit

The nursing audit in the hospital setting includes debt items, credit items, nursing auditors, quality, nursing standards, defined activities, and resources (**Fig. 52.1**).

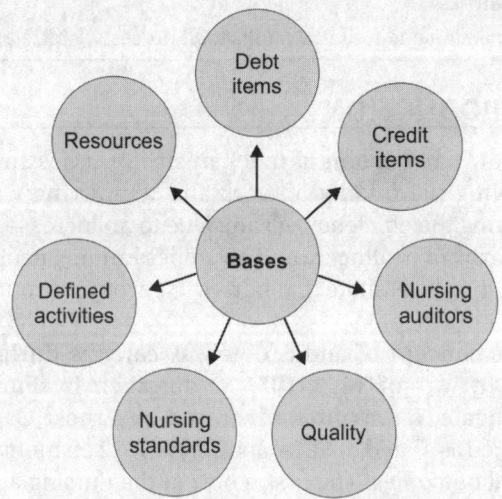

Fig. 52.1: Bases of nursing audit.

1. **Debit items:** These are items that give discredit to institutes, e.g. several deaths, complications of the disease, hospital infections, errors in treatment, patients left against medical advice, untoward reactions, etc. These variables are against the quality of care and hence referred as debit items.
2. **Credit items:** These are the items or the variables that give credit to the care rendered, e.g. several recovered/discharge patients, expansion in patients' knowledge, a shorter stay of patients, etc. are the examples of this type of item.
3. **Nursing auditors:** These are the personnel trained as auditors. They are both internal and external. Internal auditors work within an organization and responsible for internal auditing. External auditors are external parties.
4. **Quality:** It is a degree of excellence that needs to define and predetermine based on the nursing audit.
5. **Nursing standards:** The nursing standards are valid and explicit statements about the quality of facts of nursing care. These are structure, process, and outcome standards. The structure standards relate to characteristics of health-care institutions, men, money, material, methods required for the nursing organization; process standard is the performance of nursing care delivered by the care providers, and outcome standard indicates results about objectives of the nursing organization and that of the health-care institution.
6. **Defined activities:** These are the goal-oriented transactions required to carry out for auditing.
7. **Resources:** Resources include human and material required for auditing and desired healthcare.

Types of Nursing Audit

There are various ways of classifying audits in the literature. The essential methods of categorizing audits are according to the methodology adopted for auditing and according to the type of agency carried out **(Fig. 52.2)**.

According to Methodology

a. **Retrospective audit:** It is a type of inspection conducted after an event takes place. It means looking back at what has happened in the past. It carries out after the discharge of patients, usually through observations and analyzing patient records, nursing care plans, questionnaires, interviews, and surveys of the patients, administrative, and other documents.

Advantages
1. It relies on records; hence it is easy to gather information and analyze data.
2. It needs less time as compared to concurrent audit.
3. It is less costly than a parallel review, and at one time total data can be gathered.

Disadvantages
1. It may not get accurate, and up to date information if documentation not done properly.
2. The records may not be error free.
3. This type of audit will not reveal actual care received by the client.
4. Chance of having manipulative data.

b. **Concurrent audit:** Concurrent auditing is also called prospective verification. Concurrent means were happening at the same time. It is a method of evaluating ongoing nursing care rendered by nurses to the individual patient. The information gathered simultaneously with the nursing care given to the patient by the caregivers or through observing patients directly during ongoing nursing care or interviewing nurse for the care rendered to the patient. The tools used for auditing include observation checklist, interview guide, rating scales, opinionnaire, etc.

Advantages
1. It is easy to pinpoint deficiencies in the caring patient in the actual situation.
2. It provides a mechanism to identify, meeting client needs, and communicating with the client.

Disadvantages
1. It is costly and needs prior preparation as compared to retrospective audit.
2. It is time consuming and required well-trained auditors.
3. There are chances of introducing the halo effect.

c. **Mixed methods audit:** These are both retrospective and concurrent. Both methods used for auditing patient care. Observation, interviewing, questionnaires, and record analysis are the techniques used for this purpose.

According to Agency

a. **Internal audit:** The peers or nursing personnel conduct internal audits continuously. They are the employees of an organization and appointed by the authority in the audit committee. The internal auditors abstract and classify clinical records and evaluate the quality of nursing care. Internal auditing is desirable. There are norms and standards for auditing. Concurrent auditing is also an internal audit.

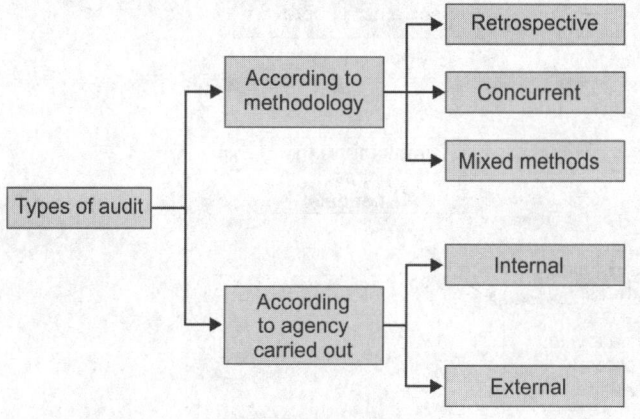

Fig. 52.2: Types of audit.

b. **External audit:** The outside agency conducts the external audit. Usually, periodically tests, completeness, and accuracy of internal audits are done by external auditors annually. Sometimes nonprofessional administrators conduct an audit.

NURSING AUDIT PROCESS

The nursing audit process undergoes six phases: the planning phase, the preparation phase, implementing phase, analysis and finding gap phase, improvement phase, and sustaining improvement phase **(Fig. 52.3)**.

1. **Planning phase:** The describing step includes activities like identification of a topic, constituting audit committee, setting criteria and standards, and developing audit protocol.
   a. *Identify subject:* It involves identifying or selecting a topic for auditing. Select an essential or significant issue. Use various sources to find out multiple matters of importance from numerous sources such as:
      ♦ Indian Nursing Council or hospital standards
      ♦ Problem encountering in practice
      ♦ Patients and public recommendation
      ♦ Scope for improving service delivery
      ♦ Area of high volume, high risk, or high cost
   b. *Constitute audit committee:* Audit committees comprising a minimum of five competent and interested members either from interdisciplinary or multidisciplinary. They should work together in a group.

The audit committee should have chairman, clinical consultants, representative of the hospital administrator, statistical record officer, nursing personnel, specialized experts. Make sure who all involved in auditing, agree with the topic selected, and also make sure that no other team is working on the same issue.

   c. *Set criteria and standards:* Criteria are measurable outcomes of care written in a statement form and used to evaluate the quality. A standard is a level or degree of the expected compliance or outcome for each criterion. These are generally expressed in percentages and represent the minimum level of acceptable performance for that criterion. The evidence and research studies must support, if not available, should develop on a consensus agreement by members of the team. Try to take up one or two criteria at one time for auditing. The established standards should have objectivity, verifiability, uniformity, specificity, and acceptability.

The elements contain criteria, which should be reliable, understandable, measurable, and acceptable (Kitson et al. 1990).

   d. *Develop an audit protocol:* A protocol is a type of document intended for general reference outlines the broad view and work plan for auditing. It is the checklist to be used by the auditors as a guide for conducting audit activities. An audit protocol should include the following:
   1. Audit objectives: The aims and objectives should be noticeable, specific, and measurable.

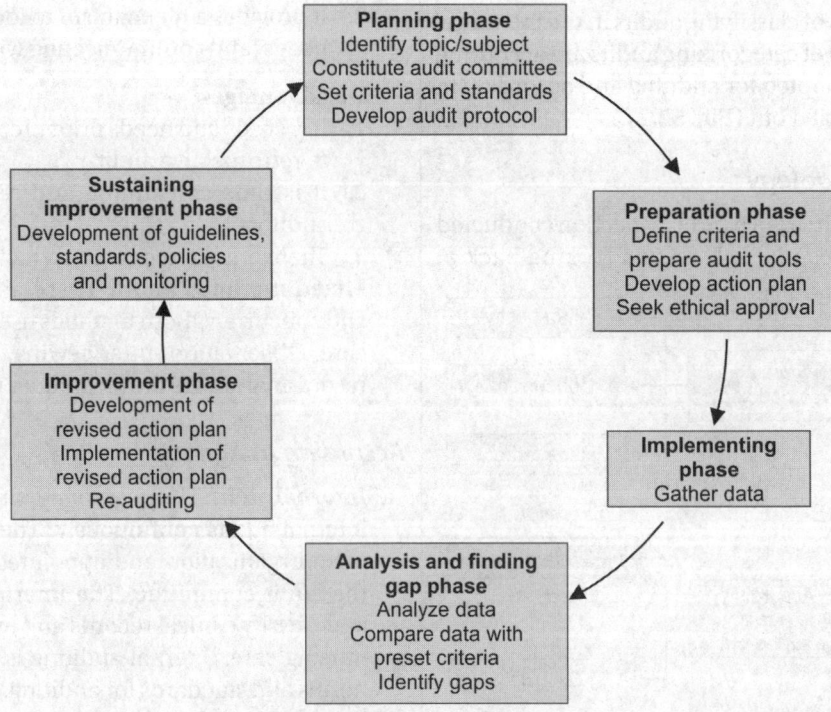

Fig. 52.3: Audit process.

2. The target group: Identify the target group for auditing.
 3. Selection of audit sample: Out of the target group, select the sample size, the sample should be representative of the target group, and sample size should also be sufficient to generalize the findings.
 4. Method of data collection: Questioning, observation, checking the record, measurement, computer, and paper record, data collection sheets. The electronic data are preferred as they are likely to be quicker and more accurate.
 5. Development of tools: Develop tools on the basis of information gathered related to staff, standards of care, patient satisfaction, and effect on organization through patient satisfaction survey, staff satisfaction survey, nursing records audit, throughput and bed occupancy, length of stay of patients, supply and demand study, staff development, sickness and absenteeism, and medical review of postoperative complications.
 6. Data collection procedure: The procedure to be followed for data gathering need to discuss and finalize.
 7. Plan for analysis: Include the appropriate methods: descriptive and inferential analysis in the protocol.

2. **Preparation phase**
   a. *Define criteria and prepare audit tools*
      - Select criteria
      - Define criteria
      - Prepare a rough draft of audit tools
      - Check content validity of tools
      - Check reliability of devices
      - Check reliability of electronic audit tools.
   b. *Develop an action plan*
      The plan should include the following:
      - Who is going to gather information? Select auditors, trained auditors, plan orientation programs for them before they do auditing. They need to skilled and thorough with the subject matter and handle the problem if it arises while gathering information.
      - The period of gathering information. Specify the period.
      - The size of the target group at one time.
   c. *Seek ethical approval*
      - Seek clearance from the ethical committee of the institute for clinical/nursing audit.
      - Get permission from the subjects per the criteria laid down.

3. **Implementation phase**
   a. *Gather data:*
      - Collect the audit data per the developed action plan and protocol.
      - Use tools and audit forms carefully.
      - Be transparent and honest in gathering information.

4. **Analysis and finding gap phase**
   a. *Analyze data:* After collection, analyze the data. Apply appropriate statistics; usually, calculated in percentage to determine the level standard.
   b. *Compare data:* Compare data with set or predetermined criteria and standard.
   c. *Identify gaps and make an audit summary:* Specify the standards achieved and the reasons for failure to meet the criteria in some cases. Make a brief report and give recommendations after a discussion with the audit team.

5. **Improvement phase:** This stage is one of the most crucial and the most difficult. After analyzing, the audit committee needs to make improvements and sustain improvements made.
   a. *Development of a revised action plan:* Decide areas requiring improvement. Make a detailed action plan.
   b. *Implementation of the revised action plan:* Put the plan into action and monitor changes made.
   c. *Re-auditing:* Plan and do re-auditing to find out how far nursing practices are improved.

6. **Sustaining improvement phase:** This phase describes the ways of continuing improvement in nursing practice. It needs the development of guidelines, standards, policies, and monitoring.

ROLE OF NURSE MANAGERS IN NURSING AUDIT

Nurse managers in the hospital setting can play an essential role in initiating and implementing nursing audits. These are as follows:

1. Appoint an audit committee with approval from an appropriate authority
2. Constitute audit committee; select members
3. Conduct regular meetings with members
4. Have a grand round with audit committee members
5. Make a priority list of problems and issues
6. Follow all steps of the audit process
7. Plan and conduct an orientation program for auditors
8. Make sure that auditors are honest in data gathering and sensitive to attitude and feelings of subjects
9. Make realistic recommendations for improvement if required
10. Ready with the action plan
11. Implement change if required and monitor the progress
12. Make audit a continuous process by implementing and re-auditing
13. Use the guiding approach rather than fault finding
14. Keep a record of all information and remedial action taken.

The purpose of the nursing audit should be for planning, evaluation, education, and research and overall improving nursing practices and procedures up to the satisfaction of patients. It needs to be introduced in all the hospitals, institutions by trained experts, and motivating administrators at all levels.

CHAPTER HIGHLIGHTS

- The concept of audit rooted as early as during the Crimean war of 1853–1855 by Florence Nightingale.
- In India, Mudaliar Committee Report (1961) reported the concept of the medical audit.
- An audit is an official examination of quality or standard of something; clinical review is the systematic and critical analysis of the nursing care.
- A nursing audit is a formal, detailed systematic review of records or observation of nursing actions to assess the quality of nursing care.
- The nursing audit in the hospital setting includes debt items, credit items, nursing auditors, quality, nursing standards, defined activities, and resources.
- Audits classified based on methodology as retrospective, concurrent, and mixed methods, and according to the type of audit: internal or external audits.
- The nursing audit process undergoes describing, preparing and implementing, and analysis and concluding phases.
- Nurse managers in the hospital setting can play an essential role in initiating and implementing nursing audits and can introduce in all clinical settings.

REVIEW QUESTIONS

I. Essay Type Questions
1. Define nursing audits and enlist objectives of nursing audits.
2. Discuss the importance of nursing audit.
3. Write the advantages and disadvantages of having nursing audits in the clinical area.
4. What are the different types of audit? Discuss.
5. Describe the nursing audit process.

II. Short Notes
1. Basis of nursing audit
2. Retrospective audit
3. Role of nurse managers in nursing audit
4. Bases of a nursing audit

III. Multiple Choice Questions
1. Which of the following year, the concept of audit rooted?
   a. 1850
   b. 1853
   c. 860
   d. 1872
2. The systematic and critical analysis of the procedure used for diagnosis, care, and treatment, utilizing available resources, and quality of life for the patient is:
   a. Clinical audit
   b. Management audit
   c. Financial audit
   d. Nursing audit
3. The issues like increase in death rate, complications of the disease, hospital infections, errors in treatment, patients left against medical advice, untoward reactions, etc. indicate:
   a. Process items
   b. Standard items
   c. Credit items
   d. Debit items
4. The measurable outcome of care written in a statement form and used to evaluate the quality is:
   a. Standard
   b. Criterion
   c. Protocol
   d. Procedure
5. In an audit process, the area of high volume, high risk or high cost, etc. are considered for:
   a. Setting criteria
   b. Developing standard
   c. Identifying a topic
   d. Developing an audit protocol

Answer Keys
1. b 2. a 3. d 4. b 5. c

SUGGESTED READING

1. Audit. [Online] Available from http://medical-dictionary.thefreedictionary.com/retrospective+audit.
2. Benjamin A. Audit: how to do it in practice. BMJ. 2008, 336:1241.
3. Cheater FM, Keane M. Nurses' participation in an audit: a regional study. Qual Health Care. 1998;7(1):27-36.
4. Donabedian A. Criteria and standards for quality monitoring. Qual Rev Bull. 1986;12(3):99-100.
5. Donabedian A. The quality of care: how can it be assessed? JAMA. 1988;260(12):1743-8.
6. Fraser RC, Khunti K, Baker R, Lakhani M. Effective audit in general practice: a method for systematically developing audit protocols containing evidence-based audit criteria. Br J Gen Pract. 1997;47(424):743-6.
7. Gillies DA. Nursing Management—A System Approach. Philadelphia: WB Saunders; 1994.
8. Griffiths P, Debbage S, Smith A. A comprehensive audit of nursing record-keeping practice. Br J Nurs. 2007;16(21); 1324-7.
9. Hearnshaw H, Baker R, Cooper A. A survey of audit activity in general practice. Br J Gen Pract. 1998;48(427):979-81.
10. Huntington J, Gillam S, Rosen R. Clinical governance in primary care: organizational development for clinical management. BMJ. 2000;321(7262):679-82.
11. Jamtvedt GM, Young JM, Kristofferson DT, O'Brien MA, Oxman AD. Cochrane Database Syst Rev. 2012;2:CD000259.
12. Kaur K, Vati J, Kalia R. A descriptive study on the maintenance of intake and output documents at Nehru Hospital, PGIMER, Chandigarh. Nurs Midwifery Res J. 2005;1(2):115-23.
13. Kitson A, Hyndman S, Harvey G, Yerrell P. Quality Patient Care: The Dynamic Standard-Setting System. London: Scutari Press; 1990.
14. Lomas C. How to carry out a clinical audit. Nurs Times. 2005;101(7):46-47.
15. Roberts C. Improving nursing records with an audit. Nurs Standard. 1993;51(7):37-9.
16. Walker L, Minchin A, Pickard J. Setting standards for planning off duty and audit of practice. Nurs Times. 2006;102(21):30-2.
17. Younger D, Martin GW. Dementia care mappings: an approach to the quality audit of services for people with dementia in two health districts. J Adv Nurs. 2000;32(5):1206-12.

53
CHAPTER

Accreditation

CHAPTER OUTLINE

- Accreditation
  - Meaning
  - Definitions
  - Characteristics of Accreditation
  - Scope of Accreditation
  - Aims of Accreditation
  - Benefits of Accreditation
  - Accreditation Process
  - Models for Accreditation
- Types of Accrediting Agencies in India
- National Assessment and Accreditation Council
- INC as an Accreditation Body
- Accreditation of Hospitals
  - Umbrella Accreditation Organizations
  - International Health-Care Accreditation Organizations
  - Hospital Accreditation System in India
  - National Hospital Accreditation Organization: National Accreditation Board for Hospitals and Health Care Providers

LEARNING OUTCOMES

After completion of this chapter, the learner will be able to:
- Understand the concept of accreditation
- Discuss the characteristics and benefits of accreditation
- Enumerate aims and purposes of accreditation
- Discuss various types of accrediting agencies
- Describe the accreditation process
- Discuss the accreditation process of National Assessment and Accreditation Council (NAAC), Indian Nursing Council (INC), and National Accreditation Board for Hospitals and Healthcare Providers (NABH)

KEY TERMS

Accreditation, accreditation agencies, accreditation process, National Assessment and Accreditation Council, NABH

INTRODUCTION

Quality of the health-care delivery system has become a focus all around the world. Accreditation has gained worldwide attention as a practical quality evaluation and management tool. Moreover, the demand for quality health-care services is increasing as consumers have been becoming increasingly aware of their rights, demanding a better quality of healthcare; the cost of health-care services is rising, and there is a lack of enforcement in the existing legislation for health-care services.

In India, the quality of health-care delivery systems in public as well as in private sector through questionable and has remained mostly fragmented and uncontrolled, but the focus on accreditation movement is gearing up, not just the achievement of a certificate or award or merely assuring compliance with minimum acceptable standards. There are three integral aspects of assuming a flow of competent practitioners into a profession: high-quality preparing programs, accreditation of the programs, and licensure of graduates. Accreditation of application is an essential aspect, whereby institution also needs to be accredited.

ACCREDITATION

Meaning

Accreditation is the mark of quality given, after evaluation, by an external body. The dictionary meaning of this term is "official recognition, general acceptance, and assurance of quality" and certificate of meeting all the requirements. Generally, the definition of accreditation "to trust," "to give authority to," and "to give credit to" is accepted.

Accreditation is a process to certify competency, authority, or credibility. It is a voluntary process to have optimal and achievable standards. It is an indicator of professional achievement and quality of care. It differs from licensure and certification.

Licensure is a necessary process that requires health-care institutions to meet established minimum standards to operate. Certification is a voluntary governmental or nongovernmental process that grants recognition to health-care institutions that meet specific standards and qualifies them to advertise services or to receive payment or funding for services provided.

Definitions

- John Braithwaite (2001) defines accreditation as a process of assessment to evaluate the level of performance in health institutions through self and by the external peer to establish standards and to implement ways to improve.
- According to Tempus (2001), it is a formal procedure used to determine competence. Harvey (2004) considered it as the establishment of the status, legitimacy or appropriateness of an institution, program, or module of study.
- In the context of medical education, it is a self-regulatory process to grant recognition to health institutions or organizations. The governmental, nongovernmental, voluntary associations or other statutory bodies give formal recognition to health-care institutions that meet specific stated criteria of educational quality. It is usually optional, time limited, and based on periodic assessments by the accrediting body.

Characteristics of Accreditation

1. Accreditation is a process applied to applicant organizations.
2. It is the label that institutions or programs may acquire as a result of accreditation procedures.
3. It is a formal authorizing power about recognition.
4. It is a legal, voluntary, and time limited.
5. It is an overall assessment of the institution and its programs.
6. It needs to meet at least minimum requirements.
7. It concerns a yes/no/conditional decision.

Scope of Accreditation

1. **Service**
   - Accreditation ensures a level of quality and thus results in high quality of care and patient safety.
   - It provides public recognition in terms of the level of performance about the standards.
   - The patients get services by credential staff and thus protecting the rights of patients.
   - It attracts foreign patients by ensuring the delivery of best services.
   - It helps to improve the quality of patient care, to ensure a safe environment, and to reduce risks to patients and staff.
   - It helps in elevating effectiveness, efficiency and cost containment, and accountability, and the need to reduce errors and increase safety in the system.
   - It helps to bring a fundamental change in the technical procedures of service delivery and ensure social participation.
   - Accreditation to a hospital stimulates continuous improvement and enables hospitals to demonstrate a commitment to quality care.
   - It also provides an opportunity for health-care units to benchmark with the best.
   - It brings satisfaction among staff and provides continuous learning, a pleasant working environment, leadership for them, and thus improve the overall professional development of staff and provides guidance for quality improvement within nursing.

2. **Education**
   - Accreditation offers a base for both quantity and quality (relevance and excellence of academic programs offered) of higher education.
   - It helps the institution to know its strengths, weaknesses, and opportunities through an informed review process.
   - It helps institutions to identify internal areas of planning and resource allocation, innovative, and modern methods of pedagogy.
   - The outcome provides objective data to funding agencies for performance funding.
   - It provides reliable information on the quality of education offered.
   - Employers have access to information on the quality of education offered to potential recruiters.
   - Promotes intra- and inter-institutional interactions.
   - It provides greater efficiency and more accountability and prevents negligence.

Aims of Accreditation

1. To gain citizen and employee confidence in the goals, objectives, policies, and nursing practices.
2. To maintain minimum standards.
3. To increase institutional capabilities to prevent and control errors.
4. To increase departmental effectiveness and efficiency in the delivery of nursing services.
5. To enhance cooperation and coordination among staff.

Benefits of Accreditation

1. Provides a yardstick to measure the effectiveness of the programs and services.
2. Defines services provided and ensure uniformity of services offered.

Chapter 53: Accreditation

3. Streamlines operations and continually get feedbacks.
4. Provides more effective infrastructure.
5. Creates high morale and a positive attitude among hospital staff.

Accreditation Process

The steps for accreditation program are as follows (**Fig. 53.1**):
1. Application for accreditation and registration
2. Self-appraisal
3. On the site visit
4. Report preparation
5. Awarding certification
6. Maintaining accreditation status.

Models of Accreditation

1. **Standard oriented:** The standard oriented model of assessment gives priority to standards related to available facility norms, equipment requirements, human resources, and space specifications.
2. **Quality assurance oriented:** The quality assurance-oriented model of accreditation gives priority to quality assurance. It sets criteria and indicators for institutions striving to attain an expected level of quality care.
3. **Health service oriented:** According to the health service-oriented model, the accreditation criteria are accessible and acceptable health systems to health seekers. It gives priority to health consumers to evaluate health systems. The leading indicators for assessing health systems are by providing user-friendly services, providing information about the services available, having redressing grievance procedures, etc. These are patient-centric indicators and bring accountability of the health system to the health seekers.

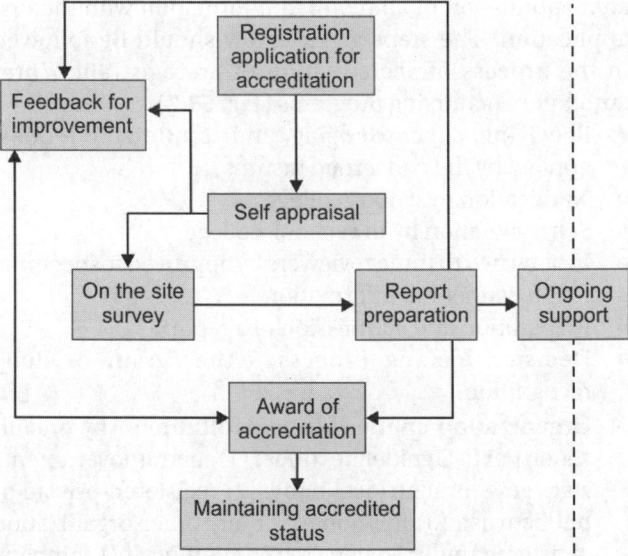

Fig. 53.1: Steps of the accreditation process.

TYPES OF ACCREDITATION AGENCIES IN INDIA

1. **For education**
   i. *National educational accrediting agencies*
      There are many national accrediting agencies such as Central Advisory Board of Education (CABS), All India Council for Elementary Education, All India Council for Secondary Education, University Grants Commission (UGC), and All India Council for Technical Education, National Assessment and Accreditation Council (NAAC), etc.
   ii. *National professional accrediting agencies*
      These are Medical Council of India, Dental Council of India, Pharmacy Council of India, Indian Nursing Council, etc.
2. **Healthcare**
   i. *Health-care accrediting agencies*
      It includes the National Accreditation Board of Hospitals and Health Care Providers, Quality Council of India (QCI), Indian Hospitals Association (IHA), The Bureau of Indian Standards, Joint Commission International (JCI), etc.

NATIONAL ASSESSMENT AND ACCREDITATION COUNCIL

National Assessment and Accreditation Council (NAAC) is an autonomous institution established in 1994 by the UGC. It is engaged in assessment, accreditation, and academic audit of universities, constituent, and affiliated colleges.

Assessment Process

National Assessment and Accreditation Council has formulated a three-stage process for assessment and accreditation as follows:
1. **Institutional eligibility for quality assessment:** The applicant institution applies for Institutional Eligibility for Quality Assessment (IEQA) at the planning stage. It helps institution in various ways as (1) to get recognized as eligible, (2) to use next accreditation process, (3) to get feedback from NAAC if it does not qualify in the first attempt by making specific improvements to achieve required quality level, and (4) to receive assistance and suitable mentoring from NAAC in the latter case to qualify for IEQA in due course of time.
2. **Preparation of self-study report by the institution:** After getting IEQA, the applicant institution prepares self-study report (SSR) per the guidelines of the NAAC and submits it to NAAC.
3. **Peer team visit to the institution:** National Assessment and Accreditation Council does an in-house analysis of data sent by the institution and prepares a report. After that, the NAAC selects a peer team comprising trained members and chairperson to visit the

institution and fixes dates for a visit. NAAC informs the applicant institution about a visit. The group, per plan, does physical verification, which is followed by a presentation of a comprehensive assessment report to the institution. After clarifying any queries by the institution, peer team assigns grade per NAAC guidelines.

Evaluation Framework

1. **Criteria for assessment:** There are seven criteria to serve as the basis of its assessment procedures. Each approach has key aspects, highlights, and tentative grades. These criteria are concerning with curriculum development and implementation process and verified by peer group. Standards and its key elements are as follows:
    i. *Curricular aspects:* It covers four key aspects, i.e. curriculum design and development, academic flexibility, curriculum enrichment, and feedback system.
    ii. *Teaching, learning and evaluation:* This criterion covers six key aspects as student enrollment and profile, catering to student diversity, teaching-learning process, teacher quality, evaluation process and reforms, and student performance and learning outcomes.
    iii. *Research, consultancy, and extension:* It also has six key aspects as promotion of research, resource mobilization, research facilities, research publications and awards, consultancy, and extension activities and institutional social responsibilities.
    iv. *Infrastructure and learning resources:* This criterion covers four/five key aspects, i.e. physical facilities, clinical and laboratory learning facilities, library as a learning resource, IT infrastructure, and maintenance of campus facilities.
    v. *Student support and progression:* It has three aspects, i.e. student mentoring and support, student progression, student participation, and activities.
    vi. *Governance and leadership and management:* It concerns five significant key aspects, i.e. institution vision and leadership, strategy development and deployment, faculty empowerment strategies, financial management and resource management, and internal quality assurance system.
    vii. *Innovative practices:* It covers three significant vital aspects, which are environment consciousness, innovations, and best practices.
2. **Grading system:** Usually, three steps are undertaken to assign a grade to institute/program. These are as follows:
    i. *Key aspect-wise grade points:* Identify each key aspects with strengths/weaknesses and issues. Based on the identified key aspects, assign tentative KAGPs on a five-point Likert scale ranging from 0 to 4. Based on the weightage assigned to each key aspect, calculate key aspect-wise weighted grade points.
    ii. *Criterion-wise grade point average:* Based on all identified KAGPs for a particular criterion, calculate criterion-wise weighted grade point (CrWGP). (Each measure has weight (W), and all total score of all seven measures is 1000.)
    iii. *Cumulative grade point average and assigning institutional grade:* Cumulative grade point average (CGPA) is calculated using formula. Based on result, the letter grade is assigned according to CGPA achieved by institution. The letter grades are classified as A++ (CGPA= 3.76 - 4.00) or A+ (CGPA= 3.51 - 3.75) or A (CGPA= 3.01 - 3.50) or B++ (CGPA= 2.76 - 3.00) or B+ (CGPA = 2.51 - 2.75) or B (CGPA=2.01 - 2.50) or C (CGPA= 1.51 - 2.00) (all stands for accredited) or D stands for not accredited.

INC AS AN ACCREDITATION BODY

The INC is an autonomous statutory body that regulates the functioning of all nursing programs. Its main objectives are to assess and accredit institutions based on the minimum laid down standards for nursing institutions, to assist in improving quality of education, to revise curriculum, and to recognize various nursing qualifications.

Process of Accreditation

The purpose of accreditation is to give official recognition to the nursing institute/organization to start a General Nursing/BSc Nursing and other nursing programs against prescribed standards at the time of establishing school/college of nursing. In contrast, accreditation at the time of renewal/validation of program/upgradation of school to college of nursing is a must for quality assurance. The accreditation process takes at least 9 months to complete after submission of all required information with the first application. The steps given below should be followed in the process of accreditation of preregistration/pre-enrollment of nursing programs **(Fig. 53.2)**:

- Receiving, acknowledging, and scrutinizing request applied by the concerned institute
- Notification to school/college
- Self-evaluation by the school/college
- Visit by two to three reviewers by approved inspector of INC to gather the information
- Preparation and submission of a report
- Decision-making process: either grant or deny recognition.

1. **Organization applies for accreditation:** Any organization per INC guidelines under (1) central government/state government/local body, (2) registered private or public trust, (3) missionary or any other organization registered under Society Registration Act, (4) company incorporated under section 25 of company's act submits online application along with a proposal of an SSR, which is in the format as specified in the "Handbook

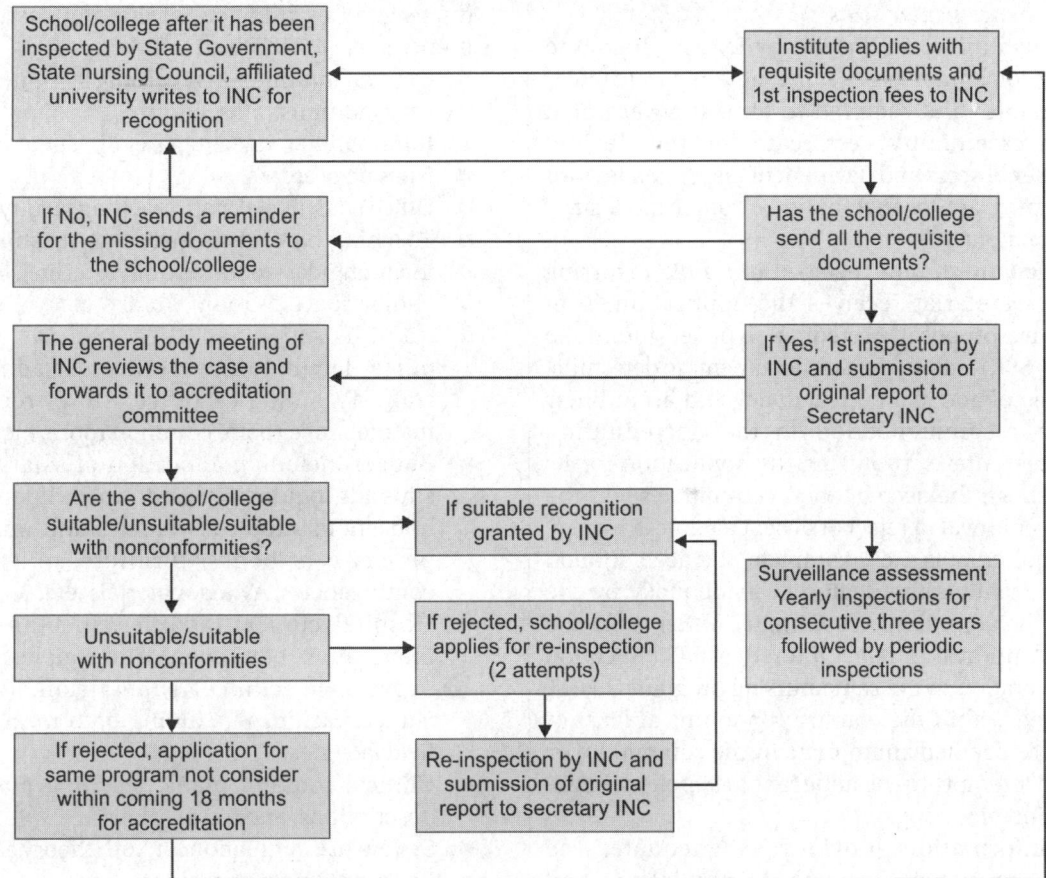

Fig. 53.2: Process for accreditation for the nursing institution by INC.

for Accreditation of Training Institutions and required documents and prescribed fees. The requested records are as follows:

a. *For a new proposal*
   The institute is required to submit the necessary documents with the proposal for starting the School of Nursing/college of nursing:
   - Particulars of the institute including offering courses
   - No objection certificate from state government for the offering courses
   - Government order/essentiality certificate for the desired nursing programs
   - Land details indicating the total area, land of ownership, registration number, etc.
   - Building details showing land deed, totally covered area, completion certificate, fire safety certificate, blueprint, water and sewerage system, electricity connection, pollution certificate, etc.
   - Finance backup, valuation certificate, FDRs balance, PAN/DAN, etc.
   - Consent letter from the university only for starting a college of nursing offering graduate/postgraduate nursing program
   - A consent letter from the respective State Nursing Registration Council to start the desired nursing program
   - Teaching, clinical, and physical facility details including budget. It includes administrative wing, library, labs, AV aids, facilities for staff, teaching staff, nonteaching staff, paramedical staff, hostel, etc.
   - One hundred (100)-bedded parent/own hospital for all areas except for hilly areas, namely J& K, Uttarakhand, and the North Eastern States and Scheduled Notified Tribal areas.
   - Documents related to parent hospital such as (1) registered deed of hospital (trust/society/company) (hospital name) along with members, (2) notary-attested registered resolution of governing body (name of trustee) and name of hospital would be the parent hospital of institution for the next 3 years, (3) CMHO certification about owner of hospital of the hospital location and number of beds, (4) income tax return for the last 3 years, (5) registration of hospital under shop and establishment act, and (6) a certificate from Pollution Control Board for both parent and affiliated hospitals.
   - Payment of the first inspection through online/bank draft for School/College of Nursing in favor of Secretary, INC, New Delhi (ANM, GNM, post-basic diploma course, PB BSc (N), BSc (N), MSc (N), MPhil (N), PhD (N).

b. *For enhancement of seats*
The institution recognized by INC is eligible to apply for enhancement of seats for a particular program(s) and required to furnish government order/essentiality certificate for the desired number of seats and payment of inspection fees for each program through online or other modes per requirement.

2. **Acknowledgment and registration:** Indian Nursing Council secretariat receives the application form along with a proposal. Accreditation panel studies the proposal (SSR) and supporting documents to determine the degree of adequacy/inadequacy and accordingly makes a recommendation to the Accreditation Committee. After scrutinizing the application for its completeness, the accreditation committee seeks the council's approval to reject or accept a request.

   If the requirements are incomplete, the accreditation panel determines the degree of inadequacy by the criteria. The accreditation committee *either* seeks the council's approval to reject the request. (Application for accreditation of the same nursing program is NOT considered within the coming 18 months at least or duration as deemed appropriate by the committee) *or* gives two attempts to the applicant to supplement the information in writing.

   If the information provided is adequate, the accreditation panel considers the application and makes a recommendation as appropriate to the accreditation committee. Indian Nursing Council acknowledges the request and assigns a registration code in a case to accept the demand for a new proposal.

3. **Notification to institution/organization**
   Notification for new proposal/enhancement of seats: Indian Nursing Council based on recommendation notifies institutions to check their status of the application on web site by logging in. It also notifies institutions that submit new proposals/proposals for enhancement of seats. These documents are as follows:
   - Self-attested passport size photographs of teaching faculty along with their original certificates and Aadhar cards
   - Sale/lease deed of the lane or building
   - Permission letters of hospitals (affiliated/parent)
   - Parent hospital documents if applicable
   - Yearly and last month census of hospitals.

4. **Appointment of inspectors:** The accreditation committee reviews the proposal made by the accreditation panel, in case accept the application for the new proposal, appoints two approved inspectors to conduct the inspection.

5. **Inspection by INC inspection team:** Indian Nursing Council notifies the institutions for inspection. The appointed inspectors visit the institution, observe, and physically verify the documents and submit a report in a prescribed format along with supporting documents duly signed by principal of the proposed institution immediately to INC that include:
   - General information regarding institution, name of trust, administrative control
   - Information related to parent hospital
   - Nursing program
   - Office staff, hostel staff, teaching faculty
   - Teaching block, infrastructure teaching facilities including classroom, examination hall, laboratories, audiovisual aids room, library, etc.
   - Administrative facilities such as principal's office, faculty offices, offices of administrative staff, accountant's office, store, record room, maintenance room, common room, etc.
   - Budget including allocation of salary, students' stipends, equipment and repair, linen and other household supplies, vehicles and maintenance, purchase of books, furniture, office supplies, contingencies, AV aid materials, etc.
   - Hospital clinical facilities, including hospital information, equipment, and supplies for clinical experience, clinical supervision. Community clinical facilities including both rural and urban field facilities.
   - Clinical rotation plans, teaching plans, course descriptions, and lesson plans
   - System of examination for both theory and practical
   - Bond system for nursing students
   - Records of students and college
   - Hostel facilities including building area, sale deed/building completion certificate, provision of separate hostel for boys and girls, infrastructure facilities, facilities for indoor and outdoor games, other recreational facilities, availability of the guest room, sick room, dining room

   The inspectors check, verify, and annex the following documents:
   - Duly filled inspection performa
   - Inspection report related to teaching staff, clinical facilities, hostel building, building, equipment, library, etc.
   - Consent letter of State Nursing Registration Council
   - Land deed documents
   - Government order/essentiality certificate for the desired nursing program
   - Consent letter from the university
   - Documents related to parent hospital if applicable
   - Permission letters of the affiliated hospital
   - Permission letter of CHC/PHC
   - Teaching faculty original certificate and photos (self-attested)
   - Relieving order of teachers
   - Transportation registration certificates.

5. **Scrutiny and review of inspection report:** Indian Nursing Council scrutinizes the inspection report and sends it to its accreditation committee. The committee decides to grant the accreditation, depending on

the observation made by inspectors. Indian Nursing Council informs the proposed institute to correct nonconformities, if any, within the stipulated time. The proposed institute requires to correct the deficiencies pointed out during the first inspection.

6. **Approval and notification by INC:** The accreditation committee of INC, based on a report of the inspection team and documentary evidence, decides either to give permission or not and accordingly notifies to the institution. If the institution gets permission/approval from INC to start the program and sanction of seats for admission of students, the institution is required to take approval from the State Nursing Council and affiliated university.

   If INC does not grant approval
   a. *Re-inspection:* The institute takes necessary corrective actions and submits the compliance report with documentary proof per the report of the first inspection along with the duly-filled application and prescribed fees for consideration. The accreditation committee reviews the report and plans for re-inspection. The INC inspectors go for site visits to review the status and submit a report of the inspection in a prescribed format along with supporting documents.
   b. *Inspection for enhancement of seats:* For the enhancement of seats, the institution is required to submit the proposal along with the fees for inspection. Usually, it inspects institutions after 1 year from the last inspection subject to the students admitted.
   c. *Scrutiny and review of re-inspection report:* Indian Nursing Council scrutinizes the inspection report and sends it to its accreditation committee. The committee decides to grant the accreditation, depending on the observation made by inspectors. If found suitable, INC grants recognition and informs institute accordingly.
   d. *Approval and notification by INC*
      The accreditation committee of INC, based on a report of the inspection team and documentary evidence, decides either to give permission or not and accordingly notifies to the institution. If the institution gets permission/approval from INC to start program and sanction of seats for admission of students, the institution is required to take approval from the State Nursing Council and affiliated university.

7. **Surveillance assessment:** Indian Nursing Council conducts surveillance assessment by inspecting institutions usually yearly for consecutive 3 years, followed by periodic and surprise inspections. It approves if it fulfills the requirement. The assigned inspectors conduct the inspection and prepare a detailed report in a prescribed format and submit to INC. Indian Nursing Council reviews the report, and if any nonconformities, informs the institution to correct the deficiencies. The institute needs to fix the shortcomings and needs to submit a compliance report.

8. **Validity/Renewal assessment and notification:** The approved institutions need to apply every year for renewal with supporting documents online and prescribed fees. Indian Nursing Council notifies institutions to check their status of an application for approval of renewal/validity on web site by logging in with their user ID and password. It is mandatory for institution before the beginning of academic session every year. The institutions found deficient of documents are further notified to submit their compliance documents through online only.

Guidelines for Conducting Inspection

The following suggestions can contribute to the effective and efficient implementation of an evaluation activity:
- Keep those who are involved well informed
- Try to be sensitive to the institution and their needs about data collection
- Provide complete directions for all data gathering instruments
- Do not promise what you cannot deliver
- Do not be casual in your approach
- Try to avoid being continuously negative
- Consider carefully the possible impact—both intended and unintended on asking the questions
- Strive to achieve and maintain objectivity and credibility
- Maintain anonymity and confidentiality and be honest in gathering the data.

How to Make Accreditation Successful

Following should be taken into account if accreditation has to be successful:
- By sound designing of the evaluation procedure
- Development of realistic criteria or standards for gathering data
- Secure and sound methods of gathering evidence
- Honesty in gathering evidence
- Proper judgment
- Accurate reporting
- Providing feedback
- Approving only for institutions met the minimal requirement.

ACCREDITATION OF HOSPITALS

Accreditation of hospitals is essential to have a high quality of care and safety of patients. It enables the hospital to continuous improvement in patient care and provides an opportunity to benchmark its best. It creates a learning and sound working environment for the staff to improve their knowledge and skills and to develop leadership in quality management. It provides a certified database and other information regarding the health-care organization regarding its infrastructure and level of care.

The United States of America led the first initiative toward accreditation in early 1910. Over some time after several experiments, the Joint Commission on Accreditation of Healthcare Organisation (JCAHO), a national accreditation program, established itself as an esteemed accreditation body by 1987. JCAHO has high standards of quality assurance and rigorous process of evaluation, which makes it a much-esteemed agency for accreditation. Health services certified by JCAHO give "deemed status."

A decade ago, accreditation was the concern in the American process, but it was also widespread in Central and South America and Eastern Europe and now has moved into the European Union as part of the Bologna Process. In India, accreditation of hospitals initiated at the local and national levels since 1986.

Umbrella Accreditation Organizations

These organizations comprise the following:
- The International Society for Quality in Health Care (ISQua) is an umbrella organization for organizations providing international health-care accreditation. Its offices are in the Republic of Ireland.
- The United Kingdom Accreditation Forum (UKAF) is a UK-based umbrella organization for organizations providing health-care accreditation. Its offices are in London.
- The Society for International Healthcare Accreditation (SOFIHA) is an organization devoted toward the development and promulgation of high-quality certification of hospitals and health-care facilities across international borders.

International Healthcare Accreditation Organizations

The following list shows the international organizations:
- The JCAHO, USA
- The Canadian Council on Health Service Accreditation (CCHSA), Canada.
- The Australian Council on Healthcare Standards (ACHS), Australia.
- Health Quality Services (HQS). The King's Fund Centre, England.
- Council on Health Services Accreditation for South Africa (COHSASA).
- The Malcolm Baldrige National Quality Award, USA. (Including the Swedish and European versions and the version modified for health-care evaluation, USA.)
- Trent Accreditation Scheme or Trent (based in UK-Europe, Hong Kong, the Philippines, and Malta) was the first scheme to accredit a hospital in Asia, in Hong Kong in 2000.
- Joint Commission International (based in the USA), the first hospital to be certified in Asia by JCI was Bumrungrad International Hospital in 2002.
- Malaysian Society for Quality in Health (MSQH) based in Malaysia
- Health-Care Quality Association on Accreditation (HQAA) based in the USA.

Hospital Accreditation System in India

The list below should be followed for hospital accreditation system:
- Indian Hospitals Association at Bombay and Delhi made efforts to promote a voluntary accreditation system in 1993.
- The Bureau of Indian Standards laid down standards for 30, 100, and 250 beds (BIS 1988).
- The National Institute for Health and Family Welfare laid down criteria for more than 50 beds, only for the equipment (NIHFW 1992).
- Encouragement of self-regulation through the association of private medical schools, doctors, and hospitals after World Development Report in 1993.
- In 1997, a committee presently named "Health Care Accreditation Council" formed with the support of the World Health Organization (WHO), Geneva to study Self-Regulation of Private Hospitals and Nursing Homes in Mumbai City: Need for an Accreditation System. It developed standards for the wards, labor room, operation theater, essential drugs, waiting for the area or reception room, consulting room, changing room, pantry, medical records, and waste management for smaller hospitals.
- In Andhra Pradesh, Vaidya Vidhya Parishad laid down standards for secondary level hospitals in the government sector.
- In Pune, the health committee of Lok Vignyan Sangathana came up with routine preoperative investigations before minor surgery.
- In Bombay, Cehat, a nonprofit health research organization, has come up with a document "proposed minimum standards for 30-bedded private nursing homes." In Maharashtra, the government hospitals follow the Hospital Administration Manual.
- The MOHFW, Government of India, constituted a National Panel to define a plan for developing accreditation for hospitals in India and make recommendations for other institutional mechanisms. There are four subpanels constituted, namely Organizational Options for Quality Assurance, Clinical Standards, Quality Systems, and Physical Standards.
- Joint Commission International, the leading health-care accreditation agency in the United States accredits hospitals in India to date.

National Hospital Accreditation Organization: National Accreditation Board for Hospitals and Health Care Providers

National Accreditation Board for Hospitals and Health Care Providers (NABH), a national hospital accreditation organization, is a constituent body under the QCI. Both the NABH and QCI are the partners of many accreditation bodies such as the Indian Medical Association and stakeholders. MOHFW and the health industry aid in establishing NABH that operates an accreditation program for the health-care organization and fulfills the needs of the health clients. It is under the Ministry of Commerce and Industry and handles the accreditation process in the Indian health-care sector. The entry-level process has become easy, faster, and user-friendly digital. Now it has operated through a new portal, namely "HOPE. It stands for Health care Organizations Platform for Entry-level certification."

Composition

The board sets benchmarks for the health industry progression, quality care, and safety of patients. All stakeholders, including industry, consumers, and government, provide support to the board. It works independently. It is an institutional, board member and member of the ISQua. It is a founder member of the proposed Asian Society for Quality in Health Care (ASQua) registered in Malaysia. It has the Appeals Committee, the Accreditation Committee, the Technical Committee, the secretariat, and a panel of over 100 assessors and experts selected among clinicians, hospital administrators, and nursing supervisors.

Focus

The main focus is on patient rights and benefits, patient safety, control and prevention of infections in hospitals, practicing suitable patient care protocols, e.g. specialized care for vulnerable groups, critically ill patients, and better and controlled clinical outcomes and at the same time benchmarked with the best international standards.

It focuses on accreditation of all health-care organizations and to provide a platform for online registration to promote the quality of healthcare. It has developed standards for hospitals and health-care providers and accredited by the apex body of the ISQua.

Objectives

1. To accredit both large and small health-care organizations.
2. To promote quality in every patient and all aspects of hospital.
3. To provide a framework for quality assurance and quality improvement in the hospitals.
4. To build a working team and a quality culture.
5. It provides a platform for education and training for quality and patient safety.
6. To focus on continuous quality monitoring and implementing a corrective action plan to improve quality patient care and safety.
7. It gives recognition by endorsing many health-care quality courses.

NABH Standards

NABH standards for hospitals: There are two types of standards in NABH: patient centered and organization centered. The patient-centered standards are regarding access, assessment, information, patient care, management of medication, patients' rights and education, and hospital infection control. The organization-centered standards are on continuous quality improvement, the responsibility of management, facility management and safety, human resource management, and information management system. There are a total of 102 standards and 636 objective elements or indicators compiled under 10 headings or chapters.

Nursing excellence standards: These are standards that focus on professional, administrative, and governance. There is a total of 48 standards and 216 indicators categorized under seven areas. These areas are nursing resource management, nursing care of patients, medicine management, education, communication, guidance, infection control practices, empowerment and governance, and nursing quality indicators.

Lab standards: All labs, including clinical biochemistry, pathology, microbiology, serology, genetics, and nuclear medicine, must fulfill the requirements. The standards are related to organization and management, documentation control, personnel, lab equipment, procurement of external supplies and services, process control, and continual quality improvement. All labs should comply with minimum standards for certification.

Standards for emergency department care: These are a total of eight standards; four related to patients and four to organizations.

The patient-related standards are on access, assessment and information, patient care and rights, management of medication, and hospital infection control. The organization's relevant standards are on continuous quality improvement, the responsibility of administration, facility management and safety, and human resource management.

Common Programs Required for Accreditation

Following programs required to start, maintain, and review periodically for accreditation purpose:
1. A quality assurance program: It should include lab, radiology, surgical, and intensive care services.
2. A hospital infection control program.
3. A continuous quality improvement program with clinical and management indicators.
4. A hospital safety program for labs, radiology, organization, and patient safety.
5. Internal audit.
6. Medical record audit program.
7. A medical audit program.
8. A nursing audit program.
9. An induction training program.
10. An in-service training program.

Steps in Quality Management for Accreditation

1. Find out and correct structural requirement.
2. Development and document policies and standard operative procedures.
3. Allocation of resources.
4. Behavioral change practices.
5. Development of fair culture in the organization.
6. Building team and implantation of teamwork.
7. Monitoring of performance.
8. Gather information based on developed performance indicators.
9. Impart training and monitor its effectiveness.
10. Identify the trend by using root cause analysis.
11. Apply the Plan- Do- Check- Act (PDCA) cycle.

Accreditation Process

The accreditation process takes at least 1 year after the submission of all required information with the first application. The following steps should be adhered in the process of accreditation of hospitals:

I. **Health-care organization preparedness for accreditation**

   The organization decides to get accreditation. It should define a plan of action and select a person to coordinate all the seeking accreditation. The nominated person must know about the organization and its functioning and quality management. The organization procures the relevant documents from the secretariat of NABH on payment and gets well acquainted with all requirements. The team of the organization conducts a self assessment to check either fulfilled all the criteria at least 3 months before the submission of the application.

II. **Applying for accreditation by the organization**

   The health-care organization fills the prescribed application, downloaded from the NABH website, and submits all the required documents with application fees. The documents include a signed copy of terms and conditions, self-assessment tool kit, hospital manual, and documents per NABH requirement.

III. **Accreditation process**

   1. **Acknowledgment and registration:** NABH secretariat receives the application form. After scrutinizing the application for its completeness, acknowledges the request and assigns a registration code.
   2. **Appointment of principal assessor and assessment team:** National Accreditation Board for Hospitals and Health Care Providers appoint the principal assessor and assessment team comprising one or two members to conduct preassessment of health-care organization.
   3. **Preassessment:** The appointed team visits the assigned organization within 3 months of submission application along with the fee to check its feasibility and preparedness for final assessment and review the documentation system. It judges the time required for accreditation, assessors needed, and explains the methodology adopted for assessment. The organization requires depositing the annual fees before the final assessment. It points out any deficiencies observed during a visit to the organization and suggests it correct.
   4. **Final assessment:** The final evaluation carries out within the 6 months of preassessment. The organization requires to correct the deficiencies pointed out during the preassessment. If needed, the assessment team, along with technical expertise, can go for site visits to review the status and sends a report within 7 days of the site visit to the assigned organization. The team then submits the detailed report to NABH within 10 days of site visit.

   The organization takes necessary corrective actions and sends the report to NABH within 3 months of the assessment date. NABH appoints an assessment committee comprising principal assessor and assessors, depending on the number of beds and services provided to conduct a final assessment. The final assessment involves reviewing of functions and services of the organization. NABH finalizes date for the final evaluation with the organization. The assessment team prepares a detailed report observed during visit in a prescribed format and submits to NABH and nonconformities to the organization. The organization corrects the deficiencies and needs to send the complete report within 3 months of final assessment to NABH secretariat.

   5. **Scrutiny and review of assessment report:** NABH scrutinizes the assessment report and sends it to its accreditation committee. The committee decides the accreditation award, depending on the score and compliance of standards. The committee may do verification assessments.

      a. *The conditions for qualifying pre-entry accreditation:* The organization must fulfill all legal requirements. The specific standards should not have more than two zeros; the average score for a single standard should not be less than five. The average rating for each chapter should be more than 5. The overall average score for all standards must exceed 5.

      b. *The conditions for pre-entry progressive accreditation:* The organization must fulfill all legal requirements. The specific standards should not have more than two zeros; the average score for a single standard should not be less than five. The average rating for each chapter should be more than 6. The overall average score for all standards must exceed 6. The validity is from 3 months to a maximum of 12 months.

      c. *The conditions for accreditation:* The organization must fulfill all legal requirements. The specific standards should not have more than two zeros; the average score for an individual standard should not be less than five. The average rating for each chapter should be more than 7. The overall average score for all standards must exceed 7. The

validity is from 3 years with specific terms and conditions.
6. **Surveillance assessment:** NABH conducts surveillance within 3 years, usually plans a visit after one and a half years of accreditation. The assessment team prepares a detailed report observed during the visit in a prescribed format and submits to NABH and nonconformities to the organization. The organization corrects the deficiencies and needs to send the complete report within 1.5 months of surveillance visit to the NABH secretariat.
7. **Reassessment:** NABH reassesses the accreditation status. The organization needs to apply for accreditation before 6 months of the expiry.

CHAPTER HIGHLIGHTS

- Accreditation is a self-regulatory process to grant recognition to health institutions or organizations. It is a voluntary process to certify competency, authority, or credibility by achieving optimal standards.
- The accreditation models are standard oriented, quality assurance oriented, and health service oriented.
- There are many educational, professional, and health-care national accrediting agencies. NAAC, INC, and NABH are examples of these types of accrediting agencies in India.
- NAAC is an autonomous institution established in 1994 by the UGC, engaged in assessment, accreditation, and academic audit of universities, constituent, and affiliated colleges.
- The INC is an autonomous statutory body that regulates the functioning of all nursing programs by assessing and accrediting nursing institutions. It assists in improving the quality of education and recognizes various nursing qualifications.
- NABH, a national hospital accreditation organization, is a constituent body under the QCI. It accredits both large and small health-care organizations and provides a framework for quality assurance and quality improvement in the hospitals.

REVIEW QUESTIONS

I. Essay Type Questions
1. Define the term "Accreditation." Describe its aims and characteristics.
2. Enlist different types of national accreditation agencies. Discuss the role of NAAC in the accreditation of academic universities.
3. Describe in detail the accreditation process followed by INC.
4. Discuss the accreditation system of hospitals.

II. Short Notes
1. Scope of accreditation
2. NAAC evaluation framework
3. Guidelines for conducting inspections
4. NABH standards.

III. Multiple Choice Questions
1. Which one of the followings is a necessary process that requires health-care institutions to meet minimum standards?
   a. Accreditation   b. Certification
   c. Licensure   d. Affiliation
2. The National Assessment and Accreditation Council is which type of accreditation agency?
   a. Educational   b. Professional
   c. Administrative   d. Healthcare
3. Which accreditation agency follows a three-stage process for assessment and accreditation?
   a. INC   b. NABH
   c. JCAHO   d. NAAC
4. How many attempts INC provides to the applicant to supplement the information in case of the adequacy of requirements to start a nursing institution?
   a. No attempt   b. Two
   c. Three   d. Four
5. How many overall average scores are mandatory for a health-care organization to qualify pre-entry accreditation?
   a. Less than 5   b. Must exceed 5
   c. Must exceed 6   d. Must exceed 7

Answer Keys
1. c   2. a   3. d   4. b   5. b

SUGGESTED READING

1. Accreditation. [Online] Available from https://www.ncsbn.org/357.htm. [Accessed July 2019].
2. Asian Hospital & Healthcare Management. [Online] Available from http://www.asianhhm.com/Knowledge_bank/articles/healthcare_accreditations_india.htm. [Accessed July 2019].
3. Available from http://www.achs.org.au. [Accessed July 2019].
4. Available from http://www.jointcommissioninternational.comhttp://en.wikipedia.org/wiki/Accreditation. [Accessed August 2019].
5. Available from http://www.planningcommision.nic.in. [Accessed August 2019].
6. European Network of Quality Agencies (ENQA), 2003, The Bologna Process, Glossary. [Online] Available from http://www.asianhhm.com/Knowledge_bank/articles/healthcare_accreditations_india.htm. [Accessed August 2019].
7. Gupta A, Gupta C. Role of National Accreditation Board of Hospitals and Healthcare Providers (NABH) core indicators monitoring in quality and safety of blood transfusion. Asian J Transfus Sci. 2016;10(1):37-41. [Accessed September 2019].
8. John Braithwaite. Regulating nursing homes: The challenge of regulating care for older people in Australia. BMJ. 2001;323:443-6.
9. NABH. [Online] Available from https://www.nabh.co/h-doc.aspx. [Accessed September 2019].
10. NABH accreditation for hospitals simplified and digitalized. [Online] Available from https://www.livemint.com/news/india/nabh-accreditation-for-hospitals-simplified-and-digitalised-1550758867046.html Updated: 21 Feb 2019, 08:22 PM IST. [Accessed September 2019].
11. Sheth S. Accreditation of hospitals. Health Care Manag. 2001;16-31Oct.

SECTION 10

Fiscal Management

54. Financial Management, Financial Planning, and Financial Audit
55. Budget and Budgetary Process
56. Cost Accounting and Health Economics
57. Economic Evaluation Techniques
58. Critical Pathways and Health Care Reforms

54 Financial Management, Financial Planning, and Financial Audit

CHAPTER OUTLINE

- Financial Management
  - Meaning and Definitions
  - Components of Financial Management
  - Objectives of Financial Management
  - Elements of Financial Management
  - Functions of Financial Management
  - Prerequisite of Financial Management
  - Health-Care Financing
  - Role of Nurse Managers in Finance Management
- Financial Planning
  - Objectives of Financial Planning
  - Importance of Financial Planning
  - Steps of Financial Planning
  - Factors Influencing Financial Planning
  - Features of a Sound Financial Plan
- Financial Audit
  - Definition
  - Purposes of Financial Audit
  - Types of Financial Audit
  - Financial Audit Process
  - Qualities of an Auditor

LEARNING OUTCOMES

After completion of this chapter, the learner will be able to:
- Understand the concept of financial management
- Describe in detail components of financial management
- Describe objectives, elements, functions, and scope of financial management
- Define financial planning and enlist its objectives
- Appreciate the importance of financial planning
- Discuss various steps of financial planning
- Elaborate on the factors affecting financial planning
- Give a note on features of a sound fiscal plan
- Describe the role of the nurse managers in finance
- Discuss financial audit, its purposes, and types

KEY TERMS

Financial management, health-care financing, nursing finance, financial planning, fiscal plan, financial audit

INTRODUCTION

Investment is a vital ingredient of any organization. As rightly said, that money makes the mare go. It is the lifeblood of the administration; without finance, the administration cannot run. Finance and administration have a direct correlation with each other. Even though funding is available, if not administered or managed correctly, it can go into waste. Hence finance and administration or management go side by side. Money is a universal lubricant for any organization, man, and machine work.

Financial administration and management in any organization are comparable with the circulatory system in the human body. As the blood circulates through the network of veins and arteries and controlled by heart, similarly, finance is spread through financial channels throughout the administrative machinery of the organization, and the top management controls it through various departments/agencies and by using multiple ways and techniques.

FINANCIAL MANAGEMENT

Meaning and Definitions

Meaning

Financial management is the planning, organizing, directing, and controlling the economic activities, including procurement and utilization of funds. It is the application of general management principles to financial resource management of the organization. It comprises business operations to have enough funds available to carry out organizational activities and to ensure efficient utilization of these funds to attain the organizational goals and objectives.

Financial management is a managerial activity concerned with planning and controlling of organizational financial resources. It was the branch of economics till 1890, but now both academicians' and managers' practice to make the most crucial decisions of the organization relates to the finance. The understanding of financial management provides them the conceptual and analytical insights to make decisions wisely.

Definitions

Harward and Upton defined financial management as a process to maximize the utilization of finance by investing rationally on funds. It applies general management principles to a particular economic operation.

According to Maheshwary, financial management is the proper management of funds. It involves managerial decisions regarding the procurement of long-term and short-term funds and adequate utilization of funds. It also deals with framing the dividend policy.

It deals with raising the financial resources and their utilization to achieve the organizational goals. It is the process of utilizing the available funds from the long-term point of view of business objectives (Richard A Brealey).

Thus financial management deals with planning, organizing, directing, and controlling the economic activities such as procurement and utilization of funds of the organization. It is concerning in assessing the need for funds, raising required funds, effective use of funds, and distribution of surplus financial controls.

Components of Financial Management

Financial management comprises three parts: planning, budgeting, and evaluation (**Fig. 54.1**). All the pieces are equally crucial for the nurse managers to gather the information used in making philosophical and operational decisions regarding the finance of the department.

1. **Planning:** Planning is the first step in the financial management triad. Planning must initiate from the unit level of the organization. It needs preparing plans before budgeting to distribute revenue properly. During preparation, identify the long-term and short-term objectives according to priority. Formulate targets based on hospital philosophy, type of patient, size, and type of organization.
   Develop a financial plan for each nursing unit. The plan must include the number of staff, type of nursing staff, nurse–patient ratio, option for staffing, and new programs for future planning. Include variable costs such as supplies, repair, and maintenance of equipment and unplanned expenses. Have a meeting with all the categories of the nursing personnel while preparing the budget for the unit.

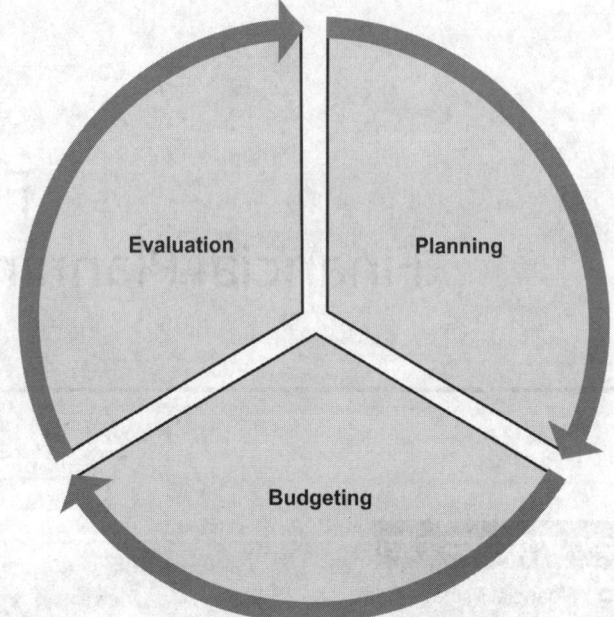

Fig. 54.1: Component of financial management.

2. **Budgeting:** Nursing managers should also be involved in the budgeting of the department. Budgeting is the allocation of human, material, and financial resources to meet nursing organizational goals and include overall revenue and expenses projections. Based on forecasts, prepare a detailed operating budget and capital budget. The operating budget contains expenses on daily activities and services such as patient care revenues, labor costs, outside purchase services, and supplies. The operating budget is a financial tool to measure daily, monthly, and yearly profitability. A capital budget is money earmarked for the purchase of permanent equipment or significant renovation and construction projects.

3. **Evaluation:** The final component of the financial management triad is evaluation. The evaluation part is critical in determining the economic success of the current budget year, as well as in identifying areas of additional attention in plans for the next fiscal year. The evaluation must be at regular intervals to keep a current view of financial status.

Objectives of Financial Management

The following list shows the objectives of financial management:
1. To implement the fiscal policies
2. To procure appropriate funds for the organizational activities
3. To ensure an adequate supply of funds
4. To ensure the optimum utilization of funds
5. To provide the fair and maximum output or health services on capital
6. To appropriate in the value of funds

7. To coordinate with different departments of the organization
8. To ensure effective financial control
9. To increase the efficiency of the departments by proper distribution of funds
10. To create goodwill of the organization.

Elements of Financial Management

The elements of financial management are as follows:
1. **Investment decisions:** The investment decision is the decision on the investment of fixed assets. It deals with investing current assets and making investment decisions or working capital decisions.
2. **Financial decisions:** The financial decision is the decision to raise finance from various resources. It depends on choice on the type of source, a period of financing, cost of investment, and the returns thereby.
3. **Dividend decision:** The dividend decision is net profit distribution. These are two types: The dividends for preserved benefits and stakeholders. The preserved or retained profit is the amount of retained profits to be finalized, which will depend on the expansion and diversification plans of the organization.

Functions of Financial Management

The functions of financial management are as follows:
1. **Estimation of capital requirements:** Financial management is concerning estimating capital requirements, which depends on its cost, profits, and future programs and policies.
2. **Determination of the capital structure:** It determines the capital structure based on the short-term and long-term debt-equity analysis.
3. **Choice of sources of funds:** The financial management aids organization in finding out alternative sources of procuring additional funds.
4. **Investment of funds:** It makes it easy to allocate and utilize the funds appropriately.
5. **Disposal of surplus:** It concerns the net profit for the expansion, innovational, and diversification plans of the organization.
6. **Management of cash:** In financial management, an account officer manages money for many purposes, such as for payment of wages and salaries, electricity, water bills, payment to creditors, meeting current liabilities, and maintaining adequate stock and purchase of raw materials.
7. **Financial controls:** Apart from planning, procuring, and utilization of funds, the finance managers exercise control over finances through control techniques such as ratio analysis, financial forecasting, and cost and profit control. They supervise cash receipt payments, safeguard cash balances, securities, records, and reports.

Prerequisite of Financial Management

The requirements of financial management are as follows:
- **Anticipation:** To forecast the requirement for the organization based on the estimated need of the organization.
- **Acquisition:** To procure the finances from different sources.
- **Allocation:** Proper distribution of available funds.
- **Appropriation:** Keep a marginal profit in terms of services.
- **Assessment:** Control the investment.

Health-care Financing

Health-care financing comprises the following:
1. **Finance:** Finance comprises providing and utilizing the money. It includes capital rights, credit, and fund operations of the organization. It is a branch of economics concerning resource allocations, resource management, acquisition, and investment.

   Finance also relates to the system that generates, regulates, and distributes the monetary resources needed for the sustenance and growth of health agency. Finance includes planning of financial resources, making of optimum capital structure, and effective utilization of financial resources by in-depth analysis of the cost of capital and capital budgeting tool.
2. **Nursing finance:** Nursing finance includes the techniques of maximizing economic output and the optimization of financial resources. Nursing financing is a science as a nurse administrator applies scientific methods to understand the intricacies and functioning of the different aspects of nursing services. Also, the income and expenditure are projected scientifically through the statistical analysis of data collected directly and indirectly. Nursing finance helps to direct and guide the nursing administrators in the formulation and implementation of the financial policies of an organization efficiently and systematically.
3. **Health-care financing:** The health-care financing is a process of mobilizing funds in health-care activities, allocating funds in different areas, population groups, and individual health-care activities, and mechanisms for paying healthcare (Hsaio, Liu, 2001). There are three significant sources of health service finance.
   a. **Public:** It includes all expenditure on health services by central and local government funds spent by the state-owned and par state enterprises as well as government and social insurance contributions.
   b. **Private:** The private source of generating finance is voluntary payments by individuals or private employers.
   c. **External sources:** The external source of funding is the foreign aid comes through bilateral aid programs and international nongovernment organizations (NGOs).

Role of Nurse Managers in Finance Managements

The role of nurse managers in financing is as follows:
- The nurse managers must involve in financial management.
- They must formulate unit goals and objectives and plans for nursing service.
- They must plan staffing costs for a particular unit during the planning phase.
- During the budgeting phase, the head nurse must determine the requirements and prepare a budget.
- The nurse manager must utilize the budget properly and give feedback monthly.

FINANCIAL PLANNING

Financial planning is an essential part of business management. It aids in determining the objectives, policies, procedures, plans, and budgets to deal with the economic activities such as procurement, investment, and administration of funds of an organization. It ensures sufficient and adequate financial and investment strategies. It is a process of estimating the capital requirements of an organization and deciding the various sources to procure.

Objectives of Financial Planning

The list below shows the objectives of financial planning:
- **To determine capital requirements:** The capital requirement depends on many factors, such as the cost of current and fixed assets, promotional expenses, and long-range planning. Estimate capital budget from short-term and long-term needs.
- **To determine capital structure:** The capital structure includes the capital details, i.e. the relative kind and proportion of money required in the business. It includes decisions of debt-equity ratio both short-term and long-term.
- **To frame financial policies:** It also concerns to develop strategies to cash control, lending, borrowings, etc.
- **To ensure maximum utilization of funds:** Utilize the scarce financial resources in the best possible manner at least cost to get maximum returns on investment.

Importance of Financial Planning

The importance of financial planning is as follows:
1. The financial planning ensures the timely funds' availability to meet day-to-day requirements of the organization and future expansion.
2. It ensures budget stability and profitability by balancing outflow and inflow of funds.
3. It aids in developing policies, procedures, plans, and expansion programs.
4. It reduces uncertainties by changing trends faced quickly through enough funds.
5. It provides direction for sound financial control and maximum utilization of funds and thus seeks to eliminate waste of funds.

Steps of Financial Planning

Figure 54.2 depicts the stages of financial planning.
1. **Determination of financial objectives:** Lay down the financial goals based on the overall organizational objectives.
2. **Estimate the capital requirements:** Assess fixed capital and working capital. Consider the needs and activities of the organization.
3. **Formulate financial policies:** Formulate financial policies related to fund procurement, cash control, and other economic activities.

Factors Influencing Financial Planning

Figure 54.3 depicts the influencing factors of financial planning. These are as follows:
1. Objectives: Formulate objectives according to the organizational goals.
2. Requirements of organization: Prepare the financial plan based on the present and future needs of the organization.
3. A balance between cost and services: The capital structure should balance the value of the funds and services.
4. Flexibility: Financial planning must ensure the flexibility for utilizing funds for maximum profitability.

Features of Sound Financial Plan

Features of sound financial plan are as follows:
- A financial plan should be simple to understand and operate.

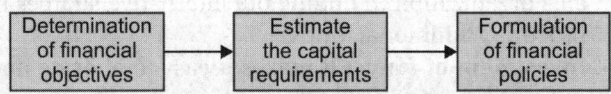

Fig. 54.2: Steps of financial planning.

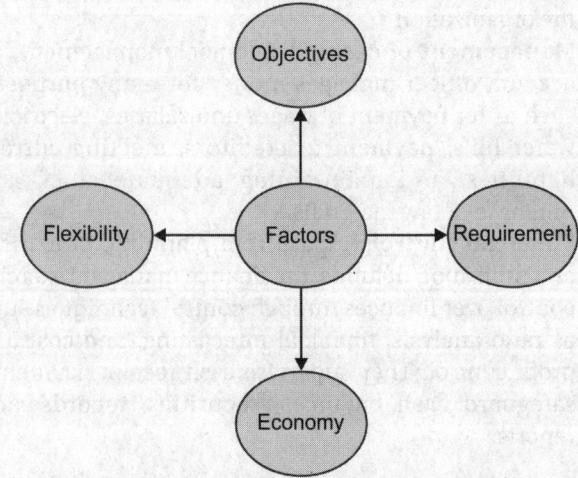

Fig. 54.3: Factors affecting financial planning.

- It should be flexible to allow deduction or expansion of funds.
- It should ensure optimum utilization of funds.

FINANCIAL AUDIT

In the global health industry, there is a need to have an adequate control system to process data belonging to their customers. Auditing is originated from accounting practices and motivated by the concept of capitalist production. It acts as a tool to control finance. In the health field, auditing had its origin in the 20th century. Auditing considered a means to verify the quality of care by analyzing medical records. Auditing is a tool to control and regulate health services in the public and private sectors. The focus was on controlling the costs of the health service.

Definitions

An audit is the assessment of the management, financial, and operations of an organization. According to the Merriam-Webster Dictionary, the audit is a formal inspection of an organization or individual's accounts or financial situation. It applies to different circumstances associated with the Internal Revenue Service (IRS).

An audit is a process of assessing the performance of a person, system, method, project or product, or organization as a whole. According to the Institute of Charted Accountants (India), a financial audit is an independent review of financial data of any organization.

Purposes of Financial Audit

The list below shows the purposes of financial audit:
- To ensure the adequacy of all the financial statements
- To provide a fair and accurate picture according to financial reports
- To increase the level of confidence among users in financial statement.

Types of Financial Audit

Financial audit is of the following types:

External Audit

The external audit is a process of reviewing the financial statements of an organization, either government or private, by an auditor from outside. It is independent in examining the financial records provided by the organization to the auditor. The regulatory body conducts the audit hired by the organization, and the auditors are generally the public accountants yearly, usually at the end of the fiscal year.

For public sectors, an external audit covers various financial documents such as budget, allocation of funds, and the actual expenses to review. It ensures the compilation of budgeted income and expenditure is correct. In private sectors, it conducts audits of all financial statements on revenue and spending quarterly and monthly to ensure its accurate compilation.

Importance of external financial audit
The significance of external financial audit is as follows:
- The external audit reviews and verifies the financial statements for its accurate compilation.
- It represents an unbiased procedure as conducted by outside expert auditors.
- It is an independent review of commercial document that ensures the taxpayers projected the revenue and spent funds accurately in public sectors.
- An external audit provides an independent assessment of organizational financial holding.

Features of an external financial audit
The features of an external financial audit are as follows:
1. It presents a summary of overall financial statements.
2. It detects any discrepancies in the financial statements of the organization.
3. It reflects the conclusion and recommendations of the audit.

Purposes of an external financial audit
The following list shows the purposes of an external financial audit:
1. To ensure the adequacy of internal control, processes, guidelines
2. To give an independent and unbiased review on financial matters of an organization
3. To verify internal procedures of control and evaluate compliance of standards and principles by the organization
4. To assess the accuracy, adequacy, and effectiveness of existing internal control.

Types of external audits
External audit is of the following types:
1. **Financial audit:** It is the verification of the financial statements of a legal entity. It is also known as the audit of financial statements. Financial statements are to ensure the accuracy of accounting records.
2. **Operations audit:** It is to detect errors in the internal control, procedures, and mechanisms.
3. **Compliance audit:** It is to evaluate how employees are abiding by regulations in performing tasks.

Internal Financial Audit

An internal financial audit is a system of monitoring the financial performance and effectiveness of various departments/units in the execution of multiple programs, schemes, and activities. It is an independent management function that involves continuous and critical evaluation of the organization's operations and to get feedback for improvements. It adds value to and strengthens the risk management and internal control system and thus improves the overall governance mechanism of the organization.

The Institute of Internal Auditors refers to it as *an independent assuring and consulting activity to meet specific objectives of the organization. It adds value to the organization and improves the internal functioning of the organization. It aids the organization in establishing an organized, systematic, and disciplined approach to assess and improve risk management, control, and governance mechanism operations.*

The audit assesses risk exposures to governance, operations, and information systems of the organization and improves the effectiveness and efficiency of its functioning, the reliability, and accuracy of financial and operational data, protecting assets, and adherence to laws and regulations.

Purpose of internal audit

The primary purpose of an internal audit is to establish standards and to guide in planning and to conduct internal audits.

Objectives of internal audit

The objectives of internal audit are as follows:
1. To improve the functioning of the organization
2. To strengthen the risk management, operations, management, internal control system, and overall governance mechanism of the organization
3. To develop and implement an internal audit action plan to prepare for the external audit.

Role of internal audit

The list below shows the role of internal audit:
1. **Regulatory and compliance functions:** It ensures the quality of public expenditure and proper implementation of rules and regulations. The organization maintains appropriate records and ensures accuracy in expenditure reporting.
2. **Efficiency cum performance roles:** It ensures efficiency and effectiveness in public expenditure. It provides compatibility with spending. It maintains proper realization, accounting, and reporting of revenue receipts.
3. **Development of overall audit plan:** Planning of internal audit is essential to ensure that appropriate attention in various financial matters, related issues, and proper utilization of skills and time. It involves the development of an overall plan and conduct of the audit. It engages managers in developing audit programs and inspection-related operations systematically.

Importance of internal financial audit

The significance of internal financial audit is as follows:
1. It aids in assessing the risk exposures and adequacies of the internal financial controls.
2. It identifies issues for improvement and strengthening the control system of the organization.
3. It ensures optimum utilization of the resources of the organization.
4. It identifies all types of liabilities of the organization.

5. It ensures compliance of the organization with regulatory laws and principles and with its guidelines and policies.
6. It safeguards the assets of the organization.
7. It reviews and guarantees the adequacy, security, relevancy, reliability, and control of management information systems.

Financial Audit Process

Internal auditing is essential to focus on deficient audit areas and their problems and appropriately utilization of skills and time. There are five phases of the audit process, as discussed in **Figure 54.4**:

1. **Preplanning/selection phase:** The preplanning step is the preaudit procedure phase. During this phase, various activities are carried out, such as:
   - Constitution of the audit committee
   - Appointing internal auditor who will undertake internal auditing independently according to bylaws and standards and per the direction of the audit committee
   - Selection of audit procedure: analytic, inquiry and confirmation, an inspection of records, observation, etc.
2. **Planning phase**
   a. Prepare an audit plan: An audit plan is a detailed comprehensive document that defines the scope and objective of audit, audit areas, risk assessment, program coverage, resources required, timings, and extent of auditing procedure over a set period. Avoid doing a review during the peak workload period. The internal auditor has the responsibility to plan and conduct internal audits.
   b. Prepare a financial checklist: The checklist includes a copy of previous audit reports, accounting requirement records, budget related, banking related, income records, purchase related, staff and salaries and bank accounts-related records, receipts,

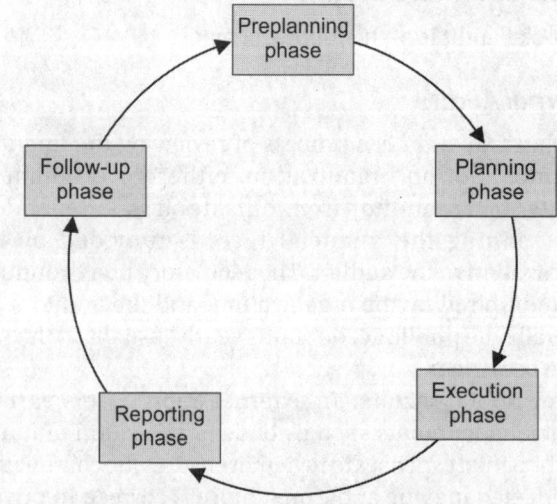

Fig. 54.4: Phases of the audit process.

ledgers, organization charts, board committee meetings, bylaws, and standards, etc.
   c. Review plan: Have a presentation and discussion in the audit committee meeting. Finalize and get approval from the audit committee.
3. **Execution phase:** The execution phase is the actual conduction of the audit. The internal auditor should conduct checks independently. It is essential to the effectiveness of internal audit functions. He should be professional and expertise and should maintain confidentiality, should clearly and timely communicate about accounting and audit issues. He should have access to records and other related resources, documents, etc.
   - Auditor should conduct audit per audit plan.
   - It should be carried out in compliance with the code of ethics and standards or bylaws and per guidelines on auditing.
   - Examine evidence-supporting documents such as financial statements according to policy and its presentation during an audit.
   - Identify potential mismatches and factors that affect the risk of material mismatches, etc.
   - Check documents for its completeness, occurrence, valuation and allocation, existence, accounting period and classification, and understandability, etc.
4. **Reporting phase:** During this phase, the internal auditor prepares a draft of the audit report.
   - The report should be factual and must specify in audit terms.
   - The report should include satisfactory performances and issues that need corrective actions.
   - It should include a summary of audit findings, conclusions, and specific recommendations.
   - Communicate officially to auditees through a draft report. Submit an action plan and give time to respond. Their responses also become a part of the final draft.
   - Finalize report and discuss with management to seek their comments and response on the summary report.
   - Prepare the final version of the audit report after incorporating the responses of management.
   - Submit the final audit report to the audit committee.
5. **Follow-up phase:** Based on the internal audit report, management does follow-up, plans, and takes corrective steps to improve upon the deficiencies. It also provides a base for external auditing.

Qualities of an Auditor

The internal auditor should:
- Be sincere, honest, and fair in his or her approach to professional work
- Have finance auditing skills; planning; analyzing; and reporting skills, research skills, and communication skills
- Prepare a checklist to check the records to (1) assess compliance with financial regulation such as general ledger, account balances, balance sheets, income statements, reports, operating practices, documentation, etc. and (2) to assess risk and internal controls by verifying assets and liabilities
- Maintain the confidentiality of the information acquired in the course of auditing
- Exercise due to professional care, competence, and diligence while performing the audit
- Delegate the work to assistants; direct, supervise, and review their work
- Plan the job well in advance and develop an audit plan
- Obtain sufficient data with his or her professional judgment to conclude reasonably
- Undertake work involving the identification of risks and recommend the design of control in existing controls
- Submit an audit report and suggest remedial actions.

CHAPTER HIGHLIGHTS

- Financial management is a managerial activity concerned with planning and controlling of organizational financial resources.
- Financial management comprises three parts: planning, budgeting, and evaluation.
- Finance planning is a process of estimating the capital requirements of an organization and deciding the various sources to procure.
- There are mainly three stages of financial planning developing financial goals, assessing capital requirements, and framing economic policies.
- Auditing is an independent examination of financial information of any organization. The external audit is a review of the financial statements or reports of an organization by someone not affiliated with the organization, usually conducted by a regulatory body.
- Internal audit is an independent management function done by appointed internal auditors to evaluate effective function of various departments in executing various programs, schemes and activities.
- Auditing requires various phases such as preplanning/selection, planning, execution, reporting, and follow-up period.

REVIEW QUESTIONS

I. Essay Type Questions
1. Define financial management. Describe its components in detail.
2. What do you mean by "financial planning?" Enumerate its objectives.
3. Define financial audit. Discuss different types of audit.
4. Describe in detail the purposes and role of internal audit.
5. Describe financial audit process in detail.

II. Short Notes
1. Functions of financial management
2. Steps of financial planning
3. External financial audit
4. Importance of internal audit
5. Qualities of an auditor

III. Multiple Choice Questions
1. Which component of financial management deals with allocating human, material, and financial resources and includes overall revenue and expense projections?
   a. Planning   b. Budgeting
   c. Controlling   d. Evaluation
2. A system of monitoring the financial performance and effectiveness of various departments in executing various programs and activities is:
   a. Financial management
   b. External audit
   c. Internal audit
   d. Operation audit
3. An external audit conducted with the purpose to detect errors in the internal control processes and mechanism is:
   a. Operation audit   b. Finance audit
   c. Compliance audit   d. Process audit
4. Internal audit must conduct independently by an internal audit because:
   a. An auditor is asked by audit committee do to so
   b. An auditor may be interested in doing so without seeking any help
   c. It is essential to the effectiveness of internal audit function
   d. It seems that auditor is the only expertise in auditing
5. In conducting an external audit in government agencies, which records an external auditor should check for its accurate usage and compilation?
   a. A review of budget and actual expenses
   b. A review of monthly budget report and allocation of funds
   c. Allocation of fund and monthly financial reports
   d. A review of the budget, allocation of funds, and actual expenses

Answer Keys
1. b   2. c   3. a   4. c   5. d

SUGGESTED READING
1. Gillies DA. Nursing Management—A System Approach. Philadelphia: WB Saunders Co.; 1989.
2. Goal SL. Financial Administration and Management. New Delhi: Sterling Publishers Pvt Ltd; 1993.
3. Mikesell JL. Fiscal Administration: Analysis and Applications for the Public Sector, 8th edition. Boston, MA: Wadsworth, Cengage Learning; 2011.
4. Patricia K. Essentials of Nursing Leadership & Management. 2nd edition, USA: Delmar Cengage Learning; 2010.
5. Swanburg RC. The nursing budget. Superv Nurse. 1978;9(6):40-7.
6. William O Cleverley. Essentials of Health Care Finance. Aspen Publishers Inc.; 1992.
7. Young LC. Nursing Administration. Philadelphia: WB Saunders Co.; 1988.

CHAPTER 55

Budget and Budgetary Process

CHAPTER OUTLINE

- Budget
  - Historical Background
  - Definitions of Budget
  - Importance of Budget
  - Purposes of Budget
  - Principles of Budget
  - Characteristics of Budget
  - Terminology of Budget
  - Typology of Budget
- Budgeting
  - Master Budget
  - Definitions
  - Principles of Budgeting
  - Purposes of Budgeting
  - Approaches to Budgeting
  - Steps in Budgeting
  - Types of Budgeting
- Budgetary Process
  - Budgetary Process
  - Nursing Budget
  - Midterm Appraisal
- Program Planning Budgeting System (PPBS)

LEARNING OUTCOMES

After completion of this chapter, the learner will be able to:
- Understand the concept of budget, budgeting, and budgetary process
- Discuss the importance of budget
- Describe the characteristics, purposes, features, and principles of budget
- Familiarize with various terminologies and typologies of budget
- Discuss the principles and elements of budgeting and budgetary process
- Enumerate the steps of the fiscal process after keeping in mind its prerequisite
- Discuss the nursing budget and its advantages
- Describe the steps followed for nursing budgeting
- Discuss the method of country budget preparation
- Explain zero-based budgeting, performance budgeting and midterm appraisal, and program planning budgeting system (PPBS)

KEY TERMS

Budget, budgeting, budgetary process, zero budgeting, performance budgeting, midterm appraisal

INTRODUCTION

Every organization has a predetermined set of goals and objectives attainable only with proper planning and execution of plans. The budgets are the plans in the form of statements. Every organization prepares the budget for its functioning. The budget expresses the plan of the hospital in health organizations to provide optimum care at a reasonable cost in financial terms. It represents the plans of a hospital in quantitative terms, evaluates the performance of finances per policy, and controls cost.

BUDGET

Historical Background

British Kings coined the word "budget" in early days from the word "bougette," which means a leather bag or pouch that held the seal of the medieval court Exchequer (former government department in charge of national revenue). After that, the chancellor of Exchequer took out papers about the government's financial scheme for ensuring a year in front of the parliament. Centuries later, the statements came popularly as budget. As early as in 1215 AD, it had constitutional exposure (Magna Carta gave the budget a political jolt), and in 1718 AD, a consolidated fund act was passed, which considered budget as a comprehensive financial statement of government activities for facilitating accountability of public fund. In 1882 AD, budget entered the parliament for first time seeking advice.

The concept of budgeting is ancient. Gradually, the word budget used for the proposals, as a statement of plans, and expectations for a future period in government, public bodies, commercial companies, or by private individuals.

Definitions of Budget

Finkler (1984) viewed a budget as a tool for planning, quantifying the plans, and controlling costs. A budget is a management tool used in planning, programming, and controlling business activity. According to Carruth et al. (2000), a budget is a plan that uses numerical data to predict the actions of an organization over some time. It is a structured plan for managing income and expenses.

A budget is a financial statement prepared before a specified period to attain a specified goal. According to Terry, budget is an estimate of future needs arranged on an orderly basis, covering all the activities of an organization for a definite period. A budget is a plan of operations for some specific coming period followed by a system of record that will serve as a check upon the program. It generally represents expected revenue as compared with anticipated expenses.

A budget is a financial plan. It forecasts the future financially on implementing strategies and decisions. Budgets are statements of anticipated results, either in monetary terms—as in revenue, expense, and capital budgets—or in nonfinancial terms—as in budgets of direct labor hours, material, physical sales volume, or units of production. It is an essential component of all the six management functions.

Budget is a part of the budgeting process developed initially and then continually monitored over time. It is a monetary declaration of action for a specific period. It is a plan of operations for a particular future period, which has a record that serves as a check upon the plan. It generally represents expected revenue against anticipated expenses.

Importance of Budget

Budget is important for the following reasons:
- Budget is an essential management tool.
- Budget provides an estimation of the money required to carry out organizational activities.
- Budget needs rigorous thinking for financial planning.
- Budget monitors income and expenses.
- It provides a base for financial accountability.

Purposes of Budget

Listed below are the purposes of budget:
- Budget is a tool of financial control exercised at various stages of financial management.
- Budget is an instrument of the organization as a policy or fiscal policy. It is a device to put plans and strategies in action.
- The budget acts as a useful tool for administration and is the principles of administration, i.e. planning, coordination, control, evaluation, reporting, and review applications, in a budgetary system.
- A budget is also a tool of accountability as it has valuable information for various activities.
- Budget is a forecast of income and expenditure in business/finance plan.
- It is a tool for decision-making. Budget provides a financial framework for the decision-making process.
- The budget is a means to monitor business performance. Once a budget is in operation, it measures the actual financial transactions against the forecast.

Principles of Budget

The various principles of budget are as follows:
- The budget plan should be according to the requirement of an organization.
- It should focus on the objectives and policies of the organization.
- It ensures appropriate utilization of scarce financial and nonfinancial resources.
- It requires planning of program activities in advance.
- The managers need to delegate responsibilities in framing and executing budget at a different level.
- It needs coordinating efforts to make managerial decisions and to develop a criterion for evaluating managerial performance.
- While setting the budget target, take utmost care to check against and balance estimates.
- Budget period and type of budget should be appropriate to the nature of service.
- Prepare and interpret budget consistently throughout the organization.
- Review performance of the previous year and evaluate its adequacy in terms of quantity and quality.
- Make the budget flexible.

Characteristics of Budget

The following list provides the characteristics of budget:
- It is a plan, framed based on experience.
- It is a comprehensive plan of action.
- Budget is a scheme for work.
- It should estimate revenues and expenditures as accurately as possible.
- It generally involves an annual plan.
- The budget should be flexible and defined clearly.
- It should be a synthesis of past, present, and future.
- The budget should be a joint venture involving different levels.
- It should be in the form of statistical standard laid down in specific numerical terms.
- The budget should represent expected revenue as compared with anticipated expenses.
- The budget should facilitate goal achievement.

Terminology of Budget

The various terminologies used with regard to budget are listed as follows:

1. **Union budget:** Union budget or annual budget is the overall finance of the Government of India. The finance minister reads a report containing revenue and expenditure for one fiscal year. The fiscal year is from April 01 to March 31. It outlines the broad direction of the budget and the economic performance of the country based on its economic survey. It comprises both revenue and capital budget, and an estimate of the next fiscal year (budgeted estimates). Finance minister presents the annual union budget in the Parliament on the last working day of February. The budget has to pass by the Lok Sabha before it can come into effect on April 01.
2. **Revenue budget:** It has revenue receipts of the government showing revenues from tax and other sources and the expenses from these revenues. Revenue receipts are tax and nontax revenues. Tax revenues include charges such as income tax, excise, customs, and other duties that the government levies. Nontax revenue is the interest and dividend on investments by government, fees, and other receipts for services rendered by the government.
3. **Revenue expenditure:** The revenue expenditure is the payment incurred for the daily running of government departments and various activities offered to its citizens. The government also has other expenses such as servicing the interest on its borrowings, subsidies, etc. The revenue expenditures generally do not result in creating assets and grants given to state governments and other parties. Usually there is no difference between revenue receipts and revenue expenditure. It means that the government spends more than it earns. The revenue deficit is the difference between revenue receipts and revenue expenditure.
4. **Capital budget:** Capital budget includes both capital receipts and payments. It incorporates transactions in the public account.
    - *Capital receipts:* The capital receipts are loans raised by the government from the public, such as market loans, borrowed from the Reserve Bank by Government, and other parties. It also includes loans from foreign governments and bodies and recoveries of loans granted by central government to state and union territories (UTs) and other parties.
    - *Capital payments:* These are the expenses acquired from assets, e.g., machinery, land, buildings, equipment, etc. and acquired by state and UT governments from the center.
5. **Plan and nonplan expenditure**
    - *Plan expenditure:* Plan expenditure includes spending from the central government's total expenditure. It also consists of the demands for grants of the various ministries, and the expense on developing "planned" projects is plan expenditure.
    - Nonplan expenditure
        - *Nonplan revenue expenditure:* It is the expenditure of interest payments, subsidies, salary, wages, pensions of government employees, police, financial and general services in various sectors, grants to states and UTs, and grants to foreign governments.
        - *Nonplan capital expenditure:* Nonplan capital expenditure mainly includes defense, loans to public enterprises, states, UTs, and foreign governments and also the nonplan expenditure incurred on the maintenance and running of the existing projects.
6. **Financial policy:** It is a plan specifying government spending changes such as taxes, spending, and budget deficit or surplus to control total economy demand to affect public expenditure.
7. **Fiscal/finance deficit:** The budgetary or finance deficit is the difference between the government's total spending and the sum of its tax and nontax revenue (revenue receipts) and nondebt capital receipts. It represents the total amount of loans required by the government to meet its cost.
8. **Hospital budget:** Hospital budget is a statement of future management policies and plans expressed in accounting terms.
    —*Charles Roswell of United Hospital Fund, New York*
9. **Nursing budget:** The nursing service budget is one of the segments of the overall hospital budget. The service budget is primarily concerned with salaries, supplies, equipment, training, and capital expenditure. But the present era, with the evolution of nursing as a business, has focused on financial management for nursing administrators. Various factors including the persistent need for nursing to have financial control as a source of professional power, the question of cost-effective nursing services, and consumers' movements for competitive pricing in the market place highlighted the importance of the financial management in nursing.

Typology of Budget

Budgets are of various types, and each is classified differently by the fiscal managers based on different criteria/bases.

1. **Based on fiscal/nonfiscal budget**
    - **Financial budget:** It includes capital budget, revenue budget, operating expenditure budget, zero-based budget, performance budget, and program budget.
        - *Capital expenditure budget:* The capital expenditure budget includes the purchases of land, buildings, major equipment of considerable expense and lifelong.
        - *Operating budget:* It provides for the cost of supplies, minor equipment repairs, and overhead expenses.
        - *Zero-based budget:* It is one of the budgets that do not utilize any historical data to determine the activity level or costs anticipated. All the

expenses are justified based on expectations or desires for the upcoming year.
- *Program budget:* Computing cost for a total program refers to the program budget.
- *Performance budget:* The budget based on functions, such as direct nursing care, supervision, in-service education, nursing audit, and so on is a performance budget.
- *Revenue and expense budget:* It is expressed in financial terms and takes the nature of proforma income statement for the future. It shows items of profit and loss under classified headings.
- **Nonfinancial budget:** It includes direct labor budget, time, space, material, and production budget, and advertising budget.
  - *Direct labor house:* Direct labor house budget includes the wages and salaries of regular employees.
  - *Time, space, material, and production budgets:* These budgets are expressed in quantities rather than in monetary terms translated into financial terms.
2. **Based on the period of coverage:** It includes the annual budget, long-term budget, current budget, and rolling budget.
   - *Annual budget:* A yearly budget is a financial plan that depicts income and expenditure for a fiscal year of an organization.
   - *Long-term budget:* A long-term budget is a financial plan depicting income and expenditure extended for more than 1 year in the future. Usually it is for a period of 5 years with strategic planning.
   - *Current budget:* A temporary or adjusted financial plan depicting the amount of money to spend in the current fiscal year that usually starts from July 1 to June 30.
   - *Rollover budget:* It is one that forecasts program, revenue, and expenses for a period higher than a year to accommodate applications that are larger than the annual budget cycle.
3. **Based on the financial position:** It consists of a balanced budget, deficit budget, and surplus budget.
   - *Cash budget:* It is prepared by the way of projecting possible cash receipts and payments over the budget period.
   - *Balanced deficit budget:* A balanced deficit budget is a type of financial plan when expenses exceed the income.
   - *Balanced budget:* A balanced budget is a financial plan having revenue and expenditure equal or nearly equal or expenses that do not exceed income, usually found in the government sector.
   - *Surplus budget:* It is a financial plan depicting expected revenue exceeding the estimated expenditure for a fiscal year.
4. **Other types of budget:**
   - Fixed budget, flexible budget, and open-ended budget:
     - *Fixed budget:* It refers to those components of budgets that will not vary regardless of changes in patient census or number of procedures.
     - *Flexible budget:* It is a variable budget and refers to those components of the budget that will determine how the budget should fluctuate based on those changes in the number of procedures or units of activity.
     - *Open-ended budget:* It is a financial plan that presents a single-cost estimate that considers the optimal activity level for each program without indicating how the policy should be scaled down if less funding is available.
   - Historical versus forecast/statistical budget and trended budget:
     - *Historical budget:* In the historical budget, the previous year's expenses are considered as a basis for costs for the next year. Most healthcare institutions use historical data to develop a budget.
     - *Forecast or statistical budget:* Forecast budget is developed by establishing a level of anticipated activity based on historical or other data such as loss or gain of a specific program.
     - *Trended budget:* Trended budget is one that is developed based on the previous year's expenditure pattern. If a specific percentage of expenses occurs in a particular month, the budget will be developed using those trends to spread the costs.

Master Budget

When the budgets of all departments are combined, it results in a "master" budget. A master budget is a comprehensive budget. It is a financial document depicting income and expenses, overhead, and production/service cost, monthly, annual averages, and total projections for a specified period. It also includes all operating budgets, such as sales, marketing, direct labor, inventory, direct material, production, overhead, capital budgets, etc.

The master budget includes an operating and financial budget plan for a specified period. The operating budget provides revenue, expenses, and profit. Profit is the expected revenue of all sources with budgeted costs. A financial plan consists of a cash budget and a capital expenditure budget. **Box 55.1** depicts operational definitions of budget terminology used in the master budget.

BUDGETING

The process of budgeting has gained importance in recent years because of rising healthcare costs and the emphasis on cost containment. The use of data from budgets to guide decision-making is essential for every level of manager in the healthcare system. It is important to budget to facilitate goal achievement.

Budgeting is an essential component of all six management functions. Budgeting is an integral part of

> **Box 55.1:** Budget terminologies.
>
> **Revenue/income:** Income includes income or revenue from all sources. It includes all interests, dividends, royalties, donations, etc.
> **Expenses:** Expenses includes production/service, material cost, and overhead cost. Expenses are those items or services necessary for the operation that costs the unit, department, or organization money, e.g. salaries, fringe benefits, utilities, and office supplies
> **Production cost:** All costs incurred for production of goods or service is known as production costs
> **Material cost:** All costs incurred for material
> **Overhead cost:** All costs incurred on department/office rent, office supplies, general and administrative cost, etc.
> **Cash flow/budget:** A prediction of future cash receipt and expenditures for a particular time period
> **Cash expenditure budget:** A process of allocating resources for major capital, long-term investment, expenditure, such as machinery, new products, new research development projects, etc.
> **Totals:** Totals refer to category-wise total income and expenses by month to determine the net income (profit) and loss per month and for a year
> **Projections:** Projections refer to projection of annual performance by averaging monthly income and expenses
> **Income statement** presents results of operating activities of the organization for a specific period of time (usually for a fiscal year). The statement summarized revenues/income and expenses and reveals net income or earnings of the organization during the period covered
> **Variance:** The difference between the budgeted amount spent and received and the actual amount paid or received
>
> $$\text{Variance} = \text{Actual amount} - \text{the budgeted amount}$$
>
> $$\text{Percentage variance} = \frac{\text{Actual amount} - \text{the budgeted amount}}{\text{Budgeted amount}} \times 100$$
>
> **Fiscal year:** It is the 12-month accounting period. In India, March 1 to February 28 is the fiscal year.
> **Contribution margin:** It is the net profit of what remains of revenue after the expenses paid.
>
> $$\text{Contribution margin} = \text{Revenue} - \text{expenses}$$
>
> $$\text{Contribution percentage} = \frac{\text{Contribution margin}}{\text{Revenue}} \times 100$$

of estimating the future while taking the management inputs, considering the internal and external factors of an organization. Budgeting is a process of expressing resource requirements that includes the amount of capital, material, and the number of people into time-phased goals and milestones.

It is a continuous process of carrying out activities to prepare a budget or a financial action plan. The budget is a document or quantitative plan for managing income and expenses. It uses numerical data to predict activities of an organization over time and provides a mechanism for planning according to the needs and contributions of each unit. It includes the amount of capital, material, and people into time-phased goals and milestones.

Principles of Budgeting

The various principles involved in budgeting are as follows:

- **Principle of comprehensiveness:** It means that budgeting should provide sound financial management by focusing per the organizational requirements. It should be objective and policy oriented.
- **Principle of flexibility:** The principle of flexibility means that there should be flexibility in budgeting.
- **Principle of annularity:** It implies that budgeting requires a review of the performance of the previous year. It is an evaluation of its adequacy both in quantity and in quality.
- **Principle of appropriateness:** It means that budgeting periods should be appropriate to the nature of business or service and the type of budget.
- **Principle of universality:** It means that the budget must be prepared and interpreted consistently throughout the organization from the planning process.
- **Principle of specificity:** It means that the budget must allocate identifiable objects and plan program activities in advance. It should contain both long-term and short-term expense items (annual operating funds).
- **Principle of exclusiveness:** According to the principle of exclusiveness, budget is concerned with money, not with issues. Setting budgeting targets requires the utmost care to check against and balance between too high or too low estimates.
- **Principle of delegation:** This principle specifies that the budgeting process needs consistent delegation. For

administrative management. It serves as a powerful tool of coordination and a useful device for eliminating duplication and wastage. It serves both planning and control functions in the process of management **(Fig. 55.1).**

Definitions

Budgeting is the allocation of scarce resources based on the forecast needs for proposed activities over some time. According to Koontz, it is the developed plans for a given future period in numerical terms. Budgeting is a process

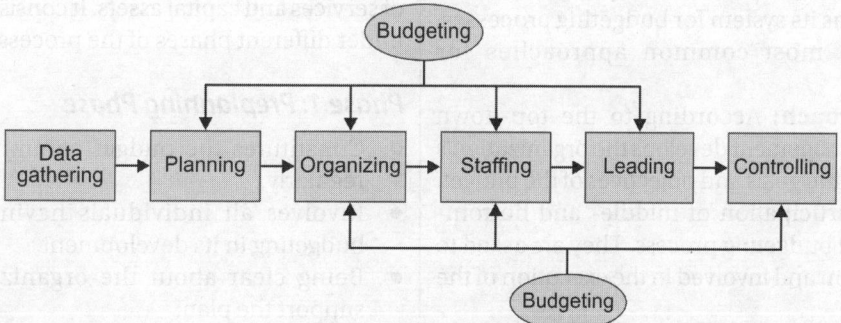

Fig. 55.1: Budgeting as planning and controlling.

that, it needs to allocate duties and responsibilities to frame and execute budget among managers at different levels.
- **Principle of coordination:** It states that coordinating efforts should be made by various departments in establishing a frame of reference for managerial decisions in budgeting and providing a criterion for evaluating managerial performance.
- **Principle of accountability:** It specifies that the managers must spend money as indicated in the budget plan. They must use scarce financial and nonfinancial resources most effectively.

Purposes of Budgeting

Primary goal: To ensure the most effective use of scarce financial and nonfinancial resources.

Specific Purposes

- It provides a detailed plan to reduce uncertainty.
- It controls expenses by an efficient and economical manner.
- It provides the mechanism for measurement of work effort on a timely basis.
- It ensures the accountability by someone for variances from budget.
- It enhances the budget planning.
- It coordinates effort among organizational departments.
- It establishes a frame of reference for management decisions.
- It provides a criterion for evaluating managerial performance.
- It allows for feedback, concerning the events to which actual spending confirm the budgetary sending.
- It offers a useful format for communication.
- It provides the best care that science can make possible on as economical a basis as possible.
- It aids in planning and controlling.
- It guides for action and future needs.
- It serves as an instrument for economic and social policies.
- It conserves the resources by regulation.

Approaches to Budgeting

Approaches for budgeting to be adopted by the organization depend on its philosophy of fiscal affairs. Various budgetary processes are used by organizations. Each organization has its system for budgeting processes. Following are the most common approaches for budgeting:

1. **Top-down approach:** According to the top-down approach, top management develops the organization's budget. They outline goals and objectives of the budget. There is little participation of middle- and bottom-level managers in budgeting process. They are asked to supply information and involved in the execution of the allocated budget.

    Advantages:
    - It is a functional approach rather than divisional.
    - The main concern is the overall growth of the organization.
    - The experienced person prepare the budget.
    - It is a fast approach wherein departmental issues are likely to miss.

    Disadvantages:
    - No or limited participation of bottom-level employees.
    - Demoralization and frustration among lower-level managers.
    - Poor communication and coordination.
    - Noncooperation at the time of execution.
    - Chances of inaccuracy in budget forecasting.

2. **Bottom-up approach:** A bottom-up approach is a participatory approach to budgeting process. Lower-level management is involved in preparing budgets under the guidance and guidelines given by the upper-level management. Each department prepares its budget. Later on, all operational budgets are combined to develop a master budget.

    Advantages:
    - It is a divisional approach rather than functional.
    - Departments prepare their budgets.
    - Managers are highly motivated and take initiative.
    - They are more committed.
    - Better coordination and communication.
    - Overall accuracy in the budget over the total budget.
    - Full cooperation from all departments for its execution.

    Disadvantages:
    - It is a slow approach and takes time in budget preparation.
    - Question of inefficiency on the part of bottom-level management.
    - May not be at par with organizational objectives.

Steps in Budgeting

Budgeting is a process of a systematic activity of creating an expenditure plan, usually for fixed resources for a given period to achieve the desired result. A method for spending is called a budget. Budget preparation is one of the activities of budgeting. The budgeting process is a sequential activity. It comprises activities that encompass the development, implementation, and evaluation of a plan for the provision of services and capital assets. It consists of many businesses under different phases of the process (**Fig. 55.2**):

Phase 1: Preplanning Phase

- Constitutes the budget committee. Have meetings regularly.
- Involves all individuals having responsibility for budgeting in its development.
- Being clear about the organizational structure to support the plan.

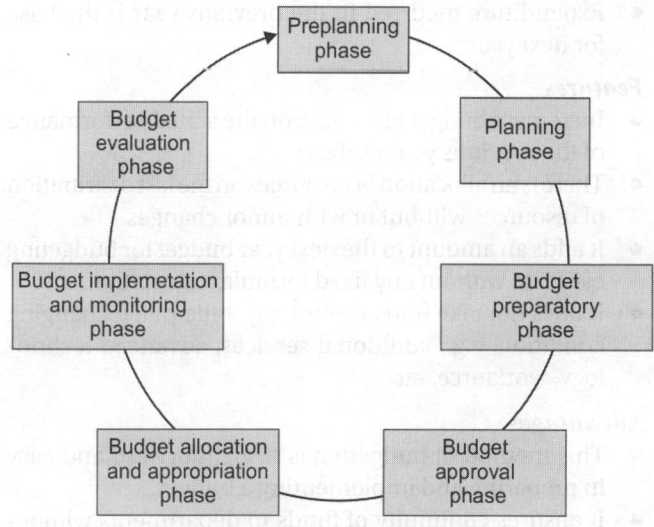

Fig. 55.2: Phases/steps in budgeting.

- Being clear about the accounting system of organization.
- Having knowledge and orientation regarding the budgeting process.
- Deciding and developing a philosophy for fiscal affairs/approaches of budgeting (either top-down or bottom-up approach) to achieve goals.
- Defining budgeting/fiscal period.
- Sending circular to departments to furnish record of money received/sanctioned, expense, and future requirements.

Phase 2: Planning Phase

1. **Plan budget foundation activities:**
   - Gather information about cost estimates, personal issues together with anticipated changes and their impact, e.g., patient's demographics, stabilization in medical practice, referral pattern, technology advancement, etc. to facilitate forecasting or projecting activity from each department.
2. **Establish broad goals and objectives:**
   - General purposes provide overall direction that serves as a basis for decision-making. The objectives should be consistent with the goals, objectives, and policies of the organization. Develop it per the guidelines of governing body or board of trustees and in consultation with the finance officer, which will constitute a tentative outline of the financial plan.
3. **Update budget assumption:**
   - Assumptions must be known and utilized throughout the process. These must be uniform and coordinated organization-wide
   - Premises must be in line with services, personnel, and materials, technology advancements, etc.
4. **Specify program priorities and plan programs:** Develop and specify programs according to preference and various ranges of possibilities with management strategies to achieve their long-term goals.
   - Plan these plans according to their importance and should be affordable within a specific period.
5. **Prepare specific measurable operating objectives:**
   - Prepare particular objectives that should be measurable, attainable, and time-bound.
6. **Plan long-range and program budgets:**
   - Plan master and different operating budgets based on (1) the approach to be used and (2) the method of budgeting to be used per policy
   - Plan monitoring methods, such as motivational tools and variance reports, etc. with their specific measures/criteria
   - Plan qualitative methods such as program evaluation review technique (PERT) and critical path method (CPM) for planning and scheduling
   - Prepare blueprint of budget activities—time frame table using the Gantt chart.

Phase 3: The Budget Preparatory Phase

1. **Develop unit and departmental budgets. Develop operating and capital budgets:**
   - Develop a master budget consistent with approaches to achieve goals
   - Prepare a financial plan and budget to achieve the overall goals within the constraints of available resources
   - Develop a draft cash flow budget
   - Forecast future
   - Anticipate changes and their impact
   - Consider the broadest possible range of alternatives
   - Plan the most effective approach using cost–benefit/effective analysis.
2. **Communicate goals, objectives, and assumption:**
   - Communicate clearly the goals, objectives, and the updated assumptions to all departments
   - Various units and departments should coordinate their plans with each other in case of a bottom-up approach
   - Have discussion and negotiations with the heads of departments and get feedback.
3. **Review and prepare the final draft:**
   - Prepare the final draft of each operating budget by the department after reviewing by the finance officer
   - Submit to authority/finance officer
   - Combine all operating budgets to prepare a master budget plan.

Phase 4: Budget Approval Phase

- Get approval from approving authority per the policy of the organization.
- Under the extramural approval system in government setup, the approving authority is the same for all government-funded hospitals, i.e. through joint secretary, health secretary, and health minister and presented in the parliament and approved by the prime minister, the chairman.

- Under the intramural approval system, approving authority is with the head of an institute through heads of departments within the organization. The finance officer in the governing body presents the final draft or board of trustees approve it.

Phase 5: Budget Allocation and Appropriation Phase

- Under the extramural approval system in government setup, the budget is allocated to organizations after the final approval of the budget voted on the account of maintenance.
- The sanctioning of finance is on funding, policy, performance, actual expenditure of last year, and plans; the finance sanction is in installment.

Phase 6: Budget Implementation and Monitoring Phase

- The departments use the sanctioned budget for the planned activities and programs, as mentioned in the Gantt chart.
- It uses motivational measures as incentives for employees to work.
- Monitor the utilization of budget by using PERT and CPM methods.
- The department prepares budget variance reports.

Phase 7: Budget Evaluation Phase

- The organization constitutes a budget monitoring committee comprising the representatives of each department; the financial advisor reviews the budget.
- The committee reviews the budget in terms of forecasting, expense, cash position, and deviation from budget.
- It evaluates the program and financial performance continually and makes adjustments to encourage progress to achieve goals.

Types of Budgeting

There are various ways of classifying budgeting. Most of the organizations classify budgeting on its policy. Important budgeting methods are as follows:

Incremental Budgeting

Incremental budgeting is a type of traditional budgeting where the budget is prepared based on the previous budget period/fiscal year or actual performance. For planning next year's budget, add the incremental amount in the last year's budget without anticipating any changing conditions. The departmental managers justify only the additional increase over the previous year's budget, and the organization automatically sanctions the spent money.

Assumptions
- All departments will continue to operate at their current expenditure level.
- Expenditure incurred in the previous year is the base for next year.

Features
- Increment budget has a base on the actual performance of the previous year budget.
- There is an allocation of resources on the last distribution of resources without or with minor changes.
- It adds an amount to the next year budget for budgeting estimate without any fixed formula/calculation.
- It does not take into account any anticipated changing condition, e.g., additional services, advanced technology, workforce, etc.

Advantages
- This method of budgeting is straightforward and easy in preparing and implementing a budget.
- It ensures continuity of funds to departments without putting much efforts to calculate.
- It is a stable budget and gradually changes budget requirements.
- It provides equal feeling among all departments and units.
- This method is more appropriate to departments having fixed funding requirements.
- One can quickly and immediately evaluate the impact of any change made in funding.
- It is easy to coordinate with all departments and to get feedback from them.

Disadvantages
- There is no objective method for calculating the incremental amount.
- Assumption of continuing to operate departments at the current expenditure is baseless.
- No effort is made to anticipate any change or advancement in the department.
- No provision to consider priority areas at the time of preparing the budget.
- Priority areas may change at the time of implementation of the budget.
- The requirement of the department is not under consideration in this type of budget.
- There is no change in the working methods of department.
- It does not focus on performance improvement.
- Activities and functions may get outdated in due course of time.
- It may encourage the highest spending of the budget for the sake of estimating the budget for the next year.
- It may create low revenue growth (income) with high expenditure (budgetary slack) to obtain the favor.
- There is no room for innovation, and cost reduction may bring inefficiency among employees.

Zero-based Budgeting

Zero-based budgeting (ZBB) was adopted in India in 1986 as a technique for determining expenditure budgets. Accordingly, the Ministry of Finance instructed all the administrative ministries to review their respective programs and activities to prepare expenditure budget estimates based on the principles of zero-based budgeting.

Meaning
Zero-based budgeting is a type of budget starting from the zero base every fiscal year. The managers need to submit detailed expenses of the approved budget with justification and start from scratch. Zero-based budgeting is a method of planning and decision-making which reverses the working process of traditional budgeting. Each department reviews budget comprehensively to seek approval for all expenditures. It ranks priority areas according to the importance and requirements. It also allocates resources according to the priority areas, without considering past performance or spending.

Assumption
No balance carried forward. Expenses of the current year need not be calculated on the previous year expenses.

Features
- Budget is prepared on a zero basis or from scratch.
- It focuses on identifying and prioritizing activities according to its importance/need.
- It needs to evaluate all possible alternative sources of fund.
- The estimation of expenses should be on cost–benefit analysis.
- The method is action oriented and dynamic.
- It works on the range of possibilities on cost reduction.

Steps
- It identifies organizational program.
- It divides the program into decision packages.
- Each decision package should have its goals, activities, and needed resources.
- It emphasizes calculating the cost for each packet from zero bases per priority.
- It focuses on calculating funds for each budget period anew according to the availability of funds and resources to various decision packages.

Advantages
- It forces the managers to plan each program package afresh.
- It avoids the prevailing tendency in the budgeting of looking at changes from a previous period.
- It allocates resources per needs and benefits.
- It includes cost-effective ways to improve operations.
- It is useful in departments that were challenging to identify the output.
- It enhances staff motivation by providing higher initiative and responsibility in decision-making.
- It improves communication and coordination within the organization.
- It tries to identify and eliminate wasteful and obsolete operations.
- The managers set priorities and use resources most efficiently.
- The managers identify opportunities for outsourcing.
- It forces cost centers to define their mission and their relationship to overall goals.

Disadvantages
- It is challenging to define decision units and decision packages.
- The process is time consuming and exhaustive.
- It forces us to justify every detail related to expenditure.
- It is comparatively expensive than traditional method as more skilled persons are required.
- It requires more administrative staff to prepare and deal with zero budgeting process.
- The honesty of the managers must be reliable and uniform.
- There is a possibility to miss critically important details.
- Sometimes, overburden may demotivate employees.
- Difference between zero-based and incremental budgeting.
- Zero-base budgeting differs from incremental budgeting in various parameters, such as basis, allocation of resources, expenses, innovation, the time factor, preparation effort, and training requirements **(Table 55.1)**.

Performance Budgeting
It is a system of presenting both inputs of resources and output of services of an organization and units. The revenue and expenditure reflected in functions, programs,

TABLE 55.1: Difference between zero-based budgeting and incremental budgeting.

Parameter	Zero-based budgeting	Incremental budgeting
Basis	Zero as a base; the starting point is zero	Previous fiscal year budget is the starting point/base
Allocation of resources	Focused on revenue generating activities/ activities beneficial to the organization	Without giving any priority to vital activities or previous year budget, it adjusts with the incremental amount
Expenses	Expense estimation is done based on cost–benefit analysis	No fixed formula to estimate the costs can lead to wasteful expenses
Innovation	Promotes innovation and range of possibilities to reduce cost	Does not encourage innovation, since budget is stable over the years with a marginal increment
Nature	It is dynamic	It is conservative
Time factor	It is time consuming and exhaustive process	It is a simple and easy method
Preparatory effort	It requires in-depth analysis and complex calculations	Easy to prepare the budget
Training requirements	Individual involved in budgeting requires specialized training regarding the budgeting process	The department can prepare a secure method easily

performance units, primarily the output, and its cost. The funds and resources are allocated to specific goals. It emphasizes accountability efficiently and economy by highlighting outcomes. The main goal is to find out and measure relative performance to achieve goal for a specified result. Work measurement studies, performance norms, indicators, monitoring methods as Gantt chart, PERT, and cost–benefit analysis methods applied to study performance budgeting.

Features
- The budget must indicate purpose and objectives for getting funds.
- It must also show the cost and output of each program and program activity.
- Each activity/program based on cost–benefit analysis regardless of fund allocation.
- It uses management tools such as work measurement, benchmarking, and cost cutting.
- It is applicable for long-term plans.
- It has performance criteria/standards.
- It requires a lot of effort in formulating objectives, identifying programs based on cost–benefit analysis, developing targets, performance indicators/criteria, method of assessing performance with planned performance budget, etc.

Process of performance budgeting
- Formulate objective.
- Identify functions, programs, activities, and projects.
- Evaluate and select program and projects based on cost–benefit analysis.
- Specify targets, performance norms, indicators for each application, and project.
- Develop a financial plan and allocate resources for each program and project and annual budget.
- Specify means of achieving them.
- Design the monitoring, recording, and evaluation system, such as PERT and CPM.
- Implement the program after getting the grants.
- Monitor the activities and regulate the flow of expenditure.
- Prepare time-phased reports showing payment and work and keep a record.
- Assess the performance of each program and compare its budgeted performance.
- Correct if any deviations.

Preparation of performance budget
1. **Allocation of resources:** Submit the requirements per program classification. Indicate its past activities, their costs, the activities to be taken up during next year, the results expected, a pattern of assignment of responsibilities, or time-phased plan for expenditure and work.
2. **Budget execution:** Initiate the action for implementation after getting the grants. Monitor the activities and regulate the flow of expenditure. Prepare the time-phased reports showing investment and work and keep a record.
3. **Appraisal and evaluation:** Evaluate each program in the light of results obtained and expenditure incurred.

Advantages
- The budget has clear goals and objectives based on performance.
- It allocates the funds on the expected performance cost.
- The method aims at improving the performance.
- It is a very objective method based on cost–effective analysis.
- Each program evaluated based on criteria and indicators.
- The outcome weighs against budgeted performance.

Disadvantages
- There is a possibility of inaccuracy in forecasting and expenses.
- It measures the results quantitatively.
- It needs a proper accounting, monitoring, and reporting system.
- It is difficult to measure the social benefit of functions.
- The process is time consuming and expensive.
- Due to its flexibility feature, programs may change at the time of implementation.
- It requires more skilled man hours to plan and implement the process.

Activity-based Budgeting

Activity-based budgeting (ABB) relies on activity framework rather than functions. It is an output-oriented approach. It is a method to (1) identify activities and estimate the cost of each event, (2) forecast unit of value for required actions, and (3) then calculate the price per unit of activity. It is a process of analyzing the operations and allocating the resources based on its outcome. It identifies overhead or nonproductive events and associates costs in proportion to operating expenses.

Features
- The budget must indicate activities requiring funds.
- It must show the cost and output of each activity.
- It needs analysis of activities on price per unit of activity.
- Cost per unit of operation is on its production.
- It draws attention to overhead activities too.
- It focuses on short-term goals.

Advantages
- This method can identify cost-effectiveness activities.
- It brings efficiency.
- Budget is prepared considering the cause and effect of cost.
- It is an activity-oriented approach to budgeting.
- Planned activities are carried out at low cost and most effectively.

Disadvantages
- It is a time-consuming process of budgeting.
- It requires knowledge of various functional areas.
- It is a complex process of analyzing each activity and its cost through cost-effective analysis.

- More working hours and skilled persons are required to plan and implement the process.
- It achieves short-term goals of an organization.

BUDGETARY PROCESS

Definitions

The budgeting process is a systematic activity that has an expenditure plan of usually fixed resources of a given period to achieve the desired result. The budgetary process is a sequential activity. The budget process activities include the development, implementation, and evaluation of a plan to provide services and capital assets.

Prerequisite of the Budgetary Process

The prerequisite of budgetary process are as follows:
- The budgetary plan should have goals or objectives.
- There should be an organizational structure to develop the budget.
- The manager should know the budget process.
- There should be enough economic data to facilitate budget planning.
- The budget period must be clearly defined.
- The accounting system must be clear.
- The departmental managers must take feedback on their performance.
- It prioritizes the organizational goals before preparing the capital budget.
- Assumptions must be uniform and coordinated organization wide.
- It prepares a statistical budget to develop an operating budget and capital budget.

Features of the Budgetary Process

Listed below are the features of budgetary process:
- Incorporates a long-term perspective
- Establishes linkages to broad goals
- Focuses on budget decisions on results and outcomes
- Involves and promotes effective communication
- Provides incentives to government management and employees.

Principles of the Budgetary Process

The principles of budgetary process are as follows:
- **Establish broad goals:** These goals guide government decision-making—broad goals provide overall direction for the government and serve as a basis for decision-making.
- **Develop strategies to achieve goals:** Define specific policies, plans, programs, and management strategies to achieve its long-term goals.
- **Develop a budget:** The budget must be consistent with the developed strategies. Prepare a financial plan and budget within the available resources.
- **Evaluate performance and make modifications:** Evaluate the program and financial performance continually and make changes accordingly.

Steps in the Budgetary Process

The four steps involved in budgetary process are as follows:
1. **Budget estimate preparation:** Usually, the account section of the institute prepares finances and budget. Most institutes have a centralized system to keep a record of revenue/income and expenditure. The head of the accounts department is usually under the head of the institution. Each department holds a record of revenue and investment. Sources of income can be many. Internal sources are revenue from different sections such as fee section, outpatient departments, indoor departments, emergency, teaching institutes, etc. The revenues generated from donations, ministries, and states are external sources **(Fig. 55.3)**.

   The institute follows a process to estimate its budget. The accounts section intimates different departments to provide departmental estimate projection well on time. The accounts section accepts the proposal and considers

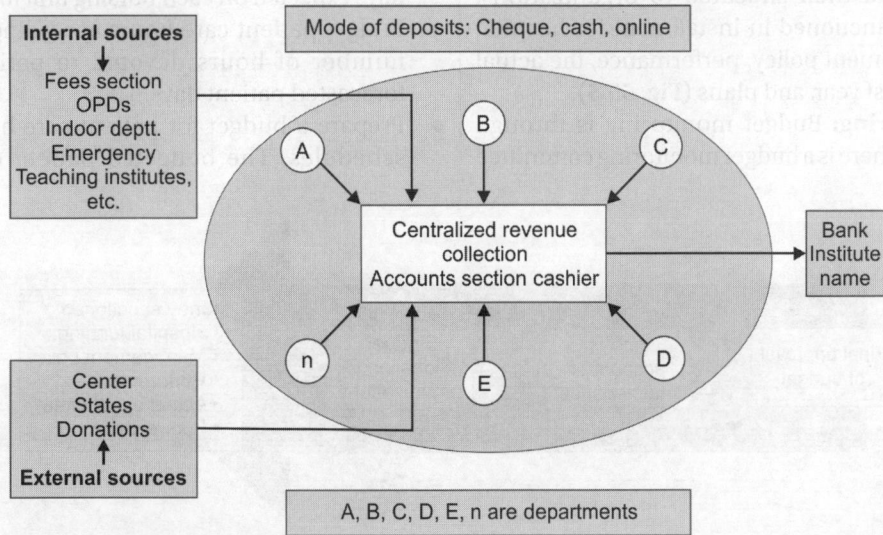

Fig. 55.3: Sources and revenue procedure of an institute.

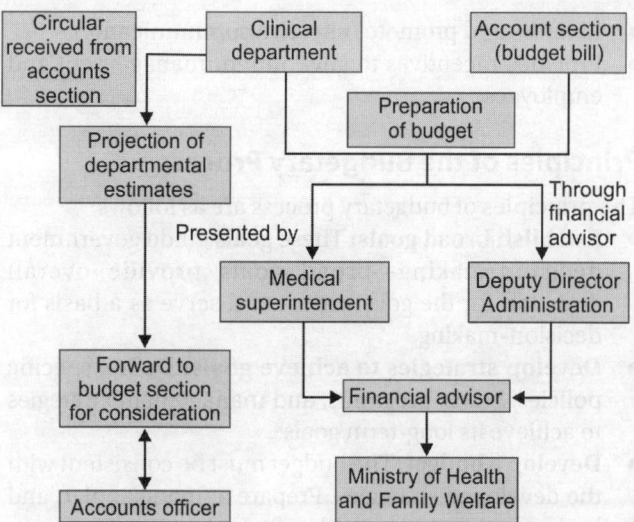

Fig. 55.4: Budget estimate preparation procedure by the government institutes.

it for discussion. The accounts section after getting the project from clinical, teaching, and other departments discusses with the medical superintendent and deputy director of the institute, through finance advisor. The finance advisor, with approval of the director, forwards the budget to the Ministry for support.

2. **Budget approval:**
   - *Extramural approval system:* The approving authority is the same for all government-funded hospitals, i.e., through joint secretary, health secretary, and health minister. The budget is presented in the parliament and signed by the prime minister for the final approval.
   - *Intramural approval system:* The intramural approval system, i.e., within the organization approval system **(Fig. 55.4)**, and it has to go in two steps: First by the head of the hospital and then by the head of the institute.

3. **Budget allocation and appropriation:** After the final approval, the budget is voted on account of maintenance and then allocated to organizations. The finance is sanctioned in installment for hospital funding, management policy, performance, the actual expenditure of last year, and plans **(Fig. 55.5)**.

4. **Budget monitoring:** Budget monitoring is through budget reports. There is a budget monitoring committee comprising representatives of each department, financial advisor to review budget prepared in terms of forecasting, expense, cash position, and deviation from budget.

NURSING BUDGET

The nursing budget is a plan of estimating revenues and expenses based on the needs for a proposed program to render patient care during one fiscal year. It is a systematic plan projecting how revenues will meet costs and a return on equity.

Advantages

The advantages of nursing budget are as follows:
- It aids in developing written broad and specific objectives for each unit and nursing organization.
- It manages the financial part in nursing through an operational budget.
- It can create a new sense of involvement for nurses.
- Effective planning eliminates the activities in case of noncompliance with goals.
- In nursing, budget plan helps to ensure that clients or patients receive the nursing services from satisfied nursing workers.
- Cost-effectiveness as a unit manager's goal.
- Cost-effectiveness does not mean inexpensive, and it means getting the most for money or that the product is worth the price.
- It takes into account factors, such as anticipated length of services, needs for such service, and availability of other alternativeness to make it cost-effective.

Steps in Nursing Budgeting

Nursing budgeting can be achieved by following the eight steps as listed below: Determine the productivity goals. The director of the nursing service and the nurse manager determine the unit's productivity goal for a fiscal year.
- Forecast the workload according to the number of patient days expected on each nursing unit for a fiscal year.
- Budget patient care hours according to the expected number of hours devoted to patient care for the forecasted patient days.
- Prepare a budget for patient care hours and staffing schedules. The budgeted patient care hours must

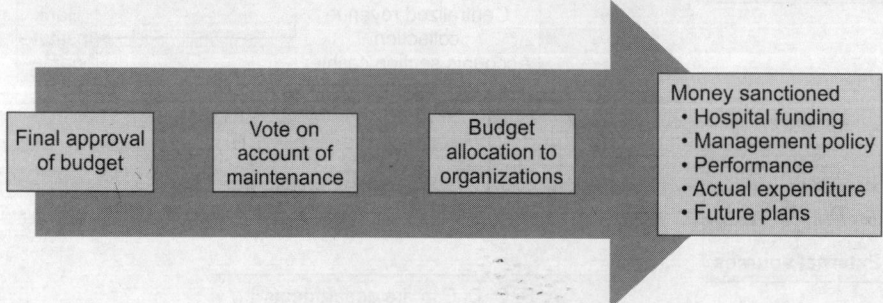

Fig. 55.5: Budget allocation procedure.

- reflect in the recommended staffing schedule by shift and by day of the week.
- Plan budget for nonproductive hours and productive hours for the coming year.
- Estimate costs of supplies and services purchased for the year.
- Anticipate capital expenses. Include the expected capital investment for the coming year in the budget.
- The nursing administrator gets a proposed budget for review. After preliminary acceptance, the nurse administrator forwards the budget to the accounting department where it translates the forecasted patient days into expected revenue. Convert the productive and nonproductive time into money and calculate the costs for supplies, services, and other operating expenses allocated to a given unit for the coming year. The accounts section sends a budget estimate indicating the operating statement to the director of nursing for reviewing which is sent back to the accounting department. The department forwards it to the rest of the head of the institute.

MIDTERM APPRAISAL

The midterm appraisal (MTA) reviews the experience in the first 3 years or midterm of the plan. Its main objective is to identify areas requiring corrective steps. It provides an opportunity for economic status and to introduce policy correctives and new initiatives in critical areas in the context of the new priorities. It monitors the progress made in utilizing available resources. It is an assessment of the resources position facing both the center and the states and the implications.

PROGRAM PLANNING BUDGETING SYSTEM

Program planning budgeting system (PPBS) involves planning and control. The PPBS concepts were first used in private industry by companies, such as the Rand cooperation, General Motors, etc. As early as 1940, the principles of PPBS were applied in World War II production control. Secretary of Defense Robert McNamara introduced it in the United States in 1961. Later, in 1965, President Lyndon Johnson mandated to use it.

Meaning and Definitions

It is a systematic method of allocating the resources to meet organizational goals and objectives. Planning is an activity to formulate and select corporate purposes and courses of action in the pursuit of goals. Programming is the process of converting plans into specific actions or operating procedures. It includes resources and measures needed to implement strategies. Budgeting is preparing an annual budget according to resources and funds available to meet the laid down objectives.

It is a management tool to provide a better analytical basis for decision-making and for putting such decisions into operation. It is an in-depth budget format to plan strategies in multiyear increments, analyze programs regularly to ensure optimal strategy in place, and develop budgets to provide resources according to those strategies. It is an integrated and analytic approach used to allocate the funds to meet the goals of operations.

Aim of Program Planning Budgeting System

The PPBS aimed at ensuring a better linkage between objectives and goals, programs, and activities. In the planning phase, system analysis was used to establish the objectives and identify related solutions. At the programming stage, means were reviewed and compared to the solutions identified at the planning stage. Sets of activities are appraised, compared, and grouped into multiyear programs. Finally, the budgeting phase translates these programs into the annual budget.

Purposes

The function of budgeting is to secure sufficient funds to put the program into operation and to implement and evaluate those operations. Based on the results, modify the current activities, if indicated, or plan the future programs. The main purposes are as follows:
- To provide management with a better analytic basis for making program decisions
- To put the decisions into operation through an integration of the planning, programming, and budgeting functions
- To unify planning, programming, and budgeting
- It is concerned primarily with major decision-making processes: Planning, programming, and budgeting
- To classify the cost by the program according to objectives
- To prepare a detailed description of preferred program activities
- To work out the alternative methods to meet the same goals
- To perform cost–benefit analysis for the selected program and alternative methods
- To select the best one in terms of cost and time. Prefer the most economical to produce the desired objective, which should be most compatible with organizational goals and resources.

Principles of PPBS

The following are the principles of PPBS:
- It examines the expenditures from a system viewpoint and analyzes resources and funds required to produce an estimated output during the process. Program planning and budgeting system analyses of investment encourage to build in feedback loops to keep the plan throughout the process as target for cost control.
- It plans for a single year in advance if the budgetary scope is limited.
- It is better to limit to a preferred program rather than an alternative method, in case financial control focuses on minute subsystems and subcomponents.

Elements of PPBS

The five elements of PPBS are as follows:
1. **A program structure:** The program structure is the heart of PPBS that makes visible both outputs and the necessary resources. A program structure is a classification of the course of action to attain the objectives of an organization. It represents a way of looking at the organization's effort that is suited to the needs of the program analysis and program decision-making. It includes the identification of objectives and courses of action to achieve those objectives. The higher level of goals and objectives are the major programs, and the courses of action constitute the elements of the program. These elements of program represent the output orientation. The course of action must possess the following features:
   - The program elements must be complete; every activity and expense should have a place in the program element.
   - It must have suitability for analysis and identification with the organization units.
   - The decision makers must have the preferences for selecting alternatives at the administrative and academic levels.
   - The program structure must reflect the goals and objectives of the program.
   - It must facilitate the quantitative and qualitative evaluation of outputs.
   - The program structure be readily understandable and compatible with legally accounting and budgeting procedures.
   - Develop and implement the program in phases.
2. **Program document:** The program document is an approved program document indicating precise, quantitative data on needs, resource inputs, and program outputs extending into the future. The program and financial plan is the document that serves the function of formalizing the program. It should also have the time horizon extending years into the future.
3. **A decision-making process:** Decision-making is an essential feature of PPBS. It establishes the functions, rules, and timetables for the actions. It involves creating the responsibilities of the organizational units engaged in planning, programming, and budget preparation.
4. **The analysis process:** An analysis process is for measuring effectiveness and for weighing alternatives. The decision-making process requires analyzing documents to select the best option. The primary function of analysis is to bring program analysis into the program formulation process. It includes various types of analysis, such as cost-effective analysis, cost-benefit analysis, and cost-utility analysis.
5. **Information system:** The information system supplies the data required to implement the system. It must satisfy the need of PPBS. It includes data on demand and output.

Characteristics of PPBS

- It focuses on the goals and objectives of a program.
- It highlights planning activities during the stage of budget preparation.
- It identifies the future implications of current budgeting decisions.
- It considers all costs and systematically analyzes and examines alternative programs in terms of utility and costs.
- It evaluates and controls activities highlighted during the stage of implementation.

Process

The four steps involved in process are as follows:
1. **Planning:** Planning is the legislative instrument that provides a rational basis for decision-making. During preparation, allocate scarce resources to ensure the availability of health services equitably. Spell out plans by programming.
2. **Programming:** It is a detailed allocation of tasks and resources and a detailed description of methods of implementing one or more specified objectives within a given time.
3. **Budgeting:** The budget is prepared to keep in mind all the activities of programs.
4. **Evaluation and control:** Specify evaluation and control activities in the programming and planning process. After implementing plans, analyze for further action.

Steps of PPBS

The various steps in PPBS are the following:
1. Develop alternate implementation program to meet the objectives.
2. Estimate the resource requirements and possible benefits of each program.
3. Selecting among alternatives.
4. Design a managerial technique to merge the planning process with the allocation of funds.
5. A planning process includes program budgeting as its primary component.

Advantages

The advantages of PPBS are as follows:
- It educates the managers to make administrative decisions.
- It clarifies cost consequences of expanding or contracting the service program.

Disadvantages

The disadvantages of PPBS are as follows:
- There is centralization of decision-making at the top level, while managing and controlling responsibilities are of the middle managers.
- It is difficult to understand the language of the program; only administration and the functional experts can understand the language of the program.

CHAPTER HIGHLIGHTS

- Budgeting is a process of allocation of scarce resources based on forecast needs for proposed activities over some time.
- The budget is a plan for an estimate of future needs arranged according to an orderly basis, covering all the activities of an enterprise for a definite period.
- Budgeting follows the principles of comprehensiveness, flexibility, annularity, universality, specificity, delegation, coordination, and accountability.
- Top-down and bottom-up are two essential approaches to the budgetary process. Both have advantages and disadvantages. Strategies for budgeting to be adopted by the organization depend on its philosophy of fiscal affairs.
- The budgeting process is a sequential activity that follows various steps. It consists of activities carried out for development, implementation, and evaluation of budget plans.
- The master budget includes an operating and financial budget plan for a specified period. The operating budget provides revenue, expenses, and profit. The business plan comprises a cash budget and capital expenditure budget as significant sections.
- Budgeting is classified according to its methodology used to prepare budgets. The many different types of budgeting are incremental, zero-based, performance-based, activity-based budgeting.
- The budgeting process is a systematic activity that has an expenditure plan of usually fixed resources of a given period to achieve the desired result.
- The nursing budget is a plan of estimating revenues and expenses based on needs for a proposed program to render patient care during one fiscal year.
- Program planning budgeting system is a system for planning and control.
- It is difficult to identify the output since quantified in financial term.

REVIEW QUESTIONS

I. Essay Type Questions
1. Define budgeting. Describe in detail the steps involved in the budgeting process.
2. What are the different types of budgeting? Discuss performance-based budgeting in detail.
3. Enumerate the principles of budgeting. Describe various approaches to budgeting.
4. What are the principles of the budgetary process? Describe in detail the steps of budgetary process.
5. "Program planning budgeting system" is a system for planning and control. Discuss it in detail.

II. Short Notes
1. Components of a master budget
2. Activity-based budgeting
3. Nursing budget
4. Preparation of performance budget
5. Difference between incremental and zero-based budgeting

III. Multiple Choice Questions
1. Which principle of budgeting focused on the requirement of the organization, its objectives, and policies?
   a. Principle of universality
   b. Principle of comprehensiveness
   c. Principle of exclusiveness
   d. Principle of appropriateness
2. Type of budgeting approach that involves department managers the least in preparing budget but exclusively in the execution of budget:
   a. Top management approach
   b. Bottom-up approach
   c. Top-down approach
   d. Bottom management approach
3. Which activities involved during the planning phase of budgeting?
   a. Updating assumptions and specifying program priorities
   b. Defining budgetary period and deciding philosophy for budgeting
   c. Developing departmental budgets and communicating goals and objectives
   d. Sanctioning budget to departments and monitoring activities
4. Which type of budget prepared on the actual performance of the previous budget with additional amount and resources allocated as of the previous year?
   a. Activity-based budget
   b. Zero-based budget
   c. Performance-based budget
   d. Incremental budget
5. The activity-based plan is usually focused on to achieve:
   a. Long-term goals
   b. Short-term goals
   c. Annual plan goals
   d. Operating plan goals

Answer Keys
1. b   2. c   3. a   4. d   5. b

SUGGESTED READING
1. Available from http://www.indiabudget.nic.in/. [Accessed March 2018].
2. Available from http://www.osbornebooks.co.uk/files/af_as_chapter_19_1.pdf. [Accessed March 2018].
3. Available from http://www.ssronline.org/ssg_a/index.cfm?id=100&p=18. [Accessed March 2018].
4. Besie LM, Carol JH. Leadership Roles and Management in Nursing: Theory and Practice, 5th edition. Lippincott Williams & Wilkins Publications. [Accessed April 2018].

5. Carruth A, Carruth P, Noto E. Financial management. Nurse managers flex their budgetary might, Nurs Manage, 2000; 31(2):16-7.
6. Finkler SA. Budgeting Concepts for Nurse Managers. New York: Grune and Stratton, 1984.
7. Mikesell JL. Fiscal Administration, 8th edition. Boston, MA: Wadsworth, Cengage Learning; 2011.
8. Patricia K. Essentials of Nursing Leadership and Management, 2nd edition. USA: Delmar Cengage Learning; 2010.
9. Rowland HS, Rowland BL (ed). Nursing Administration Handbook. 4th edition. Gaithersberg, Maryland: Aspen Publishers Inc., 1997.
10. Samuel M Greenhouse. The planning-programming-budgeting system: Rationale, language, and idea-relationships. Public Adm Rev. 1966;26(4):271-7.
11. Swanburg RC. The nursing budget. Superv Nurse. 1978;9(6): 40-7.
12. Terry GR. Principles of Management. 7th edition, Homewoods, Illinois: Richard D. Irwin, Inc, 1977.
13. WHO. Administration of environment health programmes: A system view. Public Health Papers, No. 59. Geneva: WHO; 1974.
14. WHO. Planning and programming for nursing services. Public Health Papers, No. 44. Geneva: WHO; 1971.
15. William L. Kissick. Planning, programming, and budgeting in health. Med Care. 1967;5(4):201-20.
16. William O. Cleverley. Essentials of health care finance. USA: Aspen Publishers Inc.; 1992.

56 CHAPTER

Cost Accounting and Health Economics

CHAPTER OUTLINE

- Concept of Cost
  - Definitions
  - Elements of Cost
  - Cost Classifications
  - Types of Costs in Healthcare
- Accounting
- Cost Accounting
  - Definitions
  - Objectives of Cost Accounting
  - Scope of Cost Accounting
  - Importance of Cost Accounting
  - Limitations of Cost Accounting
  - Difference Between Financial and Cost Accounting
- Health Economics
  - Definitions
  - Components of Health Economics
  - Health Economics Map
  - Need and Importance of Health Economics
  - Types of Health Economics
  - Tools for Economic Analysis
  - Economic Evaluation

LEARNING OUTCOMES

After completion of this chapter, the learner will be able to:
- Understand the concept of cost, accounting, and cost accounting
- Define cost, accounting, and cost accounting
- Enumerate various types of healthcare costs and accounting
- Enumerate objectives and discuss the scope of cost accounting
- State the importance and limitations of cost accounting
- Understand the concept of health economics
- Discuss various components and types of health economics
- Familiarize with health economics map
- Realize the need and importance of health economics
- Enumerate tools used in economic analysis
- Discuss the financial evaluation process

KEY TERMS

Cost, accounting, cost accounting, health economics, economics map, macroeconomics, economics evaluation, microeconomics

INTRODUCTION

The cost is essential to fix the price and to have the margin of profit. Costing is the process of ascertaining the expenses. It applies various principles for determining the cost of materials, services, and operations. The accounting is essential for keeping records of all receipts and payments, income, and expenditures. Accounting is an ancient science that aims at keeping records of various transactions and used to study the different aspects of cost as cost accounting.

CONCEPT OF COST

Definitions

The costs are the values of all the resources, such as labor, buildings, equipment, supplies, etc., used to produce a good or service. It is a measure of the value of all resources used in the response. The cost of intervention is an essential part of the decision to use one intervention over another. The price is the actual or estimated expenditure on given things or services.

Elements of Cost

Figure 56.1 depicts the main aspects of cost.
1. **Material cost:** The cost of material comprises direct material and indirect material costs. The direct material cost is the value of the material used directly in the manufacturing product and becomes a part of the product—direct material charges. Whereas the indirect

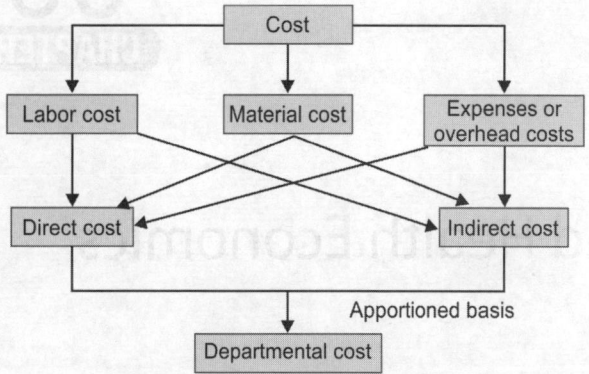

Fig. 56.1: Cost containment elements.

material cost is the cost that is indirectly required for the material but essential for the manufacturing of the equipment.

2. **Labor cost:** The labor cost is of two types: 1. Direct labor cost and 2. Indirect labor cost. The direct labor cost is applied directly to the manufacture of a product. The indirect labor cost is one that has a more general and less direct application, e.g., salaries of safaikaramcharies, electricians, etc.

3. **Expenses or overhead cost:** These include department or office rent, local rates and taxes, insurance, depreciation, etc. The following are the categories of overhead cost:
   - Departmental cost: These include all expenses chargeable to the department.
   - Administrative expenses: These include office rent, general office salaries, professional fees, etc.
   - Selling expenses: These relate to the distribution of the product.

Cost Classifications

The classification of cost helps in better control of cost and in decision-making. There are various ways of classifying cost as discussed below:

Basic Classification

1. **Classification according to elements:** The three aspects of costing are material, labor, and expenses. The total cost of services can be divided into three components to find out the contribution of each element in the total costs.
2. **Classification according to nature:** These include direct and indirect costs:
   a. *Direct costs:* Direct cost is the cost incurred exclusively on the production of a commodity, on the execution of job work, on performing a job. Direct prices are identifiable with the product or service unit. It includes expenses incurred on material, labor, and stores or incurred in the manufacture of the product.
   b. *Indirect costs:* These costs incur to carry on the business and allocate, apportion, and then added in the production or service units. These costs include departmental fees, i.e., rent, insurance, lighting, fuel, depreciation, etc. These apportions on a reasonable basis.
   c. **Direct and indirect costs:** These are materials, labors, and expenses costs.
      - *Direct and indirect material:* Direct material is the material that is identifiable with the product/service, and indirect material cannot identify with the product.
      - *Direct and indirect labor:* Direct labor is a given unit of product, such as piece rate and wages per unit. The direct wage is the remuneration paid to employees directly engaged in the service, as identified as a unit of service. Salaries paid to sweepers, gardeners, maintenance workers, etc. are indirect wages as the undefined unit of service.
      - *Direct and indirect expenses:* Direct expenses are those expenses that are acquired for a specific service, process, job, or cost unit. These expenses are chargeable. Indirect expenses do not purchase directly for a particular service, operation, or cost unit, e.g., electricity, rent, salaries, advertising, etc. The total direct expenses refer to the "prime cost," and all indirect costs involve "overheads."

3. **Classification according to behavior:**
   a. **Fixed costs:** A fixed cost that remains unchanged in total cost as the level of activity varies or changes in service. Usually, fixed costs decreased per unit with an increase in the volume of production, e.g., salaries, insurance, rent, etc.
      - *The fixed costs of a program or intervention:* The fixed costs of a program do not change in a short period and do not vary with the level of activity. Costs associated with rent, utilities, and personnel costs for support staff are the most common examples of fixed costs. These costs incurred at the beginning of program implementation and refer to "startup" costs.
      - *Facilities costs:* Compute facilities cost by adding the value of space, maintenance costs, and the costs of utilities. Costs for facilities are either the cost per unit or the total cost for the services—the equations below determine the facilities costs for programs sharing space in an existing facility.

> Facilities costs = Additional facility space used by the program × cost per square feet for space and utilities
> Or
> Facilities costs = Total facility cost for space and utilities × $\dfrac{\text{Facility time used by the program}}{\text{Facility time used by all programs}}$

   - *Cost for administrative and staff support:* Calculate the costs for administrative and staff support as a proportion of the staff time spent on this particular intervention. The equation to determine the value of administrative and staff support associated with a program is as follows:

> Administrative costs = Proportion of administrator's time spent on intervention × administrator (salary + benefits)
> Support costs = Proportion of staff's time spent on intervention × support (salary + benefits)
> Administrative costs and support costs = Administrative costs + support costs

b. **Variable costs:** Variable costs, as the name indicates, are a change in total in proportion to the level of activity. The per-unit variable cost remains the same, while the total variable costs will vary. These are the expenses incurred; indirect material, labor, and overhead vary with the volume of production—the variable costs of a program change as the level of activity changes. Examples of variable expenses include provider time, medications, tests, material, and supply costs. The typical approach to measure variable costs is to identify the quantity of the relevant resource and multiplying it with per unit price. The equation determines the provider, material, and supply costs.

> Provider cost = Provider (salary + benefits) × average duration of service × number of services provided in period
> Material and supply costs = Specific resource × cost/unit × number of units

c. **Semivariable costs:** Certain costs are partly fixed and partly variable, e.g., maintenance costs.
d. **Standard costs:** The standard cost (SC) of production/unit is the estimated cost. It is a predetermined cost of material, labor, and overhead **(Fig. 56.2)**.
The cost of production determines by fixing standards with each element of values, the standard material cost by setting the standards in terms of quality, quantity, and standard price, and the standard labor and overhead costs estimate by fixing the standard price to time and wage rate.

> Standard price = Current price + future trends + supply position
> Standard cost = Standard material cost + standard labor cost + standard overhead cost
> = (Standard quality × price + standard time × wages) (overheads − the volume of production × standard machine or workforce)

4. **Classification according to functions:**
   a. *Production costs:* All costs incurred for the production of goods are known as production costs.
   b. *Administrative costs:* The administrative cost is one that is incurred for administration, e.g., office salaries, printing, and stationery, office telephone, etc.
   c. *Selling and distribution costs:* The selling cost is to acquire for procuring an order, while all expenses incurred to execute order are distribution costs, e.g., market research expenses, advertising as selling costs and transportation expenses incurred, warehouse rent, etc., are examples of distribution costs.
   d. *Research and development costs:* Expenditure incurred for this function are called research and development costs.
5. **Classification according to time:**
   a. *Historical costs:* These are the costs which are incurred in the past or after the period is over. It has limited importance, still used for estimating the trends of the future. These aid in predicting future costs.
   b. *Predetermined costs:* The costs calculated beforehand based on a specification of all the factors affecting value and cost data are the predetermined costs. These may be either standard or estimated.
6. **Classification of costs from management decision-making:**
   a. *Average cost:* It is the total cost of the unit produced over a number of units produced. One can get the average price by dividing the total cost of production by units.

$$\text{Average cost} = \frac{\text{Total cost of production}}{\text{Number of units produced}}$$

   b. *Marginal cost:* It is the cost of marginal groups provided over a lot of production. It is the change

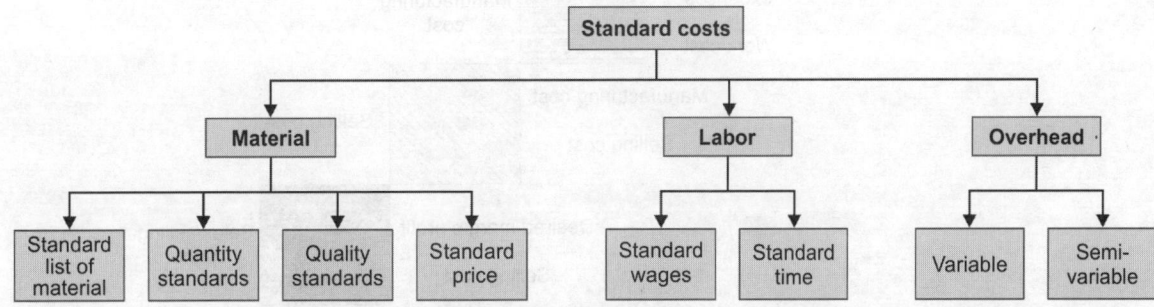

Fig. 56.2: Types of standard costs.

in the aggregate costs due to a change in the volume of output by one unit. For example, the cost of production of 99 units is ₹ 1,985, and the cost of the 100th (marginal) unit is 2,000. Marginal cost = ₹ 15.

c. *Differential costs:* Differential costs or incremental costs is the difference in total cost that arises for selecting alternatives.
d. *Opportunity costs:* The opportunity costs are the value of benefit sacrificed in selecting an alternative course of action. The opportunity cost of products or services is the revenue earned by employing that goods or services in some other alternative use.
e. *Relevant costs:* It is a cost applicable for making various managerial decisions into consideration.
f. *Replacement costs:* It is the cost incurred on the replacement of existing material or fixed assets.
g. *Abnormal costs:* It is an unexpected cost that arises due to idle time, unexpected technical fault, etc.
h. *Controllable costs:* It is a cost that is under the control of any management action in a given period, e.g., costs of telephone, printing stationery, etc. Generally, direct costs are controllable.
i. *Shutdown costs:* These are the costs that are incurred during the shutdown of the operations and disappear on continuing operations.
j. *Capacity costs:* These costs usually are fixed. These costs are like long-term costs and incurred per planning decisions.
k. *Urgent costs:* These are the costs that are incurred to continue operations.

Method of calculation of total cost (Fig. 56.3):
Direct material + direct labor = prime cost
Prime cost + work expenses = work costs
Factory cost + administrative expenses = manufacturing cost
Manufacturing cost + selling expenses = selling cost
Selling cost + desired margin of profit = sales price

Classification of Cost According to WHO

1. **Input category wise:** It consists of the expenses of all inputs, such as salaries, medical supplies, and capital.
2. **International activity wise:** It consists of the costs of all international activities, such as administration planning and supervision activities.
3. **Organizational level:** It consists of the cost of all the activities at the national, district, and hospital level and covers all the relevant costs without overlapping.

Classification of Cost According to Interventional Activities

It covers all the relevant costs of various interventional activities, such as administrative, planning, training, etc. carried out at different organizational levels **(Table 56.1)**.

Classification of Cost as per the Program Cost Sheet

1. **Recurrent expenditure**
   - *Personnel:* Personnel time used to startup and post-startup is expressed in person-months.
   - *Materials and supplies:* Quantities used for the program.
   - *Media operating cost:* This is in term of media input, e.g., radio or TV time, leaflet, posters, and advertisements in newspapers.
   - *Transport operating cost:* This cost is a total of kilometers travel using transport.
   - *Equipment operating cost:* If rented.
   - *Maintenance cost:* This is the percentage of annual fee.
   - *Utilities:* It includes the costs of utility, services, e.g. electricity, gas, water, space in square meter.

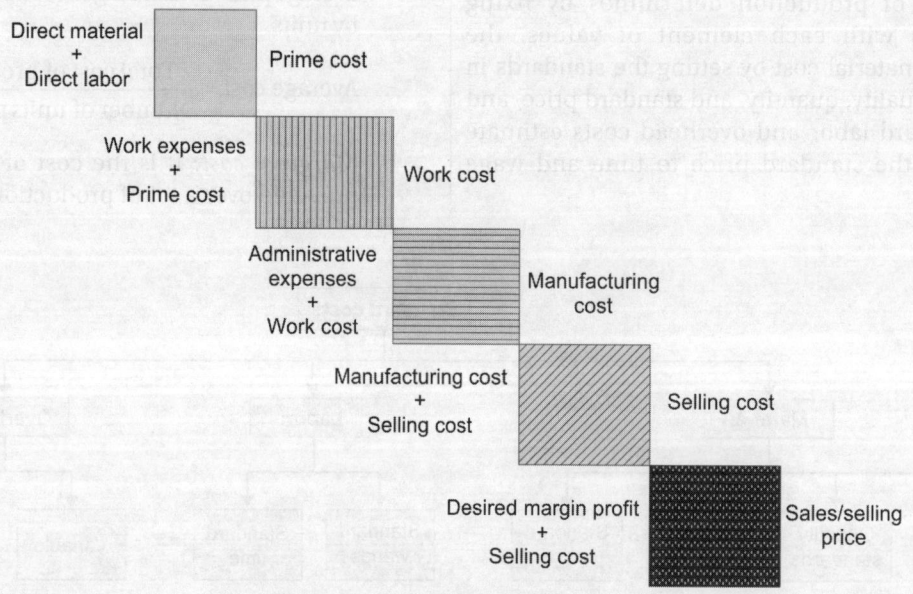

Fig. 56.3: Method for calculating the total cost.

TABLE 56.1: Types of the expenses for intervention activities at different level.

Interventional activities	Type of costs
Administration	Overhead cost: Space, furniture, equipment, utilities, and maintenance + personnel in preparation for meetings, training, and other administrative activities
Planning	Dearness allowance/travelling allowance (DA/TA) for meetings, other meeting costs, venue, supplies, transportation, etc.
Training	To develop health worker skills
Media and IEC	Development and production (information, education, communication)
Monitoring and supervision	TA/DA/personnel salaries
Social mobilization	For motivating and educating the public

- *Other charges:* These include charges for a rented building, travelling allowance/dearness allowance (TA/DA) and for other miscellaneous items.
2. **Capital cost:** It involves construction, transport, equipment and implements, furniture, and additional capital costs.

Classification of Cost on the Perspective of Analysis of Program

1. **Program costs:** Program costs include the value of all the resources incurred on the implementation and maintenance of the intervention.
2. **Cost of participants:** Costs incurred by participants are either out-of-pocket expenses or productivity losses.
3. **Costs to others:** A health intervention can cause adverse events in persons who are not directly participating in the program. If a study has a societal perspective, include the resulting costs incurred by others.

Types of Costs in Health care

Figure 56.4 depicts the different types of costs in health care.
1. **Direct costs:** Direct costs are the values of all resources expended on the design and implementation of the health intervention (e.g., personnel, lab tests, facilities, rent, and utilities). By definition, direct costs can be either medical or nonmedical.
   a. *Direct health care/medical costs:* Direct medical costs related to treatment. It includes the costs of vaccines, syringes, and nurses' salaries in direct medical expenses in a vaccination program.
   b. *Direct non-healthcare/nonmedical costs:* It is the cost incurred in health care services provided by family members' transportation to and from the site of care.
2. **Indirect cost:** Indirect costs or productivity losses are the income foregone because of changes in productivity as a result of health intervention or illness (e.g., time lost from work or decreased productivity because of health problems; the costs of lost work due to absenteeism, early retirement, and impaired productivity work).
3. **Intangible costs:** Intangible costs are the nonmaterial costs (e.g., emotional anxiety, fear, pain, and stigmatization). Intangible costs impose a significant burden on a patient. Quantifying intangible expenses is difficult as it is not included in the majority of studies. However, we must not forget to account for intangible costs because they might be a significant factor to take patients' decisions.

ACCOUNTING

Accounting is a system of gathering and aggregating information to make for decisions by administrators or decision makers including investors and the public. The accounting information has the power to influence actions.

Types of Accounting Systems

The two types of accounting systems are as follows:

National Accounting Systems

The national accounts cover the national income (NI), such as the gross national product (GNP) and gross domestic

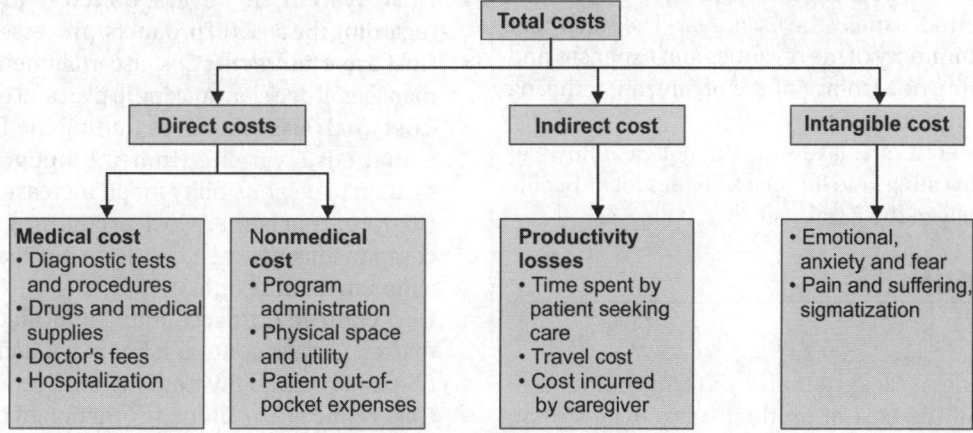

Fig. 56.4: Types of costs in health care.

product (GDP). These are adequate indicators to measure the economic health of the nation or its NI.
  a. **Gross domestic product**: It is the total production of the nation. It is the monetary value of final goods and services. It measures the expenditures on goods and services produced and the income received for products and services and the income earned on products and services.
  b. **Gross national product:** GNP refers to the total income of the nation including GDP and payments, profits, interest, etc. coming in from abroad excluding the interest, benefits, etc. going out of the country.
  c. **Per capita GDP:** Per capita GDP is the total production divided by the population. Per capita, GNP is the total income of a nation divided by its population. It is a crude estimate of the average standard of living of a country.
  d. **Net national product:** The net national product (NNP) is the GNP excluding capital depreciation.
  e. **Net income:** Net income is the NNP excluding indirect taxes paid by producers to the government.

Financial Accounting Systems

The financial accounting system aims to find the profits or losses of an accounting year. It also identifies the status of assets and liabilities through proper documentation system of transactions in a systematic manner.

Financial accounting is an art and science to classify, analyze, and document transactions in an orderly manner to get results of the accounting year by preparing a summary at the end of the year. Financial accounts use balance sheets and income statements for tracking and monitoring incomes and outflows of a business.
  a. **Balance sheet:** A balance sheet is a blueprint of the investment and finance activities of an organization at a particular period, usually the last day of the fiscal year. It presents a summary of the assets and liabilities and equity. It also reveals the sum of the assets that equalizes debts.
  b. **Shareholder's equity:** It should be per guidelines governing the estimation of assets and liabilities.
  c. **Income statement:** The income statement presents the results of the operating activities of a company for a specific period, usually the fiscal year. The statement indicates a summary of the revenues and expenses and the net income or earnings of the organization during the period covered.
  d. **Cash flow statement:** It reveals the net cash flows of operating, investing, and finance activities for a specific period, usually of the fiscal year.

COST ACCOUNTING

Definitions

Cost accounting is a systematic determination and accumulation of the cost of products or activities of an organization. It is an accounting system that provides data regarding ascertaining and controlling costs of services, operations, or products. It classifies, analyzes, and interprets the value of given products and services. It measures the operating efficiency of the organization.

Cost accounting is an accounting process of providing the cost information data, the statement, and summary reports to make managerial decisions. According to the Cost and Management Accounting Institute (London), it is a process of expenditure incurred that relate to cost units and cost centers by the organization. It deals with gathering and analyzing statistical data, applies cost control methods, and finds the profitability of planned or carried out activities. It deals with a budget, standard, and actual cost of operations, processes, events, or products. It calculates variances, profitability, or the social use of funds.

Cost accounting deals with the collection and analysis of relevant cost data to interpret and present various problems of management. It includes the cost of products, services, or operation.

Objectives of Cost Accounting

The following are the objectives of cost accounting:
- To apply budgetary control, standard costing, and inventory control techniques to control the cost of products, services, and operations
- To gather and interpret statistical information to make decisions and to develop operative procedures
- To ascertain costing profit by directing and controlling operations
- To measure the performance of managers of the organization
- To facilitate in preparing financial statements and summaries
- To estimate costs for the future.

Scope of Cost Accounting

The scope of cost accounting is as listed below:
- **Cost bookkeeping:** It is mandatory to keep and maintain a record of costs incurred on products and services by departments. Usually the organization follows a double-entry system for documentation.
- **Cost system**: It covers policies and procedures regarding the costs of products, processes, and services.
- **Cost ascertainment:** Cost ascertainment aids in taking managerial decision-making to plan and control the costs.
- **Cost analysis:** It involves finding the factors causing actual costs varying from the budgeted costs and fixation of responsibility for an increase in value.
- **Cost comparisons:** Cost accounting also includes comparisons between cost from alternative courses of action over some time.
- **Cost control:** Cost accounting information is essential to exercise cost control. It has a detailed report of each cost and profitability from the incurrence of the cost.
- **Cost reports:** The ultimate function of cost accounting is the presentation of reports for planning, controlling,

appraising performance, and making decisions by the management.

Importance of Cost Accounting

The importance of cost accounting is as follows:
1. It aids in ascertaining the cost of the process, product, and services by using different quantitative techniques.
2. It assists in fixing costs by using techniques, such as demand and supply, market competitions, and conditions. It also determines product cost and profit margin to the producer.
3. It is useful in reducing the cost of products or services by applying appropriate methods and programs of cost reduction.
4. It controls wastage by checking and monitoring time and expenses.
5. It helps in identifying unprofitable activities to employ corrective measures' action.
6. It checks the accuracy of the financial account and in estimating fixed selling prices.
7. It is useful in maintaining and controlling inventory and stock.
8. It provides data that the decision maker can use in preparing incentives and career plans for the employees.

Limitations of Cost Accounting

The limitations of cost accounting are as follows:
1. It is an expensive procedure as required analysis, allocation, and absorption of overheads.
2. The system needs a separate cost accountant and financial accountant to operate.
3. It involves the duplication of work accountancy and commercial operations.
4. The cost accounting system requires skilled managers and decision makers.

Difference between Financial and Cost Accounting

Financial accounting differs from cost accounting (**Table 56.2**).

HEALTH ECONOMICS

Health economics has developed into discipline itself due to the size and differential characteristics of the healthcare sector in economy. It is the economics applied to health. It uses the principle of economics that resources are scarce relative to the demands made on them. All the health system has the problem of how best to allocate limited resources and choices in how to allocate resources are inescapable. Health economics tries to minimize the difficulties first, increasing awareness that states resources in another different way. As Mooney states, "opportunity costs entail sacrifice" (Mooney, 2003).

Health economics developed in the 1960s as a subdiscipline of economics. It applies principles from the fields of finance, industrial organization, econometrics, labor economics, public finance, and development studies. It is a discipline, a separate area of study with its parallel development in human capital theory, social capital theory, the principal–agent theory, econometric methods, the methodology of cost-effectiveness analysis (CEA), and the theory of supplier-induced demand.

Definitions

Economics

Economics is the science of scarcity that deals with analyzing, structuring, and prioritizing the choices to maximize output within constrained resources. Lack of resources requires individuals to choose which goods and services they consume. The basis for their decision is the relative value that they place on each goods or service. The structure of these relative values is the basis for their system of prioritization.

Economics is the study of the distribution of scarce resources commonly known as goods and services across a population. It deals with the consequences of resource scarcity. It deals with the use of limited resources to satisfy human wants and needs and how best to use the resources available.

Economics is a social science to study the way individuals and organizations engage in producing, distributing, and consumption of goods and services. Economics is the study of limited resources, unlimited human wants, and selecting

TABLE 56.2: Difference between financial accounting and cost accounting.

Bases	Financial accounting	Cost accounting
Purposes	Provides information about financial performance and financial matters	Includes information of ascertainment of cost to control cost and for decision-making about cost
Nature	Classifies analyzes and records transactions in terms of money	Classify records, present, and interpret in a significant manner the material, labor, and overhead costs
Recording of data	Records historical data	Records estimated/budgeted data. Make use of both historical cost and predetermined cost
Users of information	Shareholders, financial analysts, government and its agencies	Used by internal management at different levels
Analysis	Shows the profit/loss of the organization	Provides details of the cost and profit of each product/service, etc.
Period	Usually prepared for a year	Prepares reports and statements as of and when required
Format of presentation	Set a statement format to present financial information	Has no standard format to display cost information

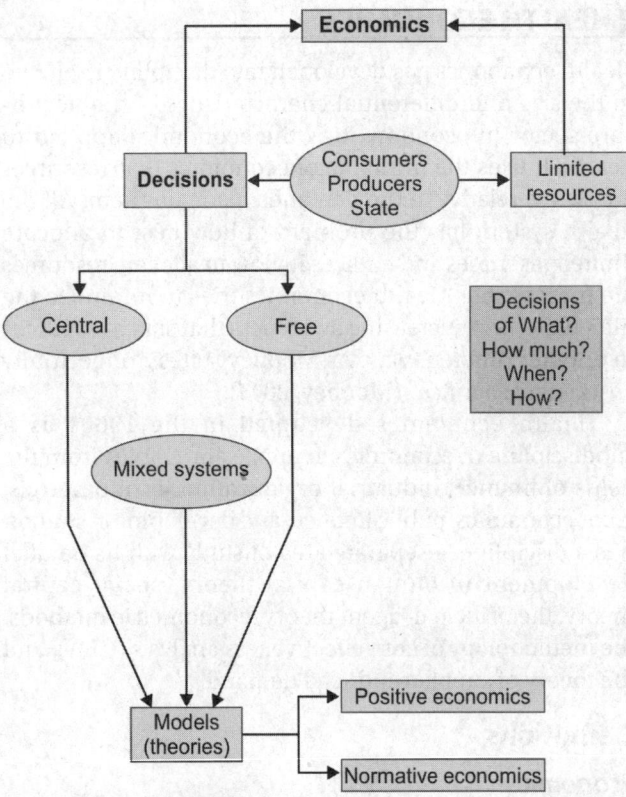

Fig. 56.5: Concept of economics.

wants that one can afford according to resources or budget available (**Fig. 56.5**).

Economics deals with costs (resource use), benefits, choice, efficiency, whereas money is a store of value, means of exchange, and accountancy relating to monitoring financial transactions. It weighs the relative benefits of each course of action and chooses the action that maximizes the well-being. All decisions have subjective value judgments; economics makes these judgments explicit.

Economics studies the ways and means used by economic agents to make decisions regarding the allocation of scarce resources. The commercial agents are the decision makers in the economy. The decisions on production/consumption, the quantity, means, and the person responsible for production depend on the organization of the economy through a central plan, free market, or mixed systems.

There are usually two models (theories): 1. Description of decision-making process-positive economics and 2. policy design, i.e., control and improvement in decision-making normative economics. Positive economics tries to establish cause and effect. Normative economics develops various methods to achieve socially desirable outcomes, whether the distribution of incomes and output is equitable health consequences for patients.

Health

Health means the absence of disease. It is a state of complete physical, mental, social, and spiritual well-being. It does not mean the absence of disease or infirmity (WHO, 1992). Health economics or healthcare economics is a study of health status using some measures.

Health from a practical point of view has been defined according to life expectancy, infant mortality, and crude death rate (Reddy, 1992). It is a function of medical care, income, education, age, sex, race, marital status, environmental pollution, and also certain personal behaviors like smoking habits, exercise, and the like.

Health Economics

Health economics is the study of the allocation of health care. It is a branch of economics concerning issues or problems related to production and consumption of health and health care in terms of its efficiency, effectiveness, value, and behavior.

It is the science to study the distribution of resources within the health system in the economy and the functioning of the healthcare market. Health system is a set of interrelated elements, e.g., environment, education, labor, etc. are the inputs which are to be transformed into a health status as the final outcome through the production of health care services (intermediate output). Health means the absence of illness, and health care is the provision of services to improve the health status of individuals (intermediate output; **Fig. 56.6**).

Health economics is the study of analyzing health costs, its benefits, and its consequences. It uses economic theory to issues and problems associated with health and health care. Health economics is the theoretical framework to help health care professionals, decision makers, or governments to make choices on how to maximize the health of the population within given constrained health producing resources.

Health economics is the study of allocating scarce resources among alternative uses to promote, cure, maintain, and improve the health of the population. It also studies the means of distributing health care and health-related services, their costs and benefits, and health itself among individuals and groups in society. It is the application of the theories, concepts, and techniques of economics to the health sector (Lee and Mills, 1983a).

Health care providers must decide whether the most efficient allocation is also socially, ethically, and morally acceptable. Health care providers including physicians, nurses, midwives, medical technologists, health aids, technicians, dieticians, etc. must take their consent from their leaders who are involved in policy making since the health care policy and economics are linked.

Concept 1: Opportunity cost—it is the value of the foregone benefit obtained from a resource in its next-best alternative use. "A" implies deciding to do and "B" deciding not to do (i.e., the value of benefits from A>B), the cost incurs without financial expenditure, and value not necessarily determined by the market.

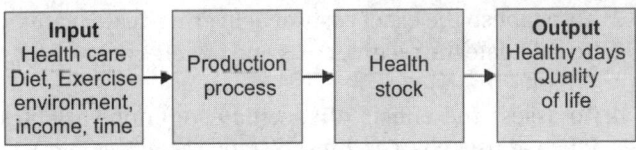

Fig. 56.6: Investing in health care.

Concept 2: Efficiency—it is maximizing the benefit of resources used. It covers technical efficiency, i.e., meeting a given objective at least cost (resources) and allocation efficiency, i.e., producing the pattern of output (supply) that matches the profile of consumer wants (demand).

Components of Health Economics

According to Culyer and Newhouse (2000), the main parts of health economics initially proposed by Williams (1987) are as listed below:
- Meaning and scope of health economics
- Determinants of health
- Demand for health and health care
- Supply of health care
- Health care markets
- The relationship between economic growth and health
- Health sector budgeting and planning
- National health systems
- Equity in health outcomes and health care
- International health.

Health Economics Map

Figure 56.7 depicts various components of the health economics map. The aspects of health economic maps are concept of health, the value of health, demand for health care, a supply of health care, market analysis, macroanalysis appraisal, planning, budgeting, regulation mechanisms, and microappraisal process.

Healthcare Market System

The health-care market is a place or situation where buyers and sellers exchange goods and services including health care. The health care market system is the interaction between providers and consumers of health-care services. Thus, a market for health care involves two groups the buyers and sellers who interact with trading health care. The organization of health care market is the crucial element of analysis of the health care system.
  a. **Buyer:** Everybody is a potential buyer or consumer of health care. A buyer is anybody who is ill or wanted preventive medical treatment/care or who wanted information about their health.
  b. **Seller:** The sellers are the providers of medical and health care services, such as doctors, nurses, physical therapists and so on in the health care field.
  c. **Price:** Price is the quantity of something requires in exchange for something else. It expresses as a monetary unit of exchange.

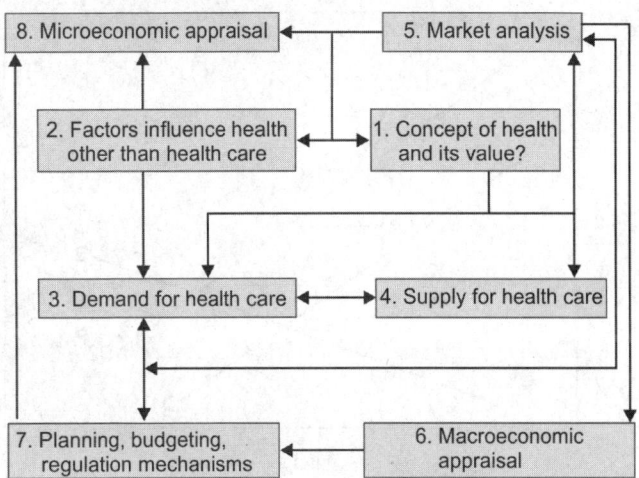

Fig. 56.7: Health economics map.

Scarce Resources

Resources are the inputs and factors of production, such as land, labor, capital (tools, machinery, etc.). Resources get limited when society demands more resources and goods/services than available resources. It covers all the inputs used to produce goods and services. The main concepts of scarcity are efficiency, opportunity cost, and production of possible frontier. Scarcity is the infinite nature of human wants and the finite or limited nature of resources available to produce goods and services. Scarcity = wants versus limited resources.

Supply and Demand

Demand is the buyer's willingness to purchase a particular product or service, and supply is the seller's willingness to supply a specific product or service for a price. In a market economy, output distributed through a system of rates. The sellers sell the goods or services produced to those buyers who are willing and able to pay the market price of the products or services. The demand for products or services in the market is the number of units to be purchased at alternative prices, without influencing other factors for the purchase decision.

A market-demand change is a shift in the market demand curve results from a change in market demand. It depends on a change in consumer preferences and their number in the market, consumer income, the price of a substitute commodity, and the amount of a complementary product. A market-supply change is a shift in the market supply curve that results from a difference in producers, in the technology, in the price or a factor of production, and the number of other commodities used in production **(Fig. 56.8)**.

The reason for the increasing demand (want) of health care by people is that people want to be healthy, and older adults require more health attention. They are in functional financial position to afford treatment. Due to the improvement in medical technology, the demand for health care by people is increasing. It also depends on the

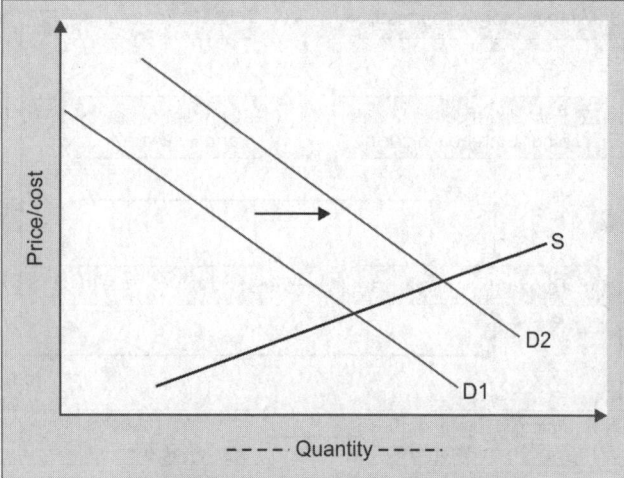

Fig. 56.8: Supplier-induced demand.

market for health and the perception of health care and health. The need for health care will also vary according to the age profile of the population.

The supply of health care refers to the availability of resources for the delivery of health services. Resources include health care facilities, human resources, and financing. Hospitals are the primary health care facility for the delivery of health care. It also consists of all other facilities providing care.

Need and Importance of Health Economics

Need

Health care is the input of producing health. Whether privately insured or dependent upon public services, everyone seeks comprehensive assistance for examination, diagnosis, treatment, and health care. Value for money that includes economy, effectiveness, and efficiency; equity; and ethical issues are essential for providing health services. Health care systems throughout the developed world have been facing the same problems of ever-increasing demand and rising costs. This increasing need for health economics on resources is due to the following:

- Medical advancements in services and treatments, such as organ transplants and gene therapy have provided new treatments and therefore created higher expectations and unique needs.
- As life expectancy increases, more resources are required for medical treatments and continuing care for the elderly.
- Changes in family structure in the developed world mean that it is ever more likely that the elderly will not be cared for by their families.
- Populations have a higher expectation about levels of health and have demanded more and better health care.

Importance

1. To formulate health services policy in the form of demand studies or by trying to discover the preferences of policy makers
2. To establish the exact costs of delivering health care
3. To calculate the relative costs and benefits of particular options
4. To assess the effects of specific economic variables (such as user charges, time, distance expenses, etc.) on the uses of health services
5. To evaluate planning and budgeting systems and make possible changes in the health care delivery system.

Role of Economics in Healthcare

Listed below are the roles of economics in health care:
1. It identifies, defines, and measures phenomena of health problem. It deals with determining the nature of the events and obtaining estimates.
2. It tries to identify the impact of change.
3. It involves explaining and predicting certain phenomena, e.g., the health status and the price of the medical services by conducting cost-effective analysis studies.
4. It studies the relative preference over situations of the population.
5. It involves judging or ranking alternative phenomena according to an acceptable standard for alternative ways of using scarce resources.

Types of Health Economics

Economics offers an overall view about understanding many problems, all of which relate to scarcity of one form or another. Economics can be macroeconomics or microeconomics.

1. **Macroeconomics:** Macroeconomics is a study of economic activities in aggregate. It includes the economic level of output, NI, employment, and general price.
   a. *The economy level of outputs:* The variables, such as GDP, rate of depression, frequency of slackness, etc. measured to find the output levels. Gross domestic product is the market value of all final goods and services produced in the domestic economy during 1 year which is measured with constant prices.
   b. *Level of NI:* NI is the income incurred due to production. Income earned, sold, or consumed GDP.
   c. *Level of employment:* It measured by calculating the rate of unemployment which is the percentage of the total labor force unemployed.
   d. *General price level:* We can measure the general price level through inflation or deflation rate. Inflation is the rate of increase in the price level annually. Deflation is the rate of decrease in the price index annually.

   The macroeconomic market covers the healthcare system of the entire country including the performance in terms of profit, loss, and efficiency. It requires answering the goods and services to be produced How many resources are allocated to different specialties? How to deliver products and services? Macroeconomics of health is concerned with parallel sets of large-scale system issuing concerning, i.e., spending for

employment; and another aspect of health care as a part of the economy and biological health status i.e., longevity/fertility/productivity.
2. **Microeconomics:** It is the study of the economic behavior of individuals, e.g., resource owners, consumers, organizations involved in making decisions about health. The individuals choose to minimize costs or maximize profit or wealth or utilities within a given health care system subject to a set of rules and prices. The major areas covered under health economics are economical and financial aspects of health status and productivity and their relationship, the economic decision-making by health organizations, and planning health development and other issues.

There are many factors influencing health economics, such as the use of extensive government interventions, uncertainty, asymmetric data, errors in data entry, and a third-party agent who insulate the price of the product or service.

Tools for Economic Analysis

The following are the tools of economic analysis:
1. **Economic variables:** The variables measured along a scale, e.g., prices, costs, incomes, and quantities of commodities are economical.
2. **Relationships between economic variables:** The economic variables depict relationships how one variable changes with another variable. Specify the links in causal or noncausal manner as well as causal relationships.
3. **Graphical representation of relationships:** This step function is a solid line relates diagrammatically to specify values. Draw a continuous curve by joining all the points specified in the link.
4. **The direction of the relationships:** The course of relationship can be positive, negative, no relation, or constant relationships (**Fig. 56.9**). It depicts the slope, position, shape, and nature of economic propositions.

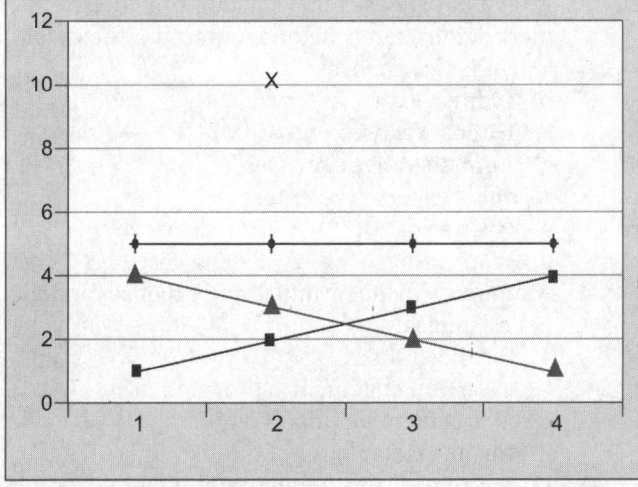

Fig. 56.9: Direction of the relationship between economic variables.

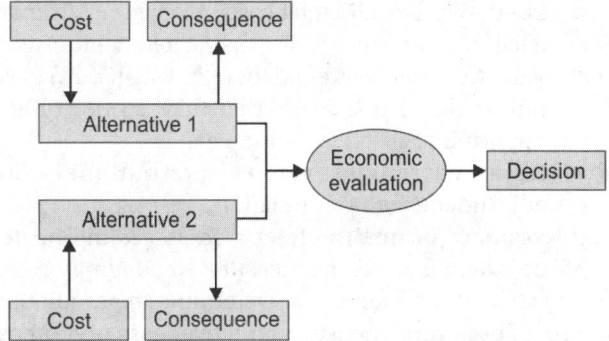

Fig. 56.10: Concept of economic evaluation.

Economic Evaluation

Economic evaluation is a comparative analysis of alternative courses of action in terms of their costs and consequences to assist policy decisions. Economic evaluation is a decision-making process to select the best alternative in terms of costs and outcomes, not choosing the cheapest (**Fig. 56.10**). It is the allocation of limited resources, equity, and ethical issues efficiently.

Steps involved in economic evaluation are the following:
1. **Deciding upon the study question:**
    - Identify the problem and aims of the assessment. Try to find out the importance of the issue. Study various aspects of the point that need to explain
    - Select alternative options. Describe the interventions accurately and define counterfactual intervention (comparator)
    - Define the audience and their needs and consider them as they use the study results
    - Define the perspective of the study, patients, providers, payers, health care system, and society and select a perspective depends on the audience
    - Specify the time frame and the analytic horizon. The analytic background must be higher than the time frame
    - Select the study format, prospective, retrospective, or model depending on data, time, and resources available.
2. **Assessment of costs:** Assess the total cost and calculate the cost by multiplying the unit of measurement by unit cost. The total cost depends on the following:
    - The type of cost—direct, indirect, or intangible
    - The value of the cost category
    - The organizational level
    - Input (capital or recurrent)
    - Intervention activities (planning, administration, media, training)
    - Time frame, startup versus postimplementation evaluation
    - Funding: National government versus nongovernmental organization (NGO) versus donor
    - Measurement: Use measure in natural physical units (e.g. hours of labor time)

- Fixed, variable, and total costs; average versus marginal costs; and marginal versus incremental costs
- Valuation and market prices (e.g., wage rates) used unless the strong belief that they do not reflect opportunity cost (e.g., volunteers)
- Local currencies versus international and adjustments for price inflation.

3. **Assessment of health effects:** To assess the health effects, identify outcome measures depending on the objective of the evaluation. Determine the evaluation procedures and measure effectiveness, outcomes, valuation, if appropriate, in terms of either utility (e.g., quality-adjusted life year (QALY), disability adjusted life years (DALY), health year equivalent (HYE) or money. e.g., willingness to pay (WTP).
4. **Adjusting for timing:** It is a sort of discount. The discount rate is the rate of time preference. It prefers to have benefits now and bear costs in the future—time preference. It allows for differential timing of costs (and profits) between programs. All future costs (and benefits) need to state in terms of their present value using a discount rate and annualize capital costs. Capital cost is an investment at a startup in an asset used and depreciated over time. Annualize the initial capital outlay over the useful life of an asset.
5. **Adjustment for uncertainty or sensitivity analysis:** It is the process of assessing the vitality of an economic appraisal by considering the effects of risk. It consists of identifying the (uncertain) variables, specifying the range of variation, and recalculating results by using appropriate statistical tests.

Types of Economic Evaluation

The essential types of economic evaluation are cost minimization analysis (CMA), cost effectiveness analysis (CEA), cost-utility analysis (CUA), and cost–benefit analysis (CBA).

CHAPTER HIGHLIGHTS

- The costs are the values of all the resources, such as labor, buildings, equipment, and supplies, etc. used to produce goods or services. The three aspects of costs are material cost, labor cost, and overhead cost.
- There are various ways of classifying value by following the basic concept per the World Health Organization, namely the types of interventional activities and program cost sheet.
- Healthcare costs include direct, indirect, and intangible costs. Intangible costs are the nonmaterial costs, such as emotional anxiety, fear, pain, and stigmatization that impose a significant burden on a patient.
- Accounting is a system of gathering and aggregating information to make decisions. The two types of accounting systems are national and financial accounting systems.
- The cost accounting measures the operating efficiency of the organization by gathering, analyzing, and interpreting the value of its given products and services. It calculates variances, profitability, or the social use of funds.
- Health economics concerns with problems related to production and consumption of health and health care in terms of its efficiency, effectiveness, value, and behavior. It studies the distribution of resources within the health system in the economy and the functioning of the health care market.
- Health economics is of two types: Macroeconomics and microeconomics. It uses various tools in economics analysis.
- Economic evaluation is a process of comparative analysis of alternative courses of action in terms of their costs and consequences to assist policy decisions.

REVIEW QUESTIONS

I. Essay Type Questions
1. What do you mean by the term "cost"? Describe different types of underlying costs.
2. Define "accounting." Differentiate between financial accounting and cost accounting.
3. Explain in detail the different types of accounting systems.
4. Define health economics. Describe its basic components.
5. Why is it important to study health economics? Describe the different types of health economics.

II. Short Notes
1. Elements of cost
2. Types of costs in healthcare
3. Financial accounting system
4. Economic evaluation

III. Multiple Choice Questions
1. A type of cost incurred on administration, office rent, stationery, and other expenses is:
   a. Material cost
   b. Labor cost
   c. Overhead cost
   d. Intangible cost
2. A type of expenses that include providers, time, medications, tests, materials, and supply cost is:
   a. Variable expenses
   b. Indirect expenses
   c. Direct expenses
   d. Administrative expenses
3. All direct expenses refer to:
   a. Overhead cost
   b. Prime cost
   c. Work cost
   d. Selling cost
4. A summary of the revenues and expenses and the net earning is:
   a. Balanced sheet
   b. Cash flow statement
   c. Shareholder's equity
   d. Income statement
5. Which one of the following is included under microeconomics?

a. The economic level of output, national income, employment, and general price
b. The health system of the entire country including performance
c. The economic behavior of resources, owners, consumers, etc. involved in decision-making regarding health
d. A parallel set of a large-scale system issuing concerns

Answer Keys

1. c 2. a 3. b 4. d 5. c

SUGGESTED READING

1. Adam T, Evans DB. Determinants of variation in the cost of inpatient stay versus outpatient visits in hospitals: A multi-country analysis. Soc Sci Med. 2006;63(7):1700-10.
2. Available from http://www.cdc.gov/owcd/eet/Cost/Glossary.html#glossarycostanalysis. [Accessed April 2018].
3. Available from http://www.rds-sc.nihr.ac.uk/planning-a-study/health-economics/economic-evaluation/. [Accessed April 2018].
4. Available from http://www.who.int/choice/publications/d_ScalingUp_MDGs_WHO_finalreport.pdf. [Accessed April 2018].
5. Brazier JE, Ratcliffe J, Tsuchiya A, Salomon J. Measuring and Valuing Health Benefits for Economic Evaluation. Oxford: Oxford University Press; 2007.
6. Culyer AJ, and Newhouse JP. (eds).Handbook of Health Economics. (Vol 1A). Amsterdam, The Netherlands: Elsevier Science BV, 2000.
7. Fallowfield L. What is a Quality of Life? London: Hayward Medical Communications; 2009.
8. Gwatkin DR. How well do health programmes reach the poor? Lancet. 2003;361(9357):540-1.
9. Hailey D. Australian economic evaluation and government decisions on pharmaceuticals, compared to the assessment of other health technologies. Soc Sci Med. 1997;45(4): 563-81.
10. Lee K, Mills A (Eds), The Economics of Health in Developing Countries. Oxford: Oxford University Press, 1983.
11. Le Pen C. Pharmaceutical economy and the economic assessment of drugs in France. Soc Sci Med. 1997;45:635-43.
12. Mooney G. Economics, Medicine, and Health Care. 3rd edition. London: Prentice Hall, 2003.
13. Phillips CJ. Health Economics: An Introduction for Health Professionals. Oxford: Blackwell Publishing; 2005.
14. Reddy KN. Health Expenditure in India. Working Paper No. 14, NIPFP, New Delhi, 1992.
15. Williams, A. (ed.), Health and Economics. London: Macmillan Press Ltd, 1987.
16. World Health Organization. Basic Document, 39th Edition, Geneva,1992.

57
CHAPTER

Economic Evaluation Techniques

CHAPTER OUTLINE

- Cost Analysis
  - Definition
  - When to use Cost Analysis?
  - Objectives of Cost Anlysis
  - Purposes of Cost Analysis
  - Principles of Cost Analysis
  - The Framework of Cost Analysis
  - Basic Steps in Cost Analysis
  - Health Valuation Methods
  - Types of Cost Analysis
- Cost-benefit Analysis
- Cost-effectiveness Analysis
- Cost-utility Analysis
- Cost Consequences Analysis

LEARNING OUTCOMES

After completion of this chapter, the learner will be able to:
- Understand the concept of cost analysis
- Discuss various steps of cost analysis
- Understand the concept of cost-benefit analysis (CBA)
- Describe purposes, importance, and features of CBA
- Familiarize with approaches of CBA
- Describe steps in social cost-benefit analysis
- Enumerate advantages and drawbacks of CBA

KEY TERMS

Cost analysis, cost-benefit analysis, cost-effectiveness, cost utility, cost consequences

INTRODUCTION

Economic evaluation techniques or quantitative control methods derive from the field of economics, operation research, and budgeting. Some of these techniques have a significant role in the management of health services, including nursing services. These are cost analysis, cost-benefit analysis (CBA), cost-effectiveness analysis (CEA), cost-utility analysis (CUA), and cost consequences analysis.

COST ANALYSIS

Cost containment is a critical issue in the healthcare system. Costing can help to assess how to better meet healthcare demands, given finite resources by identifying an approach that is the most effective, i.e. which method can achieve specified objectives of least cost. Cost is the sum of resources (labor, material, equipment, etc.) used to produce goods or services. Costing is a process of identifying and apportioning costs. A cost center is a unit, e.g. departmental or geographical, for which costs can be determined and allocated.

Costs are the values of three principle resources, i.e. (1) material costs include both direct cost and indirect cost incurred on material and supplies used in program/intervention, (2) labor costs also include both direct and indirect costs incurred on manpower, and (3) overhead costs are the cost incurred on administrative, offices rent, or departmental expenses, and other expenses.

Definition

Cost analysis is a tool used in financial management, especially for resources in an organization. It is a technique used in an economic evaluation that involves the systematic collection, categorization, and analysis of program or intervention in terms of costs and cost of illness.

When to Use Cost Analysis?

1. Cost analysis is a stand-alone evaluation method when only one program is for assessment, during nonavailability of information about the effectiveness

of the plan, or the interventions are equally effective in comparing.
2. Cost analysis can use along with CEA, CBA, or CUA. Effectiveness assessment techniques vary, depending on CEA, CBA, or CUA. Cost analysis techniques are the same for all types of economic evaluations.

Objectives of Cost Analysis

The objectives of cost analysis are as follows:
- It helps to assess the efficiency and effectiveness of function and their cost implication to contain cost.
- Its application helps to improve the policy relevance and utility through assessment, planning, and avoidance of wasteful expenditure in the hospital.
- It allows researchers to achieve cost minimization for the programs under consideration.

Purposes of Cost Analysis

The purposes of cost analysis are as follows:
- **Planning and cost projection:** Cost analysis can use as a tool to (1) develop and justify budgets and (2) to determine the funding changes necessary to achieve the desired difference in disease prevalence/incidence.
- **To assess the efficiency:** A program is considered efficient when the maximum amount of output (i.e. cases treated or persons screened) produced from the given level of inputs (i.e. resources). Cost analysis assesses the efficiency of programs by comparing the cost of equally effective programs and by identifying cost categories for further efficiency studies.
- **To assess the priorities:** Cost analysis provides information on health resource allocation. The data can be used (1) to examine how resource use reflects national, state, and local health priorities and (2) to discuss how expenditure profiles of similar programs vary from one another. Cost patterns from a cost analysis might indicate that previous preferences need to be reassessed by considering emerging trends.
- **Accountability:** Cost analysis allows us to find the method of spending the funds as intended.
- **To assess equity:** Cost analysis can help to determine the distribution of health resources among various population groups. For instance, cost analysis indicates the program spends more resources per capita in urban areas or rural areas and also compares the result of allocation mechanisms or differences in need.

Principles of Cost Analysis

- **Make explicit the analytic perspective:** It addresses who pays specific costs and who benefits from an intervention. Consider the society; third-party payers including private insurance carriers and government; service providers including hospitals, physicians and nurses; and patients.
- **Describe the anticipated benefits:** Describe the benefits of intervention as the value of the health effects, e.g. life-year gained, health-related quality of life (QOL), decreased costs, side effects, morbidity, and mortality; satisfaction; and efficiency and effectiveness.
- **Specify the components of costs:** Specify the elements of costs used, e.g. the cost of intervention, the cost of side effects or morbidity, cost averted by a response, and induced cost from the additional services. Ensure the components of cost and impact derived consistently from the stated analytic perspective.
- **Discount to adjust for differential timing:** When the costs and benefits studied accrue during significantly different periods, discount the differential timings. To control the effect of inflations, use discounting to adjust future expenses and profits to present values.
- **Perform a sensitivity analysis:** To explore the implications of alternative assumptions, preferences, and data perform a sensitivity analysis. Explore the impact of alternative hypotheses, preferences, and data. Handle uncertainty by testing the strength of conclusions against variations in premises and estimates.
- **Calculate measurement of efficiency:** Calculate a summary measurement of productivity (i.e. cost–benefit or cost-effectiveness ratio, CER). If possible, express the ratio in marginal or incremental terms unless one alternative intervention is dominant. Use incremental analysis to compare and prioritize one intervention with the next least expensive or with the most effective.

The Framework of Cost Analysis

A framework is a blueprint that guides how to go. The cost analysis framework provides the design for developing the cost inventory of the selected program or intervention. It includes the following seven steps to build:

1. **Defining the problem:** In the first step of framing a cost analysis, identify the problem and give the reasons that justify expending the limited resources on the study. Identify the question for review, its importance, the area of the problem, and gather other related information.
2. **Defining the alternatives:** Gather all relevant organizational and technological aspects of available options of interventions. Define the nature of interventions, collect baseline information for comparisons, target population, delivery site, personnel delivering the services, technology in use, and timings for the proposed interventions.
3. **Define the audiences:** The structure of the analysis depends on the type of audience that will use the outcome of the cost analysis, type of information that audience needs, and the way they will use the results.
4. **Define the perspective:** Determine which costs are relevant and should be included in the cost analysis. The perspective takes into account who bears the costs and who gains from available interventions. Analyze cost from any or all of the patient/family, provider, payer, health system, and society.

5. **Define the time frame:** It is vital to frame the time for the interventions. Have sufficient time to capture the full details of the program costs and its consequences. Plan all activities such as startup, maintenance costs, seasonal variations, and cost of intervention, including its effects.
6. **Determine the time frame and analytic horizon:** Choose an analytic background that is long enough to capture the full costs and effects of programs with an impact that occurs at different times and short if that future costs and benefits uncertain.
7. **Choose a format/methodology:** Depending on the availability of data and resources, choose one of three formats to use retrospective analyses, prospective analyses, or models based on the estimated values from other studies.

Basic Steps in Cost Analysis

The basic steps in cost analysis are as follows:
1. **Define program, treatment, or technology:** Describe program, procedure, or technology clearly. Define input and outcomes and activities; the level of facility or operation at local, district, or national; and sources of resources.
2. **Develop a plan for cost analysis:** Develop a plan of action for all the activities corresponding to cost analysis.
3. **Describe the objectives of the analysis:** Clearly formulate the purposes of cost analysis, either to compare the cost and benefits of interventions or to evaluate the health outcome.
4. **Select the type of cost analysis:** The various types of cost analysis are, e.g. CBA, cost-effectiveness analysis, cost marginal analysis, and CUA. Select the model per the objectives of cost analysis.
5. **Design methodology of cost analysis:** Decide the method for cost analysis, retrospective, prospective, or models.
6. **Apply principles of cost analysis:** Apply principles such as payers and beneficiaries, benefits, components of cost, discounting, sensitivity analysis, and efficiency measurement in cost analysis.
7. **Describe study outcomes:** Clearly describe the study outcomes of cost analysis. It should define explicitly.
8. **Develop cost inventory:** The next step involves developing an inventory of the resources required for the intervention/program. The cost inventory comprises a comprehensive list of resources with the unit and the total cost (TC) of each resource. Costs are direct, indirect, and intangible, as discussed in the previous chapter.
9. **Prepare cost summary:** Make a summary of the cost inventory. For this, prepare a comprehensive list of all resources and present them in a classification system that is most suitable for study. Include all the resources such as volunteer time, caregivers' time, patient's time, in-kind contributions/donated materials, and resources previously purchased or obtained without monetary exchange and also include resources that are hard to measure or value and supplies used in small amounts.
10. **Define the measure for evaluation of resources:** Having developed the cost inventory, measure the quantity of the resources used in the delivery of the intervention. The information can be gathered through any of the following methods. Later assign values to them and characterize costs as either fixed or variable, depending on their variation with changes in program activity level.
    - Questionnaire surveys (require a large number of survey participants to calculate unit costs)
    - Observational studies (need a large number of observations to calculate unit costs)
    - Medical records
    - Accounting and payroll systems
    - Published literature
    - Professional guidelines/practice.
11. **Calculate cost analysis results:** Calculate TCs, average costs (ACs), and marginal costs (MCs).

Total cost: It covers the cost of persons involved, the supplies, and the equipment. To find the TC of a program or intervention, add all the expenses incurred to produce output.

$$TC = \text{Quantity of Resource A} \times \text{Value of that Resource} + \ldots + \text{Quantity of Resource n} \times \text{Value of those Resources}$$

The average cost: It is the cost per unit of output, e.g. the cost per child immunized. To find the AC, divide the TC by the number of participants or other relevant intervention units.

$$AC = TC / Q \quad Q = \text{Units of output}$$

The marginal cost: MC is the cost of resources associated with producing one additional or one less unit within the same intervention/program. Because MC is an indication of the number of other resources that must be expended to serve additional patients, it is useful in making program expansion decisions. Marginal cost is usually calculated from data based on the cost of a more significant increase in outputs.

$$MC = \frac{\text{Change in total costs}}{\text{Change in quantity produced}}$$

Or

$$MC = \frac{(TC' - TC)}{(Q' - Q)}$$

Whereas,
TC' = Total costs a higher output level
TC = Total costs at the lower output level
Q' = Higher level of output
Q = Lower level of output

The MC measures the effect of making an additional investment in the intervention and is used to:
- Evaluate the change in total expenses that will result from a shift in program activity level
- Evaluate the difference in TCs that are needed to produce a change in outcomes or
- Determine the optimal activity level of a program or intervention.

Sensitivity analysis and discounting: Conduct sensitivity analysis to rule out any measurement errors, biased estimation, and omission of any cost components or inappropriate time frame. To account for time preference, convert the value of future costs and benefits accrued as a result of intervention to an equivalent present value called discounting.

Health Valuation Methods

1. **Cost-of-illness method:** The cost-of-illness (COI) method is used to estimate the direct and indirect costs of an intervention. Use the nonmarket valuation methods to calculate intangible costs.
2. **Nonmarket valuation methods:** The majority of health outcomes do not have markets; the economists developed nonmarket valuation methods for estimating the value of these nonmarket goods based on the generally accepted theories. The two primary valuation methods are revealed preference method (RPM) and the stated preference methods.
    - **Revealed preference method:** The two main types of RPMs used in health economics are hedonic pricing and averting behavior.
        - *Hedonic pricing (wage):* The hedonic is the wage that consumers pay or receive depending on the characteristics of the person. It can measure objectively, e.g. years on the job (experience) and educational level. On the labor market (which is assumed to be competitive), employees are willing and able to pay more for each characteristic, both in quality (type) and in quantity (amount); a functional relationship, therefore, exists between the wage and all the measurable characteristics. This relationship is expressed as:
        $$W = f(q, e, ex, a, g)$$
        where W is the wage rate, q is a measure of qualification, e is the education, ex is a measure of experience, a is age, and g is gender.

        This amount is the implicit price received by the worker or paid by the employee for a unit of that particular characteristic.
        - *Averting behavior:* It is the value of a small change in health status measured by the amount of money a person is willing to spend on some preventive, controlling, monitoring, or defensive action. This amount of money is the valuation of the safety of a person against a perceived risk.

        Limitations of RPM
        - It does not take into account all benefits and costs.
        - The market price might not be the actual value.
        - The behavior exhibited by the person is based on the person's perception of how the device or action will be able to control or avert the damage, rather than what it can do.
        - Other potential problems of estimation also are rooted in the empirical analysis (e.g. the correct specification of functional relationships).
    - **Stated preference or contingent valuation method:** It is a direct method of using primary surveys by asking the audience to rate the values on an intervention to achieve a level of health outcome. The advantages of contingent valuation method (CVM) are as follows:
        - It estimates both tangible and intangible benefits, thus providing a better estimate of the actual cost of the intervention (e.g. reductions in health risks, pain, and suffering).
        - It relies on survey studies to elicit individual's maximum willingness to pay or minimum willingness to accept for these intangible outcomes in hypothetical or contingent scenarios. Sophisticated regression techniques are then applied to analyze the assembled data and to estimate the population willingness to pay (WTP).

Types of Cost Analysis

The cost analysis is classified according to suitability in terms of the objective of evaluation and the data availability and other resources. It is challenging to identify and quantify all costs and benefits (or outcomes), and the units used to quantify these may differ. Different types of frameworks are used for combining costs and benefits within an economic evaluation framework. While the approach to measuring costs is the same in all contexts, they differ in terms of measuring and valuing health outcomes.

- **Cost-of-illness analysis:** The cost–benefit study is a process of determining the economic impact of an illness or condition on a given population, region, or country. It measures all the costs associated with a particular disease or condition, e.g. smoking, arthritis, or bedsores, including associated treatment costs. It is not an actual economic evaluation since it does not compare the costs and outcomes of alternative courses of action. It covers all direct costs, indirect costs, and intangible costs.
- **Cost-minimization analysis:** The cost-minimization study is a technique of determining the least cost among alternative interventions assumed to produce equivalent outcomes on comparing the

cost of alternative interventions. The alternative with the least cost that provides the same result is cost-effective.
- **Cost-effectiveness analysis:** It is a technique used to compare the cost in monetary units with outcomes in quantitative nonmonetary groups, e.g. reduced mortality or morbidity. It measures results in natural units, such as mm Hg, symptom-free days, life years gained.
- **Cost-utility analysis:** It is a technique to compare costs in monetary units with outcomes in terms of their utility, usually to the patient, measured, e.g. in quality-adjusted life years (QALYs). It measures outcomes in a composite metric of both length and QOL, i.e. the QALYs.
- **Cost consequence analysis:** It is a technique used to compare costs and outcomes in discrete categories, without aggregating or weighting them.
- **Cost-benefit analysis:** It is a technique to compare costs and benefits quantified in common monetary units. It measures costs and benefits in cash terms.

COST-BENEFIT ANALYSIS

Cost-benefit analysis is one of the economic evaluation approaches that compare costs and benefits, both of which are quantified and valued in common monetary units. It is also called a benefit–cost analysis. It evaluates all the outcomes in financial terms. The benefit-cost ratio gives monetary or welfare benefits per currency unit spent.

Costs are the values of three principle resources, i.e., (1) material costs include both direct cost and indirect cost incurred on material and supplies used in program/intervention, (2) labor costs also include both direct and indirect costs incurred on manpower, and (3) overhead costs are the cost incurred on administrative, office rent, departmental expenses, and other expenses.

Benefits are the monetary values of the expected consequences of economic decisions. These are (1) direct benefits that are the values of desirable health and nonhealth outcomes directly related to the implementation of proposed interventions that can estimate by using market-based data, (2) indirect benefits, these are averted costs and savings resulting from the responses but not related directly to them, and (3) intangible benefits that include the values of positive outcomes, e.g. reductions in health risk, pain, and suffering, which cannot be estimated from market data.

Concept of CBA

Cost-benefit analysis deals with selecting the best alternative from various alternatives in terms of costs and benefits/impacts. The benefits must be more than incurred costs for an intervention. Net profits are the costs subtracting from the total value of benefits; or in other words, the cost-benefit ratio must be more than one as depicted in equation (**Fig. 57.1**):

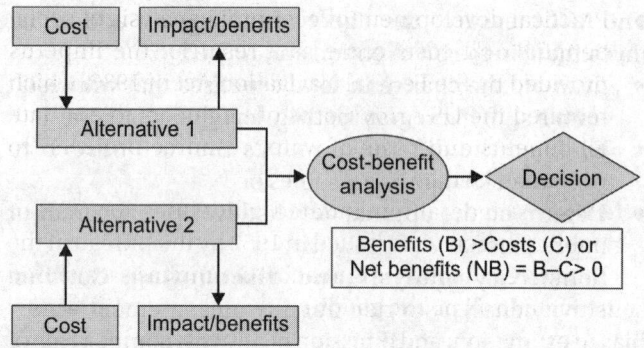

Fig. 57.1: Concept of cost–benefit analysis.

Definitions

According to the World Health Organization (WHO, 2018), CBA is a method of economic evaluation that weighs all benefits against all costs. It is a decision-making tool to consider the expenses of intervention against the benefit. Benefits and costs may be monetary or nonmonetary. The valuation of all program outcomes in monetary units allows decision makers to directly compare the health outcomes of different types of health interventions. The cost-benefit analysis is the process of analyzing the benefits of the intervention with the costs associated with it (**Fig. 57.2**).

$$\text{Benefits } (B) > \text{Costs } (C)$$
$$\text{Or}$$
$$\text{Net benefits (NB)} = B - C > 0$$

Historical Background

Listed below are the historical background of CBA:
- The idea of CBA originated from Jules Dupuit, a French engineer, and was published in 1848 in a paper on "The measurement of utility of public works."
- In early 1808, the report on "Transportation" by Albert Gallatin, the fourth US Secretary of the Treasury, recommended the comparison of costs and benefits for evaluating water-related projects.
- Alfred Marshall, a British economist, formulated some of the formal concepts that are at the foundation of CBA.

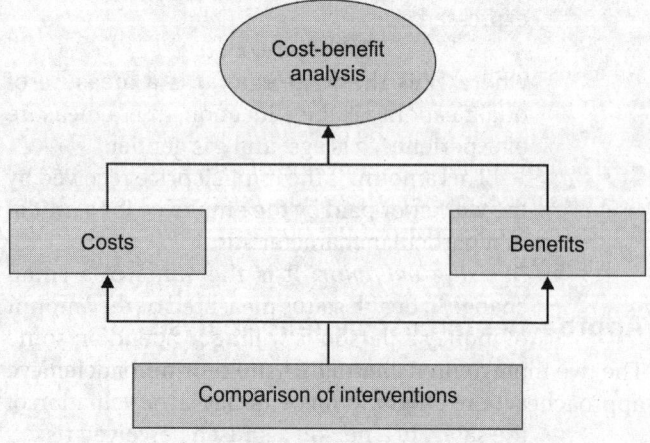

Fig. 57.2: Cost-benefit analysis.

- Practical development of economic analysis of social benefits and costs came as a result of the impetus provided by the Federal Navigation Act of 1936, which required the US Army Corps of Engineers to evaluate all benefits and costs of water resource projects "to whomsoever they accrue."
- The first federally mandated guidelines for CBA of public projects were issued in 1952 by the Bureau of the Budget. Gradually the bureaucratic emphasis expanded to include all public goods.

Purposes and Importance

The purposes and importance of CBA are as follows:
- To assess economic efficiency
- To estimate the potential value of a program/intervention
- To select and set priorities from various potential programs
- To decide whether the program is acceptable and can be implemented
- To achieve a specific health-related objective.

Features

The features of CBA are as follows:
- Cost-benefit analysis adopts a broad societal perspective.
- It includes all costs and benefits incurred.
- Cost-benefit analysis measures the outcomes in monetary terms.
- It assesses the desirability of program/intervention.
- It is a powerful and easy tool for making decisions.

Principles of Cost-benefit Analysis

Various principles of CBA are as follows:
- Benefits and costs of the program measured in terms of their equivalent money value.
- It should represent the consumer's valuation as revealed by their actual behavior.
- Gross benefits of an increased consumption should be under the demand curve.
- Valuation of human life must be on their increased or reduced risk.
- Specify alternatives explicitly and consider them in the assessment.
- Impacts of the programs must be defined.
- Avoid double counting of benefits or costs.
- The ratio of the present value of profits to the value of costs must be higher than one.
- Internal rate return must be greater than the cost of capital.

Approaches of Cost-benefit Analysis

The two main approaches of CBA are ratio and net benefit approaches:

1. **Ratio approach:** The ratio approach indicates the amount of benefit (outcomes) that is ratio per unit expenditure on technology versus a comparator. Technology is a cost-benefit to comparison if the ratio of the change in costs to the change in benefits is less than one.

$$\text{CB ratio} = \frac{\text{Rs Cost}_{\text{Intervention}} - \text{Cost}_{\text{Comparator}}}{\text{Rs Benefit}_{\text{Intervention}} - \text{Benefit}_{\text{Comparator}}}$$

Social benefit–cost ratio: The social benefit–cost ratio is the annual average economic benefits of the intervention divided by the average yearly economic net costs of the intervention.

$$\text{Benefit–cost ratio} = \frac{\text{Annual average economic benefits of the intervention}}{\text{The annual average economic net cost of the intervention}}$$

2. **Net benefit approach:** The net benefit approach indicates the absolute amount of money saved or lost due to the use of technology versus enabling comparator. A technology is cost-benefit versus a comparator if the ratio of change in benefits exceeds the net change in costs.

Cost-benefit net = (₹Cost$_{\text{Intervention}}$ − Cost$_{\text{Comparator}}$) − (₹Benefit$_{\text{Intervention}}$ − Benefit$_{\text{Comparator}}$)

In CBA of alternative programs, the expected benefits and the cost of each intervention/program are compared to determine which should receive priority funding. In the following example, intervention/program 1 (one) is preferred **(Table 57.1)**.

Steps in Social Cost-benefit Analysis

Various steps are followed for an economic evaluation in CBA **(Fig. 57.3)**.

1. **Decide study questions:**
   - *Define the problem:* Identify the study problem at the outset of any analysis. A clearly stated problem defines the objective of the study. At this initial stage of the survey, one must consider what questions need to be answered and which aspects of the problem need to be explained.
   - *Identify interventions:* Determine the scope of the study and the variety of outcomes to a large extent by the nature of the programs. Often the study

TABLE 57.1: Benefit–cost ratio of alternative interventions.

Intervention	Cost (in ₹)	Expected benefit	Benefit-cost ratio
1	400,000	12 times	12:1
2	600,000	10 times	10:1
3	200,000	9 times	9:1
4	800,000	8 times	8:1
5	100,000	4 times	4:1
6	180,000	2 times	2:1

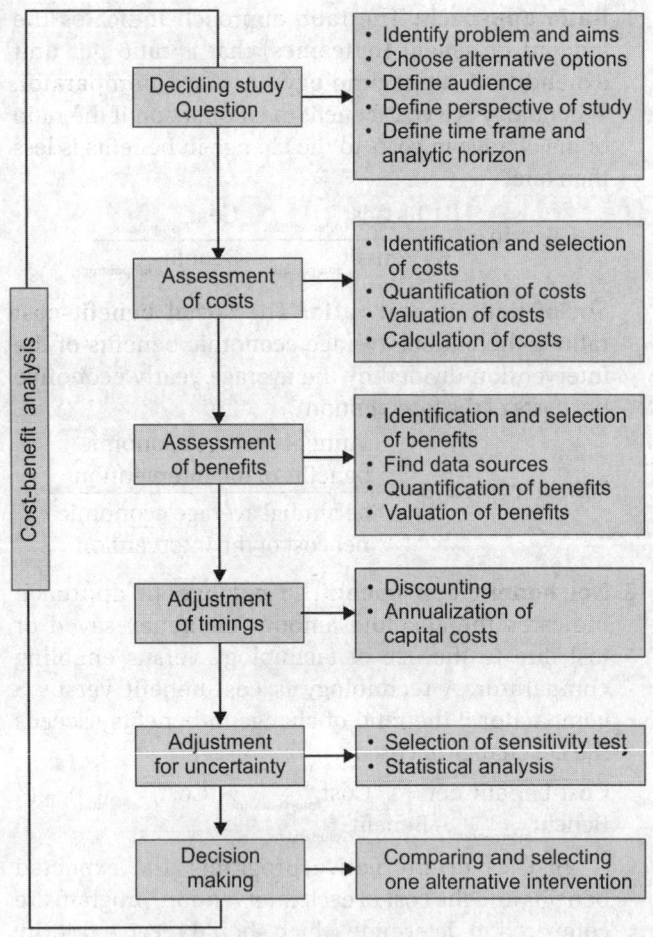

Fig. 57.3: Steps in cost-benefit analysis.

problem itself or the decisions made by policy makers specify the interventions to be analyzed. These questions highlight the various aspects that will help in identifying interventions such as what is the nature of each intervention? What is the technology used for the intervention? What are the target population, the delivery site, and the personnel for delivering the intervention? What are the options?

- *Define audience:* Understanding information the audience needs and the way the audience uses the study results are the major factors to be considered at this stage. These questions will help to identify the audience, i.e. who will be using the results of the analysis? What information does the audience need? How will the results be used?
- *Define perspective:* Usually CBAs are carried out from a societal perspective, hence all benefits and costs are considered for review. The results indicate whether the benefits to society as a whole outweigh the TCs of a proposed project. When using a narrower perspective, we should include only the benefits and costs relevant to that specific perspective. The CBA can be from any of these perspectives depending on the audience, patient perspective, provider perspective, payer perspective, healthcare system perspective, government perspective, and societal perspective.
- *Define the time frame and analytic horizon:* The time frame and the analytic background are determined by the treatments or interventions under consideration. The analytic horizon is usually longer than the time frame because the majority of interventions or treatments produce multiple health and nonhealth outcomes for periods far exceeding the duration of the interventions or treatments.

2. **Assess costs:**
   - *Identification and choice of costs:* Identify the direct, indirect or intangible cost. The cost category includes programme, patient, the level of facility costs such as national, regional, district, the cost on input categories such as capital and recurrent, on intervention activities such as planning, administration, media, training, time cost on start-up and postimplementation, source of funding from government, nongovernmental organization (NGO), donor.
   - *Measurement/quantification of cost:* Measure the value in natural physical units (e.g. hours of labor time). Quantify fixed, variable, and TCs, average and MCs, and marginal and incremental costs.
   - *Valuation of costs:* Find the market prices (e.g. wage rates) used unless there is strong belief that they do not reflect opportunity costs (e.g. volunteers). Express all values in common currency.
   - *Calculate the cost:* Calculate the cost by multiplying the unit of measurement by unit cost.

3. **Assess health effects/impact/benefits:**
   - *Identification and choice of benefits/impact:* Identity all possible results/outcomes based on the objective of evaluation; these can be positive or negative. Select relevant impacts for analysis purposes. Find the incremental effect of the intervention either by measuring the total impact of all interventions and calculate the difference between these or by identifying the difference in impact between two interventions.
   - *Find data sources:* Gather information on the effects from all sources—primary, secondary, health information system, social surveys, etc.
   - *Measurement/quantification of impacts:* Measure (count) final, not intermediate outcomes. It should be in natural physical units.
   - *Impact valuation in social CBA:* Measure the impact on monetary units. Assess the economic value of resource consequences by using different approaches such as the human capital approach, contingency valuation. Valuation should be in terms of either utility [e.g. QALYs, disability-adjusted life years (DALYs), and HYE] or money (e.g. WTP).

4. **Adjusting for differential timing:**
   - *Discounting:* The discount rate is one parameter that can be varied in a sensitivity analysis to test

its impact on the results of analysis and to make the results of studies based on different discount rates comparable. Discounting makes it possible to compare benefits and costs that occur at different times by adjusting their values according to the time preference corresponding to the chosen perspective. Centers for Disease Control and Prevention (CDC) recommends using a 3% social discount rate in analyses.

It is the value of goods at a time in the future based on the general inflation rate. To calculate the present value for the future cost, apply a discount rate to future cost. The choice of discount rate for costs varies from 0% to 10% and for the impact usually taken 3%.

- **Annualization of capital costs:** Capital cost represents an investment at a start-up in an asset that is used and depreciated over time. Annualize the initial capital outlay over the useful life of an asset.

5. **Adjustment for uncertainty or sensitivity analysis:** Identifying uncertain variables; uncertainty may be due to many factors such as differences in responses, inaccuracy in recording, missing data, instability in cost, etc. Uncertainty quantifies through sensitivity analysis. Specify a plausible range of variation. Recalculate results using one-way analysis, multiway analysis, extreme scenario analysis, and threshold analysis.

6. **Decision-making:** To make decisions, compare the net benefits of each alternative. Identify intervention outcomes. The outcomes/results of interventions are classified based on the nature of the impacts they represent. These are as follows:
   - **Health-related outcomes:** The majority of a health-related outcome includes decreased mortality, decreased morbidity, increased life expectancy, reduced disability, improved QOL, and averted medical costs.
   - **Nonhealth outcomes:** The nonhealth outcomes are those that may have impact on health-related outcome directly or indirectly such as (1) reductions in time lost from work and (2) changes in property values attributable to the provision of health services in the area, improved access to health services in the area, and other causes. These outcomes add to the correct measure of the economic value of the program.
   - **Intangible health outcomes:** These outcomes are also considered that contribute reductions in health risks, pain, and suffering in implementing an intervention or health program.

Advantages of Cost-benefit Analysis

The advantages of CBA are as listed below:
- It allocates scarce resources to programs/interventions to have a maximum societal, economic benefit.
- It studies the economic value of all potential outcomes of a response.
- It makes it possible to compare different programs having different health outcomes, or health programs to nonhealth programs.
- It allows analysts to examine its distributional aspects (e.g. who will receive these benefits and who will bear the costs).

Drawbacks of Cost-benefit Analysis

Listed are the drawbacks of CBA:
- The CBA is a technique to measure costs and outcomes in monetary terms.
- It is difficult to assign monetary values to all pertinent outcomes.
- The results of CBA depend on the assumptions and valuations.

COST-EFFECTIVENESS ANALYSIS

Till 1970, the cost-effectiveness considered as a tool for healthcare decisions making to avoid controversy regarding the assessment of health-related outcomes in monetary terms. It was applied in the clinical setting and also to evaluate health policies, programs, and interventions. It is an analysis to assess the costs and health effects of specific interventions. It compares the estimated cost-effectiveness of a single proposed new intervention either with the profitability per reported study or assuming the willingness of people to pay with a fixed price cutoff point for an additional unit of health.

Although CEA is similar to CBA, it differs from CBA in the calculation of costs for each intervention and compares alternative ways to achieve a specific level of effectiveness. The CEA is an economical technique to measure the consequences of alternative interventions by using a single outcome usually in "natural" units, e.g. case detected, increased life years, and compared in terms of cost per unit of effectiveness.

The CEA is a comparison of costs in monetary units with the outcome, qualitative nonmonetary units, e.g. reduced mortality or morbidly. It is the analysis of the benefits of expenditure of resources on a particular intervention to identify whether the resources can be utilized more effectively **(Fig. 57.4)**.

Cost-effectiveness analysis takes a predetermined objective and seeks ways to accomplish it as inexpensively as possible. Cost-effective means anything useful and productive about its cost in terms of the goods or services (health outcome) received for the money spent.

Objectives of Cost-effectiveness Analysis

The objective of CEA is to maximize the level of benefits—health effects—relative to the level of resources available.
- To measure and compare different programs or interventions with a single common outcome
- To assess the consequences of expanding an existing program

Although these are relatively simple to measure, other vital results may ignore when using such measures. For

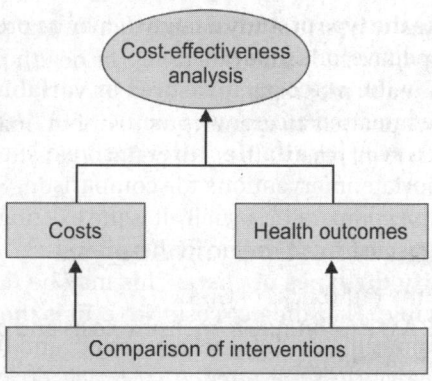

Fig. 57.4: Cost-effectiveness analysis.

example, when additional life expectancy is gained due to treatment, the quality of such years may also be necessary to patients. Another limitation of this type of analysis is that it does not facilitate comparisons across different disease areas when different outcomes have used.

Purposes of Cost-effectiveness Analysis

The main purposes of CEA are as follows:
- To identify the most cost-effective intervention from alternatives
- To provide substantial justification for a program
- To provide data on the relative costs and health benefits of different interventions
- To evaluate the programs/interventions for efficacy (cost-effective ratio), absolute health gain, and affordability (absolute cost).

Drawbacks of Cost-effectiveness Analysis

The two major drawbacks of CEA are as follows:
1. Cost data such as direct costs (such as doctors' or nurses' time and supplies used), indirect costs (such as a portion of administrative costs), and the cost of equipment are usually not readily available.
2. Cost-effectiveness is the method to judge the effect of an intervention.

Benefits of Cost-effectiveness Analysis

The benefits of CEA are as follows:
- It is easy to understand.
- It is more readily suited to decision-making.
- It provides evidence-based results regarding costs and outcomes/consequences associated with alternative interventions.

Measures for Cost-effectiveness

1. **Cost-effective ratio:** The three types of CERs are as follows:
   a. *Average CER (ACER):* It deals with a single intervention and evaluates that intervention against its baseline option (e.g. no program or current practice). To find out ACER, divide the net cost of the intervention by the total number of health outcomes prevented by the intervention.
   b. *The marginal cost-effectiveness ratio (MCER):* The marginal cost-effectiveness ratio (MCER) assesses the specific changes in cost and effect when a program expands or contracts. In general, the MCER is used in conjunction with the ACER as a tool to determine the most efficient level of program implementation.
   c. *Incremental cost-effectiveness Ratio (ICER):* It compares the differences between the costs and health outcomes of two alternative interventions that compete for the same resources and described as the additional cost per additional health outcome.

$$ICER = \frac{C_1 - C_2}{(E_1 - E_2)}$$

C_1 = Cost in the intervention group
E_1 = Impact in the intervention group
C_2 = Cost in the control/usual care group
E_2 = Effect in the control/usual care group
if, $E > 0, C < 0$, ICER < 0 = intervention is effective and cost-saving
if, $E < 0, C > 0$, ICER < 0 = intervention is worse than usual care and costs more
if, $E > 0, C > 0$, ICER < 0 = intervention is more effective than usual care and costs more

2. Net health benefits (NHBs)
   NHB = $E - C/\lambda$
   λ = a rate of substitution of money for health
   INHB(λ) = NHB$_1$(λ) − NHB$_2$(λ)

Methodological Challenges

1. Conventional 95% confidence interval
   95% confidence interval = mean ± (1.96) × (Standard Error)
   Normal distribution or large sample size.
   A good estimation of mean and variance.
2. Incremental cost-effective ratio
   The ratio is heavily skewed.
   Only approximated estimations of mean and variance are available.

Decision rule: Two programs A (comparator) and B
- If outcome of B = Outcome of A ≥ compare the costs (CMA)
- If outcome of B > Outcome of A and cost of B < cost of A, B is dominant
- If outcome of B > Outcome of A and cost of B > cost of A, make decision

Apply a cost-effectiveness ratio (CER) to select one of the interventions. The most commonly CERs used are as follows:
1. ACER

$$ACER = \frac{Cost\ B}{Effectiveness\ B}$$

2. Incremental cost-effectiveness ratio (ICER)

$$ICER = \frac{Cost\ B - Cost\ A}{Effectiveness\ B - effectiveness\ A}$$

In order to find out which intervention is effective, there is an additional requirement that the chosen alternative or combination of alternatives must also be below a ceiling ratio. A ceiling ratio is an externally-set level of the ICER that must be met if it is to be regarded as cost-effective. The ceiling ratio inferred from the amount that decision makers are willing to pay. To make a decision:
- If ICER of the program ≤ ceiling ratio → adopt the program
- If ICER of the program > ceiling ratio → do not select the program

Aspects of Cost-effectiveness Analysis

The eight aspects of CEA are as follows:
1. The study perspective, time frame, and the analytic horizon must be clear.
2. An explicitly defined study question.
3. Relevant assumptions underlying the study.
4. Detailed descriptions of the interventions.
5. Existing evidence of the interventions' effectiveness.
6. Proper identification of all applicable costs:
   - Decide whether to include or exclude productivity losses
   - Apply an appropriate discount rate
   - Confirm that added costs apply to perspective.
7. An appropriate choice of outcome
   - Calculate a suitable CER
   - Report the ICER results (unless the only comparator is baseline)
   - Conduct sensitivity analyses.
8. A comprehensive discussion of the results: Deal with issues of concern.

Procedural Steps in Cost-effectiveness Analysis

1. **Defining the problem:** Define and state the problem. Describe its significance and the areas of problems.
2. **Adopt a research strategy:** Once the study problem has identified and described, work out a research strategy. Define intervention(s) to analyze/evaluate, nature of the intervention, target population, delivery site, and personnel delivering the service, technology to be used, the timing of the intervention.
3. **Specify the audience:** Address the needs of the audience.
4. **Define perspective:** Usually the societal perspective used in CEA.
5. **Specify the time framework:** Develop the time framework during which the intervention is in effect.
6. **Prepare the analytic horizon:** Include all costs and outcomes attributable to the intervention over the entire period.
7. **Decide the type of study design:** It may be prospective, retrospective, or a model.
8. **Identify the outcome measures or variables:** These can be intermediate or outcomes.
9. **Search for available alternatives:** Select the appropriate interventions for comparison. Select the baseline comparator; usually it is the existing program and must use as an option in the analysis.
10. **Identify the types of costs:** This may be tangible or intangible. Find the net cost. Net cost is the program cost minus the cost of disease averted, and the cost of productivity losses averted.

    Net cost = Program cost – Cost of disease averted – Cost of productivity losses averted

    Include averted productivity losses in the net cost calculation from the societal perspective. Both the human capital approach and the cost of illness method can apply to assess the productivity losses.

    Disability-adjusted life years is the new metric for CEA. Disability-adjusted life years is the number of years of disability-free life that would be gained from a particular health intervention, yielding a cost per DALY where cost data are available or can be inferred.

COST-UTILITY ANALYSIS

Cost-utility analysis (CUA) is is an economic evaluation of different approaches to manage health-care costs. It compares the degree of improvement in the QOL with value spent. A quality-of-life index was applied to compare interventions, including QALYs.

Cost-utility analysis is a technique to compare different health outcomes by measuring in terms of a single unit (QALY). The utility is a value assigned to a level of health measured by the preferences of an individual or society. The CUA must take into account both the quantity of output produced and its distribution. The QALY combines quality (health status) and quantity (years) of health or life expectancy (**Fig. 57.5**).

Measures of Cost-utility Analysis

The outcomes in CUA are measured in healthy years, as it is multidimensional, and it includes QOL and quantity

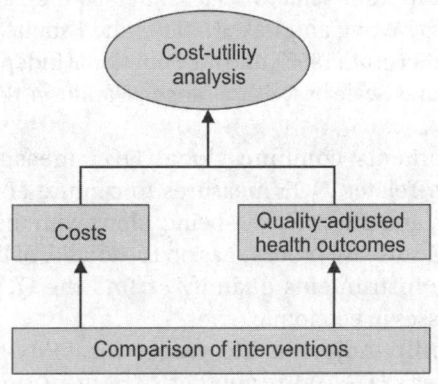

Fig. 57.5: Cost-utility analysis.

of life using a standard unit. The unit of CUA is cost/QALY (Quality-Adjusted-Life-Years) and Disability-adjusted life years (DALY).

1. **The quality-adjusted life years (QALYs):** The benefits are usually expressed in QALYs. A QALY is a mathematical measurement that combines quantity and quality of health to calculate the outcomes based on treatment or other activities that influence health. A QALY is a cost of producing 1 year of quality living. The score range of QALY is from 0 (death) to 1 (perfect health). A negative score means that a person is living a low QOL.

Components of Quality-adjusted Life Years

There are three standardized components of QALYs. The actuarial data, experimental data, or modeling are used to study a given population. The healthy life years weighted the same, and the weights for health states derived from studies of individuals with specific conditions.

Methods of Determining Quality-adjusted Life Years

- **Health rating method:** The health ratings are found by taking opinions from health experts, subjects undergoing treatment, or members of society. They are asked to assign values between 0 and 1 to various (well-described) health states.
- **Time trade-off method:** The time trade-off method is a technique to compare combinations of years and QOL by gathering responses from the respondents regarding length and QOL.
- **Health index method:** Health index is a method of assessing health status with various dimensions of well-being, such as mobility, absence from pain, etc. The Short-Form Health Survey (SF-36) of eight areas is an example of assessing the health index.

Instruments Commonly Used in Quality-adjusted Life Years

- Tools to measure the QOL globally, such as the SF-36.
- QOL tool specifically related to disease states, such as Asthma QOL Questionnaire by Juniper, Guyatt, Ferrie, and Griffith, 1993.
- The symptom-related scales, such as the Faces Pain Scale by Wong and Baker (1988), the Fatigue Scale by Chandler et al. (1993), and the Functional Independence Measures Scale by Keith, Granger, Hamilton, & Sherwin (1987).
- Instruments combine global QOL measures and health-related QOL measures to capture emotional, social, and physical well-being, along with the effect a specific disease process has on the totality of life.
- These instruments quantify or find the QOL; none expresses in economic terms.

2. **Disability-adjusted life years:** Disability-adjusted life years (DALYs) is another CUA measure used to measure the effect of ill-health regarding function and premature mortality. A DALY is a measure of one lost year of a healthy life. It is a combined measure of years in disability and years of life lost due to premature death (from the disability; Fox-Rushby & Hanson, 2001). The goal of DALY is to assess the residual burden of disease and injury as an outcome measure. It measures in two ways:

- **Years of life lost:** The number of years of life lost due to premature death is referred to as years of life lost (YLL).
- **Years lived with disability:** The number of healthy years lost due to disability from the condition until remission or death is considering years lived with disability (YLL).

> YLD = the number of incidence × disability weight × average duration of disease or infirmary until death or remission
> Disability-adjusted life years (DALY) = Years of Life Lost (YLL) + Years Lived with Disability (YLD)

The DALY scale ranges from 1 indicating death and 0 indicating the best possible state of health (it is the reverse of the QALY scale). It does not allow for negative values because 0 is equivalent to perfect health.

Advantages of cost-utility analysis
- It measures healthcare costs.
- It evaluates the effect of an intervention on QOL.
- It compares the practices/interventions improving QOL.
- It combines both quality and quantity of life measures.
- It is easy to compare across different disease areas.

Cost-utility Ratio

Cost-utility ratio compares interventions to achieve one QALY.

$$\text{Cost utility ratio} = \frac{₹\text{Cost}_{\text{Intervention}} - \text{Cost}_{\text{Comparator}}}{\text{Ulite}_{\text{Intervention}} - \text{Ulite}_{\text{Comparator}}}$$

Ulite, units of utility or preference, are often measured in QALYs.

Cost Minimization Analysis

Cost minimization analysis is a technique where the outcomes of the two or more interventions are compared based on the costs assuming similar results. The preference is for the intervention of the least cost with the same effect.

COST CONSEQUENCES ANALYSIS

Cost consequences analysis is a technique to compare alternative interventions or programs in terms of incremental costs (e.g. additional therapies, hospitalization) and consequences (e.g. health outcomes, adverse effects without aggregating these results (e.g. into a CER). It is a means to estimate whether the value of results obtained is worth the investment. In a cost consequences analysis, instead of combining the costs and effects, all the costs and outcomes are reported separately.

Advantages

The advantages of cost consequences analysis are as follows:
1. The method is simple to use.
2. It assesses costs, benefits, adjusting timings, and adjusting uncertainties to make the final decisions.

CHAPTER HIGHLIGHTS

- Cost analysis is a tool used in financial management and a technique used in an economic evaluation. Costs are the values of three principle resources, namely, material costs, labor costs, and overhead costs.
- The two health valuation methods are COI and nonmarket valuation methods. The COI method is to estimate the direct and indirect costs of an intervention. The nonmarket valuation method is to calculate intangible costs.
- Cost-benefit analysis is a technique to compare costs and benefits quantified in common monetary units. It measures costs and benefits in cash terms.
- Cost-effectiveness analysis (CEA) is a technique to compare the cost in monetary units with outcomes in quantitative nonmonetary groups.
- Cost-utility analysis (CUA) is a technique to compare costs in monetary units with outcomes in terms of their utility usually to the patient. The cost-utility ratio compares interventions to achieve one quality-adjusted life year (QALY).
- A cost consequence analysis is a technique used to compare costs and outcomes in discrete categories, without aggregating or weighting them.
- Cost minimization is a technique of determining the least cost among alternative interventions assumed to produce equivalent outcomes on comparing the cost of alternative interventions, and the alternative with the least cost provides the same result is cost-effective.

REVIEW QUESTIONS

I. Essay Type Questions
1. Define cost analysis. Discuss the principles of cost analysis.
2. Describe in detail the basic steps of cost analysis.
3. What is meant by a cost-benefit analysis? Describe steps of social cost-benefit analysis.
4. Explain the procedural steps of cost-effectiveness in detail.
5. Describe health valuation methods.

II. Short Notes
1. Approaches of cost-benefit analysis
2. Purposes of cost analysis
3. Cost-utility analysis
4. Measures of cost-effectiveness

III. Multiple Choice Questions
1. Which is an economic evaluation that involves systematic collection, categorization, and analysis of an intervention in terms of costs and cost of illness?
   a. Cost analysis
   b. Cost-effectiveness
   c. Cost utility
   d. Cost-benefit
2. The main purpose of sensitivity analysis in cost analysis is:
   a. To determine the optional activity level of a program or an intervention
   b. To rule out any measurement error, biased estimation, or omission of any cost component
   c. To evaluate the change in total expenses resulting from a shift in program activity level
   d. To evaluate the difference in total costs that require to produce a change
3. Which type of cost is associated with the production of resources one additional or one less unit within the same intervention?
   a. Total cost
   b. Average cost
   c. Induced cost
   d. Marginal cost
4. Which one of the following techniques are used to compare the cost in monetary unit with outcomes in quantitative nonmonetary groups?
   a. Cost-utility analysis
   b. Cost–benefit analysis
   c. Cost-effectiveness analysis
   d. Cost consequences analysis
5. Which one of the following mathematical measurements of CUA uses quantity and quality of health in combination to calculate outcome based on treatment?
   a. DALYs
   b. QALYs
   c. YLL
   d. YLD

Answer Keys
1. a 2. b 3. d 4. c 5. b

SUGGESTED READING

1. Available from http://www.rds-sc.nihr.ac.uk/planning-a-study/health-economics/economic-evaluation/. [Accessed July 2019].
2. Available from http://www.who.int/choice/publications/d_ScalingUp_MDGs_WHO_finalreport.pdf. [Accessed July 2019].
3. Available from https://www.who.int/choice/publications/p_2003_generalised_cea.pdf. [Accessed August 2019].
4. Available from https://www.who.int/choice/book/en/. Accessed August 2019.
5. Brazier JE, Ratcliffe J, Tsuchiya A, Salomon J. Measuring and valuing health benefits for economic evaluation. Oxford: Oxford University Press; 2007.

6. Briggs A, Claxton K, Sculpher MJ. Decision modelling for health economic evaluation. Oxford: Oxford University Press; 2006.
7. Chalder T, Berelowitz G, Pawlikowska T, Watts L, Wessely S, Wright D, Wallace EP. Development of a fatigue scale. J Psychosom Res. 1993;37(2):147-53.
8. Dolan P. The measurement of individual utility and social welfare. J Health Econ. 1998;17:39-52.
9. Elsinga E, Rutten FF. Economic evaluation in support of national health policy: The case of the Netherlands. Soc Sci Med. 1997;45:605-20.
10. Fox-Rushby JA and Hanson K. Calculating and presenting disability adjusted life years (DALYs) in cost-effectiveness analysis. Health Policy Plan 2001; 16(3): 326-31.
11. Gwatkin DR. The need for equity-oriented health sector reforms. Int J Epidemiol. 2001;30:720-23.
12. Hailey D. Australian economic evaluation and government decisions on pharmaceuticals compared to the assessment of other health technologies. Soc Sci Med. 1997;45:563-81.
13. https://www.who.int/airpollution/household/interventions/cost_benefit/en/Accessed September 2018
14. Juniper EF, Guyatt GH, Ferrie PJ, Griffith LE. Measuring quality of life in asthma. Am Rev Respir Dis 1993;127:832-8.
15. Keith RA, Granger CV, Hamilton BB, and Sherwin FS. The functional independence measure: a new tool for rehabilitation. Advances in Clinical Rehabilitation, 1987; 1: 6-18.
16. Kenneth E. Warner, Rebecca C. Hutton. Cost-benefit and cost-effectiveness analysis in health care: Growth and composition of the literature. Medical Care. 1980;18(11):1069-84. [online] Available from http://www.jstor.org/stable/3764259. [Accessed July 2019].
17. Le Pen C. Pharmaceutical economy and the economic assessment of drugs in France. Soc Sci Med. 1997;45:635-43.
18. McCabe C, Claxton K, Culyer A. The NICE cost-effectiveness threshold: What it is and what that means. Pharmacoeconomics. 2008;26:733-44.
19. McCabe C. What is the Cost-utility Analysis? London: Hayward Medical Communications; 2009.
20. McGregor M. Cost-utility analysis: Use QALYs only with great caution. CMAJ. February 18, 2003;168(4):433-34.
21. Musgrove P, Fox-Rushby J. Cost-effectiveness analysis for priority setting. In: Jamison DT et al. (Eds). Disease Control Priorities in Developing Countries, 2nd edition. New York: Oxford University Press; 2006.
22. Phillips CJ. Health Economics: An Introduction for Health Professionals. Oxford: Blackwell Publishing; 2005.
23. Vale L, et al. An economic evaluation of thrombolysis in a remote rural community. BMJ. 1997;314:570-2.
24. Wagstaff A. QALYs and the equity-efficiency trade-off. J Health Econ. 1991;10:21-41.
25. WHO. Commission on Macroeconomics and Health. Macroeconomics and health: Investing in health for economic development. Report of the Commission on Macroeconomics and Health: Executive Summary. Geneva: World Health Organization; 2001.
26. Wong DL and Baker CM. Pain in children: Comparison of assessment scales. Pediatr Nurs 1988; 14:9-17.

58 CHAPTER

Critical Pathways and Health Care Reforms

CHAPTER OUTLINE

- Critical Pathways
  - Definitions
  - Historical Perspectives
  - Goals of Critical Pathways
  - Purposes of Critical Pathways
  - Characteristics of Critical Pathways
  - Benefits of Critical Pathways
  - Steps in Developing and Implementing Critical Pathways
- Healthcare Reforms
  - Concept and Definitions
  - Historical Perspectives of Healthcare Reforms in India
  - Characteristics of Healthcare Reforms
  - Aims and Objectives of Healthcare Reforms
  - Purposes of Healthcare Reforms
  - Healthcare Reform Strategies
  - Types of Health Sector Reforms
  - Elements of Healthcare Reforms
  - Importance of Healthcare Reforms
  - Principles of Health Sector Reforms
  - Healthcare Reform Cycle
  - Factors Affecting the Design of Healthcare Reforms
  - Problems In Having Health Reforms In India

LEARNING OUTCOMES

After completion of this chapter, the learner will be able to:
- Understand the concept and historical background of critical pathways
- Discuss the goals and purposes of critical pathways
- Describe the characteristics of critical pathways
- Describe how critical pathways are beneficial in nursing
- Enumerate various steps in developing and implementing critical pathways
- Understand the concept, nature, and indicators of healthcare reforms
- Enumerate different reform strategies
- Describe the purposes and importance of healthcare reforms
- Apply the principles of health sector reforms
- Discuss the healthcare reform process and factors affecting the design of healthcare reform

KEY TERMS

Critical pathways, healthcare reform, management plan, clinical pathways, healthcare reform process

INTRODUCTION

Critical pathways are clinical pathways. These are management plans that depict the goals and objectives of care for patients. It provides the action plan in terms of sequence and timing of actions necessary to achieve those goals with optimal efficiency. Healthcare reform is a general rubric used to discuss significant health policy creation or changes. It is usually applicable in governmental policy that affects healthcare delivery.

CRITICAL PATHWAYS

Definitions

Ignatavicius and Hausman (1995) define critical pathway as an interdisciplinary plan of care that outlines the optimal sequencing and timing of interventions for patients. These are management plans having goals for patients and provide optimal care to achieve those goals with optimal efficiency. A critical pathway is a tool that details processes of care and highlights the negligence with or without evidence to changes in those processes.

A critical pathway is the sequence of events in a process that takes the most considerable length of time. It is a clinical pathway of optimal sequencing and timing of interventions by clinicians, nurses, and other healthcare professionals for a particular intervention to minimize delays and resource utilization and to maximize the quality of care.

Historical Perspectives

The concept of critical pathways originated from the theories of continuous quality improvement (CQI). Critical pathways first developed for the use in industry as a tool to identify and manage the rate-limiting steps in production processes. In healthcare, critical pathways were first developed and applied in the 1980s to improve hospital efficiency. Nurses developed most of the first critical pathways in hospitals for nursing care alone. Later on, other disciplines used to cover all the aspects.

Goals of Critical Pathways

1. To select the best practice and define the standards for the expected length of hospital stay.
2. To assess the interrelations among the different steps in the care process to find ways to coordinate.
3. To work as a team and understand their roles in the overall care process.
4. To provide a framework for collecting data on the care process.
5. To decrease documentation burdens.
6. To improve patient satisfaction by educating patients and their families about the plan of care.

Purposes of Critical Pathways

1. To examine expenses on the condition, procedure, or symptom basis.
2. To monitor and improve the quality of patient care.
3. To achieve specified patient's outcomes by a preset time frame.
4. To have an action plan in advance.
5. To shorten the hospital stays.
6. To use resources efficiently.
7. To improve communication between disciplines.
8. To utilize less expensive methods of treatment.

Characteristics of Critical Pathways

1. It is a structured multidisciplinary care plan.
2. It supports interdisciplinary care and evidence-based clinical practice.
3. It defines goals, essential elements of care, and best practices, based on evidence.
4. It guides the management for a well-defined group of patients for a defined period.
5. It sequences the actions of a multidisciplinary team.
6. It facilitates variance management and allows documenting, monitoring, and evaluating the variances.
7. It gives detailed steps in the care of patients with a specific clinical problem.
8. It facilitates translation of national guidelines into local protocols.
9. It facilitates communication with patients by providing a written summary of care.

Benefits of Critical Pathways

- It improves patient care.
- It increases the use of recommended medical therapies.
- It minimizes the use of unnecessary tests.
- It reduces the length of stay of patients by decreasing complications.
- It reduces costs and improves the quality of patient care.
- It increases participation in clinical research protocols.

Steps in Developing and Implementing Critical Pathways

According to Gordon (1995), four stages are involved in developing and implementing critical pathways:

Stage 1: Focus and recognition stage

1. Evaluate the baseline data to identify the need. Topic selection, in general, should concentrate on high-volume, high-cost diagnoses and procedures.
2. Establish preliminary goals and measurable outcomes.
3. Review research literature to obtain the latest information relevant to the pathway.

Stage 2: Evaluation and analysis stage

1. Analyze the data to determine the improvement in performance and to examine the outcome of value and to find out barriers to changing practices.
2. Implement continuous quality improvement (CQI) methods by determining the technical causes, providers, or processes for performance gap.
3. Chart review is a method of data collection to identify the most common preparations.
4. Identify additional data, such as length of hospital stay, nursing diagnoses, outcomes, critical events, etc. to focus on problem areas.
5. Evaluate benefits and harms, so that processes and practices that produce the best clinical outcomes are identified.

Stage 3: Development stage

1. Constitute a multidisciplinary team that includes all principal caregivers and affected personnel, experts, and consultants from other disciplines.
2. Develop a draft of the action plan of the pathway, indicating all actions. Begin with a blank sheet of paper with the number of columns equal to the desired length of stay and stages of care. Identify critical elements in boldface.
3. Focus on crucial elements that will clarify the characteristics necessary for the pathway. All team members should be active participants.
4. Reviewing the pathway draft by distributing it to each member of the committee to consider and select the correct intervention.
5. After reviewing the draft, check its feasibility.
6. Developing documentation forms is an essential element to the process of outcome attainment. The forms become the core for recording and managing quality assurance.

7. Develop a system for variance analysis to clarify how to document variances, who records variations and differences, so modifications to the pathway can be made accordingly for continuous improvement in the path.
8. Ensure usability of pathways by other hospital projects. It is to allow employees to involve in the educational process and improve the overall clinical care.
9. Set a timetable for 3–6 months.
10. Plan all the activities, tools, and methods of collecting data in implementing the pathway plan.
11. Plan and organize in-service education programs, so that the staff becomes confident to learn the process and consequences, minimizing difficulties during the implementation process.

Stage 4: Implementation and evaluation stage
Gather the information and analyze the data. The processes must be improved to achieve the goals of resource savings with an improvement in outcomes.
1. Check compliance frequently.
2. Compare results with baseline data and analyze.
3. Look at variances and discuss with departments.
4. Communicate results to the team and modify pathway.

Coffey et al. (1992) identified 12 steps as given below:
1. Select diagnosis or procedure.
2. Appoint a development team.
3. Choose path characteristics.
4. Document current process.
5. Study internal and external practices.
6. Develop critical path.
7. Implement critical path.
8. Define key measures of conformance and outcome.
9. Develop data collection tools and process.
10. Educate all affected staff.
11. Analyze results.
12. Improve path as required.

HEALTHCARE REFORMS

Healthcare reforms in India are taking place under the broad umbrella of structural adjustment programs (SAPs) termed as the new economic policy (NEP). The two aspects of SAPs are privatization and liberalization. The health sector reform agenda took its root during the mid-1990s with a relatively vibrant private sector. There was stagnation of public services from the mid-1980s through the 1990s due to the economy committed to socialism, economic crisis, and the oil crisis-led fiscal deficit. The highest investment declined to around 1% during the 1990s—the recession in the growth of public services depends on private sectors for its services.

Various factors in the developing countries such, investment in the health, financial constraints, poor social indicators, and privatization led healthcare reforms in India. India is regulating private healthcare services by enforcing Consumer Protection Act (COPRA) 1986, and other Acts such as the IMC Act, Code of Ethics, Dangerous Drug Act, Drugs and Cosmetics Act, Pharmacy Act, Nursing Home Act, and so on.

Concept and Definitions

Reform means a change for better or improvement. It involves the correction of errors or to do something in a better form. Health system or sector reform is a sustained and purposeful change to improve effectiveness, efficiency, and equity of the health sector. According to Cassels (1995), it is a process of defining priorities, modifying policies, and reforming the institutions to implement refined strategies.

In 2002, the World Health Organization defined healthcare reform as a sustained process of fundamental change in health policies, institutional organization of the health sector, which is guided by government. It is a process of developing a set of policy measures that cover main core functions of the health system. These are governance, provision, financing, and resource generation. The main aim of healthcare reforms is to improve the functioning and performance of the health sector and thus to improve the health status of the people at large.

Healthcare reform is a planned and deliberate process to bring about sustainable change in healthcare system. It is a process of redefining the policy objectives and restructuring the existing organization and management of health system and financing system. It is a political process that requires a consensus of all stakeholders at Ministry of Health, and other sectors, state and local government, service providers both government and nongovernmental organizations (NGOs), the population at large, resource institutions such as universities, research institutions, institutional buyers such as insurance funds, district health, and key donors.

Health system includes resources, organization, financing, and management who require to deliver the health services to the population (Roemer, 1991). The main components of healthcare reform are equity, effectiveness, efficiency, quality, sustainability, defining priorities, refining policies, and reforming/reframing institutions for policy implementation. The healthcare reforms need to complement primary healthcare, emphasizing principles of equity, collaboration, community involvement, decentralization, and research and health information to make decisions on issues to change.

Health sector reform is more than projects put together and tied to loans from the World Bank. Health sector reform is a group of projects that include communicable disease, reproductive and child health program, and health systems to promote economic efficiency, quality, and improvement of the public sector (Senior World Bank Official, Delhi, 2002).

Historical Perspectives of Healthcare Reforms in India

Traces of economic liberalization were reported in the 1980s. The healthcare reform process began in 1992 and continued to improve in the Five Year Plans. It covers areas such as reorganizing and restructuring of the existing healthcare system, the participating community, focusing on quality care, and strengthening the health management information system.

Health Survey and Development Committee (Bhore Committee) formed the landmark in developing health policy and health systems in India. It also recommended the three-tiered healthcare system to provide preventive and curative healthcare services. The National Health Policy (NHP 1983) emphasizes to encourage private initiative in healthcare service delivery. So the focus of the state policy shifted to primary healthcare, especially to the rural population.

During the Eighth Five-Year Plan (1992–1997), the concept of free medical service was initiated. User charges were levied for diagnostic and curative services on families living above poverty line. Significant reforms took place in infrastructure, strengthening of facilities, provision of essential equipment, and ensuring supply of drugs, equipment, and other materials. The Indian System of Medicine and Homeopathy and health system research were reorganized. The focus was on the health management information system and private sector involvement in healthcare delivery with proper regulation and accreditation. Free or subsidized care was committed for below poverty line (BPL) families. The family welfare services were promoted, and a check was on population growth. There was decentralization in planning and implementing health programs.

During the Ninth Five-Year Plan (1997–2002), there was horizontal integration of vertical programs and development of disease surveillance and response mechanism. Panchayat Raj institutions were involved in planning and monitoring health programs. The government included voluntary, private organizations, and self-group in the delivery of healthcare. It initiated appropriate emergency and disaster management system.

In the Tenth Five-Year Plan (2002–2007), reforms were observed in primary, secondary, and tertiary services. The focus was on equal distribution of healthcare services and near-universal coverage for meeting the cost of hospitalization, continuous care of chronic diseases, health insurance for individuals, and social protection for BPL families. Structural and functional reforms focused on human resource development and integration of health and family welfare societies at the state and district levels. There were financial, governance-related reforms. Emphasis was on public–private partnerships in national programs, capacity building, and quality assurance. There was a paradigm shift in the National Rural Health Mission (NRHM) launched in April 2005 to strengthen rural health through the Accredited Social Health Activist (ASHA) females who provide the services at the village level. There were reforms in delivery of healthcare, district health societies, the involvement of NGOs, and integration of the Indian System of Medicine.

During the Eleventh Five-Year Plan (2007–2012), time-bound targets were fixed with indicators. There was improved health equity, system approach, decentralized governance, the establishment of e-Health. The focus was on health financing, performance-based incentives to providers, Children's Behavioral Health Initiative (CBHI), and implementing food safety and standardized Act.

The Government introduced the Twelfth Five-Year Plan strategy for universal access to equitable, affordable, and quality healthcare services and to revitalize both rural and urban health sectors. The NRHM emerged into the National Health Mission (NHM) (2012–2017). The National Urban Health Mission as the sub-mission of NHM was launched on January 20, 2014, to improve the health status of urban poor, both listed and unlisted living in slums, vulnerable population by addressing in particular their health issues. It operates at national, state, and city/community levels. The focus was on effective public health administration, health financing, clinical establishment, development of human resources, developing health services master plan, and reforming private healthcare system.

The government introduced the NHP 2017 and replaced the Planning Commission with National Institute of Transforming India Aayog (NITI). The government prepared a 3-year agenda to strengthen the existing health system with the objectives to attain universal health coverage of the highest possible level, free and comprehensive and affordable primary healthcare, improved access to secondary and tertiary quality healthcare services, and reduction of poor households' out-of-pocket expenditure on healthcare.

The NHP 2017 focuses on the health finance sector, health infrastructure, and building capacity per the Indian Public Health Standards (IPHS), establishing primary and secondary healthcare facilities, health management information system, strengthening health surveillance system, developing registries for public health diseases, and integrated health information architecture

It emphasizes on universal health coverage by providing comprehensive preventive, promotive, and affordable quality healthcare services that should reach everyone. It is concerned with health security and make in India for drugs and devices to attain the highest possible level of well-being, and affordable quality healthcare services to everyone. It emphasizes on professionalism, integrity, and ethics.

The focus is on equity, affordability, universality, patient-centered quality of care. There should be financial and performance accountability and transparency in decision-making, both in public and in private. The healthcare sector must have a multistakeholder approach with partnership and participation of all nonhealth ministries and communities. There should be pluralism in access to care and an appropriate level of decentralization and community participation. The organization of healthcare should be evidence based. There are time-bound-specific goals and multiareas in the policy.

Characteristics of Healthcare Reforms

1. It covers the entire national healthcare system.
2. It includes all types of services, i.e., preventive, promotive, curative, and rehabilitative, and public and private, primary, secondary, and tertiary care.
3. It is a problem-solving process that seeks to solve the health policy and healthcare system-related major issues.
4. It involves the participation of many actors, stakeholders, institutions, and the population at large.
5. It requires ownership and commitment by local, state, and national government.

Aims and Objectives of Healthcare Reforms

The main aim of healthcare reform is to improve the health of people at large. The goals and the objectives of healthcare reforms can be achieved as follows:
1. To ensure an appropriate share to public funds to spend on healthcare especially at the local level.
2. To ensure equal distribution of health and funded healthcare among consumers.
3. To improve the organization and management of health resources to attain overall goals and objectives of health policy.
4. To enhance quality care and performance of the healthcare system.
5. To satisfy the users with the health services and health providers of healthcare.

Purposes of Healthcare Reforms

To have the population receive healthcare coverage through either public sector insurance programs or private sector insurance companies.
1. To improve access to healthcare specialists.
2. To enhance the quality of healthcare.
3. To decrease the cost of healthcare.

Healthcare Reform Strategies

1. **Health financing:** It requires the mobilization of funding and better utilization of available funding. Mobilization of health financing includes establishing alternate finance schemes such as national health insurance schemes, user fees, community financing, private sector investment, promotion of public–private mix, negotiating with donors, etc.
2. **The institutional organization, management, and decentralization:** There should be autonomy to make decision to plan, implement, monitor, and control health care reform issues at institutional, local, and state level. The primary role of Ministry of Health is to formulate policies and regulations and implementation at the government, private, and NGO level. The legislative review requires amending specific health-related laws for healthcare reform. There is also a need to train and build capacity to manage the reformed organization structure of health system. The efforts require strong advocacy regarding changes to inform public and partners. Management of resources, especially human resource planning and management, is another challenge to bring healthcare reforms to improve the performance of health service organizations. The reform also includes collaboration with the private sector (public/private partnerships, joint ventures), and public sector reforms such as civil service reforms, capacity building, productivity improvement.
3. **Health service delivery:** There should be an equitable provision of essential health services. It requires defining the priorities, proper referral and supervision mechanisms, integration of vertical programs, quality assurance mechanism, a system of improving quality care, adequate logistic support, transport and other facilities, drugs, equipment, etc.

Types of Health Sector Reforms

1. **Financial system reforms:** These reforms focus on increasing resources to health sectors, e.g. change in public health financing, new user fees, and community financing at a small scale.
2. **Change in health system organization and management:** It includes decentralization in the healthcare delivery system, contracting human resources, and public–private partnerships in the delivery of care.
3. **Public sector reforms:** These include an increased role of local government, introducing competitions, etc.

Elements of Healthcare Reforms

The main aspects of healthcare reforms are health financing, expenditure, organizational regulation, and consumers' behavior. It has undergone three generations. During the first generation, the focus was to establish national healthcare systems and the extension of social insurance. The second generation focused on the promotion of primary healthcare, and third generation is concerned with universe coverage of healthcare.

Importance of Health Sector Reforms

Health sector reforms influence the provisioning, financing, workforce, drugs, and technology in the health service system. It improves the effectiveness of national health programmes and has an impact on the availability, accessibility, quality, and cost of health services, both general and specific for reproductive and child health.

Principles of Health Sector Reforms

1. Private organizations and individuals should be responsible for healthcare.
2. Public funding must restrict to health promotion and prevention of disease.
3. Central government's role should limit to policy formulation and technical guidance.
4. The individual and nongovernmental sectors should support the key providers of health and social services.

Healthcare Reform Cycle

Healthcare reform is a problem-solving process. The healthcare reform cycle consists of the following steps (Fig. 58.1):

1. **Identification and diagnosis of the problem:** To define priorities, problems need to be identified. This can be achieved by analysing the strengths, weaknesses, opportunities, and threats of health situations (SWOT). It is at the government level and headed by the Ministry of Health.
2. **Development of vision of the reformed sector:** The next step in healthcare reform is to develop a concept. Both public and private providers' inputs are necessary to create a vision for the reformed sector.
3. **Development of health policies, strategies, strategic plans, and operational plans:** There is a need to involve resource institutions to develop strategies and plans. It requires the participation of community, families, individuals, political, and civil society groups.
4. **Sourcing of adequate funding:** To implement reformed policies and plans, it needs sufficient funding. Find the proper supply of funds through identifying donors and other partners for healthcare delivery.
5. **Implementation of operational plans:** Per policy, implement healthcare. It needs institutional buyers, other government sectors, and institutions. Here there is a need for continuous monitoring, evaluation, advocacy, and consensus building.
6. **Monitoring, evaluation, advocacy, and consensus building:** At all stages, it requires the reform process and especially at the time of development of vision and implementation.

Factors Affecting the Design of Healthcare Reforms

1. Global actors include bilateral and multilateral agencies, pharmaceutical, medical equipment industries, the insurance company, and research institutions. They can shape health policies across the world.
2. The domestic capital has a role in providing healthcare services, medical equipment, and insurance.
3. The growth of the middle class and their influence on both supply and demand of private health services (Baru, 2003).

Problems in Having Health Reforms in India

The health reforms in India face the following problems:
- The issue of the underfunding health services
- Inadequate investment by the government in healthcare to meet the demands of the people
- The scarce allocation of resources for the health sector
- Gross domestic product is short of the World Health Organization
- The minimum grants from the central government to the state governments.

CHAPTER HIGHLIGHTS

- The critical pathway is an interdisciplinary plan of care, which outlines the optimal sequencing and timing of interventions for patients.
- The main goal of critical pathways is to select the best practice and to define the standards for the expected length of hospital stay.
- Healthcare reform is a planned, deliberate, political, and sustained process of fundamental change in health policies and institutional organization of the health sector guided by the government.
- The main aim of healthcare reform is to improve the health of people at large.
- The healthcare reform process began in 1992 and continued to improve in the Five-Year Plans. Bhore Committee in 1946 formed the landmark in developing health policy and health systems in India.
- Health financing, institutional organization, management, and decentralization, and healthcare delivery are core strategies of healthcare reform.
- Healthcare reform is a problem-solving process comprising various steps to bring out changes in health policy and healthcare systems.

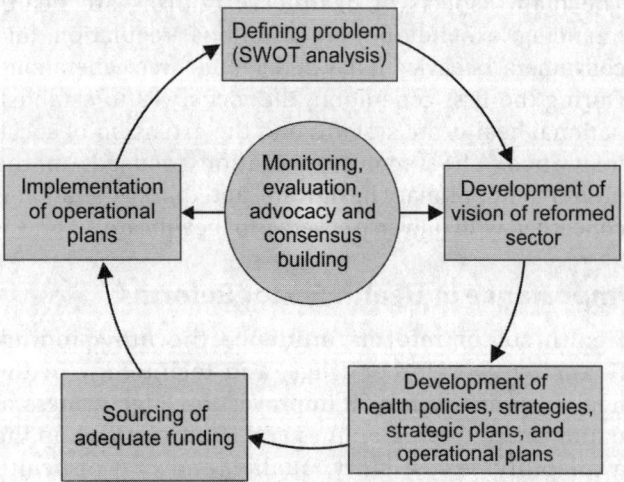

Fig. 58.1: Healthcare reform process.

REVIEW QUESTIONS

I. Essay Type Questions
1. Define critical pathways. Discuss its goals and purposes.
2. "Critical pathways is a process." Explain in detail.
3. What is meant by healthcare reform? Discuss historical perspectives of healthcare reforms in India.
4. Describe in detail the healthcare reform cycle.

II. Short Notes
1. Strategies of healthcare reform
2. Features of critical pathways
3. Importance and benefits of critical pathways
4. Types of healthcare reforms.

III. Multiple Choice Questions
1. A management plan that details the processes of care and highlights the negligence to bring a change is:
   a. Healthcare reform
   b. Quality planning
   c. Critical pathways
   d. Quality control
2. Which five-year plan focused on horizontal integration of vertical programs and development of disease surveillance and response mechanism?
   a. Eighth Five-Year Plan
   b. Ninth Five-Year Plan
   c. Tenth Five-Year Plan
   d. Eleventh Five-Year Plan
3. When was the National Urban Health Mission launched as the sub-mission of the NHM launch?
   a. April 2005
   b. March 2010
   c. November 2012
   d. January 2014
4. Which one is the most appropriate goal related to healthcare reforms?
   a. To improve organization and management of health resources to attain objectives of health policy
   b. To select the best practices and define the standards
   c. To provide a care process framework
   d. To monitor and improve the quality of patient care

Answer Keys
1. c   2. b   3. d   4. a

SUGGESTED READING

1. Available at: https://apps.who.int/iris/bitstream/handle/10665/59762/WHO_SHS_NHP_95.4.pdf?sequence=1 [Accessed Jan 2020].
2. Baru RV. Privatisation of Health Services: A South Asian Perspective. Economic and Political Weekly Oct. 18-24, 2003;38(42):4433-7.
3. Cassels A. Health sector reform: key issues in less developed countries. Geneva: World Health Organization, 1995.
4. De Bleser LDR, De Waele K, Vanhaecht K, et al. Defining pathways. J Nurs Manag. 2006;14:553-63. Pub Med.
5. Doll R. Health and the environment in the 1990s. Am J Public Health. 1992;82:933-41.
6. Health Sector Reform and District Health Systems. [online]. Available from https://www.who.int/management/HealthSectorReformDHS.pdf. [Accessed Sep 2019].
7. Health sector reform in India | World Bank | Health System Available at: https://www.scribd.com/www.scribd.com › presentation ›. [Accessed Jan 2020].
8. http://ncdrc.nic.in/bare_acts/Consumer%20Protection%20Act-1986.html. [Accessed Jan 2020].
9. Ignatavicius D, Hausman K. Critical pathways for collaborative practice. Philadelphia: WB Saunders, 1995.
10. Reddy KN. Health expenditure in India. Working Paper No. 14. New Delhi: NIPFP; 1992.
11. Vanhaecht K, De Witte K, Depreitere R, et al. Clinical pathways audit tool: A systematic review. J Nurs Manag. 2006;14:529-37. Pub Med.
12. WHO. World Health Statistics, 2009. World Health Organization.

SECTION 11

Nursing Informatics

59. Nursing Informatics, Information Technology, Use of Computers and Telecommunications
60. Documentation System: Nursing Records and Recording, Reports and Reporting, and Correspondence
61. Information Systems: Management Information and Evaluation System, Health Information and Management System, and Nursing Information System
62. Use of Communication Technology: e-Learning, Telemedicine, Telenursing

CHAPTER 59

Nursing Informatics, Information Technology, Use of Computers and Telecommunications

CHAPTER OUTLINE

- Nursing Informatics
  - History of Nursing Informatics
  - Definitions
  - Goal and Purposes of Nursing Informatics
  - Bases of Nursing Informatics
  - Computer Skills and Informatics Knowledge
  - Component Standards of Nursing Informatics
  - Importance of Nursing Informatics
  - Benefits of Nursing Informatics
  - Applications of Nursing Informatics
  - Implications for Informatics
- Difference Between Nursing Informatics and Evidence-based Practice
- Limitations of Nursing Informatics
- Information Technology
  - Purposes of Information Technology
  - Information Systems in the Clinical Setting
  - Types of Information Technology
  - Applications of ICT in Nursing
  - Barriers to Using Information Technology
- Use of Computers
- Telecommunications

LEARNING OUTCOMES

After completion of this chapter, the learner will be able to:
- Understand the concept of nursing informatics
- Define nursing informatics
- Discuss the goal and purposes of nursing informatics
- Describe bases and component standards of nursing informatics
- Explain the essentials of nursing informatics and competencies required for nurses
- Recognize the importance and benefits of nursing informatics
- Apply nursing informatics in nursing practice: clinical, management, and education and research
- Differentiate nursing informatics from evidence-based practice
- Understand the concept of information technology
- Describe the purposes of information technology
- Enumerate the different types of information technology
- Discuss the advance applications of ICT
- Describe the barriers to using information technology
- Explain computer and computer system
- Enlists the various kinds of computers and networks
- Elaborate the applications of computer use and telecommunications

KEY TERMS

Nursing informatics, competencies, evidence-based practice, information technology, computers, computer system, information and communications, telecommunication

INTRODUCTION

Nursing informatics is not a new subject. The nurses need to become computer literate and should be well versed in the dynamics of nursing informatics. Moreover, in the current information age, there is the doubling of knowledge every 5 years and the increased specialization of experience that make it imperative that nurses should know the latest technology to assist in the delivery of high-quality care. Nursing informatics is a field of integrating information and computer science with nursing. It will help nurses to gather and manage the data and can convert into data to make knowledge-based decisions about patient care. It is essentially the science and art of turning data into information. In India, nursing informatics is in the infancy stage, but it will help in the new healthcare delivery system.

NURSING INFORMATICS

A German computer scientist, Karl Steinbuch, first coined the term "informatik" in 1957 followed by Philippe Dreyfus in 1962 as "informatique," and further translated into "informatics" by Walter F Bauer. The term informatics combined the terms "information" and "automation" to name automatic information processing. The combination of words "informat" with the suffix "ics" broadened the definition and addressed the actual science and fundamental theories of information and information processing.

A Russian scientist (1966) coined the term "*informatika*" and defined it as "the discipline of science which investigates the structures and properties (not specific content) of scientific information."

Informatics is modeled after the French word *informatique* referring to "the computer milieu" by a Frenchman Francois Gramy and used as medical informatics in the late 1970s. Healthcare informatics focuses on the care of the patient, not a specific discipline. It is the science of generating, recording, and classifying the data. It also stores, retrieves, processes, and analyzes health information.

History of Nursing Informatics

The history of nursing informatics is as follows:
- Florence Nightingale was an early informatics nurse because of her use of data to inform knowledge and change nursing practices. In 1863, she was very clear in her desire to collect, retrieve, and analyze data to be able to recognize trends in illnesses and treatments to improve the quality of care.
- During the 1950s and 1960s, health care and the nursing profession in developing countries underwent many significant changes, and the analyses of nursing resources and allocations were started in the mid-60s; the nursing station was considered the center of communication activities and information exchange. Computers were used primarily in healthcare facilities for necessary financial and accounting operations.
- In the 1970s, the nursing staff became instrumental in the development of nursing applications for hospital information systems.
- In the 1970s and early 1980s, nursing informatics considered the use of computer technology to aid in nursing practice, and it was frequently confused with the computer literacy skills of the nurse.
- Scholes and Barber in 1980 first used and defined the term "nursing informatics" in their address to the MEDINFO conference the same year in Tokyo.
- During the 1990s and beyond, the Internet became the tool for web-based clinical applications, communication, was accessed to evidence-based resources, was used at the point of care where the patient was under nursing care and for other healthcare professionals.
- After that, informatics, through the use of computers, assists nurses as knowledge workers within their four domains of practice: clinical, management, education, and research.
- In 1996, Turley introduced a model that illustrates the interaction of the sciences that contribute to nursing informatics, computer science, information science,

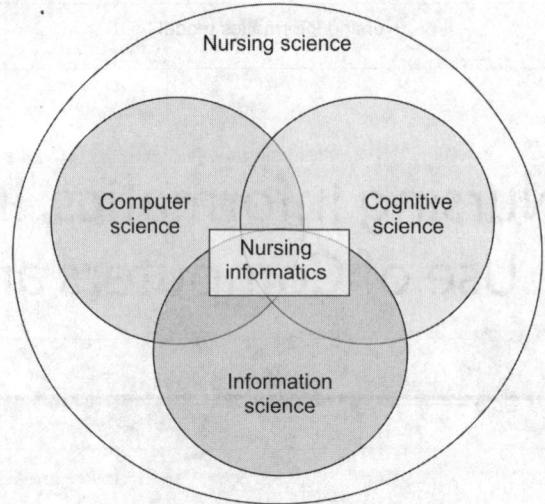

Fig. 59.1: Turley' nursing informatics model.

and cognitive science in nursing science to include topics related to cognitive science such as problem solving, memory, language processing, mental models, and visual attention **(Fig. 59.1)**.
- In 2002, Staggers and Thompson documented in one of the papers the categorization of definitions into three themes: information technology (IT)-, conceptually oriented, and role-oriented definitions.
- The definitions of informatics continue to be modified slightly to adjust for continuing advances in practice and technologies, but it has focused more on the information than on the technology.

Definitions

Scholes and Barber (1980) defined nursing informatics as the application of computer technology to all fields of nursing—nursing services, nurse education, and nursing research. It is a combination of nursing science, computer, and information science to manage, process, and communicate nursing data to deliver nursing care and enhance the quality of nursing care.

Nursing informatics is the application of computer science and information science to nursing. Nursing information promotes the generation, management, and processing of relevant data to use and develop knowledge that supports nursing in all practice domains (National Nursing Informatics Project, 1999). According to Goossen WTF (2000), it is a discipline to study the development, utility, and information system. International Council of Nurses (ICN) (2006) considered it an integration of information systems in nursing to support health efforts. It is a subspecialty of health informatics.

According to Graves and Corcoran (1989), nursing informatics is a model of the combination of computer science, information science, and nursing science in the healthcare system. It designs to assist in the management and processing of nursing data, information, and knowledge to support nursing practice, education, research, and administration **(Fig. 59.2)**.

Chapter 59: Nursing Informatics, Information Technology, Use of Computers and Telecommunications

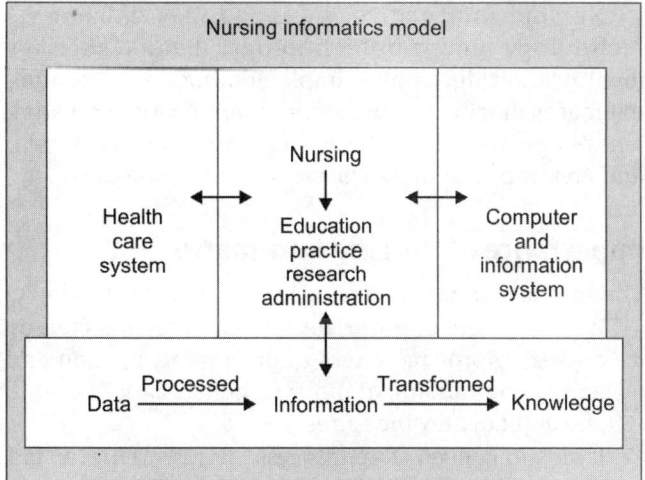

Fig. 59.2: Nursing informatics model.

Health care and nursing information science is the study of acquiring, communicating, storing, and managing healthcare data, and also the method of processing into information and knowledge. Using computer systems, networks, modems, and telecommunications, one can control and describe healthcare data.

Goal and Purposes of Nursing Informatics

The primary goal of nursing informatics is to improve the health of communities, families, and individuals by optimizing information management and communication. It includes the use of technology in direct provision of care, establishing an effective administrative system, managing and delivering education experiences, supporting lifelong learning, and nursing research. The purposes of nursing informatics are as follows:

1. To enhance all aspects of patient care and health management.
2. To study the process and structure of nursing information to support clinical decision-making and the delivery of nursing care at the micro level.
3. To help in retrieving evidence-based standards of practice, legislation acts, statistical analysis of the profession of nursing and practitioners of nursing at any given time or interval of time at the macro level.
4. To streamline data handling. The traditional method of documentation of a nurse's daily work routine consigned to paper, and it was difficult to file the massive number of documents. Computerization can make it possible to store information electronically.
5. Efficient information management to access relevant information.
6. To have easy access to sharing vital data within coworkers.
7. To safeguard personal records of patients, while at the same time allowing the most comfortable possible access to information for those who need it.
8. To develop an information-sharing network and data handling standards to work nationally and worldwide.

Bases of Nursing Informatics

Figure 59.3 depicts the bases of informatics:
- Data (objective information): Data are discrete observations not interpreted, organized, or structured
- Information (data + interpretation + organization + structure): Information is data that can be interpreted, organized, or structured to give meaning to data. Information is essential to study an information-based discipline such as nursing
- Knowledge (information + synthesis) and relationships identified: The information knowledge is the synthesis of data to identify links that provide further insight into the subject area.

All these concepts can be stored within a computer system to automate the processing of nursing data into information and the transformation of nursing information to nursing knowledge. Hence, the change of data to knowledge is the critical concept of nursing informatics' role and has a potential impact on nursing practice. As data transform into information and information into knowledge, each level increases in complexity and requires the more significant application of human intellect **(Fig. 59.4)**.

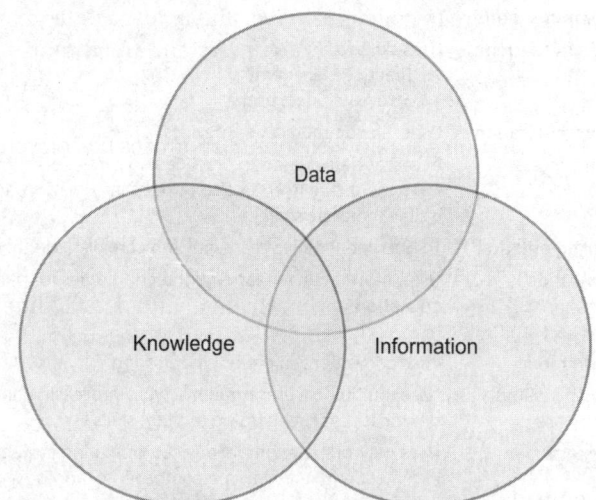

Fig. 59.3: Basic concepts of nursing informatics.

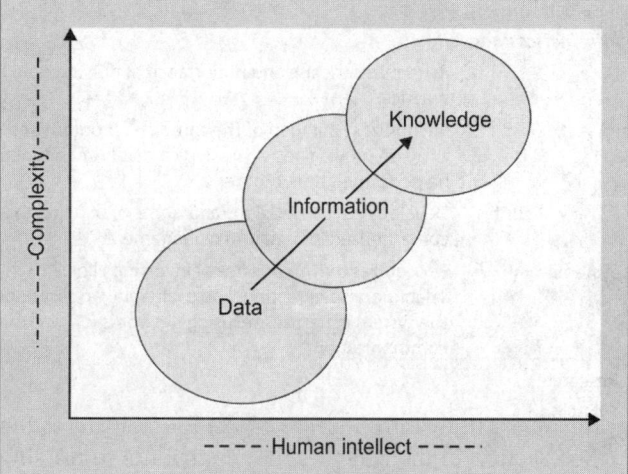

Fig. 59.4: Transformation of data into knowledge.

Computer Skills and Informatics Knowledge

According to Nancy Staggers, Carole A Gassert, and Christine Curran (2002), beginners, experienced, informatics specialists, and informatics innovator nurses require competencies (knowledge and skill) listed in **Table 59.1**.

Component Standards of Nursing Informatics

Nursing informatics' standards of practice organize around a general problem-solving framework that closely resembles the nursing process of assessment, diagnosis, and identification of outcomes, planning, implementation, and evaluation. The five major component standards of nursing informatics are as follows:
1. Problem identification
2. Alternative (or solution) identification
3. Alternative (or solution) development
4. Solution implementation
5. Solution evaluation

Nursing informatics' solutions may encompass technology and nontechnology means such as identification, developing, implementing, and evaluating databases; having a new computer application; creating a nursing vocabulary; designing informatics curricula; and creating structure, process, and outcome of IT.

Importance of Nursing Informatics

The six major values of nursing informatics are as follows:
1. It enables the appropriate flow of data collected by nurses, improving access to patient information and enhancing nursing abilities to benchmark, monitor, and audit quality measures.
2. It aids to collect, store, process, display, retrieve, and communicate timely data.
3. It facilitates to integrate data, information, and knowledge to support clients, nurses, and other providers in their decision-making in all roles and settings.

TABLE 59.1: Computer skills and informatics competencies for nursing practice.

Skills	Beginning nurse	Qualified nurse
Computer skills		
Administration	Uses skills for ➤ Practice management ➤ Structured data entry	Uses administrative application for forecasting, budgeting, managing aggregated data, staff scheduling, maintaining employee records
Communication	Uses telecommunication devices	Already acquired
Data access	Accesses data related to practice and care For patient care to enter and retrieve information, and to do online literature searches	Accesses shared data sets, extracts data and selected literature resources; integrates them to a personally usable file
Documentation	To document patient care, nursing care plan, discharge plan, etc.	–
Education	Uses information management technologies for patient education	Uses information management technologies to develop testing materials, for curriculum planning and evaluates computer-assisted instruction (CAI) as a teaching tool
Monitoring	Uses computerized patient monitoring systems	Uses monitoring system
Basic desktop software	Uses multimedia presentations, word processing and demonstrates keyboarding (typing) skills	Already acquired
Systems	Uses networks, peripheral devices, operating systems, existing external peripheral devices, computer technology safely, Demonstrates basic technology skills	Already acquired
Quality improvement	–	Uses data for statistical analysis
Research	–	Uses applications for statistical analysis and nursing research
Informatics knowledge		
Data	Recognizes the use and importance of nursing data for improving practice	Develops and use nursing data of a unified nursing language Provides for efficient data collection
Impact	Recognizes limitation of the computer program and computer as a tool to provide better nursing care as human functions cannot be performed by computer	Evaluates the effect of computerized information management on the role of the nurse
Privacy/security	Develops ethical decisions and rights of patients to access to computerized information management	Involves data integrity, professional ethics, and legal requirements and ways to protect data
Systems	Recognizes the importance of involving clinicians in designing, selecting, implementing, and evaluating applications of the system in healthcare, using networks for electronic communication	Describes general applications to support administration, clinical care, and nursing education
Research	–	Describes general applications available for research
Evaluation	–	Assesses the accuracy of health information
Role	–	Influences the attitudes of other nurses toward computer use and acts as an advocate for system users

4. It promotes to generate, manage, and process relevant data for information and to develop knowledge to improve practice and deliver better healthcare.
5. It enables nurses to make decisions at planning levels of healthcare.
6. It allows nurses to evaluate nursing practices, nursing education, and research.

Benefits of Nursing Informatics

The following are the various benefits involved in nursing informatics:

1. **In general**
   - It increases the overall efficiency and effectiveness of collection, storage, presentation, and distribution of data.
   - It aids in analyzing the massive data in a short time for decision-making and monitoring.
   - It will allow nurses to have easy access to multi-information. It will enable nurses to access health information to develop, implement, and evaluate methods of patient care or treatment.
   - It allows nurses to devote more time for clinical activities.
   - It will easily enable nurses to get logical views of services provided by the services rendered for patients.
   - It provides updated information about the accounting and finances of the organization
   - It helps in strategic and resource planning.
   - It assists in the preparation of operational documents such as treatment books, stock books, etc.
   - It will assist nurses to review all information related to a particular patient, which can lead to a more efficient communication and care.
2. **Related to the use of electronic medical record:** The nursing informatics improves access to the nursing record of nurses, leading to less time in documentation. Hence, they get more time for patient care. It facilitates data collection and improves communication. It provides them to create permanent clinical records.
3. **Use of decision support software:** The informatics offers historical and current data reports for effective data management. It provides alert to any discrepancies in inpatient medications. It provides extensive financial information and treatment-related information.
4. **Access to electronic patient records:** Point-of-care computers placed on the nursing units offer nurses and other healthcare providers error-free orders, capture of drug and food allergies, documentation of medications, nursing care measures electronically, and paperless diagnostic results from X-ray and laboratory departments and physical and respiratory therapy departments.
5. **Use the World Wide Web:** Nurses get information about current research and get experiences of publications in healthcare and nursing by using the World Wide Web.
6. **Information to consumers:** It becomes easy to inform about wellness and quality of life. They may educate them regarding the various aspects of healthcare.

Applications of Nursing Informatics

Nursing informatics is used in all areas of nursing practice: clinical practice, administration, education, and research (**Fig. 59.5**).

1. **Nursing clinical practice**
   - Computer-generated client nursing care data
   - Use of electronic medical record (EMR) and computer-based patient records
   - Automatic billing for supplies and procedures with nursing documentation
   - Client assessment and care by physiologic display parameters, storing and retrieving standardized care, monitoring client progress from plans, clinically monitoring clients, and through sophisticated diagnostic testing
   - Computer-based technologies that support clinical decision-making
   - Create an integrated computerized clinical information system
   - Integrating standardized nursing languages into clinical information systems.
2. **Nursing administration**
   - Electronic human resources database
   - Manages buildings and nonnursing services
   - Uses to facilitate billing and budget processes and cost analysis
   - Uses in preparing automated staff scheduling
   - Uses of e-mail for improving communication
   - Aids in quality assurance and conducting the nursing audit
   - Prepares leaders in the specialty.
3. **Nursing education**
   - It facilitates computerized record-keeping, computer-assisted instruction (CAI) as a teaching

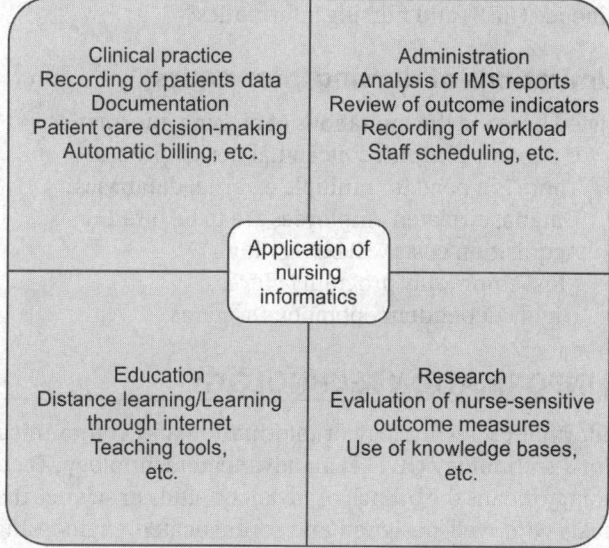

Fig. 59.5: Application of nursing informatics.

tool, interactive video technology, and distance learning.
- It aids nurses in using internet resources, PowerPoint, and MS Word for preparing slides, etc. They can access and retrieve literature.
- The nurses can utilize it as classroom technologies and strategies for distance learning.
- They can use it for examination and evaluation purpose.

4. **Nursing research:** The nurses can use informatics in computerized literature searching, such as in CINHAL, Medline, and also use statistical software such as SPSS. The informatics can of great use in disseminating the study findings. The results can be a knowledge base for nurses. It can evaluate nurse-sensitive outcome measures.

Implications of Informatics

Informatics has the following implications:
1. Nurses can work as leaders in the effective design and use of Electronic Health Records (EHRs) systems. They can integrate patients' information and make decisions. They can be care coordinators across the discipline and advocate for engaging patients and their families.
2. Nurses can create a pleasant work environment to improve quality care and coordinate and provide care through alarm/messaging, biomedical device integration, and medication administration. It gives greater nurse satisfaction, leading to higher patient satisfaction.
3. Enables nurses to incorporate data into health information, coordinate care across settings, and bring evidence for decisions to the point of care.
4. Empowers patients to be involved in the care.

Difference Between Nursing Informatics and Evidence-based Practice

Table 59.2 shows the difference between evidence-based practice (EBP) and nursing informatics:

Limitations of Nursing Informatics

Listed here are the limitations of nursing informatics:
- It needs a complex conceptual design process
- There is a need for multiple external databases
- Database-related employees are to be hired
- Acquisition costs will be very high
- Most commonly program failures
- Highly dependent operations systems.

INFORMATION TECHNOLOGY

Information technology or information and communications technology (ICT) is an advanced technology. Technology means the branch of advanced study or science that deals with well-designed and sophisticated engineering, i.e. hardware and software. The hardware includes computers, personal digital assistants, palm pilots, mobile phones, and other devices. Software is the information system that can manipulate and transmit information from one place to another. Information technology comprises computers and telecommunications networks such as e-mail, voice mail, internet, telephone, etc. The core of IT is the microprocessor, data storage devices, and data transmission elements.

TABLE 59.2: Difference between evidence-based practice (EBP) and nursing informatics.

EBP	Nursing informatics
EBP is the act of performing nursing duties based on the most recent and most accurate research/evidence available at that time	Nursing informatics uses information technologies about functions, within the scope of nursing practice carried out by nurses when performing their duties
The decision-making process in clinical nursing influenced by evidence, values, client preference, professional judgment, ethics, law, and workplace policy	It includes electronic monitors, computer charting, and web-based research
Systematic reviews, research studies, abstraction journals, and other scholarly sources are being used by nurses to facilitate their use of evidence	Technology is often used to promote a process or increase efficiency in the documentation and seeking information
EBP is the incorporation of evidence from research, expertise, and other available resources to prioritize patient care	Nursing informatics is the link between the literature and the nurse, providing access to research that is applicable to the current practice

Purposes of Information Technology

The various purposes of IT are listed below:
- To improve quality and patient safety and reduce the number of adverse events that result in death and disability.
- To reduce errors including the reduction in medication errors.
- To increase efficiency.
- To decrease time-consuming and redundant paperwork.
- To enhance communication.
- They can be used merely as a passive tool to store patient information.
- Can be used for multiple decision support functions, such as individualized patient reminders and prescribing alerts.

Information Systems in the Clinical Setting

The information systems in the clinical settings are as follows:
1. EMRs
2. Point-of-care systems
3. Decision support systems

4. Image management/communications technologies
5. Telemedicine.

Types of Information Technology

In general, various IT applications fall under main three categories:
1. **Administrative and financial systems:** These facilitate billing, accounting, and other administrative tasks.
2. **Clinical systems:** These systems facilitate or provide input into the care process. The following are the selected clinical-related IT type:
   a. *Computerized provider order entry (CPOE):* It is a system of ordering medication and a fulfillment system. More advanced CPOE includes lab orders, radiology studies, procedures, discharges, transfers, and referrals. This system reduces the errors caused due to handwriting or other communication work instructed by physicians, senior nurses, and other professionals. Under this system, they directly enter orders into a computer system.
   b. *Electronic health record (EHR):* They are the patient-centered real-time charts. It contains the patient's health history, diagnosis, treatment, medications, follow-up, and all clinical data. The healthcare providers can use evidence-based tools to make decisions about the care of the patients. It aids in automatically maintaining the workflow of the healthcare providers, and they can instantly access patient's health information. Only the authorized healthcare providers can create, manage, and share the patient's information within and with other healthcare organizations. It is beneficial to improve patient care by improving coordination among the healthcare team. It increases the patient's participation and improvement in patient's diagnosis and treatment modalities. These types of records are cost-effective and enhance efficiency in practices.
   c. *Clinical decision support system (CDSS):* It provides physicians and nurses with real-time diagnostic and treatment recommendations. The term covers a variety of technologies ranging from simple alerts and prescription drug interaction warnings to full clinical pathways and protocols. CDSS can be used as part of CPOE and EHR. It can also be used to support clinical decision-making by interfacing evidence-based clinical knowledge at the point of care with real-time clinical data at significant clinical decision points.
   The uses of CDSS in clinical decision-making are to generate alerts in response to clinical data, critique care decisions, recommend interventions at the request of a care provider, and conduct retrospective quality assurance reviews.
   d. *Infrastructure system:* This system supports both the administrative and the clinical applications. Bar coding in a healthcare environment is similar to bar code scanning in other situations: An optical scanner electronically captures information encoded on a product. Initially, it was used for the medication (e.g. matching drugs to patients by using bar codes on both the drugs and patients' arm bracelets) but may be pursued for other applications, such as medical devices, lab and radiology.

Applications of ICT in Nursing

Several areas in development demonstrate the use of ICT in nursing.
1. **Advances in education and collaborative learning:** ICT has influenced traditional and nontraditional approaches to education. Distance education programs in nursing enable outreach to geographically distributed individuals to elevate the education level of nurses for expansion, investigation, and application when there is an increased crisis for nursing workforce. Collaborative learning opportunities can be achieved via ICT, where geography becomes irrelevant. It affords exposure to the students and faculty around the world. The use of distributed e-learning and International Virtual Nursing School (IVINURS) digital repository is the example of collaborative learning using ICT for global sharing of knowledge and professional expertise. It also demonstrates the reach of IT-enabled methods in rapidly digitizing developing nations.
2. **Telenursing/telehealth:** Telenursing is the strategy of using technology to deliver nursing care and conduct nursing practice. Nurses provide telenursing, but telemedicine may be more appropriate, as the success of this modality requires multiple partners.
   Telehealth is the delivery of health services over a distance using telecommunications. Applications for telenursing include home monitoring of physiologic parameters, video consultation, and enabling self-management of chronic illness. Clinical information can be shared with other professional colleagues, including national and international experts. In developed countries, patients with chronic diseases can be cared for using telenursing services. Countries such as Canada and New Zealand, have well-developed telenursing programs.
3. **Wireless and handheld technologies:** Personal digital assistants (PDAs) are used for patient tracking, medical reference, and drug dosage in Australia. Different hardware were used to enable nurses to communicate with other nurses in the field via e-mail without having them come into the office and also provide field access to the nurses' intranet site and the Internet.
   In Africa and Asia, there is potential use of cellular telephones and PDAs for telehealth. Other methods include short message service (SMS) reminders in the treatment of tuberculosis, delivery of continuing

medical education via PDA, time-sensitive alerts to patients and healthcare workers, etc.

4. **Knowledge-based systems:** The internet offers a vast amount of information of variable quality and computer-based education for patients/clients and staff. These knowledge-based systems (KBSs) were developed to provide information to clinicians for clinical management, organizational management, research, professional development.
5. **Interoperable EHR system:** Interoperable EHR system (EHRS) is the focus for sharing data and information among various sources like a clinical information system, personal health records, public health surveillance systems, and knowledge repositories. Open medical record system (MRS) is an example of an EHRS to exchange data and to use the data in many different settings in different locales.
6. **Knowledge management and knowledge generation:** ICT has stimulated the growth of various approaches to knowledge generation and nursing research. For example, the International Council of Nursing has started an electronic International Nursing Partnership Database Project to document and share ongoing and new international partnerships as a tool to encourage similar initiatives and aid in planning new ventures. It provides the opportunity to facilitate participation and to establish collaboration using technology that connects those otherwise not connected.

Barriers to Using Information Technology

The six major categories of barriers to the adoption of IT are as follows:
1. Lack of management/stakeholder support
2. Cultural resistance toward the adoption of IT
3. Cost considerations
4. Staffing issues
5. Work practices
6. Capacity to manage change.

USE OF COMPUTERS

Computer

Computer is a device employed to compute or calculate. It is an electronic device that receives input, stores it, operates it according to a set of instructions, and gives the user the appropriate output. It is an electronic device that converts data into information. Computers can quickly and efficiently store, manipulate, and retrieve massive amounts of data. Information stored in the computers transmits links from one end to another end through telecommunication.

Computers are essential for more quantitative than qualitative data collection, storage, and retrieval. Its special features are speed, accuracy, and storage of large amounts of data. Computers can classify into large, small, and mini types based on their storage (memory) capacities and processing speeds.

Computer System

A computer system comprises hardware and software.
1. **Hardware:** The hardware device is a part of the computer that we can touch and see (e.g. keyboard, mouse, etc.). It is a group of physical equipment or devices forming the computer system. The common hardware is as follows:
   a. *Monitor* is the display screen similar to the television screen.
   b. *The keyboard* is similar to a typewriter consisting of keys on the board.
   c. *The mouse* is a small handheld device that attaches to the computer. It may have two or three buttons. The cursor (pointer) on the computer screen moves with the help of a mouse.
   d. *The computer, tower, or case:* It is the heart of the system. It is a box that contains all the parts to make the computer functional. It also has slots to put computer disks.
   e. *The printer* is a device that prints on to the paper what has been created.
   f. *The scanner* is a device that captures pictures, so that they can be seen and used on the computer, similar to a color photocopier.
2. **Software:** The software of an essential part of a computer system and cannot be touched. The software involves all the programming that makes the computer run, controlling all that the computer does. The two kinds of software are as follows:
   a. *Operating systems:* It is the base program on a computer. It reveals the functioning of the computer. The operating system allows loading other applications, e.g. Microsoft Windows, Apple's Mac OS.
   b. *Applications:* These are programs loaded in the computer to perform specific tasks, e.g. word and word perfect used to type letters and explorer and Netscape used to explore the Internet.

The computer system collects, stores, processes, retrieves, displays, and communicates timely information. It has memory and a set of states that define the relationship between a system's input and output. A computer has a simple input and output systems **(Fig. 59.6)**.

The input unit transfers the information from outside to the memory-storage unit. It performs calculations and logical operations in the arithmetic-logic unit (ALU). The output is stored in memory. The relevant information is transmitted to the output unit from memory **(Fig. 59.7)**.

The output unit transfers the data to outside documents like printed paper, terminal, etc. Each unit functions under the supervision of the control unit. The main component of

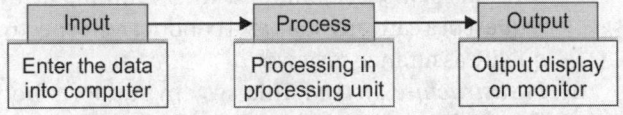

Fig. 59.6: Input/output systems of a computer.

Chapter 59: Nursing Informatics, Information Technology, Use of Computers and Telecommunications

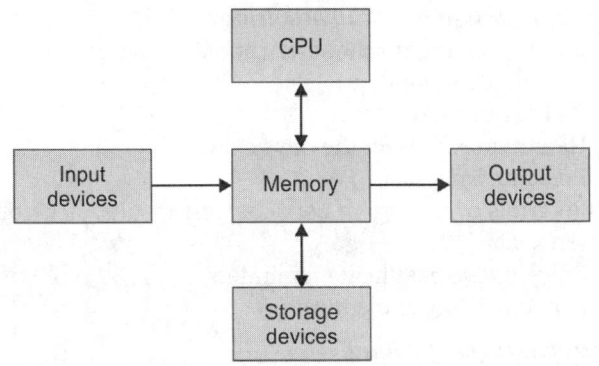

Fig. 59.7: Computer system.

a computer is the central processing unit (CPU). The CPU contains a control unit, memory unit, and an ALU.

Computer Network

A network is a link between two or more computer systems. Following are the different types of computer networks:
1. **Local-area networks (LANs):** As the name indicates, there is a link between two or more computer systems located close to each other or in the same building.
2. **Wide-area networks (WANs):** The computers are far away from each other and connected with radio waves or telephone lines.
3. **Campus-area networks (CANs):** The computers located within a limited geographic area are connected, e.g. within a campus.
4. **Metropolitan-area networks (MATs):** It is a data network designed for a town or city.
5. **Home-area networks (HANs):** It is a network contained within a user's home that connects a person's digital devices.

Computers in a network are nodes. The servers include computers and devices that allocate resources for a system.

Computer Applications

The two major areas where computers are used are listed below:
1. **Information application:** Television, virtual reality, and multimedia applications such as 3-D graphics, robotics.
2. **Telecommunication applications:** Videoconferencing, electronic fund transfers (EFTs), bulletin board system (BBS), facsimile transmission (FAX), medicine, publication, and accounting applications of telecommunication.

Uses of Computers

The various uses of computers are as follows:
1. Nurses can access important information about health or illness and treatment plans from the EHR.
2. Nurses can access information such as laboratory tests and X-ray results and health reports from other healthcare team members to give the best care possible.
3. Nurses can record health information, treatments, and progress for ready access and use by other health team members.
4. For administering the nursing services and sources in a healthcare facility.
5. To manage to standardize patient care information for the delivery of patient care.
6. To link the resource and educational application to nursing practices.
7. To assist in administering nursing services and sources.
8. To classify patient for nursing staffing.
9. To manage nursing personnel.
10. To administer quality assurance program.

Advantages of Computers in Nursing

The advantages of computers in nursing are as follows:
1. Improve and facilitate access to information
2. Reduce the redundancy of data entry
3. Decrease the time needed for nursing documentation
4. Increase the time of nursing care of patients
5. Facilitate data collection for research
6. Improve communication and reduce the risk of error
7. Work for decision-making.

Purposes of Using Computers

The computer acquires, organizes, manipulates, and presents information. The objectives of the use of computers are as follows:
1. **Administrative purposes**
   - To support management in their work by providing relevant information for their decision-making
   - To aid organizations in the processing of data into accurate, well-presented, up-to-date and cost-effective information
   - To develop strategic plans for the organization related to human resources, medical record management, facilitating management, budget and financing, quality assurance and utilization reviews, and accreditation.
2. **Clinical purposes:** Movements toward a record on the EHRs, health history, the treatments, and progress toward healthcare goals for monitoring and ready access by other team members.
   - Obtain information about past and ongoing treatments and medications and the results to ensure the best care.
   - Review data about current and past health situations and plan of care on the EHR to monitor the recovery process over time.
   - Access clinical knowledge to understand health situations and for the plan of care.
   - Helps in prescribing medication, medication cross-referencing, and the recording of patient health data.
   - Nurses can have information related to patients from other healthcare team members.

- Nurses can record patients' data, such as health history, treatments, and progress for ready access, and use by other healthcare team members.
- Nurses may use the computer to search drug databases, libraries, and best practice resources to obtain important information related to your diagnosis and care or find health education information.
- It aids in reducing nursing errors and the problems associated with such errors.

3. **In community and home health nursing practice**
   - Computer networks are used in innovative ways in home settings. A computer placed in high-risk client's homes allows them to access information on a variety of health topics.
   - They can record data about their health status and transmit to the healthcare providers at the central network computer.
   - Home alert system allows the patient to signal base station in an emergency.
   - Advances telenursing/telehealth.

4. **Computers in nursing research**
   - Computers can be used for problem identification, review literature, research design, and other steps of the research process.
   - To evaluate and determine the trends of health problems and needs for providers with specific skills.
   - Development of nursing knowledge management and knowledge generation.

5. **Computers in nursing education:** Computer-assisted and computer-based training is beneficial to teaching. Information and communications technology illustrates the growth in advanced nursing education.

TELECOMMUNICATIONS

Telecommunication is a means of one- or two-way communication to transmit messages. The examples of the combination of IT are the telephone, computer, processor, printer, etc. It saves time and money and secures data and messages.

Telecommunication Applications

E-mail Communication

E-mail communication is acknowledged as a resource to improve access, efficiency, responsiveness, patient, and the quality of healthcare. E-mail communication not only occurs between healthcare workers, but it also occurs between patients and providers.

An e-mail is a system for sending and receiving a digital message over a computer network or through a telecommunication channel or between two personal computers. An e-mail message contains two sections, the header and the body of the email. The header includes the sender's address, the receiver's address, the subject heading, and attachments if any. The body of the e-mail contains the main message and the signature block.

Uses of e-mail in the clinical setting
- For appointment schedules (booking, canceling, and automated reminders)
- Billing questions
- Health questions for the physician
- Prescription refills
- Referrals or no-urgent consults, test results, sick note renewals
- Preventative healthcare reminders
- For counseling and education.

Disadvantages of e-mail
- Increased workload
- The extra cost associated with technology
- Missing visual, auditory, and physical cues
- Not appropriate for complex issues
- The risk of inappropriate use by patients
- Privacy, security, and confidentiality issues

Advantages of e-mail
- Increased choice in the type of communication
- Increased access to remote patients and those with disabilities
- Decrease nonurgent calls
- An efficient method to disseminate and share information among professionals.
- Provides patients with written instructions
- Provides the patient and provider with time to review instructions at their own pace
- A permanent written record of communication.

Wireless Nurse Communication

In hospitals, telephones are the most commonly used communication technology. Newer technology is based on wireless solutions, i.e. Dalcon Alerts with wireless phones help nurses to easily communicate with patients, doctors, and staff. The caregiver can get various alerts, e.g. fall alerts, intravenous pump alerts, monitors, ventilators, practically anything else, and remote alert monitor at a single patient bed.

The Voice Communication System

The voice communication has two components the server software and the badge. It is a small and lightweight device that permits one-button voice access to other users on the system. It can also connect to outside telephones through private branch eXchange (PBX) integration. It is a telephone exchange, and a telephone company operates for companies or the public. The badge has voice controls and provides a hands-free ability to answer incoming calls. It can designate the individual by name, title, function, or group without knowing telephone numbers or who is on duty. It can do conference calls, broadcast messages, and voice mail messages. The benefits of voice communication are the following:
- It improves the quality and effectiveness of interactions among staff.
- It is more than five times faster than other communication methods.

- It minimizes the use of overhead paging.
- It enhances workflow and their ability to deliver quality patient care.
- It can economize time and effort and reduces the overall time.

Cellular Telephony

The use of SMS—otherwise known as text messaging—has grown in popularity as a form of communication. An SMS-based health information service offered by the San Francisco Department of Public Health is being used to educate and assist teens who have questions about sexual health. South Africa is using SMS features in cellular telephony to issue reminders to patients and caregivers in hopes of increasing adherence to antiviral therapies. Even the mobile phone is used to combat HIV/AIDs.

Videoconferencing and Teleconferencing

It is the latest buzzword in IT. It is a method of data communication, which allows people at various locations to communicate with people at different locations. A person is directly interacting with other persons, exchanging views on the screen. Thus, it is a technology that allows a person at various locations to converse, transfer data, and see each other using the standard telephone lines.

Teleconferencing is a one-way video and two-way audio conferencing system using communication satellites of the INSAT series. The communication satellite receives video signals from the sender's end using uplink earth station and transmits these signals to the receiving end through the receiver.

Facsimile Transmission

It refers to the scanning of the document and converting the shading into signals that can transmit with the help of radio waves. With the help of these signals, one can create a copy of the document.

Internet

The introduction of the internet, especially easy-to-use web, democratizes access to knowledge and provides opportunities for various organizations. The use of simulation as a learning teaching in nursing curricula has increased dramatically. The e-learning and other interactive technologies have provided excellent opportunities to expand their knowledge. The clinical information system can integrate into the simulation labs and can incorporate into nursing curricula.

CHAPTER HIGHLIGHTS

- Nursing informatics is the application of computer science and information science to nursing. Data, information, and knowledge are the bases of nursing informatics.
- Nurses require basic and advance computer skills and knowledge of informatics.
- Nursing informatics applies to all areas of nursing practice, clinical practice, administration, education, and research.
- Information technology (IT) comprises computers and telecommunications networks such as e-mail, voice mail, internet, telephone, etc.
- The different types of IT systems are administrative, clinical and infrastructure related. Several areas in development demonstrate the use of ICT in nursing.
- A computer is an electronic device that converts data into information. Computers can store, manipulate, and retrieve massive amounts of data quickly and efficiently. The hardware device is part of the computer that we can touch and see. The software is all the programming that makes the computer run and control what a computer does.
- A computer network is a link between two or more two computer systems. The different types of computer networks are LAN, WAN, MAT, CAN, and HAN.
- Telecommunication is a means of one- or two-way communication to transmit messages. A variety of uses of telecommunication in nursing is through e-mail, teleconferencing, videoconferencing, cellular telephony, FAX, internet, etc.

REVIEW QUESTIONS

I. Essay Type Questions
1. Define the term "nursing informatics." Discuss historical background of nursing informatics.
2. Differentiate between nursing informatics and evidence-based nursing practice.
3. What do you mean by information technology? Discuss the different types of information technologies.
4. Describe the purposes and advantages of the use of computers in nursing.
5. Define telecommunication. Explain telecommunication applications in nursing.

II. Short Notes
1. Bases of nursing informatics
2. Application of nursing informatics
3. Computer system
4. Uses of information technology

III. Multiple Choice Questions
1. What is the term reflecting a combination of nursing science, computer, and information science?
    a. Nursing informatics
    b. Nursing information technology
    c. Nursing communication and information technology
    d. Telecommunication
2. Who coined the term "informatik" in 1957?
    a. Philippe Dreyfus

b. Karl Steinbuch
c. Walter F Bauer
d. Francois Gramy

3. Which statement is *NOT* applicable to nursing informatics?
   a. It includes electronic monitors, computer charting, and web-based research
   b. It often uses technology to promote a process
   c. It is a link between the literature and nurse, providing access to research application to current practices
   d. It is an act of performing nursing duties on the most recent and most accurate research

4. Information technology comprises one of the following:
   a. Data, information, and knowledge
   b. Hardware and software
   c. Computers and telecommunication technology
   d. Operating systems and applications

5. A type of computer network, where the users are using computers, are far away from each other and connected with radio waves or telephone lines is:
   a. Local area network
   b. Wide area network
   c. Campus area network
   d. Home area network

Answer Keys

1. a   2. b   3. d   4. c   5. b

SUGGESTED READING

1. Available from http://www.nursing.umaryland.edu/~snewbold/skngroup.htm.
2. Available from https://nursing-informatics.com/kwantlen/National_NI_Project_Discussion_paperDRAFT.pdf. [Accessed Jan 2020].
3. Burke L, Weill B. Information Technology for Health Professions. Upper Saddle River, NJ: Prentice-Hall; 2004.
4. Carty B, Rosenfeld P. From computer information technology: Findings from a national study of nursing education. Comput Nurs. 1998;16(5):259-65.
5. Connors HR, Weaver C, Warren J, Miller KL. An academic–business partnership for advancing clinical informatics. Nurs Educ Perspect. 2002;23:228-33.
6. Goossen WTF. Nursing information management and processing: a framework and definition for systems analysis, design, and evaluation. International Journal of Biomedical Computing. 1996;40(3):187-95
7. Graves JR, Corcoran S. The study of nursing informatics. Image J Nurs Sch. 1989;21(4):227-31.
8. Graves JR and Corcoran S. The study of nursing informatics. Image J Nurs Sch. 1989;21(4):227-31.
9. Hannah KJ, Ball MJ, Edwards KJ. Introduction to Nursing Informatics, 2nd edition. New York: Springer-Verlag; 1999.
10. https://www.researchgate.net/publication/328387211_Nursing_Informatics_A_Personal_Review_of_the_Past_the_Present_and_the_Future. [Accessed Jan 2020].
11. International Council of Nurses (ICN). The ICN code of ethics for nurses, 2006. Available from: http://www.icn.ch/icncode.pdf. [Accessed Jan 2020].
12. Johntgen M, Parrinello K. Microcomputers: Turning the database into unit management information. Nurs Manag. 1987;18(2):30-8.
13. King L. Distance education: The solution for nursing and midwifery in Africa? Int Nurs Rev. 2000;47:63.
14. McGonigle E, Eggers R. Establishing a nursing informatics program. Comput Nurs. 1991;9(5):174-9.
15. Saba VK, McCornick KA. Essentials of Computers for Nursing: Informatics for the New Millennium, 3rd edition. New York: Mcgraw-Hill; 2001.
16. Sackett KM, Erdley WS. The history of health care informatics. In: Englebardt S, Nelson R (Eds). Health Care Informatics: An Interdisciplinary Approach. St Louis: Mosby; 2002.
17. Schlachta L, Sparks S. Definitions of Telenursing, Telepresence. In: Fitzpatrick J (Ed). Encyclopedia of Nursing Research. New York, NY: Springer Publishing, Inc; 1999.
18. Scholes M, Barber B. Towards nursing informatics, 1980. In: Lindberg D, Kaihara S (Eds.) MEDINFO 80. Proceedings of the 3rd World Congress on Medical Informatics. Amsterdam: North-Holland, 70-73. (Cross ref).
19. Staggers N, Gassert CA, Curran C. A Delphi study to determine informatics competencies for nurses at four levels of practice. Nurs Res 2002; 51(6): 383-90.
20. Staggers N, Gassert CA, Curran C. Informatics competencies for nurses at four levels of practice. J Nurs Educ. 2001;40(7):303-16.
21. Staggers N, Thompson CB. The Evolution of definitions for nursing informatics: a critical analysis and revised definition. J Am Med Inform Assoc. 2002;9(3): 255-61.
22. Thede LQ, Sewell J. Informatics and nursing: Competencies and applications. [online] Available from http://dlthede.net/Informatics/Informatics.html. [Accessed Sep 2019].
23. Turley JP. Toward a model for nursing informatics. Image J Nurs Sch. 1996;28:309-13.
24. William TF Goossen. Nursing information management and processing: A framework and definition for systems analysis, design, and evaluation. Int J Bio-Med Comput. 1996;40(3):186-95.
25. World Health Organization. Towards a safer future. The World Health Report 2007: Geneva. [Online] Available from http://www.who.int/whr/2007/en/. [Accessed May 2008].
26. World Health Organization. Working together for health. The World Health Report 2006: Geneva. [Online] Available from http://www.who.int/whr/2006/en/. [Accessed May 2008].
27. Young KM. Informatics for Health Professionals. Philadelphia: FA Davis; 2000.

60 CHAPTER

Documentation System: Nursing Records and Recording, Reports and Reporting, and Correspondence

CHAPTER OUTLINE

- Documentation System
  - Definitions of Documentation
  - Purposes of Documentation
  - Types of Documentation System
  - Tools for Documentation
- Records and Recording
  - Definition
  - Objectives of Records
  - Purposes of Records
- Value of Nurses Clinical Records
- Functions of Records
- Principles of Good Record Keeping
- Characteristics of Good Recording
- General Guidelines for Recording
- Steps for Designing the Record
- Reports and Reporting
- Correspondence

LEARNING OUTCOMES

After completion of this chapter, the learner will be able to:
- Understand the concept of documentation system
- Describe the purposes of documentation
- Discuss the different types of documentation system
- Explain the multiple tools for documentation
- Enlist the general guidelines for recording
- Define records, reports, and correspondence
- Describe objectives, objects, and functions of records
- Discuss how the records are valuable for nurses
- Explain the principles of good record keeping
- Discuss the purpose and types of reporting
- Discuss the importance and features of correspondence
- Describe the format and parts of correspondence

KEY TERMS

Documentation, documentation system, records, reports, correspondence

INTRODUCTION

The patient record is the most central information and communication tool for healthcare professionals. It is essential to have a standard system of documentation and to report to enhance efficient and individualized client care. Increased potential for interdisciplinary access to information is expected to increase the quality and continuity of patient care and treatment. Hospitals are increasingly relying on computer technology to improve efficiency and accuracy in the documentation since information technology has gained a more significant and fundamental role in the management, distribution, and storage of information in health care.

Nursing documentation is an essential component of nursing practice and the interprofessional documentation that occurs within the client's health record. These are the integral parts of the hospital records, which then form the central focus of all clinical activities. Even Nightingale described the need for nurses to record "the proper use of fresh air, light, warmth, cleanliness, the proper selection, and administration of diet." In Nightingale's time, documentation was a way to communicate the implementation of doctors' orders and not a means to observe or assess the patient's status. The use of computer technology in nursing documentation has been reported since the 1960s.

Nursing records, such as medical records, is an account of the quality of care provided by the nurses, and its maintenance is the contribution to good individual patient care. The patient's healthcare record is a formal, legal document that details a client's care and progresses irrespective of its format. These are the indispensable aids for monitoring, controlling, and evaluating the services rendered by the hospital. These are the legal documents and also used for statistical and research purposes.

DOCUMENTATION SYSTEM

Definitions of Documentation

Webster's dictionary defines "documents" as something written, furnishing evidence or information and "documentation" as anything written or printed, which rely on as a record of proof for authorized persons.

Documentation is a system of recording either handwritten or electronically generated information regarding the care or service provided to a patient. Health records may be paper or electronic documents, such as electronic medical records (EMRs), faxes, e-mails, audio or videotapes, etc. It provides media to communicate with nurses about their clinical actions and about their clients. It gives an accurate account of what occurred and when it happened.

"Nursing documentation" is a process of making an entry of data on a record regarding patients' care and service provided to the client.

Purposes of Documentation

The purposes of documentation are as follows:

1. **To facilitate communication:** Through documentation, nurses can communicate with other nurses and professionals in the healthcare teams, their clients' health histories, diagnosis, planning, nursing interventions, and the outcome of the responses. Thorough and accurate documentation decreases the potential for negligence and nursing errors. It facilitates communicating with the family members, and the client and family may document care provided to disclose this information with members of the healthcare team.
2. **To facilitate coordination of care:** Nurses plan interventions, make a decision about ongoing interventions, evaluate patient's progress which is used by all team members.
3. **To promote continuity of care:** Nursing documentation is a valuable tool used not only to support effective communication between providers but also to provide baseline patient information and to help continuity of care within and across settings. Practical written communication skills are essential to precisely document each of the nursing activities.
4. **To promote quality nursing care:** Documentation encourages nurses to assess client progress and determine effective interventions and record any change required in the care plan, if needed. It is a valuable source of data to make decisions about resource management and facilitating nursing research. It is a source of improving quality care and also the nursing practice. Nurses can use this information to make the clinical decision for nursing diagnosis and planning care.
5. **To achieve professional and legal standards:** Documentation is a valuable method for demonstrating that nurses are performing according to professional standards. It provides a record of a client from admission to discharge. These act as evidence in legal proceedings such as lawsuits and disciplinary hearings. The health records of patients serve as the legal record of the care or service provided.
6. **Accountability:** Nurses have the responsibility to apply nursing knowledge and skill in providing safe, competent, ethical care to the clients per the code of ethics. Nurse's professional practice concerning documentation should reflect such safe, skilled nursing care. The client record indicates the care provided to the patients and makes nurses accountable.
7. **Security:** Nurses ensure that relevant client care information is captured in the permanent record and safeguards client information by maintaining confidentiality and enacting by information retention and destruction policies and procedures that are consistent with the standard(s) and legislation.
8. **Providing quality improvement:** A healthcare record is often a tool used within quality improvement processes to evaluate services provided and outcomes achieved. Comprehensive, accurate documentation offers a sound basis to measure the quality of care and facilitates the evaluation of the patient's progress.
9. **Facilitating evidence-based practice:** The health-care record can be an essential source of data for nursing and health research and provides evidence. Hence, it is necessary to maintain accurate and thorough documentation.

Documentation Systems

Today one of the most challenging issues in nursing practice is efficient documentation system and quality documentation within the constraints imposed by regulation, resources, and finances. The ideal documentation system includes comprehensive information, address client outcomes and standards facilitate reimbursement from government and insurance company payers, serve as a legal document. Many documentation systems are available in response to changes in health-care delivery and advanced technology. Usually, there are two types of documentation systems, namely, paper-based or traditional and electronic documentation systems.

Paper-based Documentation System

The five major paper-based documentation systems are as follows:

Source–Oriented Record

It is a traditional client record where each person or department makes notations in a separate section or sections of the client's chart, for example, the admission department has an admission sheet, the physician has order sheet, a physician history sheet, progress notes, and nurse notes. All records are in narrative style.

Narrative
Narrative documentation is the traditional part of the source-oriented record for recording nursing care provided. It consists of written notes that include routine care, normal findings, and client problems. It contains patients' health, diagnosis, treatment information. There is no specific format and organization of these types of records.

Advantages: Source-oriented records are convenient because care providers from each discipline can quickly record data and trace the information specific to one's subject.

Disadvantages: Information about a particular client problem are scattered throughout the chart, so it is challenging to find chronological information on a client's issues and progress. It can lead to decreased communication among the health team, an incomplete picture of the client's care, and a lack of coordination of care.

Problem–Oriented Medical Record
The problem-oriented medical records (POMRs) focus on the specific problem of the patient. These records contain a single list of client problems generated by the healthcare team members. The nursing process forms the basis for the POMR method of documenting client problems. The data are arranged according to the problem of the patient, rather than the source of information. The healthcare team members contribute to the problem list, plan of care, and progress notes.

Advantages
- It emphasizes the client's perceptions of their problems.
- It encourages collaboration.
- It needs continuous evaluation and revision of the nursing care plan.
- It provides more excellent continuity of care among healthcare team members.
- It enhances effective communication among health-care team members.
- It increases efficiency in gathering data.
- It provides easy-to-read information in chronological order.
- It makes it easier to track the status of each problem of the patient.
- It reinforces the use of the nursing process.

Disadvantages
- It takes constant vigilance to maintain an up-to-date problem list.
- Different healthcare providers may vary in their ability to document.

Components of POMR: The POMR has four essential elements: database, problem list, plan of care, and progress notes.

a. **Database:** Consists of all information known about the client when the client first enters the healthcare agency. It includes nursing assessment, the physician's history, social and family data, and baseline diagnostic tests.
b. **Problem list:** It is a list to enter the identified problems in the order and needs to be updated continuously.
c. **Plan of care:** POMR has a provision of care plans. It generates care plans. The two types of the plan of care are medical and nursing care plans. Physicians write medical care plans, and nurses write nursing care plans.
d. **Progress notes:** These are the records of the patients, depicting progress in the health status of patients.

Formats of POMR:
a. **SOAP/IER:** SOAP format is in use frequently. It is a standard method of documentation. Using SOAP, SOAPIE, or SOAPIER format, a structured narrative progress notes are written by all health-care team members. The acronym SOAPIE provides an ideal form for a narrative patient record. SOAPIE, a systematic approach, details a goal-oriented nursing care plan in a note. The nursing process begins with an assessment that is as follows:

S refers to subjective data. It consists of information obtained from the patient and describes the patient's perceptions and experience of the problem.
O refers to objective data. It consists of information that is measured or observed by use of the senses (e.g., lab test, X-ray results).
A stands for assessment. It is the interpretation derived from the subjective and objective data. It must describe the patient's condition and level of progress in health status.
P is plan. It is the plan of care designed to resolve the stated problem.

The **SOAP** format is replaced by **SOAPIER**.
"**S**" refers to subjective data. "**O**" stands for objective data. "**A**" stands for assessment, and "**P**" for plan.
"**I**" refers to interventions, that is, specific interventions performed by the caregiver.
"**E**" stands for evaluation. It includes client responses to nursing interventions and medical treatments. It indicates the actual patient outcome or response.
"**R**" stands for revision. It reflects the care plan modifications suggested by the review.

b. **Problem, intervention, and evaluation charting (PIE):** Each client problem is labeled and numbered for easy reference. Identify the problem to take action.
c. **Focus charting (sometimes referred to as DAR):** The focus charting system of documentation makes the client and client concerns and strengths the focus of care. The progress notes are organize into data (D), which reflects the assessment phase of the nursing process; action (A), which reflects planning and implementation and includes immediate and future nursing action; the response (R), which demonstrates the evaluation phase of the nursing process and describes the client's response to any nursing and medical care.

Charting by Exception

According to Coleman (1997), most methods of documentation fall into one of the two categories: documentation by inclusion and documentation by exception. Charting by exception (CBE) is a documentation system to record only abnormal or significant findings or limitations. This type of charting prevents nursing errors, reduces repetition of documentation, saves time, and provides immediate identification of substantial changes in a client's condition.

The requirement to use documentation by exception is a practice of setting documentation policies and protocols, assessment norms, standards of care; individualized care plans; single flow sheets; and bedside accessibility of documentation forms; otherwise, this type of documentation is not acceptable.

Graphic Sheets and Flow Sheets

Graphic and flow sheets are suitable methods of depicting the pertinent information about the patient. A flow sheet or visual sheet must reflect who performs the assessment or intervention. The check mark or symbol must convey the meaning. A nursing intervention listed on the flow sheet, if not applicable, is indicated by using "N/A." Make narrative nursing notes when needed (CNPS, 1992).

Variance Charting

The variance charting (VAR) involves documenting unexpected events, cause events, actions, discharge planning, and response.

Electronic Documentation

Technology is used to support client documentation in many ways. In this system, the principles underlying documentation, access, storage, retrieval, and transmittal of information remain the same as for paper-based systems. These new ways of recording, delivering, and receiving client information, however, pose significant challenges for nurses, particularly concerning confidentiality and security of client information. It needs standardization and legibility and requires policies and procedures to ensure privacy and security.

The Electronic Health Record

The electronic health record (EHR) is the patient-centered real-time, longitudinal electronic record of patient healthcare information. It contains the patient's health history, diagnosis, treatment, medications, follow-up, and all clinical data. The health-care providers can use evidence-based tools to make decisions about the care of the patients. It aids in automatically maintaining the workflow of the health-care providers, and they can access patient's health information instantly.

The EHR is a repository of patient data in digital form, stored and exchanged securely, and accessible by multiple authorized users. It contains retrospective, concurrent, and prospective information, and its primary purpose is to support continuing, efficient, and quality integrated health care.

Only the authorized healthcare providers can create, manage, and share the patient's information within and with other healthcare organizations. It is beneficial to improve patient care by improving coordination among the healthcare team. It increases patient's participation and improves patient's diagnosis and treatment modalities. These types of records are cost-effective and enhance efficiency in practices.

Classification of EHR
1. **Per the utility of electronic devices**
    a. *The automated medical record:* This is a paper-based record with some computer-generated documents.
    b. *The computerized medical record (CMR):* This type of electronic record makes the level 1 documents electronically available.
    c. *The EMR:* This type of record restructures and optimizes the documents of the previous levels, ensuring the interoperability of all documentation systems.
    d. *The electronic patient record (EPR):* This is a patient-centered record with information from multiple institutions.
    e. *The EHR:* In this type of record, general health-related information, in addition to the EPR, is not necessarily related to a disease.
2. **According to the International Organization for Standardization (ISO)**
    a. *Electronic medical record:* An EMR is a medical record in digital format. It facilitates access to nurses about patient's health information at any place. Electronic medical record is a longitudinal collection of electronic health information for and about persons, immediate electronic access to person- and population-level information by authorized users; provision of knowledge and decision-support systems that enhance the efficiency of patient care and efficient healthcare delivery.
    b. *Departmental EMR:* It contains information entered by a single hospital department, e.g. picture archiving and communication system (PACS), anesthesia records, intensive care records, ambulatory records, emergency department systems, pathology laboratory system, oncology records, cardiology records, operation theater records, gynecology records, internal medicine records, pharmacy systems, geriatric center records, diabetes clinic records, and radiology reporting system.
    c. *Interdepartmental EMR:* These records contain information from two or more hospital departments.
    d. *Hospital EMR:* It includes all or most of the patient's clinical data from a particular hospital.

e. *Interhospital EMR:* Contains patient's medical information from two or more hospitals.
3. **The computer-based patient record:** The computer-based patient record is a clinical information system to collect, store, manipulate, and make available clinical information relevant to the care of the patient. Its central focus is on clinical data.
   a. *Electronic patient record:* It contains all or most of the patient's clinical information from a particular hospital.
   b. *Computerized patient record:* This record contains all or most of the patient's clinical data from a specific hospital.
   c. *Electronic healthcare record:* It contains all patient health information.
   d. *Personal health record:* The patient records and controls these types of documents. These contain information at least partly entered by the patient.
   e. *Computerized medical record:* These types of documents are created by image scanning of a paper-based health record.
   f. *Digital medical record:* A web-based record maintained by a healthcare provider.
   g. *Clinical data repository:* An operational data store that holds and manages clinical data collected from health service providers.
   h. *Electronic client record:* Health-care professionals other than physicians, e.g. by physiotherapists or social workers, define its scope.
   i. *Virtual EHR:* No authoritative definition.
   j. *Population health record:* These records contain aggregated and usually deidentified data.

Structure of EHRs
The structure of EHRs is time oriented, problem oriented, or source oriented; but these days, EHRs combine all these elements.
1. **Time-oriented EHRs:** Data are presented in chronological order.
2. **Problem-oriented medical record:** In the POMR, each problem of the patient is noted in this type of record, and it has a description of each problem according to the personal information, objective information, assessments, and plan (SOAP).
3. **Source-oriented record:** In the source-oriented record, the content of the document is arranged according to the method of obtaining the information, e.g., note of visits, X-ray reports, and blood tests.

The American Nurses Association (ANA) has developed a framework for nursing documentation, which also corresponds with the SOAP structure for medical documentation. The nursing process had four stages: assessment, diagnosis, planned or delivered interventions, and outcomes.

Usability of EHRs
The EHRs have been used for in-home care, self-monitoring by the patients; at primary care level where the care is provided in the community by the staff as home health care, secondary care provided by a team of specialists for both indoor and outdoor patients, and at tertiary care settings, the care provided by team of specialists in major referred hospitals for both indoor and outdoor patients.

The evidence revealed that healthcare professionals and administrative staff use EHRs. Among the healthcare professionals who use different components of the EHR are physicians, nurses, radiologists, pharmacists, laboratory technicians, and radiographers. Patients or their parents are also using EHRs.

Components of EHRs
Figure 60.1 depicts the users and components of EHRs.
1. **Medical data components:** The identified medical data component of EHR consists of referral, present complaint, i.e. symptoms, past medical history, lifestyle, physical examination, diagnosis, tests, procedures, treatment, medication, and discharge.
2. **Nursing data component:** Nursing data component of EHR comprises nursing charting area and nursing care plan; medication administration, daily charting, physical assessment, and admission nursing notes.
   - Daily charting includes patients' daily functional activities such as vital signs, food, elimination, mobility, and patient teaching
   - Physical assessment comprises all kinds of status assessments (e.g., skin status or respiratory status)
   - Admission nursing note contains information on allergies, health behavior (e.g., physical activity or smoking or sleep patterns), physical assessment (e.g., temperature and neurological status), discharge planning, and initial care plan.
3. **Multiprofessional data component:** It includes the information of patients added by another professional, e.g. consultants, referrals, tests, medications, charting, etc.
4. **Secretarial data component:** It included the information entered by secretarial staff regarding findings, procedures, diagnosis, etc.

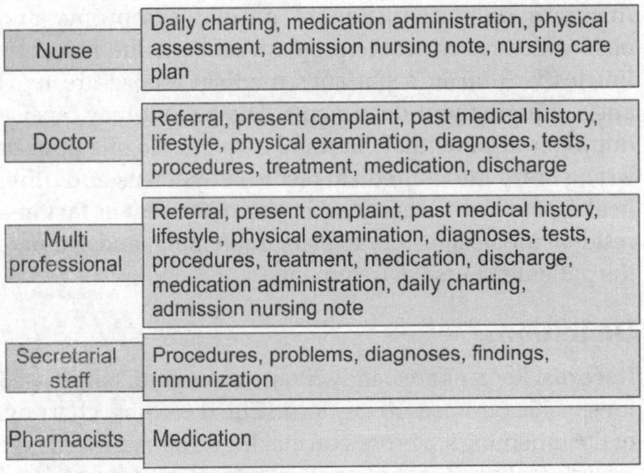

Nurse	Daily charting, medication administration, physical assessment, admission nursing note, nursing care plan
Doctor	Referral, present complaint, past medical history, lifestyle, physical examination, diagnoses, tests, procedures, treatment, medication, discharge
Multi professional	Referral, present complaint, past medical history, lifestyle, physical examination, diagnoses, tests, procedures, treatment, medication, discharge, medication administration, daily charting, admission nursing note
Secretarial staff	Procedures, problems, diagnoses, findings, immunization
Pharmacists	Medication

Fig. 60.1: Components and users of electronic health records (EHRs).

5. **Pharmacists' data component:** This component includes the data of pharmacists regarding medications, etc.

Other Electronic Record Devices

1. **Personal digital assistants (PDAs):** PDA is a handheld computer to manage patient care. This is useful to access a patient's laboratory reports and refer to the latest information on appropriate therapies, tests, and treatments. It is also used for billing and updating patient visits. It provides directions to the patient's homes.
2. **Computer-automated cancer detection:** Computer-automated cancer detection such as thin prep processor model 2000 or PAPNET are in use to identify abnormal cells from a series of digital images of the Papanicolaou test (abbreviated as Pap test, also known as Pap smear).
3. **Computerized theater management application:** This application automatically records patient information such as demographic and financial data, visit history with dates, procedures, performing and attending providers, care records with clinical highlights, and patient status. It contains operational data such as proposed, type, actual, severity, and risks, which are stored for reference in the event of future surgical procedures.

Tools for Documentation

- Initial nursing assessment
- Kardex and patient care summary
- Plan of nursing care
- Critical/collaborative pathways
- Progress notes
- Flow sheets
- Acuity charting forms
- Discharge/transfer summary
- Home healthcare documentation
- Long-term care documentation.

RECORDS AND RECORDING

Accurate documentation of patient symptoms and observations is critical to proper treatment and recovery. Entries written in a patient's medical record are legal and are permanent documents. The patient may receive improper or potentially harmful care in case of a poor or wrong entry into a medical record. Physicians and other health-care providers use what you document as fact in a resident medical history to plan, implement, and evaluate the patient's course of treatment.

Definitions

Records: Records are handwritten or computer based used for specific purposes in any form. The recording, charting, or documenting is a process of making an entry on a client's record. A clinical record or client record is a formal, legal document that provides evidence of a client's care.

1. **Hospital record:** Hospital record is the entry of events in a sequence form. It includes all activities related to the collection and utilization of clinical information. Every organization has its system of recording and maintaining hospital records.
2. **Medical record:** A medical record is a clinical and scientific record regarding patient care. It is an administrative and legal document. It provides detailed information about patient health history, diagnosis, treatment, and care written in a sequential manner.
   It is a document of facts that contains a statement by trained observers of conditions found, examinations and therapy application, and results and indicates whether the efforts of doctors, supplemented by the hospital and related facilities, are based on the reasonable expectations of the present-day scientific medicine.
4. **A nursing record:** A nursing record system is the record of nursing care planned and given to individual patients by nurses. It contains patient health history, nursing assessment, nursing diagnosis, nursing care plans, evaluation of care, and progress of patients. It reflects all the activities of the nurses regarding patient care.

Objectives of Records

1. To review patient care, make clinical decisions, and prepare treatment plans
2. To provide a legally acceptable record
3. To provide a source of information for health managers
4. It enables for hospital auditing
5. To carry out the things in the right possible manner.
6. It is useful for statistical, teaching, diagnostic, and legal purposes.

Purposes of Medical Records

The medical records are of value to patients, hospitals, caregivers, educators, and researchers.
1. **To patients**
   - To improve patient care
   - To serve to document the clinical history
   - To aid in avoiding omission or repetition
   - To assist in the continuity of care
   - To provide evidence in medicolegal cases
   - To supply the necessary information to institutes and employees.
2. **To health organization/hospital**
   - To record all activities of the healthcare providers
   - To furnish proof of kind and quality care
   - To protect hospital in legal staff
   - To evaluate the proficiency of staff
   - To help in future program planning.

Purposes of Records

1. **Communication:** The record serves as a means of communication with patients by all healthcare team members.

2. **Planning client care:** Patients records are useful in planning care and maintaining continuity of care.
3. **Auditing health organization:** The records are beneficial for auditing purposes. Auditing provides a review of client records for quality assurance purposes and helps in improving care.
4. **Statistical and research:** The information contained in a document can be a valuable source of data for research. The treatment plans for many clients with the same health problems can give information helpful in treating other clients.
5. **Education:** A clinical record provides a comprehensive view of the patients' diagnosis and treatment and is useful for educational and teaching purposes.
6. **Reimbursement:** The records can be used to obtain payment through Medicare.
7. **Lawful purposes:** The clinical record of a patient is a legal document. It provides proof as evidence in a court.
8. **Healthcare analysis and evaluation:** Patients records assist healthcare planners to identify agency needs.

Value of Nurses Clinical Records

- It provides baseline data for further plan of action and to evaluate the care given
- Nursing records, e.g. temperature chart, blood pressure record intake/output records, etc., are useful for diagnostic and treatment purposes
- These can be used to assess the workload of nurses and to evaluate the quality of care
- These records are beneficial for education, teaching, and research purposes.

Functions of Records

1. To help in improving the responsibility and accountability of healthcare providers
2. To depict decision-making related to patient care
3. To reflect the level of healthcare services and clinical judgments and decisions
4. To provide a source of patient care and communications
5. To make the continuity of care more accessible and provide evidence of services
6. To promote better discussion and coordination among team members
7. To aid in identifying risks, and early detection of complications
8. To facilitate audit, research, allocation of resources, and performance planning
9. To address complaints or legal processes.

Principles of Good Record Keeping

1. Handwriting should be legible
2. All recorded entries should be signed. Put the date and time on all documents
3. Records should be accurate and in such a way that the meaning is clear
4. Records should be readable
5. Records should be factual
6. Use professional judgment to record
7. Include only pertinent information
8. Do not alter or destroy any records without being authorized
9. Do not falsify records
10. Maintain confidentiality of the documents, follow rules governing confidentiality in respect of the supply, and use data for secondary purposes
11. Follow organizational policy and guidelines when using records for research purposes
12. Do not disclose the information and should not leave any documents, either on paper or on computer screens
13. Know how to use available information systems and tools
14. Ensure the proper use of the system, particularly about confidentiality
15. Assess the standard of record keeping and communications.

Characteristics of Good Recording

- The objectives of the records should be clear and should be able to recognize the pertinent factors like what to record, when to log, why record, how to file, who will record.
- The records should be specific and concise to the purpose. There should not be any duplicity.
- There should be enough space to record.
- The size of the record should be easily approachable, and it should be handy and such that it will be easy to record and to handle. The design should be such that it would be easy to complete and provide data that can be accessed easily.
- Record information immediately, the information should be accurate.
- The language used should be legible, simple, and understood by the team members.
- Be honest at the time of recording.
- Record specific information concisely.
- Depict important activities predominantly with some indication.
- Organize the records properly.
- Store the documents properly in a particular system. Identify each report by a number and avoid entering duplicate data.
- Follow specific instructions to complete the particular record.
- Centralize the responsibility for both control and design of the form.

General Guidelines for Recording

The documents or information are to be recorded by following the guidelines as listed below:

1. **Date and time:** Always enter the date and time of each recording. It is essential for the legal and safety of patients.

2. **Timing**: Follow the policy of organization for the frequency of documenting, and adjusting the spectrum as a client's condition indicates. Do not record anything before providing nursing care.
3. **Legibility**: The entries must be legible and easy to read to prevent interpretation errors.
4. **Permanency**: All entries are to be made in dark ink, so that the record remains legible permanently, and it will be easy to identify any change or modification.
5. **Correct spelling:** There should be accuracy in spelling while writing. Grammatical and typographical mistakes give a negative impression to the reader and, thereby, decreases the nurse's credibility.
6. **Signature:** Nurses must put signatures in each recording on all nursing documents. The signature must include the name and title.
7. **Accuracy**: Each clinical record must contain the patient's name and identifying information on each page of the clinical records with stamp and signature. Check the patient's name.
8. **Use specific descriptions**: When describing something, avoid general words, such as relevant, sound, or reasonable—accurate record information per the policy of the department.
9. **Do not erase or use corrective fluid**: When a recording mistake, draw a line through it and write the words "mistake entry" above or next to the original listing and put initials. Do not erase or use correction fluid. Write on every line.
10. **Sequence**: Record events in the order in which they occur.
11. **Appropriateness**: Document only information about the patient's health problems and care.
12. **Completeness**: Record the complete information as helpful to the client and healthcare professionals.
13. **Conciseness**: Recording needs to be brief as well as complete to save time in communication.
14. **Standard terminology**: Use only commonly accepted abbreviations and symbols. Many abbreviations are standardized and used universally.
15. **Legal cautious**: Accurate, complete documentation should give legal protection to the nurse, the client's other caregivers, the health-care facility, and the client **(Table 60.1)**.

Steps for Designing the Record

The following steps are followed for designing a record:
1. Constitute a committee. The members should be the head of the department, hospital administrator, nursing head, supervisor, and nursing staff of the operational level.
2. Call for repeated meetings to seek suggestions and prepare a rough draft of record.
3. Test for its validity and also check the feasibility and utility by conducting a pilot.
4. Periodically evaluate the record.

TABLE 60.1: Legal aspects of charting.

Do not erase, use whitener, or scribble out errors	Do not write critical comments; do not place blame
Correct all errors promptly	Spell correctly
Record all facts in objective terms	Document completely
Be accurate about time and chart as soon as possible after an event	Document omissions with reason and actions
Do not leave blank spaces	Record legibly and in black ballpoint pen
Use only approved abbreviations	Record clarification requests and corrections
Chart only for yourself	Avoid vague statement
Begin with time and end with an appropriate signature	

Records Available in Nursing Units

Various types of documents maintained in nursing units can be classified under nursing administrative records, personnel records, clinical records, and miscellaneous records **(Table 60.2)**.

REPORTS AND REPORTING

The report is oral, written, or computer-based communication intended to convey information to others. These can be formal or informal. Reporting is the process of informing the other staff about the patients and of other events. It is a summary or a statement of the information that presents facts regarding planning, coordinating,

TABLE 60.2: Records available in the nursing unit and nursing office.

Records available in the nursing unit	
Type of record	Records
Nursing administrative	Ward policies, organization chart, procedure manual, stock registers, indent books, list of equipment in use, drug book, diet book, admission–discharge books, report book, etc.
Personnel	Job descriptions personnel performance record, rotation plan, duty roster, assignment book, etc.
Clinical	Nursing care plans, nurses observation charts, nurses notes, temperature, pulse, respiration graphical record, intake/output record, drug or treatment chart, patients file, identification chart, specific charts per the unit, etc.
Miscellaneous records	Nurses errands, requisition forms, etc.
Records available in the nursing office	
Nursing administrative	Hospital policy manual, nursing policies, organization chart nursing procedure manual, etc.
Personnel	General: cumulative records, performance, personal files, etc. Personnel job descriptions of all categories Personnel duty-related records: duty roster. Duty list roll call registers, allocation and leave forms, etc.
Patients	Hospital report, census book, etc.

performing, and the general state of services in an organization.

Objectives of Reports

Listed are the objectives of record keeping:
1. It presents factual information to the management and thereby serves as a means of communication.
2. It provides valuable clinical information of patients that can be used for future reference.
3. It provides necessary information to the department, clients, and general public at large.
4. It is useful in measuring the performance of an employee.
5. It makes valuable and constructive suggestions to management.

Types of Reporting

The types of reporting are as follows:

Change-of-shift Report

It is a report by the nurses on one shift to nurses of the next shift change. It provides continuity of care of the patient to the nurses by providing a quick description of patient health status and details of care. The points that should be kept in mind while reporting:
- The information should be accurate, factual, organized.
- Avoid negativism and subjectivity while reporting.
- Use a written or printed guide to prompt thoroughness and organization.
- Be specific and avoid vague terms.
- Describe the presence of all invasive treatments.
- Focus on abnormal findings and variations from routine or the norm.

Types of change-of-shift reports

a. **Written report:** The off-going nurse records patient information, writes it down on the report book. The on-duty nurses either listen to or read the report when they arrive on the unit.
b. **Verbal report:** During the oral report, the off-going nurse gives over to the nurses on duty about the patient or other pertinent information about the ward. This report may be given in the duty room or through the bed-side round. The verbal report may be supported with a written statement.
c. **Bedside report:** The off-going nurse introduces the on-coming staff to the patient, and they discuss the plan of care. The bedside report generally lasts several minutes per patient. It benefits the on-coming nurse because it allows the nurse to meet the patient and interact with the patient. As a result, she can identify the patient's needs and prioritize for the shift. The off-going staff may even show the on-coming team how to use medical equipment in the room. When changing over work together face to face, there is teamwork spirit that allows the nursing staff to achieve common goals.

The bedside handover is a commonly used method of handing over and giving. Even patients have also perceived that bedside handover is suitable for maintaining a professional discussion and patient safety.

d. **Telephone report:** In emergency cases, the nurse may report the condition of patients or doctors may give a health description of the patient on the telephone. The nurse must document the time and date of the report given/received through telephone and name of healthcare provider delivering the report.
e. **Telephone orders:** Physicians often order treatment for a patient by telephone. The nurse must document the time and date of the message received through the phone and name of the healthcare provider giving instruction. Question any order if that is ambiguous, unusual, or contraindicated by the client's condition.
f. **Transfer report:** The reports relate to the unit-to-unit, summarized medical progress, background information, current status, current nursing diagnoses, critical assessments or interventions to be completed shortly after the transfer, special considerations, and need for special equipment report.
g. **Incident reports or occurrence reports:** These are the reports indicating unusual incidence regarding patient care such as medication errors or accidents such as falls. Incident reports can help in improving the treatment of patients. The reports should be concise and accurate. Do not explain the cause or make excuses and don't place blame in the report.
h. **Conferring:** These are consultation and referral reports such as reports of nursing care conferences, nursing care rounds.

Intradivisional Report

a. **Among nursing staff:** The reports are about patients, their condition, number of patients, census, patients with particular problems, and critical issues that need to be reported during taking and handing over.
b. **Between nursing sisters and staff nurses:** Report of patients, handing and taking over in the morning, during the rounds, reporting about any incidence, diet, etc.
c. **Between nursing sister and matron:** Reports during evening and night about patients, severe patients, census, vacant beds, events, staff on duty, any staff member admitted, ward sanitation, family planning cases, medicolegal cases, any complaints, shortage of equipment if any, absent staff, and the performance of the team.
d. **Between nursing sisters and doctors:** Nursing sisters do report, which is at the time of round about the patients, during the departmental meetings regarding the requirement of wards, and any complaints or problems.

Intradepartmental Report

It is the communication between two departments. The reports are sent from one department to another or vice versa. For example, in the hospital, the head of the nursing department sends patients' report and the staff report to the medical superintendent. Such reports include report book indicating reports of patients, VIP and acute patients, any event or disaster mishappening, accidents, complaints, staff performance reports, etc.

CORRESPONDENCE

Meaning

Correspondence is the return of communication between two persons, institutions, or departments. It can be personal or official. It is any written or digital communication exchanged by two or more parties. It may be in the form of letters, e-mails, text messages, voice mails, notes or postcards. Correspondence management is the procedure established for regular dispatch, receipt, filing, storage, retrieval, and disposition of communication records.

Importance of Correspondence

Correspondence plays a very crucial role in all domains and also in health care.
- It serves as a paper trail of events.
- It acts as a reference point for further communication.
- It helps in maintaining cordial relationships with clients, employees by using appropriate means of communication.
- It is an inexpensive and convenient mode of communication as can be provided and obtained economically and conveniently through letters, though there are other methods of communication such as telephone, telex, fax, etc.
- They create and maintain the goodwill of employees and employers.
- It serves as an evidence for legal purposes by keeping a record of all facts.

Characteristics of Correspondence

The nine characteristic features of correspondence are the following:
1. Number each correspondence subject wise, yearly wise, head-wise or dispatch/incoming number per the institute policy.
2. No communication should be left undone. Deal with all the letters within an appropriate time; however, if urgent, it has to be responded on priority wise.
3. If required, take appropriate action immediately, whatever the form it may be. Some correspondence may expect informing the senders, some may be for further action but need to inform the senders.
4. Some correspondences may be for informing the receivers. File such communications.
5. There should be a proper method of filing and storing the correspondences.
6. Treat all the correspondences as an essential document.
7. There should be separate clerical staff for keeping the records and filing all the correspondences at the appropriate places/files, so that communications can be retrieved at the time of need without any delay and wasting any time.
8. Send the official correspondence through proper channel, so that due respect is given to the seniors, not overruling the responsibilities.
9. If the correspondence is for taking action, send a reminder with or without modification in the communication, in case no action taken within 7 days.

The Format of the Correspondence

Correspondence can be achieved in the following format:
1. There should be a covering letter along with the supporting documents.
2. Mention enclosures for supporting documents.
3. Number each reminder as 1, 2, 3, etc.
4. Depending on the nature of the correspondence, give sufficient time for the authority to take action.
5. The language must be simple, clear, and easy to understand. Avoid using difficult words.
6. The statement should be accurate and the best of the sender's knowledge.
7. It should provide all the necessary information to the users and contain only essential information.
8. Show courtesy by using words like please, thank you, etc.
9. Overwriting and cutting should be avoided.
10. The correspondence must be of quality and in the paper size should be appropriate.
11. Minimize the folding of the communication, so that it can fit the size of the envelope.

Parts of Official Letter/Correspondence

An official correspondence consists of the following essential parts:
1. It should have the head with name and postal address, date, and reference number.
2. It should have the name and address of the sender.
3. It should state the subject of the correspondence in a brief.
4. It should include the salutation "Sir/Madam" below the title of the topic.
5. The body of communication should contain the actual message. It should have an introductory section, the central part, and the concluding section.
6. The correspondence should ended gracefully, e.g., "Yours faithfully/sincerely."
7. Immediately below the complimentary close, put the signature. Type the name below the signature.
8. Enclosures must be listed one by one using serial numbers.

9. Ensure carbon copy (cc) are made for copy circulation in case the copies are to be sent to other persons apart from the addressee.

CHAPTER HIGHLIGHTS

- Documentation is a system of recording either handwritten or electronically generated information regarding the care or service provided to a patient.
- Nursing documentation is a process of making an entry of data on a record, regarding patients' care and service provided to the client.
- The two types of documentation systems are paper-based or traditional and electronic documentation systems. Narrative documentation is the conventional part of the source-oriented record for recording nursing care provided.
- The problem-oriented medical records (POMRs) focus on the specific problem of the patient. It has four essential elements, namely, database, problem list, plan of care, and progress notes.
- The electronic health record (EHR) is the patient-centered real-time, longitudinal electronic record of patient healthcare information.
- Record is handwritten or computer-based used for specific purposes in any form. The recording is a process of making an entry on a client's record. A nursing record system is the record of nursing care planned and given to individual patients by nurses.
- The report is oral, written or computer-based communication intended to convey information to others. Reporting is the process of informing the other staff about the patients and of other events.
- Correspondence is any written or digital communication exchanged by two or more parties. It may be in the form of letters, e-mails, text messages, voice mails, notes, etc.

REVIEW QUESTIONS

I. Essay Type Questions
1. What is the documentation system? Discuss its purposes.
2. What are the different types of documentation systems? Describe anyone in detail.
3. Define the term "report" and "reporting." Discuss different methods of reporting.
4. What do you mean by "nursing record." Discuss its purposes and uses.
5. Elaborate on the characteristics of sound recording. Enlist the steps of designing records.

II. Short Notes
1. Problem-oriented medical record
2. Electronic health records
3. General guidelines of recording
4. Principles of good record keeping
5. Correspondence

III. Multiple Choice Questions
1. A traditional type of charting a person or department using notations in a separate section is:
    a. Problem oriented
    b. Charting by exception
    c. Graphic or flow sheet charting
    d. Source oriented
2. Which one of the following is a patient-centered electronic record of patient health information?
    a. Electronic health record
    b. Automated medical record
    c. Electronic medical record
    d. Personal health record
3. Which of the following type of records is web-based and maintained by a healthcare provider?
    a. Clinical data repository
    b. Electronic client record
    c. Digital medical record
    d. Virtual electronic health record
4. Which statement is applicable for the conferring type of reports?
    a. The reports that off-going nurses give over to ongoing nurses
    b. The reports that nurses give to other nurses regarding consultation, referral, nursing care rounds, etc.
    c. The reports that off-going nurses introduce the on-going nurses about patients and discuss their conditions
    d. The reports that nurses report on the telephone to the concerned doctors

Answer Keys
1. d   2. a   3. c   4. b

SUGGESTED READING

1. Cahill J. Patient's perceptions of bedside handovers. J Clin Nurs 1998;7(4):351-9.
2. Cheevakasemsook A, Chapman Y, Francis K, Davies C. The study of nursing documentation complexities. Int J Nurs Pract 2006;12(6):366-74.
3. Coleman A. Where do I stand? Legal implications of telephone triage. J Clin Nurs 1997; 6(3): 227-31.
4. Hendrickson G, Kovner CT. Effects of computers on nursing resource use: Do computers save nurses' time? Comput Nurs 1990;8(1):16-22.
5. Henry SB. Essential infrastructure for quality assessment and improvement in nursing. J Am Med Inform Assoc. 1995;2(3):169-82.
6. Kirkley D, Renwick D. Evaluating clinical information systems. J Nurs Adm 2003;33(12):643-51.
7. Langowski C. The times they are a changing: effects of online nursing documentation systems. Qual Manag Health Care 2005;14(2):121-5.
8. Lee T. Nurses' perceptions of their documentation experiences in a computerized nursing care planning system. J Clin Nurs 2006;15(11):1376-82.

9. Lorenzi NM, Riley RT, Blyth AJ, Southon G, and Dixon BJ. Antecedents of the people and organizational aspects of medical informatics: review of the literature. J Am Med Inform Assoc. 1997; 4(2): 79-93.
10. Minda S, Bundage DJ. Time differences in handwritten and computer documentation of nursing assessment. Comput Nurs. 1994;12(6):277-9.
11. Oroviogoicoechea C, Elliott B, Watson R. Review: evaluating information systems in nursing. J Clin Nurs. 2008;17(5);567-75.
12. Saletnik LA, Niedlinger MK, Wilson M. Nursing resource considerations for implementing an electronic documentation system. AORN J. 2008;87(3):585-96.
13. The Canadian Nurses Protective Society (CNPS). infoLAW: A legal information sheet for nurses, quality documentation, 2007 Jan, Revision of 1992; 1(1): 4-5. Available from: English infoLAW bundle - CNPS https://www.cnps.ca/upload-files/pdf_english/bundle/English%20infoLAW%20bundle.pdf. [Accessed Jan 2020].
14. Urquhart C, Currell R, Grant MJ, and Hardiker NR. Nursing record systems: effects on nursing practice and healthcare outcomes. The Cochrane Database Syst Rev 2009 Jan ;(1): D002099. doi: 10.1002/14651858.CD002099.pub2. [Accessed Jan 2020].

61 CHAPTER

Information Systems: Management Information and Evaluation System, Health Information and Management System, and Nursing Information System

CHAPTER OUTLINE

- Information System
  - Concept of Information System
  - Characteristics of Information System
  - Operating Elements of an Information System
- Management Information and Evaluation System
  - Concept of Management Information and Evaluation System
  - Classification of MIES
  - Objectives of MIES
  - Purposes of MIES
  - Advantages of MIES
- Health Management Information System
- Nursing Information System

LEARNING OUTCOMES

After completion of this chapter, the learner will be able to:
- Understand the concept of information system, management information system, health management information system, and nursing information system (NIS)
- Discuss the characteristics and operating elements of an information system
- Classify management information systems
- Describe its objectives, purposes, and advantages
- Enlist various types of health information system
- Understand how to develop a system
- Familiarize with uses, benefits, and application of NIS
- Design and implement an NIS
- Discuss the bases of a computerized NIS, nursing minimum data set (NMDS) and its uses

KEY TERMS

Information, information system, management information system, health management and information system, nursing information system, nursing minimum data set

INTRODUCTION

Information is recognized as one of the crucial corporate resources that facilitate better utilization of other essential resources, such as men, machines, materials, money, and methods. Without proper information at the right time and the right place, it is not possible to utilize resources fully. Therefore, information management becomes a necessity to make decisions regarding health care.

INFORMATION SYSTEM

Concept of Information System

Information is data that are put into a meaningful and useful context and communicate to a recipient to make decisions. Data are raw, untested facts, symbols, objects, figures, events, etc. Data are a collection of facts from secondary sources, such as census records. Information is of significance in a particular situation. It needs to communicate. It evaluates and notifies events, reduces uncertainty, reveals alternatives, aids to eliminate irrelevant ones, and encourages them to take action. An element of data constitutes information in a specific context. Useful information is relevant; cost-effectiveness has accuracy, reliability, and usability.

A system refers to a set of related components, activities, processes, and human beings interacting together to accomplish some common objectives. It is a system that provides information to aid in decision-making at all levels in the organization.

An information system is a set of related processes, activities, and individuals interacting together to provide processed data to the individual managers at various levels in different functional areas. It usually refers to a computer-based system, one that is designed to support the operations, management, and decision functions.

The information system ensures that information is available to the managers in the form they want it and when they need it. It is designed to support their work by providing relevant information for their decision-making. It was aimed to collect, store, process, retrieve, display, and communicate timely information needed in practice, education, administration, and research (Malliarou et al. 2007).

Information systems in organizations provide information support for decision makers. It encompasses transaction processing systems, management information systems (MIS), decision support systems, and strategic information systems.

Characteristics of Information System

The information system cannot generate data by itself, but it can collect, record, store, process, and retrieve data per the needs of the users. These vary according to the levels of management. The information systems facilitate electronics equipment, such as computers to integrate databases.

Operating Elements of an Information System

An information system can function with the help of the following elements:
1. **Hardware:** Hardware is the equipment and devices for input, output, secondary storage, process, and communication in the system.
2. **Software:** A set of program facilitates processing procedures. The method comprises software, application of software, and model base.
3. **Database:** The database consists of files and physical storage media.
4. **Procedures:** The operating procedures refer to documented operations or activities in the form of manuals or standing operative procedures, system manuals, and user manual. It constitutes an essential part of MIS.
5. **Operating personnel:** The system managers, system analysts, and data administrators, programmers, data entry and computer operators work using these information systems.

MANAGEMENT INFORMATION AND EVALUATION SYSTEM

Concept of Management Information and Evaluation System

The term "management information system" first appeared in a report by the US Navy regarding computers' use to build a single integrated system to manage all navy resources. It is synonymous with computer-based systems. It includes information system, information management system, and information technology. Information technology is a tool used to process data and information. An MIS, therefore, produces data that support the management functions of an organization.

Management information and evaluation system (MIES) is concerned with processing data into information. It is a system of managing information to monitor progress, measure performance, detect trends, evaluate alternatives, make decisions, and take corrective actions (Duerch).

The MIES is a system of obtaining, classifying, storing, and analyzing data to enable the management to define objectives, to plan to meet those objectives, and to complete the cycle by evaluating progress and redefine the goals. It is a formal system of gathering, integrating, comparing, analyzing, and dispensing information internal and external to the organization in a timely, effective, and efficient manner (Koontz).

Classification of MIES

1. **Databank information system:** The data information system contains observed information. It classifies and stores any observation of data potentially useful to the decision maker.
2. **Predictive information system:** The predictive information system has predictive information. It draws inferences and predictions relevant to decision-making.
3. **Decision-making information system:** The system helps in the process of decision-making. It added the criteria for choosing among alternatives and thus added value system of the organization.
4. **Decision-taking information system:** It is a decision system in which the decision-maker takes the decision as generated by the system and very confident to initiate action accordingly.

Objectives of MIES

The four main objectives of MIES are as follows:
1. To enhance communication among employees
2. To provide a method for recording and analyzing information
3. To reduce the expenses of employees-related activities
4. To support organizational goals and directions.

Purposes of MIES

The various purposes of MIES are as follows:
- To provide management information to decision makers
- To provide a base for analyzing any internal or external threats to an organization
- To regulate routine activities, thus avoiding human work in the processing tasks
- To assist management in making everyday decisions
- To provide the information necessary to make nonroutine decisions.

Advantages of MIES

The advantages of MIES are as follows:
1. It supports and enhances the overall decision-making process.

2. It improves job performance throughout the organization.
3. It provides the means to monitor activities.
4. It provides feedback on the effectiveness of risk control.

HEALTH MANAGEMENT INFORMATION SYSTEM

The health MIS (HMIS) is a system of gathering, processing, analyzing, and reporting health-related information aiming to improve the health services and its efficiency and effectiveness through better management at all levels of health services.

The clinical information management has been a paper record. There was the traditional method of documenting and keeping clinical records in practice. The health care information system reframes the strategic plan per the need for data. It can share data and networks to support communication of the information within and outside health institutes.

Historical Background

The concept of MIES in India introduced in the early 1980s and envisaged in 1983 under National Health Policy to have health information nationwide at all organizational setup. In 1983–1985, the HMIS, version 1.0, was piloted in four states, i.e. Gujarat, Rajasthan, Maharashtra, and Haryana. In 1985–1987, the National Informatics Centre, in collaboration with WHO, developed HMIS. After testing in one district of each of the four states in 1989, it was implemented in 13 states and union territories during 1990–1995. Its version was revised from 1.0 to 2.0 in 1996 after review. After continuous revisions, it was in operation. On July 1, 2019, the Ministry of Health and Family Welfare (MoHFW) launched the new real-time HIMS online portal—a digital initiative under National Health Mission, MoHFW in five states.

Objectives of HMIS

The major objectives of HMIS are as follows:
- To improve communication among health staff in the organization
- To provide a method for recording and analyzing health information
- To reduce the expenses of employee-related activities
- To support health organizational goals and directions
- To get real-time health information regarding the census, diseases, outbreaks, etc.

Purposes of HMIS

Listed below are the purposes of HMIS:
- To provide health-related management information to decision makers
- To provide a base for analyzing any internal or external threats to an organization
- To regulate routine health-related activities, thus avoiding human work in the processing tasks
- To assist health management in making everyday decisions
- To provide the necessary health information to make nonroutine decisions
- To monitor and evaluate the health services at different levels
- To develop strategies to improve the existing health services and health system.

Importance of HMIS

The HMIS is important because of the following reasons:
1. It aids in proper planning and coordinating activities in a better and systematic way.
2. It establishes a database on different aspects, such as personnel, operations, morbidity, mortality, and other health indicators, health status, census, health financing, material, quality, etc.
3. It provides real-time information regarding national health programmes and their effectiveness in promoting health.
4. It directs in selecting entry points in program interventional strategies and establishing a partnership with other organizations.
5. It provides data to develop and reform health policy to decision makers by getting, analyzing, and evaluating information regarding current national health situation.
6. It helps in prioritizing health problems, generating alternative solutions, developing indicators and performance evaluation standards, and assessing alternative interventions for its effectiveness.

Organizational Setup for HMIS in India

1. **At the central level:** At the central level, the Central Bureau of Health Intelligence (CBHI) and the statistical division Ministry of Health and Family Welfare (MoHFW) deals with the activities of HMIS. Data are received through a sample registration system, census/population survey, and health record survey.
2. **At the state level:** At the state level, the Directorate of Health and Family Welfare deals with HMIS and directs medical officers to gather information at district level.
3. **At the district level:** At the district level, civil surgeon or district/senior medical officer maintains the drug logistics and gathers statistical data and controls primary health centers and hospitals.

Types of HMIS

There are many systems under e-Health initiative in India. The major ones are as follows:
1. **Hospital management information system:** The HMIS is a part of the e-Health initiative in India. It is a health care system to provide better care to patients by addressing all functional areas of the hospital and its activities by

maintaining online electronic health records. It aids in streamlining the various operations to improve hospital services, administration, monitoring, and control. It also helps in gathering real-time data regarding state-level resource utilization, drug inventory, alerts for end users, etc.

2. **Drug logistic information and management system:** It is a system that handles procurement, storage, and distribution of drugs, medicines, injections, surgical goods, and medical equipment. *e-Aushudi* is a web-based application or an order to maintain the stocks of various drugs and surgical items. It aims to provide quality-level medicines to the people and a standardized method of procurement, storage, distribution, and the issue of drugs. Drug and Vaccine Distribution Management System (DVDMS) is a drug procurement and control system in other states.

   e-Drug intending system is another type of drug logistic information and management system to maintain annual demand for drugs and monthly inventory monitoring. It is also used to maintain offline data of institutional deliveries, census, and equipment. Drug procurement and distribution MIS is useful to monitor and control the procurement and distribution of drugs at the central level.

3. **Computerized human resource information system** It is a digital and integrated system to keep the employee's data and manages the data for the movements of the employees in the organization. It is the software system that covers all aspects of human resources. It captures the information from all vertical programs of the state of permanent and contractual staff.

4. **Admission, discharge, and transfer system:** The admission, discharge, and transfer (ADT) system is a type of information system and is the backbone of the clinical as a robust system. It includes the patient's details, such as demographic data, registration number, and so on. All the data of the patients has a link with the essential information. Laboratory results find their way to the appropriate provider or care area based on information contained in this hospital information system.

5. **Accounting or financial system:** An accounting system is another type of application under HIS. This system tracks the financial interactions and provides fiscal reporting to manage the finance of the institution.

6. **Order entry clinical oriented system:** The order entry clinical record system is a type of system where clinicians place an order by simply selecting a patient from the computer. The order is immediately transferred to the concerned department.

7. **Ancillary systems:** The ancillary system is used for other therapies, such as physical, radiology, or laboratory that shares the information with other systems.

8. **Clinical documentation system:** The clinical documentation system is a part of clinical workflow and provides communication of real-time information. The NIS uses the nursing process approach with nursing diagnoses. The clinical documentation system should provide for retrieval of data for use in research and long-range planning.

9. **Scheduling system:** The scheduling system is another vital health information system. It provides information regarding the scheduling of different staff in the organization and link with the financial system.

10. **Acuity system:** It provides information regarding the classification of patients according to their severity of illness. This system can estimate the staff and other resources required to render care. Other methods, such as ADT, staffing, etc. can integrate with this system.

11. **Specialty systems:** It provides information regarding physiological monitoring activities. These systems are capable of continuously collecting patient's data, setting off alarms, and generating decisions with an electronic information system.

12. **Pregnancy, child tracking, and health services management system:** It is a useful planning and management software tool to maintain online data of various health institutions in the state. It is an integrated system of HMIS used in tracking pregnant women, infants, and children. It facilitates health surveillance, monitoring immunization programs, institutional deliveries, and management of health institutions. It also enables to identify the cases for sterilization and maintains the directory of health institutions. It has a provision of sending short message service (SMS) alert to people and health providers. In some states, there is pregnancy and infant cohort monitoring and evaluation system used for registration till birth of the baby which is also used to identify high-risk mothers for referral and monitoring.

13. **Accredited Social Health Activist (ASHA) mobile application:** It is an application used by ASHA workers to counsel, guide, and educate pregnant, postpartum mothers and their families in their areas.

14. **Mitaan application:** It is an android-tablet web-based application used to remind virtually auxiliary nurse midwives for their work and budget monitoring, thus to improve the work efficiency and effectiveness of services. Jagaar is another android web-based app for information, education and communication (IEC) training material for teaching auxiliary nurse midwives and ASHA workers. The data flow from bottom to top level, from subcenter to primary health center to community health center/district hospital to directorate at the state level from there to central government level.

Methods of Developing a System

Take the following steps to develop a system:

Step 1: Need Assessment and Analysis

Identify information needs, analyze the present information system, flow of information, and bottlenecks. Create the first draft of an evaluation plan. Record the amount of time documentation takes, number of errors, patient safety issues, etc. Determine the cost and benefits of a new system, its impact in terms of the current workflow, and the level of training required for the staff.

Step 2: Planning

It is the second step in developing a system. Select a method according to requirements of the users and consult clinical users and information service and administrative staff. Design the features of the system and focus on security, data sharing, and screen design. Follow the standards.

Step 3: Implementation Stage

During this stage, test the features and functioning of the system including hardware, backups, downtime storage, network communication, and other related features. Plan and organize orientation training programs for the users regarding the system.

Step 4: Maintenance/Evaluation Stage

Plan and conduct periodic evaluations. Find out the difficulties faced for implementation. Do revision and replanning.

NURSING INFORMATION SYSTEM

Nursing information system, is a healthcare information system that deals with nursing, notably the maintenance of the nursing record (Currell et al., 2003). It is a computer system that manages clinical data from a variety of sources to help nurses in improving nursing care.

Uses of NIS

It has the following purposes:
- To assess patient acuity and condition
- It will aid in preparing a plan of care or a critical pathway
- It will generate specific interventions per the patients' problems and document care
- It tracks outcomes and controls the quality of the given patient care
- It will ease nurses to deliver patient care, to communicate, to conduct research, in education and ward management.

Benefits of NIS

The six main benefits of NIS are as follows:
1. The nurses can utilize maximum time for patient care.
2. It reduces paperwork/paper loss.
3. Nurses get automated tools for nursing documentation.
4. There will be uniform standards of nursing care through the nursing process.
5. It will reduce the cost of patient care.
6. It will enable nurses to measure the quality of nursing care.

Application of NIS

Nurses can use and generate a large volume of patients' related information and can also make decisions to carry out patient-related functions.

Management Applications

The nurse manager can make statistical projections of future nursing workload and staff requirements. They can make a summary and analysis of patients' classification data. It will be beneficial for staff scheduling and utilization of resources in a better way. It is helpful in budget planning and monitoring, making payroll records, and for retrieval and analysis of quality assurance information.

Nursing Practice-related Applications

The NIS facilitates the collection, transmission, analysis, and reporting of patient-related, employee-related, and process-related information among nurse managers and caregivers. Nurses can easily monitor clients by using bedside measurement of heart rate, blood pressure, blood gases, computer-controlled fluid, nutrients automated nursing audit. It will significantly help them to render care by using the nursing process strategy and documenting care given.

Nursing Research-related Applications

The nurses can use evidence-based data for further research to generate theories and models and thus to build a body of knowledge in nursing.

Designing and Implementing NIS

According to Allan and Englebright (2000), seven steps are involved in designing and implementing an NIS:

Planning Phase

During the planning phase, define the problem and state goals of the system. Determine the scope of operation and identify information needs. Prepare a time plan. Negotiate for the project definition agreement, and write the project document, allocate resources by conducting a feasibility study.

Analysis Phase

In the analysis phase, gather data through developed questionnaires, interviews, observations. Analyze data by using data flowcharts, grid charts, decision tables, organizational charts, etc. Review data before proceeding to the design phase.

Design Phase

The design phase has functional and process design. During the technical design, focus on resources, such as staff, time frame, cost and budget, facilities and equipment, data manipulation and output, operational considerations, human–computer interactions, and system validation plan. The process design focuses on design inputs, design outputs, design files and databases, and design controls.

Development Phase

The development phase includes selecting a type of hardware, developing software and test system, document system, user's manual, operator's manual, maintenance manual, etc.

Implementing Phase

It includes a detailed description of the system that specifies hardware and software implementation, training, operation, and maintenance procedures. It also includes activities, such as training to the users, installing systems, managing, and maintaining order.

Evaluation Phase

Consider the following criteria in selecting an NIS as a basis for evaluating applications, overall system performance, evaluation features, ease of system use, configuration or programming performance, security, simplification of reports, database access, hardware and software reliability, connectivity, and system cost. Various ways, such as record review, time study, user satisfaction, cost-benefit analysis are used to assess the performance.

Upgrade Phase

It will consist of new technologies. For example, bedside/point-of-care terminals, workstations, multimedia presentations, decision support system, etc.

COMPUTER-BASED NIS

The computerized-based NIS can manage a large amount of data. The NIS linked to a higher level of computer to improve the effectiveness and efficiency of information management. It is useful to store patient data, enter additional data, create, record, and re-plan nursing care of the patient.

Nursing Management Minimum Data Set

Werley in 1988 designed nursing minimum data set (NMDS) and further modified into nursing management minimum data set (NMMDS) by Delaney and Huber in 1996. It has applied internationally as i-NMDS (international NMDS) in Belgium, Canada, New Zealand, Korea, the Netherlands, Spain, Switzerland, Thailand, Britain, and the United States. It consists of three elements containing 16 groups of data:

Nursing

The nursing category includes the problem of the patient, nursing diagnosis, intervention, outcome criteria, and intensity of nursing care.

Demographic

It includes personal identification, birth date, gender, race, and culture (tribe) and shelter of patients.

Care

The care comprises institutional code of service, medical record number, registered nurse number, entry date, exit date, disposition of patient charts, and billing estimates of the cost of care.

Uses of Nursing Management Minimum Data Set

Nursing information are gathered and organized in a system that processes data into information terrapin in the database to make decisions to render care to maintain the quality of nursing care. Its uses are as follows:
1. It allows comparison of clients based on population, setting, geography, and time.
2. It describes the nursing care of clients and their families in both institutional and noninstitutional settings.
3. It demonstrates the trend of nursing care.
4. It enhances nursing research based on data already available.
5. It facilitates data to make decisions on clinical, administrative, and policy decision-making.

CHAPTER HIGHLIGHTS

- An information system is a set of related processes, activities, individuals interacting together to provide processed data to managers.
- It encompasses transaction processing systems, management information systems, decision support systems, and strategic information systems.
- The operating elements of the information system are hardware, software, database, procedures, and operating personnel.
- Management information system is a system of managing information to monitor progress, measure performance, detect trends, evaluate alternatives, make decisions, and take corrective actions.
- There are different types of MIS to store, predict, make decision, document, etc.
- Nursing information system is a health-care information system that deals with nursing, notably the maintenance of the nursing record.
- The computerized-based NIS is useful to store patient data, enter additional data, create and record, re-plan nursing care of the patient.
- Nursing Minimum Management Data Set consists of three elements containing 16 groups of data.

REVIEW QUESTIONS

I. Essay Type Questions
1. What do you understand by information system? Describe its operating elements.
2. What is the concept of management information system (MIS)? Discuss the different types of MIS.
3. Define healthcare information system. Describe the different types of healthcare information system.

4. Explain the designing and implementation of the nursing information system.
5. Describe the computer-based nursing information system.

II. Short Notes
1. Purposes and advantages of MIS
2. Nursing information system (NIS)
3. Applications of NIS
4. Nursing Management Minimum Data Set
5. Method of developing an information system

III. Multiple Choice Questions
1. Which of the following statement refers to an information system?
   a. The data that are put into a meaningful and useful context to make decisions
   b. A set of related components, activities, and human beings interact to accomplish shared objectives.
   c. A set of related processes, activities, individuals interacting together to provide processed data to make decisions.
   d. A system of managing information to monitor progress, measure performance, evaluate alternatives, and make decisions.
2. Which type of information system contains observed information, classifies, and stores any observation of data potentially useful to the decision makers?
   a. Predictive b. Databank
   c. Decision-making d. Decision taking
3. A type of health information system used for other therapies, such as physical, radiology, etc. that shares the information with other systems:
   a. Accounting system
   b. Acuity system
   c. Scheduling system
   d. Ancillary system
4. Who modified the Nursing Minimum Data Set into Nursing Management Minimum Data set?
   a. Delancy and Huber
   b. Malliarou et al.
   c. RR Duerch
   d. Warley

Answer Keys
1. c   2. b   3. d   4. a

SUGGESTED READING

1. Allan J, Englebright J. Patient-centered documentation: An effective and efficient use of clinical information systems. J Nurs Adm. 2000;30(2):90-5.
2. Available from http://www.searo.who.int/india/mediacentre/events/2019/MoHFW-launch-HMIS-Online-Portal-2019/en/.
3. Ballard EC. Improving information management in ward nurses' practice. Nurs Standard. 2006;20(50):43-8.
4. Bussing A, Herbig B. Recent developments of care information systems in Germany. Comput Nurs. 1998;16(6):307-10.
5. Goossen WT, Epping PJ, Dassen T. Criteria for nursing information systems as a component of the electronic patient record. An international Delphi study. Comput Nurs. 1997;15(6):307-15.
6. Lippeveld T. Approaches to Strengthening Health Information Systems. In: Lippeveld T, Sauerborn R, Bodart C (Eds). Design and implementation of health information systems. Geneva: WHO; 2000.
7. Mahler C, Ammenwerth E, Wagner A. et al Effects of a computer-based nursing documentation system on the quality of nursing documentation. J Med Syst. 2007;31(4)274-82.
8. Oroviogoicoechea C, Elliott B, Watson R. Review: evaluating information systems in nursing. J Clin Nurs. 2008;17(5): 567-75.
9. Schodt D, Jackson B, Borup P, et al. Implementation of hospital information system: The use of a nursing task force. Nurs Manag. 1987;18(7):39-43.
10. Tripp-Reimer T, Woodworth G, McCloskey JC, Bulechek G. The dimensional structure of nursing interventions. Nurs Res 1996 Jan-Feb; 45(1):10-7. DOI: 10.1097/00006199-199601000-00003. [Accessed Jan 2019].
11. Malliarou M and Damigou D. Information Systems in nursing practice. Health Review. Sciences Technology Policy 2007a;18(108):37-41.
12. Currell R and Urquhart C. Nursing record systems: effects on nursing practice and health care outcomes. The Cochrane Database Syst Rev 2003 July 21;(3) CD002099. DOI: 10.1002/14651858.CD002099

CHAPTER 62

Use of Communication Technology: e-Learning, Telemedicine, Telenursing

CHAPTER OUTLINE

- The e-Learning
- Modalities of e-Learning
  - Types of e-Learning
  - Elements of e-Learning
  - Importance of e-Learning
  - Theoretical Bases of e-Learning
  - Benefits of e-Learning
  - Advantages of e-Learning
  - Disadvantages of e-Learning
  - Designing a Program through e-Learning
  - Skills Required for e-Learning
- Telemedicine
- Telenursing

LEARNING OUTCOMES

After completion of this chapter, the learner will be able to:
- Understand the concept of e-Learning, telemedicine, and telenursing
- Describe the modalities, learning preferences, and styles in e-Learning
- Enumerate the different types and elements of e-Learning
- Appreciate the importance and theoretical bases of e-Learning
- Describe the benefits, advantages, disadvantages of e-Learning
- Design the program through e-Learning
- Define the terms of communication technology
- Describe the benefits of telemedicine, e-health, and health IT
- Discuss telecommunication tools
- Enlist the advantages, benefits, and applications of telenursing
- Describe the competencies for professional practice in telenursing and telenursing practice standards

KEY TERMS

Communication technology, e-Learning, e-health, telecommunication, telemedicine, telenursing, practice standards

INTRODUCTION

Human capital has become the most critical competitive advantage in hospitals and health systems. Organizations need a new strategy such as telemedicine and e-health to meet the needs of citizens, patients, healthcare professionals, healthcare providers, and policy makers and even for the learning and training of their employees. It includes the use of modern information and communication technologies. The knowledge and skills of healthcare providers are essential to the quality of care and health of the community.

The communication technology is transferring information among people or machines through the use of technology. It includes multimedia, telephone, Internet, e-mail, and other sound and video-based communication devices. The communication technology is a technical system of communication. The four modes of communication are people to people, people to machine, machine to people, and machine to machine. The machine to machine is the most advanced mode of communication that needs the use of sophisticated technological devices. It uses the latest and oldest technology inventions, i.e. the satellite, sound waves, electromagnetic carrier waves, and light waves. Most of the telecommunication systems have electronic or optoelectronic devices. The use of advanced communication technology has influenced political, social, cultural, and educational networks in many ways. It has both positive and negative impacts.

THE E-LEARNING

The e-Learning is now at the forefront of technology-based education under e-Health. It is utilizing technology to increase the effectiveness and accessibility of learning. The

Chapter 62: Use of Communication Technology: e-Learning, Telemedicine, Telenursing

utility of e-Learning is growing in healthcare professionals' knowledge and has proved in reducing costs.

Definitions of e-Learning

The letter "e" in e-Learning stands for the word "electronic." It includes all educational activities carried out by individuals or groups working online or off-line and synchronously or asynchronously through network or computers and other electronic devices.

e-Learning is a learning method that utilizes computer networks and electronic media, including a mobile phone in the teaching and learning process, to enable staff and students to learn anytime and anywhere. It involves the use of networked information and communications technology to provide training, educational, or learning the material and as a technique used to improve learning and teaching experiences in higher education. It applies to educate students with or without their instructors through any digital media.

It covers a wide range of instructional material delivered on a CD-ROM or DVD, over a local area network (LAN) or on the Internet. It includes computer-based training (CBT), Web-based training (WBT), and electronic performance support systems (EPSS), distance or online learning, online tutorials, etc.

"e-Learning" is an umbrella term that covers an extensive set of electronic educational applications and processes such as Web-based learning, computer-based learning, virtual classrooms, and digital collaboration. It includes the delivery of content via a network, audio and video recordings, satellite broadcast, interactive TV, CD-ROM, etc.

Development of e-Learning

The history behind the development of e-Learning is as follows:
- The development of the e-Learning arises from "educational revolutions." Billings and Moursund (1988) cited four such revolutionary invention of reading and writing, the emergence of the teaching profession, the development of moveable type (print or graphic technology), and the development of electronic technology.
- European schools used a Roman piece—a writing slate since 200 AC till around 1950 as an early learning aid to developing writing skills which can be now compared with new learning aids such as laptops.
- Isaac Pitman taught shorthand in Great Britain via correspondence in the 1840s and started a distance course by mail.
- In the early 1920s, Sidney Pressey, an Educational Psychology Professor at the Ohio State University, developed a machine that resembled a typewriter with a window to provide drill and practice items to students and now widely used in online systems like *"questionmark perception."*
- During the 1950s, Skinner presented the programmed instruction as (digital) self-study courses.
- In the early 1960s, Professor Patrick and Richard from Stanford University experimented with math and reading classes using computers to teach young children in elementary schools in California.
- In the 1970s and 1980s, early online courses developed at the New Jersey Institute of Technology and classes at the University of Guelph in Canada, the British Open University, and the online distance courses at the University of British Columbia.
- The introduction of the first PC (the Altair 880 in 1975) quickly followed by the Apple II and the IBM PC used for didactical purposes.
- In early 1993, William D Graziadei described an online computer-delivered lecture, tutorial, and assessment project using e-mail.
- In 1995, Harasim emphasized the use of learning networks for knowledge construction, long before the term e-Learning came into use.
- In 1997, an article published by William D. Graziadei described an overall strategy for technology-based course development and management for an educational system.
- In October 1999, during a CBT systems seminar in Los Angeles, a strange new word was used for the first time in a professional environment—e-Learning.
- The use of e-Learning is increasing in nurse education and practiced to enhance learning opportunities for students and qualified nurses in information and communication technology and to improve nursing practice and client outcome.

Modalities of e-Learning

Figure 62.1 depicts the e-Learning modalities:
1. **Individualized self-paced e-Learning online:** It refers to situations where an individual learner is accessing learning resources such as a database or course content online via an intranet or the Internet. For example, a learner studying alone or conducting some research on the Internet or a local network.
2. **Individualized self-paced e-Learning offline:** This type of modality refers to situations where an individual learner is using learning resources such as a database, offline CAL package, a hard drive, a CD, or DVD.

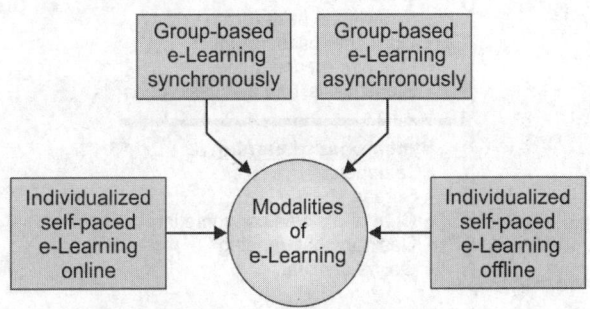

Fig. 62.1: Modalities of e-Learning.

3. **Synchronously group-based e-Learning:** Synchronously group-based e-Learning refers to an education strategy where groups of learners are working together at the same time or in real time by using an intranet or the Internet. It includes text-based conferencing and one- or two-way audio and videoconferencing. For example, learners engaged in a real-time chat, audio, or videoconference.
4. **Group-based e-Learning asynchronously:** Asynchronously group-based learning refers to an education strategy where groups of learners are working over an intranet or the Internet, and exchanges among participants occur with a time delay or not in real time, e.g. online discussions via e-mailing lists and text-based conferencing within learning management systems.

Learning Preferences and Styles in e-Learning

1. **Offline and online activities:** These are teaching–learning activities that take place while offline, not connected to the Internet but online.
2. **Synchronous and asynchronous activities:** Within synchronous learning, learning and teaching take place in real time or at the same time, while the trainer and learner sit separately from each other, e.g. watching live television broadcast and listening to a live radio broadcast, audio/videoconferencing, Internet telephony, online lectures, two ways live satellite broadcast.
Within asynchronous learning, the teaching–learning activities take place with a time delay (time shift), while the trainer and learner sit separately from each other (place shift), e.g. self-paced courses via Internet or CD-ROM, video-taped classes, Web presentations, seminars, etc. **(Fig. 62.2)**.
3. **Different multimedia:** The clients can use more than one media to carry out activities. They can combine both synchronized and asynchronized communication devices.
4. **Different didactical interactions:** Different didactical approaches can use within e-Learning, e.g. assignments, assessment, reading, presentations, video, workshop, demonstration, and simulation.

5. **Delivering lectures:** Various ways to provide the content are computers, personal digital assistants (PDAs), TVs, mobile phones, or iPods. Every device has its characteristics, advantages, and disadvantages.
6. **Self-study and collaborative learning:** Learning can be individualized and collaborative in e-Learning.
7. **Formal and informal learning:** e-Learning has every day as well as a structured learning activity. Informal learning is unstructured and unplanned, and structured learning is a planned activity with specified learning objectives, a didactical approach, and planning.

Kinds of e-Learning

Figure 62.3 depicts various forms of e-Learning:
1. Classroom aids such as overhead projectors, epidiascope, and PowerPoint slides.
2. Website courses: The learning takes place by using multiple types of websites.
3. Laptop programs: Learning takes place by using laptop educational programs.
4. Hybrid learning: Most of the time learning takes place through online.
5. Fully online learning and distance learning.

Elements of e-Learning Material

- The instructional designing of the material should be clear and consistent. It is not an area to take shortcuts. Planning is an essential element in e-Learning.
- There should be an intuitive user interface, which should be easy to navigate.
- There should be ongoing and purposeful interaction with and by the learner.
- Real-world applications, exercises, and examples are necessary.

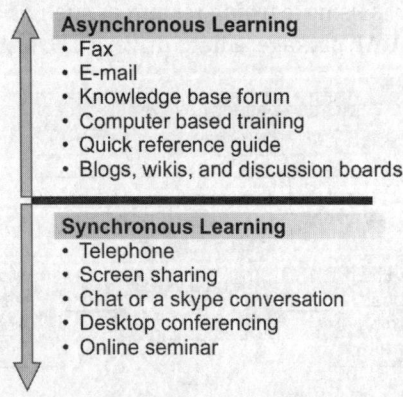

Fig. 62.2: Communication technologies used in learning.

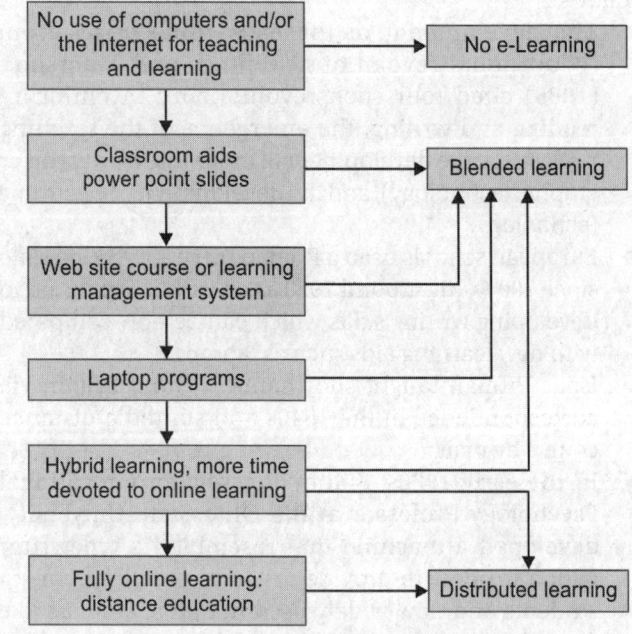

Fig. 62.3: Different forms of e-Learning.

- There must be a practical and systematic assessment of learner progress and achievement.
- Use multimedia to communicate and enhance learning.

Importance of e-Learning

1. **Importance of e-Learning to organization**
   a. *It aids in improving training costs:* Producing learning content is time-consuming, whether it's online or not, but e-Learning promotes the overall cost through decreased travel, reduced material, and hopefully improving performance.
   b. *It decreases material costs:* By creating the environment online and letting the learner practice, the costs associated with setup will be negligible.
   c. *It aids in increasing productivity:* Because e-Learning is not bound by geography or time, the learner can enhance his/her performance at any time.
   d. *It helps in maintaining standards:* e-Learning allows creating a standardized process and consistency in the delivery of content. It also compresses delivery time.
2. **Importance of e-Learning to learners or employees**
   a. *Real-time access:* e-Learning courses provide an opportunity to access anytime, anywhere even without Internet access, i.e. on-demand availability.
   b. *Use in continuing education:* Continuing nursing education (CNE) is gaining popularity without wasting time and money to attract employees to attend conferences, seminars, etc.
   c. *Improves interactivity of participants:* Due to the use of e-Learning, the participants in educational activities become active in the learning process, increase retention, and help in improving patient and employee safety and quality.
   d. *Create a pleasant learning environment:* Use of multimedia in the classroom, create an excellent learning environment, and help in getting feedback from the learners.
   e. *Improve retention:* The combination of multimedia and instructional design can produce a vibrant learning experience.
   f. *Individualized learning:* e-Learning allows learners to progress at their own pace.
3. **Importance of e-Learning in organization and community**
   a. *Ongoing access to resources:* e-Learning provides an opportunity to continue to have access to the online content and resources to brush up and to update knowledge and skills.
   b. *Knowledge management:* e-Learning includes all sorts of online technologies that allow collaboration and conversation to capture organizational knowledge.
   c. *Encourage sharing:* e-Learning mode encourages the sharing of resources among the learners.
   d. *Exploring opportunities for learners:* It allows employers to explore other opportunities in the organization.
   e. *Promotion of flexibility, autonomy, and collaboration:* It helps in promoting flexibility, independence, and coordination among users.

Theoretical Bases of e-Learning

Andragogy and constructivism are the primary theoretical bases of e-Learning.

1. **Andragogy:** Andragogy is a teaching methodology that best facilitates learning among the adult. The flexibility of anytime anywhere learning allows the adult to develop a learning plan that fits their needs related to family, vocation, and other areas of life. The dynamic interactions with other learners can demonstrate relevance as they work together to create newfound meaning.
2. **Constructivism:** Constructivism refers to the learning that occurs as a result of the learner thinking about and by interacting with the subject matter. Constructivism focuses on the concept of knowledge construction versus knowledge transmission. e-Learning is an instructional design that fits in constructivism. The flexibility of the learning may allow the learner to remain in a natural environment during the learning interaction. It also allows the instructor to bring in actual practitioners to interact with the learners. Finally, the learner can construct their plan for achieving the learning outcomes based on personal interests.

Benefits of e-Learning

- It encourages interactive, self-directed, and self-paced learning and innovative teaching.
- It is very convenient, saves time and place for education.
- It enhances data search by hyperlinks.
- It promotes Internet use as and when required.
- It builds confidence and interest among users.
- It improves learning retention and data application.
- It provides proof of completion and certification.

Advantages of e-Learning

1. It increases the flexibility of learning, and it is fast and has no geographical barriers.
2. e-Learning technology offers a wide range of opportunities for education development.
3. The use of e-Learning is independent of time and space and has easy access.
4. e-Learning is a quality-assured program and cost-effective in achieving service and learning goals.
5. It is learner centered and provides easy access to information at any time and any place.

Disadvantages of e-Learning

1. Some forms of e-Learning isolate learners from other learners.
2. Nurses may need training in IT skills to use e-Learning.

Designing a Program through e-Learning

The following steps are involved in creating e-Learning program:

1. **Strategic planning:** The essential components of strategic planning are goal development, plan development, resource analysis, plan implementation, and continuous evaluation. The goal development for e-Learning should include considerations of desired learning outcomes, organizational outcomes, and understanding of learner needs. During planning, constitute a planning team and plan instructional design. Do resource analysis for human and physical resources, physical infrastructure, and other technology. Plan for implementation, and pilot the e-Learning process before the actual implementation.
2. **Course development:** Course development can be similar to the strategic planning process. Formulate goals, plan courses, activities, learning objects, and interactions. Develop an outline for the course theory that supports the attainment of specific outcomes.
3. **Faculty development:** It includes training needs for the faculty, methodology, technology, and computer application, with e-Learning.
4. **Learner needs:** Identify learners' needs. Learners' needs should focus on technology competency, the attitude of learners, and the difficulty level of learners.
5. **Assessment and evaluation:** It includes identifying and selecting assessment and evaluation criteria for instructors and learners. It also provides the development of instructor to the learner, learner to learner, and learner to instructor feedback.
6. **Tools and skills required:** Develop the course management systems in functionality as a grade book, discussion board, chat room, e-mail, assignment submission tool, document delivery tool, Web links, calendar, and activity tracking. It also has other features that allow textbook publishers to provide materials that can be automatically integrated/uploaded into the course. Other tools needed are as follows:
    a. *Help desk:* Plan to have a help desk. A help desk is a tool vital in e-Learning. The instructor must understand the support available and make sure that learners are aware of these resources.
    b. *Administrative tools:* The administrative tools include grade book, activity tracking, assignment submission tools, and file delivery tools.
    c. *Asynchronous discussion tools:* One of the most critical tools in e-Learning is the asynchronous discussion. It requires the discussion board, bulletin board, etc.
    d. *Communication tools:* The communication tools in e-Learning include e-mail, chat, and instant messaging. E-mail can be handy in communicating with learners.
    e. *Community building tools:* Building an online learning community requires training, practice, and continuous revision.
    f. *Evaluation tools:* Exams and quizzes and paper grading can be through online and by using other mechanisms of e-Learning.
    g. *Information sources:* It requires Web sites to have access to knowledge and information.
    h. *Learning objects:* Learning objects include games, animations, case studies, simulations, etc.
    i. *Audio and video aids:* Audio and video (AV) aids can enrich e-Learning. Or record AV aids or use live programs to display on learner's computer, over the Internet, or via DVD or CD-ROM.
    j. *Simulation:* Simulation encompasses different learning modalities and objects. Simulation-based training with a human patient simulator (HPS) or computer-based simulation is beneficial in teaching–learning.
    k. *Psychomotor skill training:* It includes asynchronous discussions, sharing of experiences with admitted or discharged patients and learners.

Skills Required for e-Learning

a. **Essential computing and communication skill:** The computing skills needed are word processing, communicating via e-mail, using PowerPoint software to support presentations, using the spreadsheet to display data, or phone conferencing or video conferencing using desktop publishing packages.
b. **Use of predesigned packages:** The nursing personnel should predesign e-Learning environment tools such as Blackboard, Web Course Tools (Web CT). It supports online tools such as discussion forums, e-mail, live chat, and whiteboarding, as well as content in various formats such as html documents, Web pages, etc. It is also merged with Blackboard which is a leading provider of educational software.
c. **Assembling Internet resources:** It is essential to find the right search engine for searching clinical guidelines, the database of published articles, etc.
d. **Design courses and teaching material:** It includes courses, modules, or session materials.

TELEMEDICINE

Telemedicine is an invaluable tool in health care. It allows patients to visit physicians over video for immediate care. It can capture video/still images and store patient data and send data to physicians for diagnosis and follow-up treatment purposes.

Definitions of Related Terms

1. **Telemedicine:** Telemedicine is a strategy to provide interactive healthcare utilizing modern technology and telecommunications, including satellite links,

dedicated line connections, interactive television systems, and Internet connections to provide healthcare services to patients at some location away from the provider. It is a system of healthcare delivery in which physicians examine distant patients through the use of telecommunications technology (Preston Jane, 1993).

World Health Organization (1997) defined it as the delivery of healthcare services by healthcare professionals using information and communication technologies to people living in distant areas to exchange information for diagnosis, treatment, and prevention of disease and injuries and also for the continuing education, research, and evaluation of healthcare providers to advance the health of individuals and their communities.

It is a branch of e-Health that uses communication networks for the delivery of healthcare services, including medical specialties, such as telecardiology, etc. and medical education from a distance (Sood et al., 2007). It is the combined use of telecommunications and computer technologies to improve the efficiency and effectiveness of healthcare services. It involves the use of telephones, telehealth, internet, sensors, video, remote diagnostics, and other interactive technologies, which allow exchange between patients and healthcare providers.

2. **Telecommunication:** Telecommunication is the transmission, processing, and receiving information in the form of signs, signals, writings, images, and sounds or any other form, via satellite, sound waves, electromagnetic carrier waves, and light waves through cables, radio, visual, or other electromagnetic systems.
3. **Telehealth:** Telehealth is the strategy of providing clinical healthcare, health-related education support to patients and professionals, public health care, and health administration from the long distance by using electronic information and telecommunication technologies. It is the health services' delivering system or strategy to provide healthcare services by removing time and distance barriers using telephones, computers, interactive video transmissions, direct links to healthcare instruments, the transmission of images, and teleconferencing by telephone or video.
4. **Telehealthcare:** Telehealthcare includes all health services of all health disciplines such as radiology, pharmacy, and psychology.
5. **International Society for Telemedicine and e-Health (IsfTeH):** IsfTeH is under Swiss law and is dedicated to promoting telemedicine, telecare, telehealth, and e-Health around the world.
6. **m-Health or mobile health:** The m-health is an efficient and high-quality healthcare service for mobile citizens. It provides healthcare services by using mobiles to exchange health-related information between the user and healthcare providers.
7. **u-Health or ubiquitous health care:** It has u-Health applications to provide health care to people anywhere at any time using broadband and wireless mobile technologies.

e-Health

e-Health refers to the use of communication technology to meet the needs of people, health professionals, providers, and policy makers. It includes e-Care, e-Learning, e-Surveillance, and e-administration. It is the strategy to provide health by using information and communication technology.

The main objective of e-Health is to provide health and medical facilities available to all at any time of the day through mobile services, Web services, and short message service (SMS). It intends to cover all online medical consultations, medical records, management of supply of medicines online, and PAN (Presence Across Nation) India. It includes almost everything which is spread and related to India exchange for patient-related information.

Advantages of m-Health

The advantages of e-Health are the following:
- **Efficiency:** It brings efficiency in health care by reducing costs in unnecessary and duplicate references to diagnostic tests. It improves communication between different health organizations.
- **Enhance quality care:** The consumers can compare and analyze the cost and quality of services provided by different establishments through communication technology and decide where to seek the best quality medical services.
- **Evidence-based services:** The communication technology made it possible to evaluate the services from time to time. m-Health interventions are factual and cannot be assumed.
- **Empowerment:** Advanced communication technology such as personal electronic records made the consumers access their health records over the internet.
- **Encouragement:** The consumers and professionals develop mutual trust as they decide the health care in a shared manner.
- **Education:** The communication technology has a scope to provide health education and health-related information and to professionals to use online resources for training and education purposes.
- **Enabling:** It enables the exchange of information in a systematic and standard way between consumers and healthcare providers.
- **Extending:** The technology extended its conventional boundaries globally. Consumers can access health services online from global providers.
- **Ethics:** It involves a threat to many ethical issues such as informed consent, privacy, practices, etc.
- **Equity:** There is problem with equal distribution of health services. Many people do not have access to modern communication technologies.

Endeavors in Telemedicine

Table 62.1 depicts the landmarks in the development of telemedicine.

Benefits of Telemedicine, e-Health, and Health Information Technology

Internet Innovation Alliance (II A) has identified 10 significant benefits of telemedicine, e-Health, and health IT as listed below:

1. It helps the patient to make decisions and enhances the quality of care.
2. It saves lives through remote consultations, whether urgent or diagnostic.
3. It creates a more efficient, convenient, and potentially more cost-effective delivery of care.
4. It facilitates earlier and more accurate diagnoses.
5. It provides higher and faster access to a patient's medical history, reducing the risk of adverse drug interactions or inadequate response to a course of treatment.
6. It improves administrative efficiency and coordination.
7. It allows patients to receive expert diagnosis and treatment from distant medical centers.
8. It increases the timeliness of treatment and decreases transfer rates, while reducing medical costs through video technology.
9. It supports real-time treatment by first responders through the use of wireless devices.

TABLE 62.1: Endeavors in telemedicine.

Year	Landmark
1844	Transfer of medical information using the public telegraph
1876	Alexander Graham Bell's invention of the telephone
1897	Telephone used to diagnose a child with croup
1906	The first electrocardiograph (ECG) transmission by phone
1923	Offered medical advice to fleets of trade ships by using code in Sweden hospital
1927	The first experimental television transmission
1949	Used a television to perform X-ray data transmission in Montreal hospital
1957	First interactive video link between Psychiatric Institute in Omaha and Norfolk State
Early 1960s	The National Aeronautics and Space Administration's (NASA) effort into telemetry to monitor the physiological functions of an astronaut
1961	First radio telemetry for monitoring the patients in the intensive care unit
1965	Live transmission of an open heart surgery performed in one of the hospitals in Texas in the US
1966	Launched ATS-1, first in NASA's series of Applied Technology Satellite to investigate the use of video consultation through satellite to improve the quality of rural health care in Alaska
1967	Medical services provided for airline passengers at Boston airport clinic with an electronic link to Massachusetts General Hospital
1972–1975	Space technology delivered medical care to the Papago Indian Reservation in Arizona as a joint venture of NASA and Indian health service
Since 1977	Telemedicine center developed interactive audio networks for the educational program and transferring the medical data at Newfoundland
1984	The North West Telemedicine Project setup in Australia to provide health care to five remote towns
1989	NASA established a space bridge to Armenia to extend medical consultation for the victims of a massive earthquake in the Soviet Republic of Armenia
September 7, 2001	First complete long-distance surgery performed by a surgical team in New York by sending high-speed signals to robots operating on a patient in France

Endeavors in Telemedicine in India
1. Apollo Hospital Groups
2. Telemedicine Project by Bharat Electronics Limited
3. Telemedicine Project by National Informatics Centre (NIC), Ministry of Information Technology
   Cardiovascular Technology Institute, Hyderabad, in Association with Defense Organizations
4. Department of Information Technology at Ministry of Communication and IT (Government of India) in 1999 (as Pilot Project) to link AIIMS New Delhi, Post Graduate Institute of Medical Education and Research (PGIMER) Chandigarh, Sanjay Gandhi Post Graduate Institute of Medical Sciences (SGPGI) Lucknow, for realizing telediagnosis, teleconsultancy and tele-education
5. Telemedicine programs supported by Department of IT (DIT), Indian Space Research Organization (ISRO) North Eastern Space Applications Centre (NAC) Telemedicine Program, Apollo Hospitals, Asia Heart Foundation, state governments, some private organization

Success stories of telemedicine
- During Kumbh Mela in Uttar Pradesh (UP) through Online Telemedicine Research Institute of India (OTRI), for transferring the specific data and monitoring the level of cholera in water
- Asia Heart Foundation, Bengaluru practices interstate link between Bengaluru and eastern India and educating paramedics for lifesaving procedures through videoconferencing
- The telemedicine software system developed by the Centre for Development of Advancement Computing, The Centre for Development of Advanced Computing (C-DAC) (using Integrated Services Digital Network (ISDN), A very small aperture terminal (VSAT), POTS (plain old telephone service)) to connect them and being connected to include medical centers in Rohtak, Shimla, and Cuttack
- Telemedicine system installed in Calcutta School of Tropical Medicine (CSTM)
- First international conference organized by ISRO at Bangalore in March 2005
- There are many more telemedicine centers in the country

10. It enhances care through telemedicine and remote in-home monitoring.
11. It improves the quality of care by:
    - facilitating equitable access to our specialists for all patients regardless of their location
    - increasing active participation in inpatient/family education
    - enhancing family satisfaction by reducing the costs and time incurred traveling
    - improving quality time with their specialist
    - reducing duplicate testing
    - improving continuity of patient care by healthcare providers
    - enhancing specialist comfort by reducing the need for physician travel to underserviced areas.

TELENURSING

Tele-nursing—to boldly go where no one has gone before.
—*ICN*

Telenursing is an emerging field in nursing and gaining popularity. It uses telecommunication technology and electromagnetic channels (e.g. wire, radio, optical) to transmit voice, data, and video communications signals. Its applications enhance patient care in nursing.

Tele is a prefix meaning "at a distance" and used in telescope, the term *scope* means an instrument for viewing phenomena at a distance. The term "tele" is being used in healthcare services such as telemedicine, telehealth, telenursing, etc. The common denominators are distance and technology.

The developed countries are using the telenursing strategy to provide nursing care, which is found feasible and cost-effective. In the Indian scenario, it is still in the infancy stage. It needs to be planned carefully, keeping in mind the scope for monitoring, accreditation, and the quality of nursing practice.

Definitions

Telenursing refers to the use of telecommunication devices and information technology to provide nursing care from a distance to isolated groups of people. It is a subset of telehealth focusing on delivery, management, and coordination of services and care via telecommunications.

Telenursing is the use of telemedicine or telehealth technology to deliver nursing care and conduct nursing practice. It uses electromagnetic channels such as wire, radio, and optical to transmit voice, data, and video communications signals. It is a distance communication strategy achieved using electrical or optical transmissions between users and computers (ICN, 2001, 2007). It is the e-health application to professional nursing practice.

Telenursing is a strategy in which nurses deliver, manage, and coordinate patient care and services via telecommunication technology. Telephone nursing was first used by nurses in the late 1800s.

Communication and Information Technology Devices in Telenursing

1. **Hardware:** It includes telephone, telehealth hardware, PC or laptop, power supply, and access to Web sites.
   a. *Telephone:* The telehealth system requires the patient's telephone system for operation. There should be a working telephone to connect the monitor directly to avoid any interruption in phone service.
   b. *Telehealth hardware:* It consists of equipment such as a monitor, electronic blood pressure cuff, pulse oximeter, scale, electrocardiogram (ECG) leads, video camera, blood glucose, and peak flow capabilities. Many companies design wireless versions of these pieces of equipment for convenience.
   c. *The PC or laptop computer:* There should be a PC or laptop with Internet access to reach the patient data. It requires a power source with a wall outlet.
   d. *Power supply and Web access:* There should be a provision of an uninterrupted power supply or backup system. The users must have access to healthcare-related Web sites.
2. **Telehealth monitors:** These are vital sign monitors, pulse oximeter, and glucose monitors **(Fig. 62.4)**. There should be a provision of feeding measurements and peak flow readings monitor. The interpretations of the monitor must be easy to read by the consumers. It should have large print, some have prompted voice, the monitors should be easy to use, and user-friendly.
3. **Software:** These are the operating systems—Linux, national database, security technology and firewalls, and rewritable flash memory.
   a. *Operating system:* It is an operating system such as Windows XP; this is a free operating system that users can access. Linux system is one of the examples of such an operating system used by the telehealth companies.

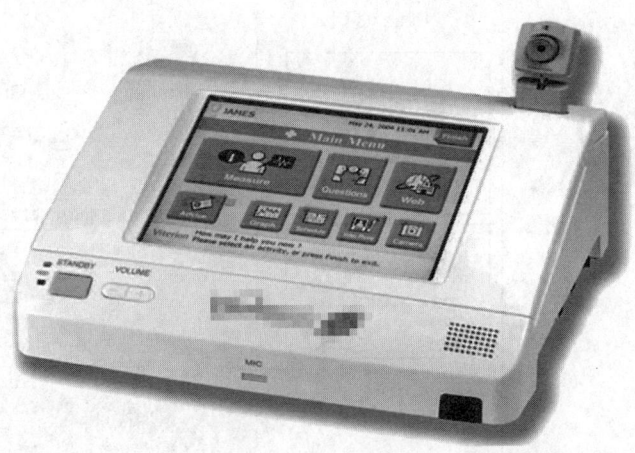

Fig. 62.4: Telehealth monitor.

b. *National database:* A national database system uses technology to ensure compliance and privacy standards. It has a user password to access the data. It stores patients' information and trends. The users can access at any time by entering passwords.
c. *Flash drive:* The flash drive can use to store data by the patient to hand over to healthcare facilities. The monitor has the facility for reprogramming the database when the patient is no longer using the system.
d. *Firewalls and other security devices:* The system has the facility of security devices as firewalls to provide security of data.
e. *Monitors:* There are two types of monitors—top monitors and bottom monitors. Multiple patients can use top monitors, and the bottom monitor is only for individual patients and the information is transmitted via POTS (old telephone system), the router, and firewalls to the Internet servers, flowing to the application server stores in the database **(Fig. 62.5)**.
4. **Software program:** Many software programs are available to us in telehealth, such as Cerner software and Misys Healthcare Systems. The Cerner software system allows users of telehealth to view patient information in a single application. It has an electronic medical record consisting of demographics, vital signs, various tests, clinical note entries, etc. sections. Misys Healthcare Systems include patient registration, discharge, and updating patient information by the healthcare provider via computer access.

Advantages of Telenursing

1. **Provide remote care:** Telehealth nursing bridges the distance between the nurse and patient and a new strategy to provide round-the-clock care. It aids in monitoring patients suffering from chronic diseases and coordinating care to patients with comorbidities from remote and distant areas. The telenursing provides an opportunity to teach patients to manage their disease symptoms, improve their compliance for treatment, and follow-up.
2. **Reduces patient visit:** Telenursing aids in reducing the hospital visits of the patient by rendering care from a distance. They can communicate with patients via many telecommunication facilities.
3. **Reduces distances:** Telenursing can provide remote care to patients. The healthcare providers and patients can talk from miles or from states to countries.
4. **Data sharing:** Telehealth provides an opportunity to render care and share data by the healthcare professionals for an individual who can share data via a secure Web-based data system. The healthcare providers can view the data collected on the Web site, and the data the patient has saved on a flash drive, fax, or e-mail.
5. **Rapid response time:** Telecommunication and information system have the provision of having fast response time according to the patient's needs to provide timely intervention to improve patient care for patients with chronic health issues.
6. **Improve access, costs, and outcomes:** Telehealth gives an avenue to provide access to needed care. It results in reducing the cost of care and improving care. It also reduces the workforce and traveling expenses to achieve the desired goal.
7. **Enhances patients' decision-making:** The patients and families get the opportunity to make their own decisions regarding their health. They can directly

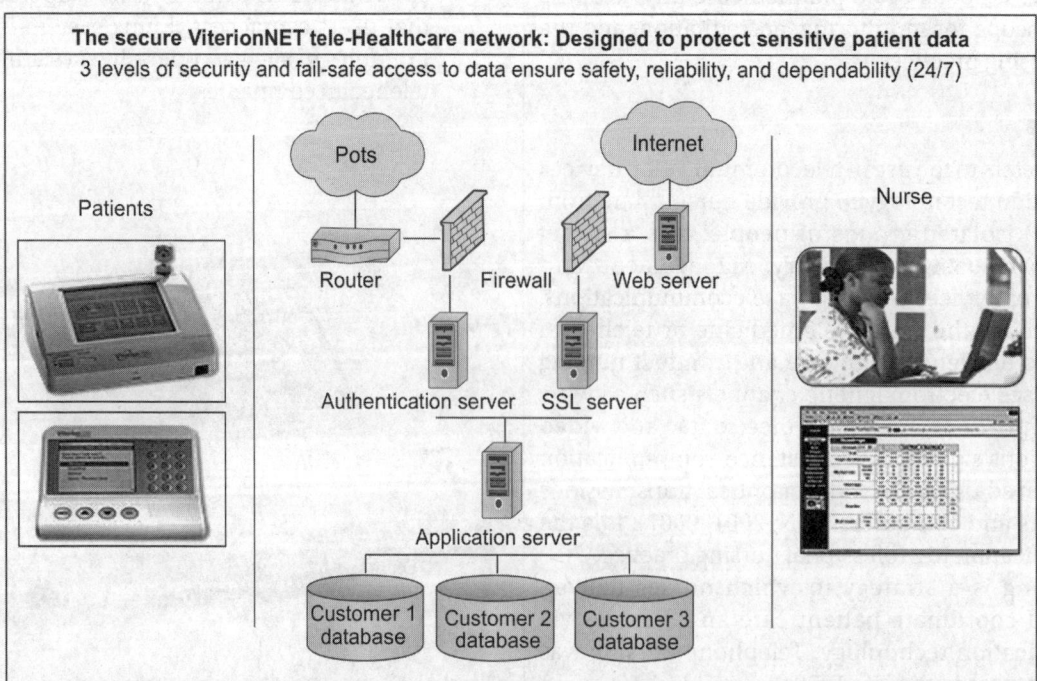

Fig. 62.5: Tele-healthcare security network.

interact with healthcare providers to make decisions on their health issues. Telenursing provides a means to educate patients and families on their illness, medications, etc.

8. **Proximity to care:** It brings closeness to the nursing care, shortens hospitalization, and reduces the workload. The telenurses can participate virtually in all the practice settings for public health, family practice, outpatient department, emergency department for providing health services to the clients using protocols, use videoconferencing, can monitor the status of early discharge patients over telephone, e-mails, by developing Web sites to provide health information.

Box 62.1 depicts evidence-based benefits documented in the literature.

Implications for Nursing

1. It helps in delivering, managing, and coordinating care to patients in many geographic areas.
2. It makes it easy to use many technologies available to view and share patient information providing prompt and effective care.
3. It plays a vital role in disease management and improving patient outcomes through distant care.

Box 62.1: Evidence-based benefits of telenursing.

Care related
- Uses triage from centralized room, thus reducing the use of emergency rooms
- Increase access to services to widely dispersed populations through videoconferencing, internet, videophone, e-mail consultation, short message service (SMS) in home nursing is especially useful
- Care of elderly, children, and adults with chronic conditions and debilitating illnesses, postsurgical situations, mothers with difficult infants reduced fatigue and distress, women with pregnancy-induced hypertension
- Home monitoring of physiologic parameters, providing accurate and timely information and support online
- Examination of test results and monitoring of daily life and symptoms for home oxygen therapy clients
- Helps patients and families to be active participants in care, particularly in the chronic illness, change a dressing, give an insulin injection, or discuss increasing shortness of breath
- Reducing the requirement for, or the length of, hospital stays

Professional education
- Sharing of clinical information with national and international experts
- Access to literature and research used extensively in continuing education
- Enhancing and practicing clinical skills through patient simulation modeling
- Offering a doctorate in nursing completely via online distance education
- Providing opportunities for senior nurses to work in the clinical arena
- Allowing a nursing student to access a clinical data repository, a faculty supervisor, and the Web.
- Disseminating educational and other materials by using Web

Increase satisfaction among nurses
By creating more collaborative and autonomous roles

Disadvantages of Telenursing

1. **Dehumanizing effects:** There are healthcare professionals who feel the telehealth system has dehumanization effects. With the lack of staff, they are providing the best nursing care possible. It is not possible to give the human touch to do an assessment. Many professionals feel without direct patient contact, triaging may be difficult.
2. **Cost:** Telenursing is quite costly due to the value of the monitor and equipment.
3. **Inability to use equipment:** Caregivers and health professionals sometimes do not feel confident to use this equipment. Many patients hesitate to use electronic equipment.
4. **Lack of telehealth knowledge of the nurses:** Sometimes nurses may not be skilled enough to handle the monitors or may lack knowledge of its functioning. The knowledge base of the nurse and clinical competence is vital to interpret data of the patient to provide appropriate interventions. Clinical guidelines are needed to ensure the consistency of care.
5. **Equipment malfunction:** Broken and malfunctioning equipment could be detrimental to our home-bound patients. The system cannot operate if the patient does not have a working phone or phone. If there is no Internet service for the nurse to retrieve the data from the Web site, the data become useless.

Problems in Implementing Telenursing

1. **Acceptability by patients:** The patients who prefer to see healthcare providers face to face. Reimbursing providers may be challenging to track and prove.
2. **Patient understanding:** Patient understanding of how to use the equipment, when to use the system, and how it may impact their health is a vital element in the success of the program. Proper patient and provider education are imperative.
3. **Software knowledge:** Problem exists with any new procedure, piece of equipment, or technology. With the implementation of telehealth, nurses must learn how to use the technology that is the foundation of the system.
4. **System errors:** System errors can occur with software applications and Internet service, and equipment malfunctions may also occur.
5. **Cost:** Cost is a factor that many do not like to consider when quality patient care is the concern. Initial cost outlay may be prohibitively high.
6. **Security and privacy of data:** There is a risk of data security, i.e. anyone can track the password to access the information. Privacy is an ongoing concern.

Issues in Telenursing

1. **Societal:** Acceptance by society, patients, specialists, administrators, and the government
2. **Technical:** Telecommunication infrastructure

TABLE 62.2: Competency-based standards for professional practice in telenursing.

Competency	Competency description
Competency 1	Telenurse demonstrates a sound level of judgment, discretion, and decision-making when communicating with each caller
Competency 2	Telenurse practices nursing in a manner that the caller determines as being culturally safe
Competency 3	Telenurse demonstrates sound clinical nursing leadership
Competency 4	Telenurse monitors and improves the standards of telenursing through active involvement in quality improvement and risk management processes
Competency 5	Telenurse develops nursing practice through research and scholarship

3. **Standards:** Safety standards standardizing, certifying, authenticating, and registering telenursing
4. **Regulatory issues:** Credentialing and certification
5. **Professional liability:** Administrative liability and civil liability
6. **Professional:** Standards of practice and competencies designed by the regulatory bodies
7. **Legal issues:** Regarding the care of patients
8. **Security:** Privacy, confidentiality, and data security
9. **Financial:** Payments and reimbursement issues.

Competencies for Professional Practice in Telenursing

Table 62.2 provides the skills required for professional practice in telenursing.

Telenursing Practicing Standards

The standards must be consistent with the Indian Nursing Council (INC) practice standards, code of ethics, state registration act. These must address the following:

1. Quality-of-care issues for providing nursing services through distance
2. Promote the safe, competent, and ethical nursing practice, in terms of structure, process, and outcome with indicators
3. License for the nurses after attaining skill in telenursing
4. There should be a plan for continuing education to update the nurses' level of performance
5. Focus on policies for the safe and ethical telenursing practice, locus of accountability, client choice regarding telenursing, informed consent to treatment/care, security, confidentiality and privacy, liability, and protection of client.

CHAPTER HIGHLIGHTS

- "e-Learning" is an umbrella term that covers an extensive set of electronic educational applications and processes.
- It has individualized self-paced e-Learning offline, individualized self-paced e-Learning online, synchronously group-based e-Learning, and group-based learning e-Learning asynchronous modalities.
- There are various forms of e-Learning, such as Web site courses, laptop programs, hybrid learning in online learning, and fully online learning—distance learning. Andragogy and constructivism are the primary theoretical bases of e-Learning.
- Telemedicine is a strategy to provide interactive medical healthcare utilizing telecommunication to improve the efficiency and effectiveness of healthcare services.
- Telehealth includes clinical healthcare, health-related education support to patients and professionals, and health administrators by using telecommunication technologies.
- Telehealthcare includes all health services of all health disciplines such as radiology, pharmacy, and psychology.
- Telenursing refers to the use of telecommunication devices and information technology to provide nursing care from a distance to isolated groups of people. There are various problems and issues in implementing telenursing in India.

REVIEW QUESTIONS

I. Essay Type Questions
1. Define e-Learning. Describe the historical perspectives of e-Learning.
2. Discuss the importance of e-Learning.
3. Define the term "telemedicine." What are the benefits of implementing telemedicine?
4. What is meant by telenursing? Discuss its advantages and disadvantages.
5. Discuss the problems and issues in implementing telenursing in India.

II. Short Notes
1. Modalities and learning preferences of e-Learning
2. Theoretical bases of e-Learning
3. Designing program through e-Learning
4. Use of communication technology devices in telenursing
5. Competencies and practice standards in telenursing

III. Multiple Choice Questions
1. Since when the European schools used a Roman piece—a writing slate till around 1950 as an early learning aid to develop writing skills?
   a. 100 AC
   b. 200 AC
   c. 300 AC
   d. 400 AC
2. Who taught a shorthand language via correspondence in the 1840s and started a distance course by mail?
   a. Billings
   b. Skinner
   c. Presley
   d. Isaac Pitman

3. In which year computer was used to teach math to young children in elementary schools in California?
   a. 1940s
   b. 1950s
   c. 1960s
   d. 1970s
4. A type of learning that takes place in real time or at the same time is:
   a. Synchronous
   b. Asynchronous
   c. Online
   d. Off-line
5. A type of strategy or application that is used to provide health care to all people at any time from any place using broadband and wireless mobile technologies:
   a. Telehealth
   b. m-Health
   c. u-Health
   d. e-Health

Answer Keys

1. b   2. d   3. c   4. a   5. c

SUGGESTED READING

1. Abbas A, Hakimeh S, Fariba Bi, Abbas H. A comparative study on the effect of e-learning versus instructor-led method on nurses' documentation competency. IJNMR 2011;16(3):235-43.
2. Idriss NZ, Alikhan A, Baba K, Armstrong A. Online, video-based patient education improves melanoma awareness: a randomized controlled trial. Telemed JE Health 2009;15(10):992-7.
3. Lamothe L, Fortin JP, Labbe F, et al. Impacts of telehomecare on patients, providers, and organizations. Telemed J E Health 2006;12:363-9. (Pub Med).
4. Lievens F, Jordanova M. International development and evolving dimensions in Telemedicine 2008.
5. McConville S, Lane A. Using on-line video clips to enhance self-efficacy toward dealing with difficult situations among nursing students. Nurse Edu Today 2006;26:200-8.
6. McKenzie K, Murray A. How e-Learning can enhance learning opportunities in nurse education. Nurs Times 2010;106:5, early online publication.
7. Schlachta-Fairchild L, Varghese SB, Deickman A, Castelli D. Telehealth and telenursing are live: APN policy and practice implications. J Nurse Pract 2010;6(2):98-106.
8. Stoepel C, Boland J, Busco R, Saal G, Oliveira M. Usefulness of remote monitoring in cardiac implantable device follow-up. Telemed JE Health 2009;15(10):1026-30.
9. Telenursing and Telehealth. [online]. Available from: http://www.icn.ch/indfact_d.pdf.
10. Timothy J Bristol, JoAnn Zerwekh. Essentials of e-learning for nurse educators. ISBN-13: 978-0-8036-2173-2©2011.
11. Varghese SB, Phillips CA. Caring in telehealth. Telemed JE Health 2009;15(10):1005-9.
12. e-Health India. <https://www.nhp.gov.in/e-health-india_mty> [accessed 29.05.17].
13. Billings K and Moursund D. Computers in education: An historical perspective. Outlook: A Publication of the Special Interest Group on Computer Uses in Education. Association for Computing Machinery 1988; 20(1), 13-24.
14. Preston J. The Telemedicine Handbook: Improving Healthcare with Interactive Video. Austin Texas: Telemedicine Consultative Services Inc, 1993.
15. Sood S, Mbarika V, Jugoo S, Dookhy R, Doarn CR, Prakash N, Merrell RC. What Is telemedicine? A collection of 104 peer-reviewed perspectives and theoretical underpinnings. Telemed J E Health. 2007;13(5):573-90.
16. 10 Benefits of Health IT - Internet Innovation Alliance, 2011 July 21. Available from: internetinnovation.org › special-reports › telemed-infographic. [Accessed Jan 2020].
17. ICN. Telenursing fact sheet, 2001. Available from URL: http://www.icn.ch/images/stories/documents/publications/fact_sheets/18b_FS-Telenursing.pdf. [Accessed Jan 2020].
18. ICN. International Competencies for Telenursing. International Council of Nurse, 2007.
19. Available from: https://ehealth.eletsonline.com/2008/06/international-development-and-evolving-dimensions-in-telemedicine/. [Accessed Jan 2020].

Glossary

Accreditation: A process to certify competency, authority, or credibility of institutions, colleges, universities to have optimal and achievable standards.

Advocacy: A mutual understanding between nurses and clients as a human being, taking into account common needs and common rights.

Annual confidential report: A detailed report about the work performance of an employee and generally prepared at the end of every year by the immediate superior.

Applied ethics: The general principles of normative ethics applied systematically to ethical issues.

Assault: A form of the crime of violence against another person.

Audit: The process by which someone looks at the result of an activity and makes a judgment about whether it carried out to the level expected, as set out by preset rules, guidelines, or standards.

Autonomy: Freedom to exercise professional judgment and can make independent decisions about their work and refers to a person's independence, self-determination, and self-reliance.

Avalanches: A mass of snow that sets in motion by its weight through violent disturbances of its equilibrium.

AYUSH: The acronym for Ayurveda, Yoga, and Naturopathy, Unani, Siddha, and Homoeopathy. Sowa Rigpa, a Tibetan system of medicine similar to Ayurveda, was also introduced under AYUSH.

Battery: An intentional touching or doing unjustified harm.

Behaviorally Anchored Rating Scale (BARS): A checklist used for critical incidents in combination with a graphic rating scale to evaluate the performance of employees.

Benchmarking: It is a systematic process of finding out, sharing, developing, and implementing excellent practices to achieve the highest level of client satisfaction.

Beneficence: It refers to do what is good and avoids harm. It also states that we should generate the largest ratio of good over evil possible in the world.

Budget: A financial statement prepared before a specified period to attain a specified goal.

Burnout: A state of exhaustion that results from repeated emotional pressure.

Career: A series of work-related activities that provide continuity, order, and meaning to a person's life.

Career planning and development: A conscious process through which a nurse becomes aware of personal career-related attributes and lifelong progression that contribute to her/his career fulfillment.

Catastrophes: A type of disaster that is exceptionally severe and requires assistance and coordination with national and international resources.

Certification: The confirmation of or certifying certain characteristics of an object, person, or organization through documentary proof.

Change-of-shift report: A report given to all nurses on the next shift to provide continuity of care.

Change management: A structured approach to modify/transition individuals, teams, and organization as a whole from current status to the desired future status.

Clinical record: A formal, legal document that provides evidence of a client's care.

Code: A collection of laws or a system of rules and regulations.

Commissioning: Refers to a process of checking and ensuring the functioning and safety of installed equipment before being used.

Communication technology: Refers to a technical system of transferring information among people or machines.

Conferring: These refer to consultation and referral reports.

Confidentiality: Refers to the privacy of the information of a person.

Constitutional law: The study of the basic laws of the nation, states, and other political organizations.

Correspondence: Any written or digital communication exchanged by two or more parties.

Consumers Protection Act: A legal instrument aims at simplification of procedures for seeking redress of grievances of consumers without any court fee.

Cost accounting: An accounting process of providing the cost information data, the statement, and summary reports making managerial decisions.

Cost analysis: A technique of systematic collection, categorization, and analysis of program or intervention in terms of costs and cost of illness.

Cost-benefit analysis: A process of analyzing the benefits of the intervention with the costs associated with it.

Credentialing: Granting formal recognition of professional or technical competence.

Credit items: Items or the variables that give credit to the care rendered.

Criminal law: Law of public rights and duties; creates and controls the wrongs committed by a person(s). It involves the imposing state sanctions for crimes committed by individuals.

Critical pathway: A clinical pathway of optimal sequencing and timing of interventions for a particular intervention to reduce delays and resource utilization and to maximize the quality of care.

Cyclones: Speedy and several winds flow in the circular band highest in the center and lowest in the periphery arise as low-pressure areas in equatorial latitude in coastal regions.

Cyclone storm surge: A large mass of water moves towards the coast and resulting flooding conditions due to high-speed wind that strikes on the surface of the sea.

Debit items: Items or variables that give discredit to institutes.

Defamation: An intentional tort or the issuance of a false statement about another person, causing harm to that person.

Demoralization: A sense of incompetence based on the inability to solve some internal conflict or external problem, coupled with feelings of distress.

Deontology: The study of duty or obligation and refers to duty and obedience at the center of all ethical decisions.

Deployment: A process of moving or shifting staff from the current place of work to another place, or position within the organization structure.

Disability Adjusted Life Year (DALY): A measure of the overall burden of disease in a defined population and effectiveness of the intervention expressed as the number of years lost due to ill-health disability or early or premature death.

Disaster: A severe event or mishap arising with little or no warning causes that affects the functioning of the community at large and has a high impact on losses and requires external resources to cope up with the injuries.

Disaster management: A process of organizing, planning, and applying all measures of preparation, responding, and initiating recovery from disaster.

Distress: A negative stress that may cause illness.

Documentation: Any written or electronically generated information about a client that describes the care or service provided to that client.

E-Learning: The educational activities carried out online or off-line, synchronously, or asynchronously through network and electronic devices.

Emergency: An event or mishap, characterized by impacts that local responders can handle by utilizing available resources.

Employee Union: The organization of employees formed to promote and protect their interests through collective action.

Epistemology: The study of knowledge about reality and existence and deals with the concept of knowledge.

Esprit de Corps: Refers to a sense of unity, team spirit, devotion, and cooperation, which unites the members of the group.

Ethics: A study of good conduct, character, and motives.

Ethical committee: A group of persons who are officially responsible for promoting ethical practices, code of ethics, and resolves ethical issues and dilemmas.

Ethical decision-making: A process of making appropriate decisions to resolve an ethical dilemma.

Ethical issue/dilemma: A situation when conflict arises to choose or select one alternative from two equal courses of action, each of which would have significant consequences for the outcome of care.

Eustress: A positive stress that stimulates a person to function better.

Feasibility: The operational efficiency of certain procedures, logistic support, and workforce and material resources.

Fidelity: It refers to an act of faithfulness or striving to keep promises or fulfilling duties and obligations honestly.

Fraud: A crime or offense of deliberately deceiving another to damage another- to obtain property or services.

Gantt chart: A simple graphical representation of an activity plan showing the relationship between tasks and time duration in the bar diagram to assess the progress of the program.

General ethics: Ethics that considers the morality of human acts in general, irrespective of any particular field of application, occupation, or profession.

Gross Domestic Product (GDP): It is the total production of the nation and the monetary value of final goods and services.

Gross National Product (GNP): the total income of the nation including GDP and payments, profits, interest, etc. coming in from abroad excluding the interest, benefits, etc. going out of the country.

Gross National Income (GNI) per capita: It is the gross national income divided by its population.

Hazards: These are trigger agents, either natural or human-induced, or a combination of both that initiate mishap.

Health Management Information System (HMIS): A system of gathering, processing, analyzing, and reporting health-related information.

Health planning: A process to plan and execute health-related issues by creating an actionable link between health needs and resources.

Indian Nursing Council: An autonomous national nursing organization and statutory body, constituted under the Indian Nursing Council Act, 1947(XLVIII of 1947) of Parliament.

Induction training: A process by which the new nurses' employees introduce to the organization.

Information system: A computer-based system designed to support the operations, management, and decision functions.

Informed consent: An agreement by a patient to accept a course of treatment or procedure after informing risks, benefits, and consequences.

Innovation: A thinking idea-generating process to create a new or something significantly different from others to improve services and products of novelty.

Invasion of privacy: The ability of an individual or group to remain unnoticed or information about themselves and thereby reveals them selectively in the public realm.

Inventory: A stock to ensure uninterrupted supplies and to have future economic value.

Job description: It is communicating a written statement of duties and responsibilities of staff.

Justice: It refers to fairness or equity in dealing and prescribes actions that are fair to those involved.

Liability: Anything that is a hindrance or puts individuals at a disadvantage.

Licensure: Granting of licenses, especially to practice a profession.

Legal liability: A legal accountability or responsibility for something or any action. If a person is found responsible for causing damage legally has to pay compensation for any damage incurred.

Malpractice: The breech (illegal, improper, or negligence) by a professional due to either professional misconduct or skill in performing standards of care.

Management Information System (MIS): A single integrated system synonymous with computer-based systems that produce data that support the management functions of an organization.

Management Information and Evaluation System (MIES): A system of managing information to monitor progress, measure performance, detect trends, evaluate alternatives, make decisions, and take corrective actions.

Mass Casualty Incidence (MCI): An unmanageable situation where the resources of the hospitals are beyond its standard capacity, and the hospital needs additional contingency measures to control the event or to provide emergency medical care.

Glossary

Material management: It refers to planning, organizing, and controlling the flow of materials such as drugs, supplies, and equipment from their initial purchase, internal operations, and to the distribution at service point to deliver healthcare services.

Medico legal case (MLC): A case requiring investigations by law enforcement agencies apart from the medical treatment to fix the responsibility to cause of injury/illness and to assess its health status.

Medical tourism: An act of attracting medical tourists or patients from other countries to India to avail of medical services.

Negligence: A tort depends on the existence of a breach of duty of care owed by one person to another.

Negotiation: A legal process in which the representative of an organization or association negotiates with employers about employment matters.

New venture: A new activity or business that involves risks and uncertainties to operationalize that needs strategic and business planning.

NITI Aayog: A national institute **of transforming India** came into existence on 15th January 2015 to replace Planning Commission to achieve sustainable development.

Nonmaleficence: It means to do no harm or choose to do the least harm possible and to do harm to the fewest people.

Norm: It refers to a standard model or pattern that guides, controls, and regulates individuals and communities.

Nurse: A person qualified as a professional nurse, has thoroughly mastered nursing technical skills and uses her emotional and technical responses in a unique design that suits the peculiar needs of the person whom she serves.

Nursing: A profession that focuses on assisting individuals, families, and communities in attaining, maintaining, and recovering optimal health and functioning.

Nursing audit: A formal, detailed systematic review of records or observation of nursing actions to evaluate the quality of nursing care by comparing documented evidence with accepted standards and criteria.

Nursing documentation: A process of making an entry on a record, data which is pertinent to patient care or services provided to the client.

Nursing ethics: An applied ethics focus on both patients' and nurses' problems related to the nursing profession: the practice of nurses, exemplified in the codes of ethics and standards of nursing practice.

Nursing informatics: A combination of nursing science, computer, and information science to manage, process, and communicate nursing data to deliver nursing care and enhance the quality of nursing care.

Nursing nomenclature: The language of nursing that addresses nursing diagnosis, nursing interventions, nursing outcomes, and classification is the systematic arrangement or a structured framework of these phenomena.

Nursing organization: A group of nursing professionals working together to maintain the quality of nursing practice, education, and research and safeguard the interest of the public and nursing community.

Nursing philosophy: A belief system of the profession and provides perspectives for practice, scholarship, and research.

Nursing regulatory bodies: Bodies to regulate the profession and play multiple roles to ensure the public right to quality health care service; and to support and assist professional members.

Nursing standard: A descriptive statement of desired quality to evaluate nursing care.

Organizing: A process of developing a system for maximum utilization of available resources.

Organization chart: A simple diagrammatic method of describing an organization structure.

Organizational climate: A normative structure of attitudes and behavior of employees towards its elements and works environment, which helps them to interpret the situation and direct them to perform.

Organizational effectiveness: A degree to which the organization realizes its goals or the ability the organization to produce the desired results.

Orientation: An activity to introduce new nurse employees to organizations, tasks, superiors, and workgroups.

Patient assignment: Delegating or assigning duties to trained nurses for the care of patients admitted in the unit.

Patient Care Unit: A unit of the hospital where the patients admitted and nursed during their illnesses for their treatment.

Patient Classification System: It is a method or a system of grouping patients.

Performance appraisal: the process of evaluating the relative worth or ability of an individual employee against predetermined job-related performance standards per job descriptions.

PDSA: An acronym for four main activities, i.e., plan, do, study, and act.

Placement: Assigning a unit or ward to candidates on the first joining.

Plan: A scheme, program, or method worked out beforehand for the accomplishment of an objective.

Planning: A decision-making process to define tasks and to plan resources.

Preamble: A written law passed by the Constituent Assembly of India having consolidated regulations that specify aims, objectives, and philosophy, including the legislative framework of the Indian Republic.

Preparedness: All the protective and proactive measures that need to take before the mishap or disaster.

Problem-Orientated Medical Record (POMR): A method of documentation having a single list of client problems generated by members of the healthcare team.

Process/performance standards: Standards that define how the services are to be carried out and define operational norms; translate organizational values into actions; and those processes in writing for which the organization will be held accountable.

Procurement: A process of obtaining equipment and supplies through purchasing or other means.

Professional body: A professional body is a group of professionals who are responsible for maintaining the legitimate practice of the profession.

Professional nursing organization: Professional nursing organization is a group of nursing professionals working together to maintain the quality of nursing practice, education, and research and safeguard the interest of the public and nursing community.

Program Evaluation and Review Technique (PERT): An advanced and recent technique for logistics (planning, scheduling and controlling) of program/project type activities.

Tsunamis: These are waves of high speed across the ocean and steeper, resulting in floods on the coastal lands.

Problem-Oriented Medical Records (POMRs): A kind of records that focus on the specific problem of the patient.

Public Interest Litigation (PIL): Filing a Writ Petition at the filing counter or addressing the letter to the Chief Justice by an individual or a group of people for the interested public at large.

Quality assurance: A process for evaluating patient care in a particular setting by developing standards of care and implementing mechanisms for ensuring to meet standards.

Quality circle: A system to identify and recognize employees, and integrate their participation with a system.

Quality control: The process of measuring actual performance and comparing it with goals and acting upon the difference, if any.

Quality improvement: The process of attaining a new level of performance or quality that is superior to any previous level of quality.

Quality management: The process of mobilizing people to achieve quality goals.

Recruitment: A process to find out and attract capable applicants for the job.

Regulation: Regulations are the rules, and restrictions need to be followed by each of the employees in an organization.

Regulatory body: A regulatory body is an external organization that has been empowered by legislation to supervise and control the educational process and outputs.

Response: It includes all the measures during or immediately before the disaster concerning the site action.

Retention: A process in which employees are encouraged to remain with the organization for a maximum period.

Scalar Chain: Refers to the chain of superiors ranging from the ultimate authority to the lowest.

Scheduling: It refers to a process of allotting or distributing staff available in different units. It is a timetable showing planned work days and shifts for nursing personnel.

Selection: A process of choosing the fit candidates or rejecting the unfit candidates or a combination of both.

Shared governance: Taking part in the decision-making to make rules, develop procedures, manuals, and standard operative procedures for nursing care.

Slander: Making defamatory statements usually an oral (spoken) representation that harms a third person's reputation.

Staffing: Refers to a strategic or long-term staff planning.

Standard: A benchmark of achievement based on a desired level of excellence.

Standard of care: Standards related to activities or outcomes of nursing activities that focus on patients' status or expectations.

Standards of nursing practice: Standards that focus on structure and process domain/ elements used by the nurse and nursing service to provide patient care.

Standards of performance: Standards relate to how well nurses must perform against identified standards of performance specified in the job description.

Strategy: An approach to meet particular aims, taking into account internal and external factors.

Stress: A state that occurs when individuals perceive that they cannot adequately cope with the demand being made on them or with the threats to their well-being.

Structural standards: Standards that establish guidelines for organizational patterns and support structures for providing health care.

Teleconferencing: A one-way video and two-way audio-conferencing system using communication satellites of the INSAT series.

Tornadoes: It is like a cyclone, but of a smaller scale.

Tort law: Law concerning a legal wrong committed intentionally or unintentionally against a person, his or her rights, or property.

Total quality management: It is a multidisciplinary, interdisciplinary, coordinated, and integrated approach to examine organizational processes for continuous improvement.

Transfer: A movement of an employee from one job to another.

Trends in nursing: Changes that take place in present days in any field of nursing, which affects the profession as a whole.

Veracity: Refers to an act of telling the truth and be honest while dealing with the person.

Vulnerability: Vulnerability is the extent of damage to society, structure and system are due to external events or hazards.

Index

Page numbers followed by *f* refer to figure, *t* refer to table and *b* refer to box.

A

ABC analysis 492
Accreditation 515, 525, 543
Act of the Sexual Harassment of Women at Workplace 42
Activity-based budgeting (ABB) 574
Activity Study Method 286
Acuity-quality 299
Adult learning 332
Anganwadi workers 274
Andragogy 332, 651
ASHA (Rural) 273
Assault 39, 49
Autonomy 29
Auxiliary Nurse Midwife/HW, (Female) 274, 278
Average cost 596
AYUSH Mission 112

B

Battery 39, 49
Behaviorally Anchored Rating Scale (BARS) 346
Benchmarking 164
Beneficence 30
Breach of contract 39
Budgetary process 486, 575
Budgeting 568
Burnout 357

C

Capital budget 567
Career 336
Case method 216
Catastrophic disaster 233
Cellular telephony 627
Certification 515
Centralization 67
Central Sterile Supply Department (CSSD) 221
Chain communication 387
Civil laws 39
Clinical audit 538
Criminal laws 39
Code of ethics 31
Coercive power 447
Commissioning 478
Committee 13, 181
Communication pattern 389
Communication process 384
Computer network 625
Computer system 624
Condemnation 472, 483

Condemnation committee 483
Conferences 399
Confidentiality 30
Constructivism 651
Consumers Protection Act 40
Consultative method 290
Continuing education 329, 338
Continuous Quality Improvement 508
Cost analysis 594
Cost-benefit analysis 598
Cost classifications 582
Cost consequences analysis 598, 604
Cost-effectiveness analysis 598, 601
Cost-utility analysis 598, 603
Credentialing 515
Custodial model 431
Cyclones 232

D

Decentralization 67
Defamation 39, 49
Delphi Method 289
Deployment practices 254
Diagonal communication 386
Dietary procurement 226
Dietary services/kitchen 224
Disability-adjusted life years (DALYs) 604
Disaster 230
Discipline 7*t*
Distress 357
District hospital 195
DMADV process 516
DMAIC process 516
Domestic Violence Act 42
Donabedian Model 513

E

Economic analysis 591
Economic evaluation 591
Economic Order Quantity 495
e-Health 653
e-Learning 648
Electronic health record (EHR) 623, 632
Electronic documentation 632
E-mail communication 626
Employee grievance 352
Employee unions 422
Empowerment of women 43
Ergonomic hazards 365
Esprit de Corps 68
Ethics 27
Equity 67
Equity theory 79, 380
Ethical committee 34

Ethical decision-making 35
Ethical issues 35
Ethical theories 28
Eustress 357
Expectancy theory 78, 380

F

Facsimile Transmission 627
False imprisonment 39
Fidelity 30
Financial accounting systems 586
Financial budget 567
Fishbone diagram 508
FOCUS–PDCA model 513
Forced choice method 347
Formal organizations 174
Fraud 50
Free flow communication 387
Functional method 217

G

Gantt chart 75, 161
General hospitals 194
Grievance Redressal Mechanism 41
Group climate 187
Group Cohesiveness 443
Group norms 442

H

Hawthorne Effect 76
Hazards 233
Health-care financing 559
Health-care laws 421
Healthcare reform cycle 612
Health economics map 589
Health valuation methods 597
Herzberg's theory 379
High Power Committee on Nursing (1987) 289
HML analysis 495
Hospital accreditation system 550
Hospital disaster management planning 236
Hospital laundry 223
Hospital management information system 643
Hospital plan 198
Human-induced disasters 232

I

Incremental budgeting 572
Indian constitution 85
Indian Nursing Council 12

Informal organization 174
Informed consent 29, 50
Innovation 149
Inspection 525, 548
Interlocation deployment 253
Intuitive method 290
Indiscipline 350
Induction training 329
Internet 627
Iowa's model 328*f*
Issues in nursing 22

K

Katz's Index 297
Kilkari 118

L

Labor cost 582
Laboratory services 226
Landslides 232
Law 38
Leadership development 408
Leadership styles 405
Legal aspect 48
Legal issues 49, 658
Legal liabilities 48
Legal safeguard 50
Legal system 38
Legitimate Power 447
Lewin's Change Model 155
Licensure 50, 514
Linen and Laundry Department 223
Lok Adalat 87

M

Macroeconomics 590
Mahila Arogya Samiti 117, 278
Malpractice 39, 49
Management 59
Management by objectives (MBO) 162
Management plan 145
Management information system 80
Marginal cost 583, 596
MARS model 378
Maslow's theory 76
Mass casualty incidence 236
Master budget 568
Master planning 198
Master rotation plan 300
Materials 469
Material cost 581
Medicolegal case 54
Microeconomics 591
Midterm appraisal 577
Mission statement 133
Modern nursing 5
Modular construction 197
Modular Nursing 218
Molestation 42
Mothers' Absolute Affection (MAA) Programme 118
Motivational theories 379
MTP Act 42
Multiple health workers (MPHWs) 274

N

National accounting systems 585
National Assessment and Accreditation Council (NAAC) 545
National Accreditation Board for Hospitals and Health Care Providers (NABH) 550
National Health Mission 113
Natural disaster 231
Negligence 39
Negotiation 51
New Venture 146
NITI Aayog 97, 118
Nightingale ward 201
Nonmaleficence/Do no harm 30
Nurses' rights 31
Nursing audit 537
Nursing budget 576
Nursing ethics 27
Nursing management 61
Nursing minimum data set (NMDS) 646
Nursing negligence 49
Nursing nomenclature 23
Nursing philosophy 134
Nursing rounds 398
Nursing standards 521
Nursing station 201
Nursing unit 200

O

Occupational hazards 364
Occupational health laws 366
Open ward 201
Operating plan 142
Operational plan 144
Organizational behavior models 431
Organization chart 177
Organizational climate 184
Organizational conflict 412
Organizational effectiveness 188
Organization structure 177
Orientation 329
Oulu patient classification (OPC) 298
Overhead cost 569*b*, 582

P

Panchayat Court 87
Pareto chart 508
Path-goal theory 81
Patient assignment 215
Patient classification system (PCS) 296
Performance budgeting 573
PCPNDT Act 42
PDSA 165
Periodic ordering method 496
Perpetual inventory system 497
Personal digital assistants (PDAs) 623, 634
Personnel management 246
Pickle Jar theory 462
Planned change 153
Planning Commission 97
POSDCORB 75

Pondy's model 413
Positive discipline 350
Postdisaster phase 234
Preamble 85
Predisaster phase 234
Primary nursing 218
Private duty nursing 216
Problem-oriented medical records (POMRs) 631
Profession 6
Procedures 143
Procurement 472, 473, 485
Professional body 11
Professional conduct 31
Program evaluation and review technique 160
Program planning budgeting system (PPBS) 577
Promotion on seniority 257
Protocol 143, 399
Psychological climate 187

Q

Quality-adjusted life years (QALYs) 604
Quality circle 456, 512
Quality evaluation systems 514

R

RAFAELA patient classification system 298
Ranking scale 347
Real-time access 651
Recruitment process 247
Recruitment policy 249
Recruitment specification 247
Referent power 447
Registrations 515
Regression method 299
Regulation 6, 10
Regulatory system 10
Regulatory body 10
Revenue budget 567
Rights of aging people/senior citizen 43
Rights of children 41
Rights of People Living with HIV/AIDS 44
Rights of Persons with Disabilities 45
Rights of Women 41
Rigs ward 201
Reorder Limit Method 496
Robbins' model 413
RPTIM model 327
Run chart 518

S

Scalar Chain 67
Schutz's three-stage model 441
SDE Analysis 494
Semantic barriers 388
Sensitivity analysis 597
Sexual harassment 42
Selection process 250
Six sigma 515
Slander 39

Index

SOAP/IER format 631
S-O-B-C model 431
Social exchange theory 440
SOS analysis 495
Source-oriented record 630
Staffing process 282
Staff Inspection Unit (SIU) 288
State Nursing Council 14
Stock inventory 472
Strategic planning 129, 140, 200
Strategic plan 144
Student Nurses Association 16
Superannuation 260
Supplies 476
Swachh Bharat Mission 118
Systems approach 80

T

Team approach 455
Team nursing 217
Telecommunication 626
Teleconferencing 627
Telemedicine 652
Telenursing 623, 655
Time schedule 210, 210t, 301
Time savers 461
Time wasters 460
360° feedback 347, 410
Tornadoes 232
Tort 39
Total quality management 511
Trained Nurses Association 14
Transactional leadership 405
Transformational leadership 405
Trended budget 568
Trends in nursing 18
Tsunamis 232
Tuckman's four-stage model 441

U

Union budget 567
Urban ASHA 277

V

VED analysis 494
Veracity 30
Videoconferencing 627
Voice Communication System 626
Volcanoes 232
Vulnerability 233

W

Ward management 208
Ward pantry 205
Ward policies 213
Ward rounds 211
Ward sister 209, 311
Wheel communication 387
Working group 455
Workload measurement 286
Work sampling study 285

X

XYZ analysis 495

Z

Zebra system 299
Zero-based budget 567, 572